PATHWAYS
of the PULP

PATHWAYS
of the PULP

Edited by

STEPHEN COHEN, M.A., D.D.S., F.I.C.D., F.A.C.D.

Clinical Professor and Chairman, Department of Endodontics,
University of the Pacific School of Dentistry, San Francisco, California;
Diplomate, American Board of Endodontics

RICHARD C. BURNS, D.D.S., F.I.C.D., F.A.C.D.

Assistant Clinical Professor, Department of Endodontics,
University of the Pacific School of Dentistry, San Francisco, California;
Diplomate, American Board of Endodontics

FOURTH EDITION

with 36 contributors,
2141 illustrations, and 1 color plate

Principal illustrator,
Richard C. Burns

The C. V. Mosby Company

ST. LOUIS • WASHINGTON D. C. • TORONTO   1987

MOSBY

A TRADITION OF PUBLISHING EXCELLENCE

Editor: Darlene Barela Cooke
Assistant editor: Melba Steube
Manuscript editor: Stephen C. Hetager, Patricia J. Milstein
Production: Debbie Wedemeier, Jeanne A. Gulledge, Kathryn Gordon

FOURTH EDITION

Printed in the United States of America

The C.V. Mosby Company
11830 Westline Industrial Drive, St. Louis, Missouri 63146

Library of Congress Cataloging-in-Publication Data

Pathways of the pulp.

   Includes bibliographies and index.
   1. Endodontics.   I. Cohen, Stephen, 1938-
II. Burns, Richard C., 1932-   [DNLM: 1. Dental
Pulp.   2. Endodontics.   WU 230 P297]
RK351.P37   1987   617.6′342   86-12558
ISBN 0-8016-1077-X

C/MV/MV 9 8 7 6 5 4 3 2 1   02/A/295

This edition is a tribute to
SAMUEL SELTZER

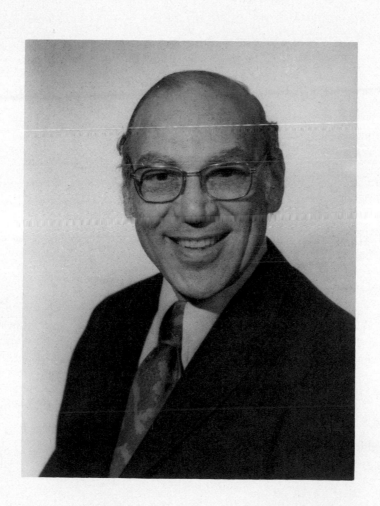

CONTRIBUTORS

Donald E. Arens, D.D.S., M.S.D., F.I.C.D., F.A.C.D.

Associate Professor, Department of Endodontics,
Indiana University School of Dentistry,
Indianapolis, Indiana;
Diplomate, American Board of Endodontics

Robert E. Averbach, D.D.S., F.I.C.D.

Professor and Chairman, Division of Endodontics,
University of Colorado School of Dentistry,
Denver, Colorado;
Diplomate, American Board of Endodontics

Richard C. Burns, D.D.S., F.I.C.D., F.A.C.D.

Assistant Clinical Professor, Department of Endodontics,
University of the Pacific School of Dentistry,
San Francisco, California;
Diplomate, American Board of Endodontics

Joe H. Camp, D.D.S., M.S.D., F.I.C.D.

Private Practice of Endodontics,
Charlotte, North Carolina

Noah Chivian, D.D.S., F.A.C.D., F.I.C.D

Director of Endodontics, Newark Beth Israel Medical
Center, Newark, New Jersey;
Diplomate, American Board of Endodontics

Stephen Cohen, M.A., D.D.S., F.I.C.D., F.A.C.D.

Clinical Professor and Chairman,
Department of Endodontics,
University of the Pacific School of Dentistry,
San Francisco, California;
Diplomate, American Board of Endodontics

Quintiliano Diniz de Deus, D.D.S.

Professor Titular, The Dental Faculty,
Federal University of Minas Gerais,
Belo Horizonte, Brazil

Thomas C. Dumsha, M.S., D.D.S.

Assistant Professor, Department of Endodontics,
The Baltimore College of Dental Surgery,
Dental School, University of Maryland at Baltimore,
Baltimore, Maryland

†Harold F. Eissmann, D.D.S., F.A.C.D.

Clinical Professor, Division of Fixed Prosthodontics,
Department of Restorative Dentistry,
University of California School of Dentistry,
San Francisco, California

Ronald A. Feinman, B.S., D.M.D.

Special Lecturer in Esthetics,
Emory University School of Dentistry,
Atlanta, Georgia

†Deceased.

Stuart B. Fountain, D.D.S., M.Sc.(Dent.), F.I.C.D., F.A.C.D.

Clinical Associate Professor, Department of Endodontics,
University of North Carolina School of Dentistry,
Chapel Hill;
Private Practice, Greensboro, North Carolina;
Diplomate, American Board of Endodontics

Albert C. Goerig, D.D.S., M.S., F.I.C.D.

Colonel, Dental Corps, U.S. Army;
Endodontic Mentor for the General Dentistry Residency,
Fort Ord, California;
Diplomate, American Board of Endodontics

Ronald E. Goldstein, D.D.S.

Clinical Professor of Restorative Dentistry,
Medical College of Georgia School of Dentistry,
Augusta, Georgia;
Associate Clinical Professor of Continuing Education,
Henry M. Goldman School of Graduate Dentistry,
Boston University, Boston, Massachusetts;
Special Lecturer in Esthetic Dentistry,
Emory University School of Dentistry,
Atlanta, Georgia

James L. Gutmann, D.D.S., F.A.C.D., F.I.C.D., F.A.I.D.S.

Professor and Chairman, Department of Endodontics,
Baylor College of Dentistry, Dallas, Texas;
Research Professor,
The Baltimore College of Dental Surgery, Dental School,
University of Maryland at Baltimore,
Baltimore, Maryland

Michael A. Heuer, D.D.S., M.S., F.A.C.D., F.I.C.D.

Professor of Endodontics,
Associate Dean for Academic Affairs,
Northwestern University Dental School,
Chicago, Illinois;
Diplomate, American Board of Endodontics

Syngcuk Kim, D.D.S., Ph.D.

Chairman, Division of Endodontics;
Director, Laboratory of Oral Physiology,
School of Dental and Oral Surgery,
Columbia University, New York, New York

Donald J. Kleier, D.M.D.

Associate Professor, Division of Endodontics,
University of Colorado School of Dentistry,
Denver, Colorado;
Diplomate, American Board of Endodontics

Anne-Li Knuut, D.D.S.

Assistant Clinical Professor, Department of Endodontics,
University of the Pacific School of Dentistry,
San Francisco, California

Stanley F. Malamed, D.D.S.

Associate Professor of Anesthesia and Medicine,
University of Southern California School of Dentistry,
Los Angeles, California

Howard Martin, D.M.D., F.A.C.D.

Clinical Associate Professor,
Georgetown University School of Dentistry,
Washington, D.C.:
Diplomate, American Board of Endodontics

Leo J. Miserendino, D.D.S., M.S.

Research Associate,
Departments of Biological Materials and Endodontics,
Northwestern University Dental School,
Chicago, Illinois;
Adjunct Clinical Assistant Professor,
Departments of Endodontics and Dental Materials,
Marquette University School of Dentistry,
Milwaukee, Wisconsin

Donald R. Morse, B.S., D.D.S., M.A.(Biol.), M.A.(Psychol.)

Professor and Research Director,
Department of Endodontology,
Temple University School of Dentistry,
Philadelphia, Pennsylvania;
Diplomate, American Board of Endodontics

Nguyen Thanh Nguyen, D.D.S., F.I.C.D., F.A.C.D., F.A.A.E.

Clinical Professor and Former Chairman,
Division of Endodontics,
University of California School of Dentistry,
San Francisco, California;
Diplomate, American Board of Endodontics

Edward M. Osetek, D.D.S., M.A., F.I.C.D., F.A.C.D.

Chairman, Department of Endodontics,
Northwestern University Dental School, Chicago, Illinois;
Diplomate, American Board of Endodontics

Ryle A. Radke, Jr., D.D.S., F.A.C.D., F.A.C.P.

Associate Clinical Professor,
Division of Fixed Prosthodontics,
Department of Restorative Dentistry,
University of California School of Dentistry,
San Francisco, California;
Diplomate, American Board of Prosthodontics

Joseph Schulz, A.B., D.D.S.

Assistant Clinical Professor, Department of Endodontics,
University of the Pacific School of Dentistry,
San Francisco, California

Stephen F. Schwartz, D.D.S., M.S., F.A.D.I.

Assistant Professor, Department of Endodontics,
University of Texas Dental Branch, San Antonio, Texas;
Visiting Lecturer, University of Texas Dental Branch,
Houston, Texas;
Diplomate, American Board of Endodontics

Samuel Seltzer, D.D.S.

Professor of Endodontology, Director,
Maxillofacial Pain Control Center,
Temple University School of Dentistry,
Philadelphia, Pennsylvania

Thomas P. Serene, D.D.S., M.S.D.

Professor and Chairman, Department of Endodontics,
College of Dental Medicine,
Medical University of South Carolina,
Charleston, South Carolina;
Diplomate, American Board of Endodontics

James H.S. Simon, A.B., D.D.S., F.I.C.D., F.A.C.D.

Chief, Endodontic Section,
Veterans Administration Medical Center,
Long Beach;
Professor of Endodontics,
Loma Linda University School of Dentistry,
Loma Linda;
Clinical Associate Professor of Endodontics,
University of Southern California School of Dentistry,
Los Angeles, California;
Diplomate, American Board of Endodontics

Henry O. Trowbridge, D.D.S., Ph.D

Professor of Pathology,
University of Pennsylvania School of Dental Medicine,
Philadelphia, Pennsylvania

Fulton S. Yee, D.D.S.

Private Practice,
San Francisco, California

Paul Eugene Zeigler, B.A., D.D.S., F.A.C.D.

Consultant, United States Navy Regional Medical Center,
San Diego, California

Edwin J. Zinman, D.D.S., J.D.

Private Law Practice, San Francisco, California

SPECIAL CONTRIBUTORS

Charles J. Cunningham, D.D.S., F.I.C.D.

Associate Professor, Department of Endodontics;
Assistant Dean for Clinical Affairs,
University of Kentucky College of Dentistry,
Lexington, Kentucky;
Diplomate, American Board of Endodontics

Shannon Wong, D.D.S., M.S.

Assistant Clinical Professor, Department of Endodontics,
University of the Pacific School of Dentistry,
San Francisco, California

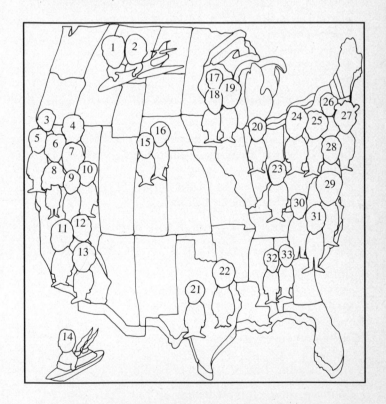

1, Richard C. Burns; **2,** Stephen Cohen; **3,** Shannon Wong; **4,** Nguyen Thanh Nguyen; **5,** Edwin J. Zinman; **6,** Fulton S. Yee; **7,** Ryle A. Radke, Jr.; **8,** Anne-Li Knuut; **9,** Albert C. Goerig; **10,** Joseph Schultz; **11,** Stanley F. Malamed; **12,** James H.S. Simon; **13,** Paul Eugene Zeigler; **14,** Quintiliano Diniz de Deus; **15,** Donald J. Kleier; **16,** Robert E. Averbach; **17,** Leo J. Miserendino; **18,** Edward M. Osetek; **19,** Michael A. Heuer; **20,** Donald E. Arens; **21,** James L. Gutmann; **22,** Stephen F. Schwartz; **23,** Charles J. Cunningham; **24,** Henry O. Trowbridge; **25,** Donald R. Morse; **26,** Syngcuk Kim; **27,** Noah Chivian; **28,** Howard Martin; **29,** Joe H. Camp; **30,** Stuart B. Fountain; **31,** Thomas P. Serene; **32,** Ronald A. Feinman; **33,** Ronald E. Goldstein.

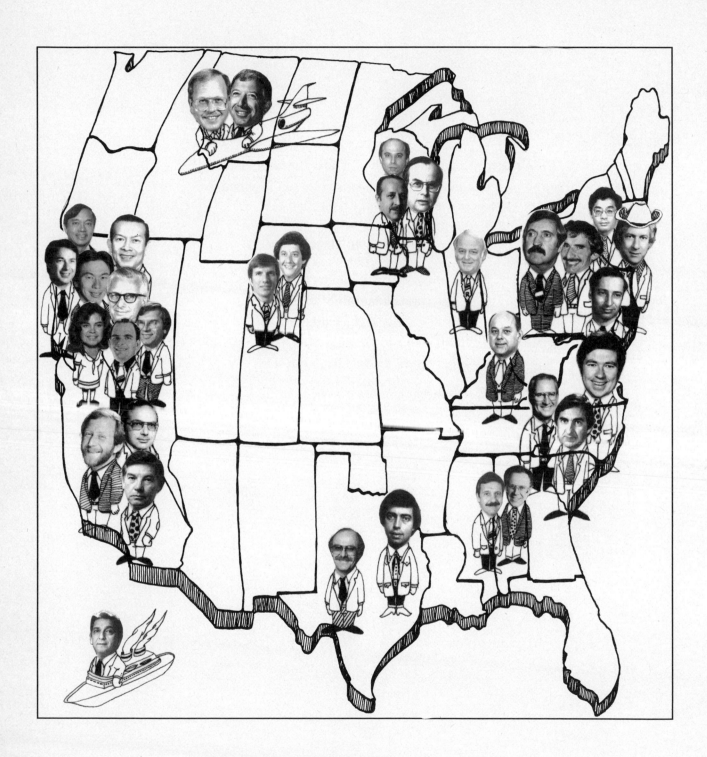

We deeply mourn the death of a dear friend of endodontics,
a role model for endodontists, and an inspiration
for this book

Dr. Irving Naidorf

His wisdom
His constant pursuit of excellence
His zest for life
His wonderful sense of humor
Have touched us deeply

Knowing him has enriched our lives

To a land that nutures excellence,
encourages achievement,
and fosters academic freedom

We dedicate this book
to America

PREFACE

The objective of this fourth edition is to impart the most current knowledge regarding the art and science of endodontics. The explosion of new information, concepts, and devices has created an avalanche of journal literature that could easily make a dentist, trying to stay abreast of the times, feel overwhelmed. This edition filters the prolific literature to provide only the most relevant papers to help the practicing dentist remain current in his or her knowledge and offer the student a generously illustrated, step-by-step guide to learn modern endodontic therapy.

As editors we are faced with the dilemma of evaluating the validity of ideas and devices that have recently been introduced in the endodontic community; after all, what may be modish is not necessarily enduring. The literature is replete with therapies, biologic interpretations, and experiments previously accepted and cited but now refuted. To accomplish this task we have been able to gather together prominent authorities as contributing authors on every aspect of endodontics, who have unselfishly agreed to devote their special talents, knowledge, and illustrative material. Most dentists will recognize the names of many of the contributors because they have written their own books, published papers in distinguished journals, directed endodontic training programs, or lectured at national and international dental meetings. The contributors have maintained the philosophy of this book, which is to present all phases of endodontic treatment in a clear and concise style and thus provide a comprehensive textbook with practical clinical application for the dental student and the general practitioner in the 1980s.

In many ways the fourth edition is virtually a new book. Twenty-two chapters have been completely rewritten or significantly revised. The remaining four chapters have been brought up to date in all respects.

To help the reader evaluate his or her own comprehension and information retention, we have provided self-assessment quizzes for each chapter. Drs. Shannon Wong and Charles Cunningham, with the help of many endodontists, general practitioners, and dental students from the University of the Pacific School of Dentistry, have carefully prepared and reviewed each question's clarity, relevance, and accuracy.

Our warmest thanks go to Bella Endzweig for typing mountains of manuscript. Her ability to read our scribbled writing, in itself, deserves a meritorious award.

We are most grateful to Darlene Cooke, Melba Steube, Myrna Oppenheim, and the rest of the editorial staff of The C. V. Mosby Company for their constructive criticism, pertinent suggestions, and encouragement. We hope this book makes it evident that the essential services of the endodontist are an integral extension of the general dentist's restorative team; for only in close cooperation with each other can both succeed.

It has been said that, in the final analysis, the process is our real product. Along the way of preparing this book we have made some lifelong friends. These friendships have been so supportive and strengthening that in many respects they represent the richest reward we could possibly receive.

Stephen Cohen
Richard C. Burns

CONTENTS

PART FOUR
HISTORY AND PHILOSOPHY OF ENDODONTICS

COLOR PLATE

INTRODUCTION

SAMUEL SELTZER

Significant changes have occurred in endodontics over the past 50 years. Prior to the early 1900s, extraction of teeth ravished by pulpal or periodontal disease was an accepted, and, in many cases, a desirable practice. Scientific investigations into the causes of dental caries and periodontal conditions were minimal. The types of continuing education courses offered were reflections of the prevailing philosophies. The most popular courses were oral surgery and prosthetics.

A scientific basis had to be established if teeth were to be saved. The pioneering studies of such superb investigators as Orban, Gottlieb, Kronfeld, Blayney, Hatton, Massler, Coolidge, and Grossman began to have an impact. In the late 1930s and early 1940s, microbiology was a major available science. It seemed to be a reasonable assumption that if microorganisms could be eliminated from root canals, the teeth could no longer be considered as "foci" of infection. Culturing of the root canal appeared to be a sure way to determine whether microorganisms had been eliminated. By this means, various studies demonstrated that infections could be eliminated from inside the teeth.

Three basic principles of root canal therapy became established: debridement, sterilization, and obturation or filling of the root canal. Debridement was accomplished with instruments and irrigating solutions. Standard files and reamers were used manually for this purpose. To ensure sterilization of the root canal, a preoperative culture was first taken. Numerous investigations were made to find the best media to support the growth of the samples. It soon became apparent that the root canals were infected with a large variety of gram-positive and gram-negative microorganisms, as well as fungi, L forms, and spirochetes. Although not known at the time, bacterial genetic variations were developing. It was not until the early 1970s that more sophisticated techniques, such as those using strictly anaerobic conditions, revealed the presence of microorganisms that hitherto had been unreported in root canals.

Numerous medicaments were advocated for killing the inhabitants of the root canal. Originally, they included powerful acids and alkalies. These were subsequently supplanted by less toxic chemicals such as metacresylacetate (Cresatin) and camphorated monochlorophenol. Soon after the advent of penicillin, it and other antibiotics, singly or in various combinations, were used for root canal sterilization.

Obtaining subsequent negative cultures was important evidence and the incentive for convincing the dental profession that endodontic therapy was indeed capable of sterilizing the root canal. It helped to negate the indictment of teeth as sources of infection for the rest of the body. It worked! More and more endodontic therapy was performed, and more and more teeth were saved.

Unfortunately, it soon became apparent that negative cultures did not necessarily reflect the true status of the root canal. Some culture reversals were detected. The emphasis on obtaining negative cultures began to be dissipated. In addition, because of culturing and other factors, treatment was time consuming. It would usually take between two and five treatments to complete endodontic therapy.

In the 1960s and 1970s, serious questions were raised about the necessity of obtaining negative cultures. The emphasis began to shift from microbiology to the emerging field of immunology. Greater emphasis was placed on the biologic aspects of endodontics. The number of patients having endodontic therapy increased. Endodontics was recognized as a specialty in 1965. Postgraduate education began to flourish, and there was a proliferation of continuing education courses in endodontics.

Single-visit endodontic therapy began to emerge as a viable and successful method of treatment. With continued interest in biologic mechanisms, investigations into various phases of endodontics proliferated. Many questions arose. How clean is the root canal after instrumentation? Which are the most efficacious irrigating solutions? What is the best method of filling the root canal? Are there better materials for filling root canals? Which root canal materials have the best biocompatibility? These and countless other questions arose and began to be investigated both by endodontists and by graduate students in endodontics.

Where are we going? I believe that in the future we will see the development of new pulp-testing modalities, computer-based diagnostic methods, biocompatible injectable root canal fillings, better ultrasonic root-cleaning instruments, more sophisticated techniques for identification of microorganisms, chemical mediators, and immunoglobulins, and the use of magnetic resonance imaging rather than x-rays to "see" inside a root canal.

The need for endodontics will gradually decline as dental caries is eliminated. However, the emerging field of pain diagnosis and management of head and neck pain will come under the purview of the endodontist. This will be reflected in the advanced educational programs by greater curricular emphasis on the diagnosis and control of maxillofacial pain.

As always, the need for advanced information on the status of endodontics exists. Such information is masterfully presented in this textbook by Stephen Cohen and Richard Burns. It emphasizes the great strides that have been made in the field and presents an authorative, up-to-date view of the "state of the art." I congratulate them for their scholarly presentation.

PART ONE

THE ART OF ENDODONTICS

1

DIAGNOSTIC PROCEDURES

STEPHEN COHEN

When I try to lie down, this tooth begins to throb.

Yesterday morning I just noticed this blister on my gum.

I got a cold last week, and since then all the upper back teeth on the left side hurt when I chew or bend over.

Doctor, ever since you put the filling in my tooth, I can't drink anything hot or cold!

For two days, the whole side of my jaw has felt swollen.

Since my teeth were cleaned by your hygienist, it hurts when I breathe in through my mouth.

Last week, while I was eating in a restaurant, I bit into a pit in a cherry pie and heard a crack; since then I can't bite on that side of my mouth.

These are a few illustrations of the common complaints dentists may encounter in practice. The purpose of this chapter is to help the clinician determine whether problems such as these are odontogenic or nonodontogenic in origin and to identify the location and cause of a patient's complaint. Endodontic diagnosis combines scientific knowledge applied to a clinical surrounding with the "art" of clinical experience and common sense.

By systematically recording a patient's presenting signs and symptoms and by properly analyzing results of clinical tests, the clinician will find that the diagnostic process is usually straightforward. The purpose of this chapter is to describe and illustrate fundamentals of gathering and interpreting clinical information yielded from common, straightforward, and nonurgent diagnostic situations. However, the patient may present with an acute situation in which there are conflicting signs and symptoms or confusing responses to clinical testing. In Chapter 2 the method of diagnosing and treating these difficult and acute cases is

discussed. Endodontic riddles provide a diagnostic challenge that, upon successful resolution, can result in a wonderful sense of personal gratification for the clinician.

HISTORY
Medical history

Even though there are virtually no systemic contraindications to endodontic treatment, a recent, succinct, and comprehensive preprinted medical history (such as the one on p. 6), signed and dated, is mandatory.

Some patients will require antibiotic prophylaxis because of systemic conditions like heart valve replacement, a history of rheumatic fever, or cancer chemotherapy and/or radiotherapy. Other patients will have diseases, such as infectious hepatitis, herpes, or acquired immune deficiency syndrome (AIDS), that require the *dentist and the assistant* to protect themselves by wearing rubber gloves, masks, and safety glasses. Only with a medical history will a clinician be able to determine that a patient or even the dentist and assistant require special protection prior to any diagnostic examination or treatment. Furthermore, to avoid a potential adverse drug interaction with a medication that might be prescribed during the course of endodontic therapy, the clinician must know about any drugs the patient may be taking. Mental disorders are not uncommon. Some patients are aware that they have a mental affliction and will inform the clinician; others may not be aware of having such illness.

If there is any question about systemic or mental ailments and how they might affect a dental treatment plan, *always consult with the patient's physician.* A brief summary of any medical advice offered by a physician should be clearly recorded and dated on the patient's record.

Dental history

After completing the medical history the clinician should develop the dental history. The goal of taking a dental history is to clearly record on the patient's chart a

---

The majority of illustrations in this chapter were prepared by Dr. Albert Goerig.

MEDICAL HISTORY

Are you in good health? _____

Are you presently under the care of a physician? _____ If so, please give reason(s) for treatment _____

_____

Physician's name and address _____

Date of last physical exam _____

Are you taking any kind of medication (prescribed or nonprescribed) or drug(s) at this time? _____ if so, please give name(s) of the medication(s) and reason(s) for taking them _____

_____

Please circle any illnesses you have ever had:

AIDS	Blood pressure	Glaucoma	Kidney or liver	Sinusitis
Alcoholism	Cancer	Head/neck injuries	Mental	Ulcers
Allergies	Diabetes	Heart trouble	Migraine	Venereal disease
Anemia	Drug/narcotic dependency	Herpes	Respiratory	Other
Asthma	Epilepsy	Infectious hepatitis	Rheumatic fever	

Do you wear a heart "pacemaker"? _____

Have you ever had any trouble with prolonged bleeding after surgery? _____

Have you ever had an unusual reaction to an anesthetic or drug (like penicillin)? _____

Is there any other information that should be known about your health? _____

_____

About previous dental visits? _____

If female, are you pregnant? _____

Have you had previous endodontic (root canal) treatment? _____

Date _____

Signature _____

---

brief summary of the chief complaint, the signs and symptoms, when the problem began, and what the patient can discern that improves or worsens the condition. The method of gathering this information is to ask the patient pertinent leading questions combined with the art of listening in a thoughtful and caring manner. For example, one might begin by simply asking the patient, "Could you tell me about your problem?" To determine the chief complaint, this question should be followed by a series of other questions, such as "When did you first notice this?" *(inception)*. Affecting factors that improve or worsen the condition should also be determined. "Does heat, cold, biting, or chewing cause pain?" *(provoking factors)*. "Does anything hot or cold relieve the pain?" *(attenuating factors)*. "How often does this occur?" *(frequency)*. "When you have pain, is it mild, moderate or severe?" *(intensity)*. The answers to these questions provide the information the dentist needs to develop a brief narrative description of the problem.

The majority of patients present with evident problems of pain or swelling, so most questions should begin to focus on these areas. For example: "Could you point to the area that you think is swelling?" *(location)*. "When cold (or heat) causes pain, does it last for a moment or for several seconds or longer?" *(duration)*. "Do you have any pain when you lie down or bend over?" *(postural)*. "Does the pain ever occur without provocation?" *(stimulated or spontaneous)*.

Questions similar to these will help the clinician establish the location, nature, quality, and urgency of the problem.

When the dentist asks a few good leading questions like the ones just described, not only are patients willing to answer but they also may volunteer additional information to help complete the verbal picture of their problem. It is fairly common that while taking a dental history the clinician may be able to formulate a tentative diagnosis; the examination and testing that follow will often corroborate the tentative diagnosis. It is then merely a matter of identifying the offending tooth.

In the taking of a dental history, common sense must prevail. These questions, along with other questions described in Chapter 2, should be asked if the diagnosis appears possibly elusive. However, if the clinician can see a grossly decayed tooth while sitting and talking with the patient and the patient points to that tooth, the dental history should be brief because of the obvious nature of the problem. Furthermore, if the patient is suffering from acute distress, with dire symptoms (Chapter 2), then taking a dental history should also be as brief as possible so the patient can obtain rapid relief.

Pain

Because pain frequently is the result of a diseased pulp, it is one of the most common symptoms a dentist is required to diagnose. The source of the pain is usually made evident by dental history, inspection, examination, and testing. However, because pain has psychobiologic components—physical, emotional, and tolerance—identifying the source is at times quite difficult. Furthermore, because of psychologic conditioning, including fear, the intensity of pain perception may not be proportional to the stimulus. When patients present with a complaint of pain that is of odontogenic origin, the vast majority of these cases reflect conditions of irreversible pulpitis with or without partial necrosis.[16]

Patients may report the pain as sharp, dull, continuous, intermittent, mild, severe, etc. Because the neural portion of the pulp contains only pain fibers, if the inflammatory state is limited to the pulp tissue it may be difficult for the patient to localize the pain. However, once the inflammatory process extends beyond the apical foramen and begins to involve the periodontal ligament, which contains proprioceptive fibers, the patient should be able to localize the source of the pain. A percussion test at this time to corroborate the patient's perception of the source might be quite helpful.

At times pain is referred to other areas within and even beyond the mouth. Most commonly it is manifested in other teeth in the same or the opposing quadrant. It almost never crosses the midline of the head. However, referred pain is not necessarily limited to just other teeth. It may, for example, be unilaterally referred to the preauricular area, or down the neck, or up to the temporal area. In these instances the source of extraorally referred pain almost invariably is a posterior tooth. Ostensible toothache of nonodontogenic origin (i.e., resulting from neurologic, cardiac, vascular, malignant or sinus disease) is described in Chapter 2.

Patients may report that their dental pain is exacerbated by lying down or bending over. This occurs because of the increase in blood pressure to the head, which therefore increases the pressure on the confined pulp.

The dentist should be alert for patients who manifest their emotional disorders as dental pain. If no apparent cause can be discovered for what appears as dental pain, the patient should be referred for medical consultation. Patients with atypical facial pain of functional rather than organic etiology may begin their long journey through the many specialties of the health sciences in the dentist's office.

If the dentist can determine the onset, duration, frequency, quality, and affecting factors that alter the perception of pain, and if the pain can be reproduced or relieved by clinical testing, then surely the pain is of odontogenic origin. The patient will usually gain immeasurable psychologic benefit if the clinician provides a caring and sincere reassurance that, once the source is discovered, appropriate treatment will be provided immediately to stop the pain.

EXAMINATION AND TESTING

The inspection phase of the extraoral and intraoral clinical examination should be performed in a systematic manner. A consistent step-by-step approach following the same procedure helps the clinician develop good working habits and minimizes the possibility of inadvertently overlooking any part of examination or testing. The extraoral visual examination should begin while the clinician is taking the patient's dental history.

Talking with the patient provides an opportunity to observe the patient's facial features. The clinician should look for facial asymmetry (Fig. 1-1, A) or distensions that might indicate swelling of odontogenic origin or a systemic ailment. The patient's eyes should be observed for the pupillary dilation or constriction that may indicate systemic disease, premedication, or fear. Additionally, the patient's skin should be observed for any lesion(s) and, if there is more than one, whether the lesions appear at random or follow a neural pathway.

After a careful external visual examination the clinician should, with the aid of a mouth mirror and the blunt-ended handle of another instrument, begin an oral examination to look for abnormalities of both hard and soft tissues. With a strong light the lips, cheek pouch, tongue, palate, and throat should be briefly examined. A high "index of suspicion" must prevail during examination for numerous types of soft-tissue lesions, as described by Eversole.[5] This also means looking for unusual changes in the color or contour of the soft tissues. For example, the clinician should look carefully for lesions of odontogenic origin such as sinus tracts ("fistulas") (Fig. 1-2) or localized redness or swelling involving the attachment apparatus. The presence of a sinus tract may indicate that periapical suppuration has resulted from a pulp that underwent complete necrosis in at least one root. The suppurative lesion has burrowed its way from the cancellous bone through the cortical plate and finally to the mucosal surface. All sinus tracts should be traced with a gutta-percha cone (Fig. 1-2) to locate their source. Because it is easier to observe abnormalities when tissues are dry, the liberal use of 2 × 2 inch gauze, cotton rolls, and a saliva ejector is strongly recommended (Fig. 1-1, B). During the visual phase of the examination the clinician should also be checking both the patient's oral hygiene and the integrity of his dentition. Poor oral hygiene and/or numerous missing teeth may indicate that the patient has minimal interest in maintaining a healthy dentition.

Visual inspection of the teeth begins with drying the quadrant under examination and looking for caries (Fig. 1-1, C) (cervical lesions occasionally are overlooked), darkened teeth (Fig. 1-1, D), observable swelling (Fig. 1-1, E) fractured or cracked crowns (Fig. 1-1, G), and defective restorations.

The clinician should observe the color and translucency of the teeth. Are the teeth intact or is there evidence of abrasion, attrition, cervical erosion, or developmental de-

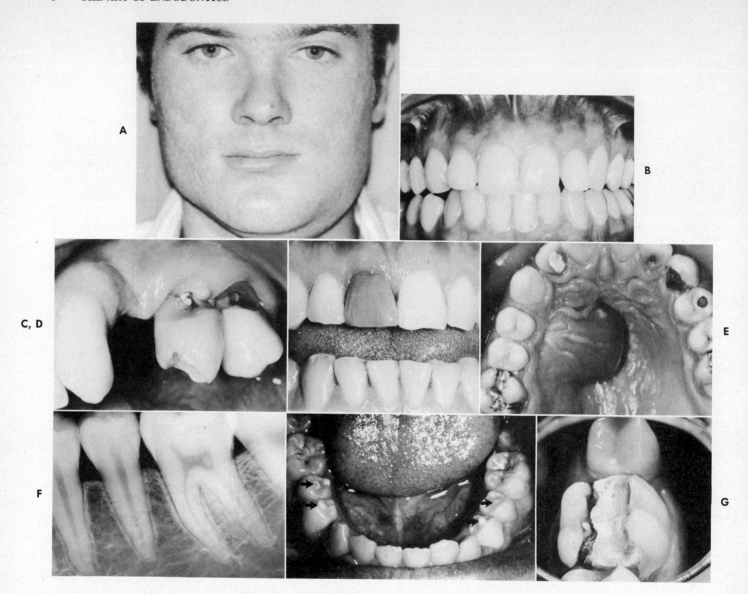

FIG. 1-1. A, Swelling around the left mandible can be readily observed by the clinician while preparing the dental history. **B,** After drying with gauze, the initial examination of the teeth and surrounding tissues is conducted with the patient's mouth closed. With good illumination and magnification, changes in color, contour, or texture can be determined by a careful visual examination. **C,** Class V caries lesion, or abrasion, not always detectable radiographically, can be observed. **D,** Tooth discolored following a traumatic incident. Although the tooth appears necrotic, vitality tests should still be conducted because the pulp could remain vital. **E,** Intraoral swelling from periapical disease usually appears around the mucobuccal fold; however, the entire mouth must be thoroughly examined, because swelling from periapical disease may occur in unusual locations, e.g., the palate. **F,** Developmental defect. *Left,* The vertical hypocalcified line between the dentin-enamel junction and the pulp chamber in the first premolar provides early evidence of a dens evaginatus. *Right,* Tubercules *(arrows)* of dens evaginatus, which provide an easy pathway to the pulp within an otherwise intact, sound tooth. **G,** With a thorough visual examination, the clinician may observe crown fractures that may not be seen radiographically. (**F,** *left,* courtesy Dr. Mitsuko Ishii.)

fects in the crowns (Fig. 1-1, *F*)? The routine use of a strong fiberoptic light is immensely helpful for the clinician in discerning defects in the teeth that might otherwise go undetected.

All observable data indicating an abnormality should be recorded on the treatment chart while the information is still fresh in the clinician's mind. If a tooth is suspected of requiring endodontic treatment, it should be assessed in terms of its restorability after endodontic treatment, its strategic importance, and its periodontal prognosis.

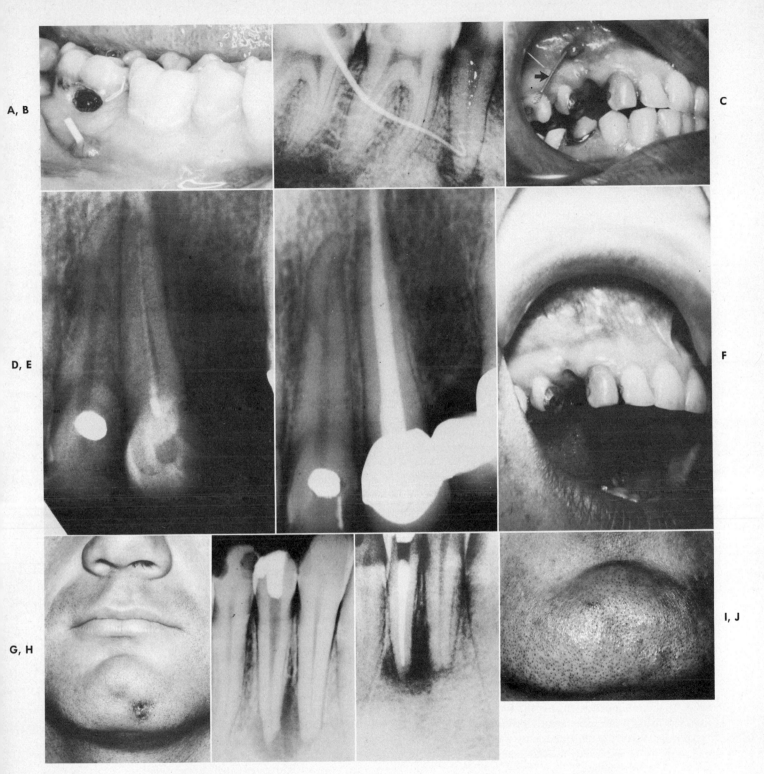

FIG. 1-2. Sinus tract ("fistula"). **A,** When a sinus tract is detected, it should always be traced with a gutta-percha cone to its source. In this case, the sinus tract appeared between the first and second molars. **B,** But the source of the sinus tract was the second premolar, as the gutta-percha probe indicates. **C,** Gutta-percha cone used to trace a sinus tract *(arrow)*. The previous dentist had extracted the first premolar 2 weeks earlier, thinking it was the source. **D,** An inadequately obturated canine was the real source of the sinus tract. **E,** Canal properly obturated. **F,** Sinus tract closed shortly after canal obturation. **G,** Sinus tracts may have extraoral exits. Root length and location of muscle attachments affect where a sinus tract will exit. A mandibular incisor caused this extraoral sinus tract, which was unsuccessfully treated for 6 months by a dermatologist. **H,** A radiograph reveals the source. **I,** Immediately following canal obturation. **J,** Two weeks later, only a slight scar remains. (**C-F** courtesy Dr. John Sapone; **G-J** courtesy Dr. Stephen Schwartz.)

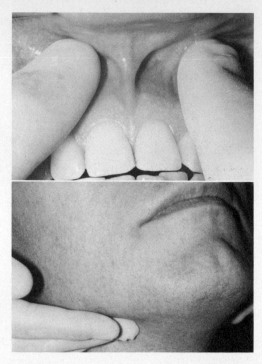

FIG. 1-3. Palpation. **A,** Bilateral intraoral digital palpation aids the clinician in detecting changes in contour or consistency of the soft tissue and underlying bone. A "mushy" feeling detected during palpation around the mucolabial fold may be the first clinical evidence of incipient swelling. For protection of the practitioner and the patient, gloves are strongly recommended. **B,** Bimanual extraoral palpation to tactilely search for the extent of lymph node involvement when there is a mandibular dental infection. Palpation should include the submandibular nodes (shown here), the angle of the mandible, and the cervical chain of nodes.

Palpation

When periapical inflammation has developed as an extension of pulpal necrosis, the inflammatory process may burrow its way through the facial cortical bone and begin to affect the overlying mucoperiosteum. Before incipient swelling becomes clinically evident, it may be discerned by both the clinician and the patient using gentle palpation with the index finger (Fig. 1-3, *A*). The index finger is rolled while it presses the mucosa against the underlying bone. If the mucoperiosteum is inflamed, this rolling motion will usually disclose sensitivity in the patient.

To improve tactile skill and learn the full extent of normal range to be expected, the clinician is urged to perform palpation testing routinely.

Other techniques involving extraoral bidigital or bimanual palpation (e.g., palpating lymph nodes or the floor of the mouth) are described in complete detail by Rose and Kaye.[14]

Occasionally a patient will be able to point to a particular facial area that felt tender when shaving or applying makeup. The clinician can follow up by palpating in the mucofacial fold, which may help reveal the area in question.

If a site that feels tender to palpation is discovered, its location and extent should be recorded as well as whether or not the area is soft or firm. This provides important information on the possible need for an incision and drainage.

If a mandibular tooth is abscessed, it would be prudent also to palpate the submandibular area bimanually to determine whether any submandibular lymph nodes have been affected by extension of the disease process (Fig. 1-3, *B*).

Finally, the cervical lymph nodes should be palpated bidigitally to discern any swollen or firm lymph nodes.

The use of extraoral, along with intraoral, palpation will help the clinician determine the furthest extent of the disease processes.

Percussion

The percussion test may reveal whether there is any inflammation around the periodontal ligament. The clinician should remember that the percussion test does *not* give any indication of the health or integrity of the pulp tissue; it indicates only whether there is inflammation around the periodontal ligament. Before the test, the patient should be instructed that a small audible sound or raising a hand is the best method to let the clinician know when a tooth feels "tender," "different," or painful with percussion.

Before tapping on the teeth with the handle of a mouth mirror, the clinician is advised to first percuss teeth in the quadrant being examined, using the index finger. Digital percussion is much less painful than percussion with a mouth mirror handle. The teeth should be tapped in a random fashion (i.e., out of sequence) so the patient cannot anticipate when "the tooth" will be percussed. If the patient cannot discern a difference of sensation with digital percussion, *then* the handle of a mouth mirror should be used to tap on the occlusal, facial, and lingual surfaces of the teeth (Fig. 1-4). The force of percussing is one of the skills that the clinician will develop as part of the "art" of endodontic diagnosis. Percussing the teeth too strongly may cause unnecessary pain and anxiety for the patient. The clinician should use the chief complaint and dental history as a guide in deciding how strongly to percuss the teeth. The force of percussion need be only great enough for the patient to discern a difference between a sound tooth and a tooth with an inflamed periodontal ligament. The proprioceptive fibers in an inflamed periodontal ligament will, when percussed, help the patient and the clinician locate the source of the pain. Tapping on each cusp has, on occasion, revealed the presence of a crown fracture.

A positive response to percussion, indicating an inflamed periodontal ligament, can be caused by a variety of reasons (e.g., teeth undergoing rapid orthodontic movement, a recent "high" restoration, a lateral periodontal abscess, and, of course, partial or total necrosis of the pulp). However, the absence of a response to percussion is quite possible when there is chronic periapical inflammation.

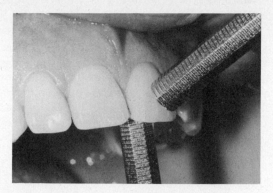

FIG. 1-5. The degree of mobility can be most effectively determined by applying lateral forces with a blunt-handled instrument in a facial-lingual direction.

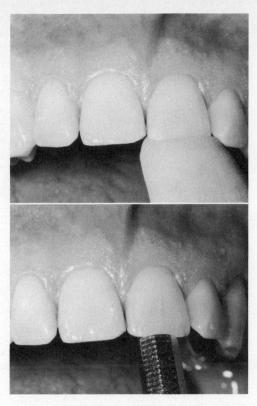

FIG. 1-4. Percussion test to determine whether there is any apical periodontitis. If the patient has reported pain during mastication, the percussion test should be conducted *very gently*. Only the index finger *(top)* should be used. The teeth should be percussed from a facial as well as an incisal direction. If the patient reports no tenderness when the teeth are percussed with the finger, a more definitive sharper percussion *(bottom)* can be conducted with the handle of the mouth mirror.

Mobility

Using the index fingers or the blunt handles of two metal instruments, the clinician applies alternating lateral forces in a facial-lingual direction to observe the degree of mobility of the tooth within the alveolus (Fig. 1-5). In addition, tests for the degree of depressibility are performed by pressing the tooth into its socket and observing if there is vertical movement. First-degree mobility is barely discernible movement; second-degree is horizontal movement of 1 mm or less; third-degree is horizontal movement of greater than 1 mm, often accompanied by a vertical component of mobility. Tooth movement usually reflects the extent of inflammation of the periodontal ligament.

The pressure exerted by the purulent exudate of an acute apical abscess may cause some mobility of a tooth. In this situation the tooth may quickly stabilize after drainage is established and the occlusion adjusted. There are additional causes for tooth mobility—including advanced periodontal disease, horizontal root fracture in the middle or coronal third, and chronic bruxism or clenching.

Radiographs

Radiographs are essential aids in endodontic diagnosis. Unfortunately, some clinicians rely exclusively on radiographs in their attempt to arrive at a diagnosis. This obviously can lead to major errors in diagnosis and treatment. Because the radiograph is a two-dimensional image of a three-dimensional object, the potential for misinterpretation is a constant risk, but with proper angulation of the cone, accurate film placement, correct processing of the exposed film, and good illumination with a magnifying glass, the hazards of misinterpretation can be substantially minimized. The benefits of periapical radiographs for diagnostic purposes can be derived by the following technique.

After correct film placement, either bisected-angle or long-cone methods are effective for film exposure. It is *imperative* to expose two diagnostic films. By maintaining the same vertical cone angulation and changing the horizontal cone angulation 10 to 15 degrees for the second diagnostic film, the clinician can obtain in subsequent film comparisons a three-dimensional impression of the teeth that will aid in discerning superimposed roots and anatomic landmarks. (Refer to Chapter 4 for further discussion of this phase of dental radiology.)

The state of pulpal health or pulpal necrosis cannot be determined radiographically; but the following findings should arouse suspicion of degenerative pulp changes: deep carious lesions, deep and extensive restorations, pulp caps, pulpotomies, pulp stones, extensive canal calcification, root resorption, radiolucencies at or near the apex, root fractures, thickened periodontal ligament, and periodontal disease that is radiographically evident.

Radiographic interpretation

Interpretation of good-quality diagnostic radiographs must be done in an orderly and consistent manner. With good illumination and magnification the clinician can detect nuances of change in the many shades of gray between black and white that may reveal early pathologic changes in or around the tooth. First, the crown of each tooth and then the root(s) are carefully observed, and then the root canal system, followed by the lamina dura, bony architecture, and finally the anatomic landmarks that may appear on the film. When posterior teeth are being investigated, a bite-wing film provides an excellent supplement for finding the extent of carious destruction, the depths of restorations, the presence of pulp caps or pulpotomies, and dens invaginatus or evaginatus. Generally it is true that the deeper the caries and the more extensive the restoration the greater is the probability of pulpal involvement. Following the lamina dura will usually reveal the number and curvature of the roots. A root canal should be readily discernible; if the canal appears to change quickly from dark to light, this indicates that it has bifurcated or trifurcated (Fig. 1-6, *A*). The presence of "extra" canals in all teeth (Fig. 1-6, *B* to *E*) is much more common than previously believed. If the outline of the root seems unclear or deviates from where it "ought" to be, an extra root should be suspected.[17] Accordingly, *the presence of at least one canal (or root) more than the radiograph shows must always be suspected until clinically proved otherwise.* Three-

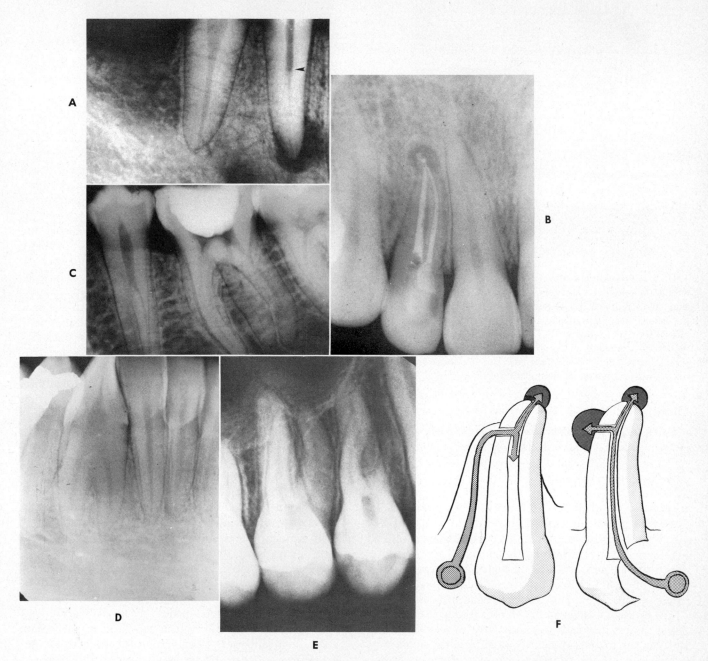

FIG. 1-6. Radiographic interpretation. **A,** A sudden change from dark to light indicates bifurcation or trifurcation of the root canal system *(arrow)*. **B,** Lateral incisor with two canals. **C,** Mandibular first molar with three roots (note the branching of the premolar root canal system in the apical half). **D,** Canine with two roots. **E,** Maxillary premolars with three roots. **F,** Radiolucent lesion indicative of pulpal inflammation or degeneration. The drawing illustrates how toxins of pulp tissue degeneration may exit from a lateral canal, causing bone destruction along the side. Conversely, this lateral canal could be a portal of entry for toxins that might destroy the pulp and create a periapical lesion.   *Continued.*

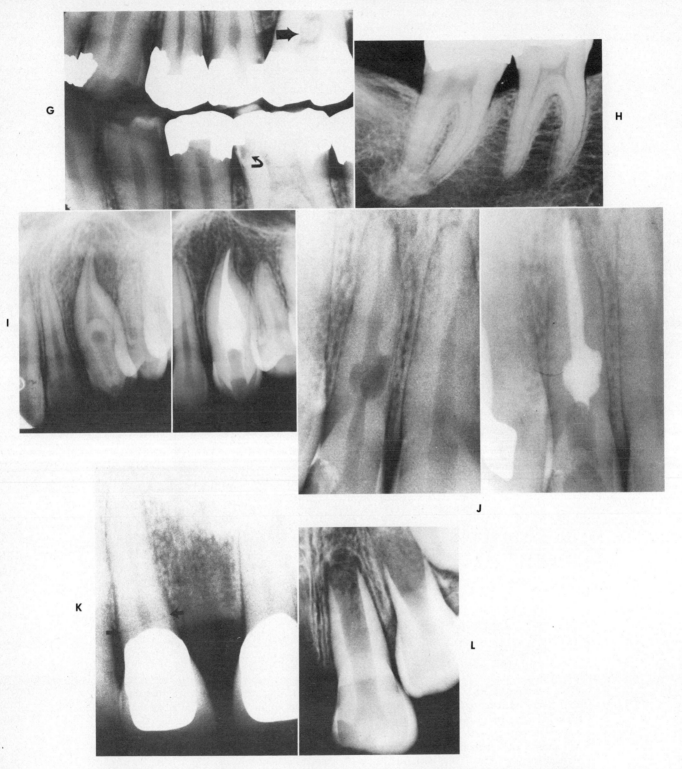

FIG. 1-6, cont'd. **G,** Pulp stones *(wide arrow),* caries *(curved arrow),* and the extent and depth of restorations can be detected more clearly with a bite-wing film. **H,** Periapical osteosclerosis, possibly caused by a mild pulp irritant. **I,** Dens in dente *(left);* following endodontic treatment *(right).* **J,** Internal resorption, once detected, must be treated promptly before it perforates the root. **K,** Horizontal root fractures can usually be detected with a good-quality radiograph. **L,** Vitality tests on a tooth with an immature apex may yield erroneous results.

Continued.

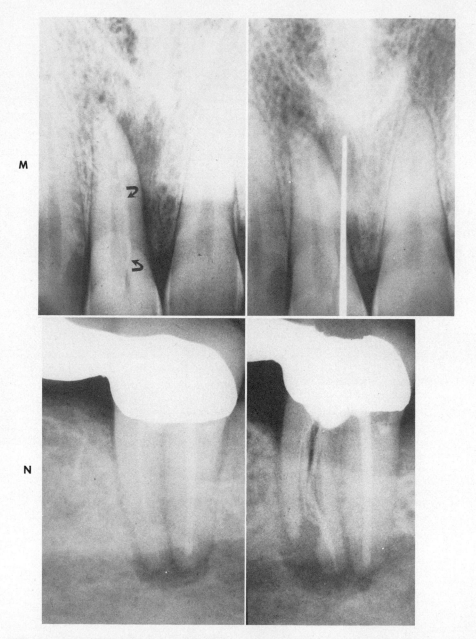

FIG. 1-6, cont'd. **M,** *Left,* Lingual developmental groove. The radiograph shows the canals of both central incisors to be distinctly different. Arrows point to the groove traced along the root. *Right,* Silver cone in the sulcular defect tracing the groove toward the apex. Although the tooth was vital, only extraction could resolve this problem. **N,** Vertical fractures are rarely evident radiographically until there is advanced root separation. *Left,* Mesial root with an undetected vertical fracture. *Right,* One year later, after advanced separation, the vertical fracture becomes evident. (**B** courtesy Dr. Irving Fried; **C** and **E** courtesy Dr. James Campbell.)

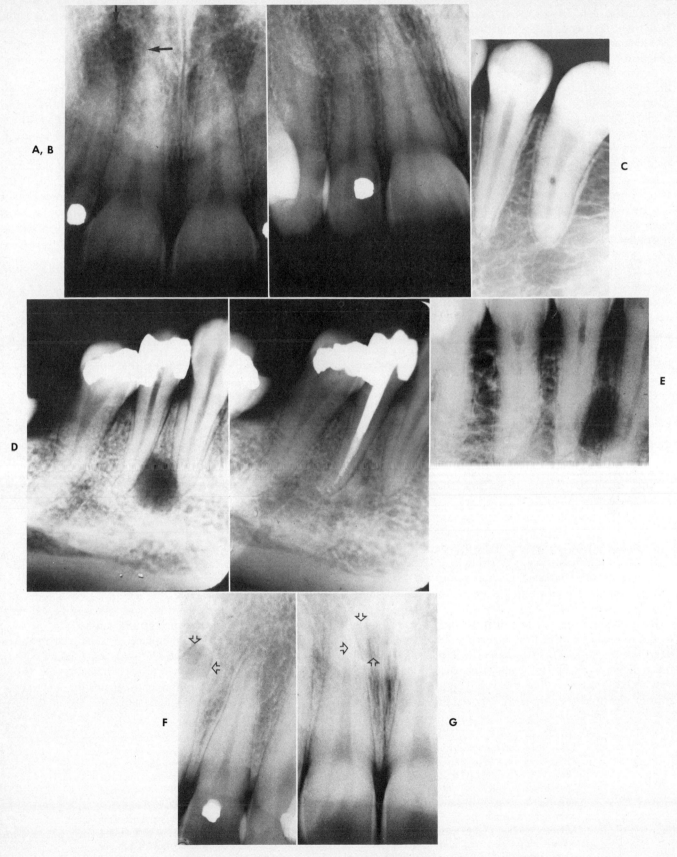

FIG. 1-7. See p. 16 for legend.

rooted mandibular molars (Fig. 1-6, *C*) and maxillary premolars (Fig. 1-6, *E*) as well as two-rooted canines (Fig. 1-6, *D*) will be found with greater frequency as the examiner's dental anatomic acumen, "index of suspicion," and diagnostic sophistication improve.

A necrotic tooth will not cause radiographic changes at the apex until the periapical pathosis has destroyed bony trabeculae at their junction with the cortical plate.[15] Thus a great deal of bone destruction may occur before any signs are radiographically evident. A radiolucent lesion need not be at the apex of the root to indicate pulpal inflammation or degeneration. Toxins of pulp tissue degeneration exiting from a lateral canal can cause bone destruction anywhere along the root. Conversely, a lateral canal can be a portal of entry for potentially harmful toxins in teeth with advanced periodontal disease (Fig. 1-6, *F*). If periodontal bone loss extends far enough apically to expose the foramen of a lateral canal, the toxins from the periodontal disease can gain entry into a vital healthy pulp via the lateral canal and cause irritation, inflammation, and even pulpal necrosis in a sound tooth. Periodontal disease extending to the apical foramen will definitely cause pathologic pulpal changes (see Chapter 17).

Pulp stones (Fig. 1-6, *G*) and canal calcifications are not necessarily pathologic; they can also be mere manifestations of degenerative aging in the pulpal tissue. Their presence can potentiate other insults to the pulp and may increase the difficulty of negotiating the root canals. The incidence of calcifications in the chamber or in the canal may increase with periodontal disease, extensive restorations, or aging. As the percentage of the population categorized as "elderly" increases, clinicians should be more atuned to detecting pulp stones and calcification of the canal space.[22]

Internal resorption (Fig. 1-6, *J*) (occasionally seen after a traumatic injury) is an indication for endodontic therapy. The inflamed pulp, expanding at the expense of the dentin, must be removed as soon as possible or a lateral perforation may occur. Untreated internal resorption leading to root perforation increases the probability of eventual tooth loss (see Chapter 16).

Root fractures may cause pulpal degeneration. Fractures of the root can be difficult to detect on a radiograph. Vertical root fractures (Fig. 1-6, *N*) are seldom identified with the radiograph except in advanced stages of root separation. Most horizontal root fractures (Fig. 1-6, *K*) can be readily identified with properly exposed and processed radiographs. However, horizontal fractures may be confused with linear patterns of bone trabeculae. The two fractures can be differentiated by noting that the lines of bone trabeculae extend beyond the border of the root whereas a root fracture often causes a thickening of the periodontal ligament.

Radiographs are important for identifying teeth with immature apices (Fig. 1-6, *L*). The clinician must have this information *before* conducting thermal and electric pulp tests because teeth with immature apices often cause erroneous readings in thermal and electric pulp testing (Chapter 22).

Finally, the clinician must realize that there are occasions when periapical, bite-wing, and panoramic films may not suffice. Other types of extraoral films, described in greater detail on p. 38, may be necessary (especially when there has been a traumatic incident) before a diagnosis can be made.

Radiographic misinterpretation

A dental humorist once claimed that if a clinician looked at a radiograph long enough he would find whatever he was looking for. This may overstate the point somewhat, but on occasion it can almost be true.

Perhaps we should begin with a general rule: be wary—but not necessarily disbelieving—of what appears to be obvious radiographically. Radiographic interpretation is often quite subjective, as illustrated by a study of more than 250 cases in which the *same* endodontists interpreted the *same* radiographs with a time lapse of 6 to 8 months. The three endodontists in this study agreed with themselves 72% to 88% of the time.[7] In an earlier study six endodontists all agreed with each other *less than half the time*.[6] Some illustrations to help develop the reasons for this "wary" rule follow:

1. Diffuse radiolucency at the apex (Fig. 1-7, *C*). At first glance this might appear to be a periapical lesion. However, a positive response to vitality tests, an intact lamina dura, the absence of symptoms and probable cause, and the anatomic location clearly show this to be the mental foramen.
2. Well-circumscribed radiolucency at or near the apex (Fig. 1-7, *D, E, F,* and *G*). At first glance (Fig. 1-7, *F*) it might appear to be a periapical lesion. However, changing the horizontal angulation and exposing a second radiograph show the lesion to have

FIG. 1-7. Radiographic misinterpretation. **A,** This radiograph suggests a periapical lesion over the apex of the lateral incisor *(arrow)*. **B,** By merely changing the vertical angulation the examiner caused the "lesion" to disappear. The effect is due to the superimposition of the nares over the lateral incisor apices. **C,** Mental foramen that might be mistaken for a periapical lesion. Thermal and electric pulp tests and an intact lamina dura revealed that the tooth was vital. **D,** *Left,* Vitality tests indicated that the first premolar was necrotic. Adjacent teeth tested vital. *Right,* One year after completion of endodontic treatment, the bone remineralized. **E,** Gingival cyst. Thermal and electric pulp tests revealed the adjacent teeth had vital pulps. **F,** Periapical radiolucency that might be mistaken for a periapical lesion *(arrows)*. **G,** Changing the horizontal cone angulation moved the radiolucency toward the midline *(arrows)*. The "lesion" was the nasopalatine foramen superimposed over the apex of the central incisor. (**B** courtesy Dr. James Campbell; **D** courtesy Dr. Nguyen T. Nguyen.)

"moved" (Fig. 1-7, *G*). Because the tooth was asymptomatic with lack of probable cause and because of a positive response to vitality tests and anatomic location, this was positively identified as the nasopalatine canal.

3. Diffuse radiolucency at the apex that appears to be a periapical lesion. However, thermal and electric pulp tests prove the tooth to be vital. By exposing a second film with a different vertical angulation, the clinician can make the radiolucency disappear (Fig. 1-7, *B*). The superimposition of the nares or the thinning of the cortical plate above the apices of the maxillary lateral incisors was creating the radiographic illusion of a periapical lesion.

Accordingly, NEVER make a clinical diagnosis based merely on the radiograph showing a periapical radiolucency; ALWAYS use thermal and electric pulp tests for clinical verification. As Grossman[9] says, "Mistake not the shadow for the substance."

Thermal tests

One of the most common symptoms associated with a symptomatic inflamed pulp is pain induced by hot or cold stimulation. Hot and cold tests are valuable diagnostic aids because with certain types of inflamed pulps, pain may be induced or relieved by a thermal application. The patient's response to thermal tests frequently provides the clinician with information about whether the pulp is healthy or inflamed; when several teeth in a quadrant are being tested, thermal tests often help pinpoint the thermally symptomatic tooth.

Before testing, the patient should be told what tests are going to be performed and why, and should be given some idea as to what to expect. Furthermore, one or two teeth on the opposite side of the mouth should be tested first so the patient has an idea of how the tests will feel. If the clinician takes the time to do this, patient anxiety and fear will be substantially reduced.

It is important to inform the patient how to respond when a sensation is experienced, so there will be no thrashing about or other untoward behavior. For example, the patient should be instructed to raise his hand as soon as any sensation is felt and should be assured that the clinician will remove the stimulus immediately if his hand is raised.

The teeth in the quadrant must first be isolated and then dried with 2 × 2 inch gauze and a saliva ejector placed. The teeth should *not* be dried with a blast of air because the room-temperature air might cause thermal shock and saliva might be sprayed on the clinician or the assistant (Fig. 1-8, *B*).

Heat test

For the heat test a stick of temporary stopping (gutta-percha) is heated for a few seconds over an alcohol flame until it becomes shiny and sags, but *before* it begins to smoke. The stopping is then immediately placed on the middle third of the facial surface of the crown (Fig. 1-9). If it is too hot (i.e., the gutta-percha appears to be "smoking"), it may cause a burn lesion in an otherwise normal pulp. This type of abuse could be the coup de grace for a debilitated pulp. If the patient has a normal pulp, the re-

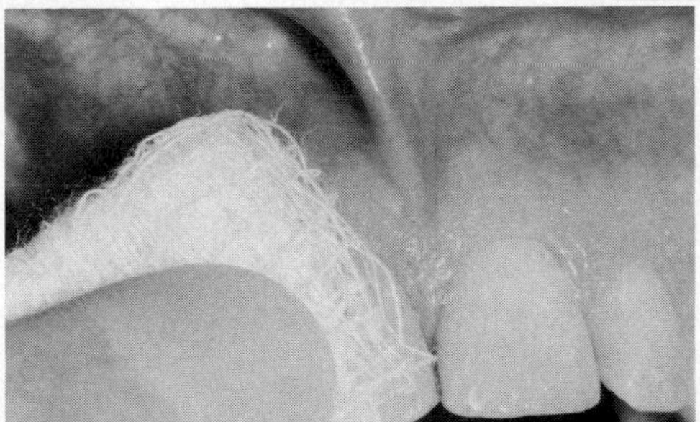

FIG. 1-8 Preparing teeth for thermal and electric pulp testing. **A,** Before testing, the teeth should be isolated with a cotton roll and dried with gauze. **B,** Air should *not* be used to dry the teeth because room temperature air may cause thermal shock. Air drying may also spray saliva on the clinician.

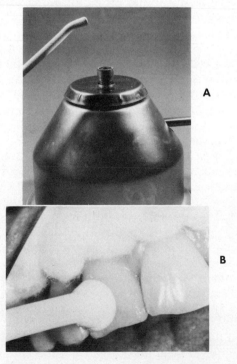

FIG. 1-9. Thermal test with heat. **A,** Temporary stopping is heated over a flame until it becomes soft and begins to bend. **B,** Temporary stopping applied to the dried tooth (lightly coated with cocoa butter to prevent sticking).

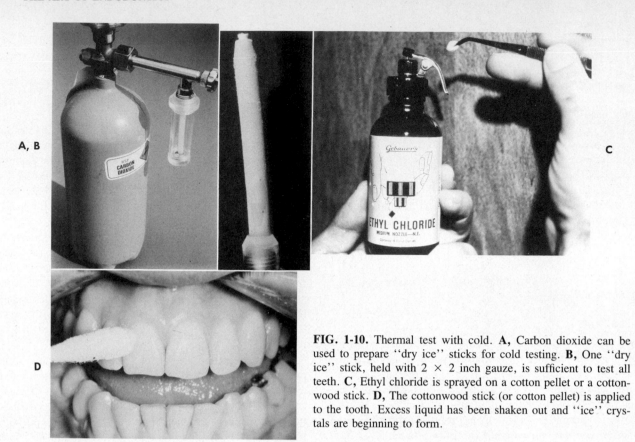

FIG. 1-10. Thermal test with cold. **A,** Carbon dioxide can be used to prepare "dry ice" sticks for cold testing. **B,** One "dry ice" stick, held with 2 × 2 inch gauze, is sufficient to test all teeth. **C,** Ethyl chloride is sprayed on a cotton pellet or a cottonwood stick. **D,** The cottonwood stick (or cotton pellet) is applied to the tooth. Excess liquid has been shaken out and "ice" crystals are beginning to form.

sponse to this test is usually mild to moderate and transient. The patient should not experience any pain. If the tooth has a full coronal coverage, the blade of a wax instrument may be heated 5 to 10 seconds in an alcohol flame and applied directly to the metal. Even porcelain-fused-to-metal crowns often have some exposed metal surface on the lingual where a heated blade can be placed directly on the metal. Another method for heating the metal of a crown sufficiently to obtain a response is by isolating the tooth with a rubber dam and bathing the tooth with very warm water (see p. 35).

Care must be used in applying these heat tests, or the pulp may be damaged by overheating. The preferred temperature for a heat test is approximately 65.5° C (150° F).

Cold test

For cold testing the teeth must remain isolated and dry. The most common techniques for cold testing utilize ethyl chloride, sticks of ice or carbon dioxide "snow," or freon 12.[19] Although all four methods are effective, ethyl chloride is the preferred technique. Sticks of ice require preparation time and, when applied to a tooth surface, may drip onto the gingiva, causing a patient's false response. Carbon dioxide "snow" or dry ice is very cold ($-77.7°$ C or $-108°$ F) and may cause infraction lines in enamel because of thermal shock[1] or may damage an otherwise healthy pulp.[2]

Ethyl chloride is sprayed liberally on a cotton pellet, and the cotton pliers holding the pellet are tapped once or twice to shake out the excess liquid. Without delay the cotton pellet is then placed on the middle third of the facial surface (Fig. 1-10). The ethyl chloride technique is effective even on teeth covered with cast metal crowns. Spraying ethyl chloride directly onto a tooth is *not* recommended, because the liquid is a general anesthetic, highly flammable, and potentially dangerous for the patient when used in this manner. The pellet should be held in close contact with the tooth surface for several seconds, or until the patient has a response.

Responses

The patient's responses to heat and cold testing are identical because the neural fibers in the pulp transmit only the sensation of pain. There are four possible reactions the patient may experience: (1) no response; (2) a moderate, transient response; (3) a painful response that subsides quickly after the stimulus is removed from the tooth; and (4) a painful response that lingers after the thermal stimulus is removed.

If there is no response, the pulp is either nonvital or possibly vital but giving a false-negative response because of excessive calcification, an immature apex, recent trauma, or patient premedication. A moderate, transient response is usually considered normal. A painful response that subsides quickly after the stimulus is removed is characteristic of reversible pulpitis. Finally, a painful response that lingers after the thermal stimulus is removed indicates a symptomatic irreversible pulpitis.

Electric pulp tests

The electric pulp tester is designed to stimulate a response by electric excitation of the neural elements within the pulp. The patient's response to the electric pulp test does *not* provide sufficient information for a diagnosis. The electric pulp test merely suggests whether the pulp is vital or nonvital and does not provide information regarding the health or integrity of a vital pulp. Restated, the electric pulp test does not provide any information about the vascular supply to the tooth, which is the *real* determinant of vitality. Additionally, a number of situations may cause a false-positive or false-negative response, *so*

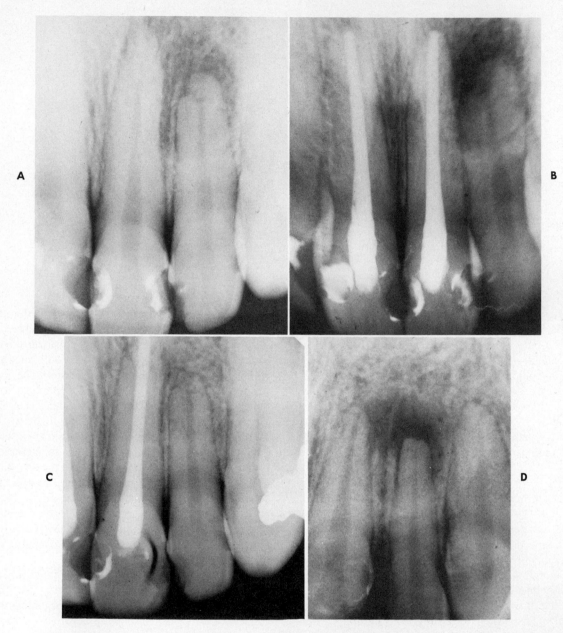

FIG. 1-11. Why thermal and electric pulp testing is so important. **A,** Demonstration of the importance of vitality testing. The maxillary left lateral incisor appears to be a candidate for endodontic treatment. A large radiolucency encompasses the apical third of the root, the root end seems to be resorbing, and the mesial-incisal angle of the crown appears to be fractured and lost. The left lateral incisor and canine responded to electric and thermal tests. The two central incisors gave no response to vitality testing. **B,** Endodontic therapy was completed on both central incisors. **C,** Eighteen-month follow-up visit. Note that the radiolucent area over the lateral incisor has remineralized. The lateral incisor and canine again responded normally to electric and thermal vitality tests. **D,** The periapical radiolucency over the lateral incisor might indicate the lateral incisors as the source of the lesion. Thermal and electric pulp tests indicated that the lateral incisor was vital and the canine was necrotic. **E,** Endodontic treatment completed for the canine. **F,** Six months after treatment the bone has completely remineralized over the apex of the lateral incisor. (Courtesy Dr. John Sapone.)   *Continued.*

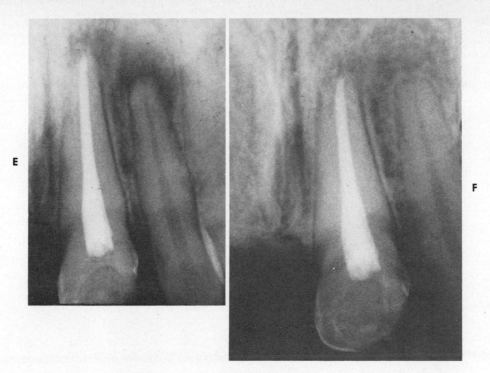

E

F

FIG. 1-11, cont'd. For legend see p. 19.

using other diagnostic tests is essential before arriving at a final diagnosis.

The electric pulp tester (Fig. 1-12) is a valuable tool for differential diagnosis. Not only does it help the clinician in determining pulp vitality, but along with thermal and periodontal tests it can also aid in differentiating among radiographic signs of pulpal, periodontal, or nonodontogenic etiologies.

The most common and convenient types of electric pulp testers used today are battery operated (Fig. 1-12).

Technique

Just as for thermal tests, the teeth must be isolated and dried with 2 × 2 inch gauze and a saliva ejector placed. Furthermore, the patient must be told about the reason for the test and how the test will be performed. One or two teeth (preferably the contralateral teeth) on the opposite side of the mouth should be tested first so that the patient becomes acquainted with the sensation. Testing the opposite side of the mouth lets the clinician know the patient's normal level of response. The electrode of the pulp tester should be generously coated with a good viscous conductor (e.g., toothpaste). The electrode/conductor is then placed on sound, dried enamel on the middle third of the facial surface.

All restorations should be avoided because they may cause a false reading. Each reading should be recorded in the patient's record. The electrode/conductor can be applied to dried dentin; however, in this situation the clinician should be most careful and the patient cautioned in advance that the sensation may be painful rather than merely warm or tingling, because dentin is an excellent conductor of electricity. The Analytic Technology pulp tester (Fig. 1-12 A) is recommended because it *always* starts at 0 current, does not require manual advancement of any rheostats, and avoids the two problems associated with other battery-operated pulp testers: an occasional painful electric shock and the inadvertent positioning of the rheostat at a high current when the test is initiated.[4] When the patient *just begins* to feel slight tingling or a sensation of heat, he should be instructed to raise his hand. The current flow should be adjusted to increase slowly, because if it increases too quickly the patient may experience pain before he has an opportunity to raise his hand. As with other pulp testers, a complete circuit between the patient and the clinician and tester must be maintained during testing or a false reading may occur. Accordingly, the clinician should not wear gloves when conducting an electric pulp test.

Each tooth should be tested two or three times and the readings averaged. The patient's response may vary slightly (which is quite common) or significantly (which suggests a false-positive or false-negative situation).

Generally, the thicker the enamel is, the more delayed will be the response. Accordingly, thin anterior teeth will yield a quicker response and broad posterior teeth a slower response because of the greater thickness of enamel and dentin. An additional function of the electric pulp tester is testing vital teeth that have been anesthetized for pulp extirpation. If the vital pulp has been profoundly anesthetized, the electric pulp tester should not be able to stimulate the pulp when maximum current is applied.

The electric pulp test is one of the *last* tests to be performed. The clinician should have a fairly good idea about

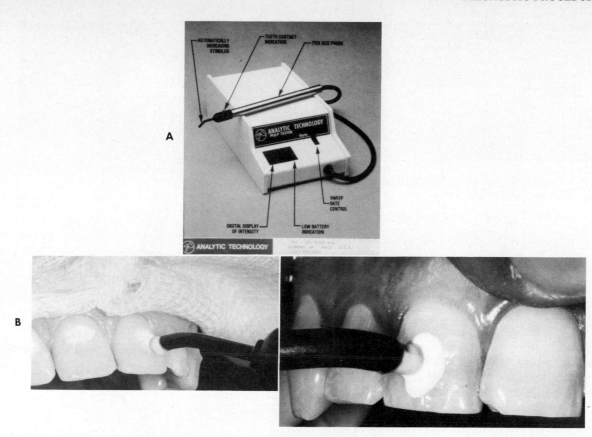

FIG. 1-12. Electric pulp testing. **A,** Analytic Technology pulp tester, a battery-operated instrument of −15 to −300 volts peak and a current from 1050 μamp. Each time the display increases one digit, one burst of 10 pulses of negative polarity is applied to the tooth. When removed and reapplied to the tooth, the tester automatically resets to 0. **B,** Electrode from the Analytic Technology pulp tester applied to dried surface. To complete the curcuit, gloves should *not* be worn by the clinician during electric pulp testing; otherwise, false readings may occur. Electric pulp testers that permit the dentist to wear gloves will soon be available.

which tooth is "suspect" before beginning the electric pulp test. This test merely corroborates what other diagnostic tests have indicated.

Precautions

If the patient's medical history indicates that a cardiac pacemaker has been installed, the use of an electric pulp tester (as well as electrosurgical units) is contraindicated because of potential interference with the pacemaker.[21]

False reading

The electric pulp tester is usually reliable for indicating pulp vitality; however, there are situations in which a false reading may occur. A *false-positive* reading means the pulp is necrotic but the patient appears to give a positive response. A *false-negative* reading means the pulp is vital but the patient appears unresponsive to electric pulp tests.

Main reasons for false-positive response

1. Conductor/electrode contact with a large metal restoration (bridge, Class II restoration) or the gingiva allowing the current to reach the attachment apparatus
2. Patient anxiety (Without proper instruction in what to expect, a hyperactive, neurotic, or frightened patient may raise his hand as soon as he thinks the electric pulp tester is turned on or may do so when asked if he "feels anything.")
3. Liquefaction necrosis (This may conduct current to the attachment apparatus, and the patient may slowly raise his hand near the highest range.)
4. Failure to isolate and dry the teeth

Main reasons for false-negative response

1. Patient heavily premedicated with analgesics, narcotics, alcohol, tranquilizers
2. Inadequate contact with the enamel (e.g., insufficient conductor or contact only with a composite restoration)
3. Recently traumatized tooth
4. Excessive calcification in the canal
5. Dead batteries or forgetting to turn the pulp tester on
6. Recently erupted tooth with an immature apex

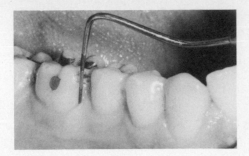

FIG. 1-13. Periodontal examination. A thin calibrated periodontal probe should be used to determine the integrity of the sulcus.

7. Partial necrosis (Although the pulp is still partially vital, ostensibly it may appear by electric pulp testing to be totally necrotic.)
8. Clinician wearing surgical gloves (prevents a complete circuit)

Periodontal examination

The periodontal probe should be an integral part of all endodontic tray setups. Using a thin, blunt, calibrated periodontal probe, the clinician examines the gingival sulcus and records the depths of all pockets (Fig. 1-13). Multirooted teeth are carefully probed to determine whether there is any furcation involvement. A lateral canal exposed to the oral cavity by periodontal disease may become the portal of entry for toxins that cause pulpal degeneration.

To distinguish lesions of periodontal origin from those of pulpal origin, thermal and electric pulp tests along with periodontal examination are essential. For further information regarding the endodontic-periodontal lesion, refer to Chapter 17.

Occasionally for diagnostic or dental-legal reasons the presence and depth of a periodontal pocket should be confirmed by placing a gutta-percha or silver cone in the sulcular defect and exposing a radiograph. This type of radiograph can be most effective in assessing periodontal repair at a later date or confirming the presence of a vertical root fracture (Fig. 1-15, *J*).

Test cavity

The test cavity involves the slow removal of enamel and dentin to determine pulp vitality. *Without anesthesia* and using a small round bur, the dentist removes dentin as the revolving high-speed bur aims directly at the pulp. If the pulp is vital, the patient will experience a quick sharp pain at or shortly beyond the dentin-enamel junction. This test quickly and accurately determines pulp vitality. However, because it frequently involves making a hole through a restoration, the test cavity is employed only when all other means of testing have yielded equivocal results. For example, with patients who have numerous porcelain-fused-to-metal crowns, thermal and electric pulp testing may be ineffective. If percussion, palpation, or radiographic examination suggests one tooth as a suspect, a test cavity to corroborate or negate the results of other tests would certainly be warranted.

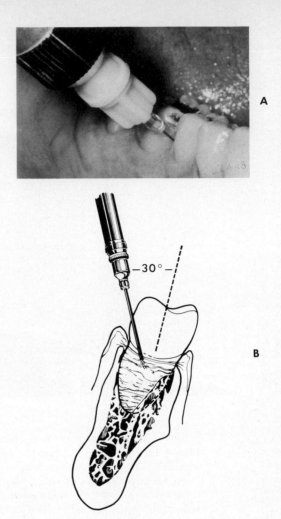

FIG. 1-14. Intraligamentary anesthesia for differential diagnosis. **A,** Administering 0.2 ml of local anesthetic (Ligmaject or Peripress) in the mesial and distal sulci will stop all pain immediately if the anesthetized tooth is the source of the pain. **B,** An ultrashort 30-gauge needle is placed into the sulcus at a 30° angle from perpendicular, with the bevel facing away from the tooth.

Anesthesia test

In the uncommon circumstance of diffuse pain of vague origin, when all other tests are inconclusive, conduction, selective infiltration, or intraligamentary anesthesia can be employed to help identify the source of the pain. The basis for this test lies in the fact that pulpal pain, even when referred, is almost invariably unilateral and stems from only one of the two branches of the trigeminal nerve supplying sensory innervation to the jaws.

For example, a patient complains of pain over the entire side of the face and no pathologic changes are evident on the radiographs. If conduction anesthesia (mandibular injection) is employed and the pain completely subsides within 2 to 3 minutes, it can be surmised that a mandibular tooth is the source of the pain. Otherwise, subperiosteal infiltration of the maxillary teeth, starting with the most distal, should be used. After each subperiosteal infiltration (0.25 ml), the clinician should wait 3 minutes. Ultimately the pain will cease completely with the onset of anesthesia around the source of the pain.

A more effective technique is intraligamentary injection administered in the mesial and distal sulci of each suspect tooth. When the offending tooth has been anesthetized by the intraligamentary injection technique, the pain will stop immediately (Fig. 1-14).[10]

On the rare occasion when pain still does not disappear and the anesthetic has been correctly administered, one must consider other possibilities. For example, pain from mandibular molars is often referred to the preauricular area. If this is truly the case, mandibular block anesthesia will quickly stop the pain. If the pain remains, one should consider the possibility, as part of a differential diagnosis, that the patient may have organic disease of nonodontogenic origin.[3]

Transillumination

The three main benefits of a strong fiberoptic light are to help the clinician distinguish between a vital and a necrotic pulp in very young patients, locate canal orifices, and diagnose vertically fractured crowns.

1. When a beam of strong fiberoptic light is passed through an anterior tooth and the room is dimly lit, a normal tooth will appear clear and slightly pink whereas a necrotic tooth may appear opaque and darker because of the breakdown of the blood within the pulp chamber. This technique may be helpful, especially with children who respond erratically to the usual diagnostic tests.
2. Shining the "cold" light in a horizontal direction toward the floor of the pulp chamber in a dimly lit room can cause an elusive canal orifice to appear as a dark spot within a well-illuminated pulpal floor.
3. Too often, a vertical crown/root fracture is identified after a tooth has been extracted as the last, desperate "treatment." Although no single method offers 100% reliability for detecting vertical crown/root fractures, transillumination, when used in combination with several other techniques, can strongly indicate the probability of a split tooth.

Techniques for detecting vertical crown/root fractures

In vital teeth the most common reason for a vertical crown/root fracture is trauma. In nonvital teeth, trauma may also be a contributory factor (if the tooth does not have metal crown protection); but endodontic treatment followed by overzealous post reinforcement[11,12,20] or a restoration tapped too firmly into place is a common cause.

1. *Fiberoptic examination.* As shown in Fig. 1-15, *A* to *E*, pointing a fiberoptic light horizontally at the level of the gingival sulcus in a dimly lit room may reveal a dark continuous line (in posterior teeth, usually oriented mesiodistally[13]) in an otherwise well-illuminated pulpal floor. This should certainly be considered as a possible vertical fracture. Most reliable results are obtained if preexisting restorations are removed from the tooth before the fiberoptic examination.

2. *Wedging and staining.* Cracks in teeth can also be discovered by a wedging and staining procedure (Fig. 1-15, *F* and *G*). Wedging force can be used to separate the two halves of the fracture. Whether the fractured tooth is vital or nonvital, there may be pain during mastication. This pain cannot always be detected with percussion at different angles; however, having the patient bite on a cotton roll as illustrated in Fig. 2-3, *A,* or a cotton-wood stick may reveal the split tooth.

If biting on a cotton roll or a cotton-wood stick still yields inconclusive results, the head of a no. 6 round bur held in cellophane tape can be applied to the occlusal surfaces of various cusps and the biting test can be gently repeated. At times this test will more readily identify the split tooth (Fig. 1-15, *F* and *G*).

The vertical fracture line can somtimes be more easily identified with food coloring placed on the dried occlusal surface moments before the wedge test. The dye solution will stain the fracture line. Immediately after the wedge test, the occlusal surface is cleaned with a cotton pellet lightly moistened with 70% isopropyl alcohol. The alcohol will wash away the food coloring on the surface, but the food coloring within the fracture line will remain and become apparent.

3. *Radiographs.* Fig. 1-15, *H,* shows a tooth with a vertical fracture that is not apparent. Fig. 1-15, *I,* shows the same tooth at a different horizontal angulation. The radiolucent halo is visible from the sulcus to the apex. Fig. 1-15, *J,* shows the periodontal examination, with diagnostic silver cones extending on the labial and palatal aspects from the sulcus to the apex. When the clinician sees a diffuse radiolucent halo around the root with diagnostic probes extending from the sulcus to the apex, there is a strong probability of a vertical fracture.

4. *Thorough dental history.* If the patient continuously complains of pain with biting (after frequent occlusal adjustments) or pain with horizontal tapping of the crown, the clinician should suspect a possible vertical fracture. These symptoms can develop any time—before, during, or after endodontic treatment. A periapical lesion that fails to resolve after a good root canal filling and repeated unsuccessful attempts at apical surgery suggests, as part of the differential diagnosis, a split root. A patient may have a hypersensitive response to thermal change in an otherwise perfectly sound tooth, may recall sudden pain after biting into an unexpected pit or bone, or may present with advanced symptoms of bruxism or clenching. Patients also may report that a restoration keeps falling out after several attempts at replacement or several recementations; before further restorative attempts are made, the remaining tooth should be carefully examined for fracture.

5. *Persistent periodontal defect.* Vertical crown/root fracture is suggested when conventional periodontal treatment does not resolve a sulcular defect.[8,13]

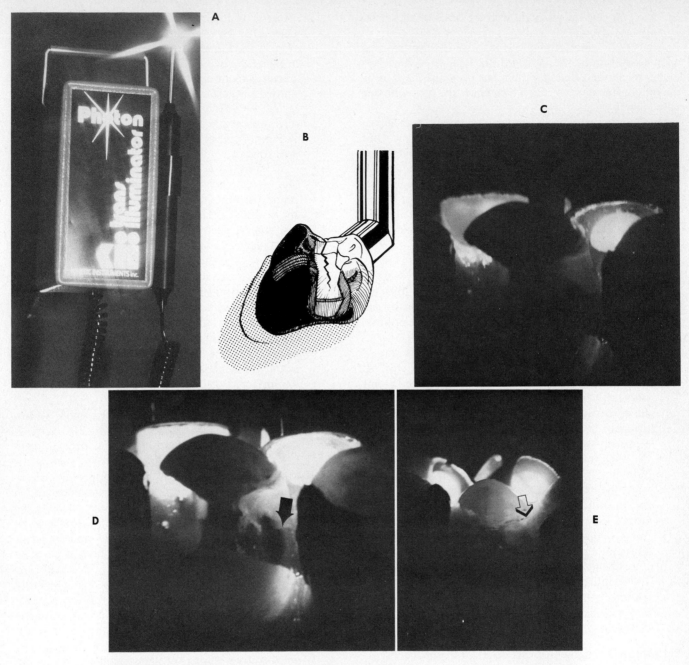

FIG. 1-15. Techniques for detecting vertical crown/root fractures. *Fiberoptic examination.* **A,** Rechargeable fiberoptic light. **B,** Transillumination. All restorations are removed. The tooth is isolated with cotton rolls and the dentin is dried with cotton pellets. A strong fiberoptic light is directed in through the buccal or lingual wall. A vertical fracture in the dentin may appear as a dark line. **C,** If the fiberoptic light is not aimed correctly, the vertical fracture may be overlooked because of poor illumination. **D,** With proper angulation of the fiberoptic light, the dark line of a fracture appears *(arrow).* **E,** Fiberoptic examination can reveal a vertical cusp fracture *(arrow).* (**A** and **C** to **E** courtesy Dr. Ronald Borer). *Continued.*

When an isolated sulcular defect continues to expand regardless of all treatment attempts and subsequent bacterial invasion hastens the periodontal breakdown around only one tooth while the other teeth appear periodontally sound, a possible vertical crown/root fracture is implicated. Reflecting a full-thickness mu-coperiosteal flap with the aid of a strong fiberoptic light may reveal the fine vertical fracture line (Fig. 1-15, *O*).

Even today the treatment of choice for a vertical fracture in a single-rooted tooth, or a mesial-distal fracture in a multirooted mandibular tooth, is still eventual extraction.

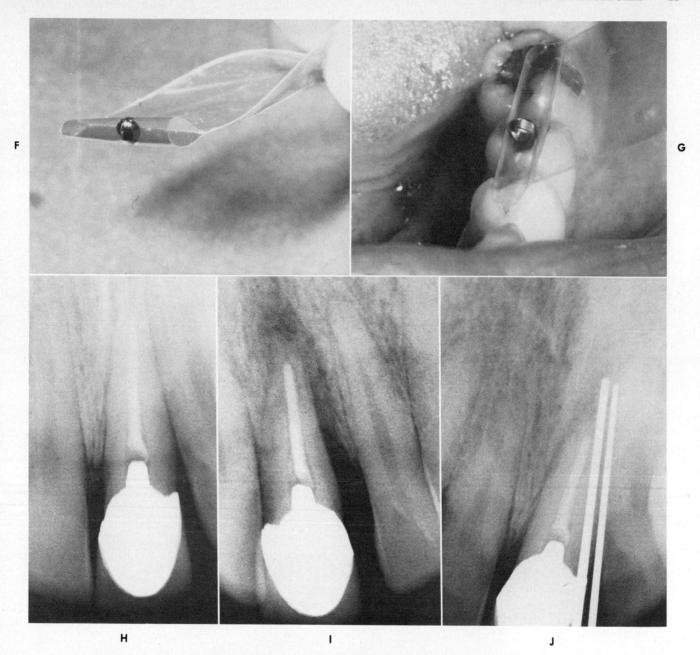

FIG. 1-15, cont'd. *Wedging and staining.* **F,** Mounting a no. 8 round bur in cellophane tape. **G,** The patient bites gently while the bur head is applied to various cusps. *Radiographs.* **H,** Vertical fracture not evident in an endodontically treated tooth. **I,** Changing the horizontal angulation revealed a characteristic diffuse demineralized "halo" around the root. **J,** Diagnostic silver cones trace the periodontal defect to the apex. *Continued.*

For some multirooted teeth, crown/root amputation may successfully resolve the fracture problem by removing the most mobile segment.

Diagnosing a crown/root fracture at early onset is far more gratifying to the clinician and kinder to the patient than is the more usual method of ultimate extraction, finally providing diagnostic hindsight.

For purposes of diagnosing vertical crown/root fractures, no one of the foregoing signs or symptoms may be conclusive; but taking them *in combination* may provide the clinician with the confirmed diagnosis of a vertical crown/root fracture.

Probable causes

Until the probable cause(s) for pulpal or periapical disease can be ascertained, the signs or symptoms that appear to indicate a dental problem should not be treated. Every dental pathologic entity should have an identifiable cause (e.g., bacterial, chemical, physical, iatrogenic, or systemic). The prudent practitioner should be extremely wary

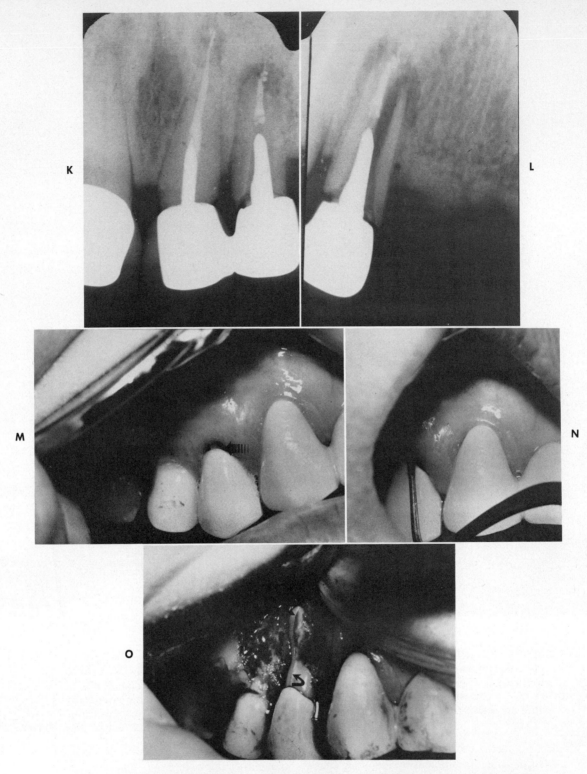

FIG. 1-15, cont'd. K, The patient complained that the two-unit bridge was constantly "falling out." The first radiograph showed a poorly fitted post in the canine root. **L,** Changing the horizontal angulation revealed the obvious vertical root fracture. (**K** and **L** courtesy Dr. Richard Cohan.) *Periodontal examination.* **M,** This patient complained of occasional "discharge" around the maxillary premolar. The clinician noted slight recession around the first premolar *(arrow).* **N,** A periodontal defect was detected. **O,** Retracting a full-thickness flap revealed a vertical fracture *(arrow).* (**M** to **O** courtesy Dr. Walter Hall.)

and cautious about treating *any* ostensible odontogenic problem until the probable cause can be determined. An error in diagnosis may lead to an error in treatment. If cause and effect are unclear, the clinician will provide the best service to the patient by referring the case for further consultation with a specialist.

CLINICAL CLASSIFICATION

A clinical classification of pulpal and periapical disease cannot list every possible variation of inflammation, ulceration, proliferation, calcification, or degeneration of the pulp and the attachment apparatus and still remain practical. Besides, this is probably unnecessary, because a clinical classification is meant to provide only a general descriptive phrase that implies the furthest extent of pulpal or periapical disease. The terms used in a clinical classification suggest the signs and symptoms of the disease process. The primary purpose of a clinical classification is to provide terms and phrases that can be used as a means of communication within the dental profession.

In the final analysis, the pulp is either healthy or not and must either be removed or not. The extent of the disease process may affect the method of treatment, from merely a palliative sedative to final pulpectomy. What follows is a series of terms that encompass the clinical signs and symptoms of the various degrees of inflammation and degeneration of the pulp or the nature, duration, and type of exudation associated with periapical inflammation. No attempt will be made to associate these terms with histopathologic findings, because with our current knowledge this cannot be done accurately.[16,18]

Normal

A normal tooth is asymptomatic and exhibits a mild to moderate transient response to thermal and electric pulpal stimuli; the response subsides almost immediately when such stimuli are removed. The tooth and its attachment apparatus do not cause a painful response when percussed or palpated. Radiographs usually reveal a clearly delineated canal that tapers toward the apex; there is no evidence of canal calcification or root resorption, and the lamina dura is intact.

Reversible pulpitis

The pulp is inflamed to the extent that thermal stimuli cause a quick, sharp, hypersensitive response that subsides as soon as the stimulus is removed; otherwise the tooth is asymptomatic. Any irritant that can affect the pulp may cause reversible pulpitis (e.g., caries, deep periodontal scaling and root planing, an unbased restoration).

Reversible pulpitis is *not* a disease, but merely a symptom. If the cause can be removed, the pulp should revert to an uninflamed state and the symptoms should subside. Conversely, if the cause remains, the symptoms may persist indefinitely or the inflammation may become more widespread, eventually leading to an irreversible pulpitis. A reversible pulpitis can be clinically distinguished from a symptomatic irreversible pulpitis by two methods:

1. With a reversible pulpitis there is a sharp, painful response to thermal stimulation that subsides almost immediately after the stimulus is removed. With an irreversible pulpitis there is a sharp painful response to thermal stimuli, but the pain *lingers* after the stimulus is removed.

2. With a reversible pulpitis there is no spontaneous pain as there often is with a symptomatic irreversible pulpitis. Most commonly, the clinician can readily diagnose a reversible pulpitis while gathering the patient's dental history (e.g., the patient may report pain when cold liquids are in contact with the tooth or when breathing through the mouth after a recent restoration or prophylaxis and scaling. Nevertheless, the diagnosis should be confirmed by thermal tests to identify the tooth or teeth involved.

Treatment consists of placing a sedative dressing or packing containing zinc oxide and eugenol in or around the tooth. If the pulp can be protected from further thermal shock, it may revert to an uninflamed state. For example, removing all caries or a recent deep amalgam and placing a temporary restoration (e.g., Intermediate Restorative Material®) in the cavity for several weeks should provide almost immediate relief. After several weeks the sedative dressing can be replaced with a well-based permanent restoration.

Irreversible pulpitis

An irreversible pulpitis may be acute, subacute, or chronic; it may be partial or total. The pulp may be infected or sterile. Clinically the acutely inflamed pulp is thought to be symptomatic, the chronically inflamed pulp asymptomatic. These thoughts are often inconsistent with histologic observations (Chapter 11). Clinically the extent of pulp inflammation, partial or total, cannot be determined. Based on present knowledge, irreversible pulpitis in any of its many forms requires endodontic therapy.

Dynamic changes in the pulp are always occurring; the change from quiescent chronicity to symptomatic acuteness may develop over a period of years or in a matter of hours. With pulp inflammation there is an exudate. If the exudate can be vented to obviate the pain that accompanies edema, the tooth may remain quiescent. Conversely, if the exudate that is being continuously formed remains within the hard confines of the root canal, pain will probably ensue.

Symptomatic irreversible pulpitis

One type of irreversible pulpitis is characterized by spontaneous intermittent or continuous paroxysms of pain.

"Spontaneous" in this context means that no stimulus is evident. Sudden temperature changes will induce prolonged episodes of pain. There may be a prolonged (i.e., remaining after the stimulus is removed) painful response to cold that can be relieved by heat. There may also be a prolonged painful response to heat that can be relieved by cold. There may even be a prolonged painful response to both heat and cold stimulation.

Continuous spontaneous pain may be excited merely by a change in posture (e.g., when the patient lies down or bends over). Commonly patients will recognize this empirically and may spend the night sleeping fitfully in an upright position.

Pain from symptomatic irreversible pulpitis tends to be moderate to severe, depending on the severity of inflammation. It may be sharp or dull, localized or referred (e.g., referred from mandibular molars toward the ear or up to the temporal area). The pain may be intermittent or constant.

Radiographs alone are of little assistance in diagnosing a symptomatic irreversible pulpitis. They are helpful in detecting suspect teeth (i.e., those with deep caries or extensive restorations). In the advanced stages of an irreversible pulpitis the inflammatory process may lead to development of a slight thickening in the periodontal ligament.

A symptomatic irreversible pulpitis can be differentially diagnosed by a thorough dental history, visual examination, radiographs, and thermal tests. The electric pulp test is of questionable value in accurately diagnosing the disease. An untreated symptomatic irreversible pulpitis may persist or abate if a vent is established for the inflammatory exudate (e.g., the removal of food packed into a deep carious pulp exposure to provide a vent for the inflammatory exudate). The inflammation of an irreversible pulpitis may become so severe as to cause ultimate necrosis. In the transition from pulpitis to necrosis the typical symptoms of irreversible pulpitis are altered according to the extent of the necrosis.

Asymptomatic irreversible pulpitis

Another type of irreversible pulpitis is asymptomatic because the inflammatory exudates are quickly vented. An asymptomatic irreversible pulpitis may develop by the conversion of a symptomatic irreversible pulpitis into a quiescent state, or it may develop initially from a low-grade pulp irritant. It is easily identified by a thorough dental history along with radiographic and visual examination.

An asymptomatic irreversible pulpitis may develop from any type of injury, but it is usually caused by a large carious exposure or by previous traumatic injury that resulted in a painless pulp exposure of long duration.

Hyperplastic pulpitis. One type of asymptomatic irreversible pulpitis is a reddish cauliflower-like overgrowth of pulp tissue through and around a carious exposure. The proliferative nature of this type of pulp is attributed to a low-grade chronic irritation and to the generous vascularity of the pulp that is characteristically found in young people. Occasionally there is some mild, transient pain during mastication. If the apices are mature, complete endodontic therapy should be provided.

Internal resorption. Another type of asymptomatic irreversible pulpitis is internal resorption. This is characterized by the presence of chronic inflammatory cells in granulation tissue and is asymptomatic (before it perforates the root). See Chapter 16 for a complete description of the various types of resorption: their causes, diagnoses, and treatments.

Internal resorption is most commonly diagnosed by ra-

diographs showing internal expansion of the pulp with evident dentinal destruction. In advanced cases of internal resorption in the crown, a pink spot may be seen through the enamel.

The treatment of internal resorption is immediate endodontic therapy; to postpone treatment may lead to an untreatable perforation of the root, resulting in possible loss of the tooth.

Canal calcification. The physical adversity of restorative procedures, periodontal therapy, attrition, abrasion, trauma, and probably some additional, idiopathic factors can cause an otherwise normal pulp to metamorphose into an irreversible pulpitis manifested by deposition of abnormally large amounts of reparative dentin throughout the canal system.[16] The condition is usually first recognized radiographically. Discrete areas of localized pulp necrosis resulting from small infarctions (e.g., caused by deep scaling that interrupts the blood supply into a lateral canal) often initiate localized calcification as a defense reaction. This abnormal calcification occurs in and around pulp vascular channels. The teeth are asymptomatic but may show a slight change in crown color. Several distinct types of calcification (denticles, pulp stones), initiated by a multitude of factors, can occur within the pulp (Chapter 10).

• • •

Irreversible pulpitis may persist for an extended time, but it is common for the inflamed pulp to succumb eventually to the pressures of inflammation and ultimately necrose.

Necrosis

Necrosis, which is death of the pulp, may result from an untreated irreversible pulpitis or may occur immediately after a traumatic injury that disrupts the blood supply to the pulp. Whether the necrotic remnants of the pulp are liquefied or coagulated, the pulp is still quite dead. Regardless of the type of necrosis, the endodontic treatment is the same. Within hours an inflamed pulp may degenerate to a necrotic state.

Pulp necrosis can be partial or total. The partial type may exhibit some of the symptoms of an irreversible pulpitis. Total necrosis, before it clinically affects the periodontal ligament, is usually asymptomatic. There is no response to thermal or electric tests. Occasionally with anterior teeth the crown will darken.

Untreated necrosis may spread beyond the apical foramen, causing inflammation of the periodontal ligament; this results in thickening of the periodontal ligament, which may be quite sensitive to percussion.

When there is more than one canal, the diagnostic skill of the clinician is tested. For example, in a molar with three canals the pulp tissue in one canal may be intact and uninflamed, that in the next canal acutely inflamed, and that in the third canal completely necrotic. This accounts for the occasional tooth that causes the patient to respond with confusing inconsistencies to vitality testing.

A natural dichotomy between health and disease does

not exist—at least not as far as the pulp is concerned. Pulp tissue may show all degrees of the spectrum from health to inflammation to necrosis. Clinically we can distinguish reversible and irreversible pulpitis from necrosis. A clinically necrotic tooth may still have vascularity in the apical third of the canal, but this can be confirmed only during chemomechanical debridement. When the pulp dies, if the tooth remains untreated the bacteria, toxins, and protein breakdown products of the pulp may extend beyond the apical foramen and involve the periapical region, thus causing periapical disease.

Periapical diseases
Acute apical periodontitis

An acute apical periodontitis implies inflammation around the apex. *Acute* means immediate and painful and *apical* tells where, at the apex. *Periodontitis* is from the Greek *peri-* (around), *odonto-* (tooth), and *-itis* (inflammation). Thus acute apical periodontitis is local painful inflammation around the apex of a tooth.

The cause may be an extension of pulpal disease into the periapical tissue. It may also be an endodontic procedure that has inadvertently extended beyond the apical foramen. The condition can even be associated with a normal vital pulp in a tooth that has suffered occlusal trauma from a high restoration or from chronic bruxism.

The clinician must therefore recognize that an acute apical periodontitis may be found around vital as well as nonvital teeth. For this reason *thermal and electric testing must be done before treatment is initiated.* Radiographically the apical periodontal ligament may appear normal or perhaps slightly widened, but the tooth is exquisitely tender to percussion. There may even be slight tenderness to palpation. Untreated, the localized acute apical periodontitis may continue to spread, additional symptoms may appear, and an acute apical abscess may develop.

If the pulp is necrotic, endodontic therapy should be started immediately. However, if the pulp is vital, removing the cause (e.g., adjusting the occlusion) should permit quick, uneventful repair.

Acute apical abscess

The term implies a painful purulent exudate around the apex. An acute apical abscess is one of the most serious dental diseases we may encounter, yet radiographically the tooth may appear perfectly normal or perhaps show a slightly widened periodontal ligament. The cause is an advanced stage of acute apical periodontitis from a necrotic tooth, resulting in extensive acute suppurative inflammation.

The acute apical abscess is easily diagnosed by its clinical signs and symptoms: a rapid onset of slight to severe swelling, slight to severe pain, pain to percussion and palpation, and possible tooth mobility. In more severe cases the patient is febrile. Radiographically the periapical tissue may appear normal because fulminating infections may not have had sufficient time to erode enough cortical bone to cause a radiolucency.

The extent and distribution of the swelling are determined by the location of the apex, the condition of the adjacent muscle attachments, and the thickness of the cortical plate.

The acute apical abscess is readily distinguishable from the lateral periodontal abscess and from the phoenix abscess.

1. With the lateral periodontal abscess there may be swelling and pain, and radiographically the tooth may appear relatively normal; however, thermal and electric pulp testing will indicate that the pulp is *vital*. Furthermore, there is almost always a periodontal pocket, which upon probing may begin to exude a purulent exudate.
2. With the phoenix abscess there will be an *apical radiolucency* around the apex of the tooth. All other signs and symptoms will be identical to those of the acute apical abscess.

Chronic apical periodontitis

The term implies long-standing, asymptomatic inflammation around the apex. Although chronic apical periodontitis tends to be asymptomatic, there may be occasional slight tenderness to palpation and percussion. Only biopsy and microscopic examination can reveal whether these apical lesions are dental granulomas, abscesses, or cysts. The dynamic equilibrium standoff between the host's defense mechanisms and the infection oozing out of the canal is manifested by a periapical radiolucency. Of course, this is a matter of radiographic interpretation; what may appear as a widened periodontal ligament to one clinician may appear as a small radiolucency to another.

Because a totally necrotic pulp provides a safe harbor (no vascularity = no defense cells) for microorganisms and their noxious allies, only complete endodontic treatment will permit these lesions to be repaired.

Diagnosis is confirmed by the general absence of symptoms, the presence of a radiolucency, and the absence of pulp vitality. Radiographically the lesions may appear large or small, and they may be either diffuse or well circumscribed.

The additional presence of a sinus tract indicates the production of frank pus. Symptoms are generally absent because the pus drains through the sinus tract as quickly as it is produced. Occasionally patients will become aware of a "gumboil."

Periapical dynamic changes are constant. Spontaneously pus production may cease for a while and the sinus tract may close. When the necrotic contents of a canal are removed during endodontic treatment, the sinus tract will permanently close shortly thereafter.

Phoenix abscess

Phoenix, the bird from Egyptian mythology that arose every 500 years from its own ashes in the desert and then consumed itself in fire, is an apt name for this lesion. A phoenix abscess is a chronic apical periodontitis that suddenly becomes symptomatic. The symptoms are identical to those of an acute apical abscess, the main difference being that the phoenix abscess is preceded by a chronic condition. Consequently there is a definite radiolucency accompanied by symptoms of an acute apical abscess. The spontaneous metamorphosis from dormant chronicity to a sudden, violent, fulminating disease gives us the analogy of the phoenix.

A phoenix abscess may develop spontaneously, almost immediately after endodontic treatment has been initiated on a tooth diagnosed as chronic apical periodontitis without a sinus tract. Initiating endodontic treatment may alter the dynamic equilibrium of a chronic apical periodontitis by the inadvertent forcing of microorganisms or other irritants into the periapical tissue. When this happens, the patient may question you closely to determine how you were able to obtain such fast results (i.e., swelling and pain) when he came to you with an asymptomatic condition!

Periapical osteosclerosis

The term implies excessive bone mineralization around the apex. Low-grade, relatively asymptomatic, chronic pulpal inflammation occasionally causes a host response of excessive bone mineralization around the apex. This is most commonly found in young people. Endodontic treatment may convert the periapical radiopacity to a normal trabecular pattern.[9] Conversely, unusual "excessive" periapical remineralization after endodontic therapy may result in osteosclerosis (Fig. 1-6, *H*). Because this condition is asymptomatic and appears to be self-limiting, whether endodontic treatment should be provided at all is arguable.

REFERENCES

1. Andreasen, J.O.: Traumatic injuries of the teeth, ed. 2, Philadelphia, 1981, W.B. Saunders Co.
2. Chambers, I.G.: The role and methods of pulp testing: a review, Int. Endod. J. **15**:10, 1982.
3. Cohen, S., et al.: Oral prodromal signs of a central nervous system malignant neoplasm—glioblastoma multiforme: report of a case, J. Am. Dent. Assoc. **112**:643, 1986.
4. Cooley, R.L., and Lubow, R.M.: Evaluation of a digital pulp tester, J. Oral Maxillofac. Surg. **58**:437, 1984.
5. Eversole, L.R.: Clinical outline of oral pathology: diagnosis and treatment, Philadelphia, 1978, Lea & Febiger.
6. Goldman, M., Pearson, A., and Darzenta, N.: Endodontic success—who's reading the radiograph? Oral Surg. **33**:432, 1972.
7. Goldman, M., Pearson, A., and Darzenta, N.: Reliability of radiographic interpretations, Oral Surg. **32**:287, 1974.
8. Goldstein, A.R.: Periodontal defects associated with root fracture, J. Am. Dent. Assoc. **102**:863, 1981.
9. Grossman, L.I.: Endodontic practice, ed. 10, Philadelphia, 1981, Lea & Febiger.
10. Littner, M.M., Tamse, A., and Kaffe, I.: A new technique of selective anesthesia for diagnosing acute pulpitis in the mandible, J. Endod. **9**:116, 1983.
11. Lommel, J.J., et al.: Alveolar bone loss associated with vertical root fractures: reports of 6 cases, Oral Surg. **45**:909, 1978.
12. Meister, F., Jr., Lommel, J.J., and Gerstein, H.: Diagnosis and possible causes of vertical root fractures, Oral Surg. **49**:243, 1980.
13. Polson, A.M.: Periodontal destruction associated with vertical root fracture, J. Periodontol. **48**:27, 1977.
14. Rose, L.F., and Kaye, D.: Internal Medicine for Dentistry, St. Louis, 1983, The C.V. Mosby Co.
15. Schwartz, S., and Foster, J.: Roentgenographic interpretation of experimentally produced bony lesions, Oral Surg. **32**:606, 1971.
16. Seltzer, S., and Bender, I.B.: The dental pulp: biologic considerations in dental procedures, ed. 3, Philadelphia, 1984, J.B. Lippincott Co.
17. Slowey, R.I.: Radiographic aids in the detection of extra root canals, Oral Surg. **37**:762, 1974.
18. Smulson, M.H.: Classification and diagnosis of pulp pathosis, Dent. Clin. North Amer. **28**:699, 1984.
19. Trowbridge, H.O.: Changing concepts in endodontic therapy, J. Am. Dent. Assoc. **110**:479, 1985.
20. Wechsler, S.M., et al.: Iatrogenic root fractures: a case report, J. Endod. **4**:251, 1978.
21. Woodley, L., Woodworth, J., and Dobbs, J.L.: A preliminary evaluation of the effects of electric pulp testers on dogs with artificial pacemakers, J. Am. Dent. Assoc. **89**:1099, 1974.
22. Zakariasen, K.L., and Walton, R.E.: Complications in endodontic therapy for the geriatric patient, Gerodontics **1**:34, 1985.

GENERAL REFERENCES

deDeus, Q.: Endodontia, ed. 4, Rio de Janeiro, 1986, Medsi Co.
Basrani, E.: Fractures of the teeth, Philadelphia, 1985. Lea & Febiger.

Self-assessment questions

1. A thorough dental history regarding the patient's chief complaint will
   a. Eliminate the need for routine clinical tests
   b. Enable the clinician to make a tentative diagnosis
   c. Identify the cause of the patient's symptoms
   d. Locate the offending tooth
2. Pain of dental origin
   a. Will usually reflect conditions of irreversible pulpitis with or without partial necrosis
   b. Can be expected to cross the midline of the head and involve other areas eventually
   c. Will respond to percussion testing even though the inflammation is pulpal only
   d. Invariably arises from an anterior tooth when referred to the periauricular area
3. The purpose of palpation is to
   a. Evaluate the gingival involvement of pulpal disease
   b. Determine if the periapical inflammatory process has penetrated the cortical bone
   c. Improve the tactile skills of the clinician relative to periapical disease
   d. Massage localized swelling of the alveolar tissue to promote drainage
4. The percussion test
   a. Indicates whether there is inflammation of the periodontal ligament
   b. Reveals the state of health of the pulp tissue
   c. Stimulates the proprioceptive fibers of an inflamed pulp
   d. Demonstrates the presence of chronic periapical periodontitis

5. Discernible movement of a tooth usually indicates
   a. Chronic pulpal disease
   b. Normal response to external pressures
   c. A need for periodontal treatment
   d. Inflammation of the periodontal ligament
6. A painful response that subsides quickly with stimulus removal is characteristic of
   a. A normal pulp
   b. A reversible pulpitis
   c. An irreversible pulpitis
   d. A nonvital pulp
7. The anesthesia test is used
   a. As another means to determine pulp vitality
   b. To eliminate the source of bilateral mandible pain
   c. Routinely for endodontic diagnosis
   d. To help determine the etiology of diffuse pain of vague origin
8. The most effective diagnostic procedure for a vertical crown/root fracture is
   a. Fiberoptic examination
   b. Radiographs
   c. A thorough dental history
   d. A periodontal defect
9. Reversible pulpitis is usually characterized by
   a. Sharp, momentary pain to thermal stimulation
   b. Palpable swelling over apex of the suspected tooth
   c. Severe, spontaneous, periodic pain
   d. Moderate pain upon percussion
10. Irreversible pulpitis may be asymptomatic when
    a. Resulting from acute pulpal infection
    b. Inflammatory exudates are vented
    c. Accompanied by a strong pulp irritant
    d. Caused by incipient caries
11. The recommended management of internal resorption is to
    a. Observe with periodic periapical radiographs
    b. Reserve definitive care until symptoms develop
    c. Institute root canal therapy immediately
    d. Assure the patient that resorption is self-limiting
12. Total pulp necrosis
    a. Will require increased stimulation by the electric pulp test
    b. Usually is asymptomatic when confined within the pulp space
    c. Is accurately diagnosed with periapical radiographs
    d. May exhibit both the reversible and the irreversible types of pulpitis
13. Acute apical periodontitis may result from
    a. Periapical extension of pulp disease
    b. Root canal procedures within the canal spaces
    c. Recently placed proximal restorations
    d. Overzealous palpation procedures opposite the apex
14. The acute apical abscess
    a. Tests the diagnositc acumen of the clinician
    b. Occurs in the initial stages of acute apical periodontitis
    c. Exhibits severe pain, tooth mobility, and positive responses to palpation and percussion
    d. Is always evident on periapical radiographs

2

ENDODONTIC EMERGENCIES

STEPHEN COHEN
ANNE-LI KNUUT
ALBERT GOERIG
FULTON S. YEE

Most individuals seeking emergency dental treatment are suffering from pain originating from the pulp or periapical area.

Dentists must be available whenever a patient is in acute distress (even during evenings and on weekends!) to relieve the signs and symptoms of dental emergencies. Patients expect no less of the dental profession, and it is one of the profession's most important responsibilities to provide this service. Managing dental emergencies is also stressful for the clinician because such urgent situations must be accommodated along with scheduled patients, the diagnosis must be made quickly and accurately, and the problem must be treated effectively. The clinician's stress may be increased further by the patient's aversion to dentists.

Considerable caution must be exercised when the clinician decides to treat after-hours dental emergencies. The validity of the emergency must first be determined, and drug abuse must be clearly ruled out. Personal safety must be considered, as well as the potential for litigation that exists when patients are treated in the absence of auxiliary personnel.[10]

This chapter describes the diagnosis and treatment of endodontic emergencies. Procedural guidelines for systematic and accurate diagnosis are presented herein, followed by a description of rapid and effective therapy for the acute dental emergency, according to the patient's presenting signs and symptoms. The chapter also includes patient and practice management techniques that should help reduce the stress level experienced by the emergency patient and the attending clinician as well.

DIAGNOSIS

Correct diagnosis of the emergency patient's orofacial signs and symptoms is a prerequisite for their proper management. As explained in Chapter 1, endodontic diagnosis is usually straightforward. The procedures and techniques described and illustrated in the preceding chapter will enable the clinician to diagnose most dental problems of a nonurgent and uncomplicated nature.

The process of endodontic diagnosis, as described in this chapter, focuses on the acute and potentially complex emergency and is divided into the following categories:

1. Procuring the diagnostic data
   a. Interrogatory examination
   b. Clinical examination
   c. Radiographic evaluation
2. Determining the diagnosis
   a. Endodontic involvement
   b. Periodontal considerations
   c. Restorative considerations
   d. Differential diagnoses

Adherence to this systematically formulated scheme for acquiring and analyzing essential data from the patient examination will enhance the diagnostic capabilities of the clinician.

Procuring the diagnostic data
Interrogatory examination

Medical history. The diagnostic sequence should begin with a comprehensive evaluation of the patient's medical history. In addition to providing medical-legal protection, a careful review of the patient's medical status will aid in identifying high-risk situations and help in deciding whether any required therapeutic procedures should be modified (e.g., scheduling brief morning appointments for the patient with coronary artery disease to minimize stress), augmented (e.g., antibiotic prophylaxis for the patient with congenital or rheumatic heart disease), or even deferred (e.g., medical consultation for the patient with uncontrolled diabetes).

From the standpoint of the differential diagnostic pro-

MEDICAL HISTORY	Physician Name: *Dr. Cohendo*	Address: *450 Sutter, SF.*	Phone: *555-1212*	Last Physical: *3 years*	Pt. Age: *38*

Heart Condition
  angina
  coronary
  surgery
  pacemaker
Rheumatic Fever/Murmur
Hypertension/Circulatory
	Anemia/Bleeding
	Diabetes/Kidney
	Hepatitis/Liver
	Herpes
	Thyroid/Hormonal
	(Asthma)/Respiratory
	Ulcers/Digestive
	Migraine/Headaches
		Epilepsy/Fainting
		Sinusitis/ENT
		Glaucoma/Visual
		Mental/Neural
		Tumor/Neoplasms
		Alcoholism/Addictions
		Infectious Diseases
		Venereal Disease
			Allergies:
			(penicillin)/antibiotics
			aspirin/Tylenol
			codeine/narcotics
			local anesthetic
			N_2O/O_2
			other:
				Major Medical Prob: *None*
				Females: Pregnant _____ mo
				Recent Hosp./Operation:
				Current Medical TX:
				Medications: *ventolin inhaler*
				Medical Status:

cess, a thorough assessment of the medical history may uncover important clues that, in turn, might facilitate identification of the etiologic factor(s) involved in the emergency patient's chief complaint. For example, a history of sickle-cell anemia or vitamin D–resistant rickets might suggest the possibility of spontaneous pulp necrosis.[2,7]

Preprinted forms that simply require a cursory survey from a provided list of specific disease entities (e.g., p. 6) represent a convenient method for taking the medical history, especially when these are completed by the patient prior to the examination. It should be emphasized, however, that the dentist must review all entries with the patient to elicit further details and to detect nondisclosures resulting from oversight or embarrassment. Furthermore, a particular disease entity that has afflicted the patient but that does not appear on the medical history form may not have been brought to the dentist's attention. The patient may simply have assumed that such a disclosure was unimportant since it was not addressed on the preprinted history.

The diagnostician should augment the medical history by leading the patient in a dialogue of detailed questions, answers, and succeeding questions. Areas of concentration should include the following:

1. Significant illness
2. Serious injuries
3. Emotional history
4. Habits (e.g., use of tobacco, alcohol, or drugs)
5. Prior hospitalizations
6. Medications
7. Current medical treatment
8. Symptoms that might indicate undiagnosed pathosis or abnormalities in the various organ systems of the body

Whenever indicated, the dentist should monitor and record the patient's vital signs (pulse rate, blood pressure, respiratory rate, and temperature). If any question exists regarding the patient's current medical status, the appropriate physician should be consulted.

Medical data of significance to the dentist should be systematically entered on the patient record. A proper medical history will include a systematic evaluation of specific disease entities and medical conditions as well as an assessment of the various somatic organ systems. The patient's current medical status should also be reviewed. (See suggested form at top of page.)

Dental history. The dental history represents the next step in the diagnostic process. Coupled with the preceding medical evaluation, a meticulous and methodical dental history will usually identify the problem and indicate the proper treatment if the patient is questioned carefully and accurate responses are analyzed correctly.

The patient should first be requested to state the present chief complaint in his own words, using a narrative format. This statement should relate as accurately as possible the main characteristics of the problem and the circumstances under which they have occurred. After recording this statement in the case history the dentist may ask the patient to provide clarification and additional pertinent information through a process of systematic questioning.

The diagnostician places much reliance on the patient's choice of words during the interrogatory phase of diagnosis. It should be remembered that the patient's account will depend on such variables as intelligence, vocabulary, psychosocial factors (e.g., ethnic origin, culture, religion), emotional state, and conception of what is taking place. The emotional component of pain can be affected by such variables as age, sex, previous dental experience, cultural development, socioeconomic level, and situational factors.[34]

The investigator must remain aware that the patient's responses may be difficult to interpret or verify, since pain is a complex, subjective phenomenon. To avoid being misled, the dentist must exercise patience, attentiveness, and perceptiveness while listening.

Several aspects of the patient's symptoms should be elucidated in the course of the interrogation:

1. Location—site(s) at which the symptoms are perceived
2. Chronology—inception, clinical course, and temporal pattern of the symptoms
3. Quality—descriptive account of the predominant complaint
4. Intensity—severity of the symptoms perceived
5. Affecting factors—stimuli that aggravate, relieve, or otherwise influence the symptoms
6. Adjunctive history—previous treatment and other details pertaining to the involved area

The purpose of this categorization is to ensure a comprehensive and logical evaluation of the chief complaint. These categories are not mutually exclusive. In fact, an adequate assessment of a particular aspect of the complaint may concurrently involve details pertaining to several categories. The examiner should adapt the line of questioning to the nature of the clinical situation. To avoid confusing the patient, all questions should be explicit and carefully formulated. If required, the dentist should be prepared to restate or rephrase any question and paraphrase any elicited response to ensure that communication is accurate.

Location. The first aspect of the complaint to be considered is its location.

The patient is asked to indicate the location of the chief complaint by pointing to it directly with one finger (Fig.

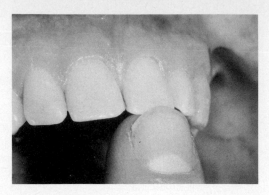

FIG. 2-1. Digital pointing by the patient is recommended for indicating the location of the chief complaint.

2-1). Pointing avoids the ambiguity or confusion that may accompany verbal delineation. Specific instructions are given to the patient to point within the mouth if the problem is manifested intraorally; and the dentist notes whether the site indicated is precise or vague, localized or diffuse. If the symptoms radiate or are referred to other regions, the patient is asked to indicate the direction and extent.

The diagnostician should bear in mind that endodontic pain from a solitary source (e.g., a mandibular left first molar with an irreversible pulpitis) may be perceived at a different unilateral site or in more than one location on the same side (single or multiple teeth, the opposing dental quadrant, the left auricular area, the left ophthalmic region, the left temporal area, or the left cervical sector). This finding is most consistent with advanced pulpitic conditions but may pertain to pulpless teeth as well.[36,46] It is axiomatic that the specific location and cause of the chief complaint must be verified by confirmatory diagnostic procedures before any irreversible palliative or therapeutic treatment is initiated.

At this preliminary stage of the investigation the dentist may have accumulated sufficient data to deduce a proper diagnosis, or further inquiries may be required.

Chronology. The temporal manifestations of endodontic symptoms are extremely variable and potentially deceptive. Therefore the dentist must question the patient in an exacting manner to establish facts that might be pertinent to a correct diagnosis.

Inception. The patient is requested to state when the symptoms associated with the chief complaint were initially perceived. After this he is guided to recount the details of any specific events (e.g., dental procedures or traumatic incidents) or conditions (e.g., emotional stress) that might be related to the onset of symptoms.

Clinical course and temporal pattern. The incipient and any succeeding episodes of pain or other symptoms are then described. The dentist should deduce and record details of the entire clinical course of symptoms, with emphasis on the following:

1. Mode—is the onset or abatement of each episode spontaneous or provoked? Is it sudden or gradual? Whenever provoking or alleviating stimuli can be associated and identified, is the induced onset immediate or delayed?

2. Periodicity—do the symptoms recur with regularity? Is the onset of symptoms predictable and reproducible, or is it sporadic and occasional?

3. Frequency—have the symptoms persisted without remission since inception, or has their occurrence been intermittent? If episodic, how often do the symptoms occur? Has the frequency remained unchanged for each symptom, or has it increased or decreased?

4. Duration—upon onset, are the symptoms momentary or lingering? Length of persistence should be stated, even if approximate, in terms of seconds, minutes, hours, or longer intervals of measured time. If provoking factors have been identified, are the induced symptoms perceived only for the duration of the stimulus, or are they protracted?

With practice the dentist should be able to describe succinctly the entire chronologic pattern of the patient's symptoms, from their inception to the present and in all temporal parameters as just defined.

Accurate results from this phase of the interrogation may be especially useful for interpreting and validating data acquired during the clinical reproduction of symptoms.

Quality. The patient is then asked to render a detailed description of each symptom associated with the presenting emergency. The character or quality of the symptoms is important in differential diagnosis because it may help the clinical investigator identify the etiology of the chief complaint.

Certain adjectives have been commonly ascribed to somatic pains of similar origin. For example, a dull, drawing, or aching quality is usually characteristic of deep tissue pains (e.g., surgery involving infrabony impactions or retrograde procedures). A throbbing, pounding, or pulsing pain generally indicates that the noxious stimuli are associated with the arterial vasculature (e.g., irreversible pulpitis, migraine headaches). Sharp, recurrent, stabbing pain is usually caused by disease involving nerve root complexes, sensory ganglia, or peripheral innervation (e.g., irreversible pulpitis, trigeminal neuralgia), whereas a single episode may be the result of injury to muscle or ligamentous tissue (e.g., mandibular subluxation, radicular fracture, iatrogenic perforation of the periodontal attachment apparatus). Anginal pain has been described as squeezing or crushing, implying a possible involuntary component of pectoral muscle contraction.

Since the dental pulp is a connective tissue composed of various elements (neural, vascular, fibrillar, cellular, and intercellular) and since pulpal tissue is contiguous with the supporting periodontal ligament and resides in close association with intraosseous structures of the craniofacial complex, it should be of no surprise that the subjective manifestations resulting from acute endodontic conditions are numerous and extremely varied. Many terms have been used to describe symptoms of endodontic origin—aching, gnawing, radiating, stabbing, flashing, dull, throbbing, shooting, and so on.

Although these descriptions may accurately convey the diverse character of endodontic pain, the investigator should bear in mind that some will also imply conditions of nonendodontic origin[5] such as muscle spasm, cardiac distress, or psychologic problems. Confusion and misinterpretation can be avoided, or at least minimized, through precise questioning to differentiate the symptoms further.

After a description of the quality of pain has been elicited, the examining dentist should instruct the patient to describe any factors that affect it. These will include all conditions that alter the spatial, temporal, or gradational character of a given pain quality. For example, a thermal stimulus may protract, intensify, radiate, and refer a throbbing ache caused by irreversible pulpitis and may even change the actual quality of the underlying pain.

It may be necessary for the dentist to reproduce and interpret these often-subtle conditions in subsequent diagnostic tests to identify the cause of the patient's complaint accurately.

Intensity. The intensity of pain in dental disease may be subject to wide variation. For instance, an asymptomatic chronic apical periodontitis may be exacerbated to manifest itself as an acute phoenix abscess.

The patient's response to pain, a function of the higher centers of the neurologic system, is also extremely variable. Pain tolerance and reaction are affected by numerous factors, depending on the individual patient and the given clinical situation.

The proliferation or gravity of a particular disease process cannot be determined solely by the severity of pain experienced by the patient. For the endodontic clinician, however, pain intensity is often the most significant factor in dictating the extent and mode of treatment in an emergency situation.

The dentist should measure the intensity level of any pains reported by the patient. Various methods may be used to accomplish this:

1. *Pain index.* The patient is asked to rate the degree of pain by assigning it a number from 0 to 10, with 0 indicating no discomfort and 10 specifying severe or intolerable pain. This system is recommended because it utilizes quantifiable units that permit subtle comparisons of pain intensity at any instance throughout its clinical course.
2. *Pain classification.* The patient is instructed to classify the level of pain into one of three categories—mild, moderate, or severe.
3. *Pain effectuation.* The degree of pain can also be evaluated in terms of (a) how it affects the patient's daily routine and (b) what measures are required to effect symptomatic relief (e.g., analgesics, rest). As a general rule, pain that interferes with occupational or leisure activities, necessitates bed rest, requires the use of potent analgesics, or awakens the patient from sound sleep may be regarded as more severe in character than that with less apparent manifestations.

The patient should also be asked to indicate whether the intensity of each type of pain is diminishing, remaining the same, or increasing.

It must be emphasized that, for a particular endodontic situation, different levels of intensity may be experienced in relation to the variable types of pain perceived. For instance, an acute apical periodontitis secondary to an irre-versible pulpitis may present clinically as a mild, dull, constant underlying ache with moderate, throbbing, lingering sensitivity to heat and a severe, sharp, protracted pain to percussion.

Whenever clinically reproducible symptoms can be identified, as in the previous example, pain intensity will frequently indicate which of the diagnostic tests should be most relevant. The examining dentist will usually attempt to reproduce those symptoms of *higher* pain intensity to help locate the source of the chief complaint. Symptoms that reflect milder differences in patient response may not be as reliably recreated or interpreted when compared to test results from dental tissues responding within normal limits.

Affecting factors. The object of this part of the dental interrogatory is to identify the factors that provoke, intensify, alleviate, or otherwise affect the patient's symptoms. The patient is asked to state all the conditions that evoke alteration in perception. The level of intensity associated with *each* modifying stimulus should be included in the answer. Special attention must also be given to the interval of elapsed time between stimulus and response (e.g., is the resultant onset immediate or delayed?). Such thorough questioning should be completed before any corroborative diagnostic tests are performed; otherwise, an inaccurate interpretation of their results could be made despite an accurate clinical reproduction of symptoms.

Assume, for example, that a 24-year-old man presents with a history of unlocalized intense radiating pain with heat stimulation. In an attempt to reproduce the patient's chief complaint, the dentist sequentially applies a local heat source to several teeth. The pain is of delayed onset (i.e., minutes), but the dentist unwisely fails to establish this fact beforehand. By the time the patient responds to the actual offending tooth, the dentist is coincidentally testing another tooth. This results in a misdiagnosis based on an erroneous interpretation of facts, and endodontic therapy is initiated on the wrong tooth. The patient returns shortly with the original complaint unchanged.

Symptoms can be more meaningfully evaluated if the investigator understands the circumstances in which they occur.

1. *Local affecting stimuli.* Stimuli such as the following are generally associated with odontogenic symptoms:
   a. Heat
   b. Cold
   c. Sweets
   d. Biting
   e. Chewing
   f. Percussion
   g. Manipulation
   h. Palpation

The significance of these factors to diagnosis of the various endodontic diseases is discussed in Chapter 1. Along with symptoms provoked by such factors, the patient may experience underlying spontaneous pain of variable quality, intensity, location, and duration.

2. *Conditional factors.* Conditional factors may also influence pain perception. All situations that predispose to or precipitate the onset of symptoms should be described by the patient:

DENTAL HISTORY	CHIEF COMPLAINT: (symptomatic) asymptomatic	*Lingering pain with hot or cold liquid began*

yesterday. Spontaneous episodes of pain; seems worse when lying down.

SYMPTOMS	Location	Chronology		Quality		Affected By		Prior Tx		
		Inception: 2-1-87		(sharp) dull	Intensity + (+) +++	(hot) ++ (cold) +++	palpation manipulation	Tx: restorative emergency RCT	(Yes) Yes Yes	No amalgam (No) 2 weeks ago (No)
	←ear	Clinical Course:			spontaneous provoked		(head position)			
localized	(referred)	constant	momentary	(pulsating) steady	reproducible	biting (chewing)	activity	Sx Pre-Tx:	Yes	(No)
(diffuse)	radiating	(intermittent)	(lingering)	enlarging	occasional	percussion	time of day	Sx Post-Tx:	(Yes)	No Initial: SC

a. Changes in posture—head pain accentuated by bending over or by forcefully blowing the nose implies involvement of the maxillary sinuses.

b. Time of day—stiffness and pain in the jaws upon waking may indicate occlusal disharmony or temporomandibular joint dysfunction.

c. Activities—pain upon exertion or vigorous physical activity may reflect endodontic pathosis or implicate coronary artery disease. A change in barometric pressure, as encountered during skin diving or flying at high altitudes, may indicate pulpal involvement or sinus disease.

d. Hormonal change—"menstrual toothache" may occur when there is an increase in body fluid retention.[5]

For the enhancement of the clinician's diagnostic acumen, a methodical approach must be coupled with perceptiveness. Systematic evaluation of affecting factors in a patient's chief complaint may enable the dentist to discern the correct location and cause of an otherwise perplexing diagnostic problem.

Adjunctive history. When an emergency arises shortly after the course of dental treatment (e.g., extreme unprecedented pain to thermal stimuli after placement of an extensive amalgam restoration), identification of the problem may be straightforward and the diagnosis uncomplicated.

However, the dentist may be challenged to diagnose and treat emergencies in which symptoms are vague and the etiology is not readily discernible. In such instances the recounting of significant incidents (e.g., trauma), previous symptoms, prior treatment, and complications involving the area of chief complaint may facilitate the diagnosis.

The disclosure of other symptoms currently or recently associated with, or apparently coincidental to, the patient's chief complaint should be elicited. They may be significant elements in determining a diagnosis.

For example, areas of depressed vision within the visual field (scotomas) may indicate classic migraine or a lesion in the optic pathways.

Any additional details pertaining to the patient's complaint, no matter how trifling, should be recorded at this time (e.g., the identification of a trigger zone, which is pathognomonic for idiopathic trigeminal neuralgia, may remain obscured in a hasty and cursory evaluation).

Familial medical disorders should also be discussed (e.g., history of headache, coronary artery disease, neoplastic conditions).

• • •

Each symptom associated with the patient's chief complaint should be evaluated in all the parameters just described. In the absence of outward clinical manifestations or observable radiographic alterations, it may be necessary to use the descriptive details gleaned from the interrogation as the sole basis for the tentative diagnosis.

All the diagnostic data acquired during the dental history phase of the patient examination should be recorded in a systematic format. (See suggested form above.)

After all the pertinent facts have been organized, analyzed, and reexamined, the dentist is ready to proceed with the diagnostic sequence.

Clinical examination

In an emergency situation the primary objective of the clinical evaluation is to identify and locate accurately the source of the patient's chief complaint.

The dentist should conduct the examination of the extraoral and intraoral hard and soft tissues in a precise and orderly manner. Establishment of a methodical approach and adherence to a formulated routine will result in the expeditious identification of features pertinent to the diagnostic process. Details of the comprehensive clinical examination should be entered on the patient record. Data acquired from the clinical examination, including results of diagnostic tests, should be recorded. (See suggested form at right.)

The clinical examination consists of two phases: (1) physical inspection followed by (2) diagnostic tests.

Physical inspection. A comprehensive regional examination should begin with a careful visual survey and is usually performed in conjunction with palpation, percussion, and periodontal evaluation.

A thorough periodontal assessment will include careful probing of pocket depths, determining the amount of attached gingiva, and noting the degree of tooth mobility.[21,41] Gingival sulcus tracts should be traced to their origin with gutta-percha points.[42] Basic techniques used in this portion of the examination are discussed in Chapter 1.

Diagnostic tests. The second phase of the clinical evaluation consists of the various diagnostic tests described in the preceding chapter. Collectively these procedures serve a dual purpose:

1. Localized reproduction of evokable symptoms that characterize the chief complaint
2. Comparative assessment of the dentoalveolar structures for detection of abnormalities accountable for the patient's symptoms

The usefulness of these diagnostic tests depends on their

CLINICAL		DIAGNOSTIC TESTS						
Tooth	Soft Tissues	Tooth No.	29	30	31			
WNL	(WNL)	perio	WNL →					
discoloration	extra-oral swelling	mobility	0	1	0			
caries	intra-oral swelling	percussion	WNL	+	WNL			
pulp exposure	sinus tract	palpation	WNL →					
prior access	lymphadenopathy	cold	WNL	+++				
attrition/abrasion	TMJ	hot	WNL	++·	WNL			
fracture	perio:	EPT	WNL	n·n·	WNL			
restoration		transillum.	WNL →					
(amalgam)	2 B	cavity						
composite	2M—D2	date:						
inlay/onlay	L 2		2-1-87					
temporary								
crown								
abutment								

correct and systematic application, as well as on the clinician's ability to interpret their results accurately. The dentist's diagnostic capabilities are significantly influenced by his or her understanding of normal and altered regional anatomy and physiology and by his or her proficiency in administration of the various clinical tests.

Just as data obtained from scientific experimentation may be disputed because of improper methodology, the conclusions deduced from a diagnostic test may be invalidated because of procedural inaccuracies. Accordingly, when attempting to reproduce the predominant symptoms of the patient's complaint, the dentist should recreate the original situational conditions as accurately as possible. This will help minimize inconsistencies in patient response and reduce the likelihood of misinterpretation.

The clinician should standardize each diagnostic stimulus in relation to duration, degree, and mode of application and, to avoid startling the patient, should make preparatory remarks regarding the nature of the test to be applied.

The patient's response to a given test can be indicated by the raising of a predesignated hand or finger immediately upon the onset and for the full duration that a reaction to an applied stimulus is perceived.

The dentist should also include adequate controls for any set of applied test procedures. Several adjacent, opposing, and contralateral teeth should be randomly tested, prior to the tooth in question, to establish the patient's normal range of response. The dentist must not bias the test results by suggesting to the patient beforehand that a particular tooth is presumably responsible for the chief complaint.

After each diagnostic test trial the patient should be asked to review the location, quality, intensity, and temporal pattern of the induced response. This information can then be compared with test results obtained from other teeth. The patient's responses to the applied diagnostic tests should also be compared with the corresponding subjective elicitations from the dental history. Only then can the diagnostician be sure that a particular symptom has been accurately recreated and its source precisely located.

The requisite fundamentals of endodontic diagnostic procedures and their interpretations are presented in Chapter 1. The discussion herein will focus on clinical considerations that may be significant in perplexing diagnostic situations.

Thermal tests. Certain established methods of thermal application (e.g., heated gutta-percha stopping,, heated instrument, rubber wheel, ethyl chloride, ice ampule or dry ice) may provide diagnostic data of limited reliability. Although these techniques afford expediency in applying the stimulus, they occasionally do not simulate the original source closely enough to be diagnostically relevant. The extent of surface coverage and actual applied temperature may be quite variable.

Whenever symptoms of pulpitis are provoked by ingestion of hot or cold liquids, the dentist should consider isolating the tooth to be tested with a rubber dam and bathing the entire coronal region in water. The temperature of the water bath should be adjusted by the patient beforehand to match the temperature responsible for the presenting symptoms.

In difficult diagnostic situations this method has proved to be more accurate than other modalities of thermal application, since it reproduces the original provoking conditions much more realistically (Fig. 2-2, p. 38).

The clinician must be aware that repeated thermal stimulation of the same tooth within a short time (i.e., seconds) may yield conflicting results. This empirical observation, presumably caused by a period of sensory refraction, underscores the need for developing a methodical diagnostic technique and emphasizes the importance of reliable patient response.

Percussion. If presenting symptoms include pain to biting or mastication, having the patient chew on a cotton roll as the dentist sequentially moves it over individual teeth may be more accurate and revealing than simple axial percussion in elusive clinical situations (Fig. 2-3, *A*, p. 39).

The excursive movements of the mandible introduced during chewing may facilitate the detection of radicular and coronal vertical fractures, occlusal disharmonies, temporomandibular arthropathies, or myofacial dysfunction as well as inflammation of the periodontal ligament secondary to endodontic or periodontal disease. After a cotton roll has been used to narrow the zone of masticatory sensitivity to two teeth (i.e., a tooth and its antagonist) selective tapping from various angles with a blunt instrument handle may then be done to isolate the individual tooth responsible for the symptoms perceived (Fig. 2-3, *B*).

Electric pulp testing. The reliability of electric pulp testing should be of concern to the clinician. The potential

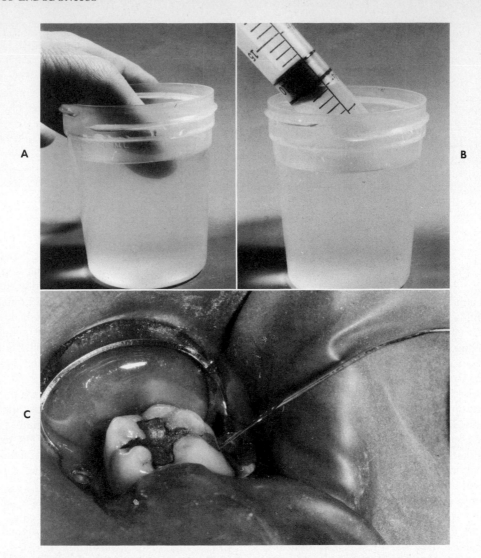

FIG. 2-2. Thermal testing in perplexing situations. **A,** The patient adjusts water to the temperature responsible for thermal symptoms reported in the dental history. **B,** A 12-ml disposable syringe is filled with water that has been adjusted to the appropriate temperature. **C,** The tooth to be tested is isolated with a rubber dam and bathed with water from the loaded syringe.

for erroneous results may be attributable to inaccuracies of the electronic apparatus, aberrant responses of individual teeth, inconsistencies in clinical technique (e.g., placement and contact angle of the electrode tip to the tooth surface),[12] and other reasons discussed on p. 21. These factors must be considered whenever results from electric pulp tests are used in formulating a diagnosis.

The electric pulp test should be regarded as an aid in detecting pulpal neural response and not as a quantifiable correlator of pulp pathoses.

Transillumination. Vertical and horizontal crown fractures are easier to detect with the new, improved fiberoptics. Transillumination should be routinely performed to search for elusive coronal fractures.

Swelling. Orofacial swelling is a common and potentially complicating manifestation of odontogenic pathosis (e.g., periapical or lateral periodontal abscess). Soft-tissue distensions associated with dental conditions may range from simple parulis formation to extensive, even life-threatening, space infections within deep tissues and fas-

cial planes and may present as the only symptom or be accompanied by other clinical manifestations, including mild to intolerable pressure-type pain.[27,49]

Most swellings of endodontic origin are precipitated by the pathologic egress of bacterial or necrotic pulpal irritants from the root canal system, which infiltrate the soft tissues via periapical or perilateral alveolar pathways.

Iatrogenic causes of endodontic swelling include indiscriminate or inadequate access preparation, cleaning and shaping, and obturation techniques as well as potentially toxic effects of certain root canal–filling materials. Acute symptoms of edema and emphysema resulting from procedural accidents (e.g., negligent use of sodium hypochlorite and hydrogen peroxide irrigants) have also been documented.[4,26,30] Swelling may be considered a routine sequela of surgical endodontic procedures and is not generally regarded as an acute emergency. (The diagnosis and management of postsurgical edema are discussed in Chapter 18.)

The cause of most orofacial swellings can be readily

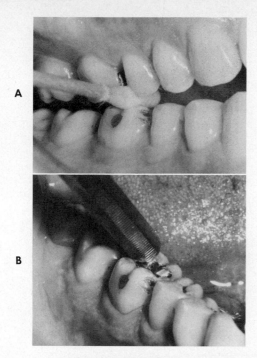

FIG. 2-3. A, If presenting symptoms include pain to chewing, the patient is instructed to chew on a cotton roll or a cotton-wood stick to reveal the zone of masticatory sensitivity. **B,** Tapping with a blunt instrument handle will usually locate the offending tooth.

identified from the dental history, correlated with clinical and radiographic examinations. However, the dentist who is confronted with an ill-defined emergency situation in which swelling is a predominant or solitary symptom must be able to distinguish tumefactions of dental origin from enlargements of alternative etiologies (e.g., systemic diseases, nondental inflammatory conditions, neoplastic alterations).[13,16,25]

The following procedural guidelines are recommended for diagnosing symptoms of orofacial swelling:

1. Identify the clinical features of the swelling. This is achieved by systematic inspection and bilateral palpation of the intraoral and extraoral tissues. Careful attention should be given to these qualities:
   a. Topology
      (1) Location
      (2) Size
      (3) Shape
   b. Physical characteristics
      (1) Consistency
      (2) Mobility
      (3) Fluctuance
      (4) Surface temperature
   c. Affected tissues
      (1) Identification of tissues involved (e.g., bone or soft tissue)
      (2) Extent of involvement within tissue planes and anatomic spaces
2. Procure required radiographs to detect the nature and entire extent of osseous involvement. It should be determined whether the lesion is osteosclerotic, os-

teogenic, or osteolytic. Supplemental radiographic views may be required to include fully the borders of extensive lesions.

3. Perform a thorough periodontal evaluation. Swellings of periodontal origin as well as those of endodontic-periodontal etiology characteristically exhibit deep sulcular or infrabony defects upon probing.
4. Perform appropriate diagnostic tests to detect endodontic involvement. All teeth in proximity to the swelling should be evaluated for pulpal vitality. As a rule, enlargements of endodontic etiology occur secondary to pulpal necrosis.
5. Usually any abnormal swelling not attributable to dental etiology should be submitted to biopsy examination for definitive histologic diagnosis.
6. The contents of soft-tissue swellings should be examined by aspiration with an anesthetic syringe immediately prior to any surgical intervention. Incision and drainage should not be performed unless the presence of accumulated purulence has been confirmed by visual inspection (Fig. 2-4, p. 40).

Radiographic evaluation

After procuring details of chief complaint from the foregoing history and physical examination, the examiner should obtain the required radiographic views. Only views that will contribute to the location and identification of the patient's stated problem should be included.

Oral radiographs can be of immense value in the differential diagnostic evaluation. It is incumbent upon the dentist, however, to avoid exposing the patient to unnecessary or excessive radiologic examinations. Xeroradiography reduces the amount of ionizing radiation required to obtain a clear, easy-to-read film of the area under investigation.

Although promiscuous use of radiation is definitely discouraged, the attending dentist is cautioned to exercise discretion in accepting prior diagnostic radiographs from the patient or another dentist, no matter how recently they were acquired. Such radiographs may not accurately reflect the present condition of the regional dental structures (e.g., the degree of pathologic involvement or the extent of healing that has occurred). Furthermore, iatrogenic alterations (e.g., ledge formation, perforation, or separation of an endodontic instrument) will not be demonstrated if they are created subsequent to these radiographs.

Diagnostic radiographs must be adequate in areal coverage as well as satisfactory in image quality. Proper film placement, exposure, processing, and handling are essential for the consistent production of high-quality radiographs. Details of the radiographic examination can be entered on the patient record (p. 40). Lapses in these techniques may result in misdiagnosis.

Diagnostic radiographs should be interpreted in a systematic and scrupulous manner. Use of an optical magnifier along with proper illumination will help the examiner discern subtle and intricate details in the radiographic image (e.g., continuity of the periodontal ligament, incipient pathologic changes involving the dentoalveolar hard tissues, evidence of ramifications within the root canal system).

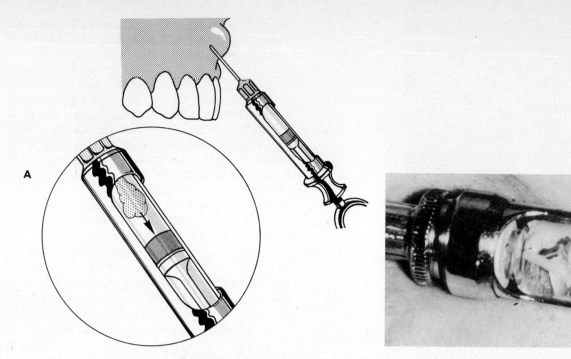

FIG. 2-4. Needle aspiration to verify the accumulation of purulence before incision and drainage is performed. **A,** An ampule of local anesthetic loaded in an aspirating syringe is half-emptied by depressing the plunger. After insertion of the needle within the site of tissue distension, the plunger is slowly withdrawn. **B,** The presence of purulent exudate in the aspirate from the swelling *(arrow)* is sufficient evidence.

EXAMINATION	RADIOGRAPHIC
Tooth	Attachment Apparatus
WNL	PDL normal
caries	PDL thickened
restoration	alveolar bone, WNL
calcification	diffuse lucency
resorption	circumscribed lucency
fracture	resorption
perforation/deviation	apical
prior RC Tx/RCF	lateral
separated instrument	hypercementosis
canal obstruction	osteosclerosis
post/build-up	perio:
open apex	

A thorough understanding of radiologic principles and limitations is essential for accurate radiographic interpretation. To correctly identify any radiologic changes that might explain the patient's symptoms, the diagnostician must also be cognizant of regional anatomic structures and their variational characteristics in health and disease.[48,52]

The dentist should be knowledgeable about the various types of radiographic examinations appropriate for differential diagnosis of orofacial pain. These are classified as follows:

1. Intraoral radiographs
   a. Periapical view
   b. Interproximal view
   c. Occlusal views
2. Panoramic radiographs
3. Extraoral radiographs
   a. Transparietal projection
   b. Transpharyngeal projection
   c. Lateral jaw projections
      (1) Oblique lateral film
      (2) Profile film
   d. Posteroanterior projections
      (1) Waters view
      (2) Caldwell view
   e. Lateral skull projection

Intraoral projections. Intraoral projections are routinely utilized by dentists and are readily obtainable:

1. *Periapical radiographs* provide high-definition views of the entire tooth, the periodontal attachment complex, and the adjacent structures. The inferior portions of the maxillary sinuses are often well detailed on periapical films of the maxillary posterior teeth. Alterations of the horizontal and/or vertical angulations may be necessary for proper differentiation of superimposed structures. Modifications in film contrast and density may also be required to enhance the diagnostic value of the radiograph. (Techniques for periapical exposures are discussed in Chapter 4.)
2. *Interproximal (bite-wing) exposures* are useful for revealing conditions of the coronal and cervical regions that might be obscured on periapical radiographs. Bite-wing films may demonstrate pulp chamber obstructions and obliterations, resorptive defects, carious lesions, and pulp cappings beneath existing restorations as well as alterations of the furcal and interproximal alveolar crests.
3. *Occlusal radiographs* permit the examination of substantial areas of the mandible or maxilla. These are useful for the detection and spatial assessment of pathologic conditions and the extent and displacement of fractures, impactions, and retained roots. Portions of the maxillary sinuses also can be seen

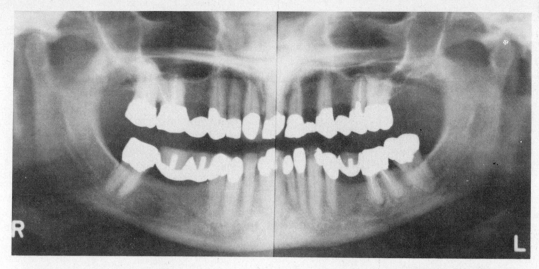

FIG. 2-5. Panoramic radiograph. This view is useful for surveying the entire dentition and contiguous structures. (Courtesy Dr. James Campbell.)

with maxillary occlusal films. Calculi in the sublingual and submaxillary glands and ducts can be detected on mandibular occlusal views.

Panoramic radiographs. Panoramic radiographs represent a versatile and important diagnostic supplement to the intraoral projections. Although limitations such as loss of detail, distortions, overlapping, shifting, and shadowing may exist, panoramic views are useful for surveying the general condition and arrangements of the entire mandibular and maxillary dentition, the alveolar bone and contiguous osseous structures, the orbital and nasal regions, and the adjacent sinuses[32] (Fig. 2-5).

Extraoral radiographs. Extraoral radiographs utilize sheet film (8 × 10 inches) loaded in flat cassettes and are occasionally required to supplement the information yielded by the various intraoral and panoramic projections. They may provide differential diagnostic information regarding the temporomandibular joints, the maxilla and mandible, and the entire craniofacial complex. The presence of foreign bodies, injury, osseous pathosis, and other conditions may be detailed with the various extraoral radiographic examinations.

Technical descriptions of the various radiographic examinations are readily available.[51,53]

Although a routine radiologic survey might detect unsuspected pathoses, the radiograph should generally be regarded as a confirmatory adjunct in the emergency diagnostic process. The dentist should always be aware of the potential for radiologic misinterpretation and should not accept the radiograph as the sole criterion for initiating treatment. Accordingly, radiographic findings should be correlated with a thorough patient history and clinical examination and confirmed by corroborative diagnostic procedures.

Determining the diagnosis

The final phase of the diagnostic sequence consists of a systematic analysis of all pertinent data accumulated from the interrogatory, clinical, and radiographic evaluations. The purpose of this exercise is to determine the precise cause of the patient's presenting signs and symptoms so that appropriate emergency care can be rendered or recommended.

Endodontic involvement

The dentist should begin by determining whether the signs and symptoms of the chief complaint are indeed consistent with an endodontic etiology. If they are diagnosed as such, the next step is to confirm the location and delineate the specific nature of the apparent endodontic problem. From the collective diagnostic findings the dentist should be able to distinguish whether the symptoms evince pulpal pathosis that is confined to the tooth or whether there has been an extension into the contiguous periapical or perilateral tissues. After this the specific etiologic factor(s) should be identified (e.g., caries, trauma, restorations, developmental anomalies). Whether or not endodontic involvement is evident, differential causes of the chief complaint should always be considered.[16]

Periodontal considerations

Sequential to the preceding endodontic analysis, the results of the periodontal examination should be evaluated. If an endodontic cause cannot be detected, it must be determined whether a periodontal condition is the reason for the patient's presenting symptoms. Even if endodontic pathosis has been categorically diagnosed, the clinician should determine whether periodontal factors are also contributory to the chief complaint (i.e., combined endodontic-periodontal lesion)[19,24] and whether such concomitant periodontal involvement adversely affects the prognosis for retaining the tooth. If a significant periodontal condition exists, the extent of involvement and the nature of the problem should be delineated. After this has been accomplished, the specific causal factors (e.g., inadequate epithelial attachment, lingual developmental groove, enamel projection) should be explicitly identified. Accurate determination of the clinical periodontal status will help define the mode of palliative and definitive therapy. For example, if extensive preexisting alveolar bone resorption indicates

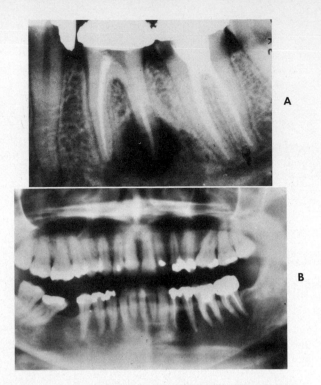

FIG. 2-6. Periapical radiolucencies of systemic origin. **A,** Eosinophilic granuloma (histiocytosis X). **B,** Osteogenic sarcoma. In each case the involved teeth would have responded within normal limits to thermal and electric pulp tests initially. Failure to establish the pulpal status of the involved dentition in both clinical situations could easily result in their misdiagnosis and unnecessary endodontic treatment.

that retention of a tooth cannot be justified, the preferred treatment may be extraction, even though the acute symptoms can be effectively alleviated by conservative endodontic procedures.

Restorative considerations

Following the periodontal examination, the future restorability of the offending tooth must be considered. If the tooth cannot be adequately restored to good function, extraction should be considered.

Differential diagnoses

Because orofacial signs and symptoms may arise from nonodontogenous etiologies (Fig. 2-6) and because such pathologic entities may coexist with confirmed endodontic and periodontal abnormalities, differential diagnoses of nondental origin should always be considered whenever the dentist evaluates symptoms for probable cause.[9,22,44] This axiom is particularly important if the presenting symptoms are inconsistent with an endodontic or periodontal etiology. The same principle applies if the symptoms seem consistent with dental etiologic factors but their location and cause cannot be positively confirmed by appropriate diagnostic procedures.

Nonodontogenous causes of orofacial symptoms can be classified into several categories:(1) organic, (2) functional, (3) vascular, (4) neuralgic, and (5) psychogenic.

On occasion, a given pathologic entity will be justifiably included in more than one of these groups, especially if the primary causative antecedents are multifactorial, unsubstantiated, or open to dispute. It should be emphasized, however, that the main purpose of categorizing the various nondentoalveolar conditions is *to facilitate* the eventual referral of the patient to the appropriate medical or dental specialist. The definitive inclusion of a disease entity in a particular organizational classification remains secondary to its accurate diagnosis and proper treatment.

The various differential diagnostic categories are described next, along with salient features of related clinical conditions most likely to confront the dentist in an emergency situation.

Organic disorders. Organic disorders involve alterations in the structure of body organs or tissues adapted to specific function(s).

Orofacial symptoms for which no dental cause can be detected should motivate the dentist to consider organic factors along with other etiologies. For example, nondental mandibular paresthesia is most suggestive of an impinging tumor.[11] Maxillary and facial paresthesia not attributable to dental origin is probably due to maxillary sinus disease.

Pathologic conditions involving the maxillary sinus (e.g., inflammations, cysts, tumors, trauma) are the *most common* nondental organic causes of odontic symptoms. The fact that the alveolar process of the maxillary posterior teeth also forms the inferior portion of the maxillary sinus helps to explain this observation.

Symptoms produced by maxillary sinus disease may involve the eyes (e.g., visual anomalies, excessive lacrimation, paresthesia, pain), the nose (e.g., drainage, epistaxis, obstruction), and the face (e.g., infraorbital, lateral nasal, or upper labial paresthesia; fullness; pain). Intraoral manifestations include pain, paresthesia, anesthesia, percussion sensitivity, and tenderness to palpation of the maxillary molar-premolar region on the involved side.[17] Vestibular and alveolar expansion may be detectable, along with crepitus of the sinus walls.

The most prevalent sinus disease is maxillary sinusitis, which may occur in chronic, subacute, and acute forms. Sinusitis is generally precipitated by an upper respiratory tract infection or allergic rhinitis; but it may also be caused by a deviated septum, cleft palate, nasal polyps, pregnancy (secondary to rhinitis),[6] and violative dental procedures. Acute symptoms of maxillary sinusitis may be accentuated when the patient occludes or bends forward. The patient may report a sensation of supererupted dentition and frontal headache pain. Concomitant symptoms may include seropurulent or mucopurulent exudate, malaise, and (if the infection has extended beyond the sinuses) fever and chills.

About 25% of the cases diagnosed as chronic maxillary sinusitis are secondary to dental infection.[8] Whenever a patient has signs and symptoms indicative of acute or chronic sinusitis, the dentist must perform a comprehensive examination to identify or rule out a dental problem. Palpation, percussion, and extensive pulp vitality tests are essential to an accurate differential diagnosis.

Functional disorders. Functional disorders affect the normal performance of an organ or tissue without apparent organic or structural changes. Considered within this category is the syndrome of myofacial pain-dysfunction (MPD), the most common disorder involving the temporomandibular joint (TMJ) region. The following components are associated with this psychophysiologic syndrome:

1. Severe emotional stress
2. Clenching and bruxism
3. Occlusal disharmonies

Major characteristics of MPD include pain of unilateral origin, limitation of jaw movement, and tenderness to palpation of the masticatory musculature. The pain perceived is usually of a dull quality and may exhibit variable intensity. Crepitus of the TMJ initiated by habits of jaw clenching and grinding, may be clinically apparent. Auscultation and palpation may facilitate the detection of such "clicking" or "popping" sounds within the TMJ.[3] Orofacial pain is the probable result of masticatory muscle spasm. Such pain may radiate or be referred to the teeth, tongue, palate, TMJ, ear, head, or neck.

The MPD syndrome is significant to the dentist because of its prevalence within the dental patient population. Approximately 20% of dental patients suffer symptoms of the condition.[45] Characteristics of the syndrome are observed much more frequently in women than in men.[36]

The diagnosis of MPD is based on clinical findings. Radiographic examinations of the TMJ are usually noncontributory, although secondary degenerative changes are occasionally detected in advanced stages.

Vascular pain syndromes. Vascular pain syndromes are clinical conditions involving symptoms of remote circulatory origin.

A significant proportion of headache pain is induced by distortion of the cranial vasculature. Of such pain-provoking disorders, the functional disturbances associated with migraine are most prevalent.

Migraine is a clinical manifestation characterized by severe, throbbing paroxysms of unilateral headache. The pain, however, may manifest itself bilaterally and is usually postocular. Nausea and vomiting are frequently experienced during the course of an attack. The duration usually is measured in hours and even days. Migraine headaches occasionally appear to emanate from the maxillary posterior dentition.

Prodromal symptoms of classic migraine include dizziness, pallor, sweating, chills, and numbness or tingling of the mouth and hands. The aura, which precedes and signals the onset of an impending attack, classically involves disturbances in the visual field (scotomas), abnormal intolerance to light (photophobia), and aversion to noise and stress.[14]

The pain associated with migraine is caused by dilation of extracranial arteries and is usually evoked by psychologic factors. Emotional anxiety and stress are frequently identified as predisposing factors.

Headache may also be a common symptom of acute intracranial or systemic infection, hypertension, craniofacial trauma, and intracranial neoplasia.[29] Diseases affecting the eyes, ears, nose, throat, and teeth may likewise cause cephalic pain. The examining dentist should consider these entities whenever headache is associated with the chief complaint.

Neuralgic disorders. Neuralgic disorders are conditions in which the dominant symptom of paroxysmal pain extends along the course of a nerve or its area of distribution.

Trigeminal neuralgia (tic douloureux) is of primary significance to the dentist because it involves the fifth cranial nerve (usually the second or third division).[20] Although the etiology of true tic douloureux is presently unclear, the most current theory suggests that the condition is due to a chronic irritation of the trigeminal nerve and a failure of inhibition in the trigeminal nucleus. This lack of inhibitory effect results in the paroxysmal discharges in the trigeminal nucleus.[18,19,39,40]

The pain of trigeminal neuralgia is distinctly perceived as a sharp, shooting, or stabbing attack similar to an electric shock. Episodes are characterized by their sudden recurrence, extreme intensity, and short duration (usually lasting several seconds). Less typically, intense pain may be followed by longer periods of vague aching or burning. The acute symptoms are perceived unilaterally in any single paroxysm.

A major pathognomonic feature of trigeminal neuralgia is the presence of a trigger zone, a localized area sensitive to touch or motion, around the mouth, face, or throat. Provoking stimuli may include light touch, talking, chewing, swallowing, washing the face, and blowing the nose.

The differential diagnosis of symptoms involving sharp radiating pain should include dental disorders (e.g., irreversible pulpitis, cracked tooth). A patient afflicted with acute neuralgic symptoms that are provoked by movement or trigger stimulation but for which no dentoalveolar cause can be found should be referred to a neurologist for definitive evaluation.

Psychogenic disorders. Psychogenic disorders are entities in which symptoms are of an emotional or psychologic origin as opposed to an organic cause.

Orofacial pain may be the predominant symptom in patients suffering psychosomatic illness. Psychogenic facial pain and headache may result from states of dejection and mental depresson. Patients suffering from hypochondriasis characteristically exhibit untoward anxiety about health and may fall victim to simulated disease states.[50] Adherence to a false belief that there is some alteration in an organ or physiologic function may lead to symptoms of somatic delusion. Psychogenic pain may also be secondary to hysterical conversion reactions, in which emotions become transformed into sensory or motor manifestations.[1]

Whenever the history reveals symptoms of a nonspecific nature and clinical and radiographic examinations fail to illuminate factors implicating an organic cause, the dentist should consider psychogenic etiologies in the differential diagnosis of orofacial pain.

• • •

In the establishment of a correct diagnosis pertinent diagnostic findings acquired from the examination must be consistent with the patient's signs and symptoms. Occasionally it will be necessary to defer the diagnosis and treatment pending further determination of symptom location or the accumulation of additional information.

If the chief complaint has been positively identified as an endodontic problem and the location has been precisely determined, the dentist should inform the patient regarding pertinent examination findings (e.g., preexisting periodontal condition, pulpal status, extent of alveolar involvement, restorative considerations), recommended treatment plan, alternative approaches, risks and prognosis. A thorough patient consultation should always be rendered before endodontic treatment is initiated.

TREATMENT

Three prudent rules apply in treating endodontic emergencies:
1. Never render dental treatment until you are certain of the diagnosis.
2. It is better to provide no treatment than to provide the wrong treatment.
3. When in doubt, refer the case out!

Keeping these three rules in mind will help the clinician to maintain a high-quality, low-stress practice. The preceding sections have shown why it is so essential to procure and document all pertinent diagnostic data through a systematic process of interrogatory, clinical, and radiographic evaluation. The clinician must be sure that all signs and symptoms are consistent with the determined diagnosis before initiating any treatment.

If the tentative diagnosis does not correspond to the patient's presenting signs and symptoms, it would be wise to refer the patient immediately. If the examination indicates that the diagnosis may be a difficult endodontic problem, it would be better for the patient, and less stressful for the clinician, to refer to an endodontist. If examination suggests that the problem may be of nondental etiology, then the patient should be referred to the most appropriate medical specialist (e.g., a neurologist, an otolaryngologist).

All treatment described below pertains to permanent teeth with mature apices; for treatment of primary teeth, refer to Chapter 22.

Treatment according to symptoms
Thermal pain

When a patient's acute symptoms involve thermal pain, the usual nature of the complaint is moderate to severe discomfort lasting for a few seconds or lingering when the tooth (or teeth) is contacted by a thermal stimulus. There are three general categories within which the patient may have such pain.

Before endodontic treatment. If pain is a symptom before endodontic therapy, its source must be determined.

When the signs, symptoms, and dental history indicate a final diagnosis of *reversible pulpitis,* the following philosophy guides the direction of treatment:
1. Placement of a sedative dressing for several weeks may allow the pulp to revert to a clinically intact and uninflamed state.
2. If a carious lesion is detected, after local anesthesia and rubber dam isolation, the caries must be thoroughly removed from the tooth.
3. If a recent restoration has preceded the development

of thermal pain symptoms, the restoration must be removed. The cavity preparation should then be filled with a sedative temporary restoration (e.g., zinc oxide–eugenol, I.R.M.). When the anesthesia subsides, the patient should notice an immediate improvement. After several weeks the sedative restoration can be replaced with a well-based final restoration if all symptoms have abated and the pulp causes a moderate, transient response to thermal and electric testing.

When the signs, symptoms, and dental history indicate a final diagnosis of *irreversible pulpitis,* the pulp should be removed immediately. Providing profound anesthesia for a tooth when an irreversibly inflamed pulp may be difficult, especially for an acutely symptomatic mandibular molar. To provide total anesthesia in these cases, if the periodontium is healthy, the use of intraligamentary injections (e.g., Ligmaject, Peripress) is strongly recommended to supplement (not replace) conventional local anesthesia. Intraligamentary injections properly administered are very helpful in providing profound anesthesia for acutely symptomatic teeth. Furthermore, this helps to reduce the anxiety of the patient and the stress for the clinician. (Please refer to Chapter 19 for further information regarding the technique for intraligamentary injections.) After profound anesthesia and rubber dam isolation, all caries, if present, should be removed. Then the access cavity should be prepared and the pulp completely extirpated. A deep pulpotomy may relieve the thermal symptoms in most cases, but the most predictable treatment (which requires complete pulp extirpation and thorough debridement of the root canal system) is described in Chapter 7. It is debatable whether intracanal medicaton should be used. If the pulp is thoroughly removed and all canals properly cleaned and shaped, there is little need for an intracanal dressing. Accordingly, it is recommended that a dry cotton pellet be placed in the access cavity and covered with Cavit. If endodontic therapy involves a posterior tooth without a cast metal restoration, the tooth should be adjusted out of occlusion to minimize symptoms of a possible apical periodontitis secondary to pulp extirpation and to reduce the chance of crown fracture. (The reader should know there is no consensus in the endodontic community regarding the need to relieve occlusion in order to minimize post-operative pain[47].) Because *all* posterior teeth require a cast metal restoration after endodontic therapy to prevent coronal fracture, the occlusal reduction should be performed at this time to provide greater assurance of patient comfort. The clinician may wish to prescribe a mild analgesic (e.g., aspirin or acetaminophen) for several days. The majority of patients should not require any analgesic medications.

After initiation of endodontic treatment but before canal obturation. If the dental history suggests a diagnosis of reversible or irreversible pulpitis *after* total pulp extirpation has been achieved, then whatever thermal symptom(s) the patient is experiencing must be caused by another tooth.

Referred pain to a tooth currently undergoing endodontic treatment is not uncommon. To prove this to the patient (patients occasionally may be somewhat disbelieving), hand the patient a mirror and allow him to watch as you attempt thermal stimulation of the tooth undergoing treatment. When the patient can see that hot and cold stimulation of the tooth does not reproduce his complaint, then examine by thermal testing the other teeth in that quadrant, or the opposing quadrant if necessary, to identify the real source of thermally stimulated pain. Once the offending tooth has been identified, pulp extirpation will promptly relieve the thermal sensitivity.

After canal obturation. The approach is identical to that immediately preceding, because in both situations another tooth must be the source of the thermally stimulated pain.

Percussion pain

When the chief complaint is pain with biting or chewing—which can be confirmed by percussion testing—this merely indicates inflammation involving the periodontal ligament. This symptom does not reveal the status of the pulp. It is therefore mandatory to perform thermal and electric pulp testing to determine the condition of the pulp before treatment is initiated. If the tooth has full coronal coverage (e.g., a ceramometal crown), a small test cavity may be required to verify the clinical status of the pulp (p. 22).

Before endodontic treatment. If percussion causes pain, the vitality of the pulp must be verified.

If the pulp is *vital* (ie., vital acute apical periodontitis), simply use articulating paper to identify occlusal prematurities on the tooth and adjust the clinical crown to normal occlusion. Complaints in this category appear to be more common following recent placement of a restoration in a posterior tooth. After the spot reduction of the occlusal prematurity, advise the patient to do all chewing on the other side for several days. Before leaving the treatment room, the patient should be somewhat aware that the tooth already feels more comfortable. Within several days the periodontal ligament should return to a state of normalcy and the patient should feel completely comfortable when chewing.

If the pulp is *nonvital* (i.e., necrosis with periapical extension as in early acute apical abscess or phoenix abscess), endodontic treatment should be started immediately. After local anesthesia and rubber dam isolation, the access cavity is prepared as described in Chapter 6. After determination of the length(s) of the canal(s), any remnants of pulp tissue should be completely extirpated and the canals thoroughly debrided. A dry cotton pellet is placed in the pulp chamber and covered with Cavit. As a rule the access should not be left exposed unless there is persistent drainage of exudate.[47] If a posterior tooth is involved, the clinician should relieve the occlusion. If the tooth has a cast metal restoration, spot grinding of the opposing tooth is suggested. If there was no evidence of extensive drainage upon entering a canal, there is little need for antibiotics, provided no swelling appears and the patient does not have a debilitating systemic ailment. Prescribing a mild analgesic (aspirin or acetaminophen) should be more than adequate for most cases if the canals have been thoroughly cleaned.

A good "practice builder" is to have your office call the patient the following day, because by that time he should be feeling much more comfortable. Patients are delighted by a simple telephone call. By far, most will report that they feel significant improvement; and if, by chance, any symptoms still linger they will be pleased by your close attentiveness, which shows how much you care.

After initiation of endodontic treatment but before canal obturation. A complaint of pain with biting or chewing should be confirmed by percussion tests. There are several reasons why this symptom can develop or persist postoperatively: extension of filing instruments past the apical foramen ("overinstrumentation"), periapical extension of bacterial or necrotic pulpal elements, or a premature occlusal contact.

Tooth initially vital. Since vital pulp extirpation is an amputation procedure, naturally some temporary inflammation of the periodontal ligament can be anticipated. This possibility should be clearly explained to the patient before treatment. Most patients will tolerate a little temporary inflammation with no complaint; some will require mild analgesics for a few days.

The potential for inflammation can be minimized if the patient's occlusion on the tooth has been relieved *prior to* initiating endodontic therapy. Treatment is based on the degree of discomfort the patient is experiencing. If the tooth is only slightly tender to percussion and if all canals have been *thoroughly* debrided, merely reassuring the patient should be adequate. If the tooth appears to be moderately or extremely tender to percussion, however, then after local anesthesia and rubber dam isolation, the temporary dressing must be removed and the root canal system carefully examined for any exudate. If there is an exudate, the canal(s) should be copiously irrigated with a mild solution of sodium hypochlorite. Then the length of the canal(s) should be reconfirmed and the cleaning and shaping repeated.

Before sealing the tooth, be sure that the canals are completely dried—and that they remain dry. Place a dry cotton pellet in the pulp chamber and seal with Cavit. Check the occlusion again and relieve any high spots. Mild analgesics can be prescribed, and the patient should be advised to chew on the other side of his mouth for several days. (Most patients intuitively know this.)

Tooth initially nonvital. The treatment for an initially nonvital tooth is basically the same as for a vital tooth. However, in all cases the temporary dressing should be removed after local anesthesia and rubber dam isolation. Examine carefully for any exudate; and if there is any, determine the type and volume. If the canal is devoid of exudate, merely placing a dry cotton pellet and Cavit in the pulp chamber and rechecking the occlusion should suffice. If an exudate is present, record the type and volume (e.g., "slight hemmorrhagic exudate," "considerable purulent exudate"). After copius irrigation, repeat all cleaning and shaping procedures described in Chapter 7. Confirm with paper points that the canal is completely dry.

In most cases the canals can be completely dried; however, if an exudate persists after thorough cleaning and shaping, leave the tooth open to drain for a day. Place a small cotton pellet in the pulp chamber and ask the patient to return the following day to have the canals disinfected and the tooth closed. When a tooth must be left open for drainage, the patient is advised to do all of his chewing on the opposite side, to use very warm rinses frequently, and to brush often and thoroughly. It cannot be emphasized too strongly that, whenever possible, a tooth should be closed, because leaving the tooth open to the oral flora increases the possibility of subsequent "flare-ups".[47]

After canal obturation. Mild tenderness to biting or chewing is fairly common after canal obturation. To minimize patient anxiety, it should be clearly explained that the tooth will probably feel tender to biting for several days. If the patient has been informed in advance of this mild transient symptom, it should not cause undue concern. If he has not been informed, then the mildest symptoms of biting or chewing sensitivity may cause alarm. ("How can the tooth hurt when you took out the nerve?")

The frequency of such responses can be reduced by thorough home care instructions, both verbal and written. Use articulating paper to recheck the patient's bite to be certain that there are no occlusal prematurities. Prescribing mild analgesics and warm water rinses will frequently suffice for this situation. However, if the pain to percussion is strong or lasts more than a few days, reexamine the postoperative radiograph carefully. Overextension of gutta-percha beyond the apical foramen or incomplete debridement and obturation of the canal will most likely be the source of the problem.

If the gutta-percha is underextended, then re-treating the canal(s) will be the treatment of choice. If it is overextended and pain with biting (percussion) persists, then periapical surgery is advised.

In situations in which pain with biting (percussion) persists, the extended use of analgesics is *not recommended,* for two reasons: (1) There are undesirable side effects with all analgesics and antibiotics used on a long-term basis. (2) The source of the problem has not been eliminated.

Swelling

Before endodontia. The nature, location, and extent of swelling, along with determination of pulp vitality, will indicate the type of clinical treatment.

If the preceding interrogatory, clinical, and radiographic examinations established that the swelling is of dental origin and the tooth is *vital (within normal limits),* then the diagnosis is most commonly a lateral periodontal abscess. Endodontic treatment is not indicated. Merely probing the associated periodontal pocket may allow the drainage to occur through the sulcus.

If the tooth is *nonvital,* the endodontic diagnosis can be only acute apical abscess or phoenix abscess. Palpation and visual examination will indicate whether the swelling is soft and fluctuant or firm and indurated, close to the apex or somewhat remote from the dental source, spread out broadly under the mucoperiosteum along fascial planes or localized around a single tooth.

If the swelling is soft and fluctuant and a nonvital tooth has been identified, then incision and drainage (p. 47) are

indicated. Occasionally a swollen area will appear soft and ready to be lanced, but upon making an incision the clinician finds that the drainage obtained is merely hemorrhagic. This, of course, provides little immediate benefit for the patient and may even complicate the presenting acute condition.

The following procedure is recommended whenever the clinician is contemplating an incision to establish drainage in a swollen area:

1. After the administration of regional block anesthesia, place a 27-gauge needle attached to an aspirating syringe containing a half carpule of anesthetic beneath the swollen mucosa; express two or three drops of anesthetic and then aspirate.
2. If a purulent exudate is present, it will appear in the carpule (Fig. 2-4). Confirm its presence before incising and draining (I & D), because if only a hemorrhagic exudate appears the area is *not* ready to be incised.
3. If the needle aspiration technique indicates that the area is not suitable for I & D, recommend rinsing frequently with very warm water. Prescribe an appropriate antibiotic and ask the patient to return when the swelling becomes larger or feels softer.

Whether or not I & D can be performed, the tooth or teeth that are the source of the swelling should be treated immediately.

After regional block anesthesia (if possible) and rubber dam isolation the tooth is relieved out of occlusion (unless it has a cast metal restoration) and an access cavity is prepared (with a high-speed handpiece to minimize vibration). Merely unroofing the pulp chamber may allow further drainage to occur. Occasionally, after access to the pulp chamber has been established, the canal(s) will appear dry. However, upon negotiating a canal with a test file the clinician may "uncork" the blocked passage. This usually becomes evident when removal of the test file is followed within a few seconds by a purulent/hemorrhagic exudate oozing out of the canal.[47]

If drainage is occurring through the root canal(s), it should be allowed to continue for several minutes. In most cases it will stop shortly. When it has ceased, the canal(s) should be thoroughly cleaned and shaped—provided the necessary time is available and the patient can tolerate sitting in the dental chair for complete canal debridement. If the drainage or exudate through the canals does not stop within 5 to 10 minutes, the tooth can be left open to drain until the next day.

The type, dosage, and quantity of antibiotics to use for the patient who has a swelling are described in Chapter 12. When a patient's chief complaint is swelling of dental origin, strong analgesics are usually unnecessary. Obviously this type of emergency requires close supervision by the clinician. If possible, the patient should be examined the following day so the dentist can assess the degree of improvement. In the vast majority of cases, the treatment just recommended will be sufficient to relieve the swelling. However, because more microorganisms are developing resistance to the most commonly used antibiotics, taking a culture from the exudate could be most helpful

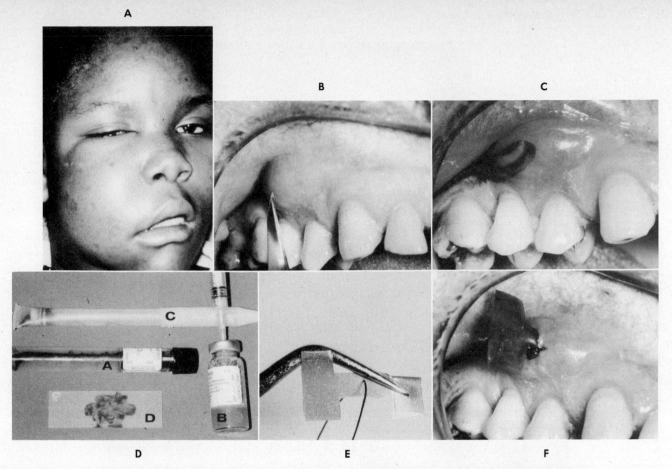

FIG. 2-7. Management of soft fluctuant swelling secondary to a phoenix abscess above a second premolar. **A,** Obvious facial distention. **B,** After confirmation of the presence of a purulent exudate by needle aspiration, incision and drainage will be established with a scalpel. **C,** Immediately after the incision is made, a purulent/hemorrhagic exudate relieves the pressure and allows the swelling to subside. **D,** Disposable supplies to aid the clinician in identifying the pathogens by antibiotic-sensitivity testing include the following: *A,* aerobic culture tube; *B,* anaerobic culture tube; *C,* transport tube containing cotton swab and transport medium; *D,* glass slide for Gram stain. **E,** Preparing a shaped rubber dam drain for suturing into the incision site. **F,** Rubber-dam drain sutured. Note that the swelling has already subsided.

when a patient does not respond to conventional antibiotic chemotherapy (e.g., penicillin or erythromycin). What often happens is that the clinician will switch from one broad-spectrum antibiotic to the next until, eventually, the patient responds and the swelling subsides. Fortunately, this empirical antibiotic roulette is usually ultimately successful; but for the unlucky, hapless patient who is hosting virulent and resistant microorganisms, this empirical use (abuse?) of antibiotics may merely postpone effective treatment. *Accordingly, whenever a purulent/hemorrhagic exudate is discovered, preparing a culture sample for antibiotic-sensitivity testing is strongly recommended.*

After initiation of endodontic treatment but before canal obturation. The main situations that predispose to this type of emergency are as follows:

1. Chronic apical periodontitis *without* a sinus tract
2. Re-treating an "old" root canal
3. Incomplete debridement of necrotic teeth
4. Inadvertently locking an irrigation needle in a canal when expressing irrigant (e.g., sodium hypochlorite)

In the first three situations the common denominator appears to be a disturbance of the dynamic equilibrium be-

tween the microorganisms, toxins, and necrotic debris within the root canal system and the chronic inflammatory cells surrounding the apex. This type of emergency is particularly unsettling to patients. After all, when the patient presented for treatment, he was essentially without symptoms. Then, following canal debridement and sealing of the access cavity, he began to experience swelling—usually within a few hours after leaving the office. Some patients may even inquire half-sarcastically, "How did you get such fast results?" The clinical management of the swelling is the same as just described. However, the dentist is cautioned to (1) check the vitality of the adjacent teeth, because there is always the possibility that by coincidence an adjacent tooth is the source of the swelling, and (2) check the periodontium, because there is also the possibility that by coincidence a lateral periodontal abscess has developed around the tooth receiving endodontic treatment. When endodontic emergencies are clinically managed in this way, the patient will often experience significant relief within a matter of minutes (Fig. 2-7).

Another type of emergency involving swelling, along with pain, may occur on rare occasions while the patient

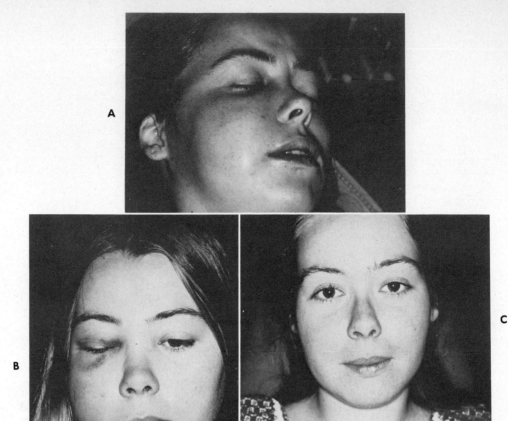

FIG. 2-8. Hypochlorite accident. **A,** Immediately following the mishap. Swelling began within minutes after the injection of 0.5 ml of 5.25% sodium hypochlorite. Within 20 minutes the edema had extended to the infraorbital region and caused further distension of the subzygomatic area. **B,** Twenty-four hours after the accident. Swelling and ecchymosis evident. **C,** One month later. Facial features have returned to normal.

is sitting in the dental chair. He may experience the following symptoms while the clinician is irrigating the root canal: (1) sudden, extreme pain (even though anesthesia has been previously induced); (2) swelling within minutes; (3) profuse, prolonged hemorrhage through the root canal. These are pathognomonic of a hypochlorite accident (Fig. 2-8). The cause is evidently locking of the irrigating needle in the root canal while the irrigant is being expressed. This causes the irrigant to be forced beyond the canal into the periapical tissues. The clinician will have no trouble making this diagnosis. The patient's reaction is so fast, so intense, and so alarming (to the patient as well as to the clinician) that it may require self-discipline on the clinician's part to avoid the first reaction, panic!

Managing this rare event requires the following:
1. Maintain self-control; don't panic!
2. Summon some type of assistance if more people are needed to keep the patient seated so you can administer regional block anesthesia to help attenuate the pain. An intramuscular injection of a sedative and an analgesic would be beneficial.
3. Allow the bleeding to continue. The body is attempting to dilute and rid itself of the toxic fluid. Continue high-volume aspiration until the bleeding begins to

subside. Depending on the amount, concentration, and temperature of the irrigant forced past the apex, this may take anywhere from 5 to 20 minutes.
4. Administer an appropriate strong antibiotic intramuscularly (preferred) or orally.
5. Refer the patient to an oral surgeon or endodontist immediately for continued management.

Of course, this type of emergency is completely avoidable if two simple rules are followed during irrigation of a root canal: (1) Do *not* lock the needle in the canal. (2) Express the irrigant *slowly*.

After canal obturation. Although several factors may precipitate this situation, the most common include filing instruments and filling materials that inoculate the periapical tissues with microorganisms or their toxins.

Because the canals have been obturated, the treatment plan is now somewhat more limited. If the canals have been filled thoroughly in three dimensions to the apical foramen, there is little to be gained by removing the canal-filling material. If the swelling is mild and localized, merely encouraging the patient to rinse frequently with warm water rinses may allow the body to resolve the swelling without need for any further treatment or systemic medications. If the swelling persists for more than a few days or gets larger or becomes soft and fluctuant, the clinician should use needle aspiration to check the nature of the exudate. Many clinicians will prescribe antibiotics at this time, especially if the swollen area seems to be increasing in size, just as a precaution. Again, preparing a culture sample of the exudate for antibiotic sensitivity testing in case rapid relief is not obtained is strongly recommended.

Treatment of this problem depends primarily on the firmness of the swelling (soft or indurated), the location of the swelling, and the quality and extension of the canal filling. Treatment based upon firmness and location of the swelling has been described. Assessment of the filling of the root canal can strongly influence treatment planning. If the canal(s) is filled well (dense in all three dimensions and extending to the apical foramen), then surgical intervention may be avoidable. If there is evidence of an inadequate root canal obturation or gross overextension of the filling material beyond the apical foramen, then nonsurgical retreatment or surgical intervention may be the only way to resolve the problem. If surgery is the only alternative, the clinician should carefully study the location of the apex vis-à-vis anatomic landmarks. If surgical access is difficult or if the mental foramen, mandibular canal, or sinuses are close to the apex, the general practitioner is advised to refer the case to an endodontist or oral surgeon rather than attempt surgery that may cause damage to anatomic structures.

As stated earlier—and it must be emphasized—be sure the adjacent teeth and the periodontium are not the source of the swelling.

Spontaneous pain

Pain as the chief complaint may occur at any time: before, during, or after completion of endodontic treatment. The diagnostic methods used to assess the various parameters of the pain were described in Chapter 1 and earlier in this chapter. The following comments regarding treatment are based on the assumption that the source of the pain has been accurately determined. The primary purpose here is to describe methods that provide simple, rapid, and effective relief of pain.

Before endodontia. If the patient presents with pain of endodontic origin as the chief complaint, the diagnosis must be symptomatic irreversible pulpitis, partial necrosis, or necrosis with periapical involvement. Considerable clinical experience, combined with research studies, indicates that approximately 90% of patients requiring emergency treatment because of pain have pain of pulpal origin.[28,35] The best assurance for relief of pain is to debride the root canal system in its entirety—regardless of the extent of pulpal inflammation or necrosis.[15] This treatment goal was described well by Natkin[37] when he stated, "As one retreats by degrees from the optimum treatment procedure, i.e., complete instrumentation, the chances of successfully eliminating pain are reduced."

Some patients may have not slept or eaten for extended periods because of their acute conditions. Exhausted and fasting, they may be difficult to manage. If they were experiencing prolonged, intense, unremitting pain prior to

entering the office, it is not uncommon for tears of relief to follow the abatement of pain by the local anesthetic. Considerable clinical challenge and positive rewards await the clinician and chairside assistant who can extend to the patient a generous amount of empathy. Professional hand contact and verbal reassurance may be of significant benefit. Offering the patient a warm liquid refreshment like hot chocolate (before starting treatment but after the anesthetic has stopped the pain) can demonstrate a caring attitude (psychologic support) as well as be a temporary source of energy (sugar).

When the diagnosis has been made, the clinician should administer profound anesthesia, adjust the tooth out of occlusion, apply a rubber dam, and remove the pulp or its remnants by thorough cleaning and shaping. Prescribing a moderate analgesic (e.g., Ibuprofen) may be helpful because some temporary pain after the treatment is likely. Prescribing a moderate analgesic when the chief complaint was pain is analgous to an insurance policy. The patient probably will not need it, but it is good to have, "just in case." Home care should include rest, frequent warm rinses for the next few days, and full meals to help the patient regain strength.

After initiation of endodontic treatment but prior to canal obturation. The most likely reason for this situation is incomplete extirpation of the pulp because of inadequate debridement or because of an "extra" canal that was overlooked. In a survey of 1000 teeth Schilder[43] reported that flare-ups after partial instrumentation were more than twice as frequent as flare-ups after complete instrumentation. When the patient comes to the office with pain immediately after the initiation of endodontic therapy, the first step is to confirm that its source is the tooth under treatment. By mere coincidence, an adjacent or opposing tooth may actually be the new source of pain. Possibly, from the quality of symptoms, it may only *appear* to the patient that the pain is originating from the tooth currently under treatment. When it has been verified that the source of pain is the tooth under treatment, local anesthetic should be administered to stop the pain.

After placing a rubber dam, remove the temporary dressing. Examine each canal with a fine paper point to determine whether there is any exudate. Also reexamine the radiographs and check the pulp chamber, looking carefully for "extra" canals. A serous or hemorrhagic exudate may be the result of residual pulp tissue or extension of instruments beyond the apical foramen. If the canal is exuding a serous/hemorrhagic fluid, repeat the steps for thorough cleaning and shaping (Chapter 7). After thorough debridement dry the canal with paper points. If the pain was due to pulp remnants, the canal should be easy to dry. If the source of the pain is of periapical origin, the exudate may continue regardless of how often cleaning and shaping steps are repeated. Calcium hydroxide paste, forced into the canal(s) with narrow pluggers and files, can act as an intracanal medication that can stop this exudation.

After removing the dressing, the clinician may find that the canals are dry. Seltzer and Naidorf suggest that if the original diagnosis was irreversible pulpitis and the canals appear dry upon reentry, and if there are no specific contraindications, a single application of a topical corticosteroid may quickly relieve the pain without any side effects.[47] For example, pumping Metimyd Ophthalmic Solution or Neo-Cortef Eye-Ear Drops (hydrocortisone plus neomycin) into and beyond the canal with a small sterile file or paper point may provide symptomatic relief within a matter of minutes. With careful case selection there is strong clinical evidence to demonstrate the validity of this treatment modality. Some investigators believe steroids serve no useful purpose. It is advised that one thoroughly acquaint oneself with the literature on this subject.

After canal obturation. Extending filing instruments beyond the apical foramen (''overinstrumentation'') and forcing sealer or solid cone filling materials beyond the apex are the primary reasons for pain after canal obturation. However, the dentist should always have a high ''index of suspicion'' regarding the possibility that either another tooth or a nondental condition may be the source of the pain. If the canals are filled well and there is no evident material impinging on the periapical tissue, then antiinflammatory analgesics will often suffice to control the pain until it subsides. If the canal obturation appears to be underextended by more than 1 mm from the radiographic apex or the canal appears to be otherwise underfilled (an incomplete apical seal), it would be advisable to refill the canals.

If the canals are filled well but the filling material is extended beyond the apex, the patient should be informed. If the patient knows that there will probably be some postobturation pain, this may help to minimize anxiety. Usually only mild analgesics are required to control the temporary pain that often follows canal obturation. If there is slight overextension of the filling material (i.e., less than 1 mm), more than likely the body will be able to accommodate to it after several days of mild pain. However, if a significant amount of filling material is impinging on the periapical tissues and the pain persists more than a few days, then apical surgery will probably be necessary to eliminate the chronic inflammation.

In all cases of postobturation pain the occlusion should be checked. It is not uncommon for mild periapical inflammation to force the tooth into hyperocclusion. Of course, any necessary occlusal adjustment should be made immediately.

Occasionally, moderate to strong analgesics will be required to ease the pain. Because of the unfortunate increase in the number of people who have become drug abusers, narcotic prescriptions should be closely monitored by the dentist. Such prescriptions are seldom required for more than 3 or 4 days. Refilling narcotic prescriptions to manage postobturation pain is like stopping a clock to save time. The dentist should be wary of the patient asking for strong narcotics or requesting refills.

The use of systemic steroid-antibiotic combinations to relieve postobturation pain has been recommended by Grossman[23] and Marshall and Walton[33] in the absence of specific contraindications. Because of its controversial nature, readers are urged to acquaint themselves thoroughly

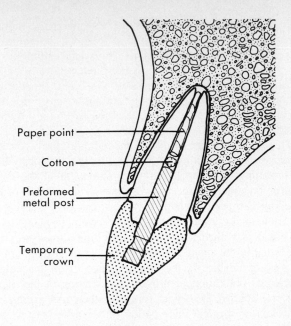

FIG. 2-9. Provisional management of a coronal fracture that occurred prior to root canal obturation.

with the literature on this subject prior to prescribing steroid-antibiotics systemically.

In summary, postobturation pain necessitates a critical assessment of the quality and extension of the canal filling before a determination of the treatment plan. If the canal is filled properly, analgesics or radicular surgery are the only remaining alternatives to extraction.

Esthetic emergency

An esthetic problem occurs when a portion of the crown, or the entire crown, fractures off the remaining tooth that is undergoing or has undergone endodontic treatment. This problem becomes an emergency when it involves an anterior tooth. Even though there may be no symptoms, the situation is quite distressing, especially with impending social and business engagements.

If only a portion of a tooth has fractured off, simply placing a temporary plastic crown with a temporary cement (e.g., Temp-Bond) should correct the problem.

If the entire crown has fractured off, the type of treatment depends on whether the canal has been filled.

1. *Canal not yet filled.* Ideally (if office time permits) the root canal should be completed, as long as the criteria for obturation are met (Chapter 8). A temporary plastic crown should then be cemented upon a preformed metal post that is cemented into a dowel preparation (Fig. 2-9).
2. *Canal previously filled.* If the entire crown has fractured off, a simple dowel preparation made with a Peeso bur can retain a preformed stainless steel post (e.g., Unitek or Parkell). These preformed posts are excellent for supporting temporary plastic crowns or the permanent porcelain-fused-to-metal crowns. Another alternative in this situation is to take a snap impression and have a laboratory prepare a tempo-

rary acrylic ''flipper'' to replace the fractured crown.

3. *Canal not filled, and patient just ''squeezed in.''* For this situation the following procedure is recommended:

   a. Place a fine paper point into the canal; cut off the blunt end so the point occupies only the apical half of the canal.

   b. Place a few wisps of cotton fibers into the canal on top of the paper point.

   c. Temporarily cement an appropriate preformed stainless steel post of suitable length and diameter into the canal.

   d. Cement a temporary plastic crown on the head of the post (Fig. 2-9).

   e. Instruct the patient to refrain from chewing with this tooth until permanent endodontic and restorative treatment has been completed.

• • •

The accurate diagnosis and effective treatment of acute situations are an important responsibility and privilege of dental practice. Effective, caring management of endodontic emergencies not only represents a service to the public, which a dentist and his or her staff can be proud of, but also enhances the positive image of dentistry.

REFERENCES

1. Alling, C.C., editor: Facial pain, Philadelphia, 1977, Lea & Febiger.
2. Andrews, C.H., England, M.C., and Kemp, W.B.: Sickle cell anemia: an etiological factor in pulp necrosis, J. Endod. **9:**249, 1983.
3. Auvenshine, R.C.: Etiology, diagnosis and treatment of temporomandibular joint derangements, J. Calif. Dent. Assoc. **13:**64, 1985.
4. Becker, G.L., Cohen, S., and Borer, R.: The sequence of accidentally injecting sodium hypochlorite beyond the root apex: report of a case, Oral Surg. **38:**633, 1974.
5. Bell, W.E.: Orofacial pains, ed. 3, Chicago, 1985, Year Book Medical Publishers, Inc.
6. Bellizzi, R., et al.: Sinusitis secondary to pregnancy rhinitis, mimicking pain of endodontic origin: a case report, J. Endod. **9:**60, 1983.
7. Bender, I.B., and Naidorf, I.J.: Dental observations in Vitamin D–resistant rickets with special reference to periapical lesions, J. Endod. **11:**514, 1985.
8. Berkow, R., editor: The Merck manual of diagnosis and therapy, ed. 14, Rahway, N.J., 1982, Merck Sharpe & Dohme Research Laboratories.
9. Burkes, E.J., Jr.: Adenoid cystic carcinoma masquerading as periapical inflammation, J. Endod. **1:**76, 1975.
10. Case, J.: The best way to handle after-hours emergencies, Dent. Manage. **25:**26, 1985.
11. Cohen, S., et al.: Oral prodromal signs of a central nervous system malignant neoplasm, J. Am. Dent. Assoc. **112:**643, 1986.
12. Cooley, R.L., and Robinson, S.F.: Variables associated with electric pulp testing, Oral Surg. **50:**66, 1980.
13. Copeland, R.R.: Carcinoma of the antrum mimicking periapical pathology of pulpal origin: a case report, J. Endod. **6:**655, 1980.
14. Dalessio, D.J., editor: Wolff's headache and other head pain, ed. 4, New York, 1980, Oxford University Press, Inc.
15. Dorn, S.O., et al.: Treatment of the endodontic emergency: a report based on a questionaire, part I, J. Endod. **3:**94, 1977.
16. Eversole, L.R.: Clinical outline of oral pathology: diagnosis and treatment, ed. 2, Philadelphia, 1984, Lea & Febiger.
17. Farb, S.N.: Otorhinolaryngology, ed. 2, New York, 1980, Medical Examination Publishing Company, Inc.
18. Fromm, G.H., Terrence, C.F., and Maroon, J.C.: Trigeminal neuralgia: current concepts regarding etiology and pathogenesis, Arch. Neurol. **41:**1204, 1984.
19. Gargiulo, A.V.: Endodontic-periodontic interrelationships: diagnosis and treatment, Dent. Clin. North Am. **28:**767, 1984.
20. Gayford, J.J., and Haskell, R.: Clinical oral medicine, ed. 2, Bristol, 1979, John Wright & Sons, Ltd.
21. Goldman, H.M., and Cohen, D.W.: Periodontal therapy, ed. 6, St. Louis, 1980, The C.V. Mosby Co.
22. Gregory, W.B., Brooks, L.E., and Penick, E.C.: Herpes zoster associated with pulpless teeth, J. Endod. **1:**32, 1975.
23. Grossman, L.I.: Endodontic practice. ed. 10, Philadelphia, 1981, Lea & Febiger.
24. Guldener, P.N.A.: The relationship between periodontal and pulpal disease, Int. Endod. J. **18:**41, 1985.
25. Gutmann, J.L., and Tillman, J.L.: Rhabdomyosarcoma: report of a case, J. Endod. **2:**250, 1976.
26. Hermann, J.W., and Heicht, R.C.: Complications in therapeutic use of sodium hypochlorite, J. Endod. **5:**160, 1979.
27. Hought, R.T., et al.: Ludwig's angina: report of two cases and review of the literature from 1945 to January 1979, J. Oral Surg. **38:**849, 1980.
28. Husler, J.F., and Mitchell, D.F.: Analysis of 1628 cases of odontolgia: a corroborative study, J. Indianapolis Dist. Dent. Soc. **17:**23, 1963.
29. Isselbacher, K.J., et al., editors: Harrison's principles of internal medicine, ed. 9, New York, 1980, McGraw-Hill Book Co.
30. Kaufman, A.Y.: Facial emphysema caused by hydrogen peroxide irrigation: report of a case, J. Endod. **7:**470, 1981.
31. Kerr, D.A., Ash, M.M., and Millard, H.D.: Oral diagnosis, ed. 6, St. Louis, 1983, The C.V. Mosby Co.
32. Manson-Hing, L.R.: Panoramic dental radiography, Springfield, Ill., 1976, Charles C Thomas, Publisher.
33. Marshall, J.G., and Walton, R.E.: The effect of intramuscular injection of steroid on posttreatment endodontic pain, J. Endod. **10:**584, 1984.
34. McGrath, P.A.: Pain control in dentistry: psychologic factors that modify the perception of pain, Comp. Contin. Educ. **8:**574, 1985.
35. Mitchell, D.F., and Tarplee, R.E.: Painful pulpitis: a clinical and microscopic study, Oral Surg. **13:**1360, 1960.
36. Mumford, J.M.: Toothache and related pain, Edinburgh, 1973, Churchill Livingstone.
37. Natkin, E.: Treatment of endodontic emergencies, Dent. Clin. North Am. **18:**243, 1974.
38. Pitts, D.L., and Natkin, E.: Diagnosis and treatment of vertical root fractures, J. Endod. **9:**338, 1983.
39. Ratner, E.J., et al.: Jawbone cavities and trigeminal and atypical facial neuralgias, Oral Surg. **48:**3, 1979.
40. Roberts, A.M., and Person, P.: Etiology and treatment of idiopathic trigeminal and atypical facial neuralgias, Oral Surg. **48:**298, 1979.
41. Robinson, P.J., and Vitek, R.M.: Periodontal examination, Dent. Clin. North Am. **24:**597, 1980.
42. Rossman, L.E., Rossman, S.R., and Garber, D.A.: The endodontic-periodontic fistula, Oral Surg. **53:**78, 1982.
43. Schilder, H.: Cleaning and shaping the root canal, Dent. Clin. North Am. **18:**269, 1974.
44. Selden, H.S.: The endo-antral syndrome, J. Endod. **3:**462, 1977.
45. Seltzer, S.: Pain control in dentistry, Philadelphia, 1978, J.B. Lippincott Co.
46. Seltzer, S., and Bender, I.B.: The dental pulp, ed. 3, Philadelphia, 1984, J.B. Lippincott Co.
47. Seltzer, S., and Naidorf, I.J.: Flare-ups in endodontics. II. Therapeutic measures, J. Endod. **11:**559, 1985.
48. Stafne, E.C.: Oral roentgenographic diagnosis, ed. 3, Philadelphia, 1969, W.B. Saunders Co.
49. Topazian, R.G., and Goldberg, M.H.: Management of infections of the oral and maxillofacial regions, Philadelphia, 1981, W.B. Saunders Co.

50. Usdin, G., and Lewis, J.M.: Psychiatry in general medical practice, New York, 1979, McGraw-Hill Book Co.
51. Wood, N.K., and Goaz, P.W.: Differential diagnosis of oral lesions, ed. 3, St. Louis, 1985, The C.V. Mosby Co.
52. Wuehrmann, A.H., and Manson-Hing, L.R.: Dental radiology, ed. 5, St. Louis, 1981, The C.V. Mosby Co.
53. X-rays in dentistry, Rochester, N.Y., 1977, Eastman Kodak Co.

Self-assessment questions

1. The most significant factor in dictating the extent and mode of treatment in an endodontic emergency is
   a. Intensity of the pain
   b. Response to thermal stimulation
   c. Duration of discomfort
   d. Localized swelling

2. A mandibular left first molar may cause pain that is perceived at a different unilateral site when the pulp-related status is
   a. Chronic apical periodontitis
   b. Phoenix abscess
   c. Reversible pulpitis
   d. Irreversible pulpitis

3. As a general rule, orofacial swellings of endodontic etiology
   a. Require biopsy for definitive treatment planning
   b. Exhibit deep infrabony defects upon probing
   c. Result from bacterial or necrotic pulpal irritants
   d. Require incision and drainage for relief

4. One of the following is not a manifestation of maxillary sinus disease:
   a. Tenderness to palpation of the maxillary molar-premolar region
   b. Radiating pain to the ear
   c. Symptoms accentuated upon bending forward
   d. Pain to percussion of the maxillary molars

5. The attending dentist is encouraged to obtain his or her own diagnostic radiographs because previous radiographs
   a. May not accurately reflect the present condition
   b. Have no value to the subsequent clinician
   c. Will not show the degree of periapical pathology
   d. Will reveal separation of an endodontic instrument

6. The characteristic symptom of trigeminal neuralgia that must be considered in the differential diagnosis of a dental disorder is
   a. Pain to cold stimulation
   b. Sharp radiating pain
   c. A trigger zone
   d. Pain to heat stimulation

7. Which of the following constitutes emergency treatment for thermal pain resulting from a reversible pulpitis following a recent restoration?
   a. Replace the restoration with a sedative dressing
   b. Re-restore the tooth permanently using a larger insulating base
   c. Prescribe an analgesic and assure the patient that the symptoms will subside
   d. Remove the tooth from functional occlusion

8. The most predictable treatment for a tooth with irreversible pulpitis is
   a. Excavation of caries and placement of a sedative dressing
   b. Complete pulp extirpation and thorough debridement of the root canal system
   c. A deep pulpotomy with dry cotton pellets over the canal orifices
   d. Occlusal reduction of involved tooth to prevent coronal fractures

9. Percussion pain before endodontic treatment is an indication of
   a. Reversible pulpitis
   b. Irreversible pulpitis
   c. Pulp necrosis
   d. Inflammation of the periodontal ligament

10. A common cause of tenderness upon mastication with a recently instrumented tooth is
    a. Instrumentation within the canal
    b. Instrumentation through the apical foramen
    c. An undetected vertical crown fracture
    d. Overirrigation with 5.25% sodium hypochlorite

11. A nonvital tooth with a firm swelling of the overlying buccal mucosa requires
    a. An incision and drainage immediately
    b. An excision biopsy for emergency treatment
    c. Access and canal instrumentation
    d. Probing of the gingival sulcus for a sinus tract

12. Emergency endodontic treatment of a symptomatic nonvital pulp with periapical extension is
    a. Opening the tooth and allowing drainage until symptoms subside
    b. Occlusal adjustment, prescribing of analgesics and antibiotics
    c. Coronal pulpotomy and temporary restoration
    d. Extirpation of pulp remnants, cleaning and shaping of the canals, and closing of the access cavity

13. Recommended treatment for a tooth with persistent exudate after thorough cleaning and shaping is
    a. Closing with a saturated formocresol cotton dressing
    b. Removing the temporary dressing and leaving open until symptoms subside
    c. Closing and prescribing an antibiotic medication
    d. Closing and prescribing an antiinflammatory agent

14. A nonvital tooth with an acute apical access may be left open until the next day if
    a. Drainage through the canals does not stop within 10 minutes
    b. The exudate is purulent or hemorrhagic
    c. An incision with drainage has been accomplished
    d. The clinician does not prescribe antibiotics

3

CASE SELECTION AND TREATMENT PLANNING

EDWARD M. OSETEK

In clinical practice, diagnosis, case selection, and treatment planning involve simultaneous thought processes that begin with the clinicians first contact with the patient, be it a telephone conversation, routine examination, emergency treatment, or other encounter.

Diagnosis, case selection, and treatment planning, as a process, is designed to provide answers to a myriad of questions: What is this entity that we are dealing with? Does it represent healthy tissue? Does it represent inflamed or diseased tissue? If it represents inflamed or diseased tissue, is the condition reversible? Or is it irreversible? Can the condition be corrected? What treatment is needed to correct the condition? What alternative treatment plans might be taken? These questions help us focus on the purpose of this chapter: case selection and treatment planning.

CASE SELECTION

Case selection in endodontics is the procedure whereby the clinician arrives at a decision with the patient's consent regarding the appropriate treatment for the patient's condition. It is the act of choosing appropriate treatment on the basis of analysis of the signs and symptoms; this could span the extremes from observation to extraction. Case selection simply requires the best answer to each of two fundamental questions: (1) Can endodontic therapy be done? (2) Should endodontic therapy be done?

Can endodontic therapy be done?
Limitations of the clinician

The first of these questions is directed to the clinician and relates to his experience and expertise. In addressing this question, the clinician must ask, "What are my limitations in providing endodontic treatment?" The answer to this question is influenced by such factors as the extent of training received, the level of experience of the clinician, and the degree of interest the clinician has in providing endodontic services. A clinician who completes an ad-

vanced training program in endodontics has far fewer limitations than a recent graduate who occasionally will treat an uncomplicated endodontically involved tooth.

Amenability of the tooth to treatment

The issue of the limitations of the clinician, however, does not stand alone; it is affected by a second, modifying issue—the amenability of the tooth to treatment.

Anatomic considerations. Teeth with extremely curved or dilacerated roots (Fig. 3-1) obviously present a challenge to any clinician. These cases may be selected for treatment by a highly experienced and skilled dentist, while others with less expertise with such cases should consider referring the patient to an endodontist.

Pathologic conditions. This same reasoning holds true for teeth with extremely calcified canals (Fig. 3-2) as well as for teeth that exhibit internal or external resorption (Figs. 3-3 and 3-4) and for teeth that have sustained horizontal root fractures (Fig. 3-5).

Re-treatments. Some cases require re-treatment because the initial root canal therapy was unsuccessful. Failure of initial treatment may be due to incomplete cleaning or shaping as a result of canal blockage, ledging, or instrument separation (Figs. 3-6 and 3-7). In other cases the initial treatment may fail because of the clinician's inability to adequately seal the apex during initial obturation (e.g., because of incomplete root end formation or because the apex was transported during instrumentation) (Figs. 3-8 and 3-9).

Isolation, access, and availability. The amenability of the tooth to treatment is also determined by such factors as isolation, access, and availability. Can the tooth be isolated with a rubber dam (Fig. 3-10)? If not, endodontic therapy should not be attempted until isolation is made possible by some corrective action such as crown lengthening, forced eruption, or amalgam or composite buildup. Is the tooth accessible? This issue also must be considered, along with the clinician's level of experience and exper-

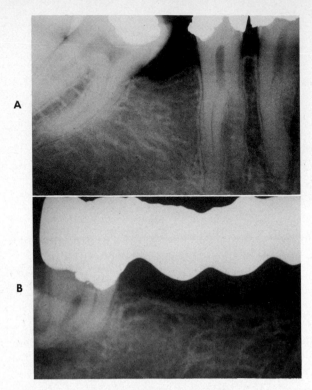

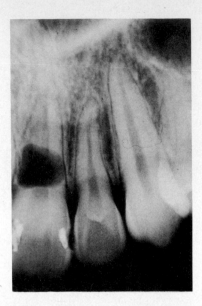

FIG. 3-1. A, Mandibular first premolar exhibiting extremely complicated anatomy. **B,** Mandibular second molar with severely curved roots. Both situations present clinical challenges requiring superior endodontic skills.

FIG. 3-3. Maxillary central incisor exhibiting extensive internal resorption that has perforated to the periodontium.

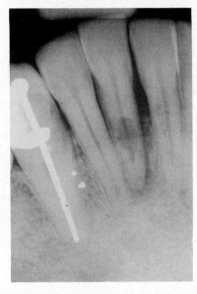

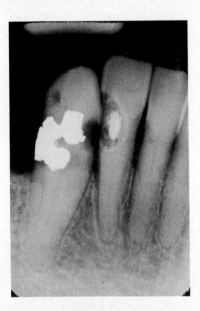

FIG. 3-2. Mandibular lateral incisor with radiographic evidence of canal narrowing by dystrophic calcification.

FIG. 3-4. Mandibular central incisor with radiographic evidence of external resorption 2 years after a traumatic injury.

tise. Occasionally, a clinician will determine, by viewing a radiograph, that a tooth presents no technical difficulties in terms of performing an endodontic service, only to discover on clinical examination that the patient exhibits extremely limited opening. Sometimes this limitation is temporary, such as in trismus, and the patient can be maintained by treatment such as pulpotomy or chemother-

apy. In other cases this limitation of opening is permanent because of microstomia, radiation therapy, radical surgery, an accident, temporomandibular joint ankylosis, or some other condition. These latter cases pose a significant challenge to the clinician's expertise. Sometimes they are best referred to an endodontist, and sometimes they are not amenable to nonsurgical root canal therapy. Alternative treatment such as replantation is a compromise but may be the best service that can be offered to the patient.

Is the patient available for treatment? Is the patient cooperative? These are two often-overlooked considerations in regard to answering the question "Can endodontic therapy be done?" Too frequently a case meets all the criteria

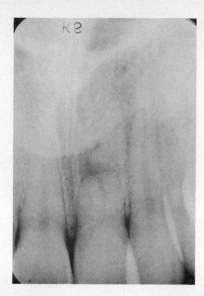

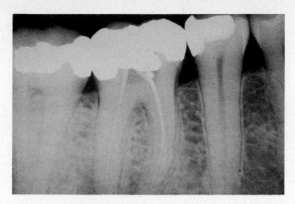

FIG. 3-7. Mandibular first molar exhibiting a separated instrument in the mesiobuccal canal, resulting in incomplete debridement.

FIG. 3-5. Horizontal root fracture of maxillary central incisor also exhibiting canal obliteration by dystrophic calcification.

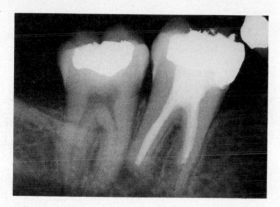

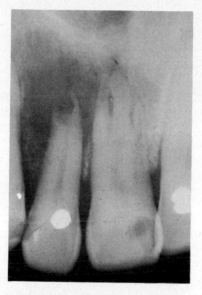

FIG. 3-6. Failure of endodontically treated mandibular first molar because of incomplete debridement of the root canal spaces in the mesial canals.

FIG. 3-8. Maxillary lateral incisor with extensive apical resorption, making an apical seal difficult to achieve.

for selection for endodontic therapy but the patient has severe scheduling conflicts that he cannot or will not resolve. The patient must be informed of the time commitment for treatment before treatment is started. Here again the clinician's limitations have an influence. A highly experienced specialist may be able to treat the case much more quickly than a less experienced clinician.

Patient cooperation, availability and financial commitment to treatment cannot be overstressed. Many problems in patient management can be avoided when the patient has a clear understanding of his responsibilities in the treatment procedure.

Once all factors have been considered and it has been determined that root canal treatment can be done, the next fundamental question must be addressed.

Should endodontic therapy be done?

Even when endodontics is technically possible, treatment might be contraindicated in some cases. The considerations are as follows.

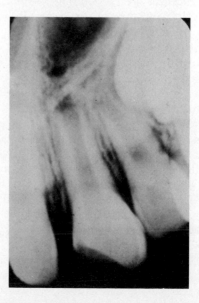

FIG. 3-9. Maxillary central incisor with an incompletely formed root, also making an apical seal difficult to achieve.

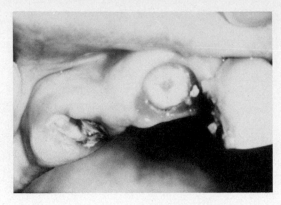

FIG. 3-10. Maxillary central incisor and canine that had served as abutments for a fixed partial denture. Fracture of these teeth below the level of the gingiva requires special procedures in order to gain rubber dam isolation for root canal treatment.

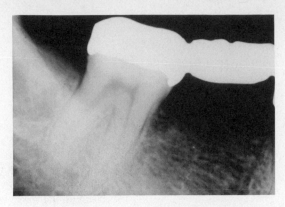

FIG. 3-11. A mandibular second molar serving as an abutment for a fixed partial denture. Loss of this tooth would require prosthetic escalation to a tissue-borne removable partial denture.

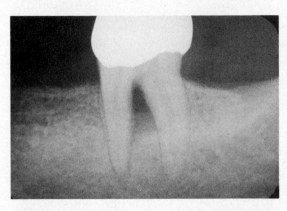

FIG. 3-12. A mandibular second molar serving as an abutment for a tooth-borne removable partial denture. Loss of this tooth would result in escalation to a tissue-borne removable partial denture.

Strategic value of the tooth

How important is it to save any given tooth? Obviously, not every tooth has the same strategic value, and in some cases, such as poorly positioned teeth, or teeth that have significantly shifted, drifted, or supererupted, the most desirable results may in fact be achieved by extraction. Just what determines the strategic value of a tooth?

Dental arch integrity. Any tooth in the dental arch that, if lost, would result in the loss of arch integrity represents the highest degree of strategic value. If a patient's dentition is intact and one tooth in the arch exhibits irreversible pulpal involvement, every effort should be made to preserve that tooth. If, for example, a first molar is extracted from an intact arch, that tooth must then be replaced with a fixed bridge, usually with adjacent teeth being used as abutments. This situation not only places the abutments at risk but burdens the patient with an oral hygiene maintenance problem. If the tooth is not replaced, severe consequences such as shifting, drifting, supereruption, and periodontal disease can occur. In addition, the masticatory function becomes compromised.

Prosthetic escalation. Patients may present with a masticatory apparatus that has already been compromised by tooth loss and consequent loss of arch integrity. What effect do these conditions have on determining the strategic value of a tooth?

If a tooth is serving as an abutment for a fixed partial denture, and its loss would necessitate escalation to a longer-span fixed partial denture or a removable partial denture, it assumes considerable strategic value. In this instance endodontic therapy should certainly be done if possible. If the tooth is the terminal tooth in the arch and serves as an abutment for a fixed or removable partial denture, it assumes even greater strategic value, since its loss would cause prosthetic escalation to a tissue-borne, free-end removable partial denture (Fig. 3-11).

Similarly, if a tooth is serving as an abutment for a removable partial denture and its loss would lead to a more extensive removable partial denture, or possibly a full denture, the tooth is of great strategic value (Figs. 3-12 and 3-13).

Esthetics. Esthetic considerations are important in regard to the issue of whether a tooth should be selected for endodontic treatment. An example is a case in which the patient presents with a diastema (Fig. 3-14). If a tooth adjacent to the diastema is lost, the practitioner is faced with a restorative dilemma. Replacing the tooth with a fixed partial denture will require the use of an oversize crown abutment and oversize pontic, which eliminates the diastema but severely compromises the esthetics of the case. Alternative replacement with a hybrid fixed partial denture or a removable partial denture in order to maintain the diastema and preserve the natural esthetics is also a compromise. It would be far better to retain the tooth by providing endodontic services.

Local clinical considerations

Local factors to be weighed in case selection for root canal treatment include restorative, prosthetic, and periodontal considerations.

Restorative considerations. *Is the tooth restorable?* A determination regarding a tooth's restorability *must* be made *prior to* selection for root canal treatment.

Another restorative consideration relative to selection of a tooth for endodontic treatment concerns "interceptive" or "prophylactic" endodontics. Patients in need of exten-

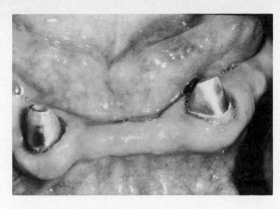

FIG. 3-13. Two mandibular canines serving as the only abutments for a removable partial denture. Loss of these teeth would result in a full denture.

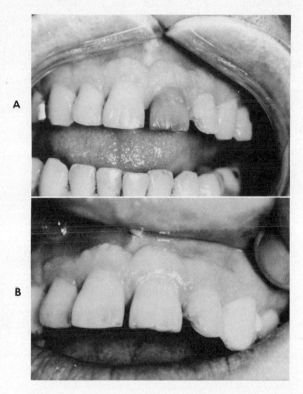

FIG. 3-14. A, A discolored maxillary central incisor. Because of the diastema, loss of this tooth would create an extremely challenging restorative situation. **B,** Root canal treatment followed by bleaching offers a better result.

sive restorative dentistry often have had some degree of pulpal injury; additional restorative procedures add to the injury to the pulp.[1,14] This "stressed pulp condition" must be considered.[1] A judgment must be made concerning the ability of a "stressed pulp" to respond to further restorative insult. If it is determined that the pulp has a significantly reduced capacity to respond favorably to the myriad restorative procedures that can be potentially damaging to the pulp (e.g., dentin cutting, drying, dentin "sterilization," impressions [see Chapter 14 for further explanation]), prophylactic or interceptive endodontic therapy may be indicated. It certainly must be considered in regard to the risk-benefit ratio. The question of whether to use pro-

phylactic endodontic treatment is perplexing because it requires prognostication based on the limited and often circumstantial evidence available. Sometimes the prognostication is an "educated guess" based upon the experience and common sense of the clinician.

No ethical dentist wishes to recommend unnecessary treatment. However, it is upsetting to both the patient and the practitioner (and no small embarrassment as well) when a tooth recently restored with a beautiful and costly porcelain/metal veneer crown exhibits irreversible pulp damage necessitating root canal treatment. Certainly endodontic treatment is significantly *less complicated* to perform prior to restoration than after the tooth has been restored with pins and amalgam/composite cores and crowns.

No matter how careful the clinician is in case selection, sometimes decisions will be made that ultimately prove to be wrong. If endodontic therapy is not performed, some cases will later require root canal treatment. Because this problem is so perplexing, it is important that the patient play a major role in the decision of whether endodontic treatment should be provided prior to placement of a permanent restoration. In order for the patient to be able to intelligently enter the decision process, all factors necessary to informed consent must be carefully explained by the clinician and clearly understood by the patient.

Prosthetic considerations. Other variables must be considered in case selection when the tooth in question is intended to serve as an abutment for a prosthesis. Extensive clinical research has demonstrated that the success rate for an endodontically treated tooth restored with a single crown is significantly greater than for an endodontically treated tooth that is required to serve as an abutment for a fixed or removable partial denture.[26] Thus it is important to exercise good judgment during case selection of teeth intended to serve as abutments. A critical consideration in these cases is the adequacy of the remaining tooth structure to provide support and retention for the restoration; if it is inadequate, the clinician must consider whether adequate support and retention can be provided by a post and/or core.

The most significant factor in providing good post retention is the length of the post; therefore, there must be sufficient root length to retain a post while at the same time ensuring that the apical seal is not compromised. Insufficient post space may contribute to the failure of the restoration, and an inadequate apical seal may lead to endodontic failure. Research has shown that a minimum of 4 mm of root canal filling ensures an apical seal and that the best seal[29] will be consistently achieved if 7 mm of root canal filling remains.[17] In certain clinical situations a compromise between post length and apical seal might be necessary; however, when such a compromise is made the success of the entire case is also compromised.

On occasion a tooth that has an intact and healthy pulp but that has insufficient remaining structure for an adequate restoration (Fig. 3-15) will become a candidate for a root canal treatment simply *because* post space is needed to provide retention.

The same considerations relative to the "stressed pulp"

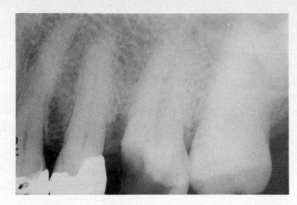

FIG. 3-15. A vital asymptomatic maxillary second molar that requires root canal therapy to facilitate restoration with a post and core with a full crown.

condition and prophylactic endodontics must be taken into account for teeth that will undergo prosthetic reconstruction.

Periodontal considerations. As with local restorative and prosthetic considerations, periodontal considerations also enter into the case selection process. Teeth with questionable periodontal conditions should be assessed in terms of their periodontal prognosis *before* they are selected for endodontic treatment. If the clinician is unable to make this determination, he or she should refer the patient to a specialist for further consultation.

As described in Chapter 17, periodontal disease and/or periodontal treatment have an effect on the pulp; these, too, contribute to the "stressed pulp" condition.

Root canal therapy is often an adjunct procedure to periodontal therapy, most notably when a root resection or hemisection is indicated as part of the periodontal treatment. The sequence of the treatment in these cases is of great importance and will be discussed later, in the treatment planning section.

Systemic considerations

A number of systemic conditions were once thought to be contraindications to root canal treatment. Advances in the art and science of endodontics have virtually eliminated systemic conditions as contraindications to root canal treatment. Indeed, the only systemic conditions that contraindicate any elective dental procedure, endodontics included, are recent (within 6 months) myocardial infarction and uncontrolled disease processes (e.g., hypertension, diabetes, tuberculosis, or syphilis).

Whereas systemic conditions once contraindicated root canal treatment, many conditions today are strong indications for endodontic treatment rather than extraction.

Bacteremia and infection. It has been clearly demonstrated that endodontic treatment poses a significantly lower threat of bacteremia than does extraction.[4,5] Consequently root canal treatment is the *treatment of choice* for patients who are placed at risk by transient bacteremias. This category includes patients who have or are undergoing any of the following:[7,12,15,16]

1. History of rheumatic heart disease
2. Prosthetic heart valve

3. Prosthetic joint replacement
4. Prosthetic repair of a congenital heart defect
5. Certain congenital heart diseases
6. Exteriorized transverse cardiac pacemaker
7. Kidney transplant
8. Immunosuppressive therapy
9. Cancer chemotherapy and severely neutrapenic
10. Surgically constructed systemic-pulmonary shunt
11. Idiopathic hypertrophic subaortic stenosis (IHSS)
12. History of bacterial endocarditis
13. Mitral valve prolapse
14. Poorly controlled or brittle diabetes
15. Systemic corticosteroid therapy.

Similarly, certain systemic conditions dictate that every effort to avoid extraction be made because of predictable adverse sequelae following extraction. If a patient has undergone radiation therapy to the head and neck area, extraction could result in osteoradionecrosis; root canal treatment greatly minimizes this risk. Patients with bleeding diatheses are placed at risk during surgical procedures. Again, root canal treatment eliminates many of the risks that would be posed by extraction in these cases.

Cardiovascular disease. The principal contraindications to elective endodontic procedures for patients with cardiovascular disease are recent myocardial infarction (within 6 months) and uncontrolled hypertension. When a clinician is treating patients with a history of cardiovascular disease, it is imperative that a stress reduction protocol, such as the following adaptation of the protocol recommended by Malamed[16] be instituted:

1. Recognition of the medical risk
2. Medical consultation prior to treatment
3. Morning appointments
4. Monitoring of vital signs preoperatively and postoperatively
5. Psychosedation during therapy
6. Short appointments
7. Pain and anxiety control during and following treatment.

This stress reduction protocol should also be employed for all significantly medically compromised patients.

Diabetes mellitus. A diabetic, even if the disease is well controlled, is a medically compromised patient, and the stress reduction protocol must be followed. If the condition is being controlled with insulin, the dentist must ascertain that the patient has received his insulin and has had a recent meal prior to treatment. The patient should be instructed to alert the dentist if during the appointment he experiences any symptoms of hypoglycemia. A source of sugar such as Glucola or orange juice should be readily available in the dental office to quickly reverse these symptoms.

Diabetics, because of their compromised microvasculature, are susceptible to infections; therefore, the clinician should prescribe broad-spectrum antibiotics in the presence of active infections, such as an acute apical abscess. All diabetics have an altered metabolism, which will slow the rate of healing following root canal treatment.

Adrenal insufficiency and corticosteroid therapy. The condition of a patient with adrenal insufficiency who is receiving corticosteroid therapy may be well controlled, but he is susceptible to adrenal crisis when stressed. Therefore, the stress reduction protocol must be followed. Root canal therapy is not contraindicated in such a patient, but the clinician must be aware that in addition to the risk associated with stress the patient may be susceptible to infections; consultation with the patient's physician is important.

Malamed[16] suggests that the "rule of twos" be applied to determine if a patient is at risk because of adrenal insufficiency: adrenocortical suppression should be suspected if the patient has received glucocorticosteroid therapy in a dose of 20 mg of cortisone (or its equivalent) daily for a continuous period of 2 weeks or longer within the last 2 years. In such an instance consultation with the patient's physician is imperative to determine if supplemental steroid therapy is indicated.

Bleeding diatheses. Patients who have bleeding disorders should receive no dental treatment without prior consultation with the patient's physician; this will minimize the risk to the patient. Treatment planning includes avoiding dental surgical procedures, if possible. Endodontic treatment is preferred in favor of extraction in virtually every instance, unless medical treatment to correct the bleeding disorder is instituted. In addition to clearly identified hemophilia, there are a number of clinical situations that should alert the clinician to suspect a bleeding disorder, including the following[15]:

1. Long-term, high-dose aspirin therapy
2. Coumarin therapy
3. Liver disease
4. History of alcohol abuse
5. Leukemia
6. Long-term antibiotic therapy or other conditions that interfere with vitamin K absorption
7. Renal dialysis
8. Autoimmune deficiency

Radiation therapy. Extraction of teeth in patients who have received radiation therapy to the head and neck region must be avoided if at all possible. The risk of osteoradionecrosis[28] following extraction is high; therefore endodontic therapy is strongly recommended.

Pregnancy. There is no contraindication to endodontic treatment during pregnancy. However, it is prudent to avoid elective treatment during the first and third trimesters when possible. The fetus is at greatest risk during the first trimester; treatment rendered at this time should be limited to emergency care only. It is advised that the patient's physician be consulted prior to the administration of any drug likely to cross the placental barrier. The patient is likely to experience the greatest discomfort during the third trimester. When the patient is placed in the supine position in the dental chair, the enlarged uterus presses against her diaphragm, which increases her postural discomfort.

TREATMENT PLANNING

Too often, endodontic therapy is the first dental treatment rendered, regardless of the need for comprehensive care, because many patients present in pain requiring immediate attention. The clinician must train himself to focus on comprehensive patient care and to put the endodontic treatment in its proper perspective, when possible. In clinical practice, when a patient presents with pulpal pain it is best to provide that patient with emergency treatment only, to relieve the patient's discomfort. Once that is accomplished, a thorough treatment plan should be developed. The proper sequencing of treatment will lead to successful management of the case, whereas improper sequencing can lead to failure, embarrassment, and patient dissatisfaction.

In the normal course of developing a comprehensive treatment plan following a thorough examination and diagnosis (and emergency care if necessary), treatment should be customized for each patient and should be done in the following sequence[27]:

1. Oral surgery for the extraction of nonsalvageable teeth
2. Caries control of deep lesions that may be a threat to the pulp
3. Periodontic procedures for the management of soft-tissue disease
4. Endodontic procedures for asymptomatic teeth with necrotic pulps, and retreatment of failing previously treated teeth
5. Restorative and prosthetic procedures

This sequence can be altered to respond to changing clinical situations. For example, if periodontal therapy is to include root resection or hemisection, endodontic therapy should be initiated before the periodontal surgery; or the need for endodontic therapy may arise during restorative or prosthetic procedures. However, as a general rule the above sequence should be followed.

Some important considerations that can alter the treatment plan and sequencing are the patient's systemic health, his dental attitude and priorities, and his financial situation.

Once endodontics has been placed with the appropriate sequence in the comprehensive plan, the clinician must then focus specifically on the endodontic treatment plan. Thus, it is a specific treatment plan within a comprehensive treatment plan. There are several approaches to providing endodontic services to patients. These approaches are modified, to a great extent, by circumstances surrounding each case.

Emergency care

Frequently when a patient presents in pain of pulpal origin requiring emergency care, the clinician is faced with a situation in which there is insufficient time to conduct a comprehensive examination in order to develop a treatment plan. In these situations it is best to first relieve the patient's chief complaint. This could include pulpotomy, pulpectomy, incision and drainage, or chemotherapy. Whatever the situation, one must resist the temptation to overtreat during an emergency procedure. Too many routine cases have been converted to extremely difficult and complicated cases by clinicians rushing through an emergency procedure and doing more than is really necessary to alleviate the patient's pain.

As described in Chapter 2, complete cleansing and

shaping of the root canal spaces should be completed at the first appointment. However, hurrying to accomplish these procedures in the face of severe time constraints can potentially result in perforation, ledging or blocking of the canal, instrument breakage, or other iatrogenic problems that can complicate an otherwise routine case. Once symptomatic relief has been provided, the patient can make an appointment for a thorough clinical examination, at which time many of the important decisions relative to case selection and treatment planning can be made.

One visit versus multiple visits

One controversy that has been debated among endodontists for decades is that of single-visit versus multiple-visit root canal treatment. Traditionalists have categorically (and empirically) associated one-visit endodontics with increased incidence of adverse posttreatment sequelae, such as pain. However, there is no sound scientific basis to support this position.

A number of clinical studies have been undertaken in an attempt to clarify the questions relative to posttreatment pain as well as the rate of success following one-visit root canal treatment as compared with multiple-visit root canal treatment.[2,3,8,9,18-25] The findings of these studies are summarized in Table 3-1. It is clear that interest in one-appointment endodontics is increasing. It is also obvious from reviewing these studies that there has been a misconception that one-sitting endodontics results in a significantly greater incidence of posttreatment pain. This simply does not appear to be true.

In a nationwide survey of endodontists,[6] 90% of those responding indicated that they treat certain types of cases in one appointment; 67% indicated that they treat teeth with vital pulps in one appointment, whereas only 16.8% would treat teeth with necrotic pulp in one appointment.

There is sufficient evidence in the aforementioned studies to support the contention that *one-visit endodontics can be successful, and that it does not necessarily result in a greater incidence of posttreatment pain.*

However, the clinician would be well advised to establish guidelines for selection of teeth to be treated in one visit. Oliet's criteria[20] for selection of cases will certainly minimize postoperative complications; these include: (1) positive patient acceptance, (2) sufficient treatment time available to properly complete the procedure, (3) absence of acute symptoms requiring drainage via the canal, as well as an absence of persistent continuous flow of exudate, and (4) absence of anatomic difficulties (calcified canals, fine tortuous canals, bifurcated canals) and procedural difficulties (ledge formation, blockage, perforation, inadequate fills). Ashkenaz[3] identifies specific contraindications to one-appointment endodontics:

1. Periapical symptoms in teeth with either vital or nonvital pulps
2. Anatomic problems (receded pulp chambers, calcified canals, sharply curved canals, bifurcated canals, and dilacerations)
3. Multirooted teeth. Although not an absolute contraindication, multirooted teeth most frequently present complex procedural challenges, such as extra canals, extreme curvatures, pulp stones, and calcifications, that render one-treatment endodontics for molars and some premolars inadvisable for the majority of general practitioners.

TABLE 3-1. One-visit versus multiple-visit endodontics

Investigator	Total number of teeth	Pulp status*	One visit			Multiple visits		
			Pain (percent)		Healing (percent)	Pain (percent)		Healing (percent)
			None or slight	Moderate to severe		None or slight	Moderate to severe	
Ferranti[8]	340	N	91	9	—	96.2	3	—
Fox et al.[9]	270	V-N	90	10	—	—	—	—
O'Keefe[19]	125	V-N	98	2	—	91	9	—
Soltanoff[25]	282	V-N	81	19	85	86	14	88
Ashkenaz[2,3]	195	V	96	4	97†	—	—	—
Rudner and Oliet[24]	283	V-N	88.7	11.2	89.7	88.6	11.4	88.6
Pekruhn[21]	102	V-N	84.4	15.6	—	84.4	15.6	—
Mulhern et al.[18]	60	N	76.7	23.3	—	73.3	26.7	—
Roane J. et al.[23]	359	V-N	84.8	15.2	—	68.8	31.2	—
Oliet S.[20]	387	V-N	89.3	18.7	89‡	93.5	6.5	89
Pekruhn[22]	925	V-N	—	—	94.7 (96.4)§	—	—	—

*V, Vital; N, nonvital.
†Percentages based on 101 recalls.
‡Percentages based on 338 recalls.
§Figure in parenthesis represents 3.6% failures attributable to endodontic causes.

Multiple teeth

Occasionally a patient needs root canal treatment on several teeth. This raises the question, "Can two or more teeth be treated at the same visit?" Basically the answer is "yes"; however, it is probably not prudent to treat more than one multirooted tooth per visit. Multirooted teeth usually present the clinician with his or her greatest technical challenges, and care must be taken to avoid rushing through the procedure.

It is probably appropriate to treat more than one single-rooted tooth at the same appointment; however, the clinician must assess the difficulties of individual cases and weigh them against his experience and expertise and the time available. It would be imprudent to attempt treatment of more than one tooth if the case involves anatomic or pathologic difficulties, such as severely dilacerated roots or calcified canals.

One disadvantage of treating two adjacent teeth at the same appointment arises when the patient experiences a posttreatment "flare-up." In these instances it is sometimes difficult to determine which of the two teeth is associated with the flare-up.

If more than one tooth is to be treated at the same appointment, it is prudent to complete instrumentation on one before preparing access to the other. However, there is an advantage to preparing for access cavities to both teeth (if they are adjacent), thereby allowing determination of working lengths with a single radiograph. Once the working length has been determined, instrumentation should first be completed on one tooth, that tooth should be sealed, and then a separate set of sterile instruments should be used to complete the second tooth.

PROGNOSIS

Endodontic therapy is one of the most highly successful dental services. If we provide thorough debridement, cleansing, shaping, and obturation of the root canal system, we can expect to enjoy success in about 90% of cases.[10,13]

There is a direct correlation between prognosis, case selection, and treatment planning. This should be recalled during the process of case selection and treatment planning. A case that is too difficult for a general practitioner (based on the total assessment of the answer to the question "Can the tooth be treated?") may have a more favorable prognosis if it is referred to an endodontist.

Many endodontically treated teeth fail not for endodontic reasons but for periodontal reasons or because they were not properly restored following root canal treatment. These failures are avoidable if clinicians broaden their focus to the entire treatment plan and place endodontics in its proper perspective in comprehensive oral health care delivery.

REFERENCES

1. Abou-Rass, M.: The stressed pulp condition: an endodontic-restorative diagnostic concept, J. Prosthet. Dent. **48:**264, 1982.
2. Ashkenaz, P.J.: One visit endodontics: a preliminary report, Dent. Surv. **55:**62, 1979.
3. Ashkenaz, P.J.: One-visit endodontics, Dent. Clin. North Am. **28:**853, 1984.
4. Baumgartner, J.C., and Harrison, J.W.: The incidence of bacteremias related to endodontic procedures. I. Nonsurgical endodontics, J. Endod. **2:**135, 1976.
5. Bender, I.B., Seltzer, S. and Yermish, M.: Incidence of bacteremia in endodontic manipulation, Oral Surg. **13:**350, 1960.
6. Calhoun, R.L., and Landers, R.R.: One-appointment endodontic therapy: a nationwide survey of endodontists, J. Endod. **8** (1):35, 1982.
7. Council on Cardiovascular Disease in the Young: Prevention of bacterial endocarditis, Circulation **70:**1123A, 1984.
8. Ferranti, P.: Treatment of the root canal of an infected tooth in one appointment: a report of 340 cases, Dent. Diag. **65:**490, 1959.
9. Fox, J., et al.: Incidence of pain following one-visit endodontic treatment, Oral Surg. **30:**123, 1970.
10. Grossman, L.I., Shepard, L.I., and Pearson, L.A.: Roentgenologic and clinical evaluation of endodontically treated teeth, Oral Surg. **17:**367, March 1964.
11. Harrison, J.W., Baumgartner, J.C., and Svec, T.A.: Incidence of pain associated with clinical factors during and after root canal therapy. II. Postobturation pain, J. Endod. **9:**434, 1983.
12. Holroyd, S.V., and Wynn, R.L.: Clinical pharmacology in dental practice, ed. 3, 1983, St. Louis, The C.V. Mosby Co.
13. Kerekes, K., and Tronstad, L.: Long term results of endodontic treatment performed with a standardized technique, J. Endod. **5:**83, March 1979.
14. Langeland, K., and Langeland, L.: Pulp reactions to crown preparation, impression, temporary crown fixation and permanent cementation, J. Prosthet. Dent. **15:**129, 1965.
15. Little, J.W., and Falace, D.A.: Dental management of the medically compromised patient, ed. 2, 1984, St. Louis, The C.V. Mosby Co.
16. Malamed, S.F.: Handbook of medical emergencies in the dental office, ed. 3, 1986, St. Louis, The C.V. Mosby Co.
17. Mattison, G.D., et al.: Effect of post preparation on the apical seal, J. Prosthet. Dent. **51:**785, 1984.
18. Mulhern, J., et al.: Incidence of postoperative pain after one-appointment endodontic treatment of asymptomatic pulpal necrosis in single-rooted teeth, J. Endod. **8:**370, 1982.
19. O'Keefe, E.: Pain in endodontic therapy: preliminary study, J. Endod. **2:**315, 1976.
20. Oliet, S.: Single-visit endodontics: a clinical study, J. Endod. **9:**147, 1983.
21. Pekruhn, R.: Single-visit endodontics: a preliminary clinical study, J. Am. Dent. Assoc. **103:**875, 1981.
22. Pekruhn, R.B.: The incidence of failure following single-visit endodontic therapy, J. Endod. **12:**68, 1986.
23. Roane, J.B., Dryden, J.A., and Grimes, E.W.: Incidence of postoperative pain after single- and multiple-visit endodontic procedures, Oral Surg. **55:**68, 1983.
24. Rudner, W.L., and Oliet, S.: Single-visit endodontics: a concept and clinical study, Compend. Contin. Educ. **2:**63, 1981.
25. Soltanoff, W., A comparative study of single-visit and multiple-visit endodontic procedures, J. Endod. **9:**278, 1978.
26. Sorensen, J.A., and Martinoff, J.T.: Endodontically treated teeth as abutments, J. Prosthet. Dent. **53:**631, 1985.
27. Wood, N.K.: Treatment planning: a pragmatic approach, St. Louis, 1978, The C.V. Mosby Co.
28. Wright, W.E., et al.: An oral disease prevention program for patients receiving radiation and chemotherapy, J. Am. Dent. Assoc. **110:**43, 1985.
29. Zmener, O.: Effect of dowel preparation on the apical seal of endodontically treated teeth, J. Endod. **6:**687, 1980.

Self-assessment questions

1. A nonvital tooth with extremely curved roots
   a. Requires a high degree of clinical skill to treat
   b. Cannot be treated
   c. Usually requires crown lengthening to improve canal access
   d. Presents no significant challenge to the clinician

2. A tooth is considered of highest strategic value when its extraction would result in
   a. Stabilization of occlusal forces
   b. Prosthetic escalation
   c. Loss of arch integrity
   d. Compromise of esthetics

3. When extensive restorative procedures are planned on a tooth with a "stressed pulp-condition," root canal therapy should be
   a. Delayed if the tooth is asymptomatic
   b. Completed prior to restorative treatment
   c. Initiated only if symptoms develop
   d. Completed following the restorative procedures

4. A nonvital tooth intended to be used as a fixed partial denture abutment must have
   a. Adequate remaining tooth structure for support and retention
   b. A crown-root of 1:1
   c. Sufficient crown structure to avoid removal of any root filling material
   d. A straight, single-canaled root

5. To maintain an adequate apical seal after post-space preparation, the remaining length of the root canal filling should be at least
   a. 3 mm
   b. 4 mm
   c. 5 mm
   d. 6 mm

6. A stress-reduction protocol for significantly medically compromised patients should include
   a. Long appointments to reduce the number of visits
   b. Afternoon appointments to avoid morning stress
   c. Medical consultation prior to treatment
   d. Anxiety control only with extensive treatment

7. A specific contraindication to elective endodontic procedures is
   a. Diabetes mellitus
   b. Adrenal insufficiency
   c. Radiation therapy
   d. Recent history of myocardial infarction

8. In a comprehensive treatment plan, the treatment sequence (other than an emergency case) would begin with
   a. Periodontics
   b. Caries control
   c. Endodontics
   d. Extraction of nonsalvageable teeth

9. Because of the limited time available to develop a comprehensive treatment plan in an emergency situation, the author recommends that the clinician
   a. Complete as much therapy as possible
   b. Undertreat rather than overtreat the patient
   c. Provide symptomatic relief for the chief complaint
   d. Avoid treatment until a definitive plan is finalized

10. All other factors being equal, the principles of root canal therapy for a tooth with a vital pulp and a tooth with a necrotic pulp are
    a. Quite different
    b. Essentially the same
    c. Immaterial to treatment planning
    d. Variable depending on the clinician

11. An important criterion for selecting a tooth for a one-visit root canal filling is that the tooth must be
    a. Asymptomatic
    b. Single rooted
    c. Multirooted
    d. Nonvital

12. Sufficient evidence exists to support the contention that, compared with multiple-root canal fillings, one-sitting root canal fillings
    a. Are usually more painful
    b. Have a poorer prognosis
    c. Are not recommended
    d. Can be quite successful

13. When a clinician is treating multiple teeth at the same appointment, the author recommends
    a. Sequential instrumentation of all canals
    b. Separate sterile instruments for each tooth
    c. Individual radiographs of adjacent teeth
    d. Separate sterile instruments for each canal

14. On the basis of clinical studies, root canal therapy
    a. Enjoys a very favorable prognosis overall
    b. Is independent of the periodontal condition
    c. Can be expected to be 100% successful
    d. Has a questionable prognosis in difficult cases

4

PREPARATION FOR TREATMENT

STEPHEN F. SCHWARTZ

PATIENT PREPARATION

Preparation for endodontic therapy extends far beyond the intricate diagnostic techniques and assembling the proper armamentarium. An important factor in the dentist's ability to treat teeth successfully is the patient's attitude. This attitude must be developed not only toward the proposed treatment plan but also toward the dentist. The patient must be convinced of the dentist's ability and of the value of the treatment. A positive attitude is essential to eliminate anxieties and to overcome the fears that many patients associate with the removal of the "nerve."

Public opinion surveys have verified that endodontic treatment is steeped in myth, mystery, and widespread fear. This undesirable and certainly undeserved stigma that surrounds modern endodontics stems from two causes. First, from a historical perspective endodontic treatment preceded the advent of effective local anesthesia, adequate radiographic techniques, and the sophistication and standardization of endodontic instruments. Unpleasant tales still circulate about treatments rendered under those circumstances. Second, there is often a failure on the part of the patient to differentiate between the painful disease process that brings him to the dental office and the treatment, which almost always provides prompt relief from that pain. The dentist must be sensitive to the misgivings the patient may have concerning the impending treatment.

The dentist's relationship with the patient must be built on a foundation of empathy, concern and sincerity. The patient deserves to know what is involved in his treatment. A concise, well-organized presentation may allay many fears and anxieties and answer the questions that are undoubtedly in the patient's mind: "What's wrong?" "How do we correct it?" "What's the alternative?" "How long will it take?" "Will it hurt?" "How much will it cost?" The answers require that certain information be presented to the patient with the use of various patient educational aids.

Case presentation should relate a story beginning with the identification of the problem and continuing through to its resolution. As with any other story, visual aids play an important role and may include printed patient educational material, the patient's own radiographs, drawings, models, and videotapes. Utilization of the patient's own radiographs is a most effective method of providing a more direct, personalized involvement.

Following is a typical case presentation covering the most important considerations:

What's the pulp?

Do I need the pulp?

What happens to the pulp?

Mr. Jones, I see you've had a chance to glance over our printed material; you may now have a better understanding of the meaning of root canal treatment. Now, to consider your particular situation, let's look at the x-ray. Our diagnostic procedures indicate this is the tooth that is going to require endodontic therapy [pointing to radiograph]. These fine gray lines running down the roots of the tooth are the root canals, and inside these canals is the pulp tissue. The pulp tissue is what some people call the "nerve," but it's much more than the nerve. The pulp is composed of highly specialized tissues that are responsible for the formation of the tooth. Once the tooth is formed the tissue's importance is greatly reduced. Deep fillings, the bacteria from decay, or injuries to the tooth can damage the pulp tissue. Often, this damage is only slight and the pulp can recover, but if the damage is too severe or there's an accumulation of irritations to the pulp over a period of time, the pulp may become diseased and begin to deteriorate. The breakdown products from this diseased pulp can extend beyond the end of the root and destroy the bone. This is what is commonly referred to as an abscess. [If a radiolucency is present, it is pointed out at this time on the radiograph. If there is no radiolucency, the explanation is given that endodontic trreatment will very likely prevent it from occurring.]

What has to be done?

Therefore, Mr. Jones, to prevent any further deterioration and to create a favorable environment for healing to take place, as well as to alleviate your symptoms, this diseased pulp tissue must be removed. After administering an effective local anesthetic, we'll make an opening through the top of the tooth to gain access to the root canals. the diseased pulp tissue will then be removed with very fine instruments all the way to the end of the root. After this diseased tissue has been removed and the canals disinfected, the root canals will be sealed to prevent any further irritation to the surrounding bone. Thorough filling, or sealing, of the canal system will eliminate the pathway and "safe harbor" for bacteria, and new bone will replace that destroyed by the diseased pulp tissue.

How are you going to do it?

How long will it take?

This procedure can often be accomplished in one visit but may require one or two additional visits to allow time for complete elimination of infection, for the medication (if any) in the canals to be effective, and finally for the tissues that surround the root to respond to our treatment. This procedure shouldn't be painful, because we will use a local anesthetic similar to the type used for a filling. Once the root canal treatment has been completed and the crown of the tooth has been properly restored, there is an excellent chance that the tooth will remain as a useful member of your dentition. Mr. Jones, if you don't have endodontic treatment, the tooth must be extracted. [At this point, the economic and functional advantages of saving the tooth in comparison to replacement by a prosthetic appliance must be discussed. In addition, the functional inefficiency and disharmony that could develop if the tooth were simply extracted with no intent of replacement must be thoroughly explained.]

Will it hurt?

Will it last?

What's the alternative?

Is it worth it?

Adequate answers must be given to commonly asked questions, such as "Will the tooth be dead?" or "Will it turn dark?" The clinician must explain that the tooth still maintains a vital communication to the surrounding tissues, having lost only its ability to respond to sensations, such as heat, cold, and sweets, and that a pulpless tooth still must receive the same oral hygiene as the other teeth. The patient must be assured that various precautions are taken during treatment to prevent any discoloration of the tooth but that in the unlikely event discoloration occurs or is already present, the tooth may be bleached or restored with an esthetic crown or veneer. The patient must also have a clear understanding that after endodontic therapy the tooth may be less structurally sound and slightly more brittle; therefore posterior teeth must be protected with an onlay or crown to prevent fracture.

At the conclusion of the appointment, printed educational material can be given to the patient to take home. It serves as a good source of reinforcement for the interested patient or for the patient who was too apprehensive to fully understand the oral presentation.

RADIOGRAPHIC PREPARATION

The sophistication of endodontics has closely paralleled the sophistication of radiographic techniques. Improvements in the physical machinery and photographic quality of the films have directly improved the results of endodonitc therapy from both a diagnostic and a treatment standpoint. To gather the maximum amount of information from the radiograph, however, the clinician must understand the factors affecting its production as well as its interpretation.

Film placement, proper exposure, and correct processing may affect the ultimate diagnosis as much as the scientific acumen necessary to interpret the resultant images. In addition to the production of films of high technical quality, interpretation depends on the ability to recognize changes from normal (Chapter 1). Wide structural variations may exist within normal limits. Finally the limitations of the radiographic technique must be appreciated and considered during film interpretation.

Production of radiographs
Film and cone placement

Properly used, either the bisecting-angle technique or the right-angle (paralleling) technique will provide the clinician with films free of excessive distortion or superimposition (Fig. 4-1).

A major disadvantage of the bisecting-angle technique is some unavoidable dimensional distortion. This characteristic creates difficulties in length determination and in accurate anatomic reproduction.

The right-angle technique reduces distortion. The film is positioned parallel to the long axis of the tooth and the rays are projected perpendicular to the film. With the paralleling technique the object-film distance is increased, which requires a greater source-image distance (16 to 20 inches) to reduce (or minimize) enlargement of the image. This technique permits a more accurate reproduction of the tooth in all its dimensions, thus enhancing a determination of the tooth's length and relationship to surrounding anatomic structures. In addition, the vertical angulation required for maxillary posterior teeth is less than in the bisecting-angle technique, and superimposition of the zygomatic process over the apices of the teeth is often avoided.

Variations in size and shape of the oral structures often make absolutely parallel placement of the film unlikely. To compensate for difficult placement, it has been demonstrated that the film may diverge from the long axis of the tooth up to 20 degrees with minimal longitudinal distortion.[3]

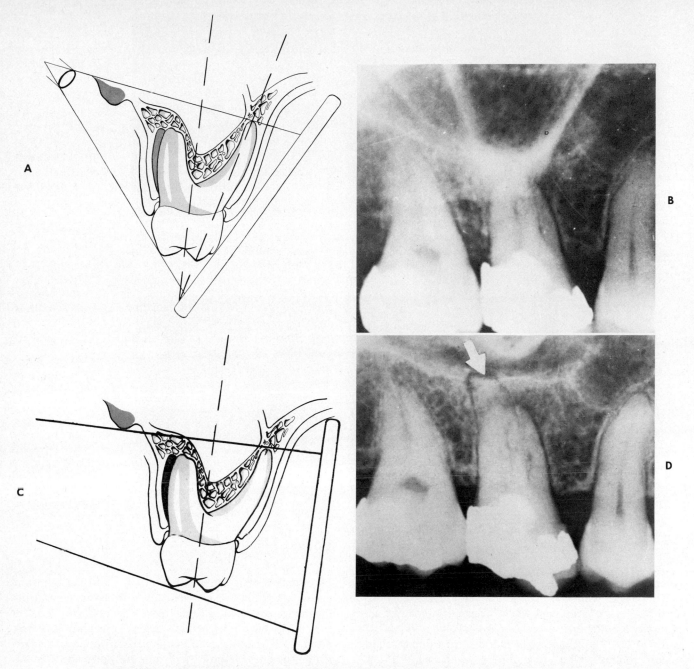

FIG. 4-1. A, Bisecting-angle technique. **B,** Superimposition of the zygomatic process over the root apices of the maxillary first molar with the bisecting-angle technique. **C,** Right-angle technique. **D,** Projection of the zygomatic process above the root apices with the right-angle technique, allowing visualization of periapical pathosis *(arrow).*

Proper exposure

The intricacies of proper kilovoltage, milliamperage, and time selection are mentioned here as examples of how the diagnostic quality of a film may be altered by changes in the film's density and contrast.

Density. Density is the degree of darkening of the film. The amount of darkening depends on the *quantity* and *quality* of radiation delivered to the film. Since milliamperage controls the electron flow from cathode to anode,

the greater the electron flow per unit time the greater will be the quantity of radiation produced. Proper density is primarily a function of milliamperage and time. Kilovoltage also affects film density, by controlling the quality and penetrability of the rays. Higher kilovoltage settings produce shorter wavelengths, which in turn are more penetrating than the longer wavelengths produced at lower settings. The ability to control the penetrability of the rays by alterations in kilovoltage effects the amount of radiation

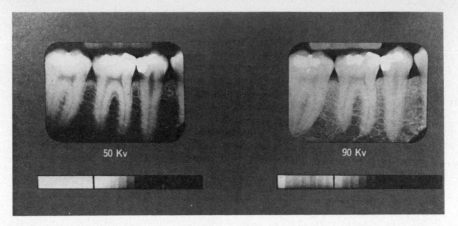

FIG. 4-2. Comparison of short-scale and long-scale contrast produced by increasing the kilovoltage. Note the increased shades of gray in the film produced at 90 kV. (Courtesy Rinn Corporation, Elgin, Ill.)

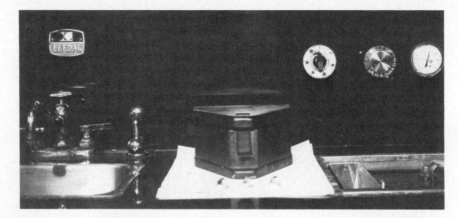

FIG. 4-3. Darkroom setup for the processing of endodontic films. The standard tank is used for pretreatment and posttreatment films. The minitank can be used for rapid processing of working films.

reaching the film and the degree of darkening or density.

Contrast. Contrast refers to the differences between shades of black, gray, and white. Changes in contrast are primarily a function of alterations in kilovoltage. Films exposed at low kilovoltage settings (60 kVp) exhibit "short scale" contrast, with sharp differences between a few shades of black, gray, and white. Films exposed at high kilovoltage settings (90 kVp) produce a "long scale" contrast as a result of the increased penetrating power of the rays. This results in images with many more shades of gray and less-sharp differences[12] (Fig. 4-2). Although more difficult to read, films exposed at higher kilovoltage settings make possible a greater degree of discrimination between images, often enhancing their diagnostic qualities.

Processing

Proper darkroom organization, film handling, and adherence to the time-temperature method of film processing play important roles in producing films of high quality. The empirical "sight developing" method is often substituted for a controlled time-temperature method for the sake of expediency in the production of "working" films in endodontics. Ingle and associates[18] demonstrated that radiographs processed in Kodak developer and fixer at 33° C (92° F) produce films of high quality in slightly less than 1 minute. The time saved in comparison with the standard 4 to 5 minutes of processing time recommended by the manufacturer can certainly expedite the endodontic procedure to the benefit of the patient, as well as the dentist. Rapid-processing solutions are also available commercially, but they tend to vary in shelf life and tank life and in the production of films of permanent quality.

It is recommended that a controlled time-temperature method be utilized for the diagnostic qualities desired in pretreatment and posttreatment films. A more rapid method may be utilized effectively for length determination and trial fitting of root canal filling materials (Fig. 4-3).

Basic principles of interpretation

Accurate radiographic interpretation is undoubtedly one of the most valuable sources of information for endodontic

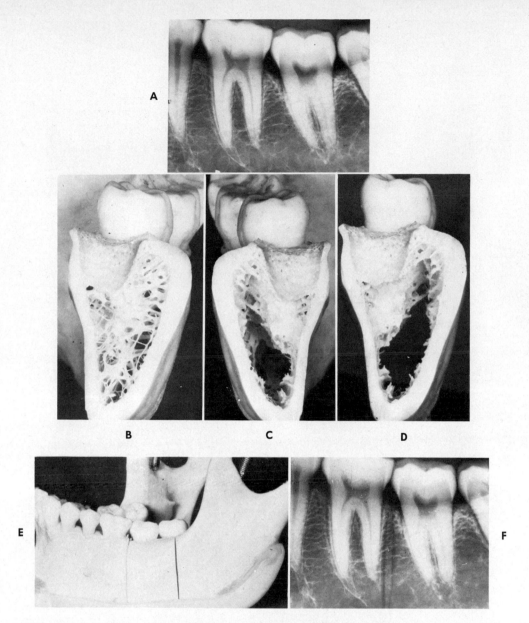

FIG. 4-4. A, Prior to any bone removal. **B,** After buccal-lingual section to demonstrate cortical and cancellous bone. **C,** After removal of cancellous bone without infringement on the junctional trabeculae or cortical bone. **D,** Block section removed to demonstrate the extent of destruction. **E,** Block section rearticulated to the mandible with an acrylic splint. **F,** After removal of cancellous bone.

diagnosis. However, the radiograph is an adjunctive tool; information gleaned from its proper inspection is not always absolute and must be integrated with information gathered from a thorough medical and dental history, a clinical examination. and pulp-testing procedures.

Utilization of the radiograph depends on an understanding of its limitations and advantages. The advantages are obvious, in that the radiograph allows a privileged insight beyond the limitations of our eyes. The information it furnishes is essential and cannot be obtained from any other source; yet its value is not diminished by a critcal appraisal of its limitations.[28]

Limitations of the radiograph

An important and often incompletely understood principle of radiography is the amount of bone destruction undetected by routine x-ray procedures. This has been demonstrated by numerous investigators,[1,5,26,29,31] and definite criteria for the production of radiographic changes have evolved.

Destruction confined to the cancellous portion of the bone cannot be detected radiographically. Although a slight increase in radiodensity may be detected, radiolucencies appear only when there is internal or external erosion or destruction of the bone cortex (Fig. 4-4).

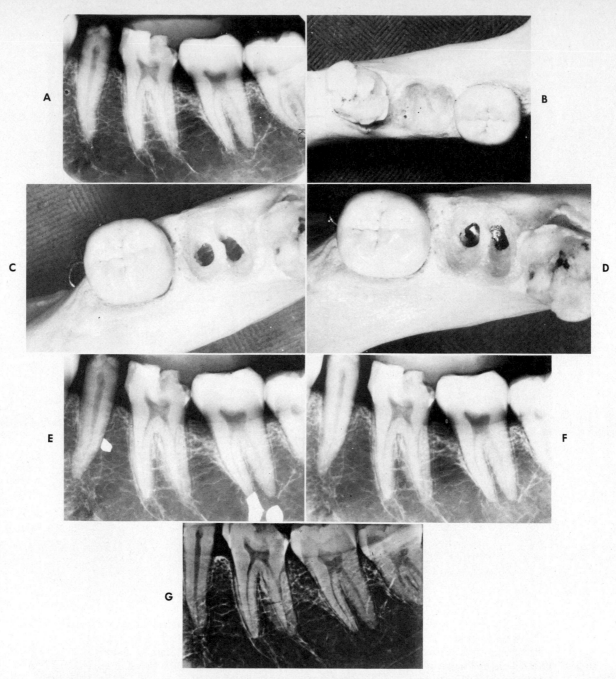

FIG. 4-5. A, Preexperimental radiograph. **B,** Second molar removed to allow creation of periapical defects. **C,** Periapical defects extending through the apical extent of the socket into underlying cancellous bone. **D,** Metallic markers inserted into the defects. **E,** Markers in the defects. **F,** Markers removed for comparison with the preexperimental radiograph. **G,** Xeroradiograph of specimen in **F.**

This radiographic limitation is especially important in endodontic diagnosis (Chapter 1). It is possible for periapical destruction to be present (but confined to cancellous bone) without obvious radiographic evidence (Fig. 4-5). Not until the cortical plate of the alveolar process becomes involved in the disease process will this destruction become visible on the radiograph. This axiom explains the development of previously undetected radiolucencies either during treatment or shortly after treatment has been insti-

tuted (Fig. 4-6). The bone destruction is present but undetected. Only after the destruction extends to the cortex is the radiographic image produced. This factor must also be considered in the evaluation of teeth that become symptomatic after treatment without any radiographic changes. The seeds of destruction may be planted, and in time the disease may sprout through the bony cortex.

It is fortunate that, from a diagnostic standpoint, the apices of most teeth are situated in or near the cortical plate.[2]

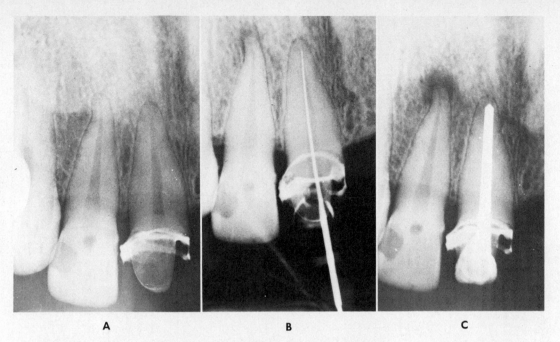

FIG. 4-6. A, Nonvital maxillary left central incisor with a jacket crown in place. **B,** Previously undetected periapical radiolucency on the left lateral incisor 10 days after the initial radiograph. **C,** Periapical bone destruction around the lateral incisor 3 weeks after the initial radiograph.

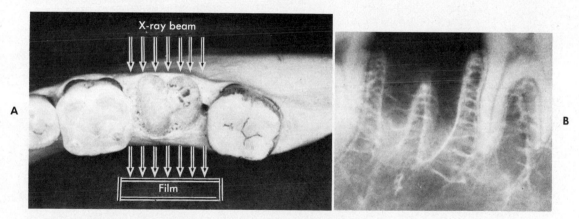

FIG. 4-7. A, Attenuation of x-rays passing tangentially through the socket by the greater thickness of bone on the periphery of the socket. This results in a greater radiopacity of the periphery as compared with the adjacent alveolar bone. **B,** White lines (lamina dura) produced by these attenuated rays.

Therefore very little bone need be destroyed before the cortex is encroached on and radiolucencies become evident.

Lamina dura: a question of integrity. The integrity, or lack of integrity, of the lamina dura is of major concern, especially in its relationship to the health of the pulp. The lamina dura represents a layer of compact bone lining the tooth socket.[11,19] Noxious products emanating from the root canal can effect a change in this structure that will be radiographically visible. Manson[24] has shown graphically that the lamina dura simply reflects a plate of bone which lines the tooth socket. X-rays passing tangentially through an oblong socket must pass through many times the width of the adjacent alveolus and are attenuated by this greater thickness of bone, producing the characteristic "white line" (Fig. 4-7). Therefore the presence, absence, or integrity of the lamina dura is determined largely by the shape and position of the root, and in turn by its bony crypt, in relation to the x-ray beam. This explanation is consistent with the radiographic and clinical finding of teeth with perfectly healthy pulps and no definite lamina dura.

Integrity changes in the periodontal ligament space, the lamina dura, and the surrounding periradicular bone can certainly be of diagnostic value, especially when compared with previous radiographs. The significance given to these changes must be tempered by a thorough understanding of the features giving rise to these images. Studies of radio-

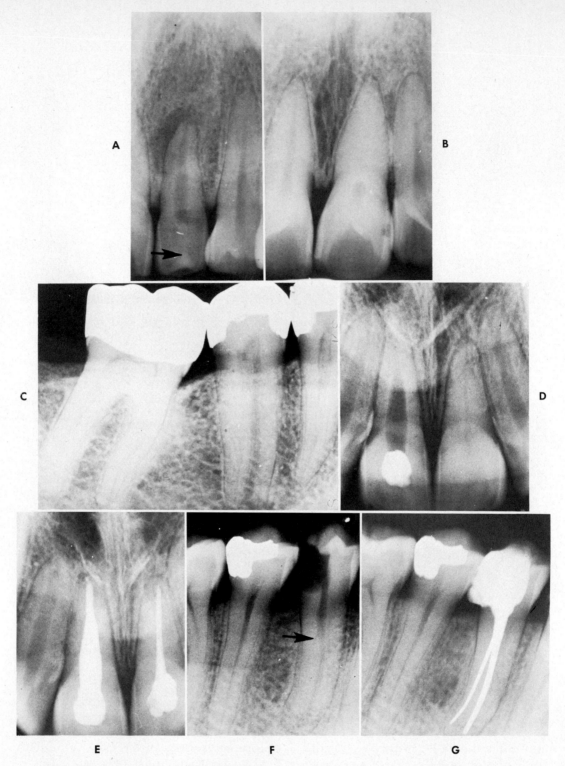

FIG. 4-8. Cases requiring careful interpretation. **A,** Enamel invagination on the incisal aspect of the maxillary lateral incisor *(arrow),* which must be sealed following endodontic therapy to prevent coronal leakage through the invaginated channel. **B,** Calcification of the root canal of the maxillary central incisor as a result of traumatic injury. **C,** Extensive calcification of the canals of the mandibular molar and bifurcation of the root of the second premolar. **D,** Opposite reactions to traumatic injury to the maxillary central incisors. The right incisor exhibts almost complete calcification of the canal, whereas the left exhibits an excessively large canal in the coronal two thirds as a result of pulpal necrosis and cessation of dentin deposition. **E,** Completed endodontic therapy. **F,** Bifurcation *(arrow)* of the root canal in a mandibular first premolar. **G,** Completed endodontic therapy; verification of the presence of two canals.

graphs of maxillary incisors and histologic sections of their apical areas were undertaken to determine whether, and to what extent, histologic changes are reflected in conventional radiographs.[7-9] A sign-analyzing method assigning a grade to various changes in structures such as the bone, lamina dura, and periodontal ligament space was effective in distinguishing normal teeth from those with pulp-related periapical changes in 98% of the cases studied. This method of radiographic interpretation shows promise for more accurate radiographic diagnosis, but clinical acceptance of the method must await further confirmation of its validity by other researchers.

Radiographic hints

Careful examination. Radiographic interpretation is not strictly the identification of a problem and the establishment of a diagnosis. The dentist must read the radiograph with an eye toward diagnosis and treatment. Frequently overlooked are the small areas of resorption, the invaginated enamel, the minute fracture, the extra canal, the calcified canal, and in turn the potential problems they may create during treatment (Fig. 4-8). Complicated treatment, time, and expense can be avoided or at least anticipated if a thorough examination of the radiograph is made; it is often desirable to have at least two exposures at various horizontal angulations for comparison (Figs. 1-14, *H* and *I*, 3-22, and 4-9).

Buccal object rule. When taking films at various horizontal angulations, one must employ the buccal object rule to differentiate the buccal-lingual relationship of structures. According to this rule the object farthest (most buccal) from the film moves the greatest distance on the film with respect to a change in the horizontal angulation of the x-ray cone. In a two-rooted premolar, if the cone is angled mesial to distal, the buccal root will move distally with respect to the palatal root on the radiogrpah. A distal-to-mesial angulation of the cone will move the buccal root mesially (Fig. 4-9). This rule affords differentiation of canals and roots for the purposes of determining length, fitting canal filling material and locating additional canals.

Differential interpretation. There are many anatomic structures and osteolytic lesions that may be mistaken for pulpoperiapical lesions.

Among the more commonly misinterpreted anatomic structures are the mental foramen (Fig. 4-10) and the incisive foramen. These radiolucencies can be differentiated from pathologic conditions by additional exposures at a different angulation and by pulp-testing procedures. Radiolucencies unassociated with a root apex can be projected away from the apex by altering the horizontal angulation.

A commonly misinterpreted osteolytic lesion is the cementoma (Fig. 4-11). The use of pulp-testing procedures and follow-up radiographic examinations will prevent the mistake of diagnosing this as a pulpoperiapical lesion. The development of a cementoma can be followed radiographically from its osteolytic through its osteogenic stage.

Other anatomic radiolucencies that must be differentiated from pulpoperiapical lesions are the posterior palatine foramen, which may project near the lingual root of the maxillary first molar; nutrient canals; unusual arborization of the trabecular framework; and depression in the mandible created by a the submandibular gland.

Many systemic conditions can affect the radiographic appearance of the alveolar process. A discussion of these is beyond the scope of the present chapter, but the reader can find complete descriptions in a book by Bhaskar.[6]

Radiation hygiene

The goal of any radiographic procedure is to gain maximum diagnostic information with minimum risk to the patient. There exists today an ever-growing concern by the public over the harmful effects of radiation exposure. A patient may question the necessity of an x-ray examination or even refuse it completely. This fear or concern is based on the extensive, but not always factual, coverage of the subject by various public media.

It therefore becomes incumbent on the dentist to educate these patients adequately about the valuable information that only the radiograph can supply and about the minimal risk in the radiograph's production. To overcome patient concern, the dentist must be familiar with the biologic effects of radiation exposure.

The roentgen (R) is the unit of measure for radiation. The National Research Council of the National Academy of Sciences recommends that the average radiation dose for the general population not exceed 10 R of man-made radiation between conception and age 30. This refers to *whole body* or somatic exposure. Although every effort should be made to minimize somatic exposure, the main concern is the effect on the reproductive organs or "gonadal exposure" for the procreative segment of the population.

Dental radiography is limited to specific areas of the head and neck; almost negligible amounts of radiation are received by the gonads. A full-mouth survey utilizing high-speed film at 65 kV, 10 mA, has been reported to cause no observable effects on the gonads.[27] In a given exposure of the face, about 1 ten-thousandth of the radiation is scattered to the gonadal region.[30] Therefore a full-mouth survey as previously described would result in an exposure to the gonads of 0.0005 R.

These facts lead to an interesting comparison between man-made radiation and exposure from natural background radiation composed of radioactive elements in the earth, water, and air and cosmic rays. Background radiation has been estimated at 0.1 R per year, or 0.00027 R per day.[12,22] Therefore, if attention is given to proper radiographic technique and processing, the gonadal exposure resulting from a full-month survey is equivalent to about 2 days of natural background radiation or a level equivalent to a day of sunbathing at the beach.[27] Endodontic procedures usually require only four to six films, thus minimizing radiation exposure to an almost insignificant point.

Although these facts mean that the advantages derived from the radiographic examination far outweigh any potential hazard, we owe it to our patients to take every measure to minimize tissue injury from radiation exposure. The danger of the cumulative effects of radiation exists as long

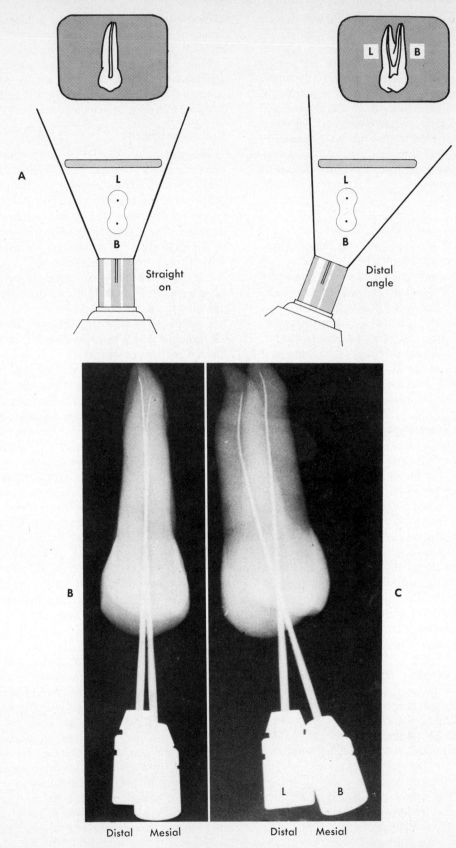

FIG. 4-9. A, Comparison of straight-on and distal-angle views of a two-rooted premolar. Viewed straight on, this tooth appears to have only one root. When the cone is angled distally, the two roots can be differentiated. **B,** Straight-on view of a maxillary premolar with a root canal instrument in the buccal and palatal canals. **C,** Mesial-to-distal angulation producing separation of the roots. The buccal root is moved distally with respect to the palatal root.

as each user dismisses his or her contributions as having a negligible risk. The practitioner must be responsible for deciding need, for ensuring technical competence, and for developing a high level of interpretive ability.[22]

Factors over which the dentist has control are proper filtration to absorb the less penetrating rays and elimination of peripheral radiation by the use of a lead diaphragm. The diameter of the useful beam should be limited to 69.8 mm (2.75 inches) at the end of the cone, regardless of the length of the cone. Proper cone size and shape are also important in reducing exposure. The use of an open-ended cone lined with lead or stainless steel is recommended.[33]

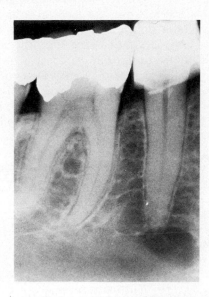

FIG. 4-10. A mandibular second premolar with an apparent periapical radiolucency. Pulp-testing procedures verified the vitality of the pulp and the fact that the radiolucency was the mental foramen.

Film speed is one of the most important factors in the reduction of exposure to the patient. Films of the lowest speed require about 12 times as much exposure as high-speed films. The better image definition attributed to the lower-speed films has been largely counter-balanced by great improvements in the higher-speed films. This improved quality, coupled with the tremendous reduction in exposure time, would seem to favor the use of high-speed films.

Last, but certainly not of lesser importance in reducing radiation exposure, is proper processing. Careful handling of the film and adherence to the manufacturer's directions will produce films of high quality and eliminate unnecessary additional exposures.

Xeroradiography

Xeroradiography, a recent advancement, is a radiographic process utilizing a conventional radiographic machine along with special intraoral film cassettes and a photoprocessor that have been developed by Xerox Corporation. This system allows for up to a two-thirds reduction in the amount of radiation exposure to the patient as compared with conventional radiography.

The resulting image appears on a dry, laminated film within 20 seconds after being placed into the photoprocessor. The technical aspects of the production of the xeroradiographic image, along with the confirmation of the ability of the process to produce images exhibiting extremely fine detail and sharply defined boundaries, have been described by many investigators.[13-16,21,32] Although the images produced by this technique exhibit an enhancement of fine detail when compared with conventional radiographs, in terms of diagnostic value the two techniques appear to be equal[23] (Fig. 4-5, G).

The standards for proper cone and film placement are

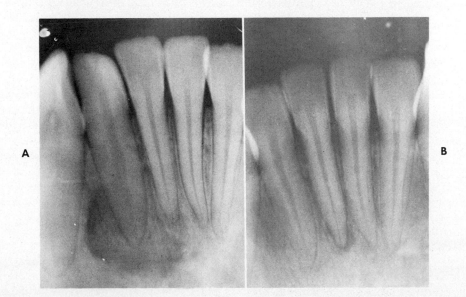

FIG. 4-11. Variations in appearance of a cementoma. **A,** Osteolytic stage, **B,** One year later. Regeneration of bone around the apex of the left lateral incisor and appearance of a radiolucency around the left central incisor.

the same as for conventional radiography, but the size and inflexibility of the film cassette can make proper intraoral placement difficult in certain situations. The lack of a double film pack and the inability to project the xeroradiograph onto a screen constitute other minor drawbacks to this technique along with the initial expense of the cassettes and the photoprocessor.

The ability to produce high-quality diagnostic films at less than half of the conventional exposure time is a significant advancement in an era of increased concern over the potentially harmful effects of radiation exposure.

TOOTH PREPARATION
Advantages of the rubber dam

Using a rubber dam is axiomatic in endodontics. The advantages and absolute necessity for the rubber dam must always take precedence over expediency and convenience. The statement has been made that "the most time-consuming thing about the rubber dam is the time required to convince the dentist to use it."[10] Proper preparation and placement of the rubber dam can be done quickly and will enhance the entire procedure.

Use of the rubber dam in endodontics provides for the following:

1. Patient protection from aspiration or swallowing of instruments, tooth debris, medicaments, and irrigants (Grossman,[17] Cohen,[9a] and Zinman, Chapter 9, have discussed the obvious legal complications that may result from the ingestion and aspiration of materials by the patient as a result of omission of the rubber dam.)
2. A surgically clean operating field
3. Retraction and protection of the soft tissues—gingiva, tongue, lips, and cheek
4. Improved vision for the work area
5. Improved efficiency—prevents patient conversation during the dental procedure and the need for frequent rinsing

Rubber dam technique

Various types of rubber dams, rubber dam clamps, rubber dam frames, and rubber dam forceps are described in Chapter 5.

Methods of rubber dam placement

An expedient method of dam placement is to position the bow of the clamp distally through the hole in the dam. This requires the use of a winged clamp. The clamp is then stretched by forceps to maintain the position of the clamp in the dam, and the dam is positioned on the frame, allowing for the placement of the dam, clamp, and frame in one motion (Fig. 4-12). After the clamp is secured on the tooth, the dam is teased under the wings of the clamp with a plastic instrument.

Another method is to place the clamp on the tooth and then stretch the dam over the clamped tooth. This method offers the advantage of enabling the clinician to see exactly where the jaws of the clamp engage the tooth, thus avoiding impingement on the gingival tissues. Gentle finger pressure on the buccal and lingual apron of the clamp before the dam is placed can be used to test how securely the clamp fits (Fig. 4-13).

A third method, the *split-dam* technique, may be used for isolation of anterior teeth without employing a rubber dam clamp. Not only is this technique useful when there is insufficient crown structure, as in the case of horizontal fractures, but it also prevents possible chipping of margins of teeth restored with porcelain or acrylic crowns by the jaws of the clamp.

In the split-dam method two overlapping holes are punched in the dam. A cotton roll is placed under the lip in the mucobuccal fold over the tooth to be treated. The rubber dam is then stretched over the tooth to be treated and over the tooth adjacent on each side. The edge of the dam is carefully teased through the contacts on the distal sides of the two adjacent teeth. Dental floss will assist in carrying the dam down around the gingiva. The tension produced by the stretched dam, assisted by the rubber dam frame, secures the dam in place. The tight fit and the cotton roll produce a completely dry field (Fig. 4-14). If the dam has a tendency to slip, a premolar clamp may be used on the tooth distal to the three isolated teeth. The clamp is placed over the rubber dam, which then acts as a cushion against the jaws of the clamp.

Regardless of the method used, after the tooth is isolated, the tooth and dam should be swabbed with a disinfectant before treatment.

Aids in rubber dam placement

Punching and positioning of holes. The rubber dam may be divided into four equal quadrants and the placement of the hole estimated according to the tooth under treatment. The more distal the tooth, the closer to the center is the placement of the hole. This method becomes easier as the clinician gains experience. An alternate method involves the use of a template (Fig. 4-15). The template enables the assistant, as well as the dentist, to position the hole accurately. The hole must be punched cleanly, without tags or tears. If the dam is torn, it may leak or permit continued tearing when stretched for application to the tooth.

Preventing bunching of the dam. To prevent bunching of the dam in the occlusal embrasure, only the edge of the interseptal portion of the dam is teased between the teeth. Dental floss is then used to carry the dam through the contacts. These contacts should always be tested with dental floss before the dam is placed.

Leakage. If small tears or holes do occur, they may be patched with an application of Orabase or Cavit. When abutment teeth of a fixed bridge are being isolated, peridontal packing may be used around the clamp and dam to prevent leakage.

Correct orientation of the dam. Two holes may be punched in the top of the dam before it is placed. These holes serve as reference points for the proper repositioning of the dam when the frame has been removed for exposing x-ray films. This prevents twisting and wrinkling of the

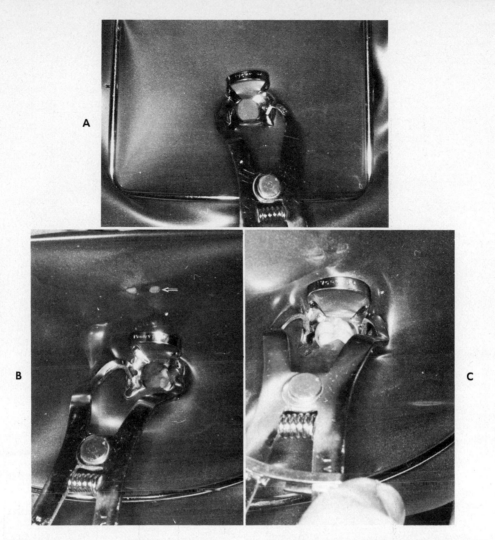

FIG. 4-12. A, Clamp positioned in the dam and held in place with the rubber dam forceps. **B** and **C,** Dam, clamp, and frame carried to the mouth as one unit and placed over the tooth. Holes in the top of the dam *(arrow)* serve as reference points for repositioning the dam on the frame.

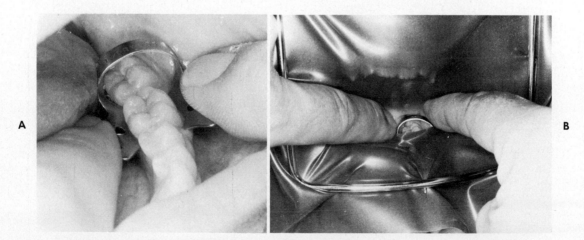

FIG. 4-13. A, Clamp positioned on the tooth and tested for a secure fit with gentle finger pressure alternately on the buccal and lingual aspects of the clamp apron. **B,** The dam is then positioned on the frame and gently stretched over the clamped tooth with the index finger of each hand.

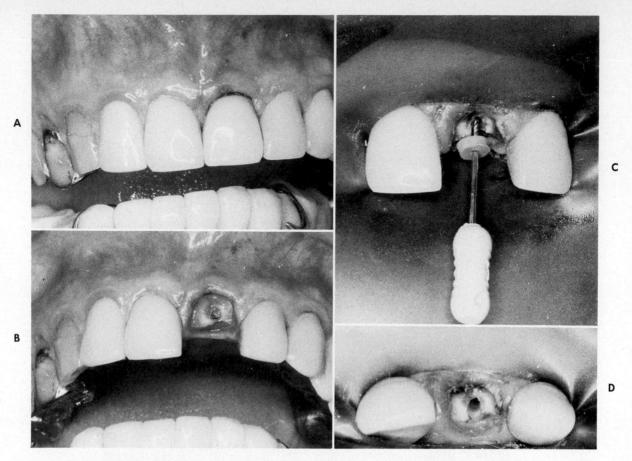

FIG. 4-14. A, Maxillary central incisor with a horizontal fracture through the cervical line. B, Appearance after removal of the coronal fragment. C, Cotton roll in place in the mucobuccal fold and rubber dam stretched over the two adjacent teeth. D, Appearance after pulp extirpation.

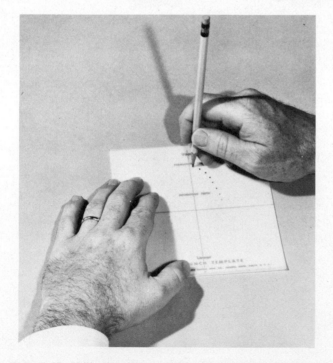

FIG. 4-15. Utilization of a template for correct positioning of holes in the rubber dam. (Courtesy Hygienic Corp., Akron, Ohio.)

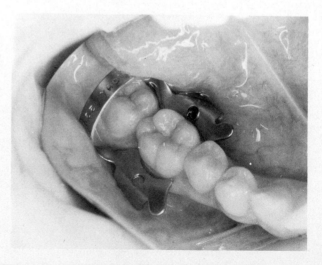

FIG. 4-16. Four-point contact between the jaws of the clamp and the tooth.

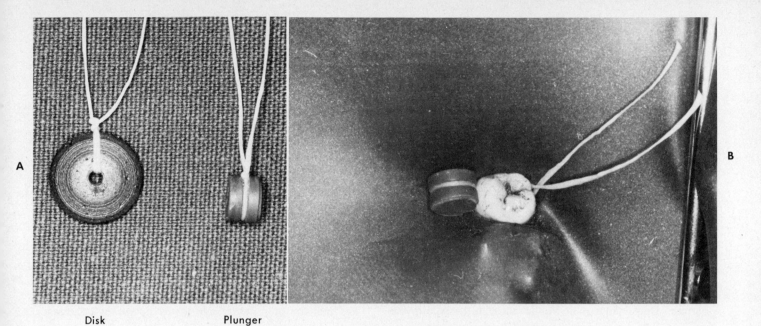

Disk   Plunger

FIG. 4-17. A, Beads may be made from a used rubber polishing disk and from the rubber plunger of an anesthetic carpule. **B,** A bead positioned on the lingual aspect of the tooth, securing the rubber dam in place.

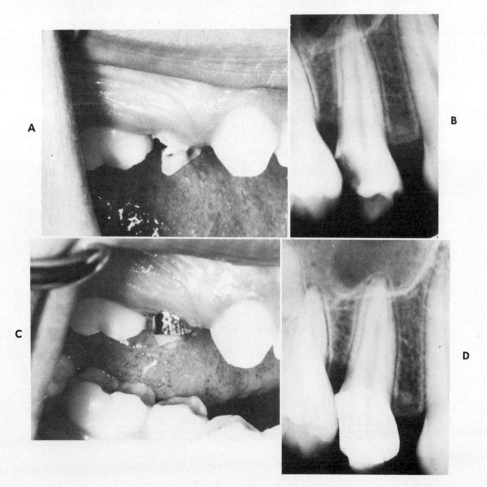

FIG. 4-18. A, Extensive carious destruction of the crown of a maxillary premolar. **B,** Note the carious involvement. **C,** Preformed contoured band adapted and cemented to the remaining crown. **D,** Band in place. (Courtesy Dr. Frank B. Trice.)

dam when it is repositioned on the frame (Fig. 4-12, *B* and *C*).

Correct seating of the clamp. Four-point contact of the rubber dam clamp against the tooth to be isolated must be confirmed (Fig. 4-16).

Situations requiring special handling

Occasionally a tooth may require modification or special preparation to facilitate dam placement. These circumstances result from unusual tooth position or shape, excessive loss of tooth structure from caries or trauma, and overgrowth of gingival tissues.

Unusual tooth position or shape. Certain teeth do not conform to the variety of clamps available. Aside from the customizing of standard clamps, an alternate method may be employed.

Ireland[20] refers to this as the bead method. The "bead" may be the type found on a woman's necklace, a rubber polishing disk, or the rubber plunger from an anesthetic carpule. Dental floss is tied either through the hole in the bead or disk or around the rubber plunger, leaving the two ends of floss long enough to encompass the tooth. The bead is positioned on the lingual side of the tooth, and the two ends of floss are tied securely on the buccal side. The dam is then placed over the tooth and under the bead (Fig. 4-17).

Loss of tooth structure. If insufficient tooth structure prevents the placement of a clamp, a preformed contoured band or a temporary crown may be cemented over the remaining natural crown. Not only will the band or crown enable the clamp to be successfully retained, but it will also serve as a seal for the retention of intracanal medication and the temporary filling. Because of the availability of numerous sizes and shapes of preformed bands, adaptation time is minimal (Fig. 4-18).

Occasionally there is so little remaining tooth structure that even band placement is not possible. In these cases it is necessary to replace the missing tooth structure to facilitate placement of the rubber dam clamp and prevent leakage into the pulp cavity during the course of treatment.

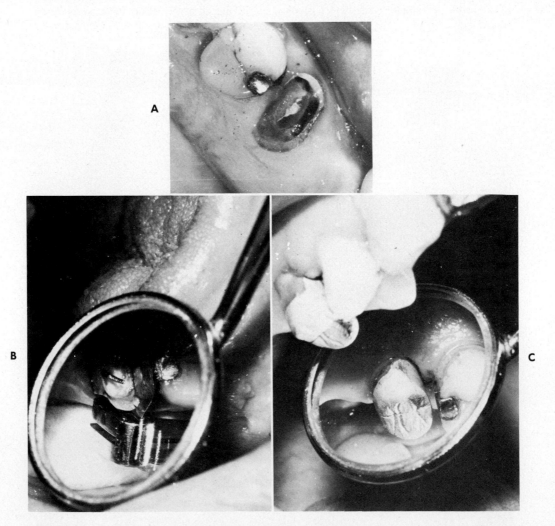

FIG. 4-19. A, Maxillary premolar with extensive destruction of coronal tooth structure. **B,** Pin placement and matrix retainer positioned for amalgam buildup. **C,** Completed amalgam buildup ready for rubber dam clamp placement. (Courtesy Dr. Fred Simmons).

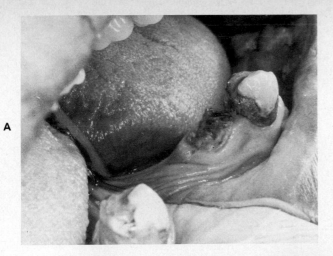

FIG. 4-20. **A,** Mandibular second premolar with extensive carious destruction of the crown and overgrowth of the surrounding gingiva. **B,** Immediately after gingivoplasty with a scalpel to expose additional tooth structure. **C,** Increased exposure of tooth structure allowed for rubber dam isolation.

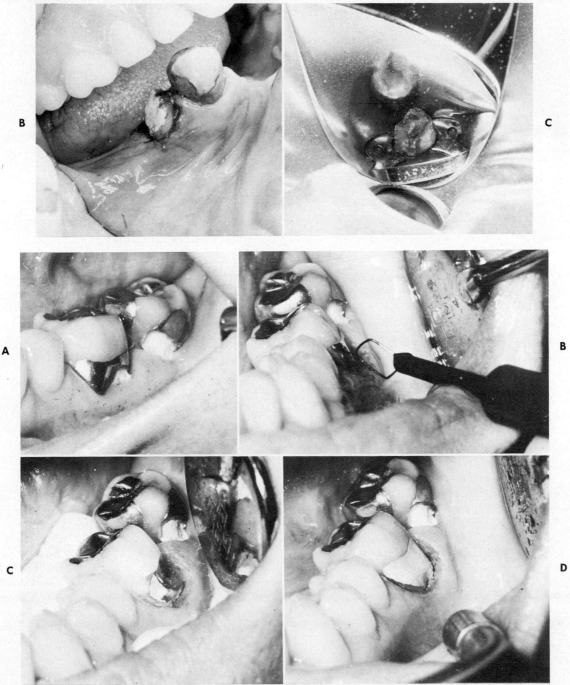

FIG. 4-21. **A,** Class V lesion extending below the marginal gingiva. **B,** Removal of the marginal gingiva with electrosurgery to expose the lesion. **C,** Exposure of the lesion with complete hemostasis, providing unobstructed access to seal off the exposed pulp. **D,** Completed amalgam restoration. (Courtesy Dr. Fred Simmons.)

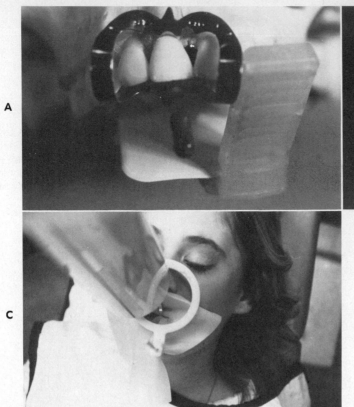

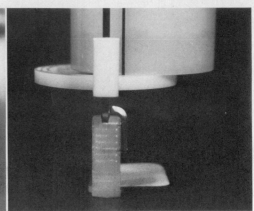

FIG. 4-22. **A,** Placement of a bite block on the tooth adjacent to the rubber dam clamp. **B,** Placement of the film off center in the bite block. **C,** Alignment of the x-ray cone.

This can be accomplished with pin-retained amalgam restorations (Fig. 4-19), composites, or crown and bridge cement.

Interference of gingival tissue. As a result of excessive crown destruction or incomplete eruption, the presence of gingival tissue may preclude the use of a clamp without gingival impingement. In such instances a gingivectomy or gingivoplasty procedure, utilizing either a scalpel or electrosurgery, is indicated (Fig. 4-20).

The latter method offers the advantage of leaving a virtually bloodless site for immediate rubber dam placement. Electrosurgery and electrosurgical equipment have become highly sophisticated. Machinery that delivers fully rectified current of undamped waveform is now available. These units are capable of providing cutting and coagulating currents that, when used properly, will not cause cellular coagulation.[25] The wide variety of sizes and shapes of surgical electrodes enables the clinician to reach areas inaccessible to the traditional scalpel. Furthermore, electrosurgery facilitates the removal of unwanted tissue in such a manner as to recreate normal gingival architecture. This, combined with controlled hemostasis, makes the "radioknife" extremely useful in the preparation of some teeth for placement of the rubber dam clamp (Fig. 4-21).

Interference of the rubber dam clamp with placement of the film. Variations in the use of the extension cone paralleling (EXP) device can prevent displacement of the rubber dam clamp and increase periapical coverage

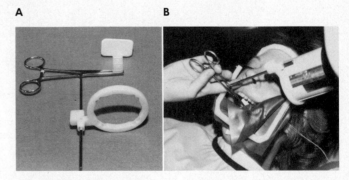

FIG. 4-23. **A,** Components of Crawford Film Holder System; Kelly hemostat with aiming rod attached, aiming ring, and bite block. **B,** Patient maintains position of film by holding handle of attached hemostat (note that bite block is not used when rubber dam clamp is in place). (**A** courtesy C.F.H. Co., Fort Worth, Texas.)

during endodontic procedures.* The film is placed off center in the bite block and the cone is similarly placed off center with respect to the aiming ring. This allows for placement of the bite block adjacent to the rubber dam clamp without altering the parallel relation of the cone to the film (Fig. 4-22).

---

*The extension cone paralleling technique uses Rinn's extension paralleling instrument.

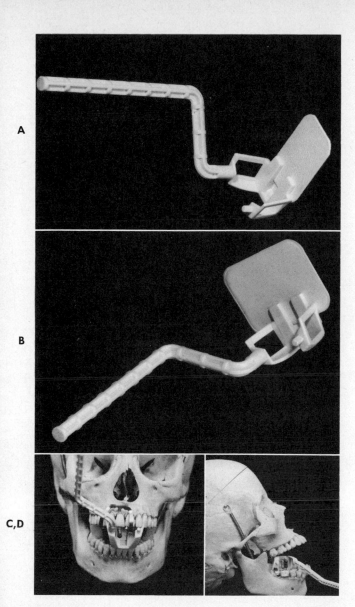

FIG. 4-24. A and **B,** Endo Ray anterior and posterior film holders. **C** and **D,** Anterior and posterior film holders in place over the rubber dam clamp. Handle aids in determining cone position and angulation. (**A** and **B** courtesy Demac, Ltd., St. Charles, Ill.)

Other specialized film holders have been disigned to assist the dentist in securing parallel "working films" with the rubber dam clamp in place. These holders generally have in common an x-ray beam guiding device for proper beam-film relationship and a modified bite block and film holder for proper positioning over or around the rubber dam clamp (Figs. 4-23 and 4-24).

REFERENCES

1. Ardran, C.M.: Bone destruction not demonstrable by radiograph, Br. J. Radiol. **24**: 107, 1951.
2. Arens, D.E.: Endodontic surgery, New York, 1981, Harper & Row, Publishers, Inc.
3. Barr, J.H., and Gron, P.: Palatal contour as a limiting factor in intraoral x-ray technique, Oral Surg. **12**:459, 1959.
4. Barr, J.H., and Stephens, R.G.: Dental radiology, Philadelphia, 1980, W.B. Saunders Co.
5. Bender, I.B., and Seltzer, S.: Roentgenographic and direct observation of experimental lesions in bone, parts I and II, J. Am. Dent. Assoc. **62:** 152, 708, 1961.
6. Bhaskar, S.N.: Radiographic interpretation for the dentist, ed 3. St. Louis, 1979, The C.V. Mosby Co.
7. Brynolf, I.: A histologic and roentgenological study of the periapical region of upper incisors, Odont. Revy. **18** (suppl. 11):7, 1967.
8. Brynolf, I.: Radiography of the periapical region as a diagnostic aid. I. Diagnosis of marginal changes, Dent. Radiogr. Photogr. **51**:21, 1978.
9. Brynolf, I.: Radiography of the periapical region as a diagnostic aid. II. Diagnosis of pulp-related changes, Dent. Radiogr. Photogr. **52**:25, 1979.
9a. Cohen, S., and Schwartz, S.: Endodontic complications and the law, J. Endod., 1987. (In press.)
10. Cragg, I.K.: The use of rubber dam in endodontics, J. Can. Dent. Assoc. **38**:376, 1972.
11. Elfenbaum, A.: Alveolar lamina dura, Dent. Radiogr. Photogr. **31**:21, 1958.
12. Ennis, L.M., Berry, H.M., and Phillips, J.E.: Dental roentgenology, Philadelphia, 1967, Lea & Febiger.
13. Gratt, B.M.: Xeroradiography of dental structures. III. Pilot clinical studies, Oral Surg. **48**:276, 1979.
14. Gratt, B.M., Sickles, E.A., and Nguyen, N.T.: Dental xeroradiography for endodontics: a rapid x-ray system that produces high quality images, J. Endod. **5**:266, 1979.
15. Gratt, B.M., Sickles, E.A., and Parks, C.P.: Xeroradiography of dental structures. II. Image analysis, Oral Surg. **46**:156, 1978.
16. Gratt, B.M., et al.: Xeroradiography of dental structures. IV. Image properties of a dedicated intra-oral system, Oral Surg. **50**:572, 1980.
17. Grossman, L.I.: Prevention in endodontic practice, J. Am. Dent. Assoc. **82**:395, 1971.
18. Ingle, J.I., Beveridge, E.E., and Olson, C.: Rapid processing of endodontic "working films," Oral Surg. **19**:101, 1965.
19. Ingram, F.L.: Radiology of the teeth and jaws, London, 1950, Edward Arnold (Publishers), Ltd.
20. Ireland, L.: The rubber dam—its advantages and application, Tex. Dent. J. **80**:6, 1962.
21. Jeromin, L.S., et al.: Xeroradiography for intra-oral dental radiology, Oral Surg. **49**:178, 1980.
22. Karen, K., and Wuehrmann, A.H.: Manual on radiation protection in hospitals and general practice, vol. 4, Geneva, 1977, World Health Organization.
23. Leff, G.S., Schwartz, S.F., and del Rio, C.E.: Xeroradiographic interpretation of experimentally induced jaw lesions, J. Endod. **10**:188, 1984.
24. Manson, J.lD.: The lamina dura, Oral Surg. **16**:432, 1963.
25. Oringer, M.J.: Electrosurgery in dentistry, ed. 2, Philadelphia, 1975, W.B. Saunders Co.
26. Pauls, V., and Trott, J.R.: A radiological study of experimentally produced lesions in bone, Dent. Pract. **16**:254, 1966.
27. Philips, J.D.: Dental x-rays: a justifiable public concern? J. Ky. Dent. Assoc. **25**:11, 1973.
28. Prichard, J.F.: Advanced periodontal disease: surgical and prosthetic management, Philadelphia, 1965, W.B. Saunders Co.
29. Ramadan, A.E., and Mitchell, D.F.: A roentgenographic study of experimental bone destruction, Oral Surg. **15**:934, 1962.
30. Richards, A.G.: Roentgen-ray doses in dental roentgenography, J. Am. Dent. Assoc. **56**:35, 1958.
31. Schwartz, S.F., and Foster, J.K.: Roentgenographic interpretation of experimentally produced boney lesions, part I, Oral Surg. **32**:606, 1971.
32. White, S.C., Stafford, M.L., and Boeninga, L.R.: Intraoral xeroradiography, Oral Surg. **46**:862, 1978.
33. Wuehrmann, A.H., and Manson-Hing, L.R.: Dental radiology, ed. 5, St. Louis, 1981, The C.V. Mosby Co.

Self-Assessment Questions

1. A well-organized case presentation identifying the patient's needs, the general procedures, and the desired outcome will
   a. Ensure the success of the proposed treatment
   b. Establish a positive relationship between the patient and the clinician
   c. Usually make the patient more apprehensive toward root canal therapy
   d. Eliminate the need for providing printed material describing endodontic therapy

2. The right-angle (paralleling) technique of film and cone placement is favored over the bisecting-angle technique because
   a. The object-film distance can be decreased
   b. Vertical angulation on maxillary placement is greater
   c. The resulting tooth image will have less distortion
   d. The x-rays are projected parallel to the film

3. To correct the superimposition of the zygomatic arch over the apical area of roots, it is suggested to
   a. Increase the vertical angulation of the beam
   b. Change the horizontal angulation by 20 degrees
   c. Increase the kilovoltage to improve contrast
   d. Increase the object-film distance with the paralleling technique

4. Films exposed at higher kilovoltage are preferred for diagnostic value because the shorter wave lengths
   a. Result in a greater degree of discrimination between images
   b. Produce a "short scale" contrast of images
   c. Allow for less tissue penetration than the long wave length
   d. Produce films that are easier to read

5. Radiographic evidence of bone destruction can be detected when
   a. The radiograph is properly exposed and processed
   b. The cancellous bone is resorbed in the periapical area
   c. Controlled time-temperature developing is employed
   d. Erosion of the internal or external bone cortex occurs

6. The radiographic integrity (continuity) of the lamina dura
   a. Is evidence of a healthy pulp
   b. Depends on the shape and position of the root relative to the x-ray beam
   c. Indicates the need for root canal therapy
   d. Is demonstrated by a thin dark image bordering the alveolus

7. According to the buccal object rule and a mesial-to-distal horizontal angulation of the x-ray cone, the image of
   a. The mesial-buccal canal will be mesial to the image of the mesial-lingual canal
   b. The distal-buccal canal will be mesial to the image of the distal-lingual canal
   c. The mesial-buccal canal will be distal to the image of the mesial-lingual canal
   d. The mesial-buccal canal will overlay the image of the mesial-lingual canal

8. A radiolucency that is commonly misinterpreted as a pulpo-periapical lesion is
   a. The mental foramen
   b. The mandibular foramen
   c. The mental synthesis
   d. The mylohyoid ridge

9. Endodontic procedures are associated with multiple radiograph exposures. Therefore, the clinician must
   a. Assure the patient that x-rays contain no radiation
   b. Minimize whole-body (somatic) exposure
   c. Utilize slower-speed films for better images
   d. Use a closed-ended cone for patient safety

10. The use of the rubber dam is
    a. Complicated and time consuming
    b. Highly undesirable for most patients
    c. Recommended particularly for posterior teeth
    d. Axiomatic in root canal therapy

11. To place the rubber dam, clamp, and frame in one motion, the clinician must use a
    a. Winged clamp
    b. Butterfly clamp
    c. Wingless clamp
    d. Gingival retraction clamp

12. To avoid placing a clamp on an anteior tooth restored with porcelain or acrylic crowns, the clinician may
    a. Elect to use no rubber dam
    b. Place the clamp on gingival tissue
    c. Use the split-dam technique
    d. Remove the crown prior to treatment

13. A quick and efficient method of patching a leak in a rubber dam is by using
    a. A silk suture
    b. Cavit or Orabase
    c. Cavity varnish
    d. Clamp adjustment

14. When gingival tissue interferes with rubber dam placement, it is recommended to
    a. Extract the tooth as untreatable
    b. Place the clamp on the gingival tissue
    c. Retract the gingiva with caustic materials
    d. Perform a gingivectomy or gingivoplasty first

5

ENDODONTIC ARMAMENTARIUM AND STERILIZATION

ROBERT E. AVERBACH
DONALD J. KLEIER

Armamentarium

ROBERT E. AVERBACH

Faster, cleaner and smoother root canal preparations

The most effective glutaraldehyde disinfectant

An exciting new breakthrough in technology

The most significant advance in endodontics in over 65 years

These quotes from recent dental advertising graphically demonstrate the furious pace at which new endodontic instruments, materials, and techniques are currently being introduced. The number of endodontic cases performed each year continues to increase in quantum leaps. As endodontic therapy becomes a steadily more routine part of general dental practice, the clinician is bombarded with an assortment of new products designed to make treatment faster and more effective. The age of high technology has arrived in endodontics, and this chapter will provide an overview of contemporary trends, describing the most current endodontic armamentarium. The explosion of knowledge and concern in the area of clinical asepsis and infection control will be detailed in the second part of this chapter.

All the technologic advances and manufacturer's marketing messages cannot replace careful attention to basic biologic principles of high-quality endodontic treatment. Technical advances must be supported with sound experimental and clinical evidence if endodontics is to continue to make strides as a scientific discipline. The keynote of the contemporary endodontic armamentarium is the acronym KISSS—"Keep It Simple, Streamlined, and Sterile." Effective organization will minimize frustration and expedite treatment.

RADIOGRAPHS

A high-quality preoperative radiograph is critical prior to initiation of endodontic treatment. As described in Chapter 4, the paralleling technique, utilizing special film holders, produces radiographs with minimal image distortion. Tooth length measurements and diagnostic information from the radiograph tend to be more accurate when the paralleling technique is used.

The radiographs obtained during endodontic treatment pose a different set of problems. These views include root length determination, verification of filling cone placement, and other procedures in which the rubber dam is in place. The rubber dam may make the positioning of these "working" radiographs more difficult. A variety of film holders have recently been introduced to overcome radiograph distortion problems (Figs. 4-22 to 4-24). All these devices are specifically designed to aid in the placement of the film and tube head in proper relationship to the tooth undergoing endodontic treatment. These devices are of considerable value in obtaining an accurate and distortion-free "working film" with files or filling points protruding from the tooth and with the rubber dam in place.

The choice of dental x-ray film for endodontic radiographs should be limited to Ultraspeed* and Ektaspeed.* Although Ektaspeed is twice as fast and consequently requires one-half the x-ray exposure, it is reported to be more grainy and less sharp in imaging characteristics compared to Ultraspeed film.[22] In a subsequent double-blind clinical trial utilizing endodontic patients in a dental school clinic, 30 dentists were asked to rate the two films by judging identical endodontic views, mounted side-by-side. These raters judged Ultraspeed film superior to Ektaspeed film in terms of contrast, image quality, and rater satisfaction.[27]

Variations in film processing for endodontics have been described in Chapter 4. Once the film has been exposed and processed, careful viewing and interpretation will yield the most information. The clinician's ability to discern subtle variations in the radiograph will be enhanced

---

*Eastman Kodak Co., Rochester, N.Y.

by two factors: magnification and peripheral light shielding. Any high-quality magnifying glass of 2 to 5 power will often clarify an extra canal or hard-to-visualize apex. The use of a cutout of black construction paper on the viewbox will effectively mask peripheral light and permit the perception of subtle differences in film density (Fig. 5-1).

DIAGNOSIS

The armamentarium for diagnosis has been detailed in Chapter 1. The technology of pulp testing continues to become more sophisticated and reliable. Examination techniques for disclosing tooth fractures with a fiberoptic light source also have been shown in Chapter 1. This transillumination technique is also of value in determining the extent of a pulpal "blush" following extensive tooth preparation. The operatory lights are dimmed, and the transilluminator is placed on the lingual surface of the preparation (Fig. 5-2).

The technique of detecting a cracked tooth by wedging

cusps with a cotton roll, round bur head or the equivalent, has been discribed in Chapter 1. An additional wedging modality for the diagnosis of fractured teeth is the "Tooth Slooth,"* pictured in Fig. 5-3. This plastic device is used as a selective wedge on or between the cusps as the patient bites. Sharp pain on *release* of biting pressure often indicates a cracked tooth.

Organization Systems

The trend toward preset trays and towel packs in endodontics has simplified and streamlined the organization, storage, and delivery of endodontic instruments. Particular instruments and tray setups are the choice of the individual clinician, but certain basic principles are common to all systems. A basic tray setup contains most of the commonly used long-handled instruments, such as mouth mirror, endodontic explorer, long spoon excavator, plastic instrument, and locking forceps (Fig. 5-4). This simple pack is often supplemented by a "tub" system containing items such as irrigating syringe and needles, ruler, sterile paper points, burs, and rubber dam clamps. A sample setup is shown in Fig. 5-5. A wide variety of file stands and file boxes are now available, facilitating organizational simplicity and sterility (Fig. 5-6). Whatever system is chosen, the emphasis is on keeping the setup easy for the staff to

*"Tooth Slooth," Encino, Calif.

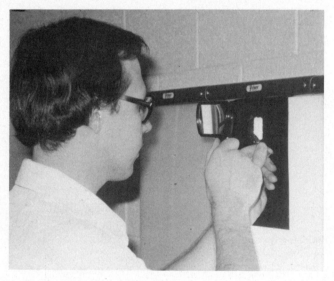

FIG. 5-1. Peripheral light blockout and magnifier for radiographic interpretation.

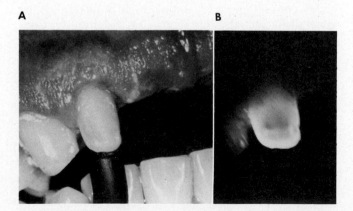

A   **B**

FIG. 5-2. Transillumination of pulpal "blush." **A,** Transilluminator on lingual of full-crown preparation. **B,** Operatory lights out—demonstration of "blush."

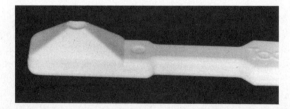

FIG. 5-3. "Tooth Slooth" for detection of a cracked tooth.

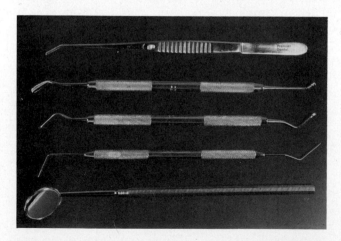

FIG. 5-4. Basic endodontic instruments (from top): locking endodontic forceps (courtesy Premier Dental Products Co., Norristown, Pa.); Woodson plastic instrument (courtesy Hu-Friedy Co., Chicago, Ill.); double-ended long spoon excavator (courtesy Hu-Friedy Co., Chicago, Ill.); DG-16 endodontic explorer (courtesy Hu-Friedy Co., Chicago, Ill.); front-surface mouth mirror.

restock and sterilize and convenient for the clinician, whether working alone or with a chairside assistant.

RUBBER DAM

Rubber dam material for endodontic therapy is currently available in a variety of sizes, colors, and thicknesses—and, yes, even scents! Advocates of the heavy-weight dam prefer its close adaptation to the crown of the tooth under

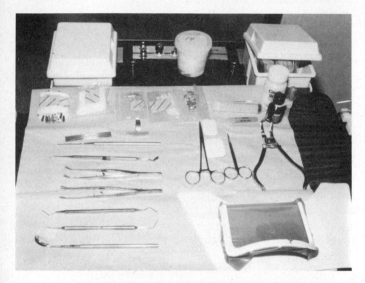

FIG. 5-5. Sample endodontic setup.

treatment and its resistance to tearing. However, many clinicians prefer the medium- or light-weight dam material, citing its increased resilience and ease of application. Color is also a matter of personal preference. Dark-colored dam material provides sharp contrast between the tooth and the dam, while the light-colored dam permits visualization of the x-ray film holder's position when a working radiograph is being exposed. Options include a green dam scented with wintergreen and a royal blue dam, which yields good visual contrast plus "eye appeal." Regardless of which color and thickness are chosen, all dam material should be stored away from strong heat and light to prevent the latex from drying and becoming less flexible. Tearing of the dam upon application usually indicates that the material is dried out and should be discarded. Refrigeration of dam material seems to extend its shelf life.

An almost endless array of rubber dam clamps are available to isolate special problem situations. However, the vast majority of teeth can be isolated by means of the three clamps shown in Fig. 5-7. The winged style of clamp is preferred, since it provides better tissue retraction and allows the use of the "unit" placement technique described in Chapter 4.

Any good-quality rubber dam punch will accomplish the goal of creating a clean hole for the tooth. Care must be taken to punch a hole without "nicks" in the rim, to prevent accidental tearing and leakage. The Ivory-design clamp forceps are preferred in endodontics because they

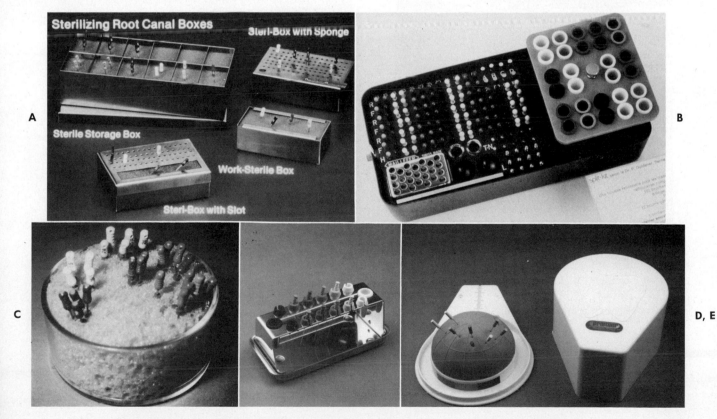

FIG. 5-6. File storage, sterilization, and delivery. **A,** Sterilizing boxes. **B,** Split-Kit. **C,** Banker's sponge. **D,** File stand. **E,** File sponge. (A courtesy Union Broach, New York, N.Y.; **B** courtesy Star Dental Products, Valley Forge, Pa.; **D** and **E** courtesy Premier Dental Products Co., Norristown, Pa.)

allow the dentist to apply gingival force when seating a clamp. This pressure is sometimes needed to engage undercuts on a broken-down tooth, allowing the clamp to be stable. A radiolucent plastic rubber dam frame eliminates the need for removing the frame during the exposure of working radiographs (Fig. 5-8).

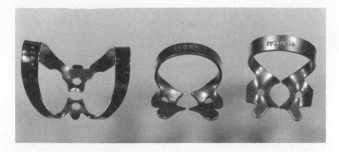

FIG. 5-7. Rubber dam clamps (from left): no. 9—anterior teeth; no. 1—premolar teeth; no. 14—molar teeth.

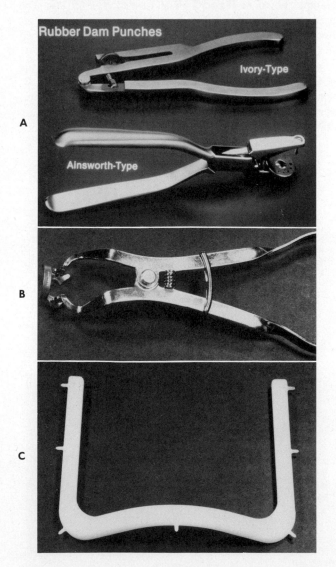

FIG. 5-8. Rubber dam armamentarium. **A,** Rubber dam punches. **B,** Ivory clamp forceps. **C,** Plastic radiolucent rubber dam frame. (**A** courtesy Union Broach Co., New York, N.Y.)

ACCESS PREPARATION THROUGH A CROWN

Gaining access through a porcelain-fused-to-metal crown is more difficult than gaining access through natural tooth structure or other restorative materials. One approach is to use a small round diamond with copious water spray to create the outline form in the porcelain. The metal substructure is then penetrated with either a tungsten-tipped or a new carbide-end-cutting bur (Fig. 5-9). This two-stage technique reduces the possibility of porcelain fracture or chipping.

HAND INSTRUMENTS

A sample setup for endodontics was shown in Fig. 5-5. The long, double-ended spoon excavator is specifically designed for endodontic therapy. It allows the clinician to remove coronal pulp tissue, caries, or cotton pellets that may be deep in the tooth's crown. The double-ended endodontic explorer is used to locate and probe the orifice of the root canal as it joins the pulp chamber. Locking en-

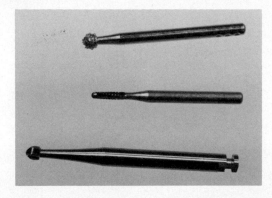

FIG. 5-9. Burs for endodontic access (from top): high-speed round diamond; high-speed no. 1557; surgical-length round bur.

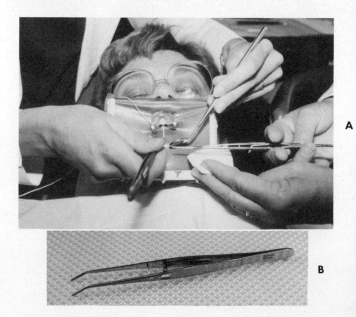

FIG. 5-10. **A,** Four-handed paper point transfer with locking forceps. **B,** Locking endodontic forceps. (Courtesy Premier Dental Products Co., Norristown, Pa.)

dodontic forceps facilitate the transfer of paper points and gutta-percha cones from assistant to dentist (Fig. 5-10). Plastic instruments are designed to place and condense temporary restorations (Fig. 5-11). A periodontal probe completes the basic setup.

CANAL PREPARATION

Techniques for determining the ''working length'' of the root canal prior to instrumentation are described in Chapter 7. Various types of silicone stops, special millimeter rulers, and stop dispensers are shown in Figs. 5-12 and 5-13. The use of electronic apex locators as an adjunct to radiographic length determination is still controversial because they are not always accurate, but they are gradually becoming more accepted (Fig. 5-14). As they improve, the accuracy of these devices is becoming more predictable.[6]

Cleaning, shaping, and sealing of the root canal, as described in Chapter 7, are primary components of clinical success.[8] The most commonly used hand instruments in canal preparation are broaches, reamers, and files. The barbed broach is used primarily for the removal of pulp tissue from large canals (Fig. 5-15). The broach is introduced into the canal and rotated to engage the tissue. Because these instruments are fragile and prone to breakage,

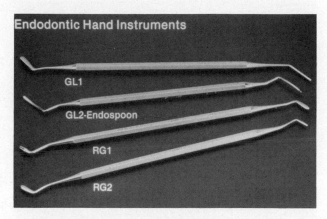

FIG. 5-11 Plastic filling instruments and Endospoon. (Courtesy Union Broach Co., New York, N.Y.)

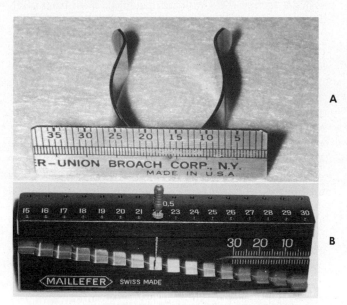

FIG. 5-13. A, Thumb ruler. **B,** Measuring stand.

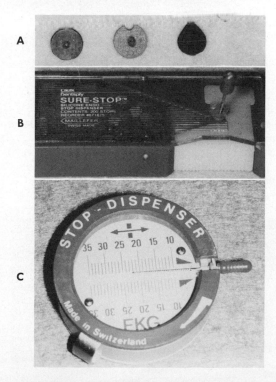

FIG. 5-12. Silicone stops and dispensers. **A,** Round and directionally oriented stops. **B,** Sure-Stop. **C,** Stop dispenser. (**B** courtesy Caulk-Dentsply, Milford, Del.; **C** courtesy Union Broach Co., New York, N.Y.)

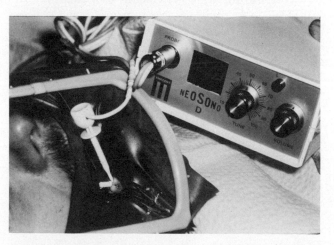

FIG. 5-14. Electronic apex locator in use. (Courtesy Dr. Stephen Cohen.)

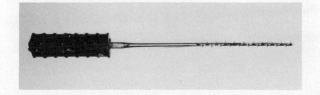

FIG. 5-15. Barbed broach.

great care must be exercised in their use.[18] Variations in reamer and file design have dramatically increased during the past few years. Triangular, square, and rhomboid blanks are usually used in the manufacturing of these hand instruments (Fig. 5-16). Variations in cutting blade angle, degree of twist, flute spacing, and cutting or noncutting tip have complicated the clinician's choice of instruments (Fig. 5-17). A detailed description of these variations will be found in Chapter 13.

The introduction of automated systems for canal preparation is also progressing at a dizzying rate. Mechanical systems such as the Giromatic handpiece have been available for many years and are described in Chapter 7.

The introduction of sonic and ultrasonic systems for canal preparation seems to be a promising development in the endodontic armamentarium.[15] All these devices more or less share certain basic principles that allow the instrument to effectively clean the canal while maintaining the natural root curvature[17] (see Chapter 7). The devices oscillate or vibrate at various frequencies when energized. The energy is then transferred to the intracanal instruments used in cleaning and shaping process. No actual rotation of the instrument is used, thus theoretically preserving the canal shape and natural anatomic constriction as described in Chapter 7. In addition, all the sonic and ultrasonic devices deliver copious streams of irrigant into the canal space during instrumentation, providing enhanced flushing action and debris removal[14] Controversy is still abundant concerning these devices and whether or not they are living up to their proponents' claims.[28]

Rotary instruments are used primarily as flaring devices for the coronal portion of the canal (Fig. 5-18). The two most common are the Gates-Glidden drill and the Peeso drill (Fig. 5-19). Both are sized in increasing diameters from the narrowest no. 1 through the widest no. 6. Both the Gates-Glidden and Peeso should be used in a passive manner to enlarge the canal orifice and flare the prepared root canal. The use of excessive force may either perforate the canal or fracture the instrument. The Gates-Glidden is designed to break high on the shaft if excessive resistance is encountered, allowing the clinician to easily remove the fragment (Fig. 5-20).

IRRIGATION

Irrigation of the canal during instrumentation is described in Chapter 7.

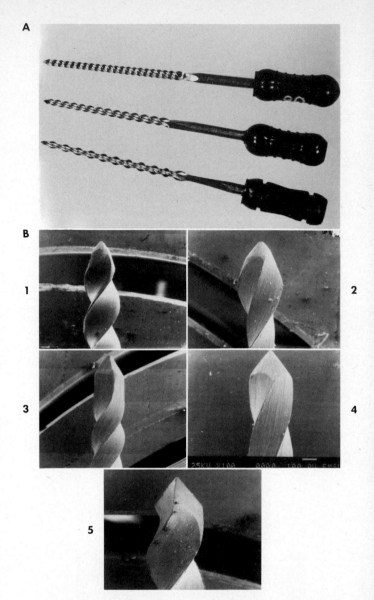

FIG. 5-17. **A,** Variations of K-file design. **B,** Composite scanning electron microscopic view of five different file tips. *1,* Flex R (Union Broach); *2,* K-Flex (Kerr); *3,* Kerr standard; *4,* Maillefer; *5,* Vereinigte Dentalwerke. (**B** Courtesy Union Broach Co., New York, N.Y.)

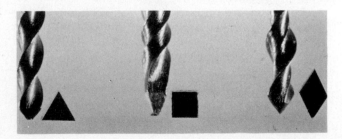

FIG. 5-16. Triangular, square, and rhomboid blanks with resulting instrument shapes. (Courtesy Kerr Manufacturing Co., Romulus, Mich.)

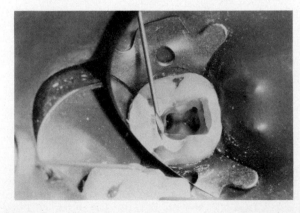

FIG. 5-18. Root canal orifices (seen through a reflector) flared with Gates-Glidden drill. (Courtesy Dr. Stephen Cohen.)

Systems for the delivery of irrigating solution into the root canal range from simple disposable syringes to complex devices capable of irrigating and aspirating simultaneously. The choice for the clinician is one of convenience and cost. The smaller syringe barrels (less than 10 ml) require frequent refilling during the instrumentation phase of therapy. Plastic syringes in the 10- to 20-ml range may offer the best combination of sufficient solution volume and ease of handling. "Back filling" of the syringe from a 500-ml laboratory plastic wash bottle filled with the irrigant of choice will save time and effort, as opposed to aspirating the solution into the barrel from a container (Fig. 5-21). The barrel tip should be a Luer-Lok design rather than friction fit, in order to prevent accidental needle dislodgment during irrigation (Fig. 5-22).

Three basic types of needle tip designs are shown in Fig. 5-

23: the standard beveled hypodermic tip, the notched tip, and the closed tip with lateral perforations. The latter two designs help prevent accidental forcing of irrigating solution into periapical tissues should the needle bind in the canal. Severe reactions have been reported if this occurs.[5]

Various sizes of paper points are available to dry the canal following irrigation. Paper points are used sequentially in the locking forceps until no moisture is evident on the paper point. Presterilized "cell" packaging is preferred over bulk packaging to maintain asepsis (Fig. 5-24).

OBTURATION

Most root canal filling methods employ root canal sealer as an integral part of the obturation technique. The most popular class of sealer-cements used in endodontics is based on zinc oxide–eugenol formulations. These products require a glass slab and cement spatula for mixing to the desired consistency. Two recently introduced products contain calcium hydroxide as a therapeutic ingredient (Fig. 5-25). Reports on the leakage characteristics of these products compared to traditional zinc oxide–eugenol formulations are just beginning to appear in the scientific literature.[38] Root canal obturation techniques are discussed in Chapter 8. Gutta-percha is the most commonly used canal-

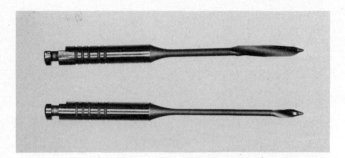

FIG. 5-19. *Top,* No. 5 Peeso drill. *Bottom,* No. 5 Gates Glidden drill. The number of rings on the shank indicate the size of the instrument.

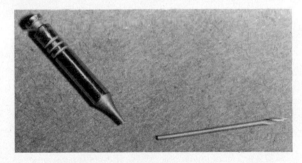

FIG. 5-20. Fractured Gates-Glidden drill.

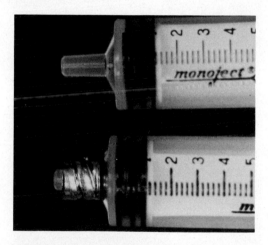

FIG. 5-22. Irrigating syringes. *Top,* Friction-fit tip. *Bottom,* Luer-Lock tip.

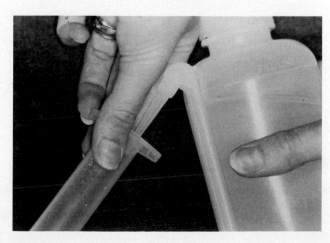

FIG. 5-21. Back-filling of irrigating syringe from wash bottle.

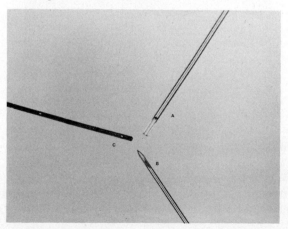

FIG. 5-23. Irrigating needles: *A,* blunt, notched tip; *B,* standard hypodermic; *C,* closed end, perforated.

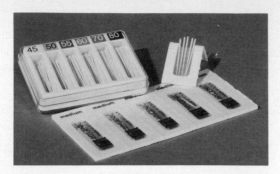

FIG. 5-24. Paper points—bulk versus "cell" packaging. (Courtesy Hygienic Corp., Akron, Ohio.)

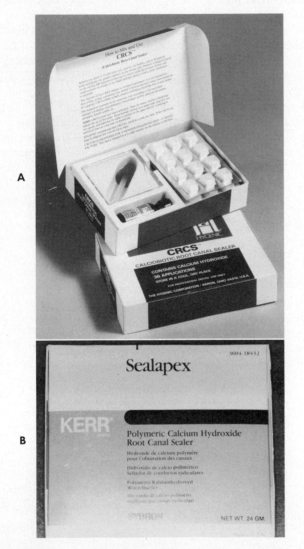

FIG. 5-25. Calcium hydroxide sealers. **A,** CRCS. **B,** Kerr Sealapex. (**A** courtesy of Hygienic Corp., Akron, Ohio.)

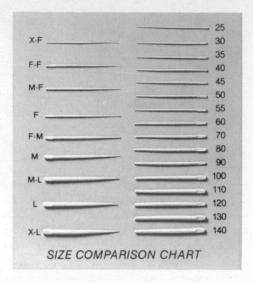

SIZE COMPARISON CHART

FIG. 5-26. Nonstandardized versus standardized gutta-percha cones. (Courtesy Hygienic Corp., Akron, Ohio).

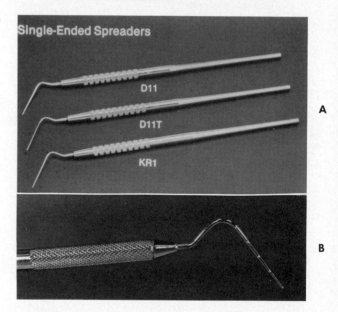

FIG. 5-27. A, Root canal spreaders. **B,** Calibrated root canal plugger. (**A** courtesy Union Broach, New York, N.Y.; **B** courtesy Hu-Friedy, Chicago, Ill.)

filling material in contemporary endodontics. Gutta-percha is available as standardized cones corresponding to the approximate size of root canal instruments (nos. 15 to 140). Nonstandardized cones are more tapered, and are designated in size from extra fine through extra large. The two styles are compared in Fig. 5-26.

Specialized instruments used in obturating the root canal with gutta-percha include spreaders and pluggers (Fig. 5-27). Spreaders are available in a wide variety of lengths and tapers and are used primarily in the lateral condensation technique to compact gutta-percha filling material. Pluggers, also called condensers, are flat ended rather than pointed, and are used primarily to compact filling materials in a vertical fashion.

On the "high-tech" front, devices for the heating, delivery, and compaction of gutta-percha into the prepared root canal have recently become available. A detailed description of these devices is found in Chapter 8; they include the Obtura system by Unitek and the Ultrafil system by Hygienic (Fig. 5-28).

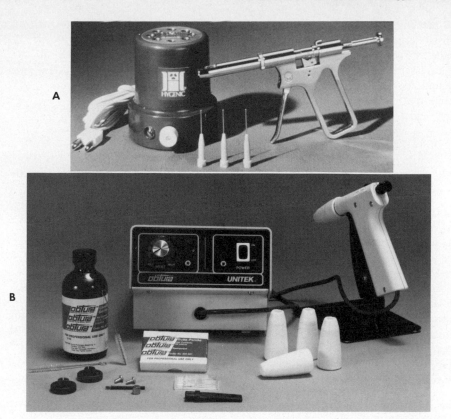

FIG. 5-28. Warm gutta-percha systems. **A,** Ultrafil. **B,** Obtura. (**A** courtesy Hygienic Corp., Akron, Ohio; **B** courtesy Unitek Corp., Monrovia, Calif.)

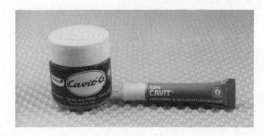

FIG. 5-29. Cavit-G and Cavit temporary filling materials. (Courtesy Premier Dental Products Co., Norristown, Pa.)

Temporary restorative materials used in endodontics must provide a high-quality seal of the access preparation to prevent microbial contamination of the root canal. Premixed products such as Cavit (Fig. 5-29) have become popular for temporary access cavity sealing because of their ease of insertion and removal, plus their demonstrated resistance to marginal leakage when a minimum thickness of 3.5 mm is placed in the preparation.[41]

Sterilization

DONALD J. KLEIER

Dentistry is in the midst of a critical self-examination process concerning office infection control. The dentist and the dental staff may be exposed to serious infectious diseases on a daily basis.[12,29,35] The public is very aware and fearful of contracting acquired immune deficiency syn-

drome (AIDS) or hepatitis, and wants to be reassured that such diseases will not be passed on to them by health practitioners or health care equipment. The purpose of this section is to describe how contaminated endodontic instruments may be safely cleaned and sterilized in order to prevent cross infection of dentists and their patients.

The two diseases of greatest concern to the dentist and the dental staff are AIDS and hepatitis B. AIDS is transmitted by the retrovirus HTLV III (human t-lymphotrophic virus type III.[19] There is evidence that this agent is transmitted through blood and other body fluids.[36] Hepatitis B is caused by the hepatitis B virus (HBV), which can be transmitted through blood or blood products and a variety of other body fluids including saliva. The carrier state of hepatitis B develops in 5% to 10% of patients, commonly following an asymptomatic infection. Estimates are that 800,000 hepatitis B carriers live in the United States today.[11] In a 1978 epidemiologic study of endodontists, Goldstein[23] found serologic evidence that 9% of the endodontists tested had a history of hepatitis B infection. Most could not recall any symptoms associated with their infections. In another study, 13% of dentists in general were found to have a history of hepatitis B infection.[32] The hepatitis B virus, the herpes simplex virus, and numerous pathogenic bacteria can infect the dentist or be passed on through the dentist to family and friends. Many diseases can be spread unknowingly by asymptomatic carriers or by patients who knowingly withhold information when completing their medical histories.

The dentist has the responsibility to thoroughly understand disease transmission and prevent cross infection. Knowing how to handle and sterilize contaminated endodontic instruments is an essential part of this responsibility. The American Dental Association and its Council on Denta Therapeutics state that all instruments coming into contact with blood or saliva must be *sterilized* or discarded.[1,3]

DEFINITION OF TERMS

The purpose of this section is to help clarify certain terms that are used in reference to office infection control.

sterilization The use of a physical or chemical procedure to destroy all microbial life, including highly resistant bacterial endospores. Sterilization is a verifiable procedure.

disinfection A less lethal process than sterilization. It eliminates virtually all pathogenic vegetative microorganisms, but not necessarily all microbial forms (e.g., spores). This process usually is reserved for large environmental surfaces that cannot be sterilized (e.g., a dental chair). Disinfection lacks the margin of safety achieved by sterilization procedures. Disinfection is nonverifiable.

carrier A person who has had a disease and recovered but who retains the pathogenic organism, potentially causing disease in another person

bacterial vegetative form Active, multiplying microorganisms

bacterial spore form (endospore) A more complex structure than the vegetative cell from which it forms. Spores form in response to environmental conditions and are more highly resistant to sterilization methods than vegetative forms.

virus An extremely small agent that grows and reproduces only in living host cells. The virus particle consists of a central core of nucleic acid and an outer coat of protein. It is generally agreed that virus particles are much *less* resistant to thermal inactivation than bacterial spores.[7]

pathogenic microorganisms A microorganism that causes or is associated with disease

cross infection Transmission of infectious material from one person to another

biologic indicator A preparation of microorganisms, usually bacterial spores, that serves as a challenge to the efficiency of a given sterilization process or cycle. Negative bacterial growth from a biologic indicator verifies sterilization.

process indicator Strips, tapes, or tabs applied to or packaged in a sterilizer load. Special inks or chemicals within the indicator change color when subjected to heat, steam, or chemical vapor and indicate that the load has been cycled through the sterilizer. Process indicators do *not* verify sterilization.

INSTRUMENT PREPARATION

The postoperative handling, cleaning, and packaging of contaminated instruments is frequently a source of injury and possible infection. Dental staff members performing such procedures should wear reusable heavy rubber work gloves similar to household cleaning gloves.[1] Contaminated instruments that will not be cleaned immediately should be placed in a holding solution so that blood, saliva, and tissue will not dry on the instrument surfaces. A basin of ultrasonic cleaner detergent or iodophor solution is an effective holding solution.

An ultrasonic cleaner (Fig. 5-30), which is many times

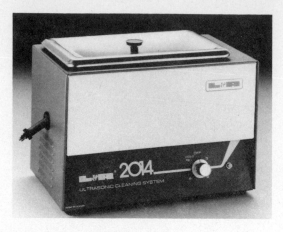

FIG 5-30. Ultrasonic cleaner. (Courtesy L & R Co., Kearny, N.J.)

more effective and safer than hand scrubbing, should be used for definitive instrument cleaning. Ultrasonic cleaners produce high-frequency vibrations that induce the rapid formation and collapse of microscopic cavities in a liquid medium. This cavitation produces hydraulic shocks, which are responsible for the cleaning action of these machines. Instruments cleaned in an ultrasonic device should be suspended in a perforated basket. Machines with the greatest efficiency have plastic lids and baskets with polished stainless steel bottoms. When an ultrasonic cleaner is on, nothing should come into contact with the tank's bottom and its lid should be in place.[20] The cleaner should be run for at least 5 minutes per load. Once the cycle is complete, the clean instruments are rinsed under a high volume of cool water, placed on a clean dry towel and rolled or patted and then air dried. The ultrasonic solution should be discarded daily, and the tub of the ultrasonic machine cleaned. The contaminated instruments are now clean but not sterile. Continued precautions are necessary until the instruments have been sterilized.

When precleaning of instruments may be hazardous, such as when instruments have been contaminated with hepatitis B virus, the contaminated instruments may be presterilized prior to cleaning.[3] Stainless steel instruments may be placed in a tray containing hot trisodium phosphate solution (1 tablespoon per quart of hot water) to cover them while they are autoclaved. The steam should then be discharged rapidly after the sterilization cycle. The sterile instruments will now be ready for more thorough cleaning and resterilization.

Clean instruments ready for sterilization should be packaged in containers designed for the specific sterilization process to be employed (Fig. 5-31). The sterilizing agent must be able to penetrate the instrument package and come into intimate contact with microorganisms.

METHODS OF STERILIZATION

The oldest and most reliable agent for destroying microorganisms is heat. The most commonly used means of sterilization in endodontic practice include steam under pressure, chemical vapor, prolonged dry heat, intense dry heat, and glutaraldehyde solutions. Ethylene oxide gas will

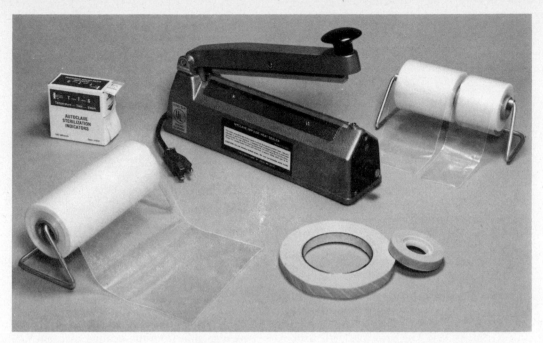

FIG. 5-31. Instrument packaging system. (Courtesy The Lorvic Co., St. Louis, Mo.)

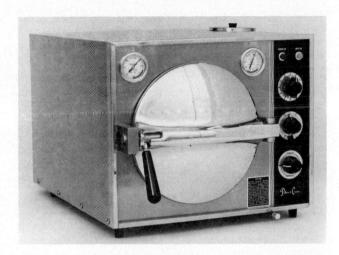

FIG. 5-32. Autoclave. (Courtesy Pelton & Crane Co., Charlotte, N.C.)

be briefly discussed but is not practical for most dental office environments.

Steam under pressure

The steam autoclave (Fig. 5-32) is considered the most common method of sterilization except when penetration is limited or heat and moisture damage is a problem. Moist heat kills microorganisms through protein coagulation, RNA and DNA breakdown, and release of low-molecular-weight intracellular constituents.[7] The autoclave sterilizes in 15 to 40 minutes at 121° C (249.8° F), at a pressure of 15 pounds per square inch. The time required depends on the type of load placed in the autoclave and its permeability. Once the entire load has reached temperature 249.8° F (121° C), it will be rendered sterile in 15 minutes. An adequate margin of safety for load warm-up and steam penetration requires an autoclave time of at least 30 minutes. The clinician should always allow more time for load warm-up if any doubt exists. Existing chamber air is the most detrimental factor to efficient steam sterilization. Modern autoclaves utilize a gravity displacement method to evacuate this air, thus providing a fully saturated chamber with no cold or hot spots. Instruments and packages placed in an autoclave must be properly arranged so that the pressurized steam may circulate freely around and through the load. Since recirculation of water tends to concentrate contaminants in an autoclave, only fresh deionized (distilled) water should be used for each cycle.[10] When instruments are heated in a steam autoclave, rust and corrosion can occur. Chemical corrosion inhibitors are commercially available, which will protect sharp instruments.

Advantages

1. Relatively quick turnaround time for instruments.
2. Offers excellent penetration of packages.
3. Will not destroy cotton or cloth products.
4. Sterilization is verifiable.

Disadvantages

1. Materials must be air dried at completion of cycle.
2. Corrosion and dulling of certain materials such as carbon steel. Most stainless steels are resistant to autoclave damage.
3. Certain metal instruments may require antirust pretreatment.

Unsaturated chemical vapor

The 1928 patent of Dr. George Hollenback and the work of Hollenback and Harvey in the 1940s culminated in the development of an unsaturated chemical vapor sterilization system. This system, which utilizes a device that is similar

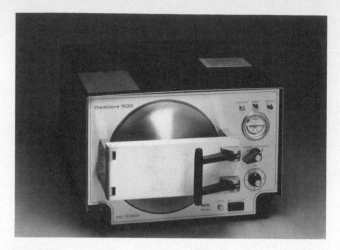

FIG. 5-33. Chemical vapor sterilizer. (Courtesy MDT Co., Gardena, Calif.)

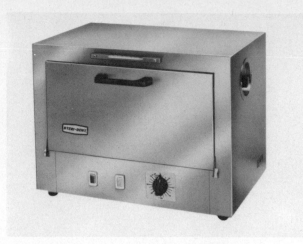

FIG. 5-34. Dry heat sterilizer. (Courtesy Sterident Co., Copiague, N.Y.)

to an autoclave, is named a Harvey Chemiclave or chemical vapor sterilizer (Fig. 5-33). The principle of Chemiclave sterilization is that, while some water is necessary to catalyze the destruction of all microorganisms in a relatively short period of time, water saturation is not necessary. Like the autoclave, chemical vapor sterilization kills microorganisms by destroying vital protein systems. Unsaturated chemical vapor sterilization utilizes a solution containing specific amounts of various alcohols, acetone, ketone, and formaldehyde, and a water content well below the 15% level at which rust and corrosion occur. When the Chemiclave is heated to 132° C (270° F) and pressurized to at least 20 pounds per square inch, sterilization occurs in 20 minutes. As with the autoclave, sterilization in the Chemiclave requires careful arrangement of the load to be sterilized. The vapor must be allowed to circulate freely within the Chemiclave and penetrate instrument wrapping material. Chemiclave solution is not recirculated; a fresh mixture of the solution is used for each cycle. The Chemiclave loses over half of its solution to ambient air as vapor. Although it has been shown that this vapor does not contain formaldehyde and is environmentally safe, the vapor has a definite characteristic odor.[9] Adequate ventilation is a necessity when a chemical vapor sterilizer is being used. A filter unit is available from the manufacturer and is reported to remove the odor of the residual vapors.

Advantages

1. Will not corrode metals.
2. Relatively quick turnaround time for instruments.
3. Load comes out dry.
4. Sterilization is verifiable.

Disadvantages

Vapor odor may be offensive, requiring increased ventilation.

Prolonged dry heat

There are complicating factors associated with sterilization by dry heat. The time and temperature factors may vary considerably, according to heat diffusion, amount of heat available from the heating medium, amount of available moisture present, and heat loss through the heating container's walls. Dry heat kills microorganisms primarily through an oxidation process. Protein coagulation also takes place, depending on the water content of the protein and the temperature of sterilization. Dry-heat sterilization, like chemical vapor and autoclave sterilization, is verifiable. Dry heat is very slow to penetrate instrument loads. Dry heat sterilizes at 160° C (320° F) in 30 minutes, but instrument loads may take 30 to 90 minutes to reach that temperature.[13] A margin of safety requires instruments to be sterilized at 160° C (320° F) for 2 hours. Small dry-heat sterilizers (Fig. 5-34) are available from a number of manufacturers.[34] An internal means of determining and calibrating temperature is an essential component of any dry-heat sterilizer. If the sterilizer has multiple heating elements on different surfaces, together with an internal fan to circulate air, heat transfer becomes much more efficient. It is important that loads be positioned within the dry-heat sterilizer so that they do not touch each other. Instrument cases must not be stacked one upon the other. The hot air must be allowed to circulate freely within the sterilizer.

Mercury vapor in high concentrations can develop in a dry heat sterilizer that has been used to sterilize amalgam instruments. Great care must be exercised to keep scrap amalgam out of any sterilizing device. Once contaminated with mercury or amalgam, a sterilizer will continue to produce mercury vapor for many cycles.

Advantages

1. Large load capability.
2. Complete corrosion protection for dry instruments.
3. Low initial cost of equipment.
4. Sterilization verifiable.

Disadvantages

1. Slow instrument turnaround because of poor heat exchange.

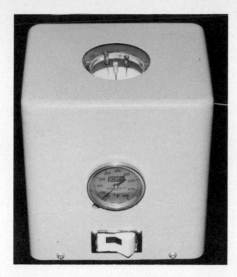

FIG. 5-35. High-temperature endodontic sterilizer. (Courtesy Pulpdent Co. of America, Brookline, Mass.)

2. Sterilization cycles not as exact as moist-heat sterilization.
3. Dry-heat sterilizer must be calibrated and monitored.
4. If sterilizer temperature is too high, instruments may be damaged.

Intense dry heat

Chairside sterilization of endodontic files can be accomplished by using a glass-bead or salt sterilizer (Fig. 5-35). This device is a metal crucible that heats a transfer medium of glass beads or salt. Clean endodontic instruments of small mass are positioned in the transfer medium and allowed to remain for a specific time interval. During this time the transfer medium heats the endodontic instrument through heat convection and kills any adherent microorganisms. At a temperature of 220° C (428° F) contaminated endodontic instruments require 15 seconds to be sterilized. Several studies have shown this method of sterilization to be effective but to have certain limitations.[16,24,42] Endodontic chairside sterilizers often require extensive warm-up times, with some requiring 3 hours to reach full operating temperature. The sterilizers often require calibration adjustment to reach a specific desired temperature. A wide range of temperature gradients may exist within the transfer medium. This process should only be used as a backup to the previously described methods of bulk sterilization.

Advantages

1. Small size and convenience of the sterilizer.
2. Serves as emergency backup to other methods of sterilization.

Disadvantages

1. Only instruments of small mass can be sterilized.
2. Only a few instruments can be sterilized at a time.
3. Sterilization is nonverifiable.

Ethylene oxide gas

Ethylene oxide (ETO) was first used as a sterilizing agent in the late 1940s by the Army Chemical Corps. Since then ETO has become an increasingly popular method of sterilization, especially within the hospital environment. The extreme penetrability of the ETO molecule, together with its effectiveness at low temperatures (70° F to 140° F), make it ideal for sterilizing heat-sensitive materials. Ethylene oxide kills mircoorganisms by chemically reacting with nucleic acids.[7] The basic reaction is alkylation of hydroxyl groups. Sterilization requires several hours, with an extended aeration time for soft goods.

Even though ETO sterilization seems an ideal solution for some dental instruments, such as nonautoclavable handpieces, it is best used in a hospital or strictly controlled environment. Ethylene oxide is thought to be potentially mutagenic and carcinogenic. The use of such a potentially dangerous substance must be weighed against the potential benefits.

Advantages

1. Operates effectively at low temperature.
2. Gas is extremely penetrating.
3. Can be used to sterilize sensitive equipment such as dental handpieces.
4. Sterilization is verifiable.

Disadvantages

1. Gas is potentially mutagenic and carcinogenic.
2. Requires an acration chamber.
3. Cycle time lasts many hours (often overnight).
4. Usually only hospital based.

Glutaraldehyde solutions

Sterilization by heat should always be the first method of choice whenever possible. However, the use of glutaraldehyde preparations (Fig. 5-36) for the chemical sterilization of heat-sensitive equipment has become a widespread practice. Glutaraldehyde kills microorganisms by altering essential protein components.[39] The glutaraldehyde molecule has two active carbonyl groups, which react with proteins through cross-linking reactions. Many 2% aqueous glutaraldehyde solutions are mildly acidic. In the acidic state the glutaraldehyde molecule is stable but not sporicidal. When the glutaraldehyde solution is "activated" by a suitable alkaline buffer, full antimicrobial activity occurs. Unfortunately, when the glutaraldehyde solution is rendered alkaline, a slow polymerization reaction takes place and the glutaraldehyde loses its biocidal capability with time. Because of this polymerization reaction, activated glutaraldehyde solutions in normal clinical practice usually have a shelf life of 14 days. Some new preparations have been formulated at less alkaline pH values or at an acid pH to lower the rate of polymerization and therefore extend the useful life of the solution. In these extended-life products, the addition of a surfactant maintains biocidal activity. There is some evidence that acid glutaraldehydes are less effective sporicides and tend to be more corrosive to instruments.[4]

In clinical practice glutaraldehyde can be used in small

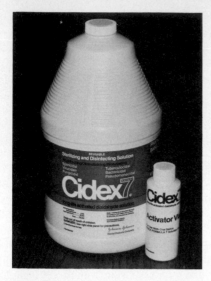

FIG. 5-36. Glutaraldehyde solution with separate alkaline buffer activator. (Courtesy Johnson & Johnson Co., East Windsor, N.J.)

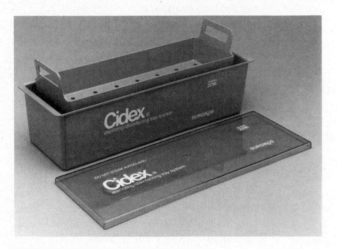

FIG. 5-37. Glutaraldehyde container designed specifically for dental instruments. (Courtesy Johnson & Johnson Co., East Windsor, N.J.)

containers specifically designed to hold dental instruments (Fig. 5-37). The solution should be discarded at least once a week. The biocidal activity of glutaraldehyde may be adversely affected by substandard preparation of "activated" glutaraldehyde, contamination of the solution by protein debris, failure to change the solution at proper time intervals, water dilution of residual glutaraldehyde by washed instruments that have not been dried, and the slow but continuous polymerization of the glutaraldehyde molecule. Indicator strips are now available to help determine what percentage of glutaraldehyde still remains in the solution. Any drop in glutaraldehyde concentration below 2% significantly decreases the biocidal nature of the solution. Instruments contaminated with blood or saliva must remain submerged in glutaraldehyde long enough for spore forms to be killed. Sterilization may require 6 to 10 hours, depending on the product used.

Advantages

1. Can sterilize heat-sensitive equipment.
2. Is relatively noncorrosive and nontoxic.

Disadvantages

1. Requires long immersion time.
2. Has some odor, which may be objectionable, especially if the solution is heated.
3. Sterilization is nonverifiable.
4. Irritating to mucous membranes (e.g., eyes).

Other methods of sterilization

A number of other methods of sterilization are available but at this time are not considered practical for the dental office. These methods either are too expensive or dangerous for dental practice, or have not been developed to a point where they can be used for the routine bulk sterilization of dental instruments. These other means of sterilization include the following:

1. Formaldehyde gas
2. Aqueous solutions of formaldehyde
3. Laser beam
4. Microwave radiation
5. Ultraviolet radiation
6. Gamma rays
7. X-rays
8. Electron bombardment

MONITORING STERILIZATION

Two methods are commonly used to monitor in-office sterilization: process indicators and biologic indicators. Both types of indicators are necessary parts of infection control.

Process indicators are usually strips—tape or paper products marked with special ink that changes color with exposure to heat, steam, chemical vapor, or gas (Fig. 5-38). The ink changes color when the items being processed have been subjected to sterilizing conditions, but a process indicator usually does not monitor the length of time that such conditions were present. There are specific process indicators for different methods of sterilization. The process indicator's main role in infection control is to prevent accidental use of materials that have not been circulated through the sterilizer. A color-change in a process indicator does not ensure proper function of the equipment or that sterilization has been achieved.

Biologic indicators are usually preparations of nonpathogenic bacterial spores that serve as a challenge to a specific method of sterilization (Fig. 5-39). Each method of sterilization is challenged by a spore form that is considered highly resistant to it. In theory, spores are the most difficult life forms to destroy. If a sterilization method destroys spore forms that are highly resistant to that method, then it is logical to assume that all other life forms have also been destroyed. The bacterial spores are usually attached to a paper strip within a biologically protected packet. The spore packet is placed between instrument packages or within an instrument package itself. After the sterilizer has cycled, the spore strip is cultured for a specific time. Lack of culture growth ensures sterility.

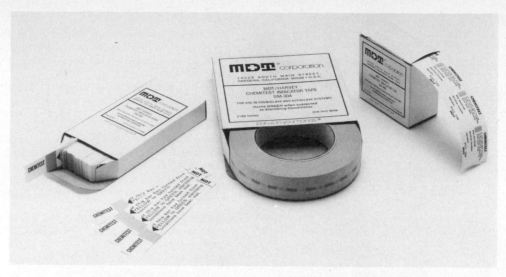

FIG. 5-38. Process indicators. (Courtesy MDT Co., Gardena, Calif.)

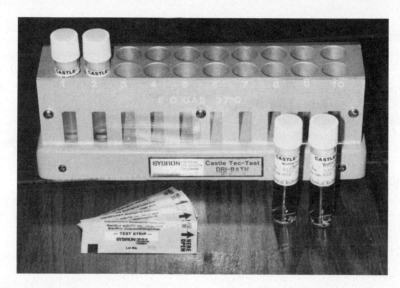

FIG. 5-39. Biologic indicator system consisting of spore packets, culture media, and an incubator.

Every sterilizer load should contain at least one process indicator. A safer method is to attach a process indicator to each item sterilized. Each sterilizer should be checked every 1 or 2 weeks with a biologic indicator to ensure proper functioning of sterilizer equipment and proper loading technique. Records should be maintained, especially of the biologic indicator results.

METHODS OF DISINFECTION

Disinfection, which does not kill spore forms, should be reserved for the wiping down of large surfaces such as cart tops and dental chairs. Solutions of sodium hypochlorite and iodophors are two liquid disinfectants well suited for this purpose. Both of these chemical solutions are broad spectrum and capable of killing many microorganisms. These disinfectants are superior to alcohols, phenolics, and quaternary ammonium compounds. Quaternary ammonium compounds have been judged unacceptable for disinfection

of instruments or environmental surfaces by the American Dental Association.[2]

Sodium hypochlorite, or household bleach, in a dilute solution (¼ cup bleach to 1 gallon tap water) can be used to wipe down environmental surfaces. The surfaces to be disinfected should be kept moist for a minimum of 10 minutes, with 30 minutes being an ideal.[7,13,35] The free chlorine in sodium hypochlorite solutions is thought to inactivate sulfyhdryl enzymes and nucleic acids and to denature proteins. Sodium hypochlorite is very biocidal against bacterial vegetative forms, viruses, and some spore forms. Unfortunately, hypochlorite is corrosive to metals, irritating to skin and eyes, and has a strong odor.

Iodophors are combinations of iodine and a solubilizing agent (Fig. 5-40). When diluted with water, this combination continuously releases a small amount of free iodine. The manufacturer's recommendations for dilution must be strictly followed to achieve the optimal amount of free io-

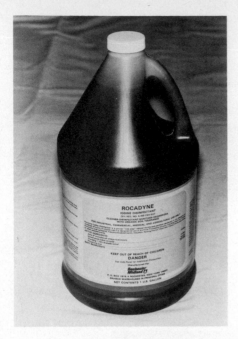

FIG. 5-40. Iodophor concentrate.

dine. Iodophors are inactivated by hard water, heat, and organic contamination. Iodophor solutions have a built-in color indicator that changes when the free iodine molecules have been exhausted. Areas or equipment to be disinfected with iodophors should be kept moist for 10 to 30 minutes. Iodophors are biocidal against vegetative bacteria, viruses, and some spore forms. They are less corrosive to metals and less irritating than hypochlorite. This method of disinfecting offers an effective, practical approach without the problems associated with other disinfectants.[7,13,35]

STERILIZATION OF GUTTA-PERCHA CONES

The sterilization of gutta-percha cones is of great importance in endodontic practice because gutta-percha is the material of choice for root canal obturation. Since this material may come into intimate contact with the periapical tissue during obturation, it should not serve as a vehicle for pathogenic microorganisms. It has been shown that 8% of commercially available gutta-percha cones, when removed from their packages, are contaminated with pathogens.[31] Gutta-percha cannot be heat sterilized and yet requires rapid sterilization chairside. *Immersing gutta-percha cones in 5.25% sodium hypochlorite (full-strength household bleach) for 1 minute is very effective in killing vegetative microorganisms and spore forms.*[21,37]

EFFECT OF REPEATED STERILIZATION ON INSTRUMENTS

Several studies have investigated the effect of repeated sterilization on the physical characteristics of endodontic files.[26,30,33] Repeated sterilization of stainless steel endodontic files by means of any heat method described in this chapter will not cause corrosion, weakness, or an increased rate of rotational failure.

REFERENCES

1. American Dental Association, Council on Dental Materials, Instruments, and Equipment: Current status of sterilization instruments, devices, and methods for the dental office, J. Am. Dent. Assoc. **103**:683, 1981.
2. American Dental Association, Council on Dental Therapeutics: Quaternary ammonium compounds not accepted for disinfection of instruments, and environmental surfaces in dentistry, J. Am. Dent. Assoc. **97**:855, 1978.
3. American Dental Association, Council on Dental Therapeutics: Accepted dental therapeutics, ed. 40, Chicago 1984, The Association.
4. Babb, J.R., Bradley, C.R., and Ayliffe, G.A.J.: Sporicidal activity of glutaraldehydes and hypochlorites and other factors influencing their selection for the treatment of medical equipment, J. Hosp. Infect. **1**:63, 1980.
5. Becker, G.L., Cohen, S., and Borer, R.: The sequelae of accidently injecting sodium hypochlorite beyond the root apex, Oral Surg. **38**:633, 1974.
6. Berman, L.H., and Fleischman, S.B.: Evaluation of the accuracy of the Neosono-D electronic apex locator, J. Endod. **10**:164, 1984.
7. Block, S., et al.: Disinfection, sterilization and preservation, ed. 3, Philadelphia, 1983, Lea & Febiger.
8. Chivian, N.: Endodontics: an overview, Dent. Clin. North Am. **28**(4):637, 1984.
9. Cooley, R.L., Stilley, J., and Lubow, R.M.: Formaldehyde emitted by chemical vapor sterilizers, Oral Surg. **57**:28, 1984.
10. Cooley, R.L., Stilley, J., and Lubow, R.M.: Mercury vapor produced during sterilization of amalgam-contaminated instruments, J. Prosthet. Dent. **53**:304, 1985.
11. Cottone, J.A., and Goebel, W.M.: Hepatitis B: the clinical detection of the chronic carrier dental patient and the effects of immunization via vaccine, Oral Surg.**56**:449, 1983.
12. Cottone, J., et al.: Hepatitis B and the dental profession, J. Am. Dent. Assoc. **110**:614, 1985.
13. Crawford, J.: Clinical asepsis in dentistry, ed. 2, Dallas, 1978, R.A. Kolstad.
14. Cunningham, W.T., and Martin, H.: A scanning electron microscope evaluation of root canal debridement with the endosonic ultrasonic synergistic system, Oral Surg. **53**:527, 1982.
15. Cunningham, W.T., et al.: Changing concepts in endodontic therapy, J. Am. Dent. Assoc. **110**(4):471, 1985.
16. Dayoub, M.: Endodontic dry heat sterilizer effectiveness, J. Endod. **2**:343, 1976.
17. DeDeus, Q., and Cohen, S.: A comparison of ultrasonic, sonic and manual instrumentation of curved root canals, J. Endod., 1987. (In press.)
18. Dentists' Desk Reference, ed. 2, Chicago, 1983, American Dental Association, p. 318.
19. Department of Health and Human Services: Progress on AIDS, FDA Drug Bull. **15**:27, 1985.
20. Eames, W.B., Bryington, S.Q., and Neal, S.B.: A comparison of eight ultrasonic cleaners, Gen. Dent. **30**:242, 1982.
21. Frank, R.J., and Pelleu, G.B.: Glutaraldehyde decontamination of gutta-percha cones, J. Endod. **9**:368, 1983.
22. Girsch, W.J., Matteson, S.R., and McKee, M.N.: An evaluation of Kodak Ektaspeed periapical film for use in endodontics, J. Endod. **9**:282, 1983.
23. Goldstein, J., Morse, K., and Gullen, W.: Epidemiology of hepatitis B among endodontists, J. Endod. **4**:336, 1978.
24. Grossman, L.: Dental instrument sterilization by glass bead conduction of heat, J. Dent. Res.**57**:72, 1978.
25. Harty, F.J., and Stock, C.J.R.: The Giromatic system compared with hand instruments in endodontics, Br. Dent. J. **137**:239, 1974.
26. Iverson, G.W, von Fraunhofer, J.A., and Herrmann, J.W.: The effects of various sterilization methods on the torsional strength of endodontic files, J. Endod. **11**:266, 1985.

27. Kleier, D.J., Benner, S.J., and Averbach, R.E.: Two dental x-ray films compared for rater preference using endodontic views, Oral Surg. **2**:201, 1985.

28. Langeland, K., Liao, K., and Pascon, E.: Work-saving devices in endodontics: efficacy of sonic and ultrasonic techniques, J. Endod. **11**:499, 1985.

29. Merchant, V.A., Molinari, J.A., and Sabes, W.R.: Herpetic whitlow: report of a case with multiple recurrences, Oral Surg.**55**:568, 1983.

30. Mitchell, B.F., James, G.A., and Nelson, R.C.: The effect of autoclave sterilization on endodontic files, Oral Surg. **55**:204, 1983.

31. Montgomery, S.: Chemical decontamination of gutta percha cones with polyvinyl pyrrolidone-iodine, Oral Surg. **31**:258, 1971.

32. Mosley, J.W., and White, E.: Viral hepatitis as an occupational hazard of dentists, J. Am. Dent. Assoc. **90**:992, 1975.

33. Neal, R.G., Craig, R.G., and Powers, J.M.: Effect of sterilization and irrigants on the cutting ability of stainless steel files, J. Endod. **9**:93, 1983.

34. Rabin, A.N., and Crawford, J.J.: Use of a home oven in a dental office for instrument sterilization, N. C. Dent. J. **57**:12, 1974.

35. Runnells, R.: Infection control in the wet finger environment, Salt Lake City, 1984, Publishers Press.

36. Seligmann, et al.: Immunologic reevaluation of AIDS, New Engl. J. Med. **311**:1286, 1984.

37. Senia, S.E., et al.: Rapid sterilization of gutta percha cones with 5.25% sodium hypochlorite, J. Endod.**1**:136, 1975.

38. Shiveley, J., et al.: In vitro autoradiographic study comparing the apical seal of uncatalyzed Dycal to Grossman's sealer, J. Endod. **11**:62, 1985.

39. Stonehill, A.: Buffered glutaraldehyde, a new chemical sterilizing solution, Am. J. Hosp. Pharm. **20**:458, 1963.

40. Turek, T., and Langeland, K.: A light microscopic study of the efficacy of the telescope and the Giromatic preparation of root canals, J. Endod. **8**:437, 1982.

41. Webber, R., et al.: Sealing quality of a temporary filling material, Oral Surg. **46**:123, 1978.

42. Windeler, S.A., and Walter, R.G.: The sporicidal activity of glass bead sterilizers, J. Endod. **1**:273, 1975.

Self-assessment questions

1. Endodontic radiographs are easier to read with
   a. Ultraspeed film
   b. Ektaspeed film
   c. No magnification
   d. Available peripheral light

2. Rubber dam material has the following characteristic:
   a. One thickness
   b. A variety of colors
   c. Unaffected by heat or light
   d. A single size

3. Sonic and ultrasonic systems for canal preparation
   a. Are used primarily as coronal flaring instruments
   b. Rotate in the canal when activated
   c. Deliver copious streams of irrigant
   d. Are scientifically proven instruments for canal preparation

4. Which of the following rotary instruments is designed primarily for flaring the coronal portion of the canal?
   a. Round bur
   b. Gates-Glidden bur
   c. Inverted cone bur
   d. Dentated fissure bur

5. The disease or diseases of greatest concern to the dentist and the dental staff is (are)
   a. Influenza
   b. Common cold
   c. AIDS and hepatitis B
   d. Strep throat

6. Which of the following definitions is correct?
   a. Disinfection—a verifiable method or process that eliminates all forms of microbial life
   b. Sterilization—a verifiable physical or chemical procedure that destroys all microbial life forms
   c. Carrier—a person who is presently in a state of acute infectious disease
   d. Pathogens—microorganisms that do *not* cause and are *not* associated with disease

7. An ultrasonic cleaner
   a. Utilizes cold water as its liquid medium
   b. Should run for at least 10 minutes
   c. Sterilizes contaminated instruments
   d. Is many times more effective and safer than hand scrubbing

8. The steam autoclave
   a. Offers excellent penetration of packages
   b. Destroys cotton or cloth products
   c. Is noncorrosive to carbon steel instruments
   d. Sterilizes in 15 to 40 minutes at 121° C (249.8° F) and 5 pounds pressure

9. The chemical vapor or Chemiclave sterilization system
   a. Corrodes metal instruments
   b. Requires that the load be air dried prior to use
   c. Sterilizes in 20 minutes at 132° C (270° F) and 20 pounds pressure
   d. Is not verifiable as to its sterilizing ability

10. Dry heat sterilization
    a. Requires instruments to be sterilized at 320° F for 2 hours
    b. Allows stacking of loads upon each other
    c. Involves no special precaution in regard to amalgam instruments
    d. Is limited by a small-load capacity

11. One of the disadvantages of the glass-bead or salt sterilizer is
    a. Its small size
    b. That it serves as an emergency backup to other methods of sterilization
    c. That it can be calibrated for correct temperature
    d. That only instruments of small mass can be sterilized

12. Which statement about sterilization indicators is true?
    a. They are not considered an absolute necessity.
    b. A process indicator ensures that sterilization has been achieved.
    c. Biologic indicators will determine if instruments are sterile.
    d. Process indicators should be used every 1 or 2 weeks.

13. Disinfectants
    a. Will kill all spore forms
    b. Include solutions of sodium hypochlorite and iodophors
    c. Are used primarily to sterilize instruments
    d. All of the above

14. Chairside sterilization of gutta-percha cones is best achieved by
    a. 90% alcohol
    b. 3% hydrogen peroxide
    c. 70% alcohol
    d. 5.25% sodium hypochlorite

6

ACCESS OPENINGS AND TOOTH MORPHOLOGY

RICHARD C. BURNS

RELATIONSHIP OF TOOTH MORPHOLOGY AND ACCESS CAVITY PREPARATION

Endodontic textbooks have tended to concentrate on the preparation of access cavities in ideal anatomic crowns in teeth with ideal root canals. The thrust of this chapter is to emphasize the practical world of canal morphology with the proved complexities that exist.

From the early work of Hess to the recent studies demonstrating anatomic complexities of the root canal system, it has been established that the root with a graceful tapering canal and a single apical foramen is the exception rather than the rule.[8] Investigators have shown multiple foramina, fins, deltas, loops, furcation accessory canals, etc., in most teeth. The student and the clinician must approach the tooth to be treated assuming that these "aberrations" occur so often that they must now be considered normal anatomy.

Access preparations can be divided into visual and the assumed. The coronal anatomy, in whatever state it exists, is the first indication of the assumed and is the first key to the root position and root canal system.

A thorough investigation of the sulcus, coronal clefts, restorations, tooth angulation, cusp position, occlusion, and contacts is mandatory before access is begun. Palpation of buccal or labial soft tissue will aid in determining root position (Fig. 6-14, *E*). Some clinicians advocate access cavity preparation prior to rubber dam placement as a visual aid to prevent disorientation.

Before entry the clinician must visualize the expected location of the coronal pulp chamber and canal orifice position. Unnecessary tooth removal may compromise the final restoration. It is important at this time to call upon one's knowledge of tooth morphology.

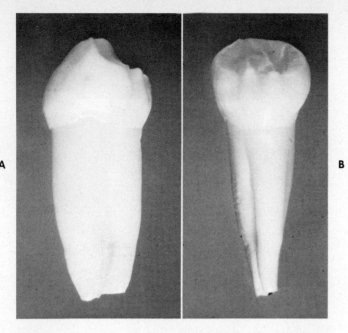

FIG. 6-1. Mandibular first premolar. **A,** Distal view. **B,** Lingual view. (From Gher, M.E., and Vernino, A.R.: Int. J. Period. Restor. Dent. **1:**53, 1981.)

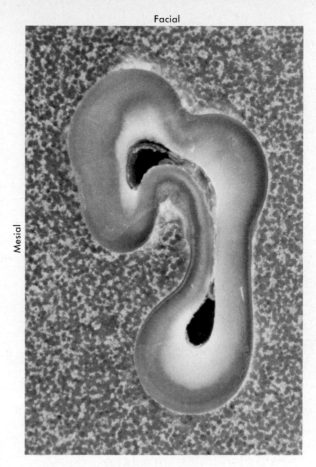

FIG. 6-2. Root section of the premolar in Fig. 6-1.

COMPLEX ANATOMY

A sagittal section of the mandibular first premolar (Figs. 6-1 to 6-3) reveals one of the truly difficult situations facing the clinician. Instead of distinct individual canals, this tooth presents a fine ribbon-shaped canal system that is almost impossible to clean and shape thoroughly, much less obturate (Fig. 6-3). The section shown in Fig. 6-2 was located 8 mm apical to the cementum-enamel junction. The root was 14 mm long.[5]

This example of anatomic complexity can be the preamble to this chapter, which is dedicated to the clear understanding of the fact that internal morphology is far from predictable, but nevertheless is conquerable in the great majority of cases.

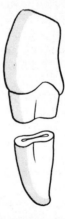

FIG. 6-3. Flat bladelike canals.

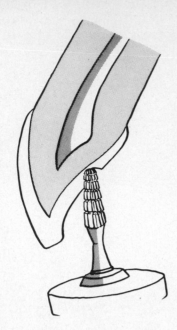

FIG. 6-4. End-cutting fissure bur in a high-speed handpiece.

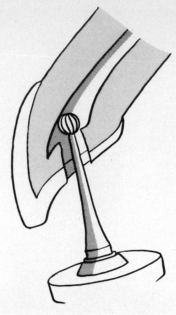

FIG. 6-5. After ''dropping through'' the roof of the chamber, the clinician switches to a long-shanked no. 2 or 4 round bur. With a ''sweeping outward motion'' he or she cleans and shapes the walls of the upper chamber.

ENTERING THE PULP CHAMBER

Initial entry is best made through enamel or restorative materials with an end-cutting fissure bur or inverted cone bur (Fig. 6-4). A proper outline form, as shown in Plates I to XVI, is prepared well into the dentin. If doubt exists as to the location of the pulp chamber and canal orifice(s), the outline form may be made conservatively until the chamber is unroofed.

The next step is done with a no. 4 or 6 surgical-length round bur. When the bur has dropped through the roof of the chamber (Fig. 6-5), no further cutting in an apical direction should be attempted. All action must be in a ''sweeping-out motion'' (Fig. 6-6) until clear access is gained to the canal orifice(s) with no impairment of future instrumentation.

Any pulp stones, loose calcifications, restorative materials, and/or debris must be removed at this time.

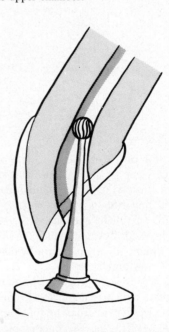

FIG. 6-6. Completed shaping of the upper pulp chamber.

USE OF THE PATHFINDER FOR LOCATING ORIFICES

After the pulp chamber is opened, the canal orifices are located with the endodontic pathfinder (Fig. 6-7). This instrument is to the endodontist what a probe is to the periodontist. Reaching, feeling, often digging at the hard tissue, it is the extension of the clinician's fingers. Natural anatomy dictates the usual places for orifices; but restorations, dentinal protrusions, and dystrophic calcifications can alter the actual configuration encountered. While probing the chamber floor, the pathfinder often penetrates or dislodges calcific deposits blocking an orifice.

Positioning the instrument in the orifice enables the clinician to check the shaft for clearance of the orifice walls. Additionally, the pathfinder is used to determine the angle at which the canals depart the main chamber (Figs. 6-7 and 6-12, *C*).

The endodontic pathfinder is preferred over the rotating bur as the instrument for locating canal orifices. The double-ended design offers two angles of approach.

High-speed handpieces (Fig. 6-8)

True-running high-rpm turbine handpieces are mandatory for gaining access into the endodontically involved tooth. The addition of fiberoptics improves the visibility during probing of the deeper reaches of the pulp chambers.

TABLE 6-1. Tooth length determination

Maxillary	Length (mm)	Mandibular	Length (mm)
Central incisor		Central incisor	
Average	22.5	Average	20.7
Greatest	27.0	Greatest	24.0
Least	18.0	Least	16.0
Lateral incisor		Lateral incisor	
Average	22.0	Average	21.1
Greatest	26.0	Greatest	27.0
Least	17.0	Least	18.0
Canine		Canine	
Average	26.5	Average	25.6
Greatest	32.0	Greatest	32.5
Least	20.0	Least	18.0
First premolar		First premolar	
Average	20.6	Average	21.6
Greatest	22.5	Greatest	26.0
Least	17.0	Least	18.0
Second premolar		Second premolar	
Average	21.5	Average	22.3
Greatest	27.0	Greatest	26.0
Least	16.0	Least	18.0
First molar		First molar	
Average	20.8	Average	21.0
Greatest	24.0	Greatest	24.0
Least	17.0	Least	18.0
Second molar		Second molar	
Average	20.0	Average	19.8
Greatest	24.0	Greatest	22.0
Least	16.0	Least	18.0
Third molar		Third molar	
Average	17.1	Average	18.3
Greatest	22.0	Greatest	20.0
Least	14.0	Least	16.0

Modified from Black. G.V.: Descriptive anatomy of the human teeth, ed. 4, Philadelphia, 1897, S.S. White Dental Manufacturing Co.

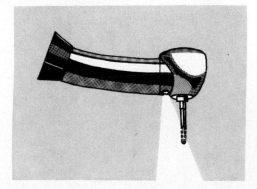

FIG. 6-8. Fiberoptic illumination incorporated in the high-speed turbine Lares handpiece. (Courtesy Lares Research, San Carlos, Calif.)

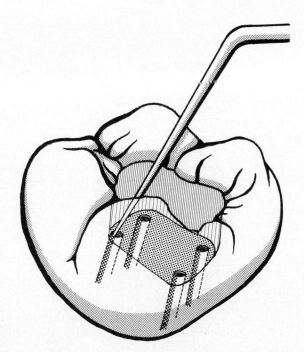

FIG. 6-7. Indispensable in endodontic treatment, the endodontic pathfinder serves as an explorer to locate orifices, as an indicator of canal angulation, and often as a chipping tool to remove calcification.

ACCESS CAVITY PREPARATION IN INCISORS
(Fig. 6-9)

Incisors, particularly mandibular incisors, are often weakened coronally by excessive removal of tooth structure. The mesial-distal width of the pulp chamber is often narrower than the bur used to make the initial access. Because of the ease of visibility and clear definition of external anatomy, lateral perforations (toward the cervical or root surface) are rare.

Labial perforations (cervical or root surface), however, are common, especially in calcified situations. To prevent this occurrence, the clinician must consider the relationship between the incisal edge and the location of the pulp chamber. If the incisal edge is intact, it is almost impossible to perforate *lingually*. Therefore in calcified cases when the bur does not drop easily into the chamber, the clinician should change to smaller-diameter burs and, keeping the long axis in mind, direct the cutting action in apical-lingual version. If the canal orifice still does not materialize after cutting in a apical direction, the clinician should remove the bur, place it in the access cavity, and expose a radiograph; the resultant film will reveal the depth of cutting and the angulation of cutting from mesial to distal (Fig. 6-15, *E*).

BASIC ACCESS CAVITY PREPARATION (Fig. 6-10)

The steps followed in preparing to enter the root canal system parallel those involved in preparing a cavity for a restoration:

The coronal anatomy is examined (A_1) and the site of initial opening visualized. The bur of choice is an end-cutting fissure bur (B_1).

The initial access starts in the central groove, extending through the enamel and well into the dentin (A_2), with the angle of cutting directed toward the center of the crown.

The long-shanked round bur drops through the roof of the pulp chamber (B_2) and gradually sweeps outward, completely removing the roof of the chamber (B_3).

The occlusal opening is extended for convenience form (B_3). Portions of the cusps are removed if necessary to establish unimpeded access to the canal orifices $(A_4$ and $B_4)$.

Testing the access with the endodontic pathfinder for clearance will assure ease of passage of hand and engine-driven instruments.

Buccal views $(C_1$ to $C_4)$ illustrate the proper extension of the access cavity mesially and distally.

Beyond the visual access lies the radicular canal anatomy, which can vary tremendously as illustrated in D_1 to D_4. To gain maximum information on suspected anatomy, refer to Fig. 6-12.

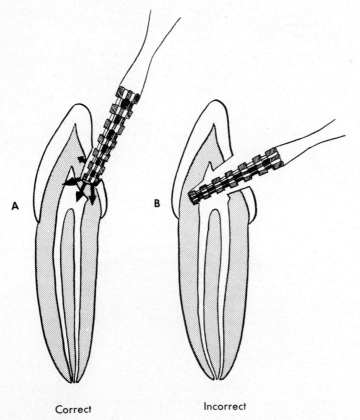

Correct   Incorrect

FIG. 6-9. A, Sweeping motion in a slightly downward lingual-to-labial direction *(arrows),* until the chamber is engaged, to obtain the best access to the lingual canal. **B,** Incorrect approach: directing the end-cutting bur in a straight lingual-to-labial direction. Mutilation of tooth structure and perforation will be the result in this small and narrow incisor.

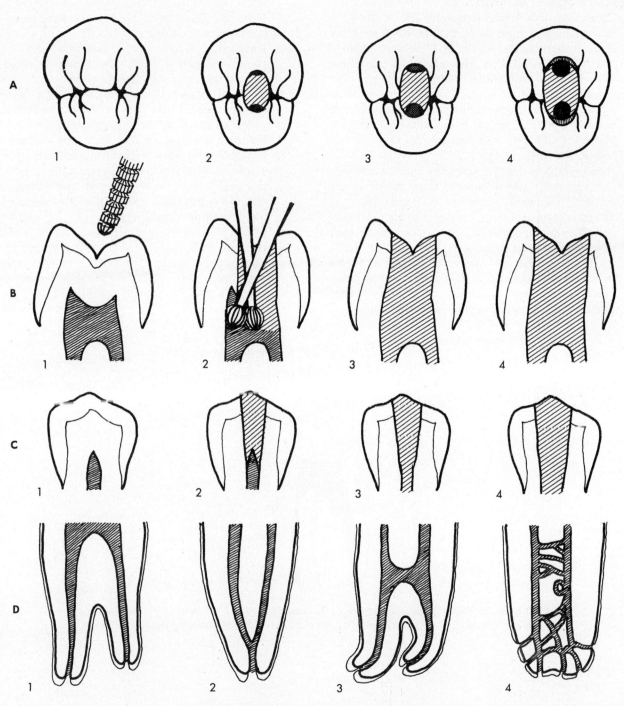

FIG. 6-10. Basic access cavity preparation.

METHODS OF DETERMINING ANATOMIC CONFIGURATION

Beyond the visual perception is the often complex anatomy of the root canal system (Fig. 6-11). The clinician must use every available means to determine the anatomic configuration prior to instrumentation.

Fig. 6-12 illustrates several techniques and methods:

1. When the radiograph shows that the canal suddenly stops in the radicular region (A_1), the assumption is that it has bifurcated (or trifurcated) into much finer diameters. To confirm this division, a second radiograph is exposed from a mesial angulation of 10 to 30 degrees. The resultant film will show either more roots or multiple vertical lines indicating the peripheries of additional root surfaces (A_2) (Figs. 4-8, *F* and *G*, and 4-9).

2. A radiograph will also reveal many clues to anatomic "aberrations": lateral radiolucencies indicating the presence of lateral or accessory canals (B_1); an abrupt ending of a large canal signifying a bifurcation $(B_1$ and $B_2)$; a knoblike image indicating an apex that curves toward or away from the beam of the x-ray machine (B_3); multiple vertical lines, as shown in this curved mesial root (B_4), indicating the possibility of a thin root, which may be hourglass shaped in cross section and susceptible to perforation.

3. The endodontic pathfinder inserted into the orifice openings will reveal the direction that the canals take in leaving the main chamber *(C)*.

4. Digital perception with a hand instrument can identify curvatures, obstruction, root division, and additional canal orifices *(D)*.

5. Fiberoptic illumination can reveal calcifications, orifice location, and fractures *(E)*.

6. Knowledge of root canal anatomy will prompt the clinician always to search for additional canal orifices where they are known to occur—for instance, the usual location of a fourth canal in the maxillary first permanent molar between the mesial-buccal and palatal canals along the developmental groove *(F)*.

7. Further knowledge of root formation can save the clinician difficulties with instrumentation—for example, in what appears radiographically to be a normal palatal root of a maxillary first permanent molar (G_1) but is actually a root with a sharp apical curvature toward the buccal (G_2).

8. Ethnic characteristics as well as other physical differences can be manifested in tooth morphology—for example, the common occurrence of four canals in Asian nationalities *(H)*.

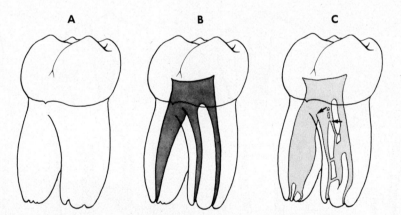

FIG. 6-11. A, Tooth appearance exteriorly. **B,** What previously was surmised as the usual anatomic configuration, **C,** Actual complex system of canals as demonstrated by Hess and Zürcher.[8]

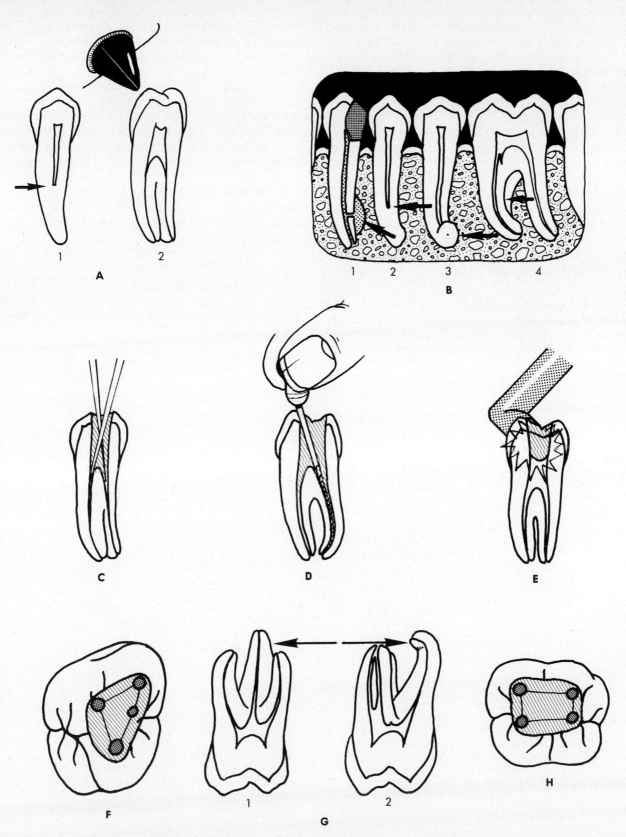

FIG. 6-12. Techniques for determining anatomic configuration.

INTRODUCTION TO PLATES I TO XVI

The anatomy presented in the following plates is as accurately illustrated as reasonably possible.* On each left-hand page is both a facial view and a proximal exterior view of the tooth. These illustrations are intended for familiarization and represent the average anatomic appearance. The lower portion of the left-hand page contains descriptive data in regard to the tooth. The right-hand page is divided into three parts.

1. The top portion illustrates in cross-sectional detail the enamel, dentin, and pulp chambers. The proximal view contains the access cavity preparation location. Between the two cross-sectional views is a lingual or occlusal exterior view with the access cavity indicated.

Experienced clinicians will note that the access openings described herein are slightly larger than those described in other textbooks. These larger sizes represent the composite opinion of several leading endodontists in the United States and reflect the changes in endodontic teaching and clinical practice.

---

*Contained in the series are many classic illustrations from Zeisz and Nuckolls.[16] All illustrations were reproduced or modified from the extremely accurate and excellent work of these authors and the talents of the artist, Mr. Walter B. Schwarz.

Within the access opening is a grid containing the location of the canal orifices of the posterior teeth. These locations are extremely important, especially when one is attempting to proceed through calcified pulp chambers. Variations in orifices exist as do any anatomic peculiarities.

2. The second division is a narrow strip illustrating a few examples of anatomic variations. These were taken from the extensive work of Dr. Quintiliano de Deus of Brazil[4] and represent actual cross sections of human teeth. They are included for the reader's information and to create an awareness of the complexities that may be present in any tooth.

3. The third division illustrates common departures from normal anatomy. When unusual anatomy is suspected, the clinician should first search for these illustrated characteristics.

. . .

The average time of eruption and average age of calcification were taken from *Anatomy of Orofacial Structures* by Brand and Isselhard.[2] The average lengths are from Table 6-1.

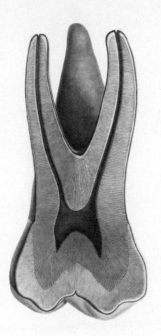

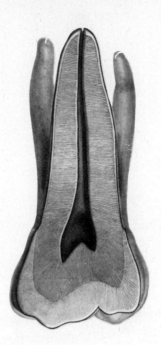

ACCESS OPENINGS
AND
TOOTH MORPHOLOGY

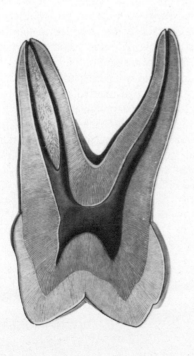

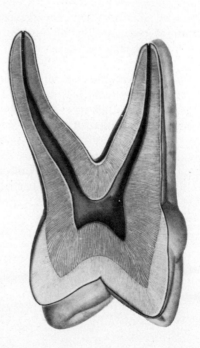

PLATE I—MAXILLARY CENTRAL INCISOR

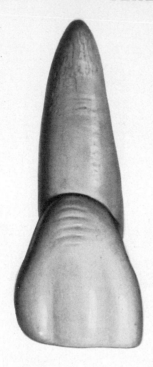
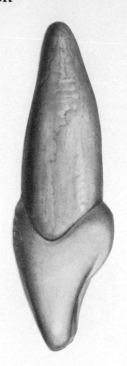

Average time of eruption: 7 to 8 years
Average age of calcification: 10 years
Average length: 22.5 mm

Somewhat rectangular from the labial and shovel shaped from the proximal, the crown of the maxillary central is more than adequate for endodontic access and is positioned ideally for direct mirror visualization. This tooth is especially suitable as the clinician's first clinical experience because over a third of its canal is directly visible. Visualization of the canal proper may be enhanced with fiberoptic illumination.

The first entry point, with the end-cutting fissure bur, is made just above the cingulum (Fig. 6-4). The direction should be in the long axis of the root. A roughly triangular opening is made in anticipation of the final shape of the access cavity. Often, penetration of the shallow pulp chamber occurs during initial entry. When the sensation of "dropping through the roof" of the pulp chamber has been felt, the long-shanked no. 4 or 6 round bur replaces the fissure bur (Fig. 6-5).

The "belly" of the round bur is utilized to sweep out toward the incisal; one must be certain to expose the entire chamber completely (Fig. 6-6). It may be necessary to return to the fissure bur to extend and refine the final shape of the access cavity. All caries, grossly discolored dentin, and pulp calcifications are removed at this time. Leaking restorations or proximal caries should be removed and an adequate temporary restoration placed.

Conical and rapidly tapering toward the apex, the root morphology is quite distinctive. Cross-sectionally the radicular canal is slightly triangular at the cervical, gradually becoming round as it approaches the apical foramen.

Multiple canals are rare; however, the incidence of accessory and lateral canals is high. The apical foramen is rarely located at the exact root apex but is usually found laterally and within the apical 2 mm.

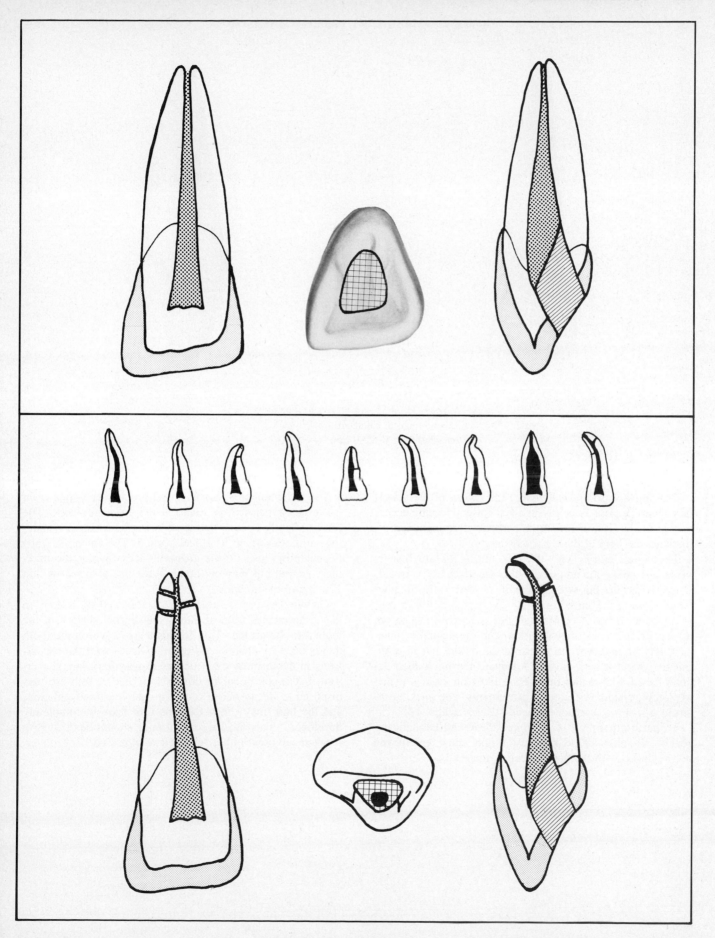

PLATE II—MAXILLARY LATERAL INCISOR

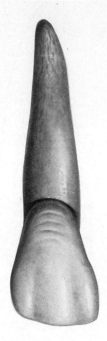
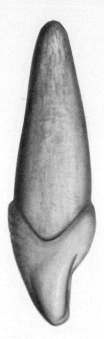

Average time of eruption: 8 to 9 years
Average age of calcification: 11 years
Average length: 22.0 mm

Tending toward an oval shape, the crown of the maxillary lateral incisor is nearly as ideal for endodontic access as that of the central incisor. Fiberoptic illumination may, likewise, be helpful during access to this tooth.

The initial entry, with the end-cutting fissure bur, is made just above the cingulum. The access cavity is ovoid. Often the fissure bur will engage the shallow pulp chamber while making the initial opening. When the chamber roof is removed, a no. 4 or 6 round bur is used to sweep out all remaining caries, discoloration, and pulp calcifications.

It may be necessary to return to the fissure bur in refining the ovoid access cavity. Adequate flaring is then accomplished with round burs. Care must be exercised that explorers, endodontic cutting instruments, and packing instruments do not contact the access cavity walls.

To ensure that the canals remain clean and hermetically sealed, all caries and leaking restorations must be removed and replaced with temporary sealing materials.

The radicular cross-sectional pulp chamber varies from ovoid at the cervical to round at the apical foramen. The root is slightly conical and tends toward curvature, usually toward the distal, in its apical portion. The apical foramen is generally closer to the anatomic apex than in the maxillary central but may be found on the lateral aspect within 1 or 2 mm of the apex.

On rare occasions, access is complicated by a dens in dente, an invagination of part of the lingual surface of the tooth into the crown. This creates a space within the tooth that is lined by enamel and communicates with the mouth. Dens in dente most often occurs in maxillary lateral incisors, but it can occur in other teeth. These teeth are predisposed to decay because of the anatomic malformation, and the pulp may die before the root apex is completely developed.[7] This mostly coronal mass should be dealt with mechanically and either removed or bypassed.

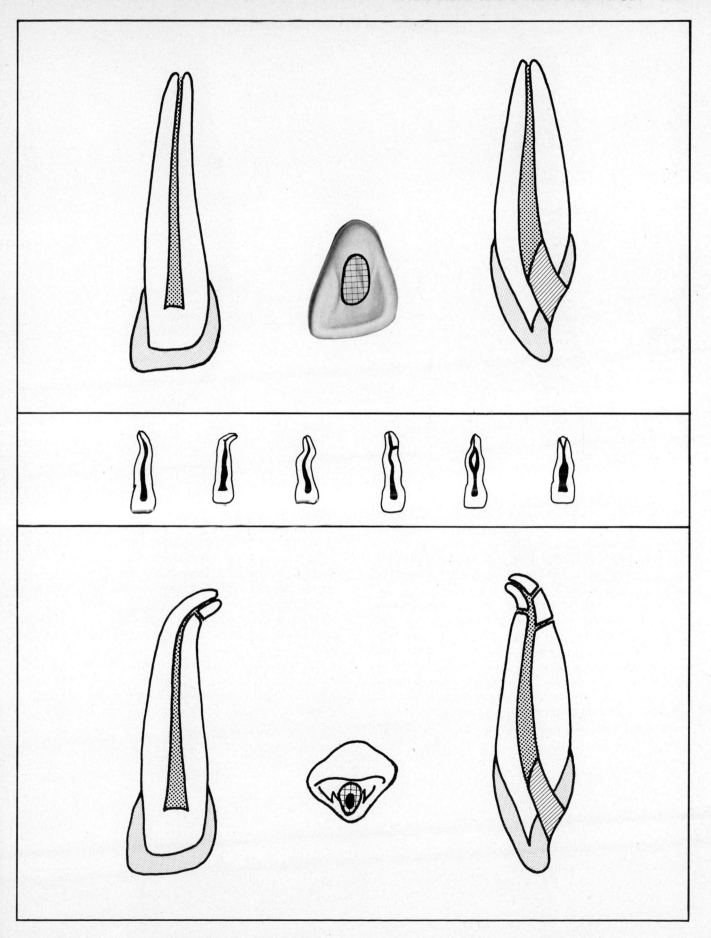

PLATE III—MAXILLARY CANINE

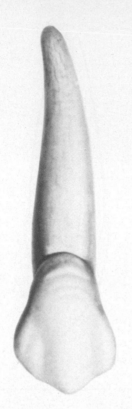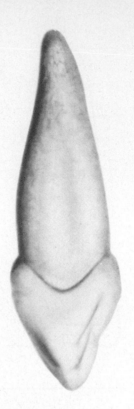

Average time of eruption: 10 to 12 years
Average age of calcification: 13 to 15 years
Average length: 26.5 mm

The longest tooth in the dental arch, the canine presents a formidable morphology designed to withstand heavy occlusal utilization. Its long, thickly enameled crown will undergo heavy incisal wear but often displays deep cervical erosion with aging.

The access cavity corresponds to the lingual crown shape and is ovoid. To achieve straight-line access, one often must extend the cavity incisally but not so far as to weaken the heavily functioning cusp. Initial access is made slightly below midcrown on the palatal. If the pulp chamber is located deeper, a no. 4 or 6 long-shanked round bur may be required. The sweeping-out motion of this bur will reveal an ovoid pulp chamber. The chamber remains ovoid as it continues apically through the cervical region and be-

low. Attention must be given to directional filing so this ovoid anatomy will be thoroughly cleaned.

The radicular canal is reasonably straight and quite long. Most canines require instruments that are 25 mm or longer. The apex will often curve any direction in the last 2 or 3 mm.

Canine morphology seldom varies radically, and lateral and accessory canals occur less frequently than in the maxillary incisors.

This buccal bone over the eminence often disintegrates, and fenestration is a common finding. The apical foramen is usually close to the anatomic apex but may be laterally positioned, especially when apical curvature is present.

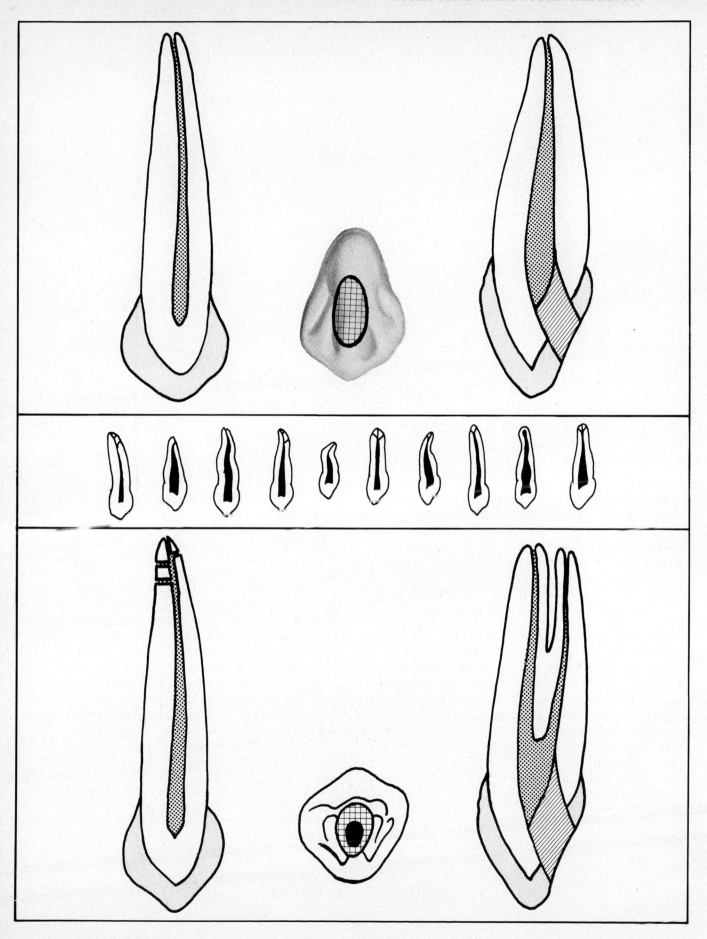

PLATE IV—MAXILLARY FIRST PREMOLAR

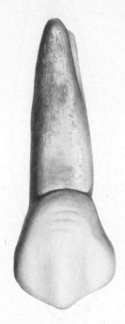
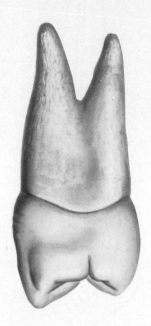

Average time of eruption: 10 to 11 years
Average age of calcification: 12 to 13 years
Average length: 20.6 mm

Most commonly birooted, the maxillary first premolar is a transitional tooth between incisor and molar. Loss of the posterior molars requires the premolars to undergo heavy occlusal function. Removable appliances increase torque on these frequently clasped teeth, and the additional forces in concert with deep carious lesions can induce heavy calcification of the pulp chambers. Early posterior tooth loss often causes rotation, which can complicate the locating of pulp chambers.

The canal orifices will be found below and slightly central to the cusp tips (Fig. 6-10, A_4). The initial opening is in the central fossa and is ovoid in the buccal-palatal. When one orifice has been located, the clinician should look carefully for a developmental groove leading to the opening of another canal. The angulation of the roots may be determined by positioning of the endodontic explorer (Fig. 6-12, C). Radiographic division of the roots on a routine periapical film will often indicate tooth rotation (Fig. 6-12, A). Divergent roots require less occlusal access extension. Conversely, parallel roots may require removal of tooth structure toward the cusp tips. All caries and leaking restorations must be removed and a suitable temporary restoration placed.

Radicular irregularities consist of fused roots with separate canals, fused roots with interconnections or "webbing," fused roots with a common apical foramen, and the unusual but always to be considered three-rooted tooth. In the last situation the buccal orifices will not be clearly visible with a mouth mirror. Directional positioning of the endodontic explorer or a small file will identify the anatomy. Carns and Skidmore[3] reported that the incidence of maxillary first premolars with three roots, three canals, and three foramina was 6% of the cases studied. The root length is considerably shorter than in the canine, and distal curvature is not uncommon. The apical foramen is usually close to the anatomic apex. Root lengths if the cusps are intact and used as reference points are usually the same. The apical portion of the roots often tapers rapidly, ending in extremely narrow and curved root tips.

The incidence of mesial-distal vertical crown/root fracture of the first premolar requires that the clinician remove all restorations at the onset of endodontic therapy and carefully inspect the coronal anatomy with a fiberoptic light.

After endodontic treatment, full occlusal coverage is mandatory to ensure against vertical or crown/root fracture.

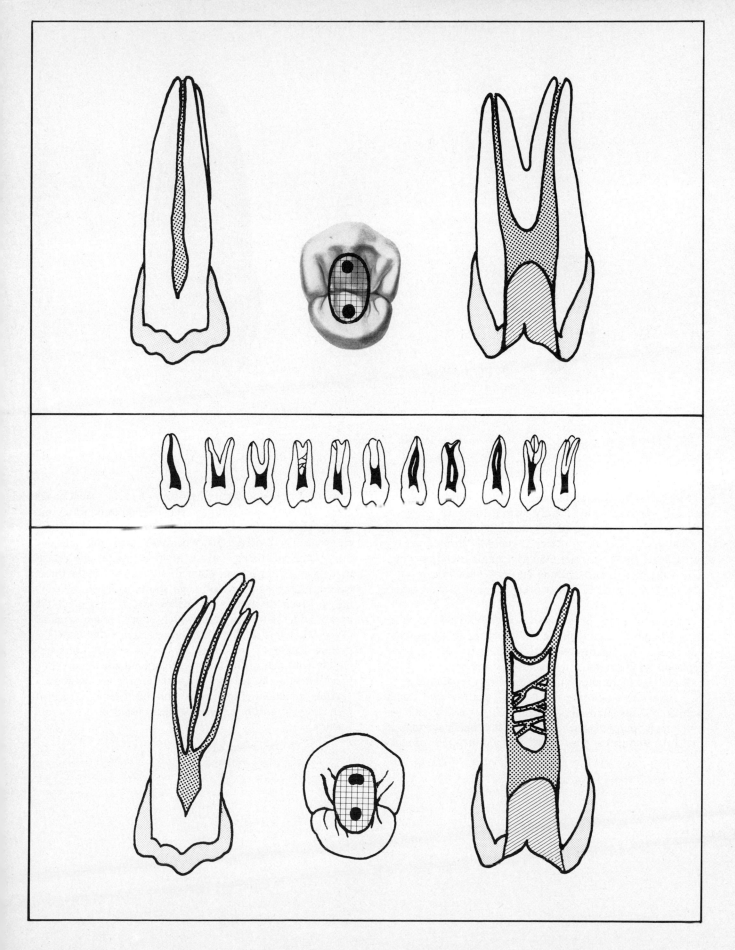

PLATE V—MAXILLARY SECOND PREMOLAR

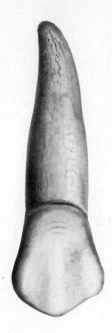
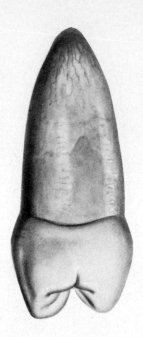

Average time of eruption: 10 to 12 years
Average age of calcification: 12 to 14 years
Average length: 21.5 mm

Similar to the first premolar in coronal morphology, the second premolar varies mainly in root form. Its crown is narrower in the buccal-palatal and slightly wider in the mesial-distal. The canal orifice is centrally located but often appears more as a slot than as a single ovoid opening. When the slot-shaped opening appears, the clinician must assume that the tooth has two canals until proved otherwise.

The basic outline of the tooth is slightly ovoid but wider from mesial to distal than the outline of the first premolar. All caries and leaking restorations must be removed and replaced with a suitable temporary restoration.

Radicular morphology may present two separate canals, two canals anastomosing to a single canal, or two canals with interconnections or "webbing." Accessory and lateral canals may be present, but with less incidence than in incisors. Vertucci and associates[14] stated that 75% of max-

illary second premolars in their study had one canal at the apex, 24% had two foramina, and 1% had three foramina. Of the teeth studied, 59.5% had accessory canals. These clinicians also reported that when two canals join into one the *palatal* canal frequently exhibits a straight-line access to the apex. They further pointed out that "if, on the direct periapical exposure, a root canal shows a sudden narrowing, or even disappears, it means that at this point the canal divides into two parts which either remain separate (Type V) or merge (Type II) before reaching the apex."

Root length of the maxillary second molar compares closely with that of the first premolar; and apical curvature is not uncommon, particularly with large sinus cavities.

After endodontic treatment, full occlusal coverage is mandatory to ensure against vertical cuspal or crown/root fracture.

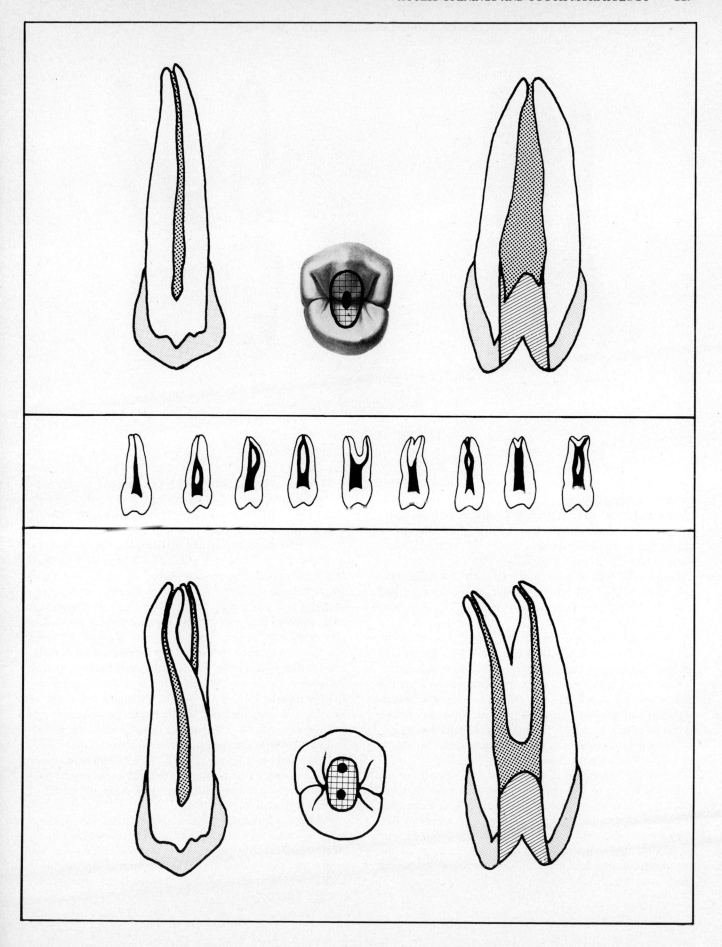

PLATE VI—MAXILLARY FIRST MOLAR

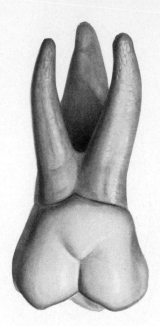 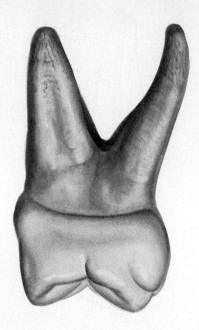

Average time of eruption: 6 to 7 years
Average age of calcification: 9 to 10 years
Average length: 20.8 mm

The tooth largest in volume and most complex in root and root canal anatomy, the "6-year molar" (Fig. 6-12, *G*) is possibly the most treated, least understood, posterior tooth. It is the posterior tooth with the highest endodontic failure rate and unquestionably one of the most important teeth.

Three individual roots of the maxillary first molar provide a tripod: the palatal root, which is the longest, and the distal-buccal and mesial-buccal roots, which are about the same length.

The palatal root is often curved buccally in its apical third. Of the three canals, it offers the easiest access and has the largest diameter. Its orifice lies well toward the palatal surface and it has a sharp angulation away from the midline. Cross-sectionally it is flat and ribbonlike, requiring close attention to debridement and instrumentation; fortunately there is rarely more than one apical foramen.

The distal-buccal root is conical and usually straight. It invariably has a single canal.

The cover illustration of this edition of *Pathways of the Pulp* was drawn to call the reader's attention to the enormous complexities of tooth morphology. New techniques of obturation capable of directing semisolid materials into spaces previously unfilled are evolving. It was the editors' decision to select the maxillary first molar to illustrate the incredibly complex and gracefully abstract forms of human dental anatomy.

The mesial-buccal root of the first molar has generated more research, clinical investigation, and pure frustration than has probably any other root in the mouth. Green[6] stated that two foramina were present in 14% of mesial-buccal roots of the maxillary first molars studied and two orifices were noted in 36% (Fig. 24-20). Pineda[10] reported that 42% of these roots manifested two canals and two apical foramina. Slowey[12] supported Pineda's conclusions within a few percentage points. The fact that almost half of these roots bear two canals, whether joining into a single foramen or not, is enough reason *always to assume that two canals exist* until careful examination proves otherwise. The extra orifice lies centrally somewhere between the mesial-buccal and palatal orifices. Searching for the extra orifice is aided by using the fiberoptic light and by locating the developmental line between the mesial-buccal and palatal orifices. The second canal within the mesial-buccal root will always be smaller than the other canals and therefore is often more difficult to clean and shape. Gaining access to the primary canal within the mesial-buccal root can be made easier by improving the angle of approach (Fig. 6-10).

All caries, leaking restorations, and pulpal calcifications must be removed prior to initiating endodontic treatment. After treatment it is mandatory to institute full coverage to ensure against vertical cuspal or crown/root fracture. It is also advisable to place internal reinforcement whenever indicated (Chapter 21).

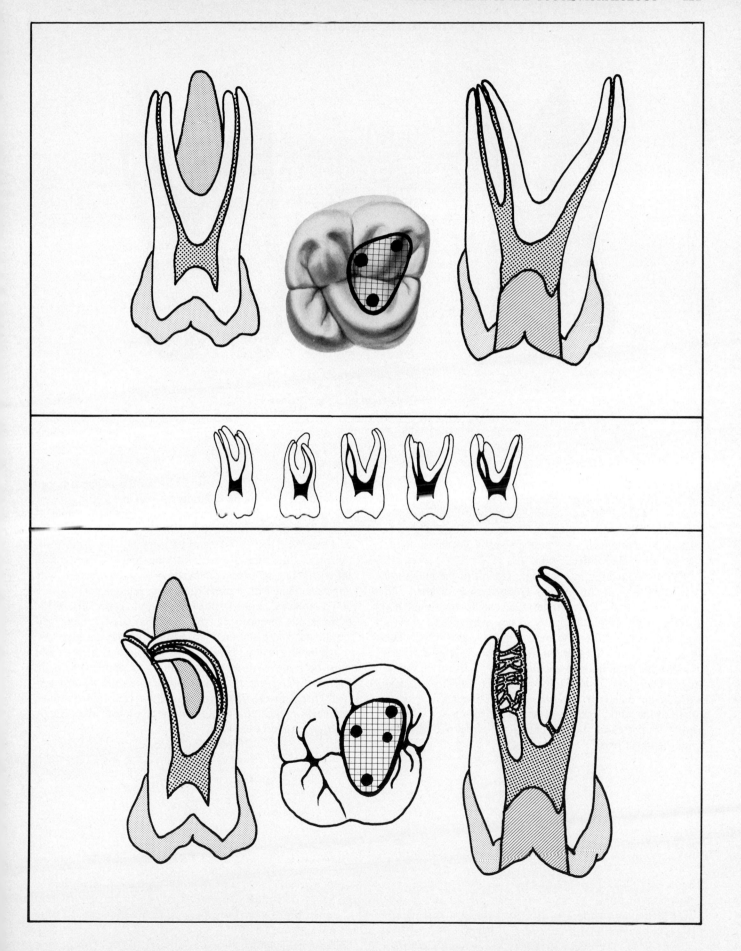

PLATE VII—MAXILLARY SECOND MOLAR

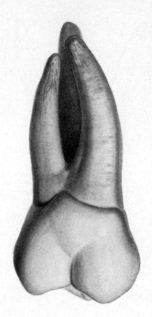
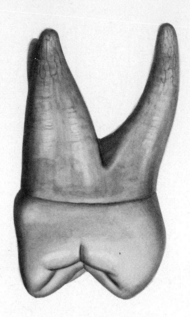

Average time of eruption: 11 to 13 years
Average age of calcification: 14 to 16 years
Average length: 20.0 mm

Coronally the maxillary second molar closely resembles the maxillary first molar, although it is not as square and massive. Access in both teeth can usually be adequately prepared without disturbing the transverse ridge. The second molar is often easier to prepare because of the straight-line across to the orifices.

The distinguishing morphologic feature of the maxillary second molar is its three roots grouped close together and sometimes fused. The parallel root canals are frequently superimposed radiographically. They are usually shorter than the roots of the first molar and not as curved. The three orifices may form a flat triangle, sometimes almost a straight line. The floor of the chamber is markedly convex, giving a slightly funnel shape to the canal orifices. Occasionally the canals will curve into the chamber at a sharp angle to the floor, making it necessary to remove a lip of dentin so the canal can be entered more in a direct line with the canal axis.[6]

Complications in access occur when the molar is tipped in distal version. Initial opening with an end-cutting fissure bur is followed by a short-shanked round bur, which is best suited to uncover the pulp chamber and shape the access cavity. Then small hand instruments are used to establish canal continuity and working length. The bulk of the cleaning and shaping may now be accomplished with engine-mounted files on reciprocating handpieces.

To enhance radiographic visibility, especially when there is interference with the malar process, a more perpendicular and distal-angular radiograph may be exposed.

All caries, leaking restorations, and pulpal calcifications must be removed prior to initiating endodontic treatment. Full occlusal coverage is mandatory to ensure against vertical cuspal or crown/root fracture. Internal reinforcement whenever indicated should be incorporated immediately after endodontic treatment.

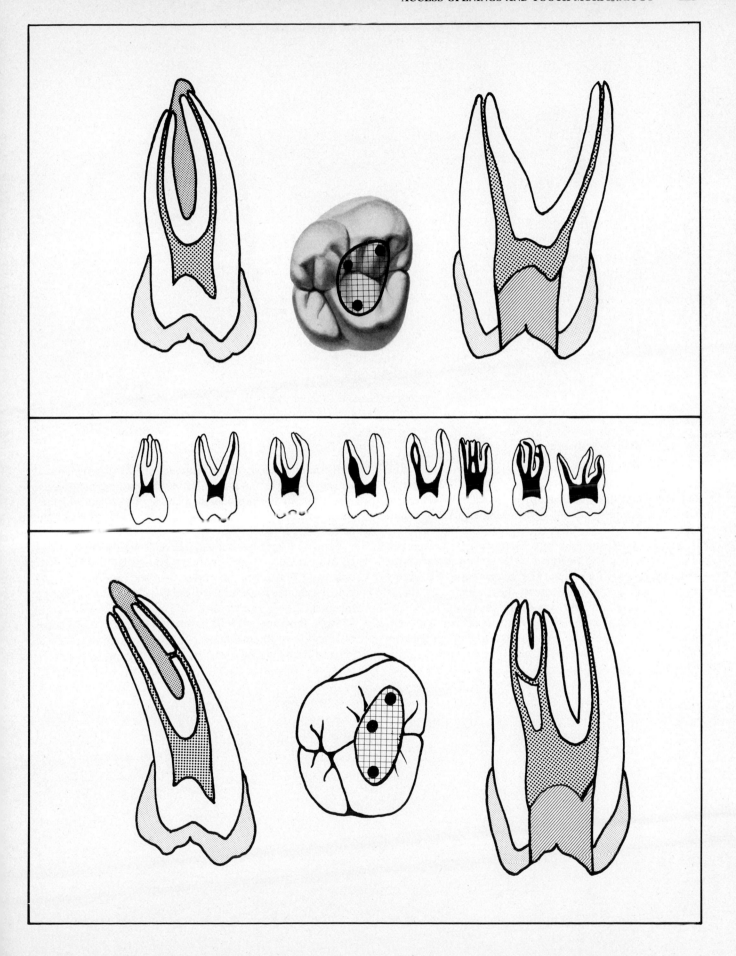

PLATE VIII—MAXILLARY THIRD MOLAR

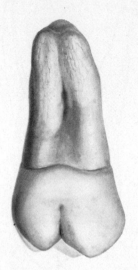
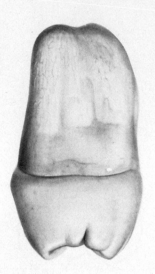

Average time of eruption: 17 to 22 years
Average age of calcification: 18 to 25 years
Average length: 17.0 mm

Loss of the maxillary first and second molars is often the reason for considering the third molar as a strategic abutment. The other indication for endodontic treatment and full coverage is a fully functioning mandibular third molar.

Careful examination of root morphology is important before recommending treatment. Many third molars present adequate root formation; and given reasonable accessibility, there is no reason why they cannot remain as functioning dentition after endodontic therapy.

The radicular anatomy of the third molar is completely unpredictable, and it may be advisable to explore the root canal morphology before promising success.

As an alternative to conventional hand instrumentation, the use of engine-mounted files in reciprocating handpieces may simplify the problem of accessibility. Precurving instruments will assist in guiding them through tortuous canals.

For visual and mechanical convenience the access may be overextended slightly with the knowledge that full coverage is mandatory. All caries, leaking restorations, and pulpal calcifications must be removed prior to instituting treatment.

Some third molars will have only a single canal, some two, and most three. The orifice openings may be made in either a triangular or a nearly straight-line arrangement.

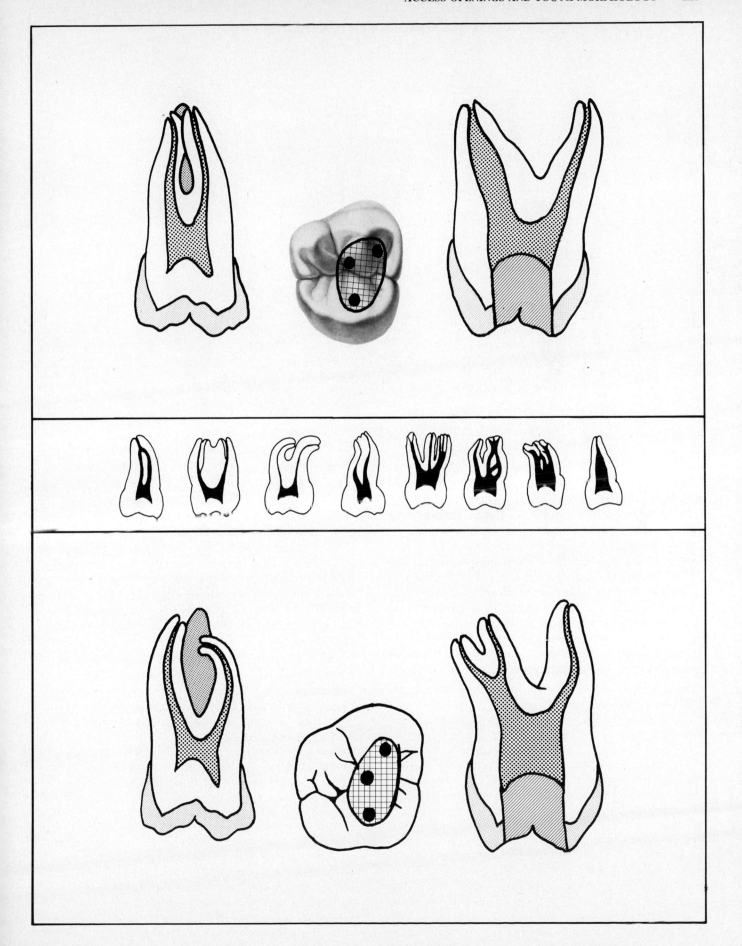

PLATE IX—MANDIBULAR CENTRAL INCISOR

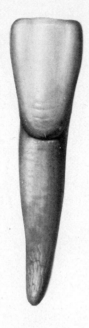

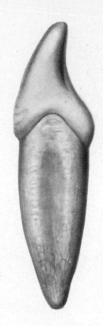

Average time of eruption: 6 to 7 years
Average age of calcification: 9 years
Average length: 20.7 mm

Narrow and flat in the labial-lingual dimension, the mandibular central incisor is the smallest human adult tooth. It is visible radiographically from only one plane and thus often appears more accessible than it really is. The narrow lingual crown offers a limited area for access. Smaller fissure burs and no. 2 round burs cause less mutilation of coronal dentition. The access cavity should be ovoid, with attention given to a lingual approach (Fig. 6-9).

Frequently the mandibular central incisor has two canals. One study[1] reported that 41.4% of mandibular incisors studied had two separate canals; of these, only 1.3% had two separate foramina. The clinician should search for the second canal immediately upon completing the access cavity. Endodontic failures in mandibular incisors usually arise from uncleaned canals, most commonly toward the lingual. Access may be extended incisally when indicated to permit maximum labial-lingual freedom.

Although labial perforations are common, they may be avoided if the clinician remembers that it is nearly impossible to perforate in a lingual direction because of the bur shank's contacting the incisal edge. The ribbon-shaped canal (Fig. 6-3) is common enough to be considered normal and demands special attention in cleaning and shaping.

Lateral perforations and pulp anatomy will be discussed in Plate XV.

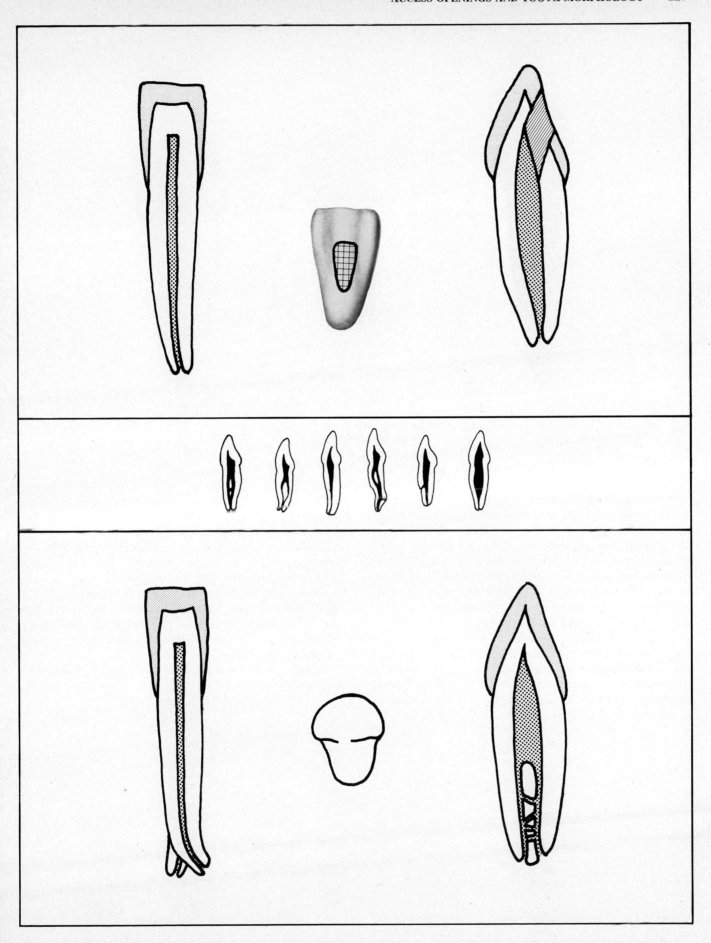

PLATE X—MANDIBULAR LATERAL INCISOR

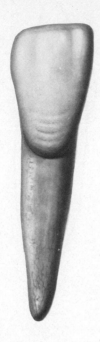

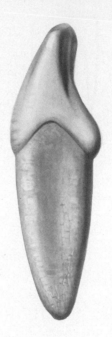

Average time of eruption: 7 to 8 years
Average age of calcification: 10 years
Average length: 21.1 mm

Nearly identical to the mandibular central incisor, the lateral incisor demands identical consideration in access cavity preparation.

The similarity can provoke a rare but serious occurrence. Hurried rubber dam placement, identical restorations, and negligence may lead to preparation of an access cavity in the wrong tooth (Fig. 6-17, *F*). Marking the labial surface of the tooth with a felt-tip pen *prior* to rubber dam isolation can prevent this problem.

Trauma, periodontal disease, caries erosion, and malocclusion may result in calcification of canal spaces. Great care must be used in reaching apically to locate the orifice. Mutilation of crown and root substance is common. Labial perforation is mentioned in Plate IX. Lateral perforation

occurs when the bur is not directed in the long axis of the tooth. The problem is further complicated by a traumatic loss of the anatomic crown. Without landmarks to follow coronally, one can easily perforate laterally. To help prevent this, the access should be made without the rubber dam so the labial root anatomy will be palpable.

Ribbon-shaped canals in narrow hourglass cross-sectional anatomy invite lateral perforation by endodontic files and Gates-Glidden drills. Minimal flaring and dowel space preparation are indicated to ensure against ripping through proximal root walls.

Apical curvatures and accessory canals are common in mandibular incisors.

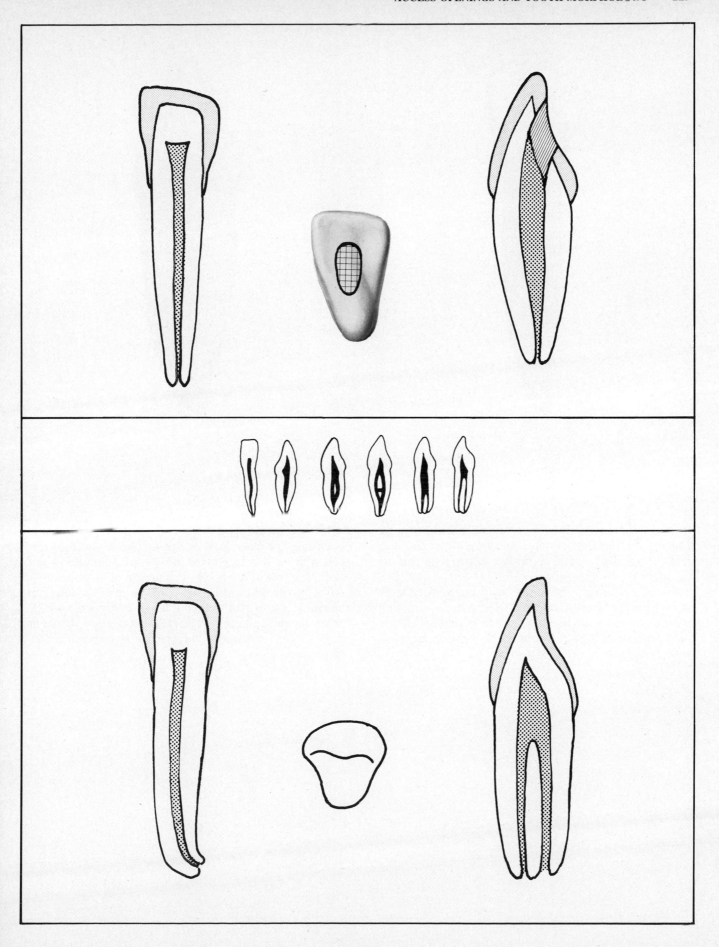

PLATE XI—MANDIBULAR CANINE

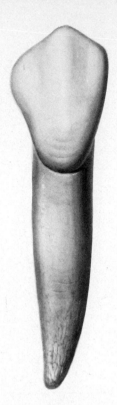

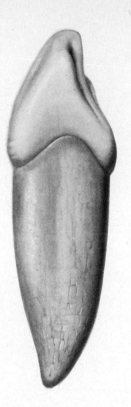

Average time of eruption: 9 to 10 years
Average age of calcification: 13 years
Average length: 25.6 mm

Sturdy and considerably wider mesial-distally than the incisors, the mandibular canine seldom presents endodontic problems. The unusual occurrence of two roots can create difficulty, but this is rare.

The access cavity is ovoid and may be extended incisally for labial-lingual accessibility. The canal is somewhat ovoid at the cervical, becoming round at midroot. Directional instrumentation is necessary to debride the canal walls completely.

If there are two roots, one will always be easier to instrument. The other must be opened and funneled in concert with the first to prevent packing of dentin debris and loss of access (Fig. 6-19). Precurving of instruments at initial access will enable the clinician to trace down the buccal or lingual root wall until the tip engages the orifice. When the difficult canal is located, every effort should be made to shape and funnel the opening to maintain continued access.

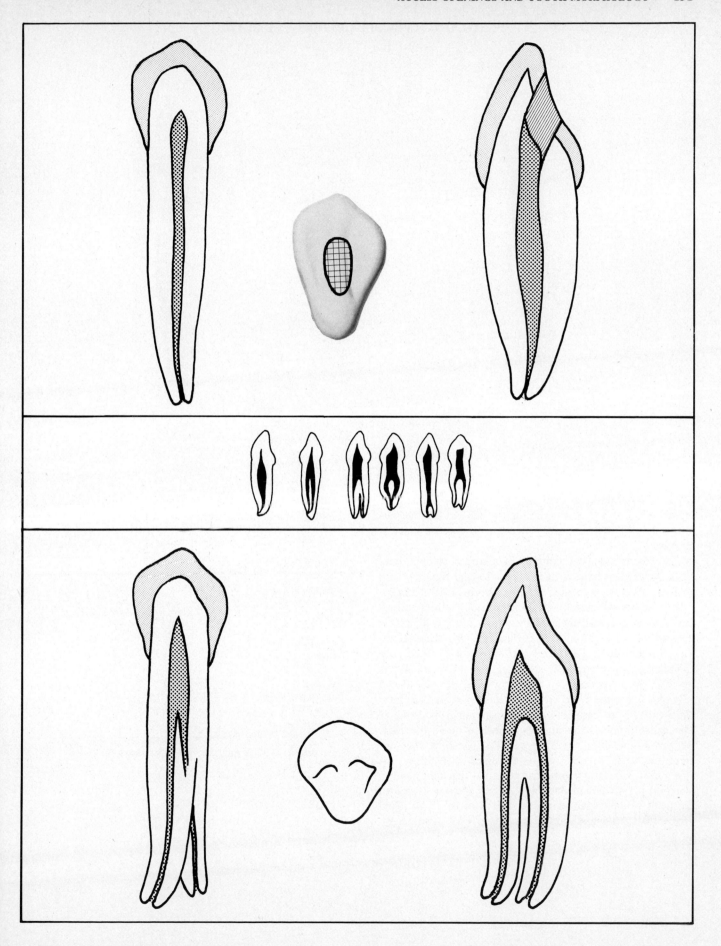

PLATE XII—MANDIBULAR FIRST PREMOLAR

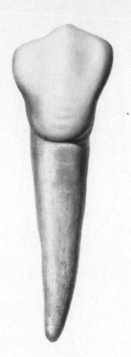
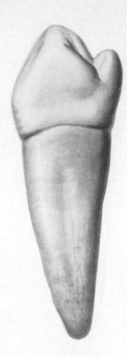

Average time of eruption: 10 to 12 years
Average age of calcification: 12 to 13 years
Average length: 21.6 mm

Often considered an enigma to the endodontist, the mandibular first premolar with dual canals dividing at various levels of the root can generate complex mechanical problems.

The coronal anatomy consists of a well-developed buccal cusp and a small or nonexistent lingual outgrowth of enamel. Access is made slightly buccal to the central groove and is directed in the long axis of the root toward the central cervical area. The ovoid pulp chamber is reached with end-cutting fissure burs and long-shanked no. 4 or 6 round burs. The cross section of the cervical pulp chamber is almost round in a single-canal tooth and is ovoid in two-canal teeth.

Another investigation[17] reported that "a second or third canal exists in at least 23% of first mandibular bicuspids." The canals may divide almost anywhere down the root. Because of the absence of direct access, cleaning, shaping, and filling of these teeth can be extremely difficult.

A recent study by Vertucci[13] revealed that the mandibular first premolar had one canal at the apex in 74.0% of the teeth studied, two canals at the apex in 25.5%, and three canals at the apex in the remaining 0.5% (Table 6-2).

TABLE 6-2. Classification and percentage of canal types found in mandibular first and second premolars

Classification	In first premolars (%)	In second premolars (%)
One canal at apex		
Type 1	70.0	97.5
Type 2	4.0	0.0
Of total	74.0	97.5
Two canals at apex		
Type 3	1.5	0.0
Type 4	24.0	2.5
Of total	25.5	2.5
Three canals at apex		
Type 5	0.5	0.0
Of total	0.5	0.0

From Vertucci, F.J.: J. Am Dent. Assoc. **97**:47, 1978.

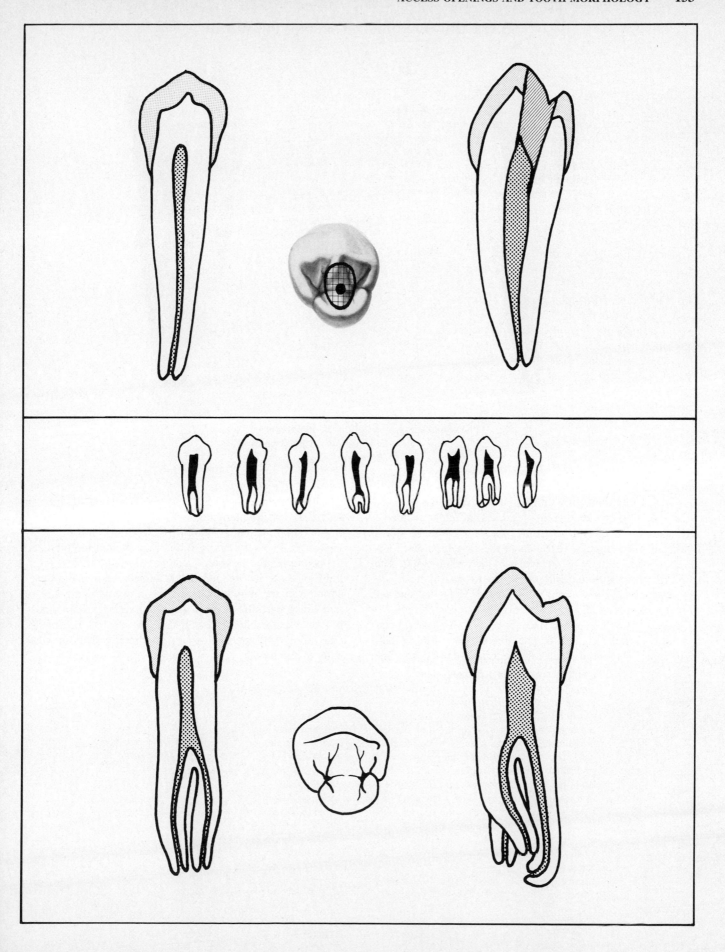

PLATE XIII—MANDIBULAR SECOND PREMOLAR

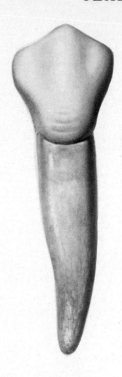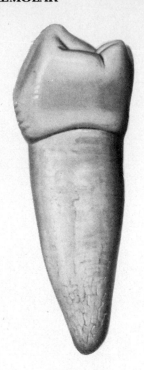

Average time of eruption: 11 to 12 years
Average age of calcification: 13 to 14 years
Average length: 22.3 mm

Very similar coronally to the first premolar, the mandibular second premolar presents less of a radicular problem.

Its crown has a well-developed buccal cusp and a much better-formed lingual cusp than in the first premolar. Access is made slightly ovoid, wider in the mesial-distal. The first opening, with the end-cutting fissure bur, is made approximately in the central groove and is extended and refined with nos. 4 and 6 round burs.

Investigators[17] reported that only 12% of mandibular second molars studied had a second or third canal. Vertucci[13] also showed that the second premolar had one canal at the apex in 97.5% and two canals at the apex in only 2.5% of the teeth studied.

An important consideration, which must not be overlooked, is the anatomic position of the mental foramen and the neurovascular structures that pass through it. The proximity of these nerves and blood vessels when acute exacerbation of the mandibular premolars occurs can result in temporary paresthesia from the fulminating inflammatory process. Exacerbations in this region seem to be intense and more resistant to nonsurgical therapy than in other parts of the mouth.

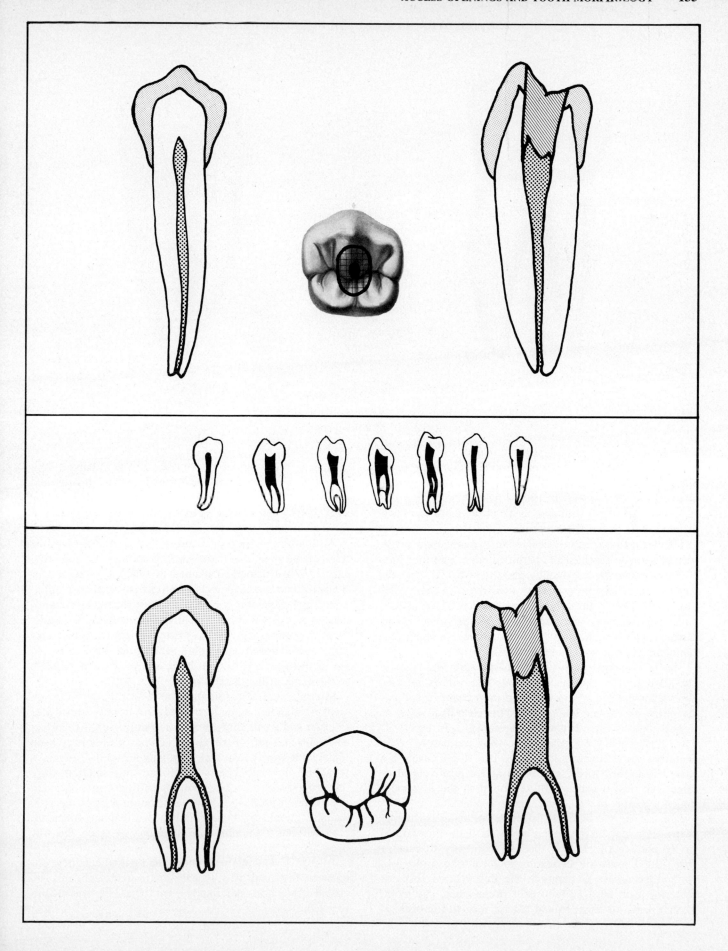

PLATE XIV—MANDIBULAR FIRST MOLAR

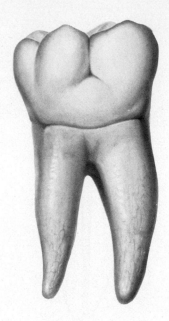 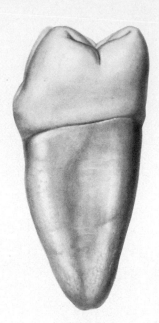

Average time of eruption: 6 years
Average age of calcification: 9 to 10 years
Average length: 21.0 mm

The earliest permanent posterior tooth to erupt, the mandibular first molar seems to be the most frequently in need of endodontic treatment. It usually has two roots but occasionally has three, with two canals in the mesial and one or two canals in the distal root.

The distal root is readily accessible to endodontic cavity preparation and mechanical instrumentation, and the clinician can frequently see directly into the orifice(s). The canals of the distal root are larger than those of the mesial root. Occasionally the orifice is wide from buccal to lingual. This anatomy indicates the possibility of a second canal or a ribbonlike canal with a complex webbing that can complicate cleaning and shaping.

The mesial roots are usually curved, with the greatest curvature in the mesial-buccal canal. The orifices are usually well separated within the main pulp chamber and occur in the buccal and lingual under the cusp tips.

This tooth is often extensively restored. It is almost always under heavy occlusal stress; thus the coronal pulp chambers are frequently calcified. The distal canals are easiest to locate; once these locations are positively identified, the mesial canals will be found in the aforementioned locations in the same horizontal plane.

Because the mesial canal openings lie under the mesial cusps, they may be impossible to locate with conventional cavity preparation. It will then be necessary to remove cuspal hard tissue or restoration to locate the orifice. As part of the access preparation, the unsupported cusps of posterior teeth must be reduced.[15] Remember, this tooth, like all posterior teeth, should always receive full occlusal coverage after endodontic therapy. (See Chapter 21.) Therefore a wider access cavity to locate landmarks and orifices is better than ignoring one or more canals for the sake of a "conservative" preparation, which may lead to failure.

Skidmore and Bjorndal[11] stated that approximately one third of the mandibular first molars studied had four root canals. When a tooth contained two canals, "they either remained two distinct canals with separate apical foramina, united and formed a common apical foramen, or communicated with each other partially or completely by transverse anastomoses. . . . If the traditional triangular outline were changed to a more rectangular one, it would permit better visualization and exploration of a possible fourth canal in the distal root."

Multiple accessory foramina are located in the furcation areas of mandibular molars.[9] They are usually impossible to clean and shape directly and are rarely seen, except occasionally, on postoperative radiographs if they have been filled with root canal sealer or warmed gutta-percha. It would be proper to assume that if irrigating solutions have the property of "seeking out" and disposing of protein degeneration products, then the furcation area of the pulp chamber should be thoroughly exposed (calcific adhesions removed, etc.) to allow the solutions to reach the tiny openings.

All caries, leaking restorations, and pulpal calcifications must be removed prior to endodontic treatment, and full cuspal protection and internal reinforcement are recommended.

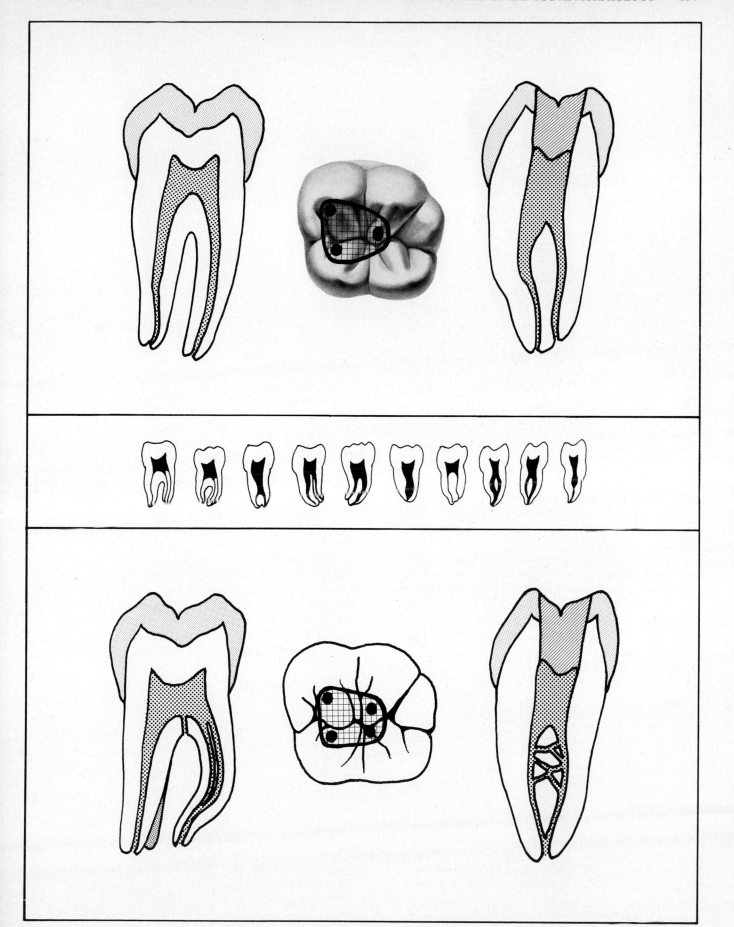

PLATE XV—MANDIBULAR SECOND MOLAR

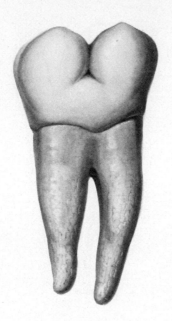 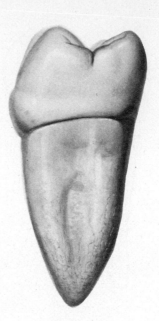

Average time of eruption: 11 to 13 years
Average age of calcification: 14 to 15 years
Average length: 19.8 mm

Somewhat smaller coronally than the mandibular first molar and tending toward more symmetry, the mandibular second molar is identified by the proximity of its roots. The roots often sweep distally in a gradual curve with the apices close together.

Access is made in the mesial of the crown, with the opening extending only slightly distal to the central groove. After penetration with the end-cutting fissure bur, the long-shanked round but is used to sweep outwardly until unobstructed access is achieved. The distal angulation of the roots often permits less extension of the opening than in the mandibular first molar.

Close attention should be given to the shape of the distal orifice. A narrow ovoid opening indicates a ribbon-shaped distal canal, requiring more directional-type filing.

All caries, leaking fillings, and pulpal calcifications must be removed and replaced with a suitable temporary restoration prior to endodontic therapy.

The mandibular second molar is the most susceptible to vertical fracture. After access preparation the clinician should utilize the fiberoptic light to search the floor of the chamber prior to endodontic treatment. The prognosis of mesial-distal crown/root fractures is highly unfavorable.

Full occlusal coverage after endodontic therapy is mandatory to ensure against future problems with vertical fracture.

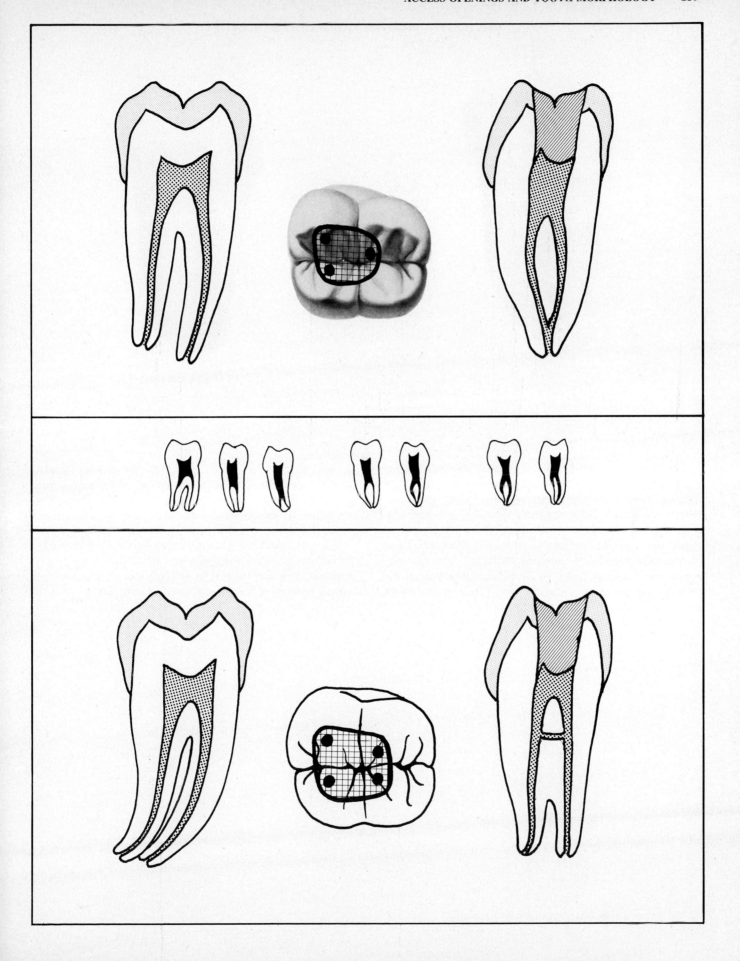

PLATE XVI—MANDIBULAR THIRD MOLAR

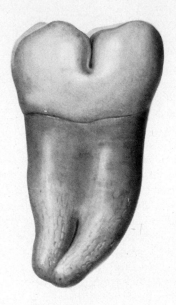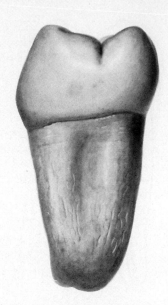

Average time of eruption: 17 to 21 years
Average age of calcification: 18 to 25 years
Average length: 18.5 mm

Anatomically unpredictable, the mandibular third molar must be evaluated on the basis of its root formation. Well-formed crowns are often supported by fused, short, severely curved, or malformed roots. Most teeth can be successfully treated endodontically regardless of anatomic irregularities, but root surface volume in contact with bone is what determines long-term prognosis.

The clinician may find a single canal that is wide at the cervical and tapers to a single apical foramen. Access is gained through the mesial aspect of the crown. Distally angled roots often permit less extension of the access cavity. Difficult accessibility in the arch occasionally can be simplified by the use of engine-mounted files on reciprocal handpieces.

All caries, leaking restorations, and pulpal calcifications should be removed and replaced with adequate temporary restoration. If the tooth is in heavy occlusal function, full cuspal protection is indicated postendodontically.

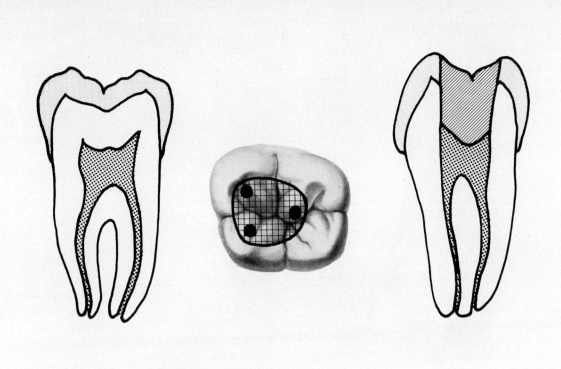

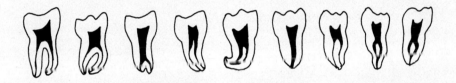

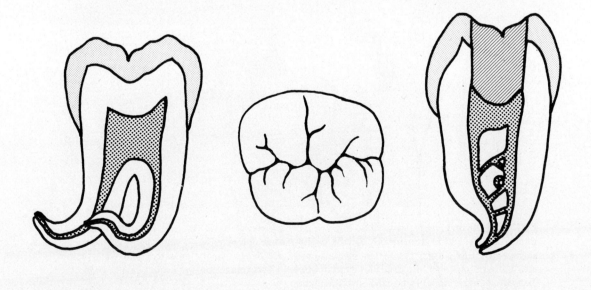

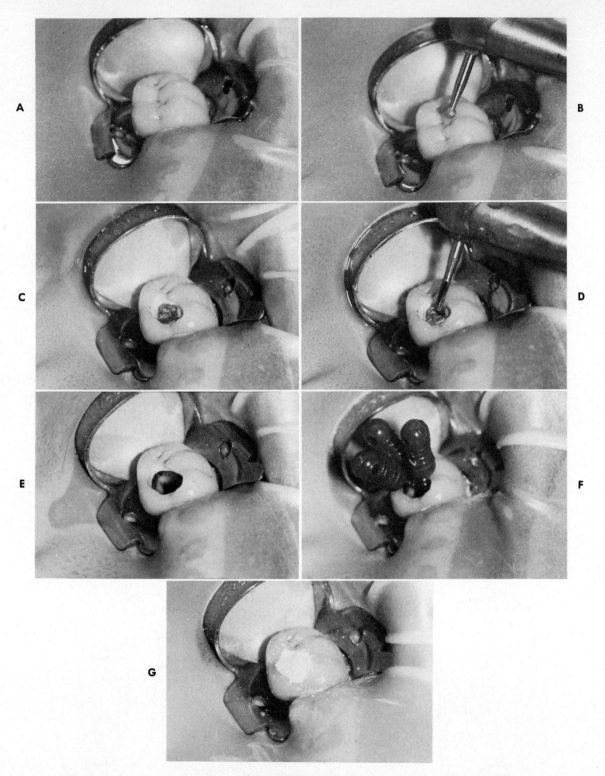

FIG. 6-13. *Access cavity preparation through a ceramometal crown.* **A,** The crown. **B,** Diamond-impregnated round instrument. **C,** Access cavity outline, prepared with water spray to the metal surface. **D,** End-cutting fissure bur in the turbine. **E,** Access cavity prepared with water spray into the pulp chamber. **F,** Test files placed without impingement on the access cavity walls. **G,** Temporary restoration placed after instrumentation.

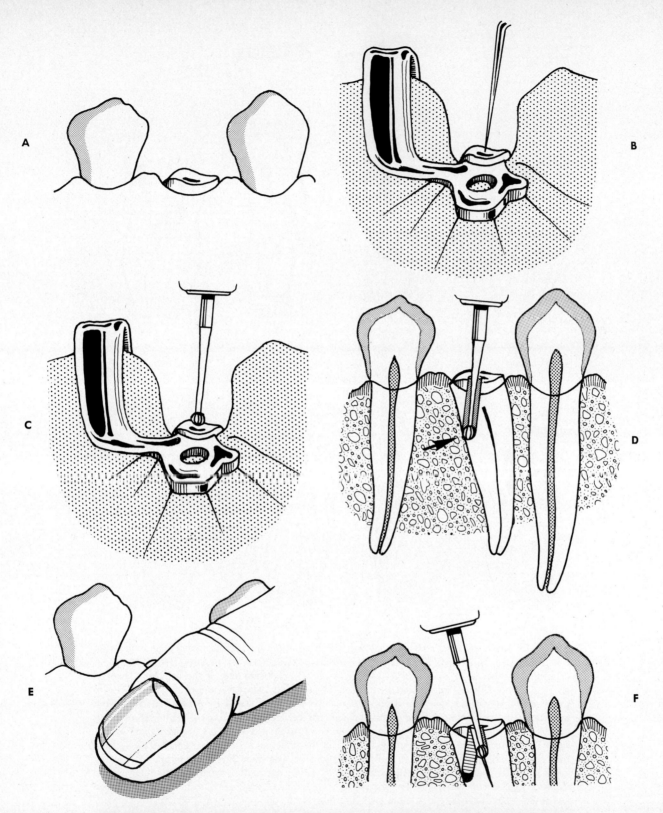

FIG. 6-14. *Errors in access cavity when the anatomic crown is missing.* **A,** Mandibular first premolar with the crown missing. **B,** An endodontic explorer fails to penetrate the calcified pulp chamber. **C,** Long-shank round bur directed in the assumed long axis of the root. **D,** Perforation of the root wall *(arrow)* because of the clinician's failure to consider root angulation. **E,** Palpation of the buccal root anatomy to determine root angulation. **F,** Correct bur angulation following repair of the perforation.

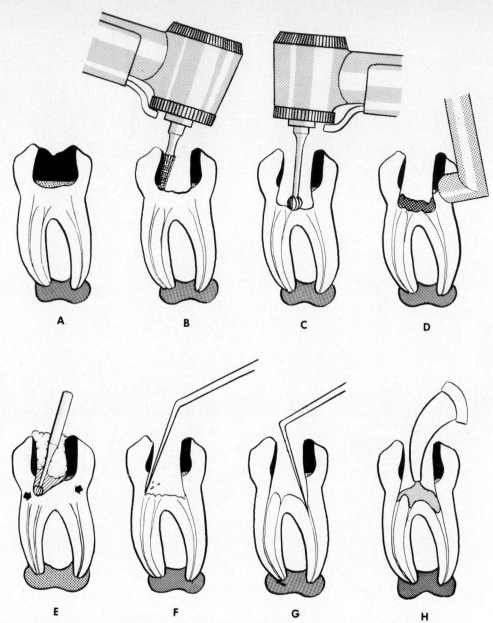

FIG. 6-15. *Complete treatment of a partially calcified tooth.* **A,** Typical mandibular molar with calcified canals. **B,** A normal access cavity is made to the depth of the existing restoration. **C,** A clear view of the cavity floor will usually reveal the old exposure site. If the bur (long-shanked no. 4) does not "drop" into the main chamber, proceed with extreme caution, cutting downward to the extent of an average pulp depth. Often, reparative dentin will be a different color from normal dentin, making the outline of the calcified chamber identifiable. **D,** The illuminating power of a fiberoptic light can assist in locating the outline of the pulp floor. If no landmarks are visible, study the external anatomy and proceed slowly in the direction of the usual canal orifices. Stop frequently to check location, since most perforations occur at this time. One means of showing depth is to place softened gutta-percha deep into the cavity and expose a radiograph. Gutta-percha is radiopaque, inexpensive, and easily removed. **E,** Another technique is to place an unattached bur in the area of deepest penetration, pack it in place with cotton pellets, and obtain a radiograph. The film will show both the depth and the direction of approach. **F,** When the pinpoint orifices are located, the endodontic explorer becomes a probe and also a chipping tool. **G,** Small calcific spicules can be teased out until a firm wedging and resistance are felt with the explorer. **H,** To facilitate cleaning and shaping, lubricate the entire chamber with RC-Prep or any calcium-chelating agent. This ointment can be stored in an impression material syringe and injected directly into the access cavity.

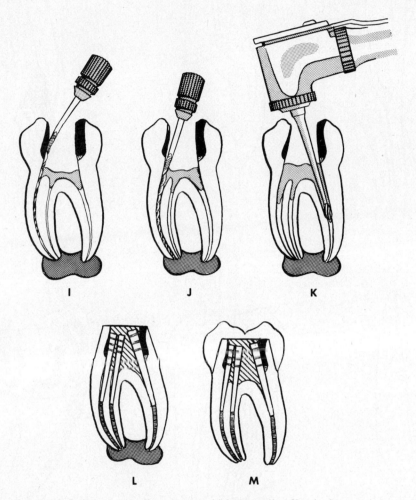

FIG. 6-15, cont'd. I, Select a small reamer to which the walls offer the least resistance and ease it into the orifice. A smooth up-and-down motion, without twisting, will provide a pathway. **J,** When reasonable penetration has been achieved, files and larger cutting instruments can be used. Continual use of a calcium-chelating solution is recommended. **K,** After a no. 35 file has reached as far as possible, the Gates-Glidden bur may be used to widen the coronal half of the canals with the chelating solution as a lubricant. An experienced clinician may use the Gates-Glidden bur to mechanically (and quickly) flare the canal orifices in the initial stages. However, the Gates-Glidden bur should not be employed as a vertical cutting tool. **L and M,** Canal obturation, dowel placement, core buildup, and a cast crown.

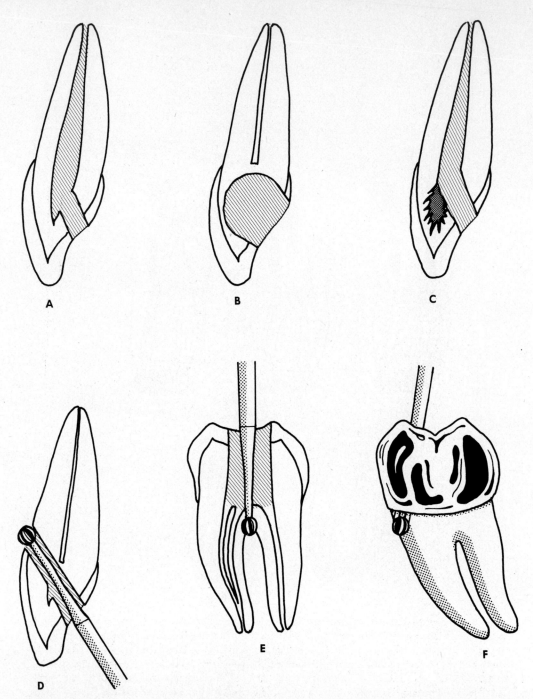

FIG. 6-16. *Difficulties encountered by poor access preparation.* **A,** Inadequate opening, which compromises instrumentation, invites coronal discoloration, and prevents good obturation. **B,** Overzealous tooth removal, resulting in mutilation of coronal tooth structure and weakening leading to coronal fracture. **C,** Inadequate caries removal, resulting in future carious destruction and discoloration. **D,** Labial perforation (lingual perforation with intact crowns is all but impossible in incisors). Surgical repair is possible, but permanent disfigurement and periodontal destruction will result. **E,** Furcal perforation of any magnitude, which (1) is difficult to repair, (2) causes periodontal destruction, and (3) weakens tooth structure, invites fracture. **F,** Misinterpretation of angulation (particularly common with full crowns) and subsequent root perforation. This is extremely difficult to repair; and even when it is repaired correctly, because it occurred in a difficult maintenance area the result is a permanent periodontal problem.

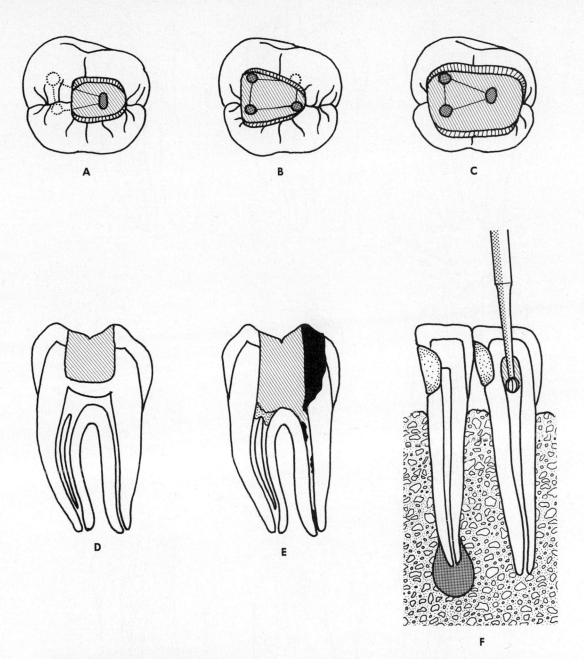

FIG. 6-17. *Common errors in access preparation.* **A,** Poor access placement and inadequate extension, leaving orifices unexposed. **B,** Better extension but not including the fourth canal orifice. **C,** Overextension, which weakens coronal tooth structure and compromises final restoration. **D,** Failure to reach the main pulp chamber is a serious error unless the space is heavily calcified. Bite-wing radiographs are excellent aids in determining vertical depth. **E,** An iatrogenic problem is allowing debris to fall into the orifices. Amalgam filings and dentin debris can block access and result in endodontic failure. **F,** The most embarrassing error, and the one with the most damaging medical-legal potential, is entering the wrong tooth. A common site of this mishap is teeth that appear identical coronally, and the simple mistake is placing the rubber dam on the wrong tooth. Initiating the access cavity *before* placement of the rubber dam will help the clinician avoid this problem.

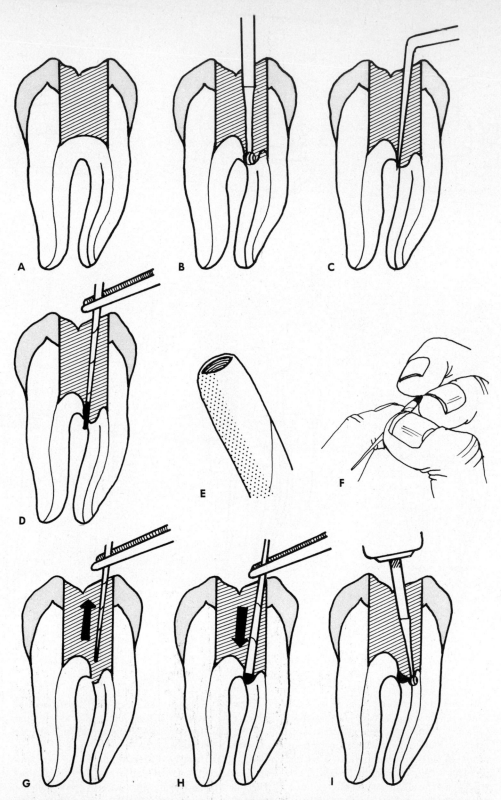

FIG. 6-18. *Perforation repair.* **A,** Access achieved in two canals but not in the calcified third canal. **B,** Minute furcal perforation during search for the elusive canal. **C,** Probing the perforation site with an endodontic pathfinder. **D,** Using absorbent point for hemorrhage control. **E,** Butt end of a paper point illustrating the recess in the tip created by the manufacturer's rolling thin paper to form the absorbent point. **F,** Placing a small bullet of fresh amalgam in the recess of the absorbent point. **G,** Removing the paper absorbent point. **H,** Inverting the point and depositing amalgam into the perforation (minimal tamping action). **I,** Adjusting the direction of the small round bur to locate the canal.

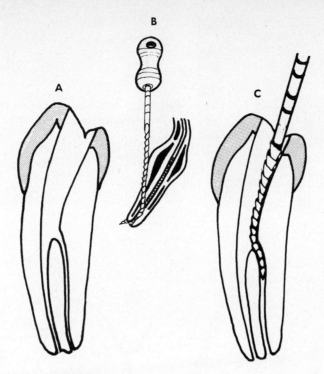

FIG. 6-19. A, Mandibular first premolar with division of the root canal system in the radicular portion of the tooth. **B,** Prebent endodontic file to facilitate access. **C,** Sliding the precurved instrument down the root wall until the tip engages the point of bifurcation.

PERIODONTAL-ENDODONTIC SITUATION

Complications of aging alone make locating canal orifices difficult. The problems of bone loss, chronic inflammation of the periodontal ligament, mobility and leakage into the root canal system are a combined periodontal-endodontic situation. The gradual closure of the internal spaces may be observed as the protective bone enclosure melts away from the root surfaces. The height of the pulp space now moves apically, making occlusal access difficult. Perforations of root walls and furcations are most common as the clinician reaches deeper and deeper with long-shanked burs. One means of locating the position of the bur tip and angle of approach is to stop, remove the bur from the handpiece and replace it in the cavity, pack the cavity around the bur with cotton, and take a periapical film (Fig. 6-15, *E*).

Periodontal patients may suffer caries on exposed root surfaces and thus require extensive Class V restorations. These restorations and the calcification often accompanying them can make obtaining occlusal access to some canals impossible. It may become necessary in unusual cases to remove the restorative material and then locate, clean, and shape the canals from the buccal (Fig. 6-20).

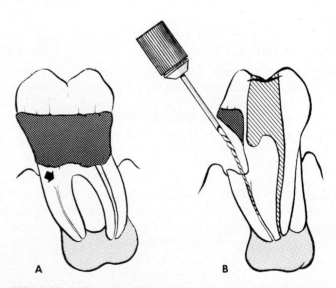

FIG. 6-20. A, Extensive Class V restoration necessitated by root caries and periodontal disease leading to canal calcification *(arrow).* **B,** Gaining access to these canals occluded by calcification may require removing the facial restoration and obtaining access from the buccal surface.

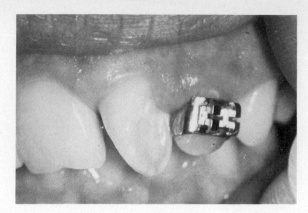

FIG. 6-21. Almost completely rotated, this central incisor offers a labial direction for straight-line access.

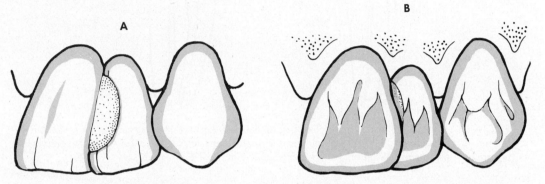

FIG. 6-22. A, Labial and, **B,** lingual views of malpositioned anteriors creating a difficult access situation.

FULL VENEER CROWNS

Properly made crowns are constructed with the occlusal relationship of the opposing tooth as a primary consideration. A cast crown may be made in any shape, diameter, height, or angle; this cast crown alteration can destroy the visual relationship to the true long axis (Fig. 6-16, *F*). Careful study of the preoperative radiograph will identify most of these situations.

Achieving access through crowns should be done with coolants, even when the rubber dam is used. Friction-generated heat can damage adjacent soft tissue, including the periodontal ligament; and with the anesthetized or nonvital tooth the patient will not be aware of pain. Once penetra-

tion of the metal is accomplished, the clinician can change to a sharp round bur and move toward the central pulp chamber. Metal filings and debris from the access cavity should be removed frequently because small slivers can cause large obstructions in the fine canal system.

When sufficient access has been gained, the clinician should search margins and internal spaces for caries and leakage and the pulpal floor for signs of fracture or perforation. Occasionally caries can be removed through the occlusal access cavity and the tooth can be properly restored (Fig. 6-25). The interior of a crown can be a surprise package, containing everything from total caries to intact dentin (as seen in periodontally induced pulp death).

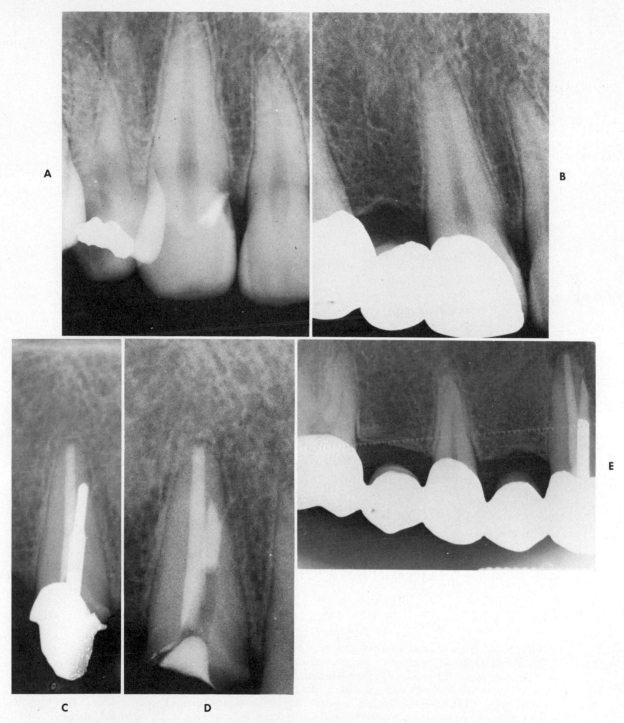

FIG. 6-23. *Dowel space perforations.* **A,** Early periapical film showing a normal maxillary canine. **B,** Fourteen months later, after the loss of the first premolar, a bridge has been constructed, utilizing the canine as an abutment. **C,** Leakage and caries under the pin-inlay abutment involved the pulp. Endodontic therapy was performed. A dowel space was prepared, and a perforation occurred. Endodontic therapy was performed on the dowel perforation, **D,** as though it were a natural root canal. A long bevel was prepared in the gutta-percha. **E,** A new dowel was placed and a fixed bridge constructed.

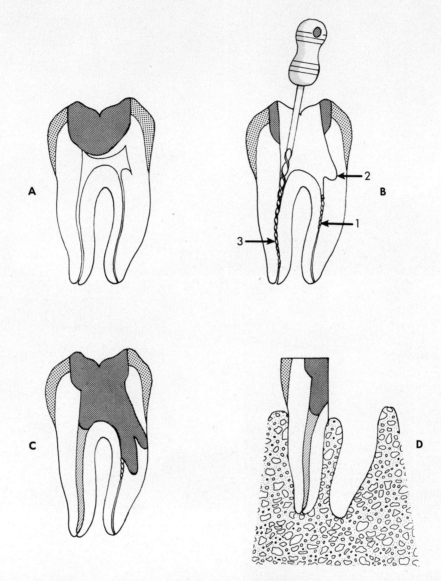

FIG. 6-24. *Hemisection as an alternative when mutilation occurs during access preparation.* **A,** Calcification after advanced caries and the application of calcium hydroxide can result in serious difficulties in making access. **B,** *1,* An instrument has fractured in the mesial canal; *2,* a second mesial canal seems totally calcified; and, *3,* the third canal, in the distal root, is navigable. **C,** Searching for canals and instrument fragments can result in mutilation of tooth structure. **D,** Obturation of one root and placement of amalgam in access areas will restore the intracanal spaces **(C)** in preparation for routine hemisection. Reinforcement with a dowel and core may be performed prior to final restoration.

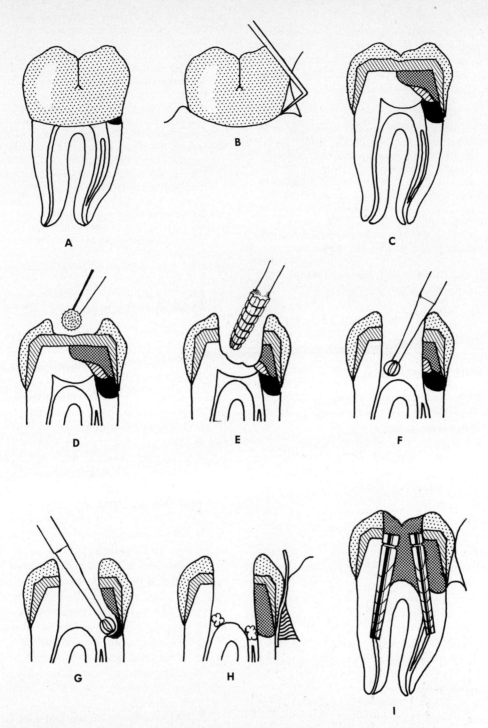

FIG. 6-25. *Retaining crowns through internal repair.* Patients with radiographic evidence of caries at the crown margin, **A,** present a difficult endodontic situation. In most cases the crown should be removed. However, sometimes it can be maintained so long as the caries is accessible and the crown repairable. Probing the crown margin, **B,** and determining the extent and depth of caries allow the clinician to determine whether the crown can be retained. The caries, **C,** has not seriously undermined the crown. Diamond instruments, **D,** are used to remove the ceramic material; and the end-cutting fissure bur, **E,** is used to penetrate the metal and the dentin above the pulp chamber. Round burs refine the access, **F,** and remove the carious dentin, **G.** A matrix is securely wedged and amalgam is packed into the void. **H,** Careful attention must be given to thorough caries removal and moisture control. Cotton pellets placed in the orifices will prevent amalgam debris from entering the canals. **I,** In a sealed environment the endodontics is completed and suitable reinforcement, including a full amalgam core, is placed.

ACKNOWLEDGEMENT

I wish to extend my appreciation to the following distinguished endodontists for helping with the preparation of the plates in this chapter: Quintiliano de Deus, Nguyen T. Nguyen, Herbert Schilder, Noah Chivian, Donald Arens, David Moore, Fulton Yee, Ronald Borer, Gerald Dietz, and Jean-Marie Laurichesse.

REFERENCES

1. Benjamin, K.A., and Dowson, J.: Incidence of two-root canals in human mandibular incisor teeth, Oral Surg. **38:**122, 1974.
2. Brand, R.W., and Isselhard, D.E.: Anatomy of orofacial structures, ed. 3, St. Louis, 1986, C.V. Mosby Co.
3. Carns, E.J., and Skidmore, A.E.: Configurations and deviations of root canals of maxillary first premolars, Oral Surg. **36:**880, 1973.
4. de Deus, Q.D.: Endodontia, ed. 4, Rio de Janeiro, 1986, Medsiedi-tôra Médica e Científica, Ltda.
5. Gher, M.E., and Vernino, A.R.: Root anatomy: a local factor in inflammatory periodontal disease, Int. J. Period. Restor. Dent. **1:**53, 1981.
6. Green, D.: Double canals in single roots, Oral Surg. **35:**689, 1973.
7. Grossman, L.I.: Endodontic practice, ed. 10, Philadelphia, 1981, Lea & Febiger.
8. Hess, W., and Zürcher, E.: The anatomy of the root canals of the teeth of the permanent and deciduous dentitions, New York, 1925, William Wood & Co.
9. Koenigs, J.F., Brilliant, J.D., and Foreman, D.W., Jr.: Preliminary scanning electron microscope investigation of accessory foramina in the furcation areas of human molar teeth. Oral Surg. **38:**773, 1974.
10. Pineda, F.: Roentgenographic investigations of the mesiobuccal root of the maxillary first molar, Oral Surg. **36:**253, 1973.
11. Skidmore, A.E., and Bjorndal, A.M.: Root canal morphology of the human mandibular first molar. Oral Surg. **32:**778, 1971.
12. Slowey, R.R.: Radiographic aids in the detection of extra root canals, Oral Surg. **37:**762, 1974.
13. Vertucci, F.J.: Root canal morphology of mandibular premolars, J. Am. Dent. Assoc. **97:**47, 1978.
14. Vertucci, F., Seelig, A., and Gillis, R.: Root canal morphology of the human maxillary second premolar, Oral Surg. **38:**456, 1974.
15. Weine, F.S., et al.: Canal configuration in the mesiobuccal root of the maxillary first molar and its endodontic significance, Oral Surg. **28:**419, 1969.
16. Zeisz, R.C., and Nuckolls, J.: Dental anatomy, St. Louis, 1949, The C.V. Mosby Co.
17. Zillich, R., and Dowson, J.: Root canal morphology of mandibular first and second premolars, Oral Surg. **36:**738, 1973.

Self-assessment questions

1. Tooth morphology and access cavity preparations are
   a. Independent factors in root canal therapy
   b. Free of variations from tooth to tooth
   c. Closely interrelated in root canal therapy
   d. Standard for similar teeth
2. The outline form of the access cavity should be prepared
   a. Well into the dentin
   b. Superficially in enamel
   c. With a no. 4 or 6 bur
   d. Into the canal orifices
3. The root canal orifices are best located by use of
   a. A periodontal probe
   b. An endodontic excavator
   c. A rotating round bur
   d. An endodontic pathfinder
4. The most common clinical error when a clinician is opening into the pulp chamber of a mandibular incisor is
   a. A lingual perforation
   b. A labial perforation
   c. An incisal fracture
   d. A lateral perforation
5. In an access cavity preparation, the occlusal (lingual) opening is extended to
   a. Include all occlusal pits and fissures
   b. Establish unimpeded access to the canal orifices
   c. Include cusps to prevent possible fractures
   d. Provide visual access to canal anatomy
6. A second radiograph from a mesial angulation of 30 degrees will assist in determining or identifying
   a. Possible additional roots
   b. Vertical root fractures
   c. The exact tooth length
   d. The location of apical foramina
7. The clinician can identify curvatures, obstructions, root divisions, and additional canal orifices by utilizing
   a. Fiberoptic illumination of the tooth crown
   b. An endodontic pathfinder in canal orifices
   c. Previous knowledge of tooth anatomy
   d. Digital perception with a hand instrument
8. The access cavity outlines of a maxillary central incisor and a maxillary lateral incisor are most often
   a. Similar because of similar crown and root form
   b. Triangular and located incisal to the cingulum
   c. Triangular and ovoid, respectively
   d. Completed with the fissure bur alone
9. From an endodontic point of view, the first and second premolars
   a. Are similar in crown and root form
   b. Vary mainly in root form
   c. Require conservative restorations following root canal therapy
   d. Have lateral, divergent canal orifices
10. The mesial-buccal root of the maxillary first molar may
    a. Contain two large canal orifices equal in size
    b. Demonstrate two canals in the majority of cases
    c. Contain a second orifice toward the distal-buccal canal orifice
    d. Have a second canal orifice toward the palatal canal

11. The distinguishing morphologic feature of the maxillary second molar is the
    a. Divergent buccal roots
    b. Nonparallel root canals
    c. Three roots grouped closely together
    d. Rectangular shape of the chamber floor
12. The root canal of the mandibular first molar with the greatest curvature is the
    a. Mesial-buccal canal
    b. Mesial-lingual canal
    c. Distal-buccal canal
    d. Distal-lingual canal
13. Inadequate access openings will
    a. Permit sufficient debridement of the chamber
    b. Compromise instrumentation of the canals
    c. Reduce the possibility of crown discoloration
    d. Aid in the obturation of the canal system
14. Access through a cast crown is best accomplished with
    a. A slow-speed cross-cut fissure bur
    b. A high-speed bur perpendicular to the occlusal surface
    c. A dry operating field to maintain visibility
    d. A coolant to reduce friction-generated heat

7

CLEANING AND SHAPING THE ROOT CANAL SYSTEM

JAMES L. GUTMANN
THOM DUMSHA

For many years the success or failure of root canal treatment resided in the philosophy that total three-dimensional obturation of the root canal system was essential to ultimate healing and tooth retention. This contention was intimately associated with the thought that percolation and stagnation of tissue fluids and/or lodgment of bacteria in spaces between the prepared root canal wall and filling would serve as sources of irritation, chronic inflammation, and ultimate failure of treatment rendered. This philosophy is presently foremost in the minds of many practitioners and serves as their guiding principle in root canal treatment. Support for this philosophy is secured from apical leakage studies[17] and long-term evaluation studies.[36] Although achievement of three-dimensional root canal obturation is desirable in all clinical situations, attainment of this goal is questionable.[6,9,69] In addition, studies have shown that tissue fluid percolation into areas of relative sterility does not necessarily result in long-term inflammation and irritation.[61,80,81] Therefore, the logical mind must focus on other potential sources of failure.

If the source of chronic inflammation does not come from outside the root canal system (i.e., stagnation of fluids or lodgment of bacteria from hematogenous sources—anachoresis), then one must look to the root canal system itself or to the oral cavity for the etiologic factors. Contaminants, from either source, leaching into the periradicular tissues will ultimately lead to failure. Therefore, while sealing the root canal system is of major importance, *proper debridement of the contaminated system is paramount as a precondition for successful treatment.*

Proper debridement of the root canal system can be achieved only through meticulous removal of the contaminants from within the anatomic irregularities of the root canal—fins, webs, cul de sacs, anastomoses, and so on. To effectively accomplish this task, not only must cleaning take place, but proper canal shaping must occur to eliminate the irregularities that may harbor debris and microorganisms.[67] This shaping not only debrides the canal system

but also prepares the canal system for a more homogeneous three-dimensional obturation—hence sealing the canal system from potential occlusal contaminants from the oral cavity, sealing within the canal small amounts of irritants inaccessible to our cleaning methods, and preventing leakage of interstitial fluids and microorganisms through the apical foramina.

This concept is not new in root canal treatment. For years the axiom in endodontics has been that what is taken out of the canal may be more important than what is put into the canal for obturation. However, for years the prevailing focus of attention was on the apical sealing of the canal, even to the point of neglecting other pathways of the pulpal space to the external environment—that is, accessory canals, lateral canals, and dentinal tubules. With the advent of sophisticated canal preparation techniques and the recognition of the importance of chemomechanical canal debridement, root canal cleaning and shaping have reached an unprecedented degree of quality, enabling total canal disinfection and an ultimate three-dimensional sealing of all the pathways of the pulp (Fig. 7-1).

The purpose of this chapter is to provide the rationale and techniques for proper cleaning and shaping of the root canal system, which will enable the clinician to obturate the system in its entirety.[67] As with many aspects of dentistry, such as a denture being no better than the initial impression, or an onlay being no better than the tooth preparation, it follows that canal obturation will be no better than the cleaning and shaping of the entire system.

Initially this discussion will center around various components of this phase of treatment, relating each to the goal to be accomplished. Finally each component will be placed in its logical progression during the thorough cleaning and shaping of the root canal system.

Three phases of canal preparation must be addressed during root canal therapy. These phases, which interrelate and overlap, consist of procedures designed to (1) initially clean the canal of its diseased tissue or foreign matter, (2)

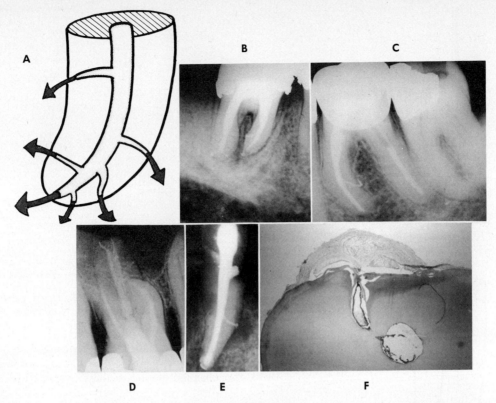

FIG. 7-1. A, Potential pathways of the pulp, which must be cleaned and sealed to ensure successful treatment. **B, C, D,** and **E,** Proper canal cleaning and shaping facilitate sealing of a myriad of pulp space configurations. **F,** Failure to effectively clean main pulp canal and large lateral canal. Note persistent lateral cystic lesion —taken from midroot mandibular premolar. (**B** and **C** courtesy Dr. David P. Rossiter, Northampton, Mass.)

both remove debris and provide an initial shape to the canal, and (3) exclusively shape the coronal two thirds of the canal to facilitate final cleaning and three-dimensional obturation. Although each phase will be discussed separately for clarity, the three are intimately related and require a goal-oriented, cognizant approach to their ultimate achievement and success.

INITIAL CLEANING

Cleaning of the canal contents implies removal of both vital and nonvital tissue remnants, associated tissue breakdown products, and microorganisms when present. This process is initially achieved by pulp extirpation (vital pulps) or canal system debridement (nonvital pulps) through the use of spoon excavators, burs, broaches, and files, along with voluminous irrigation with agents designed to dissolve tissue debris, eradicate microorganisms, and serve as lubricants.

Thorough cleaning of the gross contaminants in the root canal system is the first step in canal system disinfection, or what used to be referred to as "sterilization." However, no single procedure in the cleaning or cleaning and shaping phases can be identified as the key or sole entity in achieving canal disinfection. In years past a heavy emphasis was placed on the use of intracanal medicaments, even to the point that the medicaments were used to neutralize debris remaining in the canal system. However, modern

root canal treatment depends on a more thorough chemomechanical sanitization of the canal system rather than the use of caustic intracanal medicaments. Achievement of this goal is predicated on the proper use of both intracanal irrigants and manual cleaning procedures that will provide a thoroughly-cleaned system.[64]

Role of intracanal irrigants

Although canal cleaning is accomplished with intracanal instruments, these alone are not able to remove all the tissue remnants and debris from the canal system. Thorough flushing with effective intracanal irrigants goes hand in hand with mechanical cleaning of the canal system (chemomechanical debridement).

The literature is replete with studies that extol the various attributes of a multitude of irrigating agents: sodium hypochlorite, hydrogen peroxide, chelating agents, and so on.[36,44] However, it is generally recognized that the most important irrigating solution employed in endodontics is sodium hypochlorite (NaOCl).[67] The clinical concentrations used ranges from 0.5% to 5.25%,[82,84] with 2.5%[63] being the most common. Sodium hypochlorite possesses strong tissue-dissolution properties for fresh tissue, necrotic tissue, and fixed tissue.[32,63,76,84] It is strongly bacteriocidal, it is an excellent lubricant and bleaching agent, it has an extended shelf life, and it is quite inexpensive. In addition, its action in the root canal system is signifi-

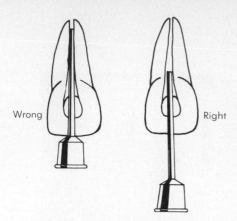

Wrong   Right

FIG. 7-2. The needle of the irrigating syringe is placed loosely into the orifice of the canal. Do not attempt to place the needle near the apex or wedge the needle in the canal.

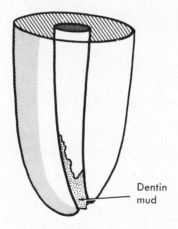

Dentin mud

FIG. 7-3. Dentin chips and tissue debris accumulated at the end of the canal.

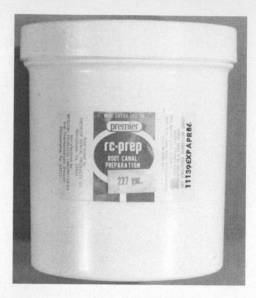

FIG. 7-4. Commonly used chelating agent RC-Prep. (Courtesy Premier Dental Products Co., Norristown, Pa.)

cantly enhanced with voluminous flushing during the cleaning and shaping phases. Once these phases take place, greater penetration of sodium hypochlorite is achieved into the depths and irregularities of the canal system, further promoting total tissue removal.

For years 3% hydrogen peroxide (H_2O_2) was recommended as a canal irrigant because of its disinfecting properties and its effervescent action.[30] The effervescent action was especially indicated in mandibular teeth, where the bubbling of the peroxide was thought to lift debris from the canal system, almost defying gravity.[67] However, hydrogen peroxide does not possess tissue-dissolution properties and is not effective as a lubricant.

The use of a combination sodium hypochlorite NaOCl and 3% hydrogen peroxide in the canal system has been recommended to effect a release of nascent oxygen, enhancing the foaming or bubbling properties desired for debris removal.[72] However, this combination of the two irrigants has been shown to inhibit their individual antibacterial properties.[33]

What must be kept in mind in regard to either of these two irrigants is that their use *must be confined to the canal space*. Forcing these irrigants beyond the canal confines, especially under pressure, will lead to severe clinical tox-

icity, tissue injury, and very acute symptoms of pain and swelling.[3,40] These fears have caused clinicians either to abandon the use of these irrigants in favor of water or saline or to significantly reduce their concentration during use. However, reductions in concentration usually result in significant reductions in the properties of the irrigants.[34] Switching to water or saline eliminates the beneficial and necessary properties of the irrigant. Therefore, although they are highly recommended, 3% hydrogen peroxide or 2.5% to 5.25% sodium hypochlorite must be used cautiously and within safe clinical parameters.

Both solutions are delivered to the canal system via irrigating syringes. Care must be exercised to prevent the placement of any needle in the canal system that would result in the delivery of the irrigants under pressure, especially beyond the confines of the canal as previously mentioned (Fig. 7-2). Various syringes are available for this purpose.

In addition to the tissue dissolution, bacteriocidal action, and lubrication achieved with the use of sodium hypochlorite, its flushing action helps to retain dentinal chips in solution, which effectively removes inorganic debris during the cleaning and shaping phase and prevents the accumulation of large amounts of dentinal debris at the apex (Fig. 7-3). This is especially crucial (1) to ensure the removal of contaminated dentin and (2) to maintain the patency of the canal from the coronal orifice to the apical foramen. The significance of this will become quite evident when recapitulation and canal shaping are discussed.

Another group of chemical agents that has been recommended during the cleaning and shaping phase of treatment is the chelating agents, primarily ethylenediaminetetraacetic acid (EDTA). Commercially, this substance is readily available as RC-Prep* (Fig. 7-4). RC-Prep, com-

---

*Premier Dental Products Co., Norristown, Pa.

posed of 15% EDTA and 10% urea peroxide in a carbo-wax water-soluble base, functions as an oxygenating agent in the presence of sodium hypochlorite and as a canal lubricant. Effectively, a softening of the calcified dentin occurs, which facilitates the negotiation, cleaning, and shaping of the canal walls, especially the radicular dentin.

When a solution of EDTA* is used subsequent to canal cleaning and shaping and in conjunction with a sodium hypochlorite rinse, there appears to be an effective removal of the dentinal smear layer that has built up on the walls as a result of instrument rubbing and burnishing during shaping procedures.[25] Removal of the smear layer effectively results in cleaner walls[53] and the potential for better adaptation of not only the root canal filling materials but also posts.[24]

By the very chemical nature and action of chelating agents they appear to be self-limiting in action[23] and therefore should be used periodically during canal cleaning procedures. Although chelating agents are effective in producing a clean canal over a period of time, the exclusive use of chelating agents should never supplant the use of sodium hypochlorite during canal cleaning and shaping procedures.

While a plethora of experimental irrigants have been evaluated for clinical use,[36] there remains a paucity of valid clinical information regarding their toxicity, biologic compatibility, and treatment effectiveness. However, critical factors for any irrigants used are canal diameter, surface tension or viscosity of the irrigant, the placement of the irrigating needle (Fig. 7-2), and the volume of flushing that occurs during clinical procedures. Maintanence of the solution within the confines of the canal is also critical. Finally, it must be remembered that no root canal should be cleaned or shaped without the use of a clinically acceptable irrigant.

Removal of vital tissue: pulp extirpation

The word "extirpation" is derived from the Latin word *ex(s)tirpare,* meaning "to pluck up by the roots." Pulp extirpation or pulpectomy is the bulk removal of a normal or diseased pulp in its initial stages of pulpitis or degeneration. Efficient and effective removal of the pulp tissue in the canal is best accomplished in larger, straighter canals through the use of a barbed broach. Smaller, curved canals will require thorough cleansing with K-files to remove the pulp tissue.

Effective use of a barbed broach to remove pulp tissue is dependent on the following factors. First, the access opening must be sufficiently large for the placement of the broach and the removal of the tissue. Second, the broach must be wide enough to engage the pulp without touching the walls of the canal. Small broaches tend to fit within a larger mass of pulp tissue without securing a sufficient grip on the tissue; the pulp is shredded into multiple segments, which if not removed in toto may result in posttreatment pain. Third, the broach should not be so wide as to have

*Roth Drug Co., Chicago, Ill.

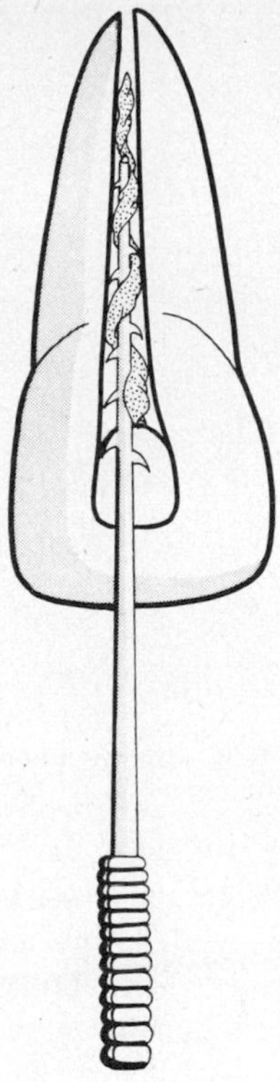

FIG. 7-5. Correct use of a barbed broach. The broach should *never* be placed in the apical third of the canal.

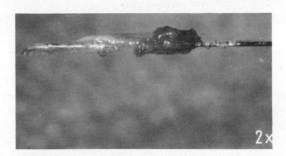

FIG. 7-6. Complete pulp properly engaged and extirpated.

its barbs engage the dentinal wall. This could lead to fracture of the narrow shaft of this instrument.

Some additional guidelines for the use of barbed broaches are as follows:

1. Confine the broach to the straight portion of the canal.
2. Do not place the broach into the canal farther than two thirds of the canal's length (Fig. 7-5).
3. Do not force the broach into the canal.
4. Avoid the use of a barbed broach when significant canal calcifications are visible radiographically.

Prior to using the barbed broach, flush the pulp chamber and canal orifices with sodium hypochlorite. Place the selected broach approximately two thirds of the way into the canal, and rotate it 180 degrees. Gently remove the broach. If the access cavity and broach are appropriately sized, a vital pulp will become entangled in the barbs without being shredded and will be detached from the walls in one piece (Fig. 7-6). Irrigate again with sodium

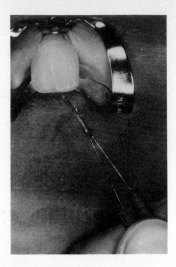

FIG. 7-7. Complete pulp enmeshed between two broaches.

hypochlorite. At this point the exact root length should be determined, followed by cleansing and shaping. In cases of very large pulp canals, two broaches may be placed mesiodistally or buccolingually within the canal at the same time. If the dentist rotates the handles of the two broaches, the pulp will become enmeshed between the shafts and easily removed (Fig. 7-7).

Caution is the key word in the use of a barbed broach. Although the instrument can be forced into the canal easily, because the barbs compress over irregularities of the canal wall with ease, removal will cause the barbs to spread, locking the instrument into the irregular dentinal wall. This may result in instrument separation and ultimate canal blockage.

An alternate method to remove the pulp would be to use a new, sharp Hedström file large enough to slip alongside the pulp. Pressure is exerted against the pulp, pressing it against the dentin wall, and the Hedström is removed, severing the pulp with the coronally angled blades of the file.

Removal of nonvital tissue: canal debridement

The word "debridement" has French, Latin, and German roots and is defined as "the surgical excision of dead and devitalized tissue and the removal of all foreign matter from a wound."[2a] Certainly this word connotes most clearly what is to be accomplished when a root canal system is replete with necrotic tissue, bacteria and their toxins, and tissue degradation products. However, in comparison with vital pulps, necrotic material is not so readily removed from the root canal system. This is especially true when advanced degeneration of the pulp negates the effective use of barbed broaches to remove the tissue intact. Broaches in such instances are useful only to remove the occasional large pieces of pulp tissue or food debris that has invaded the root canal systems open to the oral cavity. Debridement of necrotic, contaminated tissue depends primarily on the effectiveness of irrigation and its ability to flush and dissolve tissue debris, as well as the subsequent cleaning and shaping procedures. Copious irrigation with

sodium hypochlorite is strongly recommended along with mechanical cleaning and shaping, to effectively debride the canal of its irritating contents.

CLEANING AND SHAPING
Specific objectives

Generally speaking, the two main objectives in canal cleaning and shaping are biologic and mechanical. Biologically, the goal of intracanal procedures is to remove all pulp tissue remnants and microorganisms and their substrates, along with infected predentin and dentin. Mechanically, three-dimensional shaping of the canal is the objective, which must be accomplished to ensure biologic cleaning. The achievement of both of these major goals is predicated on the presence of a sufficiently large access opening to allow for direct, unimpeded entry into the canal from the orifice to the foramen. (See Chapter 6.)

Biologic objectives

From a biologic standpoint, specific objectives should be foremost with every clinician. These will enhance the ultimate success and minimize patient discomfort during and after treatment. The biologic objectives are as follows:

1. *Confine all instrumentation within the root canal space.* Attention to detail in determining the working length will establish the working parameters. Subsequently the clinician must be acutely aware of the movement of files within the canal, especially near the dentin-cementum junction. The inadvertent overextension of a fine instrument past the apical foramen while the exact length is being established, or the occasional probing of 1 mm past the apical constriction to ensure patency, is not a major irritant to the periradicular tissues. However, repeated instrumentation extending beyond the constriction is unwarranted. It causes periradicular inflammation and often destroys the normal biologic constriction of the root apex. Although rare, perforations of the floor of the nose, maxillary sinus, or mandibular canal as a result of excessive overextension of instruments can lead to severe posttreatment pain, delayed healing, and ultimate failure. Intentional overextension of small instruments past the apical constriction is warranted only when drainage must be established from the periradicular tissues (see Chapter 2), such as in an acute apical abscess or a phoenix abscess (Fig. 7-8).

2. *Avoid pushing contaminated debris past the confines of the apical constriction* (Fig. 7-9). Many instances of posttreatment pain and swelling can be attributed to necrotic tissue and microorganisms and their toxins being inoculated into the periradicular tissues as a result of indiscriminate cleaning procedures. This inoculation of the periradicular tissues will induce a rapid immunologic response[79] (see Chapter 12). Care must be taken to initially remove the gross contaminants through the copious use of sodium hypochlorite along with gross mechanical debridement. Often this is done *prior* to establishing the exact working length of the root canal.

3. *Remove all the potential irritants from the entire canal system.* This avoids recurrent periradicular inflam-

mation and creates a condition that permits prompt, uneventful healing. Because of numerous canal cul-de-sacs, copious irrigation with 2.5%-5.25% sodium hypochlorite is essential.

4. *Establish the exact working length and completely clean and shape the canal system during the first treatment visit.* The microbial and chemical factors that can provoke periapical inflammation must be eliminated. In cases involving vital pulps, where the working length has been determined but the canal has not been properly cleaned of its vital tissue remnants, exacerbations often occur as a result of the lacerated, minced pulp tissue tags left in the canal. The dentist should not approach the apical third of the root canal with a file unless he has every intent of properly measuring and thoroughly cleaning the canal space. This concept is especially true in the treatment of necrotic pulps. Leaving microorganisms, substrate, or toxins in necrotic canals predisposes the patient to posttreatment complications. Promptly removing the etiologic factors that provoke periapical inflammation permits uneventful healing.

5. *Create sufficient width in the coronal half of canal system to allow for copious flushing and debridement.* Studies have demonstrated that properly shaped canals with sufficient canal diameters and divergent walls have less remaining tissue debris[12,85] and permit the irrigating solution to go deeper into the canal.[44]

Mechanical objectives

There are five mechanical objectives in the cleaning and shaping of the root canal:

1. *Prepare a sound apical dentin matrix at the dentin-cementum junction.* The development of this matrix provides the resistance form to the intraradicular cavity preparation (Fig. 7-10, *A*). The matrix or canal narrowing prevents overextension of instruments and controls the apical movement of gutta percha and sealer during obturation.

2. *Prepare the canal to taper apically, with the narrowest cross-sectional diameter at the apical termination (apical dentin matrix).* The apical third of the canal preparation must provide a tapering or parallel, spatial configuration in order to ensure a firm seating of the gutta percha and sealer (Fig. 7-10, *B*). It is within these confines that the apical seal is obtained. The three-dimensional shape of the preparation, especially of the apical third, must provide a narrowing retentive cavity to enhance condensation procedures.

3. *Develop a continuously tapering funnel-type preparation in three dimensions within the entire root canal system.* Thorough cleaning and shaping of the canal is predicated on the funnel or flare type of preparation. Removal of bacterial substrate is ensured because of greater access to canal irregularities by both files and irrigants. In addition, this objective addresses the need to view every root canal system as a unique, individual three-dimensional

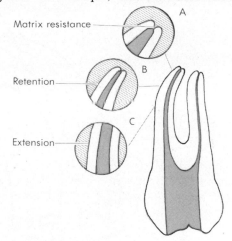

FIG. 7-10. Final shape of root canal. *A,* Apical dentin matrix. *B,* Slightly divergent walls in the apical third. *C,* Flared or funnel shaped canal that flows with the shape of the root.

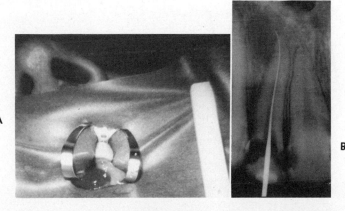

FIG. 7-8. **A,** Purulent drainage stimulated by the placement of an instrument, **B,** beyond the apical constriction.

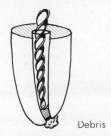

FIG. 7-9. Avoid pushing contaminated debris past the apical constriction.

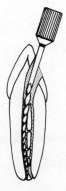

FIG. 7-11. "Boring out" of the apical third of the canal and failure to clean or shape the remainder of the irregular canal anatomy.

system. The final preparation of this system should be an exact replica of the original canal configuration in shape, taper, and flow, only larger (Fig. 7-10, *C*). Only too often canals are simply ''bored out'' with the clinician failing to consider the spatial relationship of the canal to the overall root anatomy, especially external convolutions, narrowings, and curvatures (Fig. 7-11). Root canal systems must be shaped on the basis of the original anatomy of the canal system and the objectives to be achieved. Adherence to this concept also parallels the ''extension for prevention'' concept; that is, thorough removal of the irritant enhances thorough canal obturation.

4. *Confine cleaning and shaping procedures to the canal system, thereby maintaining the spatial integrity of the apical foramen.* Adherence to this principle prevents violation of the periradicular tissues. This principle is evident when foramina are transported (i.e., moved) during excessive apical instrumentation.

Foraminal transportation can be either external or internal.

External transportation takes two forms and may occur when instrumentation is carried out beyond the apical dentin matrix (Fig. 7-12, *A*). One result is the ripping of the apical end of the canal, resulting in a teardrop, elliptical, or zipped foramen.[88] In its grosser form, external transportation leads to an outright perforation of the root (Fig. 7-12, *C*).

Internal transportation can also occur when excessively large instruments are used in the apical third of a curved canal (Fig. 7-13). Even though a perforation may not have occurred, there is a definite loss of the narrowing apical preparation and the spatial relationship of this preparation to the apical foramen.

Generally, both types of transportation of the apical fo-

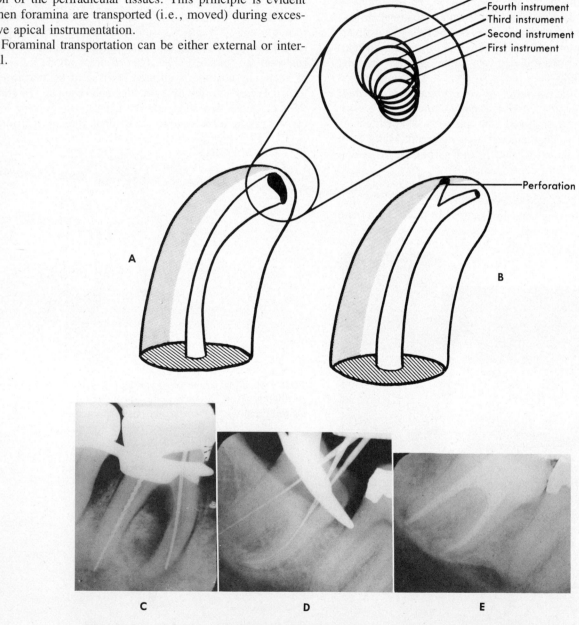

FIG. 7-12. A, Teardrop or zipped foramen resulting from large instruments cutting counter to the canal curvature and foramen position. B, Direct perforation. C, Mandibular molar showing direct perforation. D, Mandibular molar showing proper working length and canal negotiation. E, Perforation evident on mesial canals, which have excessive curves.

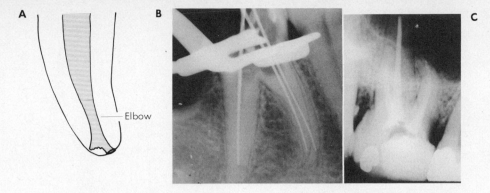

FIG. 7-13. A, Movement of the canal wall laterally and out of spatial relationship and flow with the apical foramen; this may not result in a perforation but ledging, canal blockage, and loss of canal length are common. **B** and **C,** Internal transportation evident in mandibular and maxillary molar (mesial-buccal root).

ramen can be prevented by containing cleaning and shaping procedures within the canal system, by using precurved instruments, by resisting the temptation to excessively enlarge the apical portion of the canal, by using voluminous irrigation, and by preventing a buildup of dentin shavings during instrumentation procedures by frequent recapitulation (see objective 5 below).

5. *Remove all residue of cleaning and shaping procedures that could prevent patency of the apical foramen— that is, tissue debris and dentin shavings (dentinal mud).* Thorough canal cleaning not only will ensure removal of the intracanal irritants but also will help prevent potential problems encountered during adherence to the mechanical and biologic objectives previously described. This is especially true in regard to the forcing of debris past the apical constriction or the buildup of debris in the apical third. Even with frequent irrigation, unless the apical third of the canal is kept patent, there is a tendency for the dentin mud to block the apical foramen (Figs. 7-3 and 7-9). Removal of this debris is accomplished with a no. 10 or 15 file, along with copious and frequent irrigation. This is known as *recapitulation* and is essential to all canal cleaning and shaping procedures. Ignoring this important step will often lead to the problems of ledging, loss of canal length, and development of false canals because of intracanal instrument deviation (internal transportation) or because of perforations, either lateral or apical (external transportation).

Preparatory procedures

Once the bulk of the tissue debris is removed from the canal system, the confines of the canal system must be delineated so that a more thorough cleaning procedure can be accomplished along with the initial stages of canal shaping. Delineation of the canal system implies the determination of the apical position at which intracanal cleaning procedures will be terminated, along with canal anatomy and its variations.

Years ago a smooth broach was used to determine canal curvatures, canal patency, location of the dentin-cementum junction, and location of the apical foramen. Today this is accomplished by using a small K-type file as a pathfinder (no. 10 or 15, depending on canal size, shape, and taper).

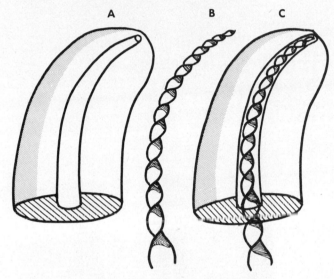

FIG. 7-14. Precurving of all intracanal instruments. **A,** Natural curvature of the canal. **B,** Precurvature of the instrument before placement into the canal. **C,** Precurved instrument in place in the canal.

Pathfinding instruments may be precurved to conform to the radiographic appearance of the canal system and to facilitate their three-dimensional movement through anticipated irregularities in the system (Fig. 7-14).

Precurving of an intracanal instrument is usually accomplished by inserting the tip into the end of a sterile cotton roll or gauze sponge and bending the instrument with the pressure of the thumb (Fig. 7-15). Cotton pliers may also be used; however, the instrument flutes may be damaged with this method. In either case direct contact of the sterile instrument with any unsterile field and the clinician's fingers must be avoided.

Using a precurved instrument provides a greater safety margin when a clinician is negotiating canals with irregularities and obstructions (Fig. 7-16). Rotations away from catches or curves in the wall are easily accomplished. Obstructions or severe deviations can be bypassed (Fig. 7-17). By controlling probing, poking, and twisting, and by turning the small, fine, precurved pathfinders, the clinician can almost always gain access to the full canal length. The

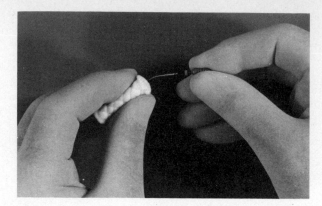

FIG. 7-15. Precurvature of an intracanal instrument by means of a sterile cotton roll.

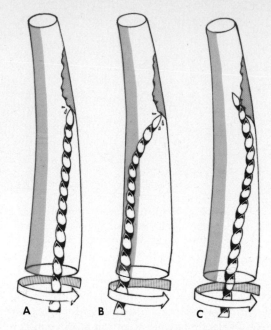

FIG. 7-17. A, Canal obstructions can often be bypassed by, B, slightly rotating the precurved instrument and, C, probing carefully for the path of least resistance.

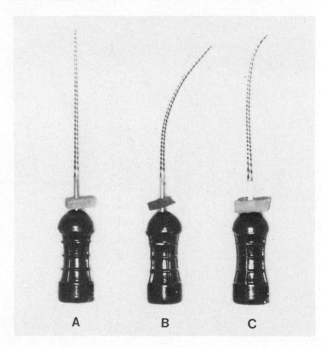

FIG. 7-16. A, Use of an uncurved instrument in the canal should be conscientiously avoided. B, Improper curvature. The working end of the instrument is straight. C, Proper curvature, with a gradual bend at the working end.

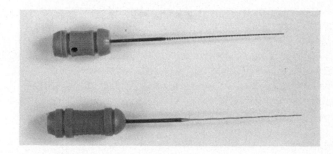

FIG. 7-18. New pathfinding instruments, small, yet with sufficient stiffness to enhance penetration of curved or partially calcified canals. (*Top* courtesy Kerr Manufacturing Co., Romulus, Mich.; *Bottom* courtesy J.S. Dental Mfg., Inc., New York, N.Y.)

clinician must make both mental and visual notations when removing the pathfinder from its position in the canal. Noting the direction of the curve and any additional changes in the instrument configuration will virtually ensure the continued insertion of files to the apical foramen.

Because of the high flexibility of the smaller files and the chance of them buckling or kinking when used to initially negotiate severely curved or calcified canals, small-diameter pathfinding instruments with a greater degree of stiffness have been developed (Fig. 7-18).

Some clinicians use the initial pathfinder to determine canal patency, curvatures, and irregularities prior to determining the actual working length of the tooth. The other option, which is recommended, is to use the initial instrument not only as a pathfinder but also to determine the working length of the tooth to be treated. This will ensure that the exact length of the canal is accurately determined prior to any instrumentation in the apical third of the canal.

Determination of working length

Select a file that corresponds to the size of the canal space visible on a good diagnostic radiographic film. Often this will be in the no. 10 to 15 size range in smaller curved roots. However, if the canal is larger, choose a larger file (Fig. 7-19). Most single-rooted teeth and larger molar canals will accomodate a size 20 to 25 or larger file. A rubber or silicone stop is placed on the instrument at right angles to the instrument shaft (Fig. 7-20). Measure the tooth length on the diagnostic film and subtract 1.0 mm. Set the rubber stop on the instrument at this length. For example:

Tooth length	22.0 mm
Subtract	1.0 mm
Set length of instrument	21.0 mm

Setting the initial file 1.0 mm short of the estimated tooth length will usually prevent penetration of the file past the apical constriction. Corrections are then easily made after the position of this file is confirmed.

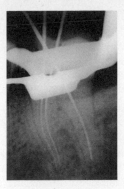

FIG. 7-19. Working length in mandibular molar. Mesial canals have No. 15 files; distal canal has no. 25 file. Radiograph exposed at 20-degree angle from the mesial.

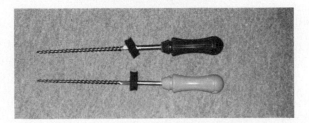

FIG. 7-20. *Bottom,* Instrument stops must be placed perpendicular to the shaft of the instrument. *Top,* Incorrect placement, resulting in inaccurate measurements.

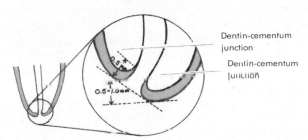

Dentin-cementum junction

Dentin-cementum junction

FIG. 7-21. The position of the dentin-cementum junction is most often 0.5-1.0 mm from the anatomic root apex.

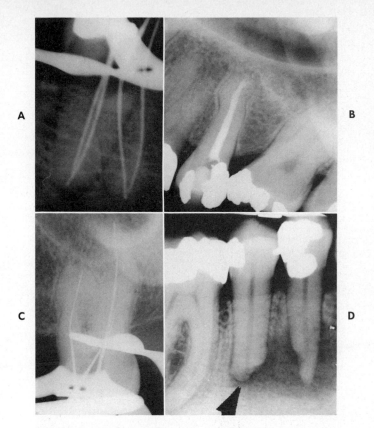

FIG. 7-22. A, Joining of canals in the apical third (mesial radiogrphic view—mandibular molar). **B,** Multiple exiting of canals in the apical third. **C,** Exiting of distalbuccal canal along distal wall of distal-buccal root, coronal to the apex. **D,** Resorptive defects, which alter the position of the foramen.

The instrument is now precurved according to previous directions. If the canal appears relatively straight, a gentle curve is imparted to the instrument before it is introduced. If the radiograph demonstrates an obviously more curved or calcified canal, the bend in the instrument should be made more pronounced and closer to the working end (Fig. 7-16). The clinician will eventually develop a tactile sensation in probing with the curved instrument, bouncing gently from wall to wall as the instrument approaches the apical foramen. The initial file should never be thrust directly at the apex, even in the simplest cases. Doing so is an invitation for the file to be hung up on the slightest canal irregularity. From the very onset, tactile finesse in the initial probing is essential.

The ideal apical termination point for all intracanal procedures is the most narrow aspect of the canal, the apical constriction or dentin-cementum junction (Fig. 7-21). However, variations in the location of this anatomic entity[18,42] have necessitated the establishment of guidelines

that must be adapted to each given situation. However, it is generally accepted that 0.5 to 1.0 mm from the radiographic apex is a sound location (within dentin) at which to terminate intracanal procedures.[86] Alterations[18] of the guidelines must be made when canals exit in a more coronal position in the root, when canals join prior to exiting the root, when multiple apical foramina exist, when calcific blockages are present, when resorption is evident, or when the roots deviate buccally or lingually in the apical third (Fig. 7-22).

Technically, termination of intracanal procedures 0.5 to 1.0 mm from the radiographic apex in sound dentin ensures the development of a firm apical dentin matrix during cleaning and shaping procedures. Also, it tends to minimize the placement of instruments beyond the apical canal confines and controls the placement of the root canal filling material.

Biologically, termination of intracanal procedures in sound dentin protects the fragile apical pulp stump in the case of a vital pulp and often precludes the occurrence of posttreatment discomfort resulting from overinstrumentation. Some authors advocate the termination of intracanal procedures 0.5 mm[70] from the radiographic apex or right at the radiographic apex, especially with necrotic pulps. However, intracanal procedures extending to the radio-

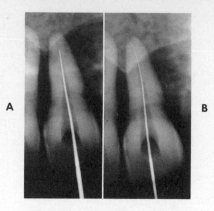

FIG. 7-23. A, Extracted tooth model with working length file greater than 1.0 mm from the ideal termination. **B,** New radiograph with working length file ideally placed.

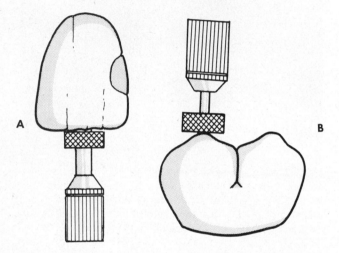

FIG. 7-24. Instrument should stop flush with the incisal edge of an anterior tooth, **A,** and the cusp height of a posterior tooth, **B.**

graphic apex are impinging on the periradicular tissues in the majority of cases. This serves no real purpose, since the body defense mechanisms have access to this area to ensure a normal physiologic debridement. In addition, in many cases in which a periradicular radiolucency is present with radiographic indication of apical resorption (Fig. 7-22, *D*), the apical preparation must end an additional 0.5 mm short of the radiographic apex (1.5 mm) or, in some cases of extensive three-dimensional resorption, as much as 2.0 mm or more from the radiographic apex.

Once the initial file reaches its predetermined depth, a radiograph is exposed according to previous guidelines (Chapter 4). The films are processed and carefully examined with good illumination and magnification. If the file is 1.0 mm or less from its ideal apical position, the correction is made and recorded, and cleaning and shaping procedures are begun. However, if the file is more than 1.0 mm from its ideal or desired position, an interpolation of the variance is made, the original length is corrected, and a new radiograph is exposed to verify the apical position of the file (Fig. 7-23). Here, again, if the correction is 1.0 mm or less, an additional simple correction is made with-

out exposing further films. Skill and experience in determining the proper length and achieving it with the initial instrument will tend to minimize the number of radiographic exposures.

In addition to the position of apical termination, there must also be a sound point of occlusal reference on which to base the working length of the tooth. In anterior teeth this is generally the incisal edge, and on posterior teeth a cusp or marginal ridge (Fig. 7-24). Care must be taken to choose a position on the tooth that is sound (not restorations) and reproducible. All canal cleaning and shaping to the apical dentin matrix are limited by approximating the instrument stop and the selected reference points. These points must also be recorded along with the working length of each canal. For example:

Canal	Reference point	Working length
MB	MB cusp	21.0 mm
DB	MB cusp	20.0 mm
P	P cusp	23.5 mm

In many situations it may be physically impossible to achieve what has arbitrarily been determined to be the ideal apical penetration of an instrument. This may be due to severe canal irregularities, curvatures, blockages, or calcifications. During undaunted, overzealous efforts to achieve the additional length, errors may occur such as instrument breakage, ledging, or canal blockage. Often it is wiser to accept the dictates of nature and proceed within the confines of what is possible.

Some authors advocate the use of mathematical formulas to determine the working length of the tooth.[36] Because of variations in the angles of radiographs, three-dimensional curves in roots, and clinician inconsistency in interpretation, the use of these formulas is *not recommended.* In addition, their use has never been shown to lead to a greater clinical success rate or to reduce the occurrence of posttreatment symptoms.

Electronic devices for determining working length.

Before the development of electronic devices for endodontics, the clinician could only use radiographs and tactile sensation to determine root canal length. There have always been inherent disadvantages to the use of radiographs.

1. Root canal systems and their apical foramina exhibit extreme morphologic variability.[27,28,42]
2. Superimpositions and distortions are common when a clinician is trying to view a three-dimensional object with a two-dimensional radiograph.
3. Observer bias is a potential error in radiographic interpretation.
4. The exposing and processing of high-quality radiographs can be time consuming.
5. Exposure to x-radiation represents a potential health hazard to patients and dental personnel.

Electronic measuring devices can be considered as viable alternatives to radiographic procedures. These devices are not new to endodontics. Suzuki[74] in 1942 described electrical resistance correlations between an endodontic in-

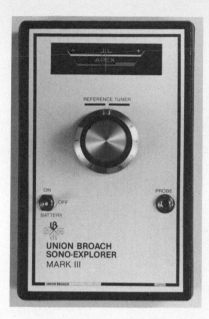

FIG. 7-25. The Mark III apex locator. (Courtesy Union Broach Co., New York, N.Y.)

strument inserted into the root canal and an electrode applied to the oral mucous membrane. Twenty years later Sunada[73] discussed the application of experimentally determined electrical resistance values between the oral mucous membrane and the periodontium to measure root canal length. In 1972 another clinical investigator[9,10] described the use of the Endometer,* which utilizes a refined meter readout system to measure the electrical potential of the periodontal ligament.

Further electronic developments led to the Sono-Explorer,†[37] for audiometrically determining canal length. One investigation showed 92% agreement between the Sono-Explorer and actual tooth lengths.[38] Other clinical researchers[7] were able to verify that in 93.3% of a patient population of 72 the Sono-Explorer gave measurements within ±0.5 mm of the radiographic apex. Another study[60] found that measurements with the Sono-Explorer were identical to direct measurements of extracted teeth in 83% of the canals and were within 0.5 mm in the remaining 17% of the canals.

Using the new Mark III‡ apex locator (newest Sono-Explorer) in a clinical study (Fig. 7-25), investigators[83] were within 1.0 mm of the radiographic apex in 94.5% of cases and beyond the apex by 1.0 mm only 2.4% of the time. In addition, they identified situations, such as unclear radiographic images of root apices, perforations, contraindications to radiographs, merging canals, and patients with strong gagging reflex, in which the use of the apex locator would be especially beneficial.

Investigative research, clinical evaluations, and additional refinements in applied technology have contributed to the development of many new-generation electronic apex locators.[5,7,60,62,68] One of the more modern developments, the Neosono,* is characterized by notably improved clinical accuracy and ease of operation.

Three versions of the Neosono have been introduced to the dental clinician (Fig. 7-26). The basic Neosono-M is a hand-held, battery-operated unit with two wired attachments: (1) a grounding clip that is hooked onto the patient's lip while the canal measurement is being taken and (2) a spring-loaded endodontic instrument holder that attaches to a file or reamer. When the unit is turned on, the audible signal volume and calibrated tuning knobs are adjusted according to the instruction manual.[57,58] An endodontic instrument with a rubber stop is attached to the spring-loaded holder, introduced within the canal, and slowly advanced toward the apex (Fig. 7-27). Three methods are used to indicate the position of the apical foramen: the positioning of the needle indicator at zero, the cessation of an audible tone, and the illumination of the apex indicator on the optional light-emitting diode (LED) panel. After the rubber stop is adjusted to an appropriate reference point, the instrument is withdrawn and measured to obtain the canal length. The newest model, the Neosono-D, operates in a similar fashion but uses an advanced digital readout system in place of a needle indicator to designate the position of the apical foramen. Another new model is the Neosono-D-SE, which relies entirely on the advanced digital readout system; that is, there is no audio component.

In one well-designed study,[4] the clinical accuracy of the Neosono D was determined using patients whose teeth were indicated for extraction. In comparing clinical length determination with radiographic evaluation and direct measurements, the investigators found that the Neosono-D consistently located the apical terminus of the canal and the beginning of the periodontal ligament with a degree of accuracy well within the limits technically possible in clinical practice.

Several operational limitations of all the Neosono devices are listed by the manufacturer:

1. During acquisition of the measurement, the instrument must not contact any metal (e.g., amalgam or cast restorations).

2. Ionic solutions such as sodium hypochlorite must be either neutralized or evacuated from the root canal before the unit is turned on. Local anesthetics should not be used as an irrigant, since they may interfere with measurement readings. The canal should be free of putrescent or hemorrhagic fluid.

3. The endodontic instrument attached to the holder should have a plastic handle or be otherwise insulated from the clinician's hand.

Despite these few procedural restrictions, the benefits of advanced integrated circuitry, convenience, and reliability make the Neosono an important clinical aid in conventional endodontic therapy.

The inherent problems with most of the studies that have evaluated electronic measurement of working length center

---

*Dentotronics Corp., San Antonio, Tex.
†Electro-Dent Corp., Cherry Hill, N.J.
‡Union Broach Co., New York, N.Y.

*Amadent, Inc., Cherry Hill, N.J.

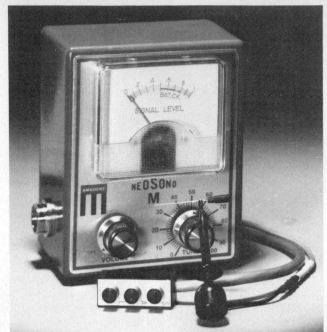

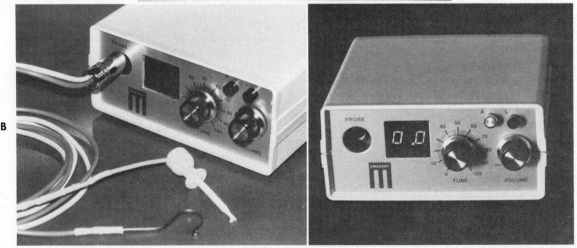

FIG. 7-26. Electronic devices for measuring the root canal. **A,** Neosono-M (miniature). **B** and **C,** Neosono-D (digital). The readout LED directly indicates the distance in millimeters (to 0.10 mm) of the instrument tip from the apical foramen.

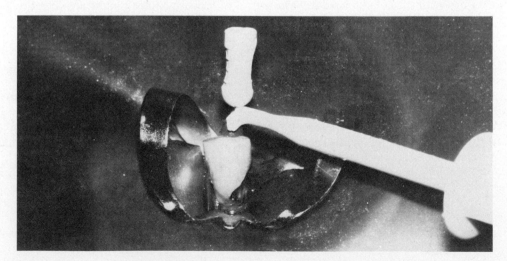

FIG. 7-27. Use of an electronic device to determine initial canal length. The endodontic instrument, with spring-loaded holder attached, is advanced to the apical foramen. The instrument stop is adjusted to correspond to the coronal reference point.

around clinician usage, adherence to manufacturer's directions, subtle differences in equipment, and ultimate clinician interpretation and extrapolation. Other investigators,[78] in comparing radiographic methods to electronic methods, astutely commented that "the electronic instruments may have a place in endodontic therapy especially if the operator is familiar with the characteristics of the particular instrument being used and the inherent variability these instruments appear to display."

Recent evaluations of techniques for length determination have focused on the comparison of conventional and xeroradiographic means.[65] This has been based on the fact that greater apical detail was reported with the use of xeroradiography[90] and that xeroradiography was qualitatively superior for visualization of dental tissues, metal instruments, and filling materials[29] (Fig. 7-28). Although no statistically significant difference between the conventional and xeroradiographic measurements has been identified, subjective evaluation of the xeroradiographic exposures resulted in a better overall visualization of bony trabeculae, bony margins, root canal configurations and morphology, root outline, and periodontal ligament space.[65] Xeroradiography is recommended primarily because of the improved image for interpretation and the decrease in ionizing radiation.

Methods of instrumentation

Many methods of instrument action within the canal system have been espoused over the years. The most common of these actions is the push-turn-pull motion, in which a K-file is inserted to the working length and given a ¹⁄₁₆, ¹⁄₈, or ¹⁄₄ turn, engaging the canal wall, and then withdrawn with pressure against the canal wall. When the file becomes loose within the canal, the next size file is used and the action is repeated until a desired size (often suggested as three times larger than the first instrument that binds in the apical third) is attained. Debris is wiped from the instrument each time it is removed from the canal (Fig. 7-29). The push-turn-pull action is referred to as the "filing action" and is often considered adequate for straight canals in larger teeth.

A "reaming action" is defined as a boring action designed to drill out an apical matrix and remove irregularities in the apical third of the canal (Fig. 7-11). As with the

filing action, this approach is limited to straight-rooted, larger-canal teeth. The motion incorporated is similar to that of an electric shop drill.

The major problem with both of these techniques is that neither takes into account the degree of irregular canal anatomy often encountered. Curves in three dimensions and canal extensions perpendicular to the radiographic pulpal confines are most difficult to anticipate. In addition, the highly irregular nature of external root anatomy and canal position in relation to it makes the strict or exclusive use of these two techniques highly questionable. Ironically, techniques of canal preparation with automated handpieces follow these same principles, and their shortcomings will be discussed later in this chapter.

"Circumferential filing" is defined as moving the file

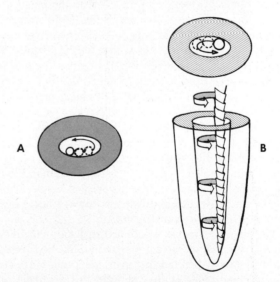

FIG. 7-29. Debris can be wiped from the instrument with a 2 × 2 gauze moistened with a disinfectant.

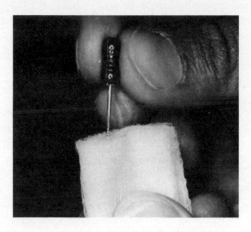

FIG. 7-30. A, Cross-sectional view of circumferential filing. The instrument is moved around the wall of the canal using a 1.0-3.0-mm amplitude stroke. B, Longitudinal view of step-back circumferential filing. The instrument cleans and shapes the wall about the circumference and in a coronal-apical plane. Gradually the entire three-dimensional aspect of the internal root wall is cleaned and shaped in a progressively increasing funnel from the dentin-cementum junction to the orifice with each file. Irrigation and recapitulation are essential with increased instrument sizes.

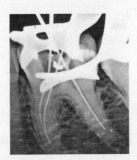

FIG. 7-28. Xeroradiograph used to determine working length. Note clarity of detail with radioopaque objects.

around the circumference of the canal space (Fig. 7-30, *A*) while at the same time stroking the instrument in a 1.0- to 3.0-mm amplitude. This approach to canal instrumentation favors the mechanical objectives of canal preparation previously discussed in that the spatial relation of the canal within the root and the location of the apical foramen are retained. When combined with a gradual movement of the instrument into more coronal levels within the canal (step-back circumferential filing), it also favors the development of a flared or funneled canal preparation (Fig. 7-30, *B*). Finally, it aids in opening the coronal confines of the canal, which facilitates easier penetration to the apical third by both instrument and irrigant.

Although all techniques of canal preparation appear to have a place in treatment, tooth anatomy should dictate the technique or combinations thereof chosen. Any course of treatment, however, must fulfill the biologic and mechanical objectives cited. The practitioner's ability and expertise and his objective assessment of those capabilities will also have a direct bearing on choice of treatment, quality of treatment, and ultimate success or failure.

Apical preparation

Once the working length of the tooth has been established, the clinician should focus on the apical preparation of the canal system. The same file used for determining the length, or a file one size smaller, is precurved and carefully teased to its determined apical position. The file is stroked against the canal walls in a circumferential fashion using a 1.0- to 3.0-mm amplitude. Care must be exercised to follow the path of the canal, especially when curves are present. Ideally, this process should proceed until the K-file fits loosely in the canal to the planned position of the apical dentin matrix. When large amounts of debris are present, the file is periodically removed and the debris is wiped from the file with a sterile, disinfectant-moistened 2 × 2 gauze (Fig. 7-29). Copious and generous irrigation is also used to keep loosened debris in solution for easy removal and to facilitate instrument lubrication.

One of two approaches may be pursued at this point. Either the apical preparation can continue in this manner, using K-files, until a desired size is attained, or the K-files can be used in a step-back circumferential manner to facilitate not only apical preparation, but also the initial funnel shape of the canal and middle to coronal canal debridement. In any case, recapitulation is always necessary in conjunction with frequent irrigation.

It has been previously mentioned that the guideline for the termination of the apical preparation has been cited as three sizes larger than the first instrument that binds at the apical terminus. One study[31] showed this approach to be adequate above a size no. 35 instrument. Some authors recommend a minimum of a size no. 40 at the apex in straight canals.[36] However, this does not address straight canals with three-dimensional, radiographically undetectable curves, the commonly encountered curved roots in maxillary lateral incisors and most posterior teeth.

The following range of sizes is recommended as a guideline for the final apical size of the canal preparation.

Tooth group	Final apical size
Maxillary centrals	35-60
Maxillary laterals	25-40
Maxillary canines	30-50
Maxillary premolars	25-40
Maxillary molars	
MB/DB	25-40
Palatal	25-50
Mandibular incisors	25-40
Mandibular canines	30-50
Mandibular premolars	30-50
Mandibular molars	
MB/ML	25-40
Distal	25-50

If the roots on a given tooth are **relatively straight,** anywhere in the range may be satisfactory with a tendency to prepare the apex at the higher end of the range.

The greater the curvature of the canal, the smaller the size of the final enlarging file to extend to the apical foramen (Fig. 7-31). However, each case will be deter-

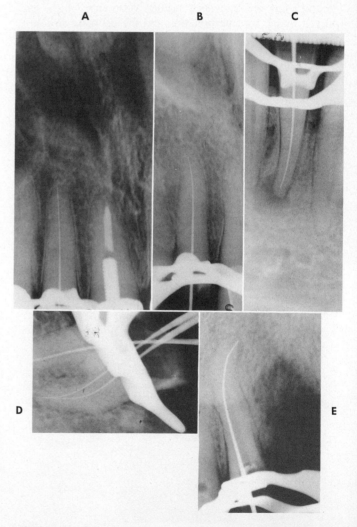

FIG. 7-31. A, Canal system with 0-degree curvature. **B,** 10-degree curvature. **C** and **D,** 10- 20-degree curvature. **E,** 20-degree curvature.

mined by the complexity of the canal system present, type and flexibility of the instrument used, and the clinician's technique and skill.

Midroot preparation

If the apical portion of the canal has been prepared without step-back circumferential filing, then the use of the classical step-back preparation or funnel-shaped preparation is now undertaken to shape and clean the transition from the apical third through the middle third or body of the canal. The use of this classical technique has been highlighted by Mullaney[56] and Tidmarsh[77] (Fig. 7-32).

With the final apical size being used as the starting point—for example, a size no. 25—the next 3 or 4 instrument sizes—nos. 30, 35, 40, and 45—are shortened by 1.0, 2.0, 3.0, and 4.0 mm, respectively, and used sequentially in the canal to produce a coronally directed taper. The step-back instruments may be either K-files or H-files. The patency of the apical canal segment must be ensured by continued use of the no. 25 file to its full length (recapitulation) along with copious irrigation after each instrument step-back.

The use of the 1.0-mm incremental step-back is not a hard-and-fast rule. Both 0.5-mm and 1.5- to 2.0-mm incremental step-backs may also be used, depending on canal anatomy and clinician preference.

If the apical portion (and middle to coronal portion) has been initially prepared by the step-back circumferential technique, then the following step-back preparation or funnel-shaped preparation is recommended. For purposes of example, a size no. 25 to 30 K-file is used to prepare the apical matrix (Fig. 7-33, A). Then a no. 25 H-file is inserted the full length of the canal and the step-back cir-

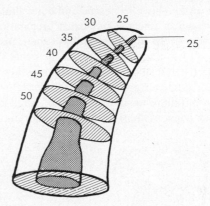

FIG. 7-32. Standard step-back technique in which the apical segment is prepared to a size 25 K-file. The next 3 or 4 instruments are shortened to limit their canal penetration and to effect a funnel or flare-shaped preparation. Recapitulation and irrigation are essential throughout the procedure.

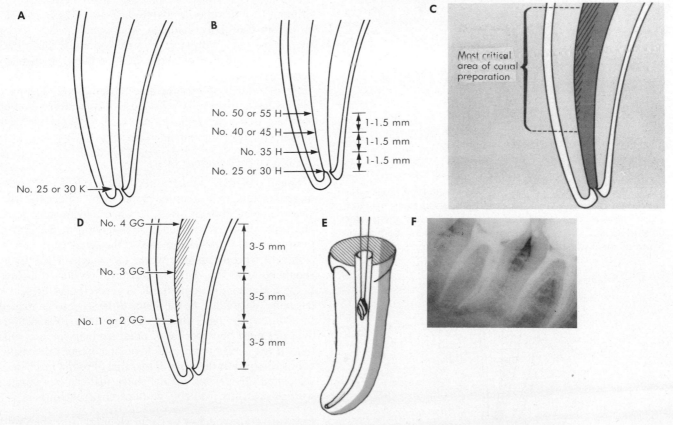

FIG. 7-33. A, Preparation of canal with 10- to 20-degree curvature to no. 25 or 30 K-file at apical matrix. **B,** Incremental step-back with H-files using a circumferential motion. **C** and **D,** Shaping the transition from the apical third through to the coronal third is crucial, with midroot shaping being the most critical. **E,** Shaping of midcoronal portions of the canal with Gates-Glidden burs cutting on the outstroke. **F,** Clinical case reflecting proper canal shape and flow.

cumferential technique is used throughout the full length of the canal. Recapitulation with the no. 25 K-file and irrigation follow. Subsequently the next 3 or 4 or more sizes of H-files are shortened in 1.0- to 1.5-mm increments and used sequentially in the canal, with emphasis of use both at their determined depth and throughout the middle to coronal canal length by means of the step-back circumferential technique (Fig. 7-33, *B*).

The use of the above technique embodies the attainment of the mechanical objectives of canal preparation. This is especially true in the crucial shaping of the transition from the apical third to the middle third of the canal (Fig. 7-33, *C* to *F*). If the transition is not continuously smooth, tapered, and patent, all gutta-percha filling techniques tend to suffer from failure to achieve depth of spreader penetration (lateral condensation),[2] plugger penetration (vertical

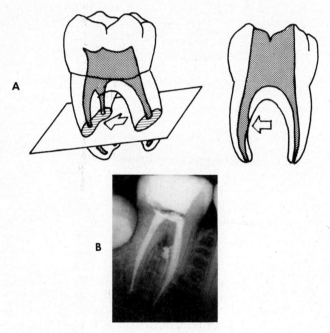

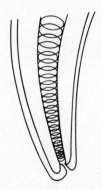

FIG. 7-34. Anticurvature filing. **A,** The proximity of root canals to external root concavities, especially in curved roots, requires a concentrated effort to direct shaping procedures to the greater bulk of dentin. **B,** Mandibular molar with lateral perforation (strip) of canal wall.

FIG. 7-35. Final canal taper must be a continuous funnel from the dentin-cementum junction to the orifice. Refer to Figs. 7-10 and 7-33, which reflect proper flow and taper of the prepared canal.

condensation),[66] or flow of the gutta-percha (diffusion technique; thermoplastic technique), as described in Chapter 8.[47]

The proper development of the apical-middle transitional area of the canal is facilitated and expedited through the use of the H-files and copious irrigation. In addition, Gates-Glidden (GG) burs may also be used in the middle portion of the root. In canals with an apical preparation of no. 25, size no. 2 or 3 GG is often used, with the clinician making sure that it passively penetrates the patent canal and cuts *only on the outstroke* in a circumferential shaving manner (Fig. 7-33, *E*). The canal should be flushed well between sizes. Often the no. 3 GG bur will penetrate only into the coronal portion of the canal, and its use should therefore be restricted to that area, especially in curved canals.

During midroot penetration in straight canals there are generally few anatomic dangers other than the external invagination of some roots in this area. Prudent and conservative preparation techniques should be carried out when this may be of concern. However, in curved roots, when these invaginations or concavities are present, extreme care must be exercised in the midroot preparation. Both files and GGs must be directed away from these root concavities, which are especially prevalent in mesial roots of molars. The cutting of tooth structure away from the curves and their concavities is known as anticurvature filing[1] and is designed to prevent lateral perforations or strippings of the root walls (Fig. 7-34). These clinician errors are especially common when small curved canals are "bored out" with large files or reamers or when there is excessive reliance on large GGs or Peeso reamers for midroot preparation.

Recent advances in ultrasonic cleaning and shaping in the midroot may minimize these errors because tooth structure is usually removed evenly throughout the canal system. (See section on endosonics, p. 174.)

Coronal preparation

Shaping of the coronal aspect of the canal is achieved in conjunction with midroot preparation, especially when Gates-Glidden burs are used. However, some authors recommend additional coronal shaping, tying in the flow of the apical and middle segments of the canal into one continuously tapered funnel. While the shape of the funnel should be relatively round in the apical portion, roundness in the middle and coronal thirds is generally not present or desirable, depending on the shape of the root to be treated. In addition, the taper that is developed in cross-sectional diameter must be wider every point from apical to coronal third (Fig. 7-35). From a biologic standpoint this ensures debris removal in the canal intracacies. From a mechanical standpoint this creates a canal shape that can be obturated with all presently available gutta-percha techniques.

Innovative approaches to canal cleaning and shaping

The "crown-down pressureless preparation" was introduced a few years ago.[48] This technique involves early canal flaring or a step-down preparation with Gates-Glidden burs, followed by the incremental removal of canal debris and dentin from the orifice to the apical foramen.

Straight files are used in a *larger to smaller sequence* with a reaming motion and no apical pressure once binding occurs. This continues until the desired length is achieved (Fig. 7-36). The rationale for this technique is twofold. First, the pressureless coronal to apical movement would minimize debris and thereby minimize the extrusion of

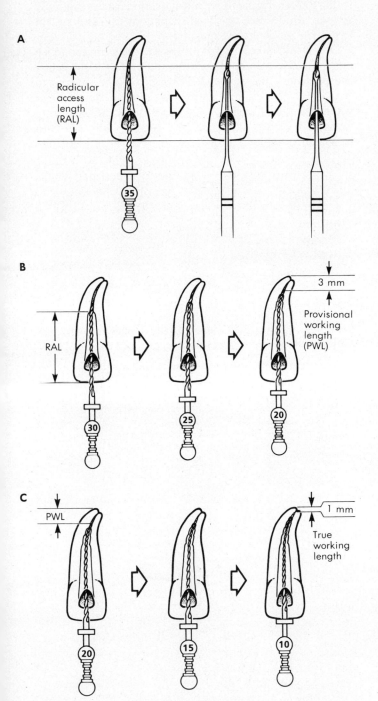

contaminants past the apical constriction. Second, it would eliminate the binding of instruments in the coronal portion of the canal, which makes controlled apical cleaning and shaping difficult.[44]

Recently the preparation of the coronal portion of the canal prior to the apical portion has received considerably more support.[19,20,22,44,54]

Goerig and co-workers[22] advocated a combination of the crown-down and step-back or flare preparation technique, especially in curved canals. A file is placed two thirds of the way down the curved canal, and lateral filing at this length is performed with Hedström files, sizes 15 through 25. Next, Gates-Glidden burs, no. 2 and no. 3 are used to enhance the coronal flare. Finally, the working length is established and the apex is enlarged to a size no. 25 K-file along with step-back instrumentation.

Morgan and Montgomery[55] compared the crown-down pressureless approach to the standard step-back preparation in curved canals. Their purpose was to determine the incidence of ledging, zipping, and perforation in using the two techniques. Five evaluators rated the effectiveness of canal instrumentation and statistical comparisons were made, with the following conclusions:

1. The crown-down pressureless technique received significantly more ''excellent'' ratings than the step-back technique.
2. The incidence of zipping (ripping the apical foramen) was similar in both techniques.
3. The incidences of ledging and perforation were questionable in either technique.

Although the use of the crown-down pressureless technique alone or in combination with the step-back technique appears to show great promise, it must be kept in mind that the biologic and mechanical objectives must be maintained to ensure success. However, the achievement of these objectives appears to be related more to the expertise of the clinician than to the preparation method itself.

Canal preparation with handpieces, sonic techniques, and ultrasonic systems
Reciprocating handpieces

The search for armamentarium to minimize the time spent in canal cleaning and shaping resulted in the development of reciprocating handpieces, such as the Giromatic.* Various authors have evaluated the Giromatic from a clinical usage standpoint,[21,35,41,87] and in terms of its ability to clean the canal,[41,84] its ability to properly shape the canal,[39,59] and its propensity for creating procedural errors.[87]

A general summary of the in vitro studies conducted would tend to support the following concepts in regard to using the original Giromatic technique:

1. Hand instrumentation requires approximately the same amount of time as automated instrumentation.
2. Flare preparations with hand instrumentation tend to remove more debris from within the canal systems than automated instrumentation.

FIG. 7-36. A, Determination of radicular access length and radicular access preparation. **B,** Determination of provisional working length during the first instrumentation sequence. **C,** Determination of true working length during the first instrumentation sequence. (From Morgan, L.F., and Montgomery, S.: An evaluation of the crown-down pressureless technique, J. Endod. **10:**491, 1984. © by American Associationn of Endodontists, 1984.)

*Micro-Mega S, Geneva, Switzerland.

3. The automated system is more difficult to use in the most posterior regions of the oral cavity.
4. There is greater propensity for the automated system to produce zipped canals, ledges, apical perforations, and debris packing.

However, recent long-term clinical observations using newer Giromatic equipment would tend to support the use of this type of automated preparation in the hands of the experienced clinician.[89]

A controlled power-assisted system designed to eliminate some of the original problems encountered with the Giromatic appeared in 1981. This system, the Dynatrak* system, uses stainless steel intracanal instruments with increased flexibility for curved canals and constant flute depth and rounded tip to minimize and control ledges, zips, and perforations. The use of the Dynatrak system in tooth models has been promising, with symmetrical and continuously tapered shapes being developed; however, in vivo studies and independent research are currently unavailable.

Sonic systems

The development of the Endostar 5† (Fig. 7-37) and the Endo Sonic Air 3000‡ (Fig. 7-38) introduced sonic vibratory canal cleaning and shaping to endodontics. Intracanal instruments vibrate at precise amplitudes to properly debride and enlarge the canal (Fig. 7-39). The sonic cutting that occurs, coupled with the sonic irrigating action, is claimed to reduce fatigue and stress during canal preparation in addition to achieving a superior result. Both systems are entirely compatible with standard delivery systems employed with handpiece and flushing attachments. Presently, however, few independent studies[43] exist that have assessed the efficiency and effectiveness of these products or their potential for creation of procedural errors. Initial clinical impressions would tend to place these instruments in the category of potentially promising.

Ultrasonic systems

Ultrasonic endodontics has brought a new era of biotechnology to root canal therapy. This technology, which uses ultrasound energy, combines the traditional endodontic concepts of debridement and irrigation with ultrasonic, biologic, chemical, and physical actions. These effects are separate, additive, and interactive. Root canal systems are rapidly and effectively cleaned, irrigated, disinfected, and shaped by the clinician using an ultrasonic system.

Ultrasound is a mechanical form of energy. With these systems, ultrasonic waves are generated and transferred to files in a handpiece (Fig. 7-40). Irrigation may come from a separate irrigation cylinder (Cavi-Endo§) or from a hook-up to a water system in the dental unit. The ultrasonic systems have flow-through components that enable the irrigant to pass along or through the file into the canal, enhancing debridement and irrigation. Diamond-coated files

have also been introduced to the combination of ultrasound-energized debridement and activated irrigation and aid in canal cleaning and disinfection[52] (Fig. 7-41).

Preparation of the root canal with ultrasonic systems for canal obturation consists of four interrelated and dependent phases: mechanical debridement of hard and soft tissue within the canal system, chemical debridement of the canal system, disinfection, and final shaping of the canal system to receive the obturating material.

One study indicates that ultrasonic files appear to be more effective than K-files for the removal of tissue debris and predentin, and diamond files appear to be superior to Hedström files in their ability to remove dentin from within the canals[51] (Fig. 7-42). Because of the energizing ultrasound waves, ultrasonic files become fully active in their cutting ability and diamond files cut even more effi-

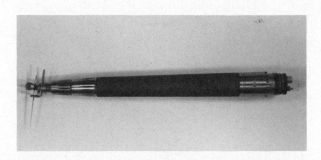

FIG. 7-37. Endostar 5. (Courtesy Syntex Dental Products, Valley Forge, Pa.)

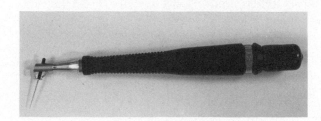

FIG. 7-38. Endo Sonic Air 3000. (Courtesy Medidenta Int., Inc., Woodside, N.Y.)

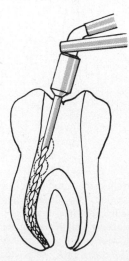

FIG. 7-39. Sonic files vibrate at precise and specific amplitudes, which enhances cutting and energizes the irrigation solution.

---

*R & R/Dentsply, Philadelphia, Pa.
†Syntex Dental Products, Valley Forge, Pa.
‡Medidenta International Inc., Woodside, N.Y.
§Caulk-Dentsply, Milford, Del.

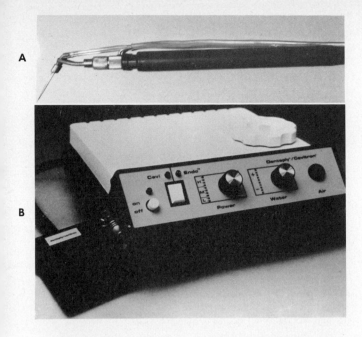

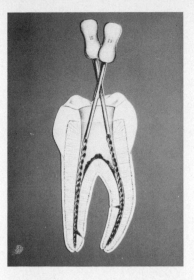

FIG. 7-43. Determination of working length and initial apical preparation are accomplished with small (no. 10 to 20) hand files. (Courtesy Dr. Howard Martin, Silver Spring, Md.)

FIG. 7-40. A, Endosonic handpiece with file and irrigation tubes attached. B, Cavi-Endo unit. (B courtesy Caulk/Dentsply Int., Inc., Milford, Del.)

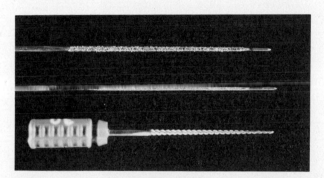

FIG. 7-41. Endosonic diamond files. Coarse *(top)*, medium *(middle)*, K-type no. 30 *(bottom)*.

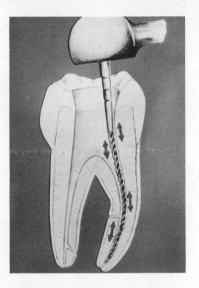

FIG. 7-44. A push-pull action of the ultrasonic file enhances dentin removal. (Courtesy Dr. Howard Martin, Silver Spring, Md.)

ciently than the Hedström files, adding the component of dimensional planing of the canal walls. This leaves the canal wall surface extremely smooth, enhancing obturation procedures. The diamond files are very hard, wear resistant, and chemically inert, displaying a keen edge. They are excellent for conducting ultrasound waves and require only a very light cutting pressure. The continuous flow-through irrigation and vibratory movement create a self-cleaning action that prevents clogging, aids disinfection, and debrides the canal simultaneously.

Initial root canal length determination and apical preparation are accomplished with small hand files (Fig. 7-43). Subsequent canal preparation is performed with smaller-sized ultrasonic files, which are precurved prior to entry into the canal. The file motion used in ultrasonic root canal preparation is essentially a push-pull action enhancing dentin removal (Fig. 7-44). Circumferential movement of the

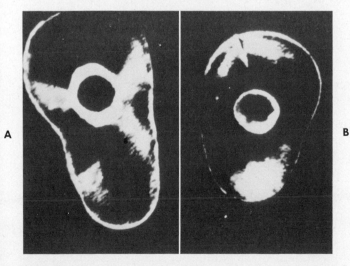

FIG. 7-42. Dentin removability of the Endosonic file. A, Endosonic treatment. B, Hand treatment. White area around the canal indicates the amount of dentin removed.

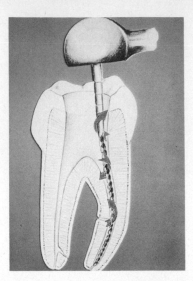

FIG. 7-45. Incorporation of a circumferential file motion enhances canal shaping. (Courtesy Dr. Howard Martin, Silver Spring, Md.)

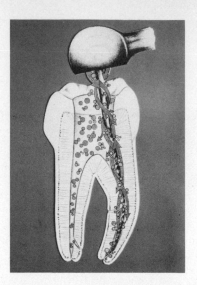

FIG. 7-46. The activated sodium hypochlorite irrigant swirls around the file during its movement in the canal, enhancing dentin and debris removal. (Courtesy Dr. Howard Martin, Silver Spring, Md.)

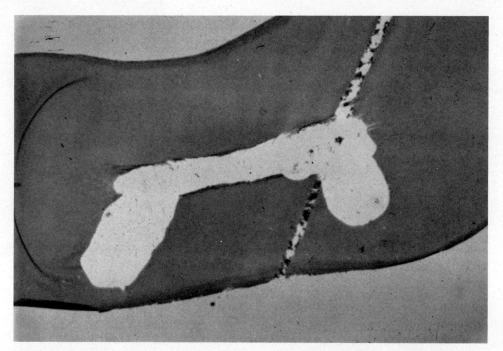

FIG. 7-47. Endosonic treatment of the mesial root of a mandibular molar. Note typically clean canals. Note that the intercanal space has been effectively debrided. However, injudicious use of the ultrasonic systems may remove tooth structure to the point of near perforation.

files is also advocated to achieve the smooth tapering canal shape that is considered optimal for obturation (Fig. 7-45). A side-to-side action or lateral movement activates the irrigant solution, which improves its disinfecting and cleaning qualities.

Irrigation, or chemical debridement, is indispensable for achieving thorough cleaning of the root canal system. Both the Endosonic system* and the Enac† use a high-volume,

continuous flow-through irrigation system with improved filing to provide a significantly cleaner canal.

The coupling of the flow-through irrigation is accomplished by connecting a separate irrigation cylinder to the Endosonic handpiece. The irrigant (water or sodium hypochlorite) passes through the handpiece and swirls completely around and beyond the file (Fig. 7-46). The principal ultrasonic effect of cavitation is accomplished by the mechanical vibratory action of stirring and agitating of the activated, energized irrigant. The debris is floated into the irrigant mainstream, where high-volume aspiration rapidly removes it. For the Endosonic system the manufacturer

---

*Caulk-Dentsply Int., Inc., Milford, Del.
†Osada Electric Co., Ltd., Tokyo, Japan.

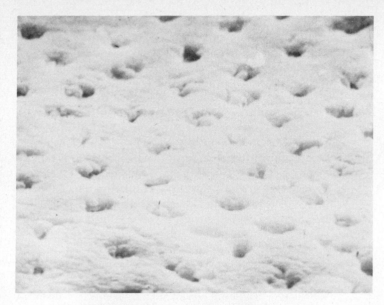

FIG. 7-48. Scanning electron microscopic photograph showing the canal walls smooth and clean after Endosonic treatment.

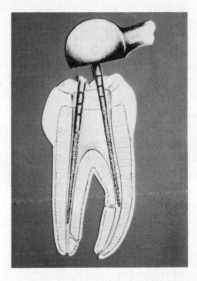

FIG. 7-49. Middle and coronal root shaping is performed with the diamond files. (Courtesy Dr. Howard Martin, Silver Spring, Md.)

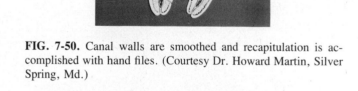

FIG. 7-50. Canal walls are smoothed and recapitulation is accomplished with hand files. (Courtesy Dr. Howard Martin, Silver Spring, Md.)

recommends that 2.5% sodium hypochlorite solution be used to derive the maximum benefit of ultrasonics.

Evaluation of cross sections prepared by hand and ultrasonic techniques demonstrates the improved cleaning ability when ultrasonic technology is used for canal debridement[14] (Fig. 7-47). Debris is effectively removed from the many canal ramifications by ultrasonic treatment.[43] Scanning electron microscopy of the root canal walls shows the smear layer greatly reduced, with exposure of dentinal tubules[13] (Fig. 7-48).

The continuous, high-volume, flow-through irrigation and aspiration, within the root canal, create the equivalent of an "ultrasonic bath." This allows three-dimensional debridement of the complex root canal morphology by the hydrodynamic action and enhanced physical chemistry of the activated irrigant. The combination of continuously activated irrigation and the energized files/diamonds produces a multidimensional synergistic system

that results in a biologically cleaner root canal system.

The effectiveness of the mechanical-chemical debridement and canal shaping by the ultrasonic systems has received mixed reviews in recent evaluative studies.* Here again, clinician variability and familiarity with techniques and variations in equipment, along with the in vitro nature of the studies, may have contributed to these diverse findings. At the same time, clinical uses for the ultrasonic instrumentation have expanded to include pathfinding, as well as removal of obstructions, silver cones, and posts.[71]

Ultrasonic chemical debridement is accomplished by the continuous high-volume flush combined with the microbiocidal effect of the activated irrigant. The mechanical lavage of the energized irrigant combined with aspiration physically removes the bulk of debris and bacteria. Ultra-

---

*References 8, 11, 16, 26, 43, and 75.

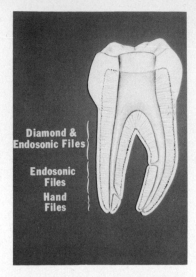

FIG. 7-51. Proper canal preparation is accomplished using hand files apically and ultrasonic files and diamonds in the middle and coronal portions of the canal. (Courtesy Dr. Howard Martin, Silver Spring, Md.)

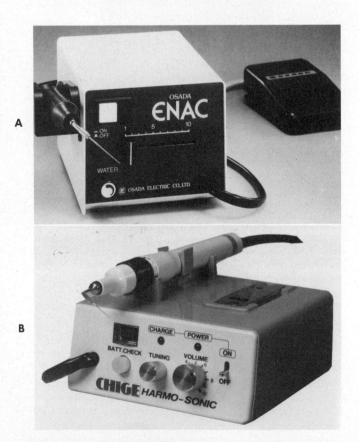

FIG. 7-52. A, Enac. **B,** Harmo-Sonic. (**A** courtesy Osada Electric Co., Tokyo, Japan; **B** courtesy Sheikosha, Tokyo, Japan.)

sonic energy has been shown to kill bacteria.[49] Therefore, ultrasonic debridement may be an even more effective means of canal disinfection.[15]

The combination of ultrasonic waves and a microbiocide (e.g., 1% to 2.5% sodium hypochlorite) results in an extremely efficient system. The improved effect is due to the agitation, acoustic streaming, and cavitation created by the ultrasonic waves emitted from the energized file and is the catalytic agent that augments, accelerates, and improves the chemical action. Bacteria are rendered more susceptible to the chemical action of the irrigant.

During chemomechanical debridement of the root canal system with ultrasonic technology, proper canal shaping also occurs in the middle and coronal thirds of the canal with ultrasonic diamond files (Fig. 7-49). This ideal canal shape, required for three-dimensional obturation, is rapidly rendered by the push-pull, circumferential, side-to-side action of the files. Once shaping is completed, final smoothing and/or recapitulation can be accomplished with hand files (Fig. 7-50). As noted in Fig. 7-51, the safe and efficient use of ultrasonic technology requires the careful application of both hand files and ultrasonic files in specific canal locations. However, extreme care must be exercised in areas of the canal system where the canal is close to the external root wall—for example, mesial roots of mandibular molars. Because of the efficiency of ultrasonic cutting, rapid perforations may occur[43] (see Fig. 7-47).

Pain from endodontic procedures is linked to the inflammatory process. The most common inflammatory agents are bacteria, necrotic debris, and chemical and mechanical irritation. In a clinical study comparing conventional and ultrasonic procedures,[50] postoperative pain did not occur with any greater frequency in either technique. Thus ultrasonic debridement does not increase intrusion of harmful agents into the periapical tissues.

Recent advances in ultrasonic root canal preparation have led to the development of newer equipment, which utilizes the ultrasonic oscillation technology not only in canal preparation but also in obturation (Fig. 7-52). There appears to be an exciting future for the use of ultrasonic technology for cleaning, shaping, and perhaps even obturating root canal systems.

CONSIDERATIONS IN REGARD TO INTRACANAL MEDICATION

After the root canal has been properly cleaned and shaped, few indications, if any, exist for the use of intracanal medication. Tissue remnants and bacteria should have been eliminated from the root canal system, with the removal of the contaminated portion of the dentinal tubules. Scanning microscopic evidence indicates that root canals can be rendered totally free of microorganisms and organic substrate after conscientious cleaning and shaping.[46] When such cleaning and shaping are coupled with thorough flushing with sufficient quantities of 2.5% to 5.25% sodium hypochlorite, root canal systems can be debrided efficiently and effectively without resorting to tissue-toxic chemicals.

Advocates of routine intracanal medication claim that (1) there is no clinical guarantee that tissue and bacteria can be completely removed or rendered harmless, (2) there is no way to clinically determine the extent of tubule penetration by necrotic debris or bacteria, and (3) the medication may play a role in controlling external contamination between visits. However, no amount of medication will disinfect a contaminated canal, overcome incomplete cleaning, or prevent leakage in a carelessly sealed access opening.

While the success rate of root canal therapy is not based on the use of intracanal medicaments, there may be a few indications for the use of volatile-type drugs, such as camphorated monochlorophenol (CMCP) or formocreosol. In cases of complete necrosis with canals open to oral contamination or in cases of a pulpotomy dressing in emergency treatment, some clinicians may still choose to use a miniscule amount of formocreosol on a cotton pellet placed in the pulp chamber.

After the final recapitulation, the root canal is thoroughly dried. If hydrogen peroxide has been used, the clinician must be certain to follow the last application with several rinses of sodium hypochlorite. Oxygen released from unspent peroxides in the closed canal theoretically may be the cause of periapical discomfort.[67]

The pulp chamber and canals are dried with sterile cotton pellets and paper points. To save time and minimize the number of paper points required, initial removal of irrigants can be achieved with a high-speed endodontic aspiration tip. If a medicament is to be used, the bottle containing the medication should be inverted to allow the liquid to cling to the side near the mouth of the bottle. The cover is removed and a sterile cotton pellet is lightly wiped on the inside, picking up some of the liquid. The cotton pellet is then squeezed dry in a sterile gauze sponge. The amount of medicament remaining in the pellet is more than sufficient to render its temporary antibacterial action.

The medicated pellet is placed only in the pulp chamber. Paper points, medicinally impregnated or not, should never be left in root canals; nor should canals be flushed or filled with medicaments between patient visits.

If the access cavity is carefully designed with proper external flaring, a simple closure with Cavit or similar cement will seal the tooth effectively between visits. The occlusion should be carefully checked to ensure there will be no unnecessary trauma to the periradicular tissues between appointments.

HOME CARE INSTRUCTIONS TO THE PATIENT

Initially, the patient should be made aware of the success rates of root canal therapy as well as the probability of some discomfort after the first or second visit.

The best home care instructions for the patient are those that include most of the more common sequelae of root canal therapy. These include mild discomfort for 24 to 72 hours after the instrumentation visit(s), sensitivity to chewing on the tooth for a day or two (which can be minimized by reducing the occlusion), and an awareness of a dull ache in the area of the treated tooth. A patient who is told to *expect* some mild to moderate discomfort is either pleasantly surprised if there is none or does not call unnecessarily if and when the temporary discomfort occurs. The potential or probability for flare-ups should be mentioned along with the importance of phoning the dentist if severe swelling, lymphadenopathy, or severe discomfort results. Although routine prophylactic antibiotic coverage is not indicated in root canal therapy, the patient should be told that the use of antibiotics occasionally may be necessary.

With the advent of over-the-counter nonsteroidal anti-inflammatory agents, patients should be advised of the benefits of such medications and their effect on the source of their discomfort, that is, inflammation. Prescription analgesics or antibiotics are not routinely indicated, and the dentist should be aware of the treatment options available when prescribing these medications.

Dentists performing root canal therapy must understand that the placement of some microorganisms or a few grains of dentin powder through the apical foramen is generally not the chief source of posttreatment inflammation. Rather, common iatrogenic causes of posttreatment discomfort include inadequate cleaning of canals, inadequate radiographic control of instrument length, external transportation of apical foramina, overmedication, and improper sealing of the access opening. When these occur, there is little that the patient can do except call the dentist for an emergency appointment for relief of pain. Calls of this nature can be minimized if the clinician spends the appropriate time necessary to properly clean and shape the canal in one visit. Not only will this minimize patient posttreatment distress, but it significantly minimizes the needless prescribing of drugs that often only manage the symptoms and do not address the source of the patient's problem.

REFERENCES

1. Abou-Rass, M., Frank, A.L., and Glick, D.H.: The anticurvature method to prepare the curved root canal, J. Am. Dent. Assoc. **101:** 792, 1980.
2. Allison, C.A., Weber, C.R., and Walton, R E.: The influence of the method of canal preparation on the quality of apical and coronal seal, J. Endod. **5:**298, 1979.
2a. American heritage dictionary of the English language (new college ed.), 1979.
3. Becker, G.L., Cohen, S., and Borer, R.: The sequelae of accidentally injecting sodium hypochlorite beyond the root apex, Oral Surg. **38:**633, 1974.
4. Berman, L.H., and Fleischman, S.B.: Evaluation of the accuracy of the Neosono-D electronic apex locator, J. Endod. **10:**164, 1984.
5. Blank, L.W., Tenca, J.I., and Pelleu, G.B., Jr.: Reliability of electronic measuring devices in endodontic therapy, J. Endod. **1:**141, 1975.
6. Brayton, S.M., Davis, S.R., and Goldman, M.: Gutta percha root canal fillings, Oral Surg. **35:**226, 1973.
7. Busch, L.R., et al.: Determination of the accuracy of the Sono-Explorer for establishing endodontic measurement control, J. Endod. **2:**295, 1976.
8. Cameron, J.A.: The use of ultrasonics in the removal of smear layer: a scanning electron microscope study, **9:**289, 1983.
9. Cash, P.W.: Electronics in endodontics—a clinical report on the Endometer, Tex. Dent. J. **90:**21, 1972.
10. Cash, P.W.: Electronics and root canals, J. Acad. Gen. Dent. **21:**20, 1973.
11. Chenail, B.L., and Teplitsky, P.E.: Endosonics in curved root canals, J. Endod. **11:**369, 1985.
12. Coffae, K.P., and Brilliant, J.D.: The effect of serial preparation versus nonserial preparation on tissue removal in the root canals of extracted mandibular human molars, J. Endod. **1:**211, 1975.
13. Cunningham, W., and Martin, H.: A scanning electron microscope evaluation of root canal debridement with the endosonic ultrasonic synergistic system, Oral Surg. **53:**527, 1982.
14. Cunningham, W., Martin, H., and Forrest, W.: Evaluation of root canal debridement by the endosonic ultrasonic synergistic system, Oral Surg. **53:**401, 1982.

15. Cunningham, W., et al.: A comparison of antibacterial effectiveness of endosonic and hand root canal therapy, Oral Surg. **54:**238, 1982.

16. Cymerman, J.J., Jerome, L.A., and Moodnik, R.M.: A scanning electron microscopic study comparing the efficacy of hand instrumentation with ultrasonic instrumentation of the root canal, J. Endod. **9:**327, 1983.

17. Dow, P.R., and Ingle, J.I.: Isotope determination of root canal failure, Oral Surg. **8:**1100, 1955.

18. Dummer, P.M.H., McGinn, J.H. and Rees, D.G.: The position and topography of the apical canal construction and apical foramen, Int. Endod. J. **17:**192, 1984.

19. Fahid, A.: Coronal root canal preparation, Dent. Stud. **61:**46, 1983.

20. Fava, L.R.G.: The double-flared technique: an alternative for biomechanical preparation, J. Endod. **9:**76, 1983.

21. Frank, A.L.: An evaluation of the Giromatic endodontic handpiece, Oral Surg. **24:**419, 1967.

22. Goerig, A.C., Michelich, R.J., and Schultz, H.H.: Instrumentation of root canals in molars using the step-down technique, J. Endod. **8:**550, 1982.

23. Goldberg, F., and Spielberg, C.: The effect of EDTAC and the variations of its working time analyzed with scanning electron microscopy, Oral Surg. **53:**74, 1982.

24. Goldman, M., DeVitre, R., and Tenca, J.: Cement distribution and bone strength in cemented posts, J. Dent. Res. **63:**1392, 1984.

25. Goldman, L.B., et al.: The efficacy of several irrigating solutions for endodontics: a scanning electron microscopic study, Oral Surg. **52:**197, 1981.

26. Goodman, A., et al.: An in vitro comparison of the efficacy of the step-back technique versus a step-back/ultrasonic technique in human mandibular molars, J. Endod. **11:**249, 1985.

27. Green, D.: A stereomicroscopic study of the root apices of 400 maxillary and mandibular anterior teeth, Oral Surg. **9:**1224, 1956.

28. Green, D.: Stereomicroscopic study of 700 root apices of maxillary and mandibular posterior teeth, Oral Surg. **13:**728, 1960.

29. Gratt, B.M., Sickles, E.A., and Nguyen, N.T.: Dental xeroradiography for endodontics: a rapid x-ray system that produces high quality images, J. Endod. **5:**266, 1979.

30. Grossman, L.I.: Irrigation of root canals, J. Am. Dent. Assoc. **30:**1915, 1943.

31. Haga, C.S.: Microscopic measurements of root canal preparations following instrumentation, J. Br. Endod. Soc. **2:**41, 1969.

32. Hand, R.E., Smith, M.L., and Harrison, J.W.: Analysis of the effect of dilution on the necrotic tissue dissolution property of sodium hypochlorite, J. Endod. **4:**60, 1978.

33. Harrison, J.W., and Hand, R.E.: The effect of dilution and organic matter on the antibacterial property of 5.25% sodium hypochlorite, J. Endod. **7:**128, 1981.

34. Harrison, J.W., Svec, T.A., and Baumgartner, J.C.: Analysis of clinical toxicity of endodontic irrigants, J. Endod. **4:**6, 1978.

35. Harty, F.J., and Stock, C.J.R.: The giromatic system compared with hand instrumentation in endodontics, Br. Dent. J. **137:**239, 1974.

36. Ingle, J.I., and Taintor, J.F.: Endodontics, ed. 3., Philadelphia, 1985, Lea & Febiger, p. 178.

37. Inoue, N.: An audiometric method for determining the length of root canals, J. Can. Dent. Assoc. **50:**544, 1955.

38. Inoue, N.: A clinico-anatomical study for the determining of root canal length by use of a novelty low frequency oscillation device, Bull. Tokyo Dent. Coll. **18:**71, 1977.

39. Jungmann, C.L., Uchin, R.A., and Buchler, J.F.: Effect of instrumentation on the shape of the root canal, J. Endod. **1:**66, 1975.

40. Kaufman, A.Y.: Facial emphysema caused by hydrogen peroxide irrigation: report of case, J. Endod. **7:**470, 1981.

41. Klayman, S.M., and Brilliant, J.D.: A comparison of the efficacy of serial preparation versus Giromatic preparation, J. Endod. **1:**334, 1975.

42. Kuttler, Y.: Microscopic investigation of root apexes, J. Am. Dent. Assoc. **50:**544, 1955.

43. Langeland, K., Liao, K., and Pascon, E.A.: Work-saving devices in endodontics: efficacy of sonic and ultrasonic techniques, J. Endod. **11:**499, 1985.

44. Leeb, J.: Canal orifice enlargement as related to biomechanical preparation, J. Endod. **9:**463, 1983.

45. Lehman J., Bell W.A., and Gerstein, H.: Sodium lauryl sulfate as an endodontic irrigant, J. Endod. **7:**381, 1981.

46. Lifshitz, J., Schilder, H., and Dameijer, C.H.: Scanning electron microscope study of the warm gutta percha technique, J. Endod. **9:**17, 1983.

47. Marlin, J., and Desilets, R.P.: Technique manual for the Obtura heated gutta percha delivery system, Monrovia, Calif., 1984, Unitek Corp.

48. Marshall, F.J., and Pappin, J.: A crown-down pressureless preparation root canal enlargement technique. In Technique manual, Portland, Ore., 1980, Oregon Health Sciences University.

49. Martin, H.: Ultrasonic disinfection of the root canal, Oral Surg. **42:**92, 1976.

50. Martin, H., and Cunningham, W.: An evaluation of postoperative pain incidence following endosonic and conventional root canal therapy, Oral Surg. **54:**74, 1982.

51. Martin, H., Cunningham, W., and Norris, J.: A quantitative comparison of the ability of diamond and K-type files to remove dentin, Oral Surg. **50:**566, 1980.

52. Martin, H., et al.: Ultrasonic versus hand filing of dentin: a quantitative study, Oral Surg. **39:**79, 1980.

53. McComb, D., and Smith, D.C.: A preliminary electron microscopic study of root canals after endodontic procedures, J. Endod. **1:**238, 1975.

54. Montgomery, S.: Root canal wall thickness of mandibular molars after biomechanical preparation, J. Endod. **11:**257, 1985.

55. Morgan, L.F., and Montgomery, S.: An evaluation of the crown-down pressureless technique, J. Endod. **10:**491, 1984.

56. Mullaney, T.: Instrumentation of finely curved canals, Dent. Clin. North. Am. **23:**575, 1979.

57. Neosono—electronic root canal measurement: instruction manual, American Medical & Dental Corp., Cherry Hill, N.J.

58. Neosono-D—electronic root canal measurement, digital readout: instruction manual, American Medical & Dental Corp., Cherry Hill, N.J.

59. O'Connell, D.G., and Brayton, S.M.: Evaluation of root canal preparation with two automated endodontic handpieces, Oral Surg. **39:**298, 1975.

60. O'Neill, L.J.: A clinical evaluation of electronic root canal measurement, Oral Surg. **38:**469, 1974.

61. Phillips, J.M.: Rat connective tissue response to hollow polyethylene tube implants, J. Can. Dent. Assoc. **33:**59, 1967.

62. Plant, J.J., and Newman, R.F.: Clinical evaluation of the Sono-Explorer, J. Endod. **2:**215, 1976.

63. Rosenfeld, E.F., James, G.A., and Burch, B.S.: Vital pulp tissue response to sodium hypochlorite, J. Endod. **4:**140, 1978.

64. Rubin, L., et al.: The effect of instrumentation and flushing of freshly extracted teeth in endodontic therapy: a scanning electron microscope study, J. Endod. **3:**194, 1977.

65. San Marco, P.A., and Montgomery, S.: Use of xeroradiography for length determination in endodontics, Oral Surg. **57:**308, 1984.

66. Schilder, H.: Filling root canals in three dimensions, Dent. Clin. North Am. **11:**723, 1967.

67. Schilder, H., and Yee, F.S.: Canal debridement and disinfection. In Cohen, S., and Burns, R.C., editors: Pathways of the pulp, ed. 3, St. Louis, 1984, The C.V. Mosby Co.

68. Seidberg, B.H., et al.: Clinical investigation of measuring working lengths of root canals with an electronic device and with digital-tactile sense, J. Am. Dent. Assoc. **90:**379, 1975.

69. Seltzer, S.: Endodontology: biologic considerations. In Endodontic procedures, New York, 1971, McGraw-Hill Book Co., pp. 318-325.

70. Serene, T.P.: Principles of preclinical endodontics, Dubuque, 1983, Kendall/Hunt, p. 76.

71. Stamos, D.G., et al.: Endosonics: clinical impressions, J. Endod. **11:**181, 1985.

72. Stewart, G., Cobe, H., and Rappaport, H.: A study of a new medicament in the chemomechanical preparation of infected root canals, J. Am. Dent. Assoc. **63:**33, 1961.

73. Sunada, I.: New method for measuring the length of the root canal, J. Dent. Res. **41:**375, 1962.

74. Suzuki, K.: Experimental study on iontophoresis, J. Jap. Stomatol. **16:**414, 1942.

75. Tauber, R., et al.: A magnifying lens comparative evaluation of conventional and ultrasonically energized filing, J. Endod. **9:**269, 1983.

76. Thé, S.D.: The solvent action of sodium hypochlorite on fixed and unfixed necrotic tissue, Oral Surg. **47:**558, 1979.

77. Tidmarsh, B.G.: Preparation of the root canal, Int. Endod. J. **15:**53, 1982.

78. Tidmarsh, B.G., Sherson, W., and Stalker, N.L.: Establishing endodontic working length: a comparison of radiographic and electronic methods, N.Z. Dent. J. **81:**93, 1985.

79. Torabinejad, M., Walton, R.E., and Ogilvie, A.L.: Periapical pathosis. In Ingle, J.I., and Taintor, J., editors: Endodontics, ed. 3, Philadelphia, 1985, Lea & Febiger, p. 421.

80. Torneck, C.D.: Reaction of rat connective tissue to polyethylene tube implants, part I, Oral Surg. **21:**379, 1966.

81. Torneck, C.D.: Reaction of rat connective tissue to polythylene tube implants, part II, Oral Surg. **24:**674, 1967.

82. Trepagnier, C.M., Madden, R.M., and Lazzari, E.P.: The effect of instrumentation and flushing of freshly extracted teeth in endodontic irrigant, Oral Surg. **49:**175, 1980.

83. Trope, M., Rabie, G., and Tronstad, L.: Accuracy of an electronic apex locater under controlled clinical conditions, Endod. Dent. Traumatol. **1:**142, 1985.

84. Turek, T., and Langeland, K.: A light microscopic study of the efficacy of the telescopic and the Giromatic preparation of root canals, J. Endod. **8:**437, 1982.

85. Walton, R.: Histologic evaluation of different methods of enlarging the pulp canal space, J. Endod. **2:**304, 1976.

86. Weine, F.: Endodontic therapy, ed. 3, St. Louis, 1982, The C.V. Mosby Co.

87. Weine, F.S., Kelly, R.F., and Bray, K.E.: Effect of preparation with endodontic handpieces on original canal shape, J. Endod. **2:**298, 1976.

88. Weine, F.S., Kelly, R.F., and Lio, P.J.: The effect of preparation procedures on original canal shape and on apical foramen shape, J. Endod. **1:**255, 1975.

89. Weisz, G.: A clinical study using automated instrumentation in root canal therapy, Int. Endod. J. **18:**203, 1985.

90. White, S.: Intraoral xeroradiography, Oral Surg. **46:**862, 1978.

Self-assessment questions

1. Modern endodontic therapy depends primarily on which of the following for a successful prognosis?
   a. Caustic medicaments
   b. Thorough mechanical sanitization
   c. Ultrasonic cleaning
   d. Sterilization of the canal

2. The most widely accepted intracanal irrigant displaying optimal cleansing and bacteriocidal properties is
   a. Formocresol
   b. Hydrogen peroxide
   c. Sterile saline
   d. Sodium hypochlorite

3. Which one of the following statements regarding the use of barbed broaches is true?
   a. The broach may be used in curved canals.
   b. The broach is to be placed to the entire length of the root canal.
   c. The broach may be forced in place.
   d. The broach must be wide enough to engage pulp without touching canal wall.

4. The standard for determining working length is
   a. To subtract 1 mm from tooth length
   b. To subtract 2 mm from tooth length
   c. To rely on the feel of a stop at the apex of the tooth
   d. Measuring from a preoperative radiograph

5. One of the biologic objectives in cleaning and shaping the canal system is
   a. Confining all instrumentation within the root canal space
   b. Preventing the pushing of contaminated debris beyond the apex
   c. Removing all potential irritants from the canal system
   d. All of the above

6. Recapitulation is
   a. Using successively larger files to flare the canal
   b. Removing debris with an instrument smaller than the instrument that goes to apical extent, with thorough irrigation
   c. Using a no. 35 file to clean the apex
   d. Circumferential filing with a Hedström file

7. The major problem with the action of "reaming" or "push-turn-pull" movement is
   a. Too slow
   b. Does not clean properly
   c. Does not take into account the degree of irregular canal anatomy
   d. Does not work well with K-files

8. When a clinician is determining proper canal working length, a second radiograph is recommended
   a. To reconfirm the established length
   b. When the initial file is 1.0 mm or less from the ideal termination
   c. When the initial file is more than 1.0 mm from the ideal termination
   d. In all cases of severely curved roots

9. Mechanical objectives in root canal cleaning and shaping include
   a. Preparation of a sound apical matrix
   b. Removal of all vital tissue
   c. Preparation of a parallel shaped canal
   d. Use of sodium hypochlorite

10. Intracanal medication is
    a. Necessary for complete canal cleansing
    b. Used to prevent posttreatment pain
    c. Generally contraindicated
    d. Placed with paper points in the canal

11. Electronic measuring devices may overcome what disadvantage of radiographic length determination?
    a. The unpredictability of the apical foramen position in relation to the radiographic apex
    b. Superimpositions and distortions
    c. The health hazard of radiation exposure
    d. All of the above
12. Why are determination of working length and canal cleaning and shaping recommended to be accomplished in one visit?
    a. To prevent midtreatment flare-ups
    b. To minimize the number of appointments
    c. To establish a sound apical matrix
    d. To provide optimum space for intracanal medication
13. External transportation is
    a. Ripping of the apical end of the canal
    b. Creating a perforation
    c. Desirable for proper canal shaping
    d. Caused by recapitulation
14. Home care instructions should include
    a. Potential sequelae of root canal treatment
    b. Emphasis on calling the dentist for any mild discomfort
    c. A prescription for antibiotics
    d. A prescription for analgesics

8

OBTURATION OF THE ROOT CANAL SYSTEM

NGUYEN THANH NGUYEN

OBJECTIVES OF CANAL OBTURATION

The final stage of endodontic treatment is to fill the entire root canal system and all its complex anatomic pathways completely and densely with nonirritating hermetic sealing agents. Total obliteration of the canal space and perfect sealing of the apical foramen at the dentin-cementum junction and accessory canals at locations other than the root apex with an inert, dimensionally stable, and biologically compatible material are the goals for consistently successful endodontic treatment (Fig. 8-1). Endodontic lesions positioned laterally to a root or asymmetrically about the root apex and periodontal sulcular defects of endodontic origin are vivid reminders of the complexity of the root canal system with its numerous and infinite variety and location of canal ramifications described by many investigations (Figs. 8-2 to 8-4).

To become accomplished and versatile, it behooves a clinician to master several sound methods of obturating the root canal system. To be "married" only to one obturation technique or material is to limit one's ability to undertake a diversity of complex cases. Not infrequently a combination of several materials and filling techniques proves most beneficial in sealing unusually complicated endodontic cases. The use of solvents, together with vertical condensation, heat, sealer hydraulic pressure, and/or mechanical compaction, improves the chance of success in sealing the complex root canal system three-dimensionally (Figs. 8-3 and 8-65). Nearly 60% of endodontic failure is apparently caused by incomplete obliteration of the canal space.[27] Unless a dense well-adapted root canal filling is achieved, the prognosis may be jeopardized regardless of how well other phases of the treatment are carried out. Although cement sealers enhance the sealing ability of the root canal filling, a serious effort should be made to maximize the volume of the core material and minimize the amount of sealer between the inert core and the dentinal wall. An excel-

lently compacted and tightly adapted endodontic filling should result in the complete closure of the dentinal wall–core material interface, achieving a perfect apical seal.*

The success of the canal obturation is dependent on the excellence of the endodontic cavity design and thorough canal shaping and cleaning. Regardless of the method employed to obturate the canal, the intensive efforts made toward obtaining total debridement and complete patency of the complex root canal system will facilitate its successful sealing three-dimensionally (Fig. 8-5).

Current studies[2,11,23,136,140] have shown that a flare-type preparation, which allows for more thorough debridement and deeper penetration of obturating instruments closer to the apex, will result in more effective condensation and a better sealing of all the pathways of the root canal system.

A three-dimensionally well-filled root canal system does the following:

1. Prevents percolation of periapical exudate into the root canal space (An incompletely filled canal allows percolation of tissue exudate into the unfilled portion of the root canal, where it would stagnate. Subsequent breakdown of tissue fluids diffusing out into the periapical tissues would act as a physiochemical irritant to produce periapical inflammation [Fig. 8-6, *A*].)
2. Prevents reinfection (Perfect sealing of the apical foramina prevents microorganisms from reinfecting the root canal during transient bacteremia. Bacteria transported to the periapical area may lodge, reenter, and reinfect the root canal and subsequently affect the periapical tissues.)
3. Creates a favorable biologic environment for the process of tissue healing to take place (Fig. 8-6, *B* and *C*).

Text continued on p. 185.

---

*References 22, 23, 27, 34, 35, 37, 39, 41, 43-46, 48, 61, 62, 65, and 71-73.

183

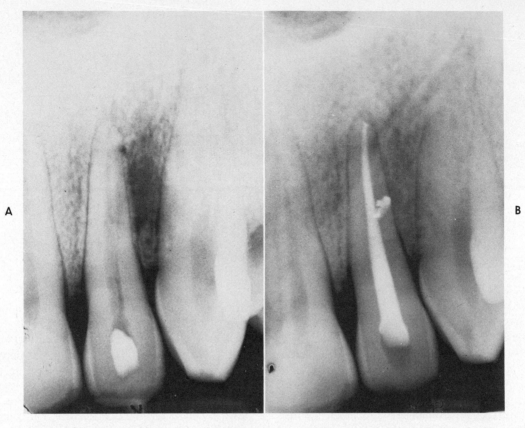

FIG. 8-1. A, Lateral incisor with a large endodontic lesion along the distal root surface. **B,** Six-month recall showing good healing. (Courtesy Dr. L. Stephen Buchanan.)

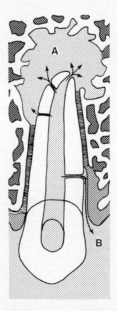

FIG. 8-2. A, Multiple portals of exit allowing egress of irritants contributing to the asymmetrical lesions. **B,** Periodontal lesion of endodontic origin. (Courtesy Drs. L. Stephen Buchanan and Clifford J. Ruddle.)

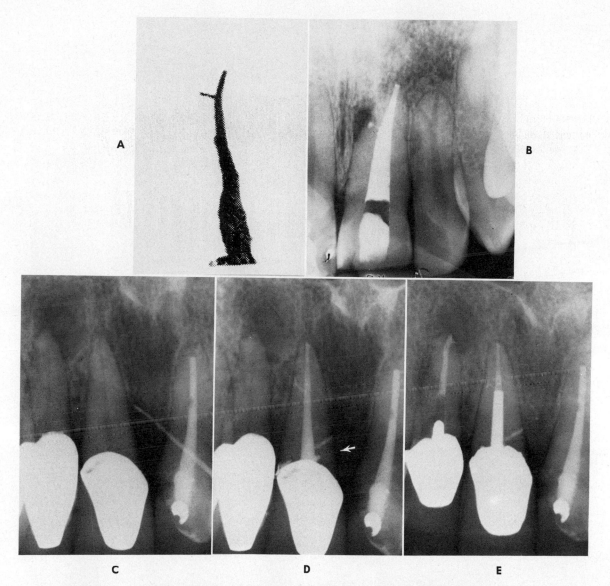

FIG. 8-3. A, Vulcanite rubber impression of a root canal system with a large lateral canal. (Walter Hess, 1925.) **B,** Similar clinical case. Note the absence of periapical pathosis and a significant lateral canal exiting to a lateral root lesion. Note also the bifurcated root canal system of the lateral incisor. **C,** Preoperative radiograph of a central incisor with a gutta-percha cone tracing the sinus tract to a large mesial crestal bone lesion. The intersulcular tissues were fortunately still intact. **D,** Postfilling radiograph demonstrating a well-obturated canal space with sealer filling the lateral canals and oozing out along the distal margin of the defective crown *(arrow).* **E,** Six-month recall radiograph showing the new crown and post and significant healing laterally and apically. (Courtesy Dr. Clifford J. Ruddle.)

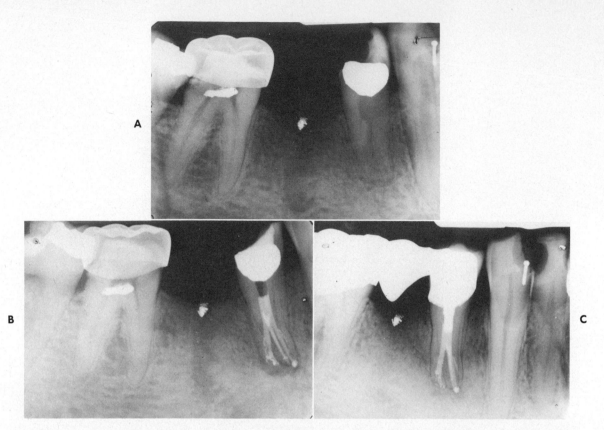

FIG. 8-4. **A,** Preoperative radiograph showing atypical root morphology of the mandibular first premolar. **B,** Postobturation radiograph. Note the three separate canals with multiple ramifications. **C,** One-year recall, good osseous repair. Warm gutta-percha with vertical condensation. (Courtesy Dr. L. Stephen Buchanan.)

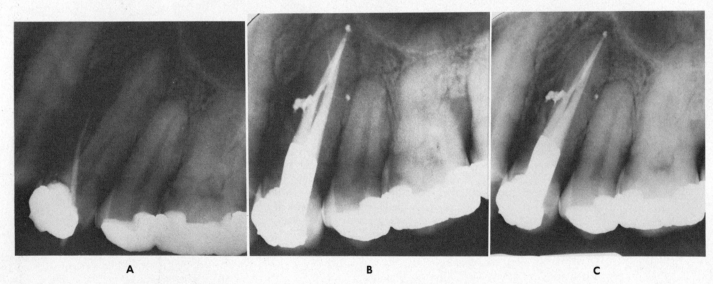

FIG. 8-5. **A,** Preoperative radiograph with extensive lateral root pathosis traced with a gutta-percha cone through the sinus tract. Atypical canal morphology suggests other internal pathologic changes. **B,** Postobturation radiograph showing early osseous repair. Note the obturation of a significant lateral canal or defect and other ramifications. **C,** Eight-month recall, good osseous repair. Warm gutta-percha with vertical condensation. (Courtesy Dr. Clifford J. Ruddle.)

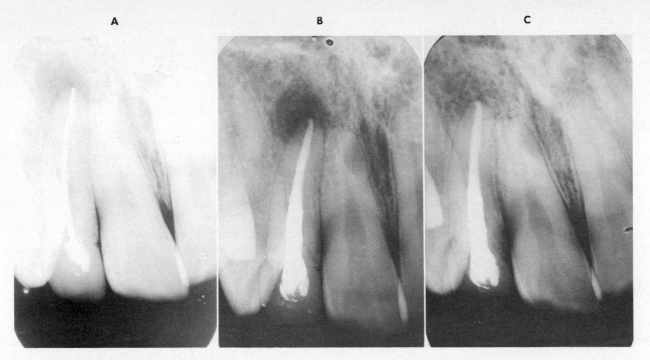

FIG. 8-6. Failure related to an incompletely filled canal. **A,** Percolation into the poorly filled portion, causing a persistent periapical lesion. **B,** After nonsurgical retreatment. The canal has been densely filled with gutta-percha. **C,** One year later, good repair.

APPROPRIATE TIME FOR OBTURATION

After the completion of root canal cleaning and shaping, the root canal is ready to be filled when the following criteria have been met:

1. The tooth is asymptomatic. There is no pain, tenderness, or apical periodontitis; the tooth is comfortable.

2. The canal is dry. There is no excessive exudate or seepage; excessive seepage of exudate is observed in wide-open canals and in cases of cysts. Grossman[45] advocates sealing with zinc iodide–iodine solution in the canal for at least 24 hours to reduce seepage.

3. There is no sinus tract. The tract (if one was previously present) should have closed.

4. There is no foul odor. A foul odor suggests the possibility of residual infection or leakage.

5. A negative culture is obtained. The question of whether or not to culture is still a source of controversy. Morse,[93] an advocate of not culturing (Chapter 12), has stated, ''Although I believe the culture is irrelevant in routine endodontic therapy, I also believe that it is essential to reduce the microbial population to as low a level as possible.'' Without a bacteriologic culture, deciding when the microbial population has been reduced to the lowest level is guesswork. Although the numerous fallibilities of a negative culture have often been raised, a positive culture suggests it might be unwise to fill the root canal at that time. Statistical clinical evidence reported by some authors* shows an average of 11% more success in healing

*References 9, 20, 45, 102, 142, and 145.

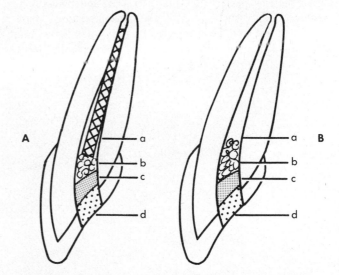

FIG. 8-7. Double-filling procedure. **A,** For contact-type nonvolatile drugs: *a,* short blunt paper point used to bring medicament into close contact with the canal wall; *b,* sterile cotton pledgets in the pulp chamber; *c,* temporary stopping; *d,* outer filling of Cavit or I.R.M. **B,** For volatile-type intracanal dressings such as camphorated parachlorophenol, the paper point is unnecessary; a cotton pledget barely moistened with medicament may be used.

when teeth are filled after a negative culture has been obtained. Furthermore, filling a root canal known to be infected increases the probability of post-filling discomfort.[62]

6. The temporary filling is intact. A broken or leaking filling causes recontamination of the canal. It is imperative

that the tooth restoration be adequately prepared before endodontic treatment. The temporary filling material must seal hermetically to prevent contamination and must be strong enough to withstand the forces of mastication. Zinc oxide–eugenol cements provide the most effective seal against marginal leakage when no particular stress is present. Commercial preparations such as Cavit or I.R.M. are satisfactory zinc oxide resin temporary fillings. Because of their slow setting time, the patient should be cautioned not to chew on the tooth for about 45 minutes after treatment. A double filling made of an inner base of gutta-percha temporary stopping and an outer filling of Cavit or I.R.M. is usually adequate. I.R.M. is used in cases of heavy occlusal stress. A double filling (Fig. 8-7) presents several advantages: (a) it provides additional support against the forces of mastication and effective protection against a broken filling or marginal leakage; (b) the potency of the medicament sealed in the canal is not affected by gutta-percha temporary stopping, which is practically insoluble and nonreactive; and (c) it prevents particles of cement from falling into the root canal system when the temporary filling is removed.

ROOT CANAL FILLING MATERIALS
Types

A large variety of root canal filling materials has been advocated throughout the years. The gamut runs from materials such as plaster of Paris, asbestos, and bamboo to precious metals such as gold and iridioplatinum. Many materials used have been rejected by the profession as impractical, irrational, or biologically unacceptable. Root canal filling materials currently in use or under clinical investigation may be grouped into the following categories.

Pastes. Paste-type filling materials include zinc oxide–eugenol cements with various additives, zinc oxide and synthetic resins (Cavit), epoxy resins (AH-26), acrylic, polyethylene, and polyvinyl resins (Diaket), polycarboxylate cements, and silicone rubber. Sometimes chloropercha paste has been used as the sole canal filling material. It is used more frequently, however, in conjunction with gutta-percha points in the Johnston-Callahan technique and the Nygaard-Østby method (p. 219). N-2 (p. 241) may be classified as a paste.

Semisolid materials. Gutta-percha (Fig. 8-8), acrylic, and gutta-percha composition cones are included in the category of semisolid materials.

Solid materials. Solid filling materials may be divided into (1) the semirigid or flexible type, including silver cones and stainless steel instruments, which can be precurved before insertion and made to follow the curvatures of a tortuous canal (Figs. 8-9 and 8-104) and (2) the rigid type. Vitallium and chrome-cobalt implant cones are inflexible and cannot follow the curvature of the canal (Fig. 8-10). They are used as endodontic endosseous implants or stabilizers and as internal strength reinforcement cones for root fractures (Chapter 15), root resorption (Chapter 16), and rebuilding of multilated crowns.

Silver amalgam. Silver amalgam is the material most widely used in endodontic surgical techniques, in cases of internal-external root resorption or perforation, in the sealing of large accessory canals, and in apical fillings (Fig. 8-11).

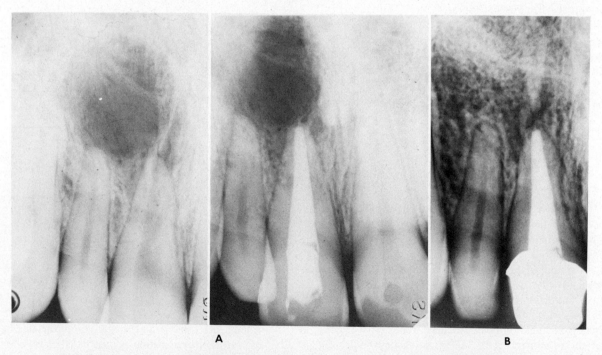

A **B**

FIG. 8-8. A, Preoperative *(left)* and postoperative *(right)* views of the left central incisor. A large periapical lesion extends over the apex of the adjacent lateral incisor. No surgery was performed. The incisor was filled with gutta-percha. **B,** Eighteen-month recall, good osseous repair. The white appearance of the filling is indicative of its density.

Role of cement-sealers

The current methods most frequently used in canal obturation employ a semisolid, solid, or rigid cone cemented in the canal with a root canal cement-sealer used as a binding agent. The sealer is needed to fill in irregularities and minor discrepancies between the filling and the canal walls. It acts as a lubricant and aids in the seating of the cones. It also fills the patent accessory canals and multiple foramina. (For a discussion of the various types of sealers available, see p. 198.)

Requirements for an ideal root canal filling material

According to Grossman,[45] an ideal root canal filling material should:

1. Provide for easy manipulation with ample working time
2. Have dimensional stability; not shrink or change form after being inserted
3. Be able to seal the canal laterally and apically, conforming and adapting to the various shapes and contours of the individual canal

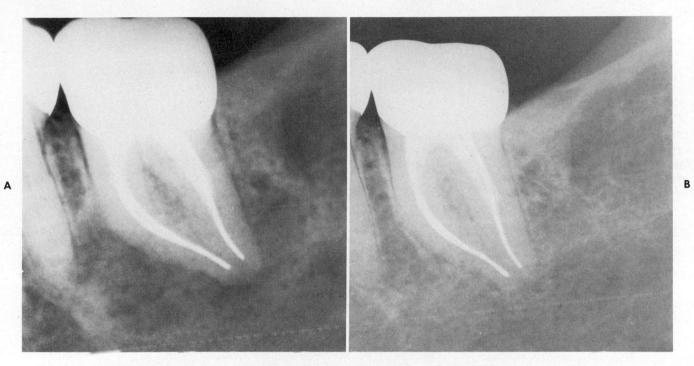

FIG. 8-9. Mandibular second molar filled with semirigid silver cones. **A,** Immediately after treatment. Note the large diffuse apical radiolucency. **B,** Complete repair 2 years later.

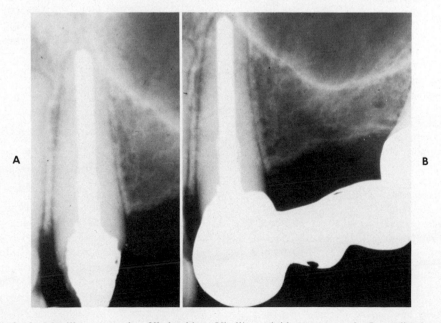

FIG. 8-10. Maxillary premolar filled with a Vitallium rigid-type cone. **A,** Immediately after treatment. The cone adds internal strength to prevent fracture. **B,** Tooth used as sound abutment for a fixed prosthesis.

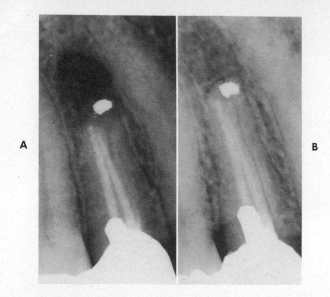

FIG. 8-11. Maxillary premolar retrofilled with non-zinc amalgam. **A,** Failure resulting from an inadequate apical seal. During surgery the apex of the palatal root was retrofilled with silver amalgam. **B,** Good repair 18 months later.

4. Not irritate periapical tissues
5. Be impervious to moisture, nonporous
6. Be unaffected by tissue fluids and insoluble in tissue fluids; not corrode or oxidize
7. Be bacteriostatic; at least, not encourage bacterial growth
8. Be radiopaque, easily discernible on radiograph
9. Not discolor the tooth structure
10. Be sterile or easily and quickly sterilized immediately before insertion
11. Be easily removed from the canal if necessary

Requirements for an ideal root canal cement-sealer

An ideal root canal sealer should:

1. Be tacky when mixed and have good adhesion to the canal wall
2. Have ample setting time, giving the clinician sufficient time to make necessary adjustments to the filling material
3. Be capable of producing a hermetic seal
4. Have very fine powder particles that will mix easily with the cement liquid
5. Be radiopaque, often revealing the existence of accessory canals, multiple foramina, resorptive areas, fracture lines, and other unusual morphologic characteristics
6. Expand while setting
7. Be bacteriostatic
8. Be biologically acceptable; not irritate periapical tissues
9. Be insoluble in tissue fluids
10. Not stain the tooth structure
11. Be soluble in common solvents if removal becomes necessary

To the above requirements one might add that an ideal root canal sealer:

12. Should not provoke an immune response in periapical tissues[13-15,131]
13. Should not be mutagenic or carcinogenic[49,77]

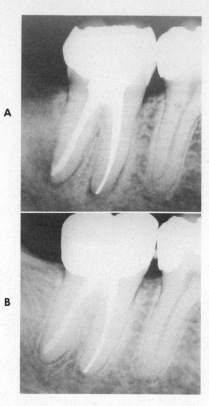

FIG. 8-12. Combination fillings on a mandibular second molar; gutta-percha packed around a silver cone on the mesial root, gutta-percha cones on the distal root. **A,** Immediately after treatment. **B,** Good repair 18 months later.

Four approaches are presently being used to scientifically evaluate the toxic effects of endodontic materials: (1) cytotoxic evaluation, (2) subcutaneous implants, (3) intraosseous implants, and (4) in vivo periapical reactions.

Primary cone selection

The selection of cone material depends on the condition of the tooth, the type and size of the canals, the necessity for partial removal of such materials, and the philosophy of the clinician.

Combination fillings are often used in filling canals. Gutta-percha cones may be packed around primary silver cones (Fig. 8-12) or coronal to a silver cone tip sealing the apical foramen. Silver cones in mesial canals and gutta-percha in the distal canals of mandibular molars are other examples of combination fillings.

CANAL OBTURATION WITH A SEMISOLID MATERIAL: GUTTA-PERCHA

Gutta-percha, popularized by Bowman in 1867,[18] is still the most widely used and accepted root canal filling material. It seems to be the least toxic, least tissue-irritating, and least allergenic root canal filling material available (Chapter 13). The composition of gutta-percha cones varies according to brand. The clinician should be aware of the possible toxicity of the additives in each brand. Gutta-percha is a rubberlike substance manufactured in two different shapes: standardized and nonstandardized (or conventional) cones (Fig. 8-13).

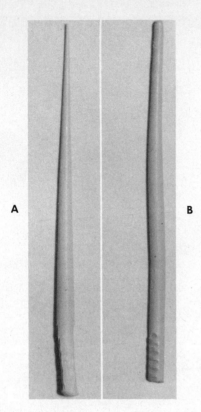

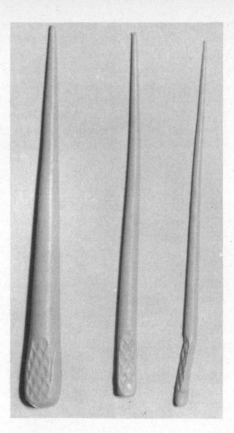

FIG. 8-13. Comparison of nonstandardized and standardized gutta-percha. **A,** Nonstandardized cones have greater taper. They may be used as auxiliary cones or as primary cones in some unusually shaped canals. **B,** Standardized cone with taper similar to that of root canal instruments.

FIG. 8-15. Nonstandardized (old style) cones of different sizes.

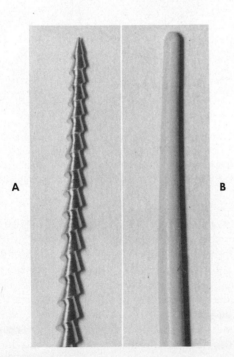

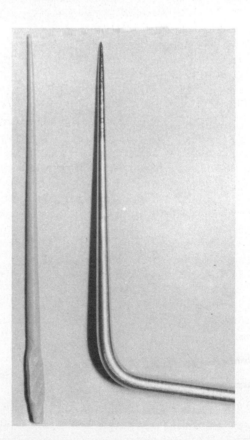

FIG. 8-14. Standardized gutta-percha cone with a taper similar to that of a Hedström file. **A,** File (largest-sized instrument, carried to working length). **B,** Corresponding size of a standardized gutta-percha cone.

FIG. 8-16. Nonstandardized (old style) cone with the same taper as a root canal spreader. This type is used in lateral and vertical condensation.

Because they approximate the diameter and taper of root canal instruments (Fig. 8-14), standardized cones (nos. 15 to 140) are normally used as *primary* cones.

Nonstandardized (or conventional) cones, more tapered in shape, are useful as *secondary* or *auxiliary* cones in lateral and vertical condensation (Figs. 8-15 and 8-16). Because of their greater flare, conventional cones in sizes *XX fine, X fine,* and *fine* make sturdier and more rigid primary cones in smaller-sized canals than do the small standardized cones.

Gutta-percha is slightly soluble in eucalyptol and freely soluble in chloroform, ether, or xylol. Gutta-percha cones may be purchased in sterilized containers and should be refrigerated for longer shelf life. When gutta-percha becomes brittle from age and oxidation, it should be discarded, although it has been shown that they can be rejuvenated by alternate heating and cooling.[122]

Gutta-percha should be the filling of choice whenever possible; its use is suggested in the following cases:

1. In teeth requiring a dowel for reinforcement of coronal restoration
2. In anterior teeth requiring bleaching or in apicoectomy cases
3. Whenever irregular walls or noncircular shapes (oval, kidney bean, ribbon-type) are present, either because of canal anatomy or as a result of preparation (Fig. 8-17)
4. When a lateral or accessory canal is anticipated (Figs. 8-18 and 8-19), when it is determined that multiple apical foramina are present (Fig. 8-20), or in cases of internal resorption (Fig. 8-21)
5. When, in extremely large canals, a customized gutta-percha cone may be fabricated for the individual case (Fig. 8-22)

Advantages

The advantages of gutta-percha as a filling material are as follows:

1. It is compactible and adapts excellently to the irregularities and contour of the canal by the lateral and vertical condensation method.
2. It can be softened and made plastic by heat or by common solvents (eucalyptol, chloroform, xylol).
3. It is inert.
4. It has dimensional stability; when unaltered by organic solvents, it will not shrink.
5. It is tissue tolerant (nonallergenic).
6. It will not discolor the tooth structure.
7. It is radiopaque.
8. It can be easily removed from the canal when necessary.

Disadvantages

The disadvantages of gutta-percha as a filling material are as follows:

1. It lacks rigidity. Gutta-percha is relatively difficult to use unless canals are enlarged above size no. 30. Because of their greater taper, nonstandardized cones of smaller sizes are more rigid than small standardized

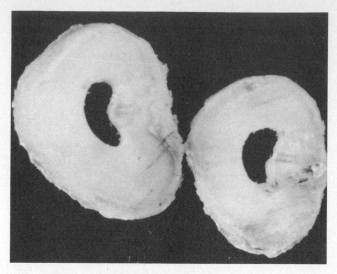

FIG. 8-17. Cross section of palatal roots of a maxillary molar. Note the kidney bean–shaped canals. (Courtesy Dr. Gery Grey.)

A   B

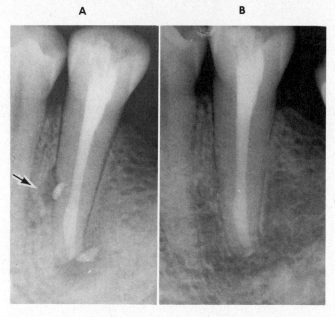

FIG. 8-18. Mandibular premolar filled with gutta-percha. **A,** Immediately after treatment. Note the well-filled lateral canal *(arrow)* and the internal resorption area. **B,** Root canal cement has been absorbed, and there is complete repair of periapical bone 2 years later.

cones and often are used to better advantage as primary cones in small canals.
2. It lacks adhesive quality. Gutta-percha does not adhere to the canal walls; consequently, sealer is required. The necessary use of a cementing agent introduces the risk of using tissue-irritating sealers.
3. It can be easily displaced by pressure. Gutta-percha permits vertical distortion by stretching. This characteristic may tend to induce overextension during the condensing process. Unless it meets an obstruction or is packed against a definite apical seat (box), it can be easily pushed beyond the apical foramen. To ensure

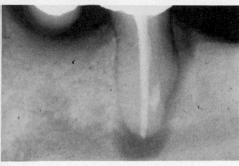

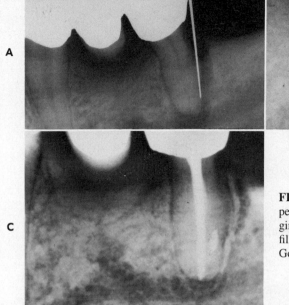

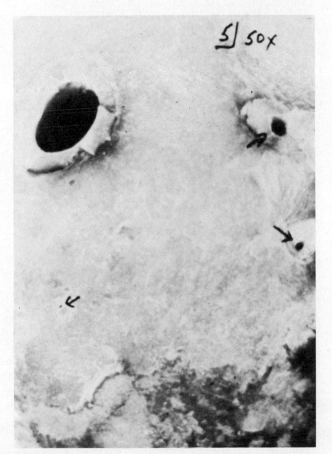

FIG. 8-19. Mandibular premolar bridge abutment. An extensive periapical lesion communicates with the oral cavity through the gingival sulcus. **A,** Note the silver cone used as a probe. **B,** After filling. Note the accessory canal filled with cement sealer. **C,** Good osseous repair 18 months later.

FIG. 8-20. Root apex of a maxillary central incisor. Note the multiple apical foramina *(arrows)*. (Courtesy Dr. Seymour Oliet.)

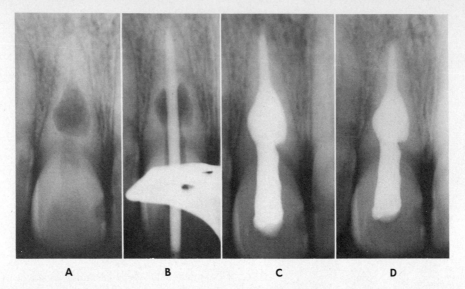

A   B   C   D

FIG. 8-21. A, Central incisor with a large area of internal resorption. **B** to **D,** Treatment using gutta-percha with the lateral and vertical condensation method to fill the canal space. (Courtesy Dr. John Sapone.)

A   B   C

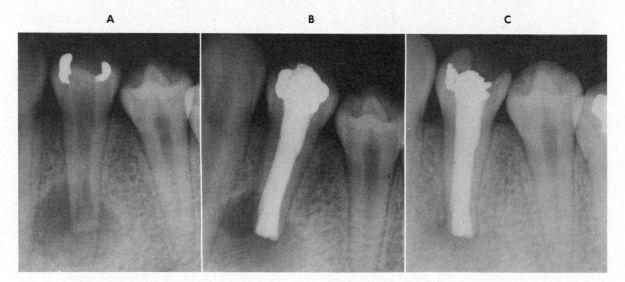

FIG. 8-22. Incompletely formed mandibular premolar with a large canal and immature apex. **A,** Apexification with calcium hydroxide for 2 years did not induce apical closure in this 22-year-old woman. **B,** Immediately after periapical surgery. The canal has been filled with a customized gutta-percha cone and Diaket cement (a nonabsorbable sealer). **C,** Almost complete osseous repair 1 year later, indicating that the canal was successfully filled.

against overextension with gutta-percha, a meticulous endodontic preparation with a definite seat or constriction in the apical portion at the dentin-cementum junction is required (Chapter 7) (Fig. 8-38).

In an effort to improve the working qualities of gutta-percha, acrylic resin has been added to its formula to increase rigidity. A group at the University of California reported that acrylic-reinforced gutta-percha has essentially the same irritational qualities as regular gutta-percha points.[99]

Procedure

The most important objective is to fill the canal system completely and densely and seal the apical foramina her-

metically. To fill the canal efficiently would be difficult if it were not designed and prepared specifically for use with gutta-percha cones. An endodontic preparation with a slight flare and a definite constriction or minimal opening at the dentin-cementum junction makes the task of condensing the gutta-percha into the canal easier and more effective. The presence of accessory canals and multiple apical foramina increases the difficulty of complete sanitization and filling of the root canal system.

Fitting of the primary gutta-percha cone

In determining the size of the primary cone, the clinician is guided by the largest reamer or file used in the final preparation of the root canal (Fig. 8-14).

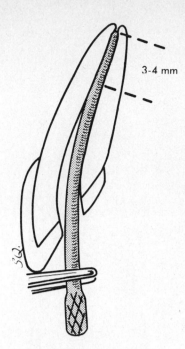

FIG. 8-23. Gutta-percha cone tightly fitted in the apical 3 to 4 mm (apical seat) of the canal.

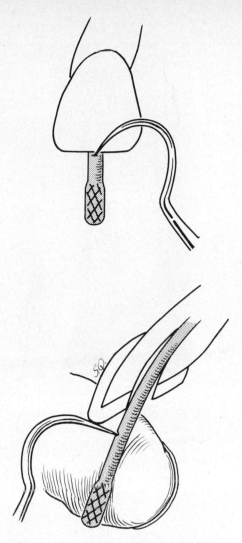

FIG. 8-24. Placement of an indentation mark on the gutta-percha cone with the tip of an explorer placed at a right angle to the incisal edge of the tooth.

The selected standardized cone is held with operating pliers at a length equivalent to the measured tooth length or working length. It is inserted into the canal until the beaks of the operating pliers touch the edge of the tooth or reference cusp (Fig. 8-23).

The primary cone must (1) fit tightly laterally in the apical third of the canal (have good tugback), (2) fit to the full length of the canal (i.e., to the dentin-cementum junction or about 1 mm from the radiographic apex), and (3) be impossible to force farther beyond the apical foramen.

A small indentation mark is made on the gutta-percha cone on the incisal edge of the tooth or reference cusp with the beaks of the operating pliers, the tip of a file, or the tip of an explorer slightly warmed over a Bunsen burner. The tip of the file or explorer is positioned at a right angle to the incisal or occlusal edge of the tooth (Fig. 8-24). Some clinicians prefer to cut the cone flush with the incisal or occlusal edge of the tooth. The technique of cutting the cone flush with the incisal edge makes the cone more difficult to grasp and handle with the pliers.

A radiograph is exposed when the cone is well stabilized with sterile cotton pellets in the canal.

If the radiograph shows the cone to be within 0.5 to 1 mm of the apex, the cone is an acceptable length. A perfect coincidence of the image of the cone with the radiographic apex will produce a cone probably protruding beyond the apical foramen. When the cone is slightly short of the radiographic apex (1 to 1.5 mm), the added pressure of condensation plus the increased lubrication provided by the sealer will be sufficient to produce complete seating (Fig. 8-25).

If the radiograph shows the cone to be too short, a correct cone fit may be obtained in one of the following ways:

1. Rechecking the working length for precise tooth length measurement and preparing the canal again accordingly
2. Enlarging the canal by filing and then trying the cone again
3. Thinning out the cone by rolling it between two sterile glass slabs or with a sterile spatula on a sterile slab or by selecting a slightly smaller cone
4. Using the chloroform-dip technique in filling the canal (next section)
5. Checking for the presence of debris clogging the canal near the apex (Debris is removed best with a reamer or a Hedström file and copious irrigation.)

If the cone is too long, it is reduced proportionally from the small or apical end (Fig. 8-26). It is reinserted tightly into the canal, and a radiograph is exposed to verify the fit.

A radiolucent line appearing between the gutta-percha cone and the wall of the canal indicates that the cone may be too small (Fig. 8-27), that the canal preparation is not round, or that an extra canal is present (Fig. 8-28).

Chloroform-dip technique. The chloroform-dip technique, as a cone-fitting method, is used in large canals

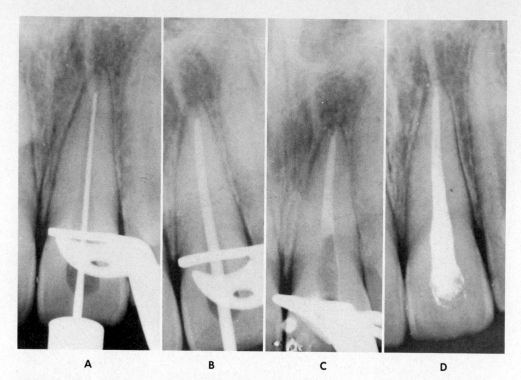

A   B   C   D

FIG. 8-25. Maxillary central incisor filled with gutta-percha. **A,** Obtaining tooth length. **B,** Primary cone with good tugback fitted 1 mm short of the apical foramen. **C,** Complete seating of the cone with condensation pressure and lubrication by sealer. Gutta-percha was removed to the apical two thirds of the apex in preparation for a dowel and core. **D,** Dowel-core reinforcement cemented.

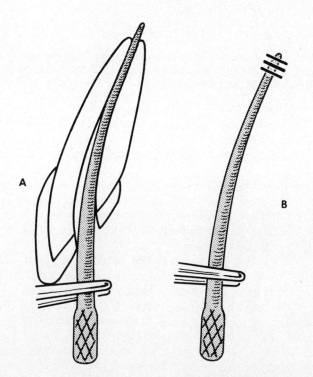

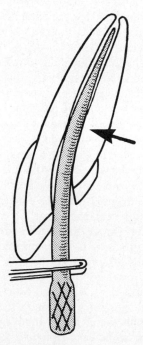

FIG. 8-26. A, Gutta-percha cone extending beyond the apex. **B,** Cone shortened a corresponding amount to improve its fit.

FIG. 8-27. Gutta-percha cone binding in the coronal half *(arrow)* but loosely fitted in the apical half, giving a false sense of a tight fit (tugback).

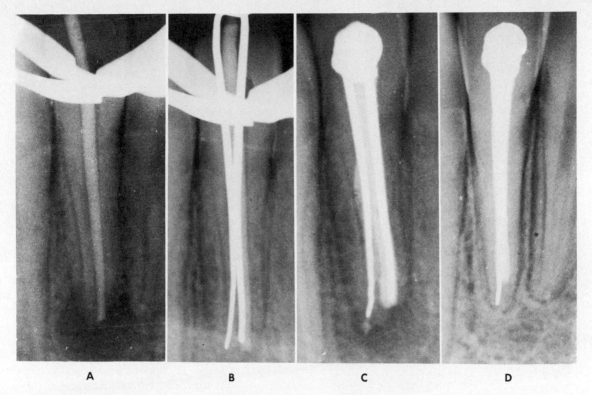

A   B   C   D

FIG. 8-28. Triple-rooted mandibular central incisor (quite rare). **A,** Tightly fitted gutta-percha cone (good tugback). Radiolucent lines on both sides reveal the presence of two extra canals. **B,** Main canal fitted with a gutta-percha cone, two smaller canals fitted with silver cones. **C,** After filling. Note the three definite canals. **D,** Complete healing 1 year later.

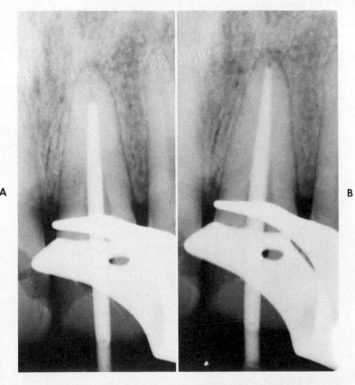

A   B

FIG. 8-29. A, Cone fitted quite short of the prepared canal length. **B,** Well-fitted cone obtained by dipping for a few seconds into chloroform and reinserting into the canal. (Note: The canal must be kept moist with irrigant to prevent the softened cone from sticking to the canal wall.)

requiring custom made gutta-percha cones or when it is desired to further seat a cone size 50 or larger that is 2 or 3 mm short of the radiographic apex (Figs. 8-29 and 8-30). This technique may be used at the time of cone fitting or cementation (below).

Note: Although investigations by the Food and Drug Administration have shown chloroform to be a potential carcinogen, I am not aware of any cases of malignancy traced to chloroform used in endodontic therapy. Other organic solvents such as eucalyptol or xylol may be used in place of chloroform.

At fitting time. An imprint of the apical portion of the prepared canal can be obtained by using chloroform to superficially soften a gutta-percha cone.

The canal should be kept moist by irrigation; otherwise, some of the softened gutta-percha might stick to the dried dentinal walls. Occasionally the softened apical section of the cone detaches from the body of the cone and adheres to the canal. The detached segment can be easily removed by a Hedström file one size smaller than the last size used in the preparation of the canal.

The cone is held with the pliers at the correct operating length. The apical 4 to 5 mm of the cone is dipped for 4 to 6 seconds into a dappen dish containing chloroform.

The softened cone is inserted into the canal with a slight apical pressure until the beaks of the pliers touch the referring landmark. It is then withdrawn slightly and reinserted a few times until a satisfactory imprint is obtained.

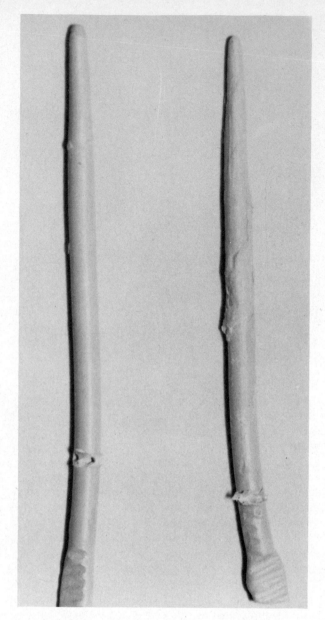

FIG. 8-30. Effect of chloroform on the gutta-percha cone in Fig. 8-29. *Left,* Before dipping. *Right,* After dipping. Note the impression of the canal space on the softened cone.

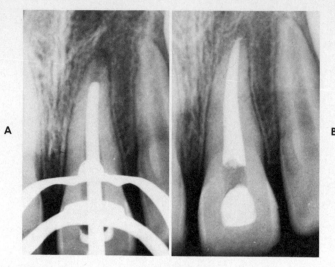

FIG. 8-31. Chloroform techinique at filling time. **A,** Primary cone fitted tightly about 2 mm short of the apex. **B,** Softened by chloroform, the cone is completely seated apically.

An indentation mark is placed on the cone at a level corresponding to the incisal edge of the crown, and a radiograph is used to verify correctness of fit.

While the radiograph is being developed, the cone should be removed from the canal and submerged in 99% isopropyl alcohol. This cone will be used later, when the canal is ready to be filled.

The canal is irrigated again to remove traces of chloroform.

At cementing time. A tight-fitting gutta-percha cone about 2 to 3 mm short of the prepared canal length may be completely seated in the following manner:

1. The canal is coated with cement sealer.
2. The cone (uncoated) is held with pliers at the correct

operating length, and the apical 4 to 5 mm of the cone is dipped into chloroform for 4 to 8 seconds. The length of dipping time depends on the amount of softening desired and the distance the cone must travel to reach the apical foramen.
3. The softened cone is inserted into the canal with steady pressure until the pliers touch the operating landmark (Fig. 8-31).

Wong and co-workers[140] in an investigation of replication properties and volumetric change of three chloroform gutta-percha filling techniques, found that the chloroform-dip technique produced fillings with significantly less shrinkage than did the chloropercha and Kloroperka N-Ø techniques. The chloroform-dip fillings showed the least volume change, with an average shrinkage of 1.40% in 2 weeks versus 12.42% for chloropercha and 4.86% for Kloroperka N-Ø fillings. If a chloroform technique is to be used, the chloroform-dip filling technique is recommended because of its low shrinkage and excellent replication qualities (Fig. 8-66).

Other recent investigations[68,104,109] on apical leakage reported that the very brief softening of the master cone with chloroform produced poor sealing results. One group of investigators[69] suggested that chloroform may affect the gutta-percha dye absorption. Also, the gutta-percha shrinkage and the physical or chemical alteration of the sealer may be responsible for the leakage. Another group of investigators[104] thought that "the surface layer of the chloroform dissolved the sealer." Although "clinical" success of the chloroform-softened gutta-percha cone technique is accepted, it certainly bears further study.

ROOT CANAL CEMENT-SEALERS AND THEIR PROPERTIES

Cements used in endodontics are often referred to as root canal cement-sealers. Most sealers are composed of zinc oxide and eugenol with various additives to render them radiopaque, antibacterial, and adhesive. Some cements contain epoxy resins (AH-26) or polyvinyl resins (Diaket).

The root canal sealer acts as (1) a *binding agent* to cement the well-fitted primary cone into a canal, much as zinc phosphate cement binds a well-fitted inlay into a cavity preparation, (2) a *filler* for the discrepancies between the cone and the canal walls, and (3) a *lubricant* to facilitate the seating of the primary cone into the canal.

Before setting, the root canal cement can be made to flow and fill the accessory canals and multiple apical foramina by the lateral and vertical condensation method.

A good sealer should be biologically compatible and well tolerated by the periapical tissues.[123,124] *All* sealers are highly toxic when freshly prepared.[126] However, their toxicity is greatly reduced after setting takes place. A few days after cementation, practically all root canal sealers produce varying degrees of periapical inflammation (usually temporary); this usually does not appear to prevent tissue healing and repair.

A root canal sealer should not provoke an immune response in periapical tissues.[13,14,15,78,131] Sealers of zinc oxide–eugenol type pastes modified with paraformaldehyde have been reported to alter dog pulp tissue, making it antigenetically active.[13,14,15] In regard to mutagenicity or carcinogenicity, investigators[49] found that eugenol and its metabolites, although suspect, were uniformly negative in a bacterial mutagenicity test. The probability of eugenol acting as a carcinogen is therefore relatively low. However, formaldehyde- and paraformaldehyde-containin sealers are highly suspect. Following a study on the subject by the National Academy of Sciences,[36] the U.S. Consumer Product Safety Commission issued warnings about the hazards of formaldehyde.[51]

In their studies of tissue reactions to root canal cements investigators[30,31] reported that although most cement sealers were highly irritating to periapical tissues, the most severe alveolar and bone destruction was caused by poor debridement and poor filling of the root canal system. Minimal tissue reaction was found when the canal was not overfilled. Their findings were confirmed by other researchers,[119] who found, using human beings and monkeys as subjects, that overinstrumentation and overfilling caused immediate periapical inflammation, which tended to persist and to cause epithelial proliferation and cyst formation. In the group of teeth filled short of the foramen, the reaction was temporary and complete repair eventually took place.

There are many sealers available commercially. The sealers most commonly used by American dentists are Rickert's, Tubliseal, Wach's, chloropercha, eucapercha, and Grossman's formula.

Some well-known root canal cement-sealers, which are less frequently used by American dentists, are zinc oxide and synthetic resins (Cavit), epoxy resins (AH-26*), acrylic polyethylene and polyvinyl resins (Diaket†) and polycarboxylate cements. Other recently advocated root canal sealers include zinc oxide–noneugenol cement (No-

genol*), calcium hydroxide–containing cement (Dycal† and Calciobiotic‡),[40] plastics-containing cements such as Silastic medical adhesive type A, silicone rubber for syringe injection (Endo-Fill§), and Fuji type I glass ionomer luting cement‖.[110,147] Researchers[108,141] have experimented with silicone rubber material sealed in the canals with cyanoacrylate, polycarboxylate or silicone adhesive, or Silastic.[66]

Rickert's sealer. Rickert's sealer contains powder—zinc oxide (41.2 parts), precipitated silver (30 parts), white resin (16 parts), and thymol iodide (12.8 parts); and liquid—oil of clove (78 parts) and Canada balsam (22 parts). It is germicidal, has excellent lubricating and adhesive qualities, and sets in about half an hour. Because of its silver content, Rickert's sealer may cause discoloration of tooth structure and must be removed meticulously from the crown and pulp chamber with xylol.

Tubliseal. Tubliseal contains zinc oxide (57.4%), bismuth trioxide (7.5%), oleoresins (21.25%), thymol iodide (3.75%), oils (7.5%), and a modifier (2.6%). This sealer is packaged in two collapsible tubes containing a base and an accelerator, which when mixed together in equal amounts form a creamy mix. Tubliseal mixes well, has excellent lubricating properties, and does not stain the tooth structure; however, it sets rather rapidly, especially in the presence of moisture.

Wach's sealer. Wach's sealer[88] contains powder—zinc oxide (10 g), calcium phosphate (2 g), bismuth subnitrate (3.5 g), bismuth subiodide (0.3 g), and heavy magnesium oxide (0.5 g)—and liquid: Canada balsam (20 ml) and oil of clove (6 ml). This sealer is germicidal, has relatively low tissue irritation, and has an adequate setting time; its lubricating qualities are limited, however. It should be mixed to a smooth, creamy consistency and should string out at least 1 inch when the spatula is raised from the glass slab. Because of its low level of tissue irritation and limited lubricating characteristics, this sealer is desirable when there is the possibility of overextension beyond the confines of the root canal.

Chloropercha and eucapercha. Chloropercha and eucapercha are made by dissolving gutta-percha in chloroform or eucalyptol, respectively. These are used by some clinicians as the sole canal filling material, but more often they are used in combination with gutta-percha cones. Shrinkage after the evaporation of the solvent and irritation of the periapical tissue by the chloroform are definite disadvantages. The chloropercha filling method (p. 217-218) can produce excellent results in the filling of unusual curvatures or in cases of perforation or ledge formation.

Grossman's sealer. Grossman's sealer is used widely and meets most of Grossman's own requirements for an ideal sealer; it presents a minimal degree of irritation and

---

*DeTrey, Ltd., Switzerland; Dentsply Distributor (U.S.A.)

†ESPE, West Germany; Premier Dental Distributor (U.S.A.).

*COE Mfg. Co., U.S.A.

†Hygienic Rubber Co., Akron, Ohio.

‡Lee Pharmaceutical, South El Monte, Calif.

§Fuji G.C., Japan.

‖L.D. Caulk Co., U.S.A.

a high level of antimicrobial activity. It contains powder—zinc oxide reagent (42 parts), staybelite resin (27 parts), bismuth subcarbonate (15 parts), barium sulfate (15 parts), and sodium borate, anhydrous (1 part)—and liquid—eugenol.

A sterile glass slab and spatula are used to mix a small amount of powder to a creamy consistency (Fig. 8-32). *No more than 3 drops of liquid should be used at a time.* Excessive time and effort would be required to spatulate a larger amount.

Tests for proper consistency include the "drop" test and the "string-out" test.

With the drop test, the mass of cement is gathered onto the spatula held edgewise. The cement should not drop off of the spatula's edge in less than 10 to 12 seconds (Fig. 8-32, *A*). A root canal instrument may also be used for this test. After a no. 25 reamer or file is rotated in the gathered mass of cement, it is withdrawn and held in a vertical position. A correctly mixed cement should remain, with very little movement, on the blade of the instrument for 5 to 10 seconds. If a teardrop forms, the mix is too thin and more powder should be added.

With the string-out test the mass of cement is returned to the slab. After touching the mass of cement with its flat surface, the spatula is raised up *slowly* from the glass slab. The cement should string out for at least 1 inch without breaking (Fig. 8-32, *B*).

Grossman's cement will not set hard on a glass slab for 6 to 8 hours. A mixed batch of cement can therefore be used for several hours. If it thickens, respatulation will break up any crystals formed and will again restore the mix to proper consistency. In the canal, because of moisture in the dentinal tubules, the cement will begin to set in about half an hour.

The popularity of this cement results from its plasticity and its slow setting time, which is due to the presence of sodium borate anhydrate. It has good sealing potential and small volumetric change upon setting. However, zinc eugenate can be decomposed by water through a continuous loss of eugenol, making zinc oxide–eugenol a weak, unstable material. Therefore, the use of Grossman's sealer in bulk as a material for retrofillings and surgical root end repairs is questionable.[121] On the other hand, this ability to be absorbed is an advantage in case of gross apical extrusion of the sealer during canal obturation.

The cement is soluble in chloroform, carbon tetrachloride, xylol, or ether. It is easily removed from the glass slab and spatula with alcohol or chloroform.

Diaket. Diaket cement, a resin-reinforced chelate formed between zinc oxide and diketone, is known for its high resistance to absorption. First reported in 1952, Diaket was found in one study[141] to be less effective as a sealer than Tubliseal, but both were found to be more effective than paraformaldyhyde zinc oxide–eugenol cement.

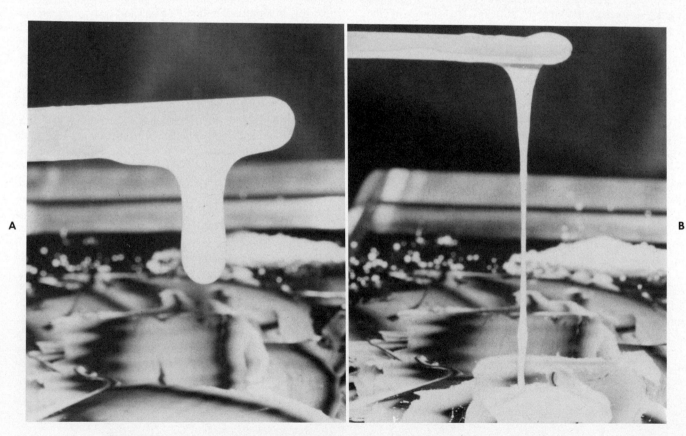

FIG. 8-32. Mixing Grossman's cement to a thick and creamy consistency. **A,** Drop test. The cement should drop off the spatula edge in 10 to 15 seconds. **B,** String-out test. The cement should string out for at least 1 inch when the spatula is raised slowly from the glass slab.

Other studies on root canal sealing cements found Diaket and AH-26 satisfactory as sealers.[32,67] These cements have been used frequently to cement endosseous implants.

AH-26. AH-26, first reported about 1957, is an epoxy resin with low solubility. It is composed of silver powder (10%), bismuth trioxide (60%) titanium dioxide (5%), and hexamethylene tetramine (25%), to be mixed to a thick creamy consistency with the liquid—bisphenol diglycidyl ether (100%). It has good adhesive property, antibacterial activity, and low toxicity and is well tolerated by periapical tissue.[30,33,103]

Two studies[47,107] tested several root canal sealers, including N-2 by implanting them into the subcutaneous connective tissue of rats. They found that AH-26 elicited

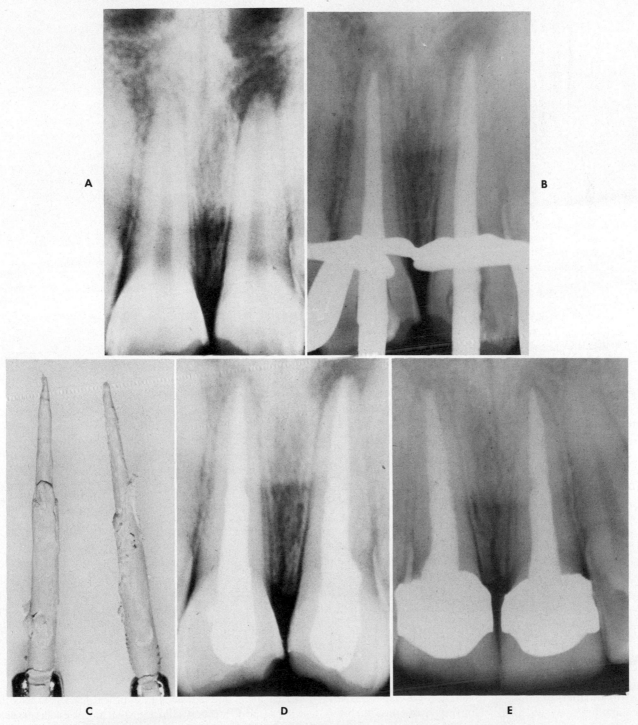

FIG. 8-33. Single-cone method with maxillary central incisors. **A,** Pretreatment. **B,** Gutta-percha primary cones fitted with chloroform. **C,** Chloroform-fitted cone showing the canal space impression. **D,** Posttreatment. **E,** Good osseous repair 1 year later. (**C** courtesy Dr. John Sapone.)

A   B   C   D

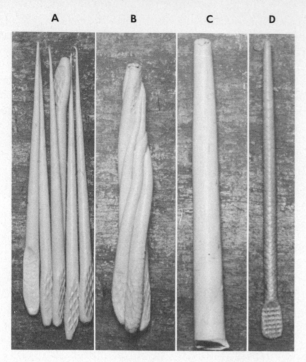

FIG. 8-34. Fabrication of a customized gutta-percha cone. **A** and **B,** Several gutta-percha points are warmed over a Bunsen burner and the tips are rolled together. **C,** Large fabricated cone. **D,** Largest-sized gutta-percha cone (no. 140) available commercially.

no response at 35 days, while N-2 provoked the "most severe inflammation elicited by any of the test materials."[107] Paresthesia following the overextension of AH-26 beyond the apex has been reported.[127,129] There was a case report[6] of paresthesia of the mental nerve resulting from gross overfilling with AH-26, but the nerve function was completely restored 14 weeks after the removal of the offending overfilled mandibular second premolar.

As with Rickert's cement, AH-26 contains silver powder, therefore, all traces of the sealer must be removed below the free gingiva level to prevent tooth discoloration.

Polycarboxylate cement. Some studies[87,121] have advocated the use of polycarboxylate cement as root canal cement. Composed of zinc oxide with polyacrylic as a liquid, polycarboxylate cement will bond to enamel and dentin. Polycarboxylates will set in a moist environment and are insoluble in water. Unfortunately, their rapid setting does not allow for ample working time. Other studies[7,112,118,138] have reported unfavorable results and have found that polycarboxylates are unsatisfactory and difficult to manipulate for endodontic use.

Nogenol. The zinc oxide–noneugenol cement Nogenol has been advocated as a less irritating sealer. One study[25] tested Nogenol subcutaneously against two eugenol-containing cements—Tubliseal and Rickert's cement—and found that "after 24 hours all sealers caused considerable inflammation." At 96 hours, Nogenol was considerably less irritating than the other two sealers, even better than the polyethylene tubing control. At 6 months Tubliseal remained significantly more of an irritant than Rickert's ce-

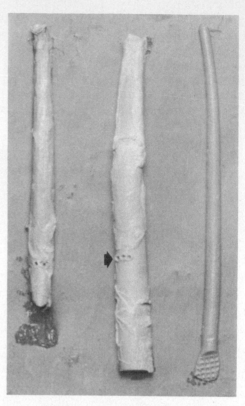

FIG. 8-35. *Left,* Customized, chloroform-fitted gutta-percha cone. *Center,* Dot marks *(arrow)* on the labial surface of the cone made by an explorer tip at the incisal edge to facilitate proper reinsertion at cementation time. *Right,* Largest-sized (no. 140) commercial cone for comparison.

ment, Nogenol, or the polyethylene control. Another study[135] found that Nogenol expands on setting and may improve its sealing efficacy with time.

Filling techniques

Single-cone method. The single-cone method may be used when (1) the canal walls are reasonably parallel and the primary cone fits snugly in the apical third of the canal and (2) the canal is too wide and commercially available gutta-percha cones will not fit the canal adequately. A customized cone is then fashioned and fitted with the chloroform technique (Fig. 8-33) (p. 195).

Fabrication of a customized gutta-percha cone. Three or more gutta-percha cones are warmed together over a flame and are pressed and twisted together into a bundle (Fig. 8-34, *A* and *B*). The slightly warmed cones are rolled between two sterile glass slabs held at an angle to make a cone with a diameter approximately the size of the canal (Fig. 8-34, *C*). If the angle of the slabs is too large for the canal, the cone is rewarmed and rerolled to a smaller diameter.

Ater the cone is allowed to cool and harden or is chilled with a spray of ethyl chloride, the apical end is softened superficially in chloroform (p. 195). The softened cone is inserted with a few gentle pumping motions until it reaches the working length.

A   B

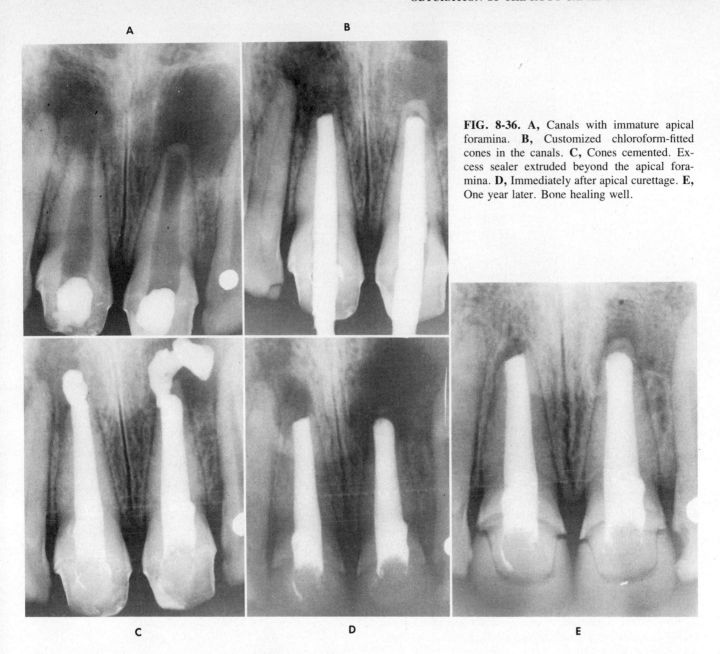

FIG. 8-36. A, Canals with immature apical foramina. **B,** Customized chloroform-fitted cones in the canals. **C,** Cones cemented. Excess sealer extruded beyond the apical foramina. **D,** Immediately after apical curettage. **E,** One year later. Bone healing well.

C   D   E

The customized cone is a replica of the internal shape of the canal (Fig. 8-35) and should be inserted in the same path and position when cemented.

When a customized cone is being cemented in the single-cone technique, it should be inserted very *slowly;* otherwise it will act as a plunger to force the cement sealer beyond the apical foramen (Fig. 8-36, *C*). Slow insertion of the customized cone will allow time for the cement to flow back coronally (Fig. 8-37). Often, the single cone method leaves some space in the occlusal half of the canal not densely filled. Lateral condensation with the addition of several fine gutta-percha cones may be required at times to obtain a densely filled canal.

Lateral condensation method. Frequently the lateral condensation method is preferred to the single-cone method because most teeth present wide canals or flares

that cannot be densely filled with a single gutta-percha or silver cone. Additional auxiliary cones inserted and condensed laterally around the primary cone can effectively fill irregularly shaped canals.

Wong and co-workers[139] in an in vitro study found that with lateral condensation the shape of a cast gold artificial root canal was notably less well replicated than with the warm gutta-percha vertical condensation, which placed a larger mass of gutta-percha into the canal (Figs. 8-61 and 8-62). The mechanical compaction technique was judged better than lateral condensation in its ability to replicate the shape of the standard cast gold artificial root canal (Fig. 8-64).

Lateral and vertical condensation method (Figs. 8-46 and 8-47). The endodontic cavity should be designed and prepared specifically for the efficient use of gutta-percha

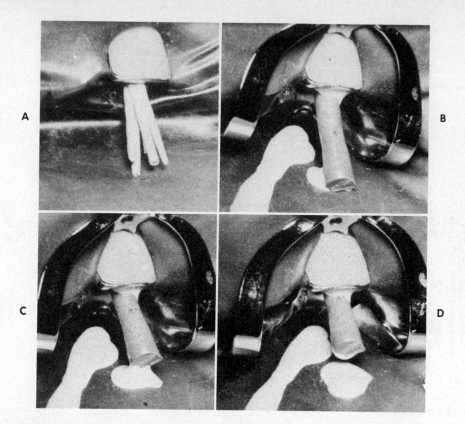

FIG. 8-37. **A,** Multiple absorbent points used to dry a large canal. **B** to **D,** Very slow insertion of a well-fitted customized cone, allowing ample time (1 to 2 minutes) for the sealer to flow out coronally.

cones as filling material. It should be so shaped that a continuously tapering funnel is created with the narrowest diameter at the dentin-cementum junction (about 1 mm from the radiographic apex) and the widest diameter at the access to the cavity. This constriction, with minimal apical opening, acts almost like a matrix against which the mass of gutta-percha is forcibly condensed. The narrow apical opening at the dentin-cementum junction prevents excess filling material from being forced beyond the apical foramen (Fig. 8-38, *A* and *B*).

Overinstrumentation destroys the apical constriction by creating an apical "zip" and making it extremely difficult to prevent overextension of the filling material during the condensing process (Fig. 8-38, *C* and *D*). The result is a poorly compacted filling with a doubtful apical seal. Invasion of periapical space by any filling material will cause periapical inflammation.

Preparation for cementation. The canal is sanitized again with irrigant solution as described in Chapter 7. With a no. 15 or 20 file the clinician rechecks the canal for patency to its full working length and to ascertain that there are no pulpal remnants or debris left at the apical terminus.

The tightly fitted primary cone with the apical tip 1 mm short of the radiographic apex is rechecked for correct fit, withdrawn, and placed into the 70% isopropyl alcohol.

To ensure the *removal of residual moisture* from the

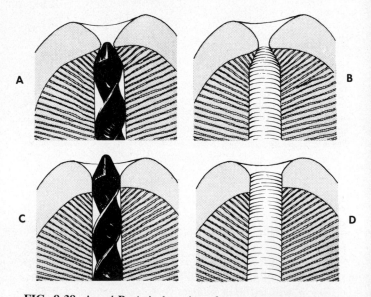

FIG. 8-38. **A** and **B,** Apical portion of a canal prepared slightly inside the apical foramen. **C** and **D,** Overinstrumentation destroys the apical constriction.

canal, it is necessary to dehydrate the canal walls before filling. This can be accomplished by flushing the canal with a solution of either 95% ethyl alchol or 99% isopropyl alcohol placed in an irrigating syringe. To be effective, the alcohol should remain 2 to 3 minutes in the canal. The

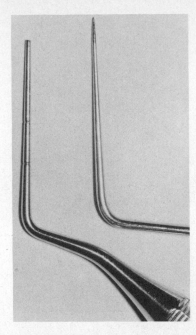

FIG. 8-39. *Left,* Root canal plugger with a flat tip and depth markings at 10 and 15 mm. *Right,* Spreader with a pointed tip.

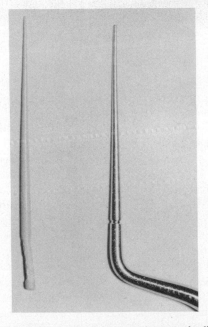

FIG. 8-40. *Left,* Fine gutta-percha cone (nonstandardized or regular type). *Right,* Fine plugger of similar size.

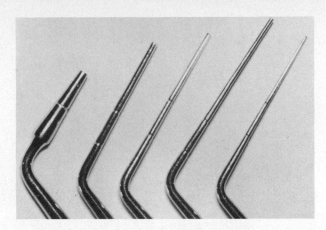

FIG. 8-41. University of California (Nguyen T. Nguyen) double-ended pluggers.

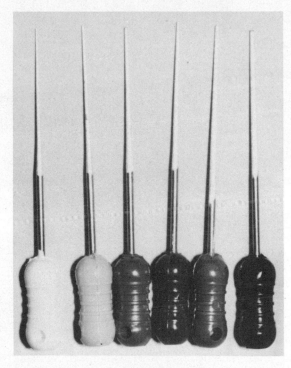

FIG. 8-42. Union Broach finger spreaders and pluggers, color coded and mounted on plastic handles.

canal is then dried with sterile absorbent points inserted to a depth 1 mm short of the working length. An absorbent point is placed in the canal to absorb exudate until the clinician is ready to obturate.

Sterile spreaders and pluggers (Fig. 8-39) are prepared for lateral and vertical condensation. *Spreaders* are long, tapered, pointed instruments used to condense the filling material laterally against the canal walls, making room for insertion of additional auxiliary cones. *Pluggers* or condensers, regardless of their width, have flat apical tips and are used to pack the gutta-percha mass vertically (Figs. 8-

40 and 8-41). Like spreaders, pluggers come in different sizes, have depth markings on the shaft, and are either long- or short-handled (Figs. 8-40 to 8-44).

Selection of pluggers. Three or four pluggers (Fig. 8-41) to be used in the coronal, middle, and apical thirds of the canal must be preselected to ensure their loose fit. During the vertical condensation phase the prefitted plugger will be compressing the gutta-percha mass apically, unimpeded by the walls of the canal.

Application of cement. The absorbent point is removed to check the moisture in the canal. If necessary, the canal is dried again with additional absorbent points.

The cement is carried to the canal in small amounts on a sterile reamer one size smaller than the last instrument used for enlargement. If very small portions of sealer are

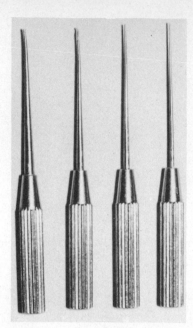

FIG. 8-43. Set of four Luks finger pluggers.

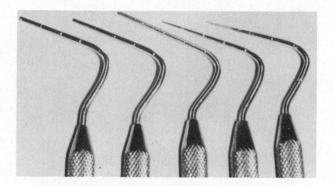

FIG. 8-44. Set of long-handled Kerr pluggers.

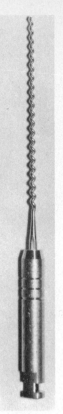

FIG. 8-45. Lentulo paste carrier.

carried in first, there will be less chance of trapping air. The reamer, set 1 mm short of the working length, is rotated *counterclockwise* as it is withdrawn, spinning the sealer into the canal; then a slow, gentle, pumping action combined with a lateral rotary motion of the instrument is used to thoroughly coat the canal walls and disperse air entrapped in the cement. The procedure is repeated until the canal walls are well coated with sealer.

An absorbent point or Lentulo paste carrier can also be used to coat the canal walls with sealer. The Lentulo, a fin-spiraled wire paste carrier (Fig. 8-45), can be rotated between thumb and index finger or mounted on a contraangle. Rotated in a *clockwise* action, it spins the sealer into the apical portion of the canal. When the Lentulo is used mechanically, a small amount of cement is first carried into the canal to a depth of 2 or 3 mm from the apex without running the engine. The Lentulo is then rotated at *very slow speed* as it is withdrawn from the canal. Experience will aid in keeping excess cement from going past the apical foramen. The Lentulo breaks if it accidentally locks in the curved or narrow canal or if the engine is

running in reverse. The spiral, once broken in the canal, is almost impossible to remove because its coiled spring binds tightly against the wall of the canal.

Lateral and vertical packing technique. The primary cone is removed from the alcohol and air dried. Its apical half is coated with sealer (Fig. 8-47, *B*) and inserted *slowly* and *gently* into the canal to the measured length (until the mark on the cone coincides with the incisal or occlusal edge) (Fig. 8-47, *C*). After a few seconds' pause the cone is inserted farther, until the full depth is reached. Slow insertion of the cone permits the excess sealer to be dispersed toward the coronal end of the tooth (Fig. 8-37).

Note: When the tooth is not anesthetized, some sensation may be experienced by the patient as the cone is being inserted apically. This slight pain may be due to entrapped air that must be given time to be absorbed or to excess cement being pushed out beyond the apical foramen.

One or two auxiliary cones can be inserted alongside the primary cone *without the use of a spreader*. If there is any doubt about the relationship of the primary cone to the apex, radiographic verification should be done immediately before more auxiliary cones are added with the aid of a spreader. If an overextension occurs, usually because of improper apical preparation, the cones can be easily removed, the primary cone shortened, and the process repeated while the sealer is still plastic. If the filling is short, the gutta-percha mass can be vertically packed farther apically.

A spreader is then inserted apically alongside the primary cone, wedging it against the canal wall and creating

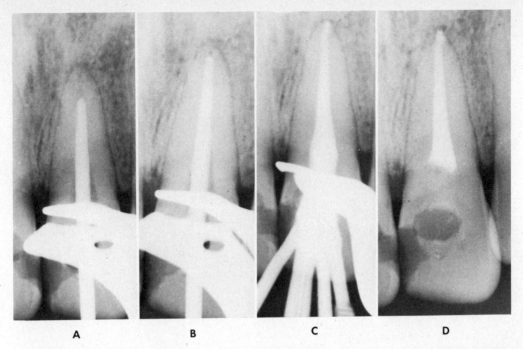

A   B   C   D

FIG. 8-46. Lateral and vertical condensation. **A,** Selected primary cone too short. **B,** Correct apical fit obtained by using the same cone dipped a few seconds into chloroform and reinserted to the working length. **C,** Cone cemented with several secondary cones inserted between the primary cone and the canal wall. **D,** Completed canal obturation after lateral and vertical condensation has been carried out.

space for an additional cone. Lateral and apical pressure is applied by revolving the spreader through half an arc (Fig. 8-47, *D*).

The spreader is removed with one hand while a gutta-percha cone of a corresponding size is inserted with the other hand in exactly the same hold just vacated by the spreader (Fig. 8-47, *E*).

Coating the auxiliary cone with sealer before insertion is optional. Some clinicians dip auxiliary cones into sealer or eucalyptol to give the cones sufficient lubrication to reach the space prepared for them.

The spreader is inserted again with apical pressure, making room for another cone. The spreading process is repeated several times until the wedged cones block further access to the canal (Figs. 8-46, *C*, and 8-47, *F*).

Vertical condensation is now combined with *lateral condensation* to obtain greater density and compactness and to force the filling material into the complex configuration and ramifications of the root canal system.

With the blade end of the spreader instrument heated *red-hot,* the butt ends of the cones are cut flush with the coronal opening (Fig. 8-47, *G*).

While the gutta-percha mass is still soft, because of the heat transmitted by the instrument, vertical compaction is done without delay. The gutta-percha mass is forcibly packed apically with a preselected *cold* plugger dipped into cement powder to prevent the still-warm gutta-percha from sticking to it and being pulled out when the instrument is removed.

With a suitable-size plugger heated red-hot, the gutta-percha mass is removed to a level 3 or 4 mm beyond the canal orifice (Fig. 8-47, *H*). While the gutta percha is still warm, a bent smaller plugger is used with vertical pressure to condense it further apically (Fig. 8-47, *I*).

To be effective, the pluggers selected must fit loosely and work at all times within the gutta-percha mass, unimpeded by the walls of the canal. This vertical packing deep in the apical third of the canal forces the gutta-percha and sealer into the irregular configurations of the canal system and improves the chances of filling patent accessory canals and foramine (Fig. 8-47, *J*).

The whole canal is then filled by continuation of the spreading process followed by the insertion of auxiliary cones. When the spreader cannot be inserted more than 3 or 4 mm beyond the canal orifice, the spreading process is terminated (Fig. 8-47, *K*).

The protruding butt ends of the cones are removed with the blade end of the spreader instrument heated red-hot, and the gutta-percha mass is firmly condensed vertically (Fig. 8-47, *L* and *M*).

A radiograph is exposed to ascertain that there is an opaque homogeneous filling to within 1 to 0.5 mm of the radiographic apex and that there are no radiolucent or fuzzy gray areas (voids) present in the canal. If the filling is short or shows voids, the gutta-percha mass is removed as far apically as needed with a red-hot plugger. A smaller-width cold plugger is used to condense the softened gutta-percha apically. The process of vertical condensation combined with lateral condensation is repeated until the canal is filled to the desired height.

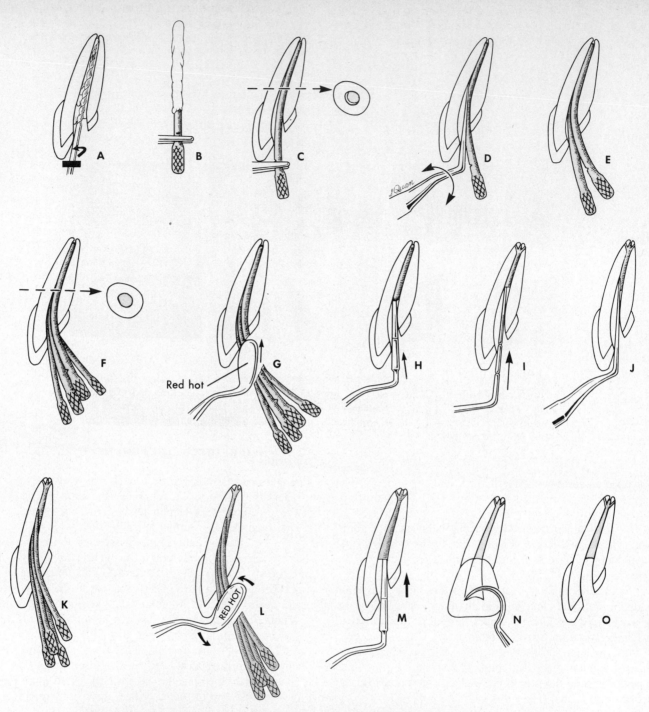

FIG. 8-47. Step-by-step procedure for lateral and vertical condensation. **A,** Cement carried into the canal with a reamer set 1 mm short of the working length. The reamer is rotated counterclockwise, spinning sealer into the canal. Note the constriction at the apex of the endodontic cavity preparation. **B,** Primary gutta-percha cone coated with cement-sealer. **C,** Cone inserted into the canal until the mark on the cone coincides with the incisal edge. Arrow points to a cross section of the middle third of the canal. **D,** Spreading to create space for an additional cone. **E,** Auxiliary cone inserted into the space created by the spreader. **F,** Spreading process with several secondary cones added. Arrow points to a cross section of the middle third of the canal. **G,** Butt ends of the cones removed with a hot instrument. **H,** Vertical condensation packing the still-warm gutta-percha mass apically. **I,** After removal of the gutta-percha to the apical third of the canal, prefitted pluggers are used to vertically pack the gutta-percha mass farther apically. **J** and **K,** Continuation of spreading and cone addition until the remainder of the canal is densely filled. **L,** Butt ends of the additional accessory cones removed with an instrument heated red hot. **M,** The still-warm plasticized gutta-percha mass is packed vertically with a prefitted cold plugger to the canal orifice's level. **N,** Filling materials removed from the pulp chamber and pulpal horns. **O,** Final fill after condensation.

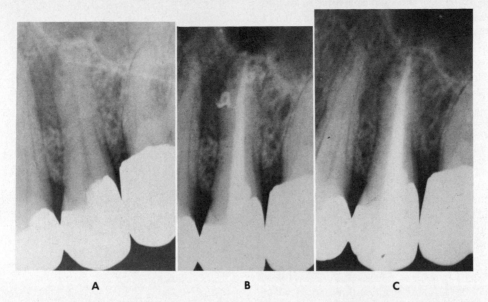

FIG. 8-48. Maxillary second premolar. **A,** Pretreatment. There is a possibility of lateral canals because of the unusual location of the radiolucency along the mesial aspect of the root. **B,** Canal filled by the lateral and vertical condensation method. Note the complex foramina and lateral canals. **C,** Two years later, complete osseous repair.

The filling procedure is completed as follows:

When the canal is densely and completely filled, as verified by the radiograph, the coronal gutta-percha is removed to the canal orifice with a red-hot instrument. With a cold plugger the gutta-percha mass is condensed farther apically, forming a clean flat surface slightly below the cervical line (Fig. 8-47, *O*). The cement is cleaned from the pulp horns and the chamber wiped with alcohol or chloroform (Fig. 8-47, *N*).

The crown is filled with a light shade of cement (the final restoration is placed at a later date). The rubber dam is now removed, the occlusion is checked, and two radiographs are exposed at different horizontal angles for future comparison.

If the need for a *dowel* is anticipated, the gutta-percha is removed a little deeper apically with a red-hot calibrated plugger or suitable rotating instruments, the chamber is packed with cotton pellets, and the access cavity is closed with a temporary cement.

The combination of lateral and vertical condensation when used well can produce filling of great density and can effectively fill the complex root canal system three dimensionally and in its entirety (Figs. 8-48 and 8-49).

Warm lateral condensation technique. Martin[84a] developed a cordless, rechargeable, battery-operated gutta-percha heat condensor for use in *warm lateral condensation*. The device (Fig. 8-50) is adapted with a replaceable and flexible spreader/plugger tip equivalent in size to approximately a no. 30-35 K-type file.

The technique follows the lateral condensation procedure and can produce a three-dimensional filling superior to that obtained with the usual cold lateral condensation. After the canal is coated with sealer and the master cone is placed to proper depth, the Martin heat condensor tip is introduced into the canal alongside the gutta-percha cone, as with an ordinary spreader. The activator switch is then depressed, causing the tip of the instrument to become warm within 2 seconds. The heat condensor is gently forced apically and laterally into the canal with a rotary penetrating motion, causing the gutta-percha to spread laterally and apically for a more complete obturation of the canal space. The heat condensor is then gently withdrawn, and an auxiliary cone is inserted in the channel just created by the condensor tip. The same procedure is repeated, adding, spreading, and condensing several gutta-percha cones until the canal is filled.

Since the gutta-percha mass has been softened by the heat condensor, little exertion is required to spread and condense the material apically and laterally. It has been shown in trial use that 3 or 4 more gutta-percha cones can be added when the heat condensor is used as compared with the regular lateral condensation technique. If stronger pressure is desired, the normal plugger or spreader may be used to compact the thermoplasticized gutta-percha.

The Martin gutta-percha heat condensor is self-contained, cordless, battery operated, and rechargeable. The tip size corresponds with a file size and has a taper to match a file/spreader/plugger. This allows the heater tip to penetrate deeply into the canal for effective condensation. A rubber stop marker can be used for depth control to correlate with the canal length.

The device can be utilized to remove gutta-percha for post preparation or for retreatment of inadequately filled canals. The Martin gutta-percha heat condensor appears to be a good instrument for use in the warm lateral condensation technique.

Sectional method. The sectional method varies slightly with different clinicians; but in essence, it consists of fill-

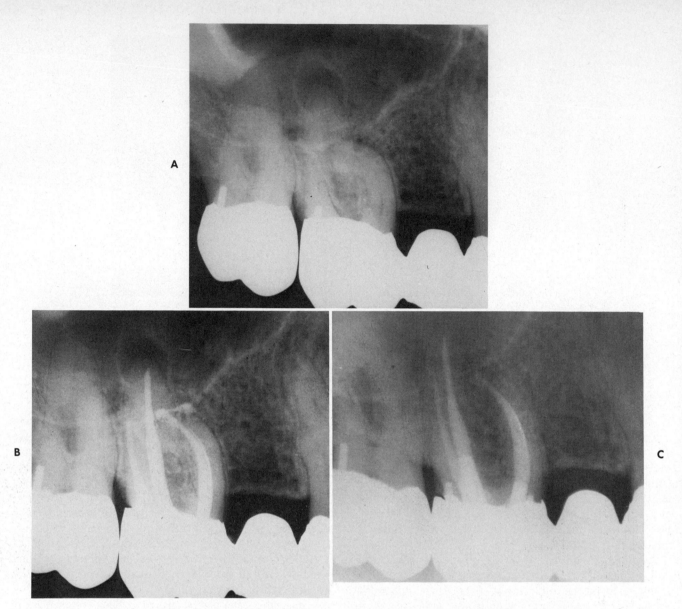

FIG. 8-49. Maxillary first molar. **A,** Bridge abutment with chronic apical periodontitis and a sinus tract. **B,** Canal filled with gutta-percha by lateral and vertical condensation. **C,** Eighteen months later, good healing.

ing the canal with sections of gutta-percha 3 to 4 mm in length (Fig. 8-51).

A plugger is selected, and a suitable marker is engaged on the instrument for length control. The plugger is introduced into the canal so it will reach a point 3 or 4 mm from the apex.

A gutta-percha cone of approximately the size of the canal is fitted a few millimeters short of the apex and cut in 3- to 4-mm sections.

After the end of the plugger is warmed over the Bunsen burner, the apical section of gutta-percha is tacked to it. The section of gutta-percha is dipped into eucalyptol and then carried to the apical foramen. Some clinicians coat the canal walls with a thin layer of sealer before inserting the gutta-percha. *Moving the plugger back and forth through a lateral arc will cause it to release from the section of gutta-percha.*

A radiograph is exposed to verify the position of the cone. If the cone is short, the next smaller plugger, with a rubber band marker for length control, may be used to pack the cone farther apically.

Additional sections of gutta-percha are inserted to fill the canal completely. If the need for a dowel is contemplated, the filling process may be stopped after the condensation of several sections of gutta-percha.

This technique is useful in filling tube-type canals or severely curved canals but requires very precise length control by the clinician. If too much pressure is used, the apical section of gutta-percha may be forced into the periapical space or vertical root fracture may result.

Vertical condensation method with warm gutta-percha. A variation of the sectional gutta-percha method introduced and popularized by Schilder[115] has been referred to as the warm gutta-percha method.

The technique involves the placement of the master cone

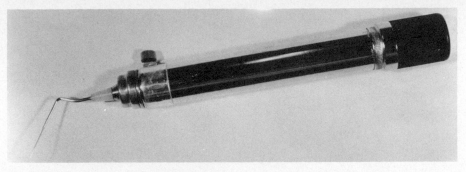

FIG. 8-50. Prototype Martin gutta-percha heat condensor for warm lateral condensation. (Courtesy Dr. H. Martin, L.D. Caulk Co.)

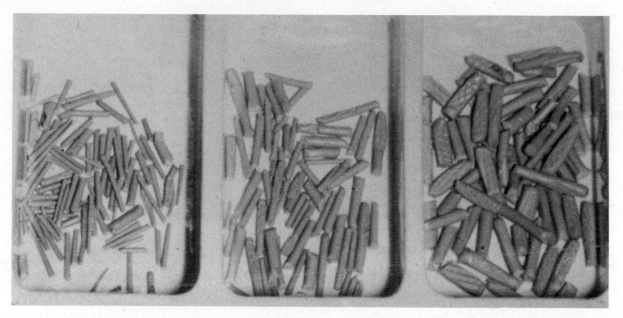

Fig. 8-51. Precut sections of gutta-percha, of different diameters, for use in the sectional method.

in the prepared canal with a minimal amount of sealer, the controlled softening of the gutta-percha with a heat transfer instrument, and the gradual vertical compaction of the softened gutta-percha with a series of prefitted pluggers to obturate the root canal system three-dimensionally.

The armamentarium consists of a series of gutta-percha pluggers, spoon excavators, and a heat-transfer instrument (Fig. 8-53).

Although gutta-percha is a poor heat conductor, it can be softened by heat over a range of approximately 4 to 6 mm and vertically condensed to fill the root canal system.

The apical extent to which the gutta-percha can be compacted is dependent upon the quantity and depth of heat transmitted and the force of condensation. The thermosoftening of the gutta-percha is governed by the amount of heat used. This varies in direct proportion to the proximity and intensity of the heat source, the frequency of the heating cycle, and the volume of gutta-percha in the canal.[42] The most effective compaction potential is obtained where the highest concentration of heat is imparted to the gutta-percha mass. The thermosoftened gutta-percha as used in this technique has been shown to expand 1% to 2%.[22] A

recent study[139] showed that the warm gutta-percha shrinkage upon cooling is on the order of 0.45%.

To counterbalance the effect of dimensional changes when the gutta-percha is thermosoftened, *continuous condensation force must be exerted during cooling*. Under forceful condensing pressure, canal ramifications are filled with softened gutta-percha or cement sealer (Fig. 8-52).

This technique requires a preparation with an optimal access cavity and a continuously tapered canal. (See Chapter 7.) Such preparation facilitates cleaning of the canal system and the subsequent introduction of a graded series of pluggers to within 4 to 6 mm of the apical foramen during the obturating procedures (Figs. 8-53 and 8-54, *B*). The cross-sectional diameter of the prepared apical terminus is usually kept as small as practical (no. 20 to 25 file) for more effective packing and greater condensation control with minimal risk of pushing the filling materials beyond the apical foramen by the force of condensation.

Technique

Cone fitting. Because their taper approximates the shape of the prepared canal, nonstandardized gutta-percha

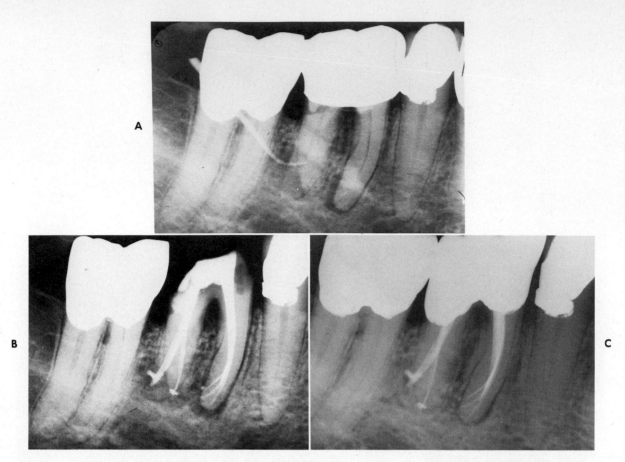

FIG. 8-52. **A,** Preoperative radiograph. Mandibular first molar with a sinus tract traced with a gutta-percha cone that points to the distal-buccal root with a large lateral root lesion. Note the asymmetric lesion along the distal aspect of the mesial root and the furcation involvement. **B,** Postobturation radiograph. Note the significant accessory canals and their positions, which explain the asymmetry of the periapical lesions. Warm gutta-percha with vertical condensation. **C,** Good progressive healing 6 months later. This case was originally planned for hemisection and bicuspidization; however, because of the patient's age (83), it was decided to open the furca from the buccal and lingual (odontoplasty) and restore the tooth with a single-unit crown. (Courtesy Dr. Clifford J. Ruddle.)

cones are used as the primary cones in this method.

The pointed tip of the cone is cut off a few millimeters to ensure a good fit. The cone is fitted to bind apically with good tugback 1 to 1.5 mm short of the length of the prepared canal. This distance is dependent on the diameter of the foramen, the apical curvature and rate of taper of the canal, the viscosity of the sealer, and the pressure of condensation. If the shape of a manufactured cone needs to be greatly modified to obtain a closer fit in an irregularly shaped foramen or unusually tapered canal, the clinician may elect to fabricate a custom-fitted cone with the aid of solvents (p. 202).

Selection of pluggers. Three or four pluggers to be used in the apical, middle, and coronal thirds of the canal must be selected ahead of time to fit loosely in the canal (Fig. 8-54). During the vertical compaction the prefitted plugger compresses the thermally softened gutta-percha mass apically without contacting the walls of the prepared canal. The appropriate plugger captures a maximum cushion of softened gutta-percha and moves the entrapped material

apically. An inappropriately large plugger binds against the canal walls and cannot possibly compact the gutta-percha toward the apex. On the other hand, a small plugger is ineffective in the wider portion of the canal. The narrow plugger pierces the softened gutta-percha without compacting it effectively.

Sealer. Although any biologically compatible sealer may be used successfully with this technique, the Kerr sealer has been advocated because of its tenacity, ability to vary viscosity, and acceleration of setting time in the presence of heat.

The canal is irrigated with 99% isopropyl alcohol solution and dried with absorbent points. The canal walls are coated with an extremely thin layer of sealer. The primary cone, lightly coated with sealer on its apical third, is gently inserted and firmly seated in the prepared canal. When the canal morphology abruptly or extremely flares in its middle and coronal thirds, supplemental gutta-percha cones may be placed alongside the primary cone to enhance the initial stages of the down-packing condensation.

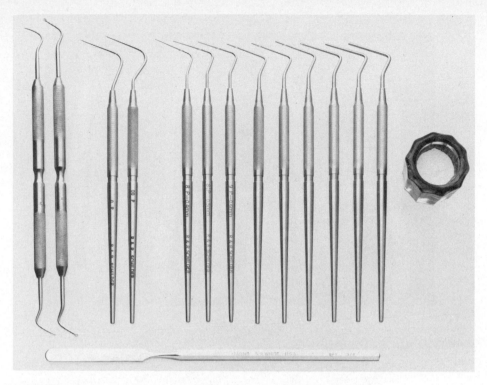

FIG. 8-53. Armamentarium for vertical condensation of warm gutta-percha. Assembled are spoon excavators, no. 0 and 00 heat carriers, a graded series of posterior root canal pluggers (Ransom & Randolf), and a Dappen dish of cement powder. (Courtesy Drs. L. Stephen Buchanan and Clifford J. Ruddle.)

Down-packing phase. With the blade of a spoon excavator heated red-hot the primary cone and supplemental cones, if present, are seared off at the canal orifice level (Fig. 8-55, *A*). A cold plugger is used to condense the still-warm gutta-percha vertically. The plugger should be dipped into cement powder to prevent the gutta-percha from sticking to it. Because the plugger used was preselected to fit loosely at the coronal third of the canal, it packs the gutta-percha unimpeded by the canal walls. During this first "wave of condensation" in the plasticized gutta-percha mass the coronal few millimeters are compacted laterally and apically, forming a cast of the canal configuration at this level (Fig. 8-55, *B*). The gutta-percha in the middle and apical sections of the canal is not much affected by heat or condensation forces.

Note: The heat source can be an alcohol lamp, a Bunsen burner, or any other heating device available commercially (Fig. 8-56). The newly formed coronal seal, together with an apically well-fitted primary cone, can generate enormous apical and lateral hydraulic forces when additional waves of condensation are carried out. This dynamic hydraulic effect causes the entrapped sealer to be forced into the complex configuration and ramifications of the root canal system.

To proceed further with packing, the heat carrier instrument heated red-hot is stabbed 3 to 4 mm into the coronal gutta-percha mass and quickly removed (Fig. 8-55, *C*). Because of dentin's poor heat conductivity, instruments heated red-hot can be introduced momentarily in the prepared canal without injuring the attachment apparatus.

Some gutta-percha is removed with the heat carrier. The thermosoftened gutta-percha mass within the canal is then immediately compacted vertically. Depending on the proximity of the heat source and the quantity of heat delivered, the gutta-percha mass can be softened over a depth of approximately 4 to 5 mm. A cold plugger that was fitted in the middle third of the canal condenses the gutta-percha vertically, delivering another forceful wave of condensation to the thermally plasticized gutta-percha mass (Fig. 8-55, *D*). The plugger moves the mass 2 or 3 mm apically. It is important to clear as much gutta-percha as possible from the sides of the canal by withdrawing and reinserting the plugger several times to ensure good compaction. The working level of the gutta-percha mass is maintained relatively even at the end of each series of vertical compactions. The heat carrier is again heated red-hot, stabbed 3 or 4 mm into the remaining gutta-percha, and immediately withdrawn (Fig. 8-55, *E*).

A cold plugger that was fitted in the apical third of the canal firmly packs the gutta-percha vertically, creating the final wave of condensation (Fig. 8-55, *F*). Under the force of vertical condensation the softened gutta-percha and entrapped sealer are compressed into the irregular configuration and canal ramifications, creating the desired sealing effect. A radiograph is exposed to check for discrepancies and to verify the apical extent of the filling. About 5 mm of gutta-percha should remain apically after the down-packing condensation (Figs. 8-55, *G,* and 8-57).

Post and dowel space. If post space is desired, the obturation procedure is ended at this stage. A cotton pellet is

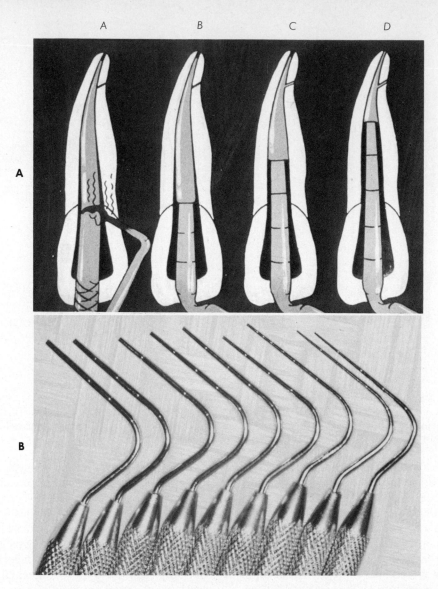

FIG. 8-54. A, Selection of pluggers for vertical condensation. *A,* Flare preparation with the apical terminus kept as small as practical. Fitted gutta-percha cone cemented in place. Coronal section of the cone removed by heated excavator, ready for vertical condensation. *B to D,* How preselected pluggers should fit in the coronal, middle, and apical thirds. Pluggers must fit loosely and not touch the walls of the canal. During vertical condensation they should be in gutta-percha at all times, unimpeded by dentinal walls. (Courtesy Dr. Frank Casanova.) **B,** Set of root canal pluggers redesigned by Schilder for the warm gutta-percha technique.

placed in the pulp chamber and Cavit or I.R.M. is used as a temporary filling until the post and final restoration can be done.

Back-packing phase. If a post is not required, the rest of the canal is filled to the desired height with the back-packing technique.

A few cones of gutta-percha of the same taper as the original primary cone are cut into 3- to 5-mm long segments and placed in sequence on a glass slab. A slightly warmed heat carrier picks each segment up (Fig. 8-58), passes it through the heat source to soften it adequately, quickly introduces it into the canal, and twists it off (Fig. 8-55, *G*). A cold plugger, prefitted in the apical third, condenses the segment of gutta-percha vertically. Systematic

and forceful stepping of the preselected plugger along the periphery of the root canal will produce a homogeneous and dense filling (Figs. 8-55, *H,* and 8-59). Some clinicians prefer the use of cotton pliers instead of the heat carrier to carry the gutta-percha segments to be introduced into the canal during the back-packing phase (Fig. 8-58, *E to I*).

This procedure is repeated until the canal space is filled to 1 mm below the orifice.

Common problems encountered with warm gutta-percha vertical condensation

1. The primary cone may adhere to the plugger and become dislodged. This can be avoided by dipping the plugger in cement powder and moving it back and

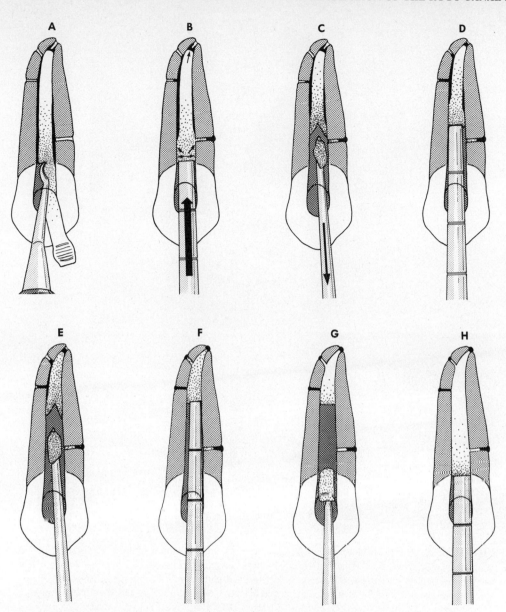

FIG. 8-55. Down-packing phase. **A,** Removal of the gutta-percha cone to the canal orifice with a spoon excavator heated red-hot. **B,** Prefitted cold plugger condensing the still-warm gutta-percha vertically. **C,** A heat carrier heated red-hot is stabbed 3 to 4 mm into the gutta-percha and quickly removed. Some gutta-percha is removed with the instrument. **D,** A preselected cold plugger that was fitted loosely into the middle third of the canal is used to compact the thermosoftened gutta-percha vertically. **E,** A heat carrier heated red-hot is stabbed again into the gutta-percha mass and quickly removed. **F,** A preselected cold plugger that was fitted loosely into the apical third of the prepared canal is used to deliver the final apical wave of vertical condensation. **G,** Back packing with addition and compaction of segments of gutta-percha. **H,** Canal filled to 1 mm below the canal orifice. (Courtesy Drs. L. Stephen Buchanan and Clifford J. Ruddle.)

forth laterally in the canal to release it from the warm gutta-percha.

2. The primary cone may be dislodged by the red-hot heat carrier. This is usually due to failure to remove the instrument quickly from the canal. If the dislodged primary cone is undamaged, it is simply detached from the instrument, reseated carefully in the canal, and condensed apically.

3. The nonrelease of gutta-percha segments is likely due to the presence of sealer on canal walls or the improper attachment of the segment to the heated instrument. Cotton pliers may also be employed to introduce the segments. A cold plugger seats them firmly in place.

4. The nonhomogeneous filling caused by voids and seams can be prevented by careful size selection of the gutta-percha segments, adequate heating, and thorough condensing waves.

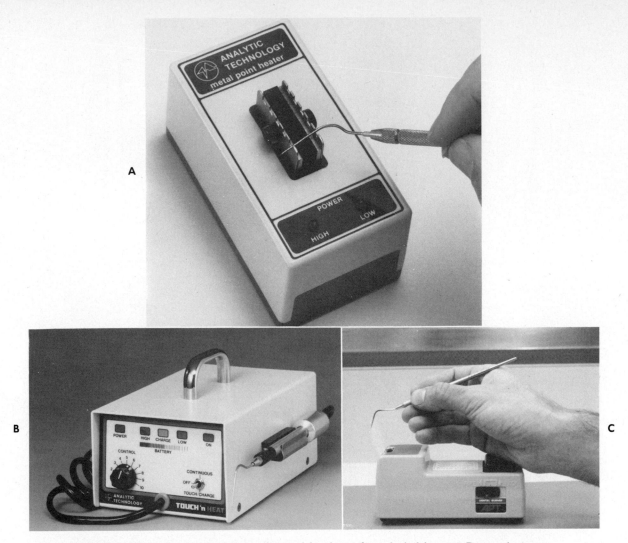

FIG. 8-56. **A,** A heating device may be used in place of an alcohol lamp or Bunsen burner to heat the heat carrier. **B,** ''Touch 'n Heat'' battery-powered (rechargeable) heating device. Heat carrier will heat to glowing within seconds for softened gutta-percha technique. **C,** Portable chairside butane gas burner APT as a convenient and effective heat source. (**A** and **B** courtesy Analytic Technology, Redmond, Wash.; **C** courtesy Phoenix-Dent Co., Ltd., Tokyo, Japan.)

5. Procedural accidents and patient harm when hot instruments are being passed during canal obturation in *four-handed* endodontics can be avoided by positioning the dental assistant on the same side as the clinician. This facilitates the rhythmic and efficient exchange of instruments.

6. Difficulty in filling unusually curved canals where small pluggers cannot be placed into the apical third of the canal for effective condensation may be overcome by meticulous cone fitting and greater reliance on sealer hydraulics (Fig. 8-60, *A* and *D*).

Wong and co-workers[139] in an in vitro study found that the warm gutta-percha vertical condensation technique (Fig. 8-61) replicated the shape of a cast gold artificial root canal (Fig. 8-62) significantly better than did lateral condensation (Fig. 8-63) or mechanical compaction (Fig. 8-64). The mechanical compaction technique was better than lateral condensation, which produced fillings consistently judged to be poor or barely acceptable by all investigators.

Vertical condensation also placed a larger mass of gutta-percha into the artificial canal space than did lateral condensation. In this study the vertically condensed warm gutta-percha showed a shrinkage of 0.45% versus 0.62% for thermomechanically compacted gutta-percha.

The warm gutta-percha vertical condensation method gives a consistently dense, homogeneous, well-adapted filling; and accessory ramifications are often filled by this procedure (Figs. 8-4, 8-5, 8-51, 8-60, and 8-65 to 8-67). Its use is recommended for most clinical cases when there is no suspected root fracture present. The technique is somewhat time consuming, however, and requires several radiographs to verify the position of the filling. Care must also be taken to prevent cracking or splitting of weak roots caused by improper plugger size selection and overzealous vertical compaction.

Chloropercha method. Chloropercha is made by dissolving gutta-percha in chloroform. The chloropercha paste has been used by some clinicians as the sole canal

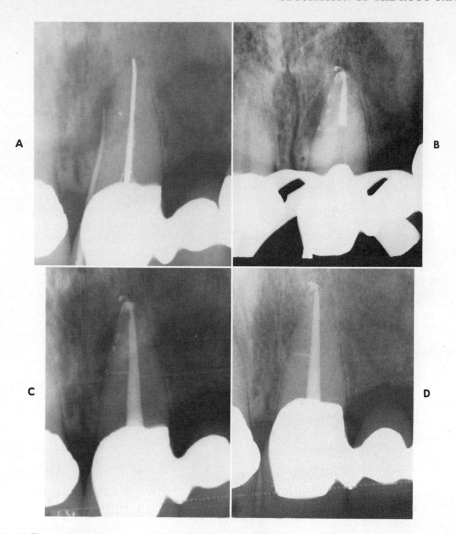

FIG. 8-57. A, Preoperative radiograph depicting a sinus tract tracing to an extensive mesial-lateral root lesion associated with a failing silver point case. **B,** Working radiograph demonstrating an obturated lateral canal coronal to the gutta-percha mass. The vertical condensation pressure during the down-packing procedure forced the softened gutta-percha and entrapped sealer into the canal ramifications along the mesial aspect of the root. **C,** Postfilling radiograph showing numerous lateral canals obturated. **D,** Excellent healing 3 years later. (Courtesy Dr. C. J. Ruddle.)

filling material. As such, the technique is unsound because of the excessive shrinkage of the filling after evaporation of the chloroform. However, used as a sealer in conjunction with a well-fitted primary cone, chloropercha can fill accessory canals and the root canal space successfully. The technique is useful in perforation cases and in filling unusually curved canals that cannot be negotiated (Fig. 8-68) or canals with ledge formation.

Modified chloropercha methods. There are two modifications of the chloropercha method: the Johnston-Callahan and the Nygaard-Østby.

Johnston[65] modified the Callahan[21] chloropercha technique to develop the *Johnston-Callahan diffusion technique*. By this method, the canal is repeatedly flooded with 95% alcohol and then dried with absorbent points. It is then flooded with Callahan's rosin chloroform solution for 2 to 3 minutes. More chloroform is added if the paste becomes too thick by diffusion or evaporation. A suitable gutta-percha cone is inserted and compressed laterally and

apically with a stirring motion of the plugger until the gutta-percha is entirely dissolved in the chloroform rosin solution in the canal. Additional points are inserted, one at a time, and dissolved in the same way. A plugger is used to apply lateral and vertical pressure to force the chloropercha into the accessory canals and multiple foramina. Care must be exercised to prevent overfilling, because freshly prepared chloropercha is toxic[126] before evaporation. As chloroform from the chloropercha evaporates, it causes a significant dimensional change of the filling and a possible loss of the apical seal.[140] If sufficient time is allowed for the chloroform to become dissipated in the course of the filling operation and the gutta-percha is compressed to form a homogeneous mass, successful fillings can be obtained by this method (Fig. 8-69).

Nygaard-Østby[100] modified the chloropercha method by adding a preparation made of finely ground gutta-percha, Canada balsam, colophonium, and zinc oxide powder mixed with chloroform in a Dappen dish or watch glass.

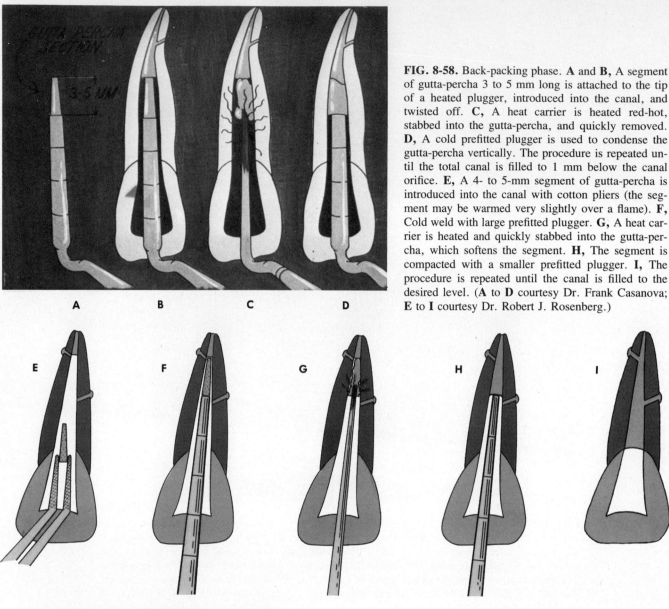

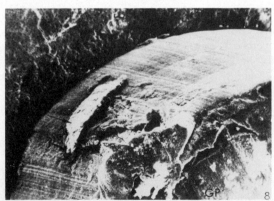

FIG. 8-58. Back-packing phase. **A** and **B,** A segment of gutta-percha 3 to 5 mm long is attached to the tip of a heated plugger, introduced into the canal, and twisted off. **C,** A heat carrier is heated red-hot, stabbed into the gutta-percha, and quickly removed. **D,** A cold prefitted plugger is used to condense the gutta-percha vertically. The procedure is repeated until the total canal is filled to 1 mm below the canal orifice. **E,** A 4- to 5-mm segment of gutta-percha is introduced into the canal with cotton pliers (the segment may be warmed very slightly over a flame). **F,** Cold weld with large prefitted plugger. **G,** A heat carrier is heated and quickly stabbed into the gutta-percha, which softens the segment. **H,** The segment is compacted with a smaller prefitted plugger. **I,** The procedure is repeated until the canal is filled to the desired level. (**A** to **D** courtesy Dr. Frank Casanova; **E** to **I** courtesy Dr. Robert J. Rosenberg.)

FIG. 8-59. Scanning electron micrograph depicting the gutta-percha–dentin interface in a canal obturated with warm gutta-percha by vertical condensation. The striations in the gutta-percha are impressions of instrumentation marks in the dentinal wall. Note also the impression of a canal cul-de-sac. (×500.) (Courtesy Dr. Clifford J. Ruddle.)

After the canal walls are coated with Kloroperka, the primary cone, dipped in sealer, is forcefully inserted apically, pushing the partially dissolved tip of the cone to its apical seat. Additional cones dipped in sealer are packed into the canal to obtain a satisfactory filling (Fig. 8-70). Nygaard-Østby suggests additional lateral condensation; but, to avoid overfilling with the chloropercha technique, the use of a spreader is delayed until a subsequent appointment. At this sitting, chloroform is used to soften and remove the coronal chloropercha to a point slightly below the apical third of the canal. Spreading is done thoroughly in the coronal two thirds of the canal. The undisturbed apical section acts as a plug to prevent overfilling. Nygaard-Østby's method is reported to greatly reduce both apical extrusions and shrinkage of the final filling.

Gutta-percha–eucapercha method. Investigations by the F.D.A.[35] have shown chloroform to be a potential carcinogen. The Council on Dental Therapeutics of the American Dental Association has decided to delete chloroform

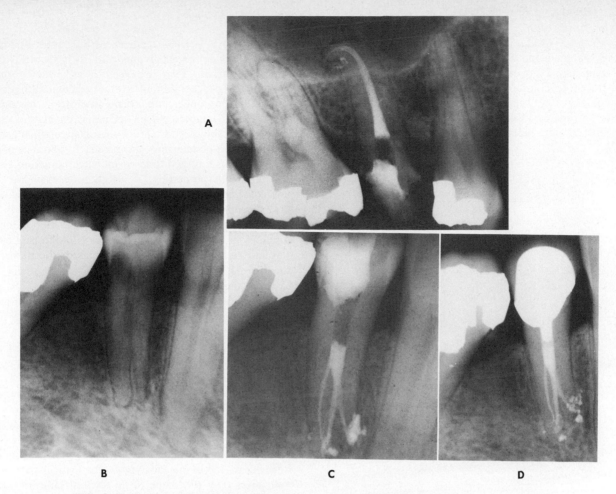

FIG. 8-60. A, Premolar with canal curvature in excess of 90 degrees. Note the sealer puff from a ramification exiting the curved portion of the obturated system. B, Preoperative radiograph. Mandibular first premolar with two roots. Note the radiolucent area along the mesial aspect of mesial root. C, Postobturation radiograph. Note the ramifications and complexity of the filled system. Warm gutta-percha with vertical condensation. D, Good healing after 18 months. (A courtesy Dr. Clifford J. Ruddle; B, C, and D courtesy Dr. Robert J. Rosenberg.)

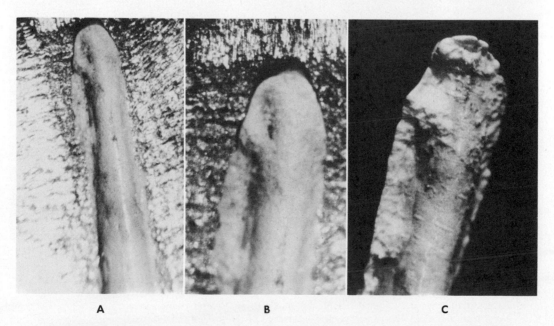

FIG. 8-61. A, Gutta-percha filling (vertical condensation) just before removal from the mold. (Original magnification ×10.) B, Higher magnification of the apical section of A. (Original magnification ×25.) C, Vertical condensation filling. The filling is homogeneous, and the surface texture smooth. Replication of the apical portion of the canal was judged excellent. (Original magnification ×25.) (Courtesy Drs. M. Wong, D.D. Peters, and L. Lorton.)

from *Accepted Dental Therapeutics*.[4] This action may serve to eliminate the clinical use of chloroform in dentistry. Although I am not aware of any cases of malignancy traced to chloroform used in endodontic therapy, many clinicians[85,94,101] have advocated the use of eucalyptol (also an organic solvent) in place of chloroform by revising the old gutta-percha–eucapercha technique.

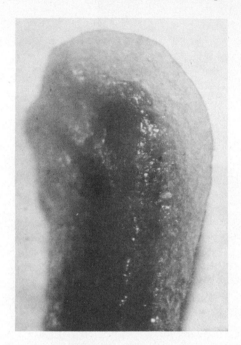

FIG. 8-62. Silicone impression of an artificial root canal. (Original magnification ×25.) (Courtesy Drs. M. Wong, D.D. Peters, L. Lorton, and W. Bernier.)

Eucalyptol is derived from eucalyptus trees and is the major constituent of eucalyptus oil.[80] It has much less local tissue toxicity than does chloroform and is used in medicine as a decongestant and rubefacient. Although it takes a much longer time than chloroform to dissolve gutta-percha (minutes versus seconds), eucalyptol can be heated up to about 30° C (86° F) in a Dappen dish and will dissolve gutta-percha into eucapercha in about a minute. Eucalyptyol is reported to have antibacterial action and antiinflammatory properties.[94,95] Both properties are desirable characteristics of a root canal filling ingredient.

Technique. The endodontic cavity preparation is done as usual to obtain a smooth tapered preparation. Since the gutta-percha–eucapercha can be diffused and made to flow into narrow and curved canals, the endodontic preparation does not have to be very extensive apically. Usually a no. 25 or 30 file at the apical foramen is adequate. The preparation should present a definite apical constriction to prevent an undue amount of eucapercha from being forced beyond the confines of the root canal system.

The primary cone should be fitted very tight to about 1 or 1.5 mm short of the radiographic apex; it should possess a definite "tugback." The canal is irrigated and dried and is then rechecked with a small file set at full working length to ensure the patency of the canal all the way to the apical foramen.

The large well of the Dappen dish is filled about two-thirds full with eucalyptol. Segments of gutta-percha (Fig. 8-50) are placed in the eucalyptol. The Dappen dish is held with pliers over the flame of an alcohol lamp or Bunsen burner for 20 to 30 seconds. This warms the eucalyptol and increases its ability to dissolve gutta-percha. The Dap-

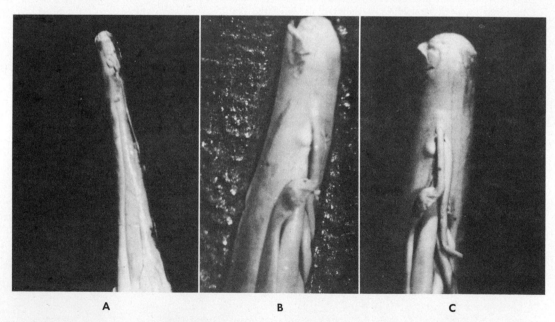

A   B   C

FIG. 8-63. A, One of the best lateral condensation fillings. Some coalescence of the master point and accessory cones can be observed. Incomplete adaptation to the apical portion of the test canal was invariably noted. (Original magnification ×10.) **B,** Lateral condensation filling before removal from the mold. There was some coalescence of the master and accessory points. Note the incomplete replication of the apical portion of the canal. (Original magnification ×25.) **C,** Same lateral endodontic filling 3 weeks later. There is a slight tendency of accessory cones to separate. (Original magnification ×25.) (Courtesy Drs. M. Wong, D.D. Peters, and L. Lorton.)

pen dish is then placed over the work counter and the contents are stirred with a plastic instrument until the gutta-percha segments are dissolved. The eucapercha mixture turns into a cloudy mass.

The prefitted primary cone is held with the cotton pliers at the full working length. The apical half of the cone is dipped into the warm eucapercha mixture and rotated for 30 to 45 seconds. The length of time depends on how short the cone was fitted; the shorter the fit at the apical foramen, the longer the gutta-percha cone must be rotated in

the eucapercha mixture. A primary cone can be dipped in the warm eucapercha for about a minute without losing its basic shape. The eucapercha-coated cone is inserted into the canal until the beaks of the pliers coincide with the operating landmark on the incisal or occlusal surface.

A radiograph is exposed to determine the position of the cone in the canal. Vertical and lateral condensation is then done to complete the filling procedure. On occasion, a few drops of warm eucalyptol can be added to the pulp cavity to help soften the filling mass and move the gutta-percha–

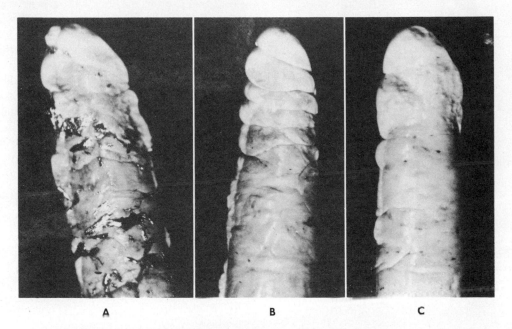

FIG. 8-64. Thermomechanical compaction filling. **A,** Gold filings are seen in this case. The overall surface is not homogeneous. Many horizontal interfaces of gutta-percha are characteristic of this filling. Replication of the apical 2 to 3 mm and mold interface superior to the lateral condensation. (Original magnification ×25.) **B,** Incomplete heat compaction has produced a spiral-like filling in the apical portion. This is an example of the best replication achieved by this technique. (Original magnification ×25.) **C,** An example of the best replication achieved by this study. (Original magnification ×25.) (Courtesy Drs. M. Wong, D.D. Peters, and L. Lorton.)

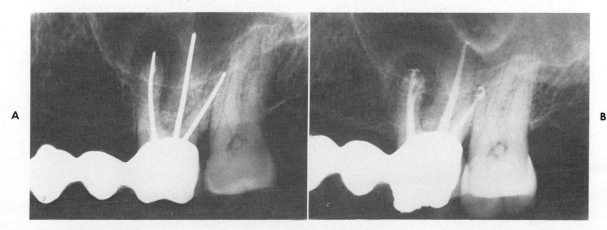

FIG. 8-65. A, Preoperative radiograph showing a fan-shaped lesion associated with the mesial-buccal root and a failing silver point filling. **B,** Postobturation radiograph with multiple fan-shaped ramifications revealing the reasons for failure of the previously underfilled mesial-buccal root and a failing silver point filling. (Courtesy Dr. L. Stephen Buchanan.)

eucapercha apically. Prefitted and premeasured pluggers are used for vertical condensation. Additional accessory cones are added and fused to the gutta-percha–eucapercha mass to fill the canal system three dimensionally.

To facilitate insertion of the accessory cones, it is best not to dip them in the eucapercha mixture. The correctness

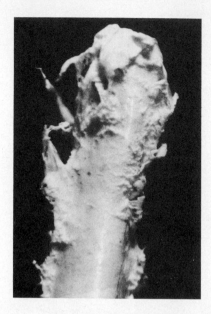

FIG. 8-66. Chloroform-dip filling. This filling is homogeneous with excellent replication of the apical portion and mold interface. (Original magnification ×25.) (Courtesy Drs. M. Wong, D.D. Peters, L. Lorton, and W. Bernier.)

and compactness of the filling are again verified with a radiograph. Gross overfilling can usually be effectively controlled if the canal was prepared with an apical constriction acting as a matrix against which the gutta-percha–eucapercha mass is condensed.

The gutta-percha–eucapercha technique, if carried out properly, can effectively fill lateral and accessory canals. However, the fine canals will not appear as radiopaque as when the gutta-percha is used in conjunction with a root canal cement-sealer containing barium sulfate.

The mixture of eucapercha in the Dappen dish can be saved by covering the dish with a paper cup. It will last an entire day without much evaporation as compared with the chloropercha, which will evaporate in a few minutes.

Thermomechanical condensation method. An automated technique using thermatic condensation of gutta-percha was introduced in 1978 by McSpadden.[117]

Principles. This innovative technique, known as thermatic condensation, uses a calibrated stainless steel McSpadden compactor.*

The mechanical condensor is available in color-coded assorted sizes and resembles a Hedström file with inverted blades (i.e., the shoulder of the blades faces the tip of the instrument instead of the shaft) (Fig. 8-71). When mounted and operated on a conventional high-torque handpiece capable of *at least* 10,000 rpm, the compactor generates adequate frictional heat to plasticize, feed, and compact gutta-percha into the root canal space. Because

---

*L.D. Caulk Co., Milford, Del.

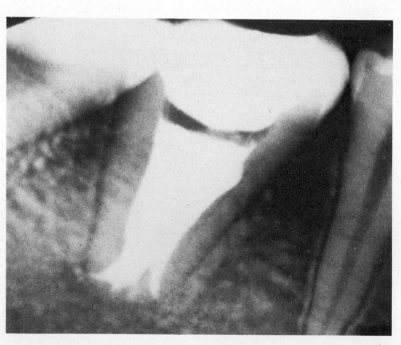

FIG. 8-67. Mandibular first molar filled by the vertical condensation method with warm gutta-percha. Note the well-filled multiple apical foramina. Whiteness of the filling is an indication of its density. (Courtesy Dr. Frank Casanova.)

compaction is effective within 1.5 mm ahead of and lateral to the shaft of the instrument, the apical extent of obturation can be controlled by adjusting the depth of the compactor in the canal (Fig. 8-72). Even with an open apex, careful control of the condensor's depth may prevent overextension beyond the confines of the root canal (Fig. 8-73). The thermatic condensation technique is very rapid and can obturate canals in seconds.

Technique. The canal, thoroughly cleaned and shaped, is irrigated and dried with absorbent points and is then thinly coated with a very small amount of sealer.

Selection of the gutta-percha point. It is important to

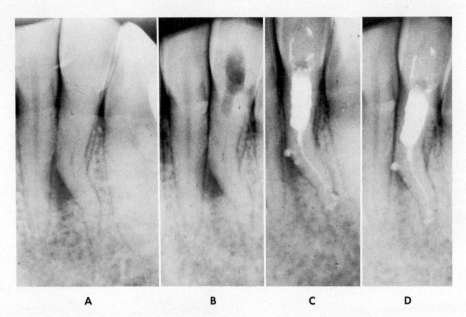

FIG. 8-68. Mandibular lateral incisor. **A,** Pretreatment. Note the calcification of the coronal half of the pulp cavity and the narrow bayonet canal. **B,** Checking the direction of the cut made by a no. 2 long-shanked round bur mounted on a miniature contraangle handpiece for better vision and access. **C,** The canal could not be negotiated but was filled in its entirety by a combination of chloropercha diffusion and forceful vertical condensation. Note the well-filled lateral canals and multiple foramina. **D,** Posttreatment. Within 5 months there was significant bone repair.

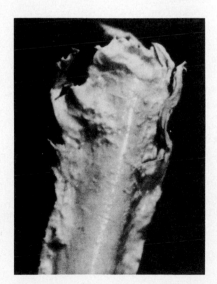

FIG. 8-69. Chloropercha filling. This filling is homogeneous with excellent replication of the apical portion and mold interface. (Original magnification ×25.) (Courtesy Drs. M. Wong, D.D. Peters, L. Lorton, and W. Bernier.)

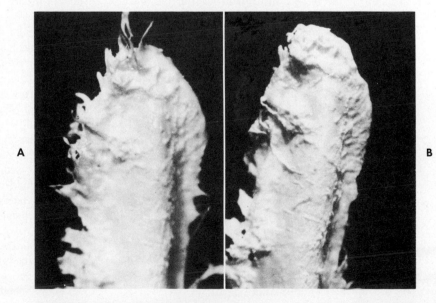

FIG. 8-70. Kloropercha filling. This filling is homogeneous with excellent replication of the apical portion and mold interface. **A,** Immediately after filling. **B,** Three weeks after filling. (Original magnification ×25.) (Courtesy Drs. M. Wong, D.D. Peters, L. Lorton, and W. Bernier.)

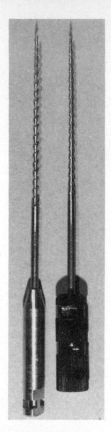

FIG. 8-71. *Left,* McSpadden condensor. *Right,* Hedström file. (Courtesy Dr. J.T. McSpadden.)

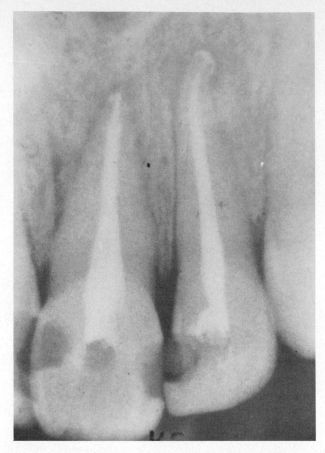

FIG. 8-72. Central and lateral incisors obturated with the thermomechanical condensation method. (Courtesy Dr. J.T. McSpadden.)

choose the proper size of gutta-percha point so the tip cannot pass through the apical foramen. This will prevent any excess plasticized gutta-percha from being extruded.

1. The tip of the largest instrument used at the apical terminus is measured with a Boley gauge (Fig. 8-74, *A*). A medium-fine gutta-percha point is inserted between the jaws of the gauge until it *binds firmly* (Fig. 8-74, *B*).
2. The gutta-percha point is clipped off at this diameter so it will be the same size as the terminus of the prepared canal (Fig. 8-74, *C*).
3. The gutta-percha cone is measured (Fig. 8-74, *D*) and then coated lightly with sealer in its apical third (Fig. 8-74, *E*).
4. Upon insertion, it will bind in the canal approximately 1.5 mm from the apical terminus.

Note: If the diameter of the gutta-percha tip is smaller than the apical foramen, the tip will be pushed through the apex when the compactor is activated (Fig. 8-75).

Selection of the compactor. The initial compactor should be the same size as the largest file used within 1 to 1.5 mm of the apical terminus (Fig. 8-76). A second and larger compactor may be required to condense the flared coronal portion of the canal.

Steps in compaction. Following is an enumeration of

steps in the thermomechanical condensation technique:

1. *The selected compactor is inserted into the canal beside the gutta-percha cone until resistance is met.* The canal should have enough flare to allow the straight insertion of the compactor to a depth of approximately 4 mm before resistance is encountered. The compactor should feel slightly wedged between the cone and the canal wall at this point (Fig. 8-77, *A*).

If the initial gutta-percha cone completely obstructs the coronal portion of the canal, preventing insertion of the compactor to an adequate depth, the excess cone will be clipped off without being fed into the canal when the engine is turned on. The compactor's direction of rotation should be checked to ensure the displacement of gutta-percha in an apical vector.

2. *The compactor must be activated full speed at the start without any apical pressure.* The frictional heat will plasticize the gutta-percha, and resistance will be minimized. *After approximately 1 second,* while rotating at maximum speed, the compactor is carried in one fluid motion apically to a level not to exceed the predetermined depth of the prepared canal (Fig. 8-77, *B* and *C*). When the compactor begins to rotate against the unplasticized

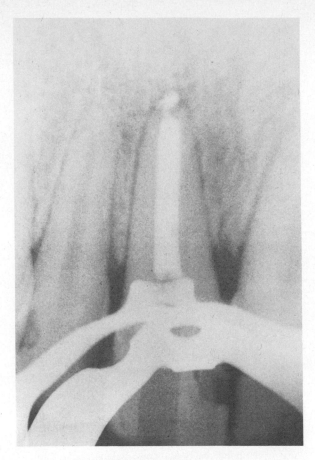

FIG. 8-73. Central incisor with a wide canal obturated compactly. There is minimal extrusion of filling materials. (Courtesy Dr. J.T. McSpadden.)

gutta-percha cone, a whipping action of the portion of the cone protruding beyond the access cavity is observed momentarily. Then the cone goes rigid and appears to be feeding down into the canal.

The most important experience is the feel of the *instrument backing itself out*. This sensation usually indicates that the canal is completely filled. At the beginning, however, a certain amount of backing-out motion is always encountered from the body of the gutta-percha cone and must be compensated for or overcome during the initial insertion of the compactor. Excessive backing out at the beginning may result if the shoulder of the compactor engages the canal wall, particularly in a canal with an acute curvature. Excessive backing out may also result from the compactor's being forced to the apical foramen. A radiograph is exposed at this point to determine whether the canal is filled.

To prevent vertical pushing of the gutta-percha, in-and-out pumping motion of the instrument should be avoided. Plasticization and compaction of the gutta-percha result from the full-speed rotation of the compactor and its movement apically in one fluid motion to the desired level, not from vertical pumping movements. A pumping motion

is used only when obturating very small and acutely curved canals that are inaccessible to the compactor.

3. *While rotating at full speed, the compactor is gradually withdrawn* (Fig. 8-77, *D*). If the compactor is withdrawn faster than the gutta-percha is being fed into the canal system, voids may develop in the body of the gutta-percha mass. Up to this point of the condensation process only 4 to 6 seconds have elapsed. If the withdrawn compactor shows plasticized gutta-percha clinging to its end, it has been left too long in the canal and voids have formed in the gutta-percha mass, resulting in an incomplete obturation. Staying too long in the canal will cause the formation of air cavitations (evidenced by the "popcorn" appearance of the gutta-percha on the radiograph).

Radiographic verification is done at this point. If the voids are found in the canal or the filling is short of the apex, recompaction can be performed immediately. If the gutta-percha was overheated, one should remove the bulk of the gutta-percha with a Gates-Glidden drill, use a new cone, and compact again.

4. *A second and larger compactor may be required to condense the flared coronal portion of the canal.* For the compactor to function effectively, it must be in contact with the gutta-percha and the canal walls. If the gutta-percha cone stops feeding into the canal and begins a whipping movement, a larger compactor may be needed. The diameter of the compactor should approximate the size of the canal. The average canal can be filled with one or two medium-fine cones. Occasionally a third cone will be required in a large canal or if internal resorption has occurred. As the compactor is brought out of the orifice, it is moved side to side against the funneled walls to allow the gutta-percha to feed more smoothly.

5. When *filling curved canals,* it is important to clean and shape the canal to the *widest possible dimension*. The compaction is done by introducing the gutta-percha and the compactor to the depth of the curvature and activating the compactor to plasticize the gutta-percha. The compactor is removed while the engine is turning, the rotation stops, and the softened material is immediately packed twice apically. In most cases the filling material will move to the extent of the prepared canal. If necessary, the engine is rotated again and the compactor pumped two to four times apically while rotating at full speed.

An alternative method consists of fitting a standardized gutta-percha cone around the curvature and cementing it in place. With a spreader, as in lateral condensation, one accessory cone is added and then the compactor is introduced and rotated at full speed. The gutta-percha near the apex does not become plasticized, but the compactor backfills the canal compactly.

With the thermatic condensation technique, certain guidelines can prevent undesirable results:

1. The compactor should approximate the canal size and be in contact with the gutta-percha and canal wall to work efficiently.

2. The compactor should be inserted into the canal beside the gutta-percha cone to a depth of at least 4

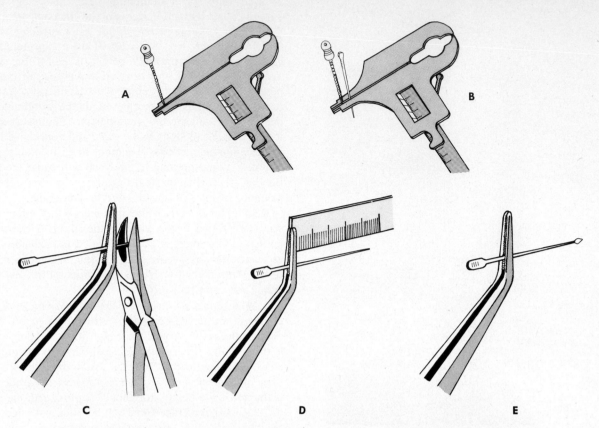

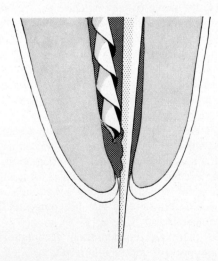

FIG. 8-74. Thermatic condensation. Selection of the gutta-percha point. A, Boley gauge holding the tip of the largest file used at the apical terminus of the prepared canal. B, A medium-fine gutta-percha cone is inserted between the jaws of the Boley gauge until it binds. C, Clipping the gutta-percha cone off at this diameter will provide a cone of the same size as the canal at the apical working length. D, The gutta-percha cone is measured. Upon insertion it should bind in the canal approximately 1 to 1.5 mm from the apical terminus, E, Sealer is applied in the apical one fourth of the cone.

FIG. 8-75. If the tip of the gutta-percha cone is smaller than the apical foramen, it will be pushed through the apex when the compactor is activated.

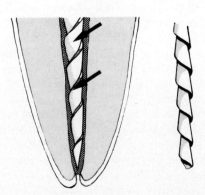

FIG. 8-76. Selection of a compactor. The initial compactor should be the same size as the largest file used within 1 to 1.5 mm of the terminus of the canal. (Courtesy Dr. J.T. McSpadden.)

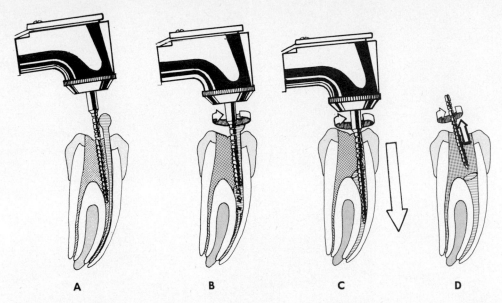

A   B   C   D

FIG. 8-77. A, Premeasured compactor inserted into the canal beside the gutta-percha cone until it is slightly wedged between the cone and the canal wall at a depth of at least 4 mm. **B,** The compactor is activated at full speed for 1 second without applying apical pressure. **C,** After approximately 1 second it is carried with one fluid motion apically to the predetermined depth. **D,** It is then withdrawn gradually while rotating at full speed.

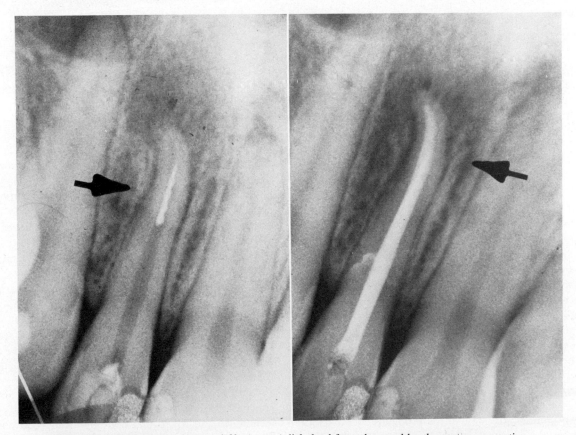

FIG. 8-78. Fragment of a fractured file *(arrow)* dislodged from the canal by thermatic compaction of gutta-percha apical to the broken instrument.

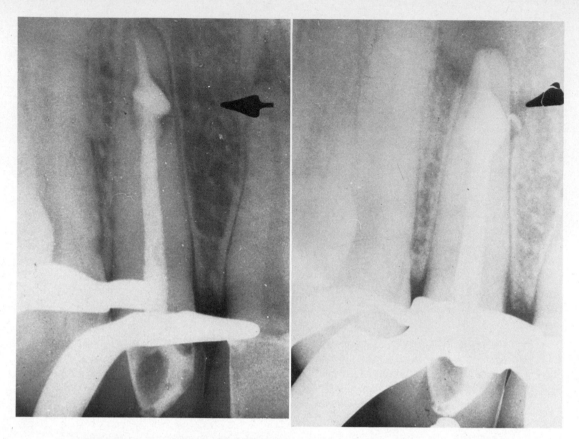

FIG. 8-79. Internal resorptive defect *(arrow)* obturated efficiently by the thermatic compaction method.

mm before resistance is met, and it must be rotating at full speed to plasticize the gutta-percha properly.

3. Never force the compactor beyond the apical working length.
4. Never resist *excessive* backing out of the compactor.
5. Attempt to stay in the canal less than 10 seconds.

Although the thermatic condensation method requires much patience, perseverance, and control to master its efficient use, several advantages can be gained by this technique: The procedure is rapid and most canals can be thermomechanically obturated in seconds (Fig. 8-72). The technique can be used to recondense inadequately filled canals without the necessity of removing the old gutta-percha. It can occasionally aid in the removal of broken instruments that are not tightly bound (the gutta-percha compacted apically to the instrument tends to dislodge the broken fragment occlusally) (Fig. 8-78). It can efficiently obturate canals with a large internal resorptive defect (Fig. 8-79). There is an economic advantage in the reduced number of gutta-percha cones needed to fill a canal three-dimensionally.

Common difficulties. McSpadden[117] suggested several causes and solutions for a few of the problems encountered by this technique (top of next page).

One study[11] used calcium 45 in a radioautographic leakage study to compare the apical seal produced by lateral and vertical (warm gutta-percha) obturation methods with the seal produced by the thermoplastic compaction (McSpadden) technique. Statistical analysis of the results indicated that there were only minor differences between the three techniques regardless of whether a root canal sealer was used and that the thermomechanical compaction method compared favorably with the lateral and vertical obturation techniques. Vertical condensation without sealer appeared to produce a better apical seal. With the thermatic compaction and lateral condensation techniques, however, the use of sealer reduced the radioisotope leakage rate and produced a better apical seal than without sealer.

Wong[139] in an in vitro investigation comparing thermatic compaction with vertical (warm) and lateral condensation techniques used without sealer, found that thermatic compaction produced a filling which replicated a standard artificial root canal better than that achieved by lateral condensation but poorer than that by vertical condensation (Figs. 8-61 to 8-64).

Another study[79] compared in vitro the vertical (warm) condensation and the automated thermatic compaction techniques and found that both produced good clinical radiographic results. The fills appeared to be dense, radiopaque, and exempt of voids (Figs. 8-80 and 8-82). By scanning electron microscopic (SEM) analysis, however,

Problem	Cause	Solution
1. Fracturing of compactor	Insufficient handpiece speed, excessive vertical pressure, acute curvature of canal	Increase air pressure, exchange handpiece, slow insertion of compactor with less vertical pressure, use modification for curved canal
2. "Popcorn" appearance of gutta-percha on radiograph	Air cavitations from staying in canal too long	Attempt to stay in canal less than 10 seconds
3. Diagonal radiolucent lines across gutta-percha on radiograph	Twist in gutta-percha from using too small a compactor	Use larger compactor in coronal portion of canal
4. Gutta-percha whipping around compactor and not feeding into canal	Inadequate contact of gutta-percha against compactor	Use larger compactor
5. Gutta-percha unplasticized to terminus of canal	Compactor insertion shy of predetermined depth	Use formula for depth of insertion
6. Unplasticized tip of gutta-percha forced through apical foramen	Gutta-percha tip smaller than apical foramen	Cut tip of gutta-percha off to diameter larger than apical foramen
7. Extrusion of gutta-percha through apical foramen	Compactor forced to depth exceeding level of desired condensation.	Refer to calibrated lines or use rubber stops to ensure against insertion to excessive depth

the gutta-percha material was not as homogeneous as expected. In the warm gutta-percha technique minor folds, voids, and inclusions were observed (Fig. 8-81) and the material that extruded into lateral canals consisted primarily of sealer. The extent to which the gutta-percha is compacted into the lateral canals is dependent on the diameter of the accessory canal, the proximity of heat, and the amount of pressure applied to the material. The major observable differences with the rotary packing method were typical convolutions and twists of the gutta-percha, oblique cold welds, large pools of sealer materials (Fig. 8-83) at various sites along the gutta-percha fill, and a relatively undisturbed apical end of the gutta-percha cone. In general, the filling showed good density and adaptation to the root canal walls.

Fisher[34] in an in vitro study investigated the effectiveness of the McSpadden thermatic condensor with regard to heat generation and sealing qualities. Thermistors were used to measure the heat generated in the gutta-percha mass and on the external surface of extracted teeth after 10 seconds of compaction. The maximum temperature produced in the gutta-percha material was 120° C when a no. 120 instrument was used. The maximum temperature recorded was over 100° C on the external surface. The larger the instrument and the higher the psi (rpm), the greater was the temperature generated after a 10-second test run.

Pelikan ink infusion methods were used in analysing the seal. Fisher[34] found that the apical seal was better with sealer than without. The larger canals, with greater accessibility to the apex, showed a greater percentage of apices sealed. In small-canal teeth only 44% of the apices were sealed. Of these, 62.5% were ones in which sealer was used in conjunction with gutta-percha. In large canals 50% of the teeth were sealed. Of these, sealer was used in 66.7%. In curved canals only 39% of the teeth tested were sealed apically. In teeth with open and divergent apices only 25% of the apices were sealed.

Kerekes and Rowe[70] found that thermomechanical compaction is superior to lateral condensation in filling irregularly-shaped canals. Other leakage studies and autoradiographic techniques showed that the McSpadden compaction technique compared favorably with the lateral condensation method.[50,51,63,104] A recent report[28] showed that lateral condensation produced significantly less gutta-percha in the apical level of the canal than vertical, mechanical, or chloroform-dip methods.

The thermatic compaction technique does not exert excessive lateral force against the root canal walls as compared with the vertical (warm) condensation method. However, as the compactor rotates 360 degree at full speed, the instrument may be susceptible to fatigue failure, particularly in dilacerated or curved canals. Indiscriminate use can cause the sharp flutes of the compactor rotating at 10,000 to 12,000 rpm to gouge and cut the dentinal walls of the canal, with a strong potential for perforation and/or fracture of small or curved canals. In selected cases, however, the automated thermatic condenser can prove to be a useful and rapid method for obturating the root canal system.

Thermoplasticized gutta-percha injection-molded method. The obturation of the canal system using a thermoplasticized injectable gutta-percha in conjunction with a pressure syringe was introduced in 1977.[142]

Heated gutta-percha was injected in vitro in teeth that had been cleaned and shaped with and without the use of a sealer. The quality of the seal was assessed by dye penetration studies. The investigation showed that effective root canal obturation could be achieved in vitro, so the technique was modified and improved for in vivo use.

Experimental technique. The root canal system of the extracted tooth is thoroughly cleaned and shaped to receive gutta-percha. The endodontic pressure syringe (Fig. 8-84) is adapted with a threaded needle selected from size 18 to 22 gauge so it will negotiate the canal to within 4 mm of

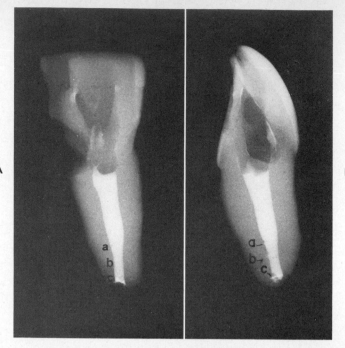

FIG. 8-80. Warm gutta-percha vertical condensation in a maxillary central incisor. **A,** Labial-lingual and, **B,** mesial-distal views. *a,* Cold weld; *b,* lateral canal; *c,* apical sealer pool. (Courtesy Drs. A.A. Lugassy and F. Yee.)

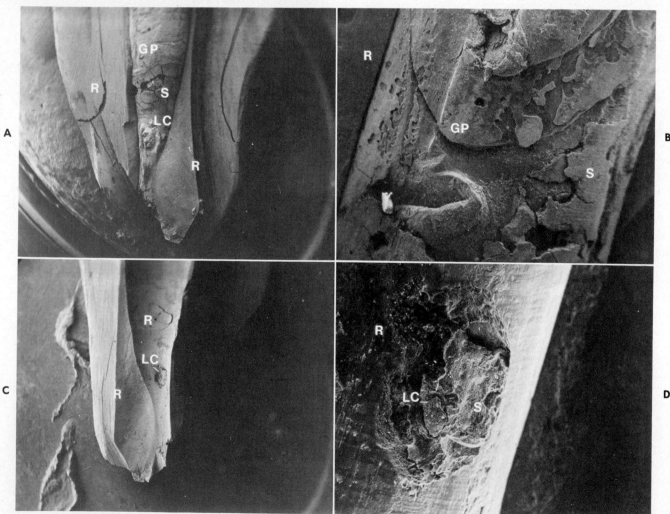

FIG. 8-81. Scanning electron micrograph. Warm gutta-percha vertical condensation filling. **A,** *GP,* Cold weld; *LC,* lateral canal gutta-percha knob; *S,* apical sealer pool; *R,* root. (IKV, original magnification ×100.) **B,** *R,* Root; *S,* sealer scale; *GP,* gutta-percha fold. (IKV, ×250.) **C,** Light band facing the cold-weld junction. *LC,* Lateral canal orifice, *R,* root. **D,** Lateral root canal orifice, showing the sealer contents. (IKV, original magnification ×200.) (Courtesy Drs. A.A. Lugassy and F. Yee.)

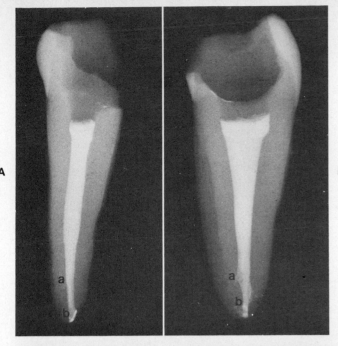

FIG. 8-82. Automated thermatic compaction in a mandibular premolar. **A,** Buccal-lingual and, **B,** mesial-distal views, *a,* Fin; *b,* spical sealer pool. (Courtesy Drs. A.A. Lugassy and F. Yee.)

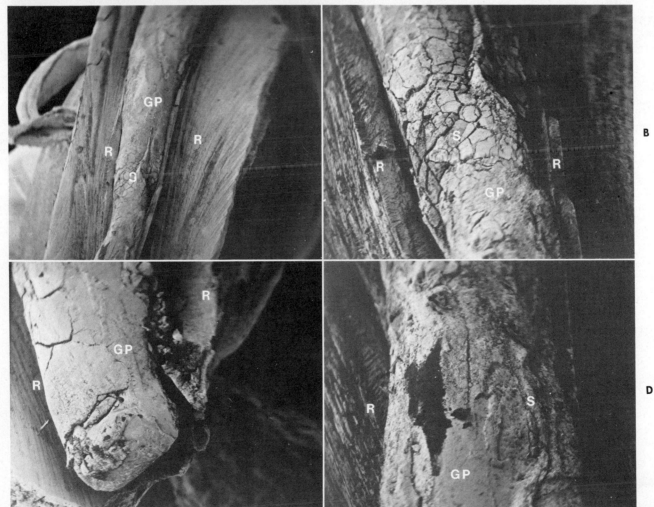

FIG. 8-83. Scanning electron micrograph (SEM). Automated thermatic compaction in a mandibular premolar. **A,** *GP,* Gutta-percha oblique cold weld; *S,* sealer pool; *R,* root, (ικν, original magnification ×100.) **B,** Sealer pool found in the fin area in the apical third of a root canal fill. (ικν, original magnification ×250.) **C,** Apical extremity. Note the angular configuration of the gutta-percha point at the apex. (ικν, original magnification ×250.) **D,** Gutta-percha tear, middle section of the filling. (ικν, original magnification ×250.) (Courtesy Drs. A.A. Lugassy and F. Yee.)

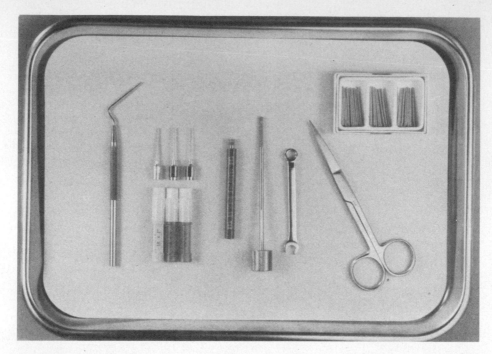

FIG. 8-84. Clinical equipment. *Left to right,* Root canal plugger, assortment of needles, disassembled pressure syringe, scissors, gutta-percha cones.

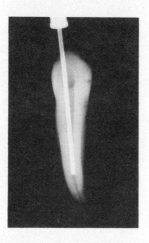

FIG. 8-85. Radiographic confirmation of the needle positioned within the apical third of the prepared root canal.

the root apex (Fig. 8-85). The syringe, loaded with gutta-percha cones (Fig. 8-86), is placed in a Thiele Dennis melting tube containing glycerin heated to 160° C over a Bunsen burner (Fig. 8-87). The thermoplasticized gutta-percha is injected into the root canal until the desired obturation level has been accomplished. Radiographic examination shows the injected gutta-percha to be of uniform density with occasional small voids caused possibly by air entrapment when no sealer was used.

Yee et al.[142] reported that no voids along the root canal walls could be detected radiographically when the sealer was used. The injection-molded gutta-percha seems to be capable of filling multiple foramina and other apical ramifications (Fig. 8-88).

The time required to inject the gutta-percha in the prepared canal was reported to be less than 20 seconds. To obliterate possible voids left by the needle, manual condensation may be used because the gutta-percha remains plastic for up to 2 minutes after injection.

Although the syringe and needle were heated to 160° C, the actual temperature of the extruded gutta-percha was lower and was tolerated well by human oral mucosa; no adverse effects were noticed in clinical tests.

The thermoplasticized injection-molded gutta-percha method appears promising as a new way to fill the root canal system.

Torabinejad et al.[132] used the SEM to evaluate in vitro the thermoplasticized injection-molded gutta-percha fillings on the basis of their adaptation to the surrounding dentinal walls, the presence of voids, and the extent and thickness of the cement sealer. Their study indicated that the root canal system was obturated at least as well by the injection of thermoplasticized gutta-percha in conjunction with sealer as by other generally accepted methods of obturation. However, the early delivery system was cumbersome. Furthermore, both patient and clinician must be protected from a device utilizing a temperature in excess of 155° C.

Marlin and associates,[83] using a simpler delivery system, evaluated 125 clinical cases of thermoplasticized injection-molded gutta-percha on the basis of clinical and radiographic findings and reported favorable results. "The method shows promise because the success rate seems comparable with the rate achieved by conventional gutta-percha obturation procedures."

Obtura and PAC-160. Recently, more convenient delivery systems (Figs. 8-89 and 8-90) have been developed.

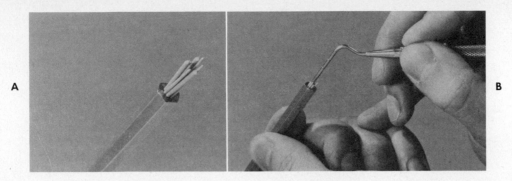

FIG. 8-86. A, Placement of gutta-percha cones in the syringe barrel. Note the interposition of the narrow tips with the broad ends. **B,** Forcing gutta-percha into the syringe barrel with a root canal plugger. (Courtesy Dr. F. Yee.)

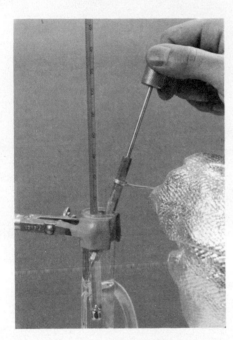

FIG. 8-87. Glycerin bath in a Thiele Dennis melting tube. Note that a protective glove is used to handle the pressure syringe. (Courtesy Dr. F. Yee.)

Relatively flexible silver needles of different sizes (18, 20, and 25 gauge) are used to introduce the plasticized gutta-percha into the prepared canal. The injection time averages less than 20 seconds. Upon completion of the injection the gutta-percha remains sufficiently plasticized for up to 2 minutes, which is adequate time for manual condensation. To counterbalance the effect of dimensional changes when the gutta-percha is thermally softened, *continuous condensation force must be exerted during cooling.*

Although the reduction of chair time is an important benefit, the presently available needle sizes make it difficult to introduce them deeply enough apically in narrow canals. The flow of the gutta-percha through the silver needle is affected by the thickness of the silver walls, which influences heat transmission, and the diameter of the lumen, which affects frictional resistance. Insufficiently heated gutta-percha will not flow properly into the prepared canal and may interfere with successful three-dimensional obturation.

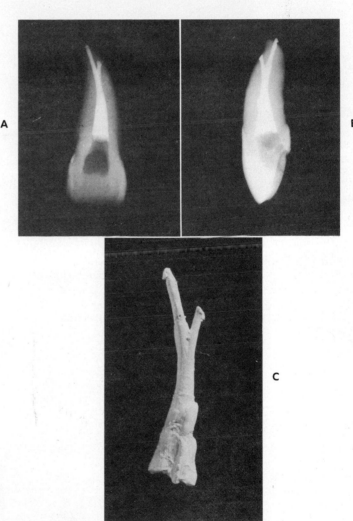

FIG. 8-88. A, Labial-lingual view of a root canal obturated with thermoplasticized gutta-percha. **B,** Mesial-distal view. **C,** Recovered root canal filling of injected thermoplasticized gutta-percha. Note the accessory canal and the irregular outline of the canal proper. (Courtesy Dr. F. Yee.)

In 1981 Schoeffel[116] designed and built a prototype delivery system (Fig. 8-90, *A*) to operate indefinitely and accurately at 160° C. This new and safer syringe facilitates the clinical application of the technique of thermo plastic injection molding. An engineering prototype incorporating

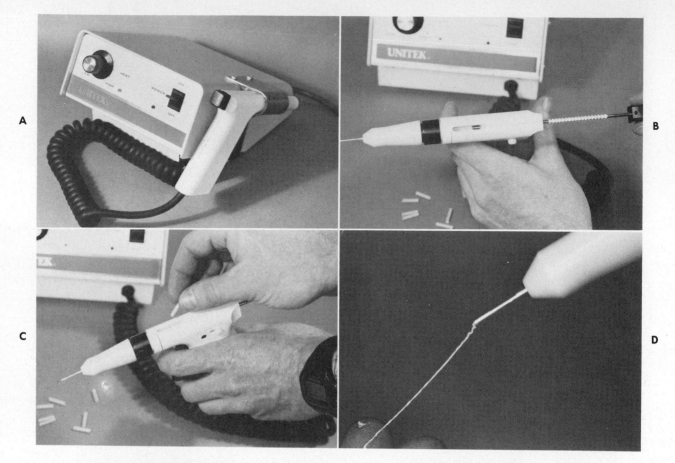

FIG. 8-89. The Obtura, a new delivery system for the thermoplasticized gutta-percha injection-molded technique. **A,** Electrical control unit with pistol-grip syringe. **B,** Loading slot exposed by pulling out the piston. **C,** Loading of the gutta-percha cylinder. **D,** At sufficient temperature the gutta-percha flows freely from the needle. It is sticky at this temperature, has good consistency, and is not uncomfortable to the touch. (Courtesy Unitek Co., Long Beach, Calif.)

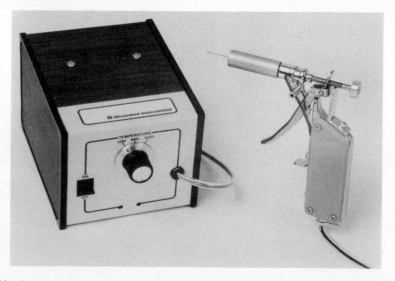

FIG. 8-90. Warm plasticized gutta-percha injection prototype development unit PAC-160 by Whaledent International (New York, N.Y.). It is designed and built to operate indefinitely and accurately at 160° C. (Courtesy Dr. C.J. Schoeffel.)

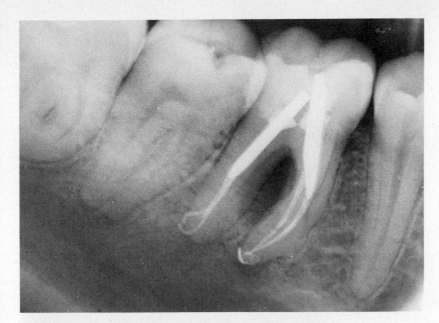

FIG. 8-91. Thermoplastic gutta-percha injection molding. Radiograph taken after filling of a mandibular molar. An accessory canal became apparent after the obturation. (Courtesy Dr. C.J. Schoeffel.)

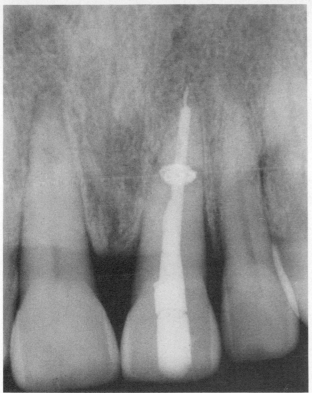

FIG. 8-92. Fractured central incisor. Both segments were successfully obturated with PAC-160 (Fig. 8-90) gutta-percha without excessive overfilling in the area of the fracture line. The apical 1.5 mm was instrumented to a size 45 file, and the remainder to a size 100 file, to accommodate the pressure dynamics necessary for thorough obturation in this unique situation. (Courtesy Dr. C.J. Schoeffel.)

the features of the delivery system developed by Schoeffel is shown in Fig. 8-90, *B*. This unit uses standard dental gutta-percha, which provides parameters clinically identical to those established experimentally.[142] The device is known as the PAC-160 (Precision Apical Control at 160°

C), and the thermoplasticized gutta-percha extruded from it is referred to as PAC-160 gutta-percha.

The thermoplasticized gutta-percha injection-molding technique seems to be capable of filling multiple foramina and other irregular configurations of the root canal system (Figs. 8-91 to 8-93, *A*). To compensate for shrinkage upon cooling, continuous manual condensation force should be exerted. Vertical condensation with selected pluggers serves also to minimize or prevent small voids caused possibly by air entrapment, thereby improving the density and compactness of the root canal filling. An endodontic cavity preparation with a slight flare and definite constriction or minimal opening at the apical terminus makes it easier to obtain a three-dimensional well-condensed gutta-percha filling with minimal apical extrusion.

Variations in gutta-percha thermoplasticizing technology. Technologic variations in the art of thermoplasticizing gutta-percha to improve and facilitate its compaction into the canal space have been suggested by several clinicians.

Use of ultrasound. Moreno[91,92] from Mexico used an ultrasonic scaling unit (Cavitron) to supply heat for plasticizing gutta-percha to obtain better compaction. The no. 25 file attached to the PR 30 insert of the ultrasonic unit is placed alongside the primary gutta-percha point and sealer to a depth of about 5 mm short of the working length. The ultrasonic unit with the rheostat set at 1 is activated for 3 to 4 seconds. The ultrasound thermal energy released by vibratory motion of the ultrasonically activated file plasticizes the gutta-percha. Upon removal of the file, the spreader is inserted immediately to create room for auxiliary cones. The softened primary cone allows a deeper penetration of the spreader, and a greater number of auxiliary cones can therefore be used to obtain better compaction.

In a leakage study using iodine 131 to compare this modified technique with regular lateral condensation, Moreno[91,92] reported that the mean leakage for regular lat-

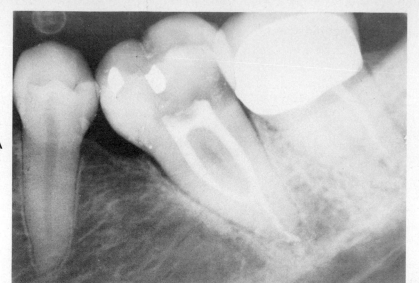

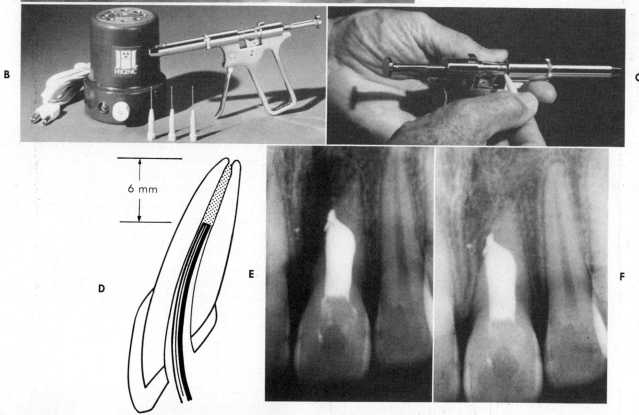

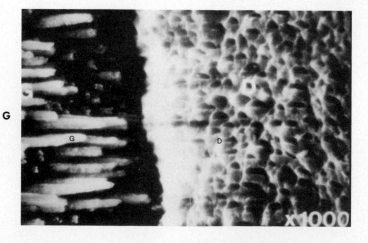

FIG. 8-93. A, Thermoplasticized injection-molded gutta-percha method in a mandibular molar with a common canal in the apical third. This case demonstrated the ability of PAC-160 gutta-percha to flow around and through intracanal obstructions. An island of dentin has been surrounded. (Courtesy Dr. C.J. Schoeffel.)

B, Prototype of low-temperature injection system. Portable heater, pressure syringe, cartridge-needles, gutta-percha cannulas. **C,** Cannula needle can be custom bent or pre-curved by drawing the needle over the syringe barrel while pressing the needle against the syringe. **D,** The cannula needle is inserted to within 6 mm of the apical terminus. Note the apical constriction of the prepared canal. Ultrafil gutta-percha injection technique. **E,** Internal resorption shown by postfilling radiograph. **F,** One-year recall radiograph showing good healing. **G,** Scanning electron micrograph showing projections of the low-temperature gutta-percha filling penetrating into dentinal tubules. *G,* Gutta-percha; *D,* dentin. (×1000.) (**B** and **C** courtesy The Hygienic Co., Akron, Ohio; **D,** redrawn from The Hygienic Co. technical bulletin; **E** to **G** courtesy Dr. A.E. Michanowicz.)

eral condensation was 2 mm (1 to 3 mm) versus a mean leakage of 0.6 mm for the modified technique.

Another clinician, Martin,[84] suggested softening the apical gutta-percha with the ultrasonic enlarging instrument that he helped develop (Dentsply Cavi-Endo device). The thermoplasticized gutta-percha allows deeper and more efficient penetration of spreaders and pluggers and a better lateral and vertical compaction of the gutta-percha mass.

Thermoplasticized low-temperature (70° C) gutta-percha injection-filling technique. As the injection technique of thermoplasticized gutta-percha to fill the root canal system gained popularity, clinicians developed ingenious injection systems. It is entirely possible that in the not-too-distant future canal obturation will consist of injecting an ideal filling material in the canal space with a well-perfected injection device.

Recently Czonstkowsky and co-workers[26] and Michanowicz and Czonstkowsky[89] developed and tested a new way to fill the root canal system; this method, which uses a low-temperature (70° C) plasticized gutta-percha, is called the *Ultrafil system.* The system consists of an injection syringe, gutta-percha cannulas with a needle attached, and a small portable 120-V heater with preset temperature (Fig. 8-93, *B*). The gutta-percha used contains the same ingredients as gutta-percha points; however, there appears to be a greater percentage of paraffin. A process developed by the Hygienic Corporation allows the gutta-percha to flow at 70° C. For convenience, the gutta-percha is packed into a prototype cartridge-needle combination or cannules (Fig. 8-93, *B*).

To gain better canal access and visibility during injection, the cannula needle is prefitted in the canal to a depth of about 6 mm from the apical terminus and custom bent or precurved accordingly prior to heating. Curving is done by placing the cannula needle over the barrel of the syringe and drawing the needle over the syringe barrel with the thumb (Fig. 8-93, *C*). Bending the needle with a pair of pliers may crimp or damage it and prevent the free flowing of gutta-percha.

The cannulas are then placed in the portable heater with the temperature preset at 90° C (194° F) and heated for a minimum of 15 minutes before use. The Ultrafil cannulas should not remain in the heater for longer than 4 hours; otherwise the properties of the gutta-percha are adversely affected. The cannulas can be reheated; however, when the cumulative time exceeds 4 hours, they should be discarded. When not in use, the cannulas are best kept under refrigeration. One cannule is ample to fill one tooth, although partially used cannulas can be reused.

The thermoplasticized gutta-percha will flow for approximately 1 minute after the cannula is removed from the heater and loaded onto the syringe. To ensure good results, the injection procedure must be smoothly and promptly executed. It takes usually 15 to 30 seconds to fill most canals without the need for manual condensation.

The trigger is squeezed slowly and released to extrude some gutta-percha through the needle before inserting it into the canal to within 6 to 8 mm from the apical terminus (Fig. 8-93, *D*). Since the gutta-percha cools faster in the needle than in the body of the cannula, constant flow must be maintained during injection. Care must be taken not to bind the needle tightly against the canal walls.

It is important to understand the concept of "passive injection" to prevent excessive internal pressure buildup within the cannule. The plasticized gutta-percha is not forced out of the cannula as in a hypodermic injection technique. It should be allowed to flow out of the needle at its own rate by means of a squeeze-release-pause-squeeze-release motion on the trigger. As the plasticized gutta-percha fills the canal, the back pressure created by the free-flowing gutta-percha will gradually "lift" or "push" the needle out of the canal. Withdrawing the needle without feeling this back pressure could result in voids or an incomplete filling.

When obturating a multi-rooted tooth, after filling one canal, the clinician may place the cannula-and-syringe combination back in the heater for a few minutes before repeating the injection procedure in other canals.

The Ultrafil technique does not advocate manual compaction. If desired, pluggers should be dipped in isopropyl alcohol before use to prevent adhesion and dislodgment of the tacky gutta-percha. Hand condensation with pluggers is done with a *light tapping pressure* rather than a forceful vertical compaction.

A sequential obturation technique, if desired, may be used. A small amount of gutta-percha is injected and condensed by light tapping with a small plugger while the syringe-cannula combination is reheated in the heater. An additional amount of gutta-percha is injected and condensed lightly with a larger plugger. The process is continued until the canal is obturated.

The Ultrafil injection technique was tested with and without a root canal sealer and was found to create a good apical seal (Fig. 8-93, *E* and *F*). As in vitro study[89] utilizing methylene blue dye to investigate the sealing properties of the low-temperature (70° C) gutta-percha injection technique showed that the injected gutta-percha sealed as well or slightly better than the lateral condensation technique using gutta-percha cones and Grossman's sealer. Another study,[26] utilizing radioactive isotopes to quantitatively determine leakage, had similar results. The low-temperature injection gutta-percha with Grossman's sealer had the least amount of leakage, followed by the lateral condensation with gutta-percha and Grossman's sealer. When used without sealer, the low-temperature injection gutta-percha showed a slightly greater isotope leakage than the other two groups. Overall, the three groups showed a good apical seal with only minimal leakage.

A recent scanning electron microscopic investigation[89a] showed that the low-temperature gutta-percha injection technique used without sealer produced a filling with close adaptation to the dentinal wall, with the gutta-percha penetrating the dentinal tubules (Fig. 8-93, *G*). Good adaptation but no gutta-percha penetration was observed when the UltraFil technique was used with a root canal sealer.

More recently, Evans and Simon[32] reported that both the lateral condensation and the injected thermoplasticized gutta-percha techniques do not provide an apical seal to ink penetration when used without a root canal sealer, even with the smear layer removed. An effective apical seal could be obtained with both techniques when they were used with a sealer. The presence or absence of the smear layer had no significant effect on the apical seal in vitro. It was recommended that the use of injected thermoplasticized gutta-percha be accompanied by the use of a sealer whether or not the smear layer has been removed.

As with all injection techniques, the Ultrafil technique stresses the importance of maintaining the integrity of the apical foramen; therefore a "stop" at the dentin-cementum junction must be maintained to restrict the flow of gutta-percha beyond the apex. The canal is flared back from the apical foramen and should be prepared to receive a 22-gauge needle inserted approximately 6 mm from the working length, since the plasticized gutta-percha will flow 6 to 8 mm to reach the apex. This size can be obtained by enlarging the middle third of the canal with a no. 2 or 3 Gates-Glidden bur or a no. 70 file.

In case of an open apex, an apical "stop" may be created by the use of either of the following two methods:

1. "Dry-file the canal walls and pack the dentin chips at the apex, using a file or a finger plugger" (Hygienic Corporation UltraFil pamphlet). Dentin chips can be produced by a Hedström file or Gates-Glidden bur. (Please see section on dentin-chips apical-plug filling technique, p. 260.)
2. Fit a primary cone very snugly at the apex. After cementation, remove most of the cone with a hot endodontic excavator spoon or a hot plugger. The remaining apical section will act as a stop. The injected thermoplasticized gutta-percha will flow around the gutta-percha point but not beyond the apex.

The Ultrafil system using low temperature (70° C) in conjunction with a sealer appears promising. The minimal amount of time required to fill the root canal system and the fact that manual condensation is not needed offer additional appeals. The technique and the device deserve further *independent clinical investigation* before practitioners adopt it for canal obturation.

CANAL OBTURATION WITH PASTES

Pastes may be either soft or semisolid. They are composed mostly of zinc oxide with various additives, to which glycerin or an essential oil (usually eugenol) is added. They can be freshly mixed before use (soft paste) or come premixed and ready for use (Cavit, a semisolid paste).

Pastes have been used as the sole canal filling material. Some paste formulas contain iodoform, which is radiopaque and absorbable. Maisto and Erausquin[81] suggested a slowly absorbable, antiseptic paste of iodoform and other additives and used it in conjunction with gutta-percha points. Overfilling can cause the patient to experience a great deal of discomfort until absorption takes place. To consistently obtain a dense nonporous filling using a creamy paste in comparison with the more reliable use of a solid cone and sealer to obturate the canal space is rather difficult. The hazard of relying on absorbable pastes as filling materials lies in the difficulty of eliminating entrapped air within the filling. If the entrapped air creates voids near the apical foramen, both leakage and percolation of exudate into the canal space may occur. Also, in

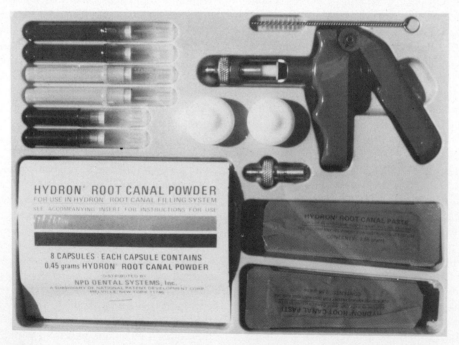

FIG. 8-94. Hydron root canal filling system. Syringe with 25-, 27-, and 30-gauge needles; mixing capsules and pestle package with Hydron root canal paste and powder and other materials. (Courtesy NPD Dental Systems, Inc., New Brunswick, N.J.)

the absence of positive pressure, pastes cannot effectively fill accessory canals.

One instance in which pastes, despite their low density and their tendency to be easily forced out beyond the apical foramen, may prove useful is in the filling of root canals of primary teeth. The paste will be absorbed along with the physiologic resorption of the roots. A thick paste made of zinc oxide and eugenol may be packed into the canals of primary molars by means of a Jiffy tube and pluggers. Radiographic verification is used to control the depth of the paste filling so as to confine it within the canal space.

Hydron, a hydrophilic plastic root canal filling material

Hydron (a gel based on products of the alcoholic reesterification of methylmethacrylate with ethylene glycol) is a hydrophilic plastic commercially available as an injectable root canal filling material.

Initially Hydron was reported to be inert, nontoxic, biocompatible, nonabsorbable, and noninflammatory and was said to fulfill the criteria for an ideal root canal filling material.[10,108] Subsequent studies,[41,72,75,126,130] however, showed different results with regard to the physical, chemical, and biologic properties of Hydron. Although the mechanical mixing of the material and a new syringe (Fig. 8-94) have simplified the delivery system, the working time of 6 to 8 minutes may prove insufficient for the correction of procedural difficulties.

Hydron's radiopacity is very low, much less than that of gutta-percha (Figs. 8-97 and 8-98). This complicates the radiographic observation of an overfill, especially in radiopaque areas (Fig. 8-99).

The syringe method used in Hydron filling makes it difficult to control the placement of the plastic gel accurately and to control the formation of voids within its structure (Figs. 8-95 and 8-100).

Hydron has been shown to be capable of penetrating fins, spurs, instrument marks, and dentinal tubules (Fig. 8-96). Other investigators,[41,72] however, did not find that the material penetrated the dentinal tubules (Fig. 8-101).

With regard to the inert property and tissue tolerance of Hydron, the opinions are controversial. Whereas some authors[10,108] have reported excellent biocompatibility, others[72,126] have shown long-term inflammation, material absorption, and transportation and have questioned Hydron's ability to effect a permanent seal (Fig. 8-102).

Observations by some investigators[72,75,126] have indicated that overfillings with Hydron cause long-term, severe periapical inflammatory responses with the activation of a large number of macrophages containing particles of Hydron. Lymphocytes were observed but to a lesser degree. After Hydron had hardened by polymerizing, its removal from the canal for post preparation or re-treatment could

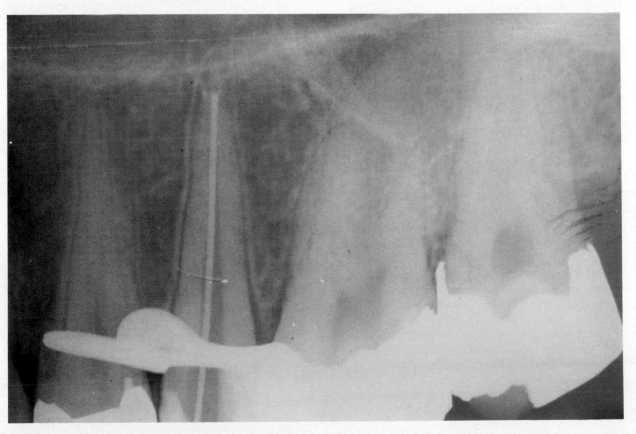

FIG. 8-95. Tip tightly fitted in the prepared canal, about 1 mm short of the working length. (Courtesy Dr. Melvin Goldman.)

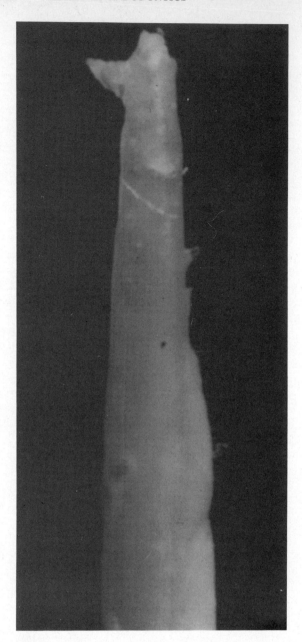

FIG. 8-96. Hydron replica of a root canal space. Note the fins and spurs.

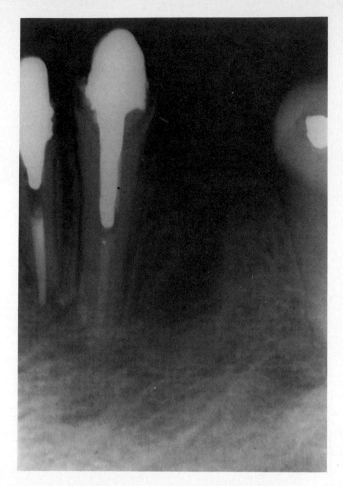

FIG. 8-97. Mandibular canine filled with Hydron and reinforced with dowel and core. Note the difference in radiopacities between the gutta-percha (lateral incisor) and the Hydron (canine). (Courtesy Dr. Melvin Goldman.)

be accomplished only by drilling with burs such as Peeso reamers.

A recent study[97] using a scanning electron microscope with energy-dispersive analysis found Hydron to be significantly more permeable to manganese ions than gutta-percha with Grossman's sealer.

In view of the foregoing controversies, further evaluation of Hydron as a root canal filling material is necessary. Radioisotope or similar tracer studies to determine whether Hydron is being transported to other parts of the body and additional studies are needed *before* clinicians can routinely use this material for canal obturation.

Pressure syringe injection technique

Krakow and Berk[71] popularized the pressure syringe developed by Greenberg[43,44] (Fig. 8-103). The pressure sy-

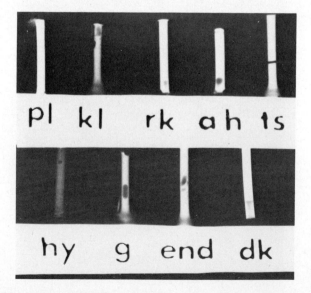

FIG. 8-98. Comparative radiopacity of nine different root canal filling materials: Maisto iodoform paste *(pl)*, Kloroperka N-Ø *(kl)*, pulp canal sealer *(rk)*, AH-26 *(ah)*, Tubliseal *(ts)*, Hydron *(hy)*, Grossman sealer *(g)*, Endomethasone *(end)*, and Diaket A *(dk)*. (Courtesy Dr. F. Goldberg.)

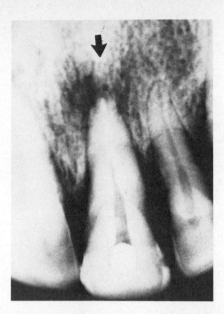

FIG. 8-99. Postoperative radiograph. Maxillary central incisor filled with Hydron in the apical third *(arrow)*. Hydron's radiopacity is very poor. (Courtesy Dr. F. Goldberg.)

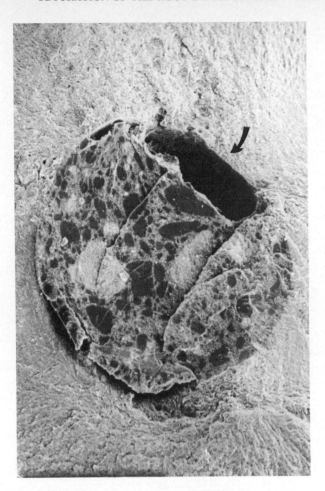

FIG. 8-100. Cross section of a root canal filled with Hydron technique. Note the presence of a big void of approximately 300 μm *(arrow)*. (×100.) (Courtesy Dr. F. Goldberg.)

ringe provides an effective method of introducing the sealer into the canal. The root canal may be filled entirely with cement without a solid core of gutta-percha or silver cone.

A modified Wach's extrafine cement is mixed, loaded in the pressure syringe, and introduced with a fine needle to about 2 mm from the apical foramen. The position of the needle is determined by a marker and verified by a radiograph. The cement is extruded by giving the handle of the syringe a quarter turn. Additional cement is extruded from the syringe into the canal by stages until the canal is completely filled with cement.

The pressure syringe injection technique seems to be useful in filling fine tortuous canals that cannot be negotiated with instruments, in filling primary teeth, and in filling some large canals. The control of excessive extrusions of cement into the periapical space can be a difficult task.

N-2 and related pastes

N-2 root canal filling material, introduced by Sargenti,[114] may be grouped as a paste. N-2 is advocated for use in "sterilizing" and filling the root canal in usually one treatment. During the past 20 years, N-2 as a root canal filling material and the N-2 method have been the objects of considerable controversial discussion. The material and technique employed appear to be a modification of the so-called "mummification" technique no longer popular in the United States but still practiced in some parts of Europe.

The composition and name of N-2 have been changed repeatedly during the last 15 years. Preparations of N-2 (R-C, RC-2B, RET-B, etc.) contain (along with zinc oxide and eugenol) paraformaldehyde (basis of many of the old mummification techniques), an organic mercury compound (phenylmercuric borate), lead oxide, and corticosteroids.

Paraformaldehyde-containing pastes are highly irritating and present a hazard if forced beyond the apical foramen. One N-2 formula (1972) consists of hydrocortisone (1.5%), titanium oxide (2%), trioxymethylene (paraformaldehyde) (7%), lead oxide (16.5%), and zinc oxide (73%) (percentages by weight). Other formulas, often with different names, differ primarily by the number and percentage of ingredients.

In June, 1962, the N-2 distributing company headed by Angelo G. Sargenti submitted a new drug application for N-2 to the Food and Drug Administration for clearance. The information submitted by the company consisted of testimonials instead of raw data supported by adequate and well-controlled clinical studies.[74,111] Consequently the application for N-2 was denied by the F.D.A. In June, 1967, AGSA (Sargenti's company) withdrew the application. The Council on Dental Therapeutics of the American Dental Association also classified N-2 as an unacceptable drug.[4]

Scientific studies[19,48,126] *have indicated the potential danger of the N-2 formulas to patients.* The material has essentially been banned in a number of countries, in California, and in several branches of the U.S. Armed Forces. Therefore, no further discussion of the techniques or their use seems appropriate in this book.

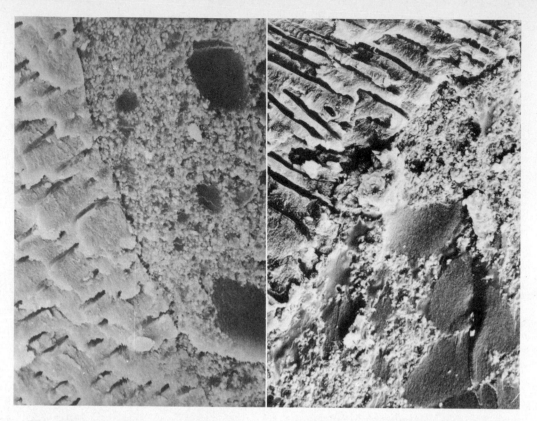

FIG. 8-101. Close adaptation of Hydron to the dentinal wall, without penetration of the material inside the dentinal tubules. ($\times 1000$.) (Courtesy Dr. F. Goldberg.)

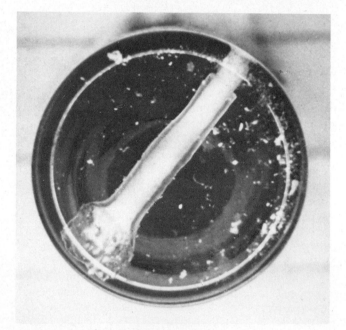

FIG. 8-102. Polyethylene tube filled with Hydron and immersed in distilled water for 3 months. Particles can be seen coming out of the material and surrounding the tube. (Courtesy Dr. F. Goldberg.)

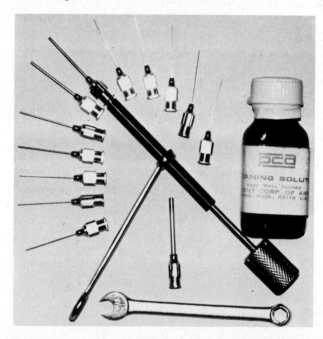

FIG. 8-103. Pressure syringe and accessories for expressing root canal cement. (Courtesy Pulpdent Corporation of America, Boston, Mass.)

Problems inherent in injection technique

All pastes, cements, plastic and plasticized materials, or resins placed into the canal space by pumping, spiraling with a Lentulo, or injection with pressure syringes share some common difficulties or problems.

1. It is difficult to control *overextension,* with its attendant tissue inflammatory responses and discomfort. The literature is replete with case histories ranging from mild reactions to severe reactions with bone loss and paresthesia.[5,90,96,125,137] Although initial re-

ports on silicone resins[76,128] appear favorable, practically all filling materials are toxic and cause inflammatory tissue responses, particularly materials containing formaldehyde and its derivatives.[24,98] Zinc oxide–eugenol, a long-time standard against which other sealers were measured, is quite toxic[5] when compared with N-2, Rickert's, and Cavit. As the cement sealers reach their final set, the initial inflammatory reaction usually subsides and healing takes place unless the material continues to break down, releasing toxic products of some of its components. In all pumping or injection filling methods the maintenance of an apical constriction is of paramount importance. Recent improvements in pressure syringe design provided some degree of control of overfillings. A pressure syringe adapted with a micrometer-type threading plunger that can inject an equal and small amount of material with each revolution of the plunger has been recently introduced by Lee Pharmaceutical (see Fig. 8-130).

2. It is difficult to control *underextension* with injection or pumping techniques. There is no assurance of sealing efficacy, since it is not easy to precisely and securely control or compact viscous or pasty materials. This may lead to incomplete obturation, with partially filled canal spaces. Underextension along with material resorption and solubility would lead to fluid percolation, with subsequent periapical inflammation. In a study using Adaptic, AH-26, Cavit, Durelon, and ZOE cement placed in canals by pressure syringe, Fogel reported that after 30 days all filling exhibited seepage, with AH-26 showing the least marginal leakage.[34a]

3. It is difficult to prevent *voids* in the body of the filling. If a void is located opposite a patent accessory canal or the foramen, fluid percolation would occur and complete healing may be in jeopardy. Sealant materials containing relatively more radiopacifiers such as lead, silver, bismuth, iodine, or barium may give the impression of compactness despite the presence of minor voids in the body of the filling. Eucapercha or chloropercha pastes pumped into the canal space will shrink substantially as the solvent evaporates. Voids are likely to develop, and the seal may be affected.[144] The Ultra-fil low-temperature (70° C) gutta-percha injection technique does not advocate hand compaction after injection. This poses a serious question of possible void development or poor density resulting from shrinkage of gutta-percha as it cools from 70° C to body temperature. Additionally, during mixing of a paste or silicone resin, a too rapid stirring or whipping motion is to be avoided because it may incorporate air bubbles in the mixture.

4. It is difficult to effectively and securely fill the complex root canal system, including accessory canals, with pastes, cements, or plastic materials because of the *lack of positive pressure.*

On the basis of the attributes and shortcomings of cements, pastes, and plastic or plasticized materials used without a solid core, one cannot help but feel a strong reservation about their routine use.

Solid core material with a cement sealant

On the basis of published studies, the most reliable and predictable endodontic seal available at present is that of a solid core compacted into the canal space with a cement sealant. The core material should be plastic or be made plastic enough to allow for as minimal a reliance on the sealant as possible. The sealant acts as cement to fill discrepancies between the core material and canal walls, including patent accessory canals. Gutta-percha is the currently recommended core material. Presently, silver points are rarely used as core material. Popular sealant cements include Rickert's and Grossman formulas and the resin AH-26; a newly introduced silicone resin or rubber sealant has also gained increasing popularity.

Silicone rubber can be used as a cement sealant or as a sole sealant and filling material to be injected into the canal space with a pressure syringe.

The choice of obturation method or a combination of methods best suited to treat and fill three-dimensionally a specific root canal system is substantially left to the discretion of the individual clinician.

However, regardless of the obturation technique used, a well-cleansed and shaped canal with a tapered flare and a definite constriction or minimal opening at the dentin-cementum junction makes it easier to obtain a well-compacted three-dimensional filling of the root canal system.

CANAL OBTURATION WITH SOLID MATERIALS

Although at present gutta-percha is by far the preferred material, other solid substances have been used with success for canal obturation. The most commonly used solid materials are silver cones. Stainless steel instruments and chrome-cobalt–type cones, although helpful in specific cases, are seldom employed.

Solid-type materials may be grouped into semirigid (flexible) types and rigid (inflexible) types. Semirigid materials, such as silver cones and stainless steel instruments, are flexible and can be easily curved to conform to severe canal curvatures. For all practical purposes, rigid material, such as Vitallium (chrome-cobalt) cones, are inflexible and cannot be easily bent to follow the curvature of the canal.

Silver cones
Advantages

Silver cones are manufactured to correspond to instrument sizes, making cone selection less time consuming. They are flexible and can be precurved before insertion to follow the curvature of the canal (Fig. 8-104). They may be used in narrow or tortuous canals, where it is not advisable or safe to enlarge the canal beyond a no. 20 or 25 instrument. Because of their relative rigidity, ease of placement, and length control, silver cones are sometimes useful in bypassing a ledge or broken instrument or in filling complicated multirooted teeth (Fig. 8-105). Silver cones may also be used in sectional filling (Fig. 8-106) or as a diagnostic probe (Fig. 8-19, *A*).

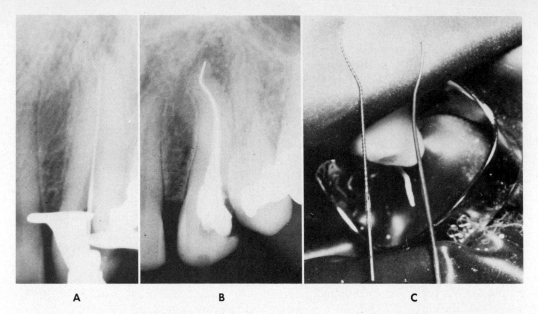

FIG. 8-104. A, Bayonet-curved maxillary canine. The file is precurved to navigate the tortuous canal. **B,** Silver cone. A solid but flexible material, silver can be precurved before insertion to follow the canal. **C,** File and precurved silver cone duplicating the canal curvature.

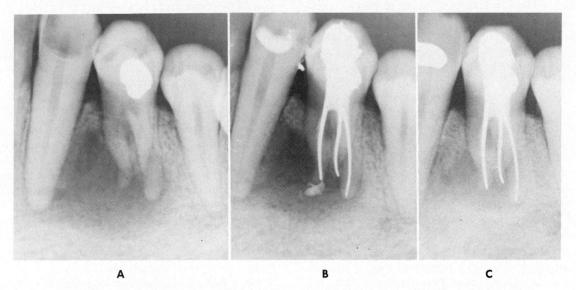

FIG. 8-105. Triple-rooted mandibular first premolar (quite rare). **A,** Pretreatment. Note the extensive, chronic, periapical bone demineralization. **B,** Postfilling. Three canal orifices are so close together that it was impractical to use gutta-percha as the filling material. No surgery was performed. **C,** Five years later, substantial osseous repair.

Disadvantages

Silver cones are difficult to use correctly and require extreme care to ensure a perfect fit. They may bind in an elliptical canal, contacting the walls at only two points and giving an illusory fit. Unlike gutta-percha, silver cones are noncompressible and cannot be packed into the irregularities of the canal. In oval canals this lack of adjustment makes it necessary for the silver cone and dentinal wall interface to be filled with a thick layer of cement (Fig. 8-107), complicating the correct sealing of the root canal system.

The removal of a silver cone for post preparation or retreatment can sometimes be a difficult task.

Corrosion from overextension and leakage (Fig. 8-108) is a potential hazard of silver cones.[16,17,39,120] The corrosion is due to the leakage of interstitial fluids into the root canal. For this reason the corrosive signs are most evident in the apical third of the silver cones (Fig. 8-109). The prevention of silver cone corrosion is therefore dependent on the thoroughness and quality of the filling technique.

In a study investigating the relation between corroded silver points and endodontic failures, Goldberg[39] found that the presence or absence of corrosion visible through the scanning electron microscope was corroborated by microanalysis. Electron probe microanalysis showed the presence of phosphorus, sulfur, chlorine, calcium, and

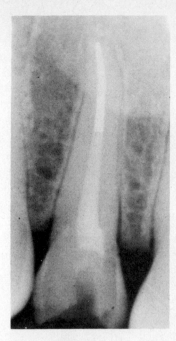

FIG. 8-106. Sectional filling after the coronal section has been twisted off. Gutta-percha was used to fill the remainder of the canal. A dowel hole can be prepared later by removing part of the gutta-percha with a heated plugger, a Girdwood bur, or a Gates-Glidden bur.

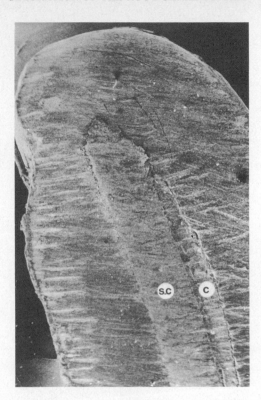

FIG. 8-107. Endodontic filling with silver cone and sealer. Note the thick layer of cement *(c)* between the silver cone *(sc)* and the dentinal wall. (×60.) (Courtesy Dr. F. Goldberg.)

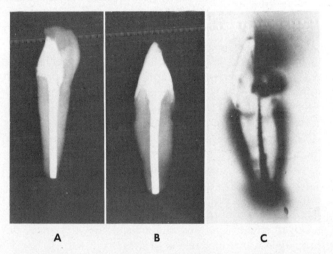

FIG. 8-108. **A** and **B,** Postoperative radiographs, buccal-lingual and mesial-distal views, of a root canal filled with silver cone and Grossman's sealer. **C,** Autoradiograph showing great penetration of the radioactive solution (^{131}I). (Courtesy Dr. F. Goldberg.)

some concentrations of sodium and potassium in the apical portion of corroded silver cones.

Using a scanning electron microscope, Seltzer and co-workers[120] found that in cases of failure, silver cones contacting tissue fluids became corroded, resulting in the formation of silver sulfide, silver sulfate, and silver carbonate. These compounds could damage the periapical tissues, although the concentration level of metal ions necessary to produce damage is unknown.

Zielke and co-workers[146] implanted silver cones in rat tibias and found that the tissue showed good tolerance in spite of corrosion. This supports Goldberg's findings[39] that certain apparently successful cases of silver cone fillings, judged by clinical and radiographic criteria, actually showed some apical corrosion of the silver cones (Fig. 8-110).

Silver cones should preferably be avoided in the following situations:

1. Large canals of maxillary anterior teeth
2. Kidney-shaped or elliptical canals of premolars, palatal roots of maxillary molars, or distal roots of mandibular molars (Fig. 8-17)
3. Teeth of young patients when the canals are incompletely formed, large, or irregular
4. Surgical cases in which root resection is anticipated
5. Teeth in which an overfilling is difficult to avoid (Gutta-percha is preferred in this case because it is better tolerated by periapical tissues.)

Selection and fitting

A silver cone of the same standardized size as the last enlarging instrument should theoretically fit the prepared canal snugly. Experience indicates, however, that this rarely occurs. Great care must therefore be exercised in the selection and fitting of silver cones.

Cone selection. A standardized micrometric gauge or a machinist gauge (Fig. 8-111) may be used as a quick screening device to select the primary silver cone. The last enlarging instrument is placed through a suitable hole in the gauge so its apical tip protrudes about 2 mm. The selected cone should be adjusted to protrude a corresponding

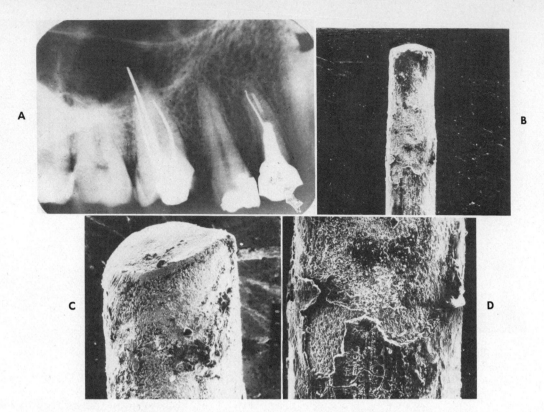

FIG. 8-109. A, Postoperative radiograph (4 years after treatment) showing overextension of the silver cone in the palatal root. **B,** Intensive corrosion at the protruded apical portion of the cone. (×80.) **C** and **D,** Higher magnification showing the peeling surface of the silver cone. (×200 and ×600.) (Courtesy Dr. F. Goldberg.)

amount through the same hole. If the apical end of the cone has been chipped off during this screening process, it is rebeveled with a fine sandpaper disk. The cone, sanitized in alcohol, in a glass bead (salt) sterilizer, or by careful flaming, is inserted into the canal with a hemostat or silver cone pliers. A radiograph should not be used until the requirements listed next are met.

1. The selected cone reaches the end of the prepared canal. If the cone is short, its apical 2 to 3 mm may be thinned down a little by rotation between the abrasive surfaces of folded-over sandpaper disk; or the canal may be enlarged slightly and irrigated meticulously to remove debris, after which the cone is tried again.

2. The cone fits snugly and requires strong force to remove it from the canal. If the cone can be easily removed, it should be shortened 0.5 mm, rebeveled, and tried again in the canal. The process is repeated until a very tight fit is obtained. Often a cone that protrudes slightly beyond the apical foramen will impart a feeling of having a tight fit. Shortening the cone so it stays inside the apical foramen will likely show that is was actually loose. The cone should be shortened further and refitted until very tight. In an elliptical canal, the cone may feel tight and binding yet contact the walls only at two points (Figs. 8-112 and 8-113). *Great care must be taken to develop a round apical preparation for the successful use of silver points.* The apical seal should not be dependent on the root canal cement

or on the compressibility of dentin and silver but on the perfect fit of the round cone in a round preparation in the last 2 or 3 mm of the canal. In the apical 2 mm, a well-fitted silver cone should fit as snugly and accurately as a well-made gold inlay.

3. The cone cannot be pushed farther with any amount of apical pressure. Ideally the apical tip of the cone should be wedged very tightly at a point 0.5 to 1 mm inside the apical foramen. When cemented, the tip will be covered with sealer, unexposed to direct contact with tissue fluids (Figs. 8-9 and 8-120). The sealer will protect the cone from being corroded.

When the foregoing three requirements of cone selection have been met, the cone is bent over the incisal or occlusal edge, resting securely and firmly on a definite landmark on the occlusal surface (Fig. 8-114). While the cone is being bent, firm apical pressure is applied through the pliers to prevent unseating at the apex. A radiograph is exposed to verify the position of the cone. If within 1 mm of the radiographic apex, the cone is acceptable for cementation.

Cone cementation. With a Carborundum disk rotating at low speed, a nick is placed on the cone at a point about 2 mm above the cervical line, halfway through the cone, to establish the point of breakage after cementation (Fig. 8-115).

After the canal is coated with cement, the cone is sanitized as mentioned previously and inserted slowly into the

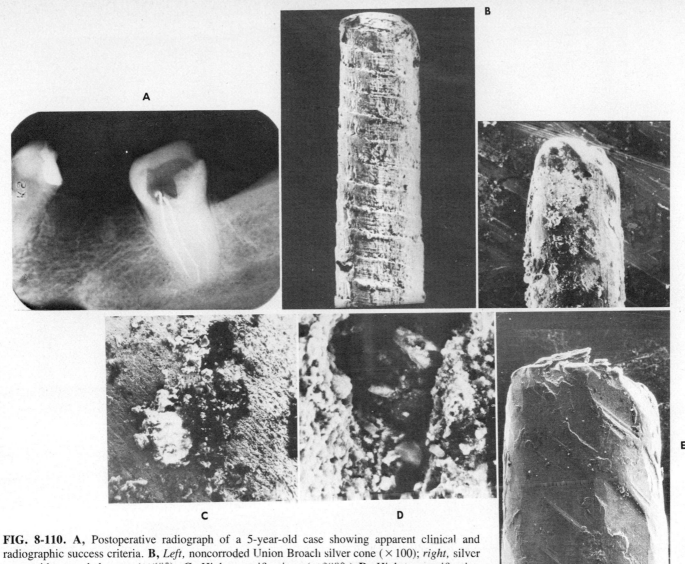

FIG. 8-110. **A,** Postoperative radiograph of a 5-year-old case showing apparent clinical and radiographic success criteria. **B,** *Left,* noncorroded Union Broach silver cone (×100); *right,* silver cone with corroded areas (×300). **C,** High magnification. (×2000.) **D,** Higher magnification showing particles of silver coming from the silver cone structure. (×4000.) **E,** New uncorroded silver cone. (×150.) (Courtesy Dr. F. Goldberg.)

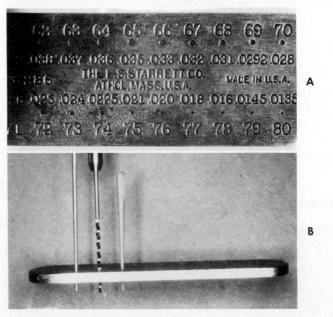

FIG. 8-111. **A,** Machinist gauge. **B,** Approximate amount of protrusion of instrument or cones (different holes only for comparison of length protruded, not for size).

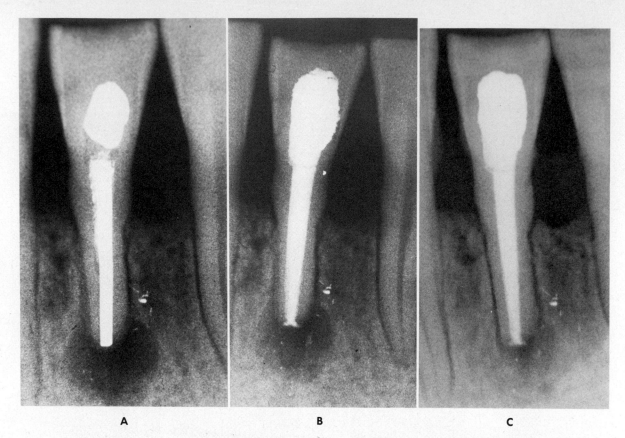

A   B   C

FIG. 8-112. A, Mandibular central incisor 4 years after apicoectomy. There was a sinus tract with a persistent periapical lesion. The dark line along the silver cone and canal wall suggests poor fit and lack of an apical seal. B, Canal refilled with gutta-percha after removal of the silver cone. C, Progressive healing 6 months later.

canal. Gentle but firm apical pressure is applied until the cone is seated and the bent section comes to rest firmly on the landmark on which it was previously bent. Lateral condensation with additional gutta-percha cones is then done to fill the void and obliterate the entire canal space. A radiograph is exposed to verify correctness of filling.

If the cone has been nicked before cementation, the coronal excess can be easily removed by working with the pliers back and forth until it breaks off. Firm apical pressure with the pliers is maintained throughout the process to prevent the cone from being unseated. The cone is bent carefully over the floor of the chamber and covered with gutta-percha and then with zinc phosphate cement (Fig. 8-116). The coronal silver excess can also be cut off with curved scissors (Fig. 8-117) and the cones bent over the pulpal floor. Another way to remove the coronal excess of silver cone is to pack zinc phosphate cement into the chamber around the cone. When the cement has set, the excess silver can be cut off with a new inverted cone; temporary cement is then placed, the rubber dam removed, and the occlusion checked with articulating paper.

Split or sectional cone technique

The split or sectional cone technique is used mainly when a dowel-and-core crown is anticipated. The silver cone is carefully fitted and notched with a Carborundum disk a few millimeters from the apical tip to establish the point of breakage after the core is firmly seated apically. The application of sealer and the cone insertion are done in the same manner as in a conventional case.

After cementation and radiographic verification, with the pliers applying firm apical pressure, the cone is rotated and twisted off, leaving the apical section tightly wedged apically (Fig. 8-118, C). Instead of being held with pliers, the fitted cone can be held tightly in a test handle to improve its maneuverability during cementation.[136] The cone can therefore be easily inserted by good tactile feeling and seated precisely and firmly with finger pressure. It is also more easily twisted off when mounted in the test handle.

The unfilled portion of the canal is prepared for a dowel-and-core crown, or gutta-percha cones are added and condensed vertically against the apical silver. This gutta-percha condensation procedure is useful and effective in cases of internal resorption or in filling lateral canals (Fig. 8-118) with positive control of extrusions of filling materials beyond the apex.

Technique with improved silver cones. Improved silver cones come mounted on color-coded handles in sizes identical to those of standardized instruments. They are handled by the thumb and index finger instead of by pliers.

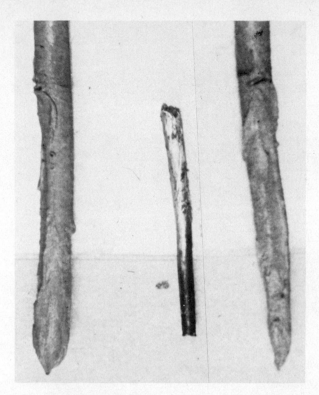

FIG. 8-113. *Left,* Mesial-distal view of a chloroform-fitted gutta-percha cone showing an elliptical canal not readily apparent from the buccal-lingual view. *Right,* Buccal-lingual view of the chloroform-fitted cone. Note the great difference in size between the gutta-percha cones and the silver cone. *Center,* Loose silver cone removed from the canal in Fig. 8-112, *A,* showing corrosion.

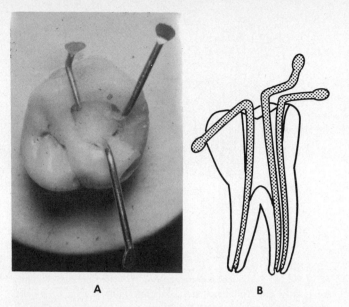

A   **B**

FIG. 8-114. Fitting of silver cones. **A,** After the cones are tightly fitted to the end of the prepared canal, they are bent firmly over a definite landmark on the occlusal surface. **B,** Fitted and bent cones. A double bend may be placed on one cone to differentiate it from other cones.

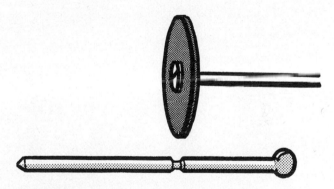

FIG. 8-115. Silver cone notched with a Carborundum disk to establish the point of breakage after cementation.

The clinician retains good tactile feeling and control during cone fitting and cementation. Well-controlled apical pressure combined with back-and-forth rotation can seat the cone firmly and strongly into the softer dentin to obtain an additional grip between the silver and dentinal walls. Being hand held, improved silver cones lend themselves well to the sectional or split cone technique.

Technique with apical silver cones. Apical cones or apical silver tips come in standardized sizes in either 3- or 5-mm lengths (Fig. 8-119). The apical silver tips are threaded to a 40-mm instrument handle. After cone fitting and cementation, the handle is unscrewed, leaving the tip wedged apically. Apical silver tips are an improvement of the sectional or split cone method and are useful when crown buildup with a dowel and core is indicated.

Role of sealers in cementation of silver cones

Gutta-percha can be rendered plastic and under strong condensation pressure can adapt itself to the complex internal morphology of the canal. The canal space is filled almost totally by a solid core of inert gutta-percha with a minimal amount of resorbable sealer. Silver cones, although flexible, are unyielding and cannot be compressed to conform to the irregularities of canal morphology. The sealers therefore play an indispensable role in filling the lateral space between the cone and the canal walls. The

development of a perfectly round preparation in the apical few millimeters of the canal so the solid cone will fit tightly against the walls is essential for the success of the silver cone filling technique.

Although any biologically compatible sealer may be used, it is preferable to cement silver cones with a sealer that has a short setting time and low solubility. Plastic resins such as Diaket A or AH-26, which are relatively nonabsorbable and very adhesive, may be used to advantage.

Gutiérrez et al.[46] filled roots of extracted teeth with silver cones using Diaket A, AH-26, or Tubliseal as sealers. The roots were subsequently implanted in the subcutaneous tissue of rabbits. The results, analyzed after 30, 90, and 150 days, indicated that when the silver cones were adequately covered with sealers corrosion was absent. The plastic resins (Diaket A, AH-26) gave better results than did Tubliseal.

For silver cone cementation the sealer should be mixed

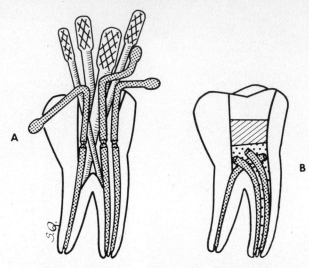

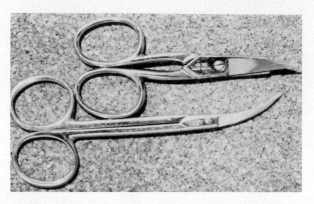

FIG. 8-116. Silver cone cementation. **A,** After the silver cones are tightly and fully seated, secondary gutta-percha cones are added to fill voids between the silver cones and the canal walls. **B,** Cones bent over the pulp chamber floor and covered with gutta-percha *(stippled area)* and zinc phosphate cement *(lines).*

FIG. 8-117. Curved scissors used to reach deep into the pulp chamber and nip off the excess coronal portion of silver cones.

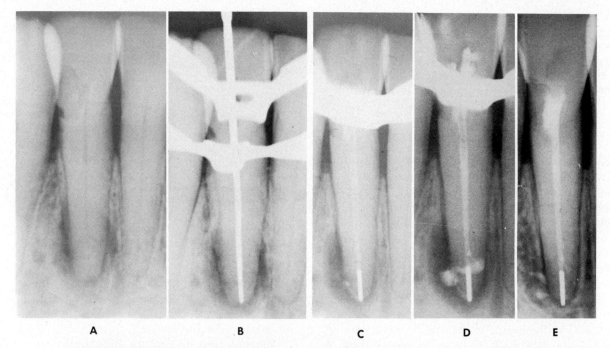

A   B   C   D   E

FIG. 8-118. Step-by-step procedure in filling lateral canals of a mandibular central incisor with the sectional silver cone method. **A,** Pretreatment. Note the presence of lateral canals suggested by the bone rarefaction on the mesial and distal aspects of the root apex. **B,** Silver cone fitted. **C,** After the notched cone is cemented in place, the coronal portion is twisted off below the level of the lateral canals. **D,** Additional cement carried into the canal with a Lentulo spiral and the remainder of the canal packed with gutta-percha. The lateral canals are overfilled with cement. **E,** Good osseous repair 1 year later.

to a heavy, creamy consistency and the canal walls well coated with the cement. Although the cone may be thoroughly coated with cement before insertion, frequently because of the tight fit the cement is wiped off the cone along the way before it reaches its apical seal. If the canal walls are not well coated with cement, the apical portion of the cone may be placed in position without sealer, resulting in possible lack of an apical seal with subsequent leakage and corrosion.

In very narrow canals the lateral space between the sil-

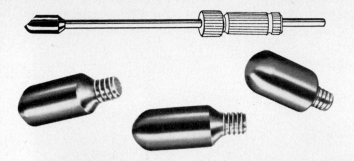

FIG. 8-119. *Top,* Apical silver tip and applicator. *Bottom,* Enlarged view of apical silver tips 3 and 5 mm long.

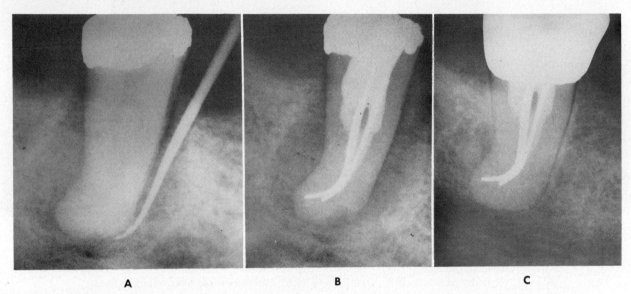

A B C

FIG. 8-120. Mandibular third molar as a partial denture abutment in a 65-year-old patient. **A,** Pretreatment. Note the extensive periapical lesion communicating with the oral cavity, as shown by a gutta-percha cone probe. **B,** After filling with silver cones and auxiliary gutta-percha cones. **C,** Two year later, complete osseous repair.

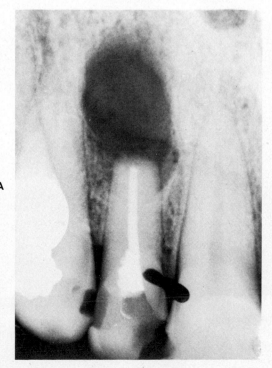

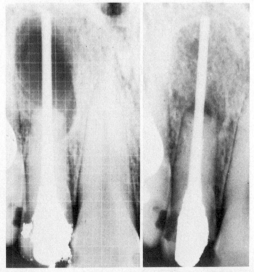

A

B

C

FIG. 8-121. Maxillary lateral incisor with endodontic endoseous stabilizer. **A,** Five-year-old root resection failure. The cystic lesion had been verified histologically. Note the poor crown/root ratio with minimal tooth retention. **B,** Postsurgical. Cemented chrome-cobalt implant. **C,** Two years later, almost complete bone repair around the implant cone. The tooth is firmly stabilized.

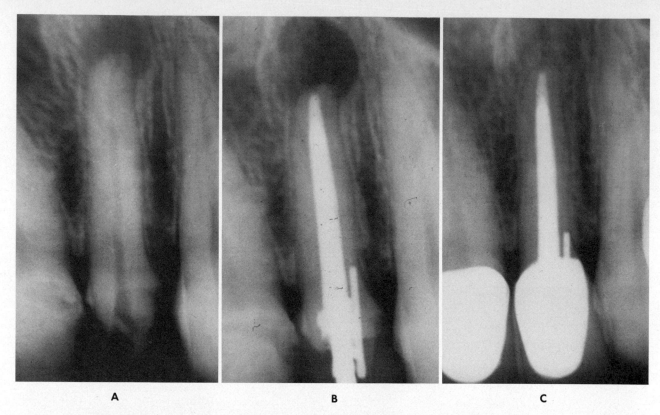

FIG. 8-122. A, Maxillary incisor mutilated by caries. **B,** Canal filled with gutta-percha and a Vitallium cone extending coronally. The crown was rebuilt with additional pins and composite material. **C,** Eighteen months later, complete bone repair and a new porcelain crown. (Courtesy Dr. John Sapone.)

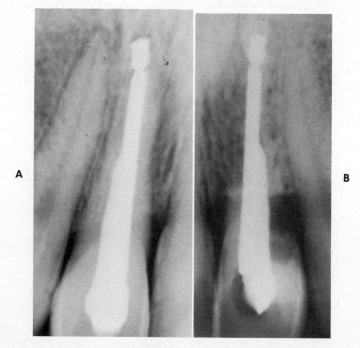

FIG. 8-123. A, Traumatically avulsed central incisor replanted after placement of apical amalgam. A rigid cone was cemented 3 months later, when root resorption was observed. **B,** Extensive root resorption 3 years later. The rigid cone is acting like an endosseous stabilizer. (Courtesy Dr. John Sapone.)

ver and the walls is filled entirely with sealer. However, wherever possible, lateral and vertical condensation with additional gutta-percha cone should be done.

In one technique the canal is filled initially with sealer and gutta-percha; a heated silver cone is then inserted until it reaches the apical foramen.[1] The silver cone may be removed, reheated, and reinserted several times until it is properly seated apically.

Another method consists of coating the silver cone with chloropercha. After the canal is coated with sealer, the silver cone, covered with a layer of dry chloropercha, is inserted into the canal. Hot forceps or pliers are brought into

contact with the silver cone as it is forced in apically. The heat softens the chloropercha and allows the cone to be inserted into its apical seat.

Gutta-percha versus silver cones

Many materials and techniques have been used to obturate root canals successfully. Silver cones correctly fitted and cemented in a canal geometrically round in its apical portion can offer successful results (Fig. 8-120). However, as mentioned previously (p. 244), silver cones present far too many disadvantages in comparison with gutta-percha. Some 15 or 20 years ago silver cones enjoyed great popu-

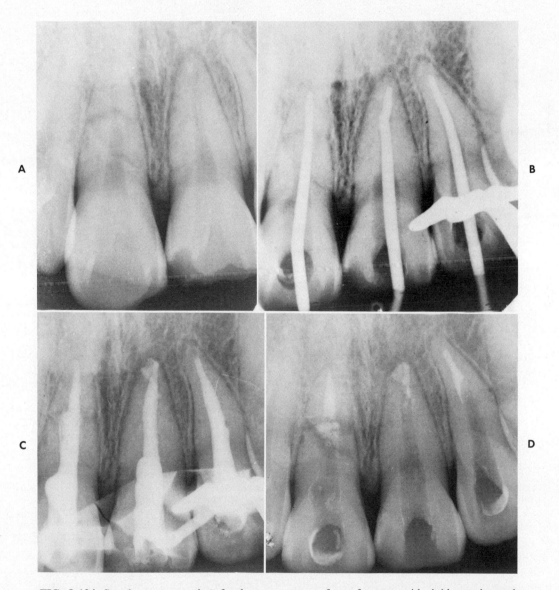

FIG. 8-124. Step-by-step procedure for the management of root fractures with rigid cone internal reinforcement. **A,** Extensive root fractures on the right central incisor and devitalization of the two adjacent teeth as a result of an impact injury. Note one fracture line in the coronal quarter of the root. The tooth had extreme mobility. Removal of fractured apical sections would leave too short a root for a successful endosseous implant procedure. **B,** Canals enlarged and gutta-percha cones fitted. **C,** Canals filled with gutta-percha and Grossman's cement. **D,** Coronal gutta-percha removed with heated pluggers. The apical quarter of the filling was left intact.

Continued.

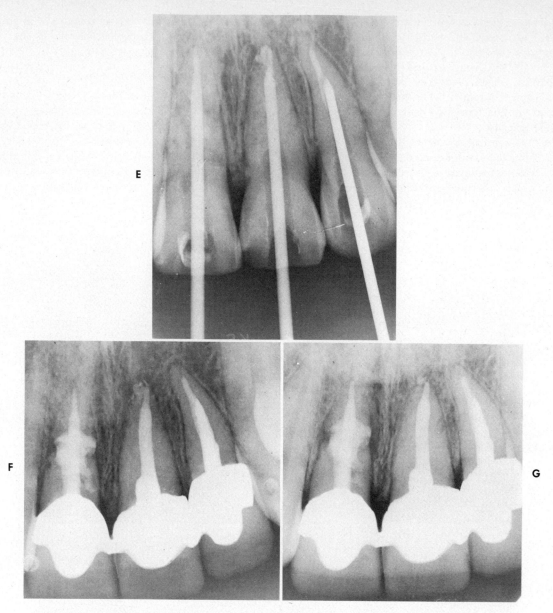

FIG. 8-124. cont'd. E, Chrome-cobalt rigid cones fitted. The cone on the right central incisor reaches past the last apical fracture line to stabilize all fractured sections. **F,** Rigid Vitallium cones cemented with Diaket. Vitallium cones are used also on the nonfractured left central and lateral incisors as endodontic stabilizers in anticipation of possible future root resorption. The three teeth were splinted with ceramometal crowns. **G,** No further root resorption 1 year later. The teeth are stable and asymptomatic.

larity in many schools and private practices. *The pendulum has presently swung toward gutta-percha, the preferred root canal filling material.*

With the use of silver cones, canals were often inadequately cleaned and shaped. Furthermore, the esthetically pleasing radiographs obtained with silver cones do not necessarily mean that a tight and true apical seal has been obtained, especially if the canal is elliptical in a buccal-lingual direction (Figs. 8-112 and 8-113). This alone can increase the rate of failure of canals filled with silver cones. Today, with the aid of orifice-opening burs (Gates-Glidden, Jovanovic, and Girdwood) (Chapters 13 and 21),

standardized files and reamers, and effective chelating agents, canal cleaning and shaping are done more completely and in less time. This greater emphasis on thorough canal cleaning and shaping to optimal size reduces the chance of leaving irritants, bacteria, and debris in the canal and makes the packing of gutta-percha in the canal simpler and more efficient. With so many well-designed pluggers, gutta-percha can be densely compressed and adapted to the irregularities and complex contour of the canal system without too much difficulty by a thorough lateral and vertical condensation method. Canals filled with gutta-percha often show accessory canals and multiple foramina well

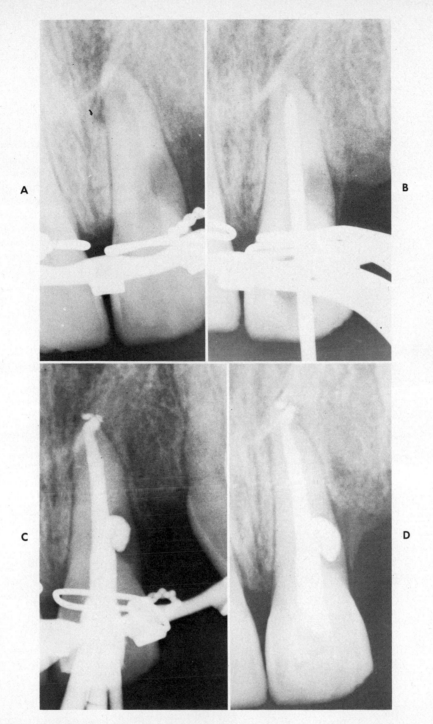

FIG. 8-125. A, Pretreatment. External root resorption 3 months after nonintentional replantation of a central incisor. **B,** Rigid Vitallium cone fitted. **C,** Cone cemented with Diaket and auxiliary gutta-percha cones. **D,** Shortly after treatment. Sealer is being absorbed. This is a recent case; recalls will be carried out for several years.

filled (Figs. 8-18, 8-48, and 8-49), thereby improving the percentage of success of endodontically treated teeth.

Rigid cones

Because of their rigidity, supposed inertness, and alleged lack of electrogalvanism, Vitallium endodontic implants may be useful for improving the crown/root ratio (Fig. 8-121). Rigid Vitallium cones may be used in conjunction with threaded pins when it is desirable to build up a mutilated crown[113] (Fig. 8-122). They may also be employed as a reinforcement core in cases of nonintentional replantation in anticipation of future root resorption (Fig.

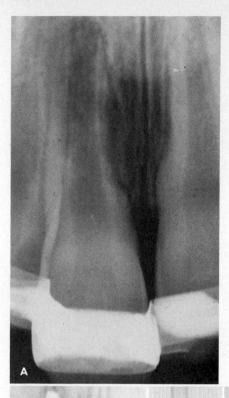

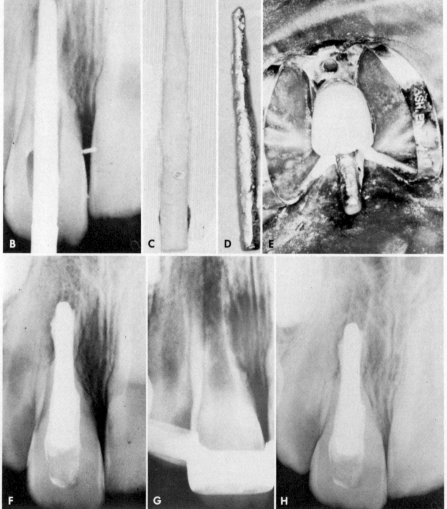

FIG. 8-126. A, Traumatically avulsed central incisor 3 months after replantation. Note the external root resorption and the large canal. **B,** Customized gutta-percha cone fitted with the chloroform technique. **C,** Gutta-percha cone outside the canal. **D,** Vitallium cast of the gutta-percha cone with a satin finish. **E,** Cone ready for cementation. **F,** Rigid cone cemented in place with Diaket, **G** and **H,** Comparison of preoperative and 2-year recall radiographs. Note the further root resorption with good osseous repair around the cone. The tooth is firm and asymptomatic.

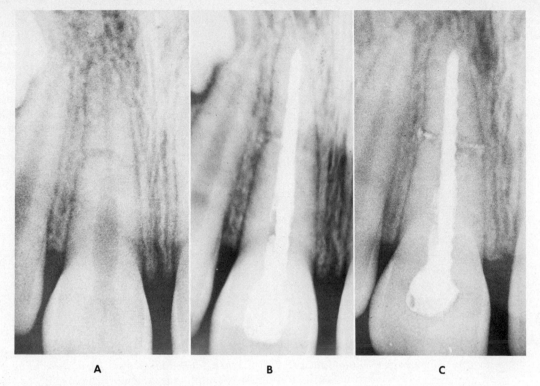

FIG. 8-127. Root fracture of a central incisor stabilized with a stainless steel file. **A,** Pretreatment. Fracture line in the middle of the root. **B,** Stainless steel file cemented with Kerr sealer. **C,** Two-year recall, no evidence of disease around the fracture area. (From Cohen, S.: Dent. Dig. **74:**162, 1968.)

8-123), root fracture (Fig. 8-124), or internal and external resorption (Fig. 8-125).

When replanting traumatically avulsed teeth, clinicians have routinely used rigid chrome-cobalt cones as a solid core in conjunction with a sealer. If root resorption occurs, the rigid cone will act as an endodontic stabilizer to retain the tooth. Usually the avulsed tooth is replanted *before* endodontic therapy. After 4 to 6 weeks have elapsed and the tooth has been stabilized in the socket, endodontic therapy may be started. In replantation cases calcium hydroxide paste may be used to advantage in controlling root resorption. (See Chapter 16.)

In extremely large canals a custom-made Vitallium casting may have to be fabricated. An impression of the canal is taken with a chloroform-fitted, customized gutta-percha cone (Fig. 8-126). The cone is sent to a dental laboratory for casting. Chloroform is used to dissolve and remove the invested gutta-percha cone, because the heat from the oven will not burn out the gutta-percha completely and a faulty casting will result. The laboratory should be instructed not to polish the cast Vitallium cone to a high shine but to leave it with a satin finish.

Stainless steel files

Stainless steel files have been used occasionally as a solid core in conjunction with a sealer in some difficult fine, tortuous canals.[111] A new file of the same size as the last small file used to enlarge the canal is selected and curved to match the canal curvature. The canal is thoroughly coated with cement sealer. The file, liberally coated with cement, is firmly seated in position by strong apical pressure. After radiographic verification, the excess part of the instrument can be cut off with a high-speed diamond bur.

Another way of removing the excess part of the instrument is to make a nick with a Carborundum disk halfway through the shaft at a point 2 mm from the canal orifice. After cementation the coronal excess is removed by working with the pliers back and forth until it breaks off.

Large-size stainless steel files have also been used as reinforcing cores in some cases of root fracture (Fig. 8-127).

Endo-Fill

A recently introduced injectable silicone resin endodontic sealant is known as Lee Endo-Fill.* The manufacturer claims it can be used as a sealer in conjunction with a core material like gutta-percha points or as a sole sealant and filling material to be injected in the canal space with a pressure syringe.

Endo-Fill, a silicone elastomer, consists essentially of a silicone monomer and a silicone-based catalyst plus bismuth subnitrate filler. The mixed silicone resin has low

---

*Lee Pharmaceutical Co., South El Monte, Calif.

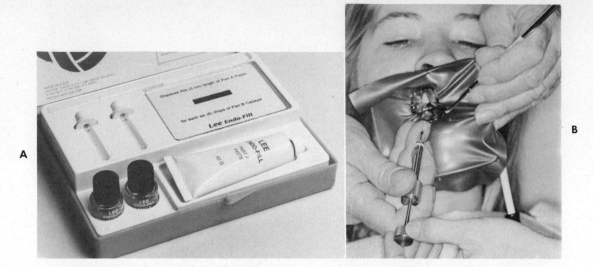

FIG. 8-128. A, Lee Endo-Fill kit of injectable silicone resin sealant. **B,** Micrometer pressure syringe injecting an equal and small amount of material with each turn of the plunger as the needle is slowly withdrawn.

working viscosity with good adaptation to tooth structure (Fig. 8-128) and good penetration of accessory canals. It cures to a pale pink rubbery solid resembling gutta-percha in properties. In regard to their involvement in tissue inflammatory response, silicon elastomers are low in toxicity and inert to tissues. Biggs and associates,[12] in their study of rat macrophage response to implanted sealer cements used a silicone rubber (Silastic 500-9, Dow Corning Corp.) as the implant control. Other studies[3,76] indicate that sealing ability is about the same as with older root canal cement sealers.

When the silicone resin is *used as sealer in conjunction with a solid core material* such as gutta-percha, the following method is suggested: A well-cleaned and well-shaped canal with the smear layer removed with EDTA or citric acid to ensure penetration of the sealant into the dentinal tubules and patent accessory canals is recommended. The gutta-percha master cone is fitted to the working length with a good "tugback." The apical 4 mm of the well-fitted gutta-percha point is cut off to be used as a positive apical seal, and the rest of the point is discarded. (Fig. 8-129, *A*) The Lee Endo-Fill is mixed according to instructions. The 4-mm segment is attached by its larger end to the tip of a slightly warmed plugger. The gutta-percha segment is dipped in the silicone mixture and introduced into the canal. It is condensed to the apical terminus (Fig. 8-129, *B*). The plugger is twisted from the segment of gutta-percha and removed. If the quick radiographic verification shows a satisfactory apical seal, the canal is filled with the silicone sealant using a Lentulo spiral or a pressure syringe. A gutta-percha point one or two sizes smaller than the largest file used to enlarge the body of the canal is selected. The apical 5 mm is cut off and discarded (Fig. 8-129, *C*). The larger section is then inserted, by hand, as far as possible into the canal. The gutta-percha will act somewhat like a plunger, forcing the silicone sealer into patent accessory canals and dentinal tubules.

When Endo-Fill is used as a sole filling material, an injection filling technique is employed: The technique uses a pressure syringe (Lee Precision Micrometer Endodontic Syringe) to inject silicone rubber into the canal space. The micrometer syringe (Fig. 8-130) provides a stable and reproducible technique, since the threaded precision plugger injects equal and small amounts of material with each revolution. As in all injection techniques, the canal must be enlarged sufficiently to accommodate the different sizes of needles used.

To be able to insert a 30-gauge needle to the apical terminus, the canal must be enlarged to a size 20 to 25 file. A 27-gauge needle requires size 30 to 40, a 25-gauge needle requires a size 50 instrument, a 22-gauge needle size 60 to 80, and an 18-gauge needle size 90. *A parabolic or flare-type cavity preparation with an apical constriction* to act as a matrix to prevent overfilling is recommended. The flare preparation provides a reservoir for pressure relief to minimize the chance of forcing material beyond the apical foramen by the powerful pressure syringe (Fig. 8-131).

The silicone resin mix is *prepared only when the canal is ready to be filled.* Its bonding ability to canal walls decreases if it is not used within about 20 minutes after mixing. Prior to filling, the canal is irrigated with sterile water and dried with absorbent points. (*Caution:* The final irrigant should not be hydrogen peroxide or sodium hypochlorite, since they may affect the polymerization of silicone.) The blunt needle is inserted to within 1 mm of the apical terminus of the preparation, and the silicone sealer is slowly expressed by turning the plunger a "nudge" (approximately 2 degrees) to deposit a plug of about 1 mm of the material (Fig. 8-131, *A*). After a *pause of a few seconds,* the needle is withdrawn slightly from the apical constricted area to the flare area and the silicone paste is expressed out again as the needle is gradually withdrawn. (Fig. 8-131, *B*). Care must be taken to turn the plunger slowly to extrude the material. *Turning the plunger too*

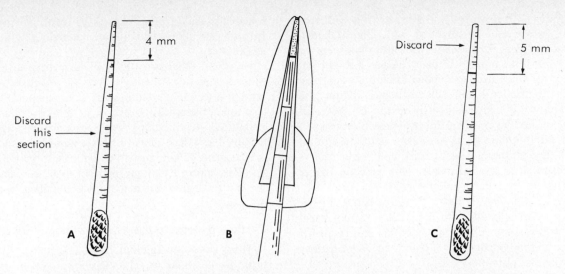

FIG. 8-129. Endo-Fill single-cone technique. **A,** Well-fitted gutta-percha master cone. Apical 4 mm is used to obtain positive apical seal. **B,** Plugger with apical segment of master cone (which has been dipped in Endo-Fill sealant) attached to it is used to condense cone to working length; then the canal is filled with silicone sealant. **C,** A gutta-percha point one or two sizes smaller than final file used to enlarge the canal body is cut off 5 mm and placed by hand as apically as possible to ensure condensation of Endo-Fill in the canal space. (Redrawn from Lee Pharmaceutical Co. technical bulletin 9085.)

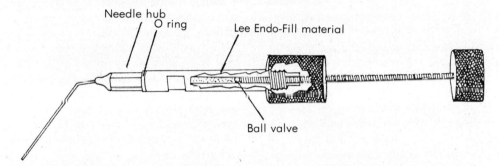

FIG. 8-130. Precision micrometer endodontic syringe, filled with silicone sealant ready for use. (Courtesy Lee Pharmaceutical Co., El Monte, Calif.)

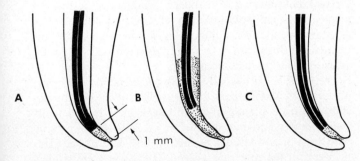

FIG. 8-131. A and **B,** "Parabolic" funnel preparation of apical third of canal, recommended for pressure syringe for silicone or other plasticized materials. **A,** Needle is inserted 1 mm short of apical terminus and a "plug" of material is deposited. **B,** After a few seconds' pause, the needle is withdrawn slowly from "neck" of preparation to flare area and more material is expressed by turning plunger slowly. Flared preparation allows material to flow up around the needle as it is slowly withdrawn. **C,** Straight-wall preparation, contraindicated in pressure syringe technique. Since needle blocks pressure relief, material will be forced out of apical foramen. (Redrawn from Lee Pharmaceutical Co. technical bulletin 9103.)

fast would create too high a local pressure, which *may force the plug at the apex past the foramen and create an overfill.* It is important to keep the needle buried in the material during injection and to withdraw the needle slowly until the canal is completely filled or until the material is seen oozing out of the pulp chamber.

A quick radiographic verification is made. Because of its high content of bismuth subnitrate, Endo-Fill is quite radiopaque. If voids are detected, the needle is reinserted to a point below the void and more material is slowly extruded. This will work the air bubble to the surface. A moist cotton pellet is used to compact the filling vertically against the mass, and the excess is cleaned from the pulp chamber. *Note:* Water markedly accelerates the setting time.

Endo-Fill setting time can be controlled—from 8 to 90 minutes—by varying the amount of catalyst used. The more drops of catalyst used, the quicker the material sets and the greater the shrinkage, which is a disadvantage. Another disadvantage is that Endo-Fill's bonding ability to the walls of the canal decreases if it is not used within about 20 minutes of mixing. Endo-Fill sets to a pink rubbery solid, which can be removed with Gates-Glidden burs, Peeso reamers, endodontic files for placement of dowels or for re-treatment. If the material has not yet cured fully, the force used to remove the top portion may dislodge the remainder, which will necessitate refilling the canal. If a dowel is anticipated, it is best to fill the canal only to the desired level. Endo-Fill is nondiscoloring upon aging and exhibits little or no shrinkage upon curing. At the present time all the cements, pastes, and plastic sealers used in endodontics are resorbable; only silicone rubber and polycarboxylate cements are not soluble.

Although *preliminary* reports[76,128] on silicone rubber (Endo-Fill) were favorable, the material as a root canal sealant or as a sole injectable filling material still needs the test of time and more extensive *independent* investigations before its popular use.

Dentin-chips apical-plug filling technique

In the perpetual search for biocompatible materials and as a result of the desire to keep irritating products from apical contact, clinicians became increasingly interested in dentin chip filling. Dentinal plugs inadvertently formed, even while clinicians were trying to avoid forming them, seemed to create an effective apical barrier against which healing could occur. A deliberate dentin-chips filling technique was born.

Essentially it consists of filling at least the apical 1 mm of the root apex with dentin chips to block the foramen. Other materials, usually gutta-percha with a sealer, are then compacted against this apical plug barrier or "biologic seal."

Dentin chips are produced only after the canal has been properly debrided and shaped, sanitized, and dried. A Hedström file, or a Gates-Glidden bur is used to produce dentin powder from the occlusal two thirds of the canal. A small plugger or the blunt end of a paper point may be utilized to push the dentin chips apically. Care must be taken to gather scattered chips raised by the file or bur around the pulp chamber floor and pack them apically. A file 1 or 2 sizes larger than the master key file or a very small plugger or a paper point may be used for this purpose. With a no. 15 or 20 file the apical plug is tested for completeness of density. A dense plug of at least 1 mm in thickness should offer resistance to perforation by the file. The canal is then obturated with gutta-percha in conjunction with a sealer or with other plastic materials or silicone rubber.

This technique is popular mostly in Europe. Investigators[86] reported 91% success on 1300 teeth filled with apical dentin and coronal canal cement fillings. In a subsequent publication Ketterl[70a] reported 95% success. Another study[8] reported apical closure with "osteodentin" proportional to the thickness of the dentin plug, with some incomplete calcification across all the serial sections. Another study[134] found healing in monkey teeth in which apical plugs had been introduced. Still another study[105] found more rapid healing where dentin plugs had been created, even when the foramen is perforated. Investigators[29]

found that dentin plugs were most effective in confining irrigating solutions and filling materials within the canal space.

However, other investigations have been less favorable to the technique. Recently it was found[64] that leakage was greater in teeth with dentin plugs than without. Others[16,143] also found the apical plug to be of dubious value.

Infected dentin chips may be a serious deterrent to healing[57] and may actually irritate and hinder repair.[133]

According to findings from published reports, the dentin-plugs filling technique appears to be a viable and favorable procedure when the apical foramen is perforated or open.

Calcium hydroxide pastes as sealers and apical plugs

The success of calcium hydroxide and calcium phosphate formulations in achieving apical closure in cases of open apices has stimulated the use of calcium compounds as sealers, paste fillings, or apical plugs.* One study[106] reported that calcium hydroxide plugs and dentin plugs resulted in significant calcification at the foramen. However, the calcification observed with the dentin plugs was more complete than that observed with calcium hydroxide plugs. Another investigation[53] found that calcium hydroxide plugs produce a periapical response that overall is indistinguishable from that produced by dentin plugs.

Calcium hydroxide or calcium compounds may be carried into the canal by means of a small amalgam carrier normally used in retrofilling. The Messing amalgam carrier may be suitable for this purpose. A small plugger or paper point is used to push and pack the material apically, forming an apical plug or barrier against which the core material, usually gutta-percha, and a sealant are condensed.

The search for the perfect filling material continues. Some clinicians have experimented with calcium compounds such as Proplast or used a cross-linked collagen–calcium phosphate gel to induce dentinogenesis and cementogenesis and apical closure. Others used silicone resin as a sole sealant and filling, delivered by a precision micrometer syringe, not to mention the use of ultrasonic devices to enhance canal obturation.

The quest for a beyond-the-space-age endodontic filling material has many ardent followers. This would be a magical material that satisfies all of Grossman's requirements and other requirements as listed on pp. 189-190; a material fluid enough and viscous enough to flow into all the ramifications of the root canal system, and form a mechanical and even chemical bond with the dentinal tubules; a perfectly biocompatible material capable of inducing dentinogenesis and cementogenesis and apical closure. When the ideal material and the perfect delivery system become a reality, the task of obturating the "pathways of the pulp" will be a joyful labor of love.

---

*See references 52, 54-56, 58-60, 77, 78, 82.

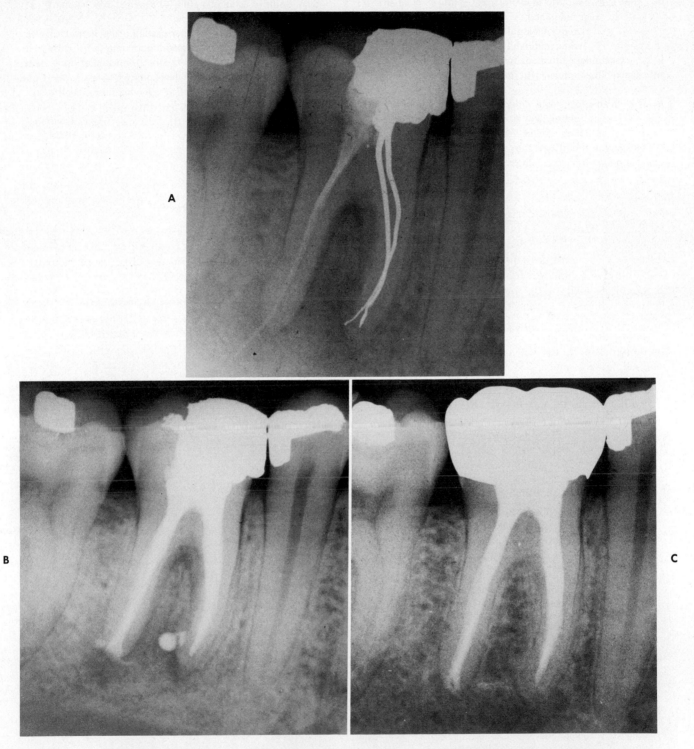

FIG. 8-132. Mandibular first molar filled with silver cones. **A,** Note the grossly overextended and underfilled distal canals and the loose cones in the mesial canals. **B,** After removal of the cones. Retreatment with gutta-percha cones as the filling material. Note the overfilling and the extruding cement. **C,** Eighteen months later, good osseous repair with complete absorption of sealer.

APICAL EXTENT OF ROOT CANAL FILLINGS

The question whether the canal should be filled flush with, short of, or beyond the radiographic apex merits clarification. The radiographic apex is where the root apex appears to join the periodontal ligament as viewed on the radiograph. The vast majority of endodontists prefer filling the canal to the dentin-cementum junction (apical foramen) so as not to impinge on the periapical tissues, permitting, hopefully, physiologic closure of the root canal by cementum. The vertical position of the dentin-cementum junction is variable with each tooth. It may be located 0.5 to 2 or 3 mm from the radiographic apex (Figs. 8-12, *A,* and 8-120, *C,* and Chapter 10). Filling the canal so it appears flush with the radiographic apex produces esthetically pleasing radiographs. However, in reality, the filling is probably overextended 0.5 to 2 mm beyond the apical foramen, especially in roots curved in a buccal-lingual direction. Because of the physics of dental radiography, the true extent of root curvature seldom appears on the radiograph (Chapter 4). The most desirable vertical extent of the root canal filling is a homogeneously dense filling extending 0.5 to 1 mm short of the radiographic apex. An overwhelming majority of successful cases have been obturated in this manner (Figs. 8-9, 8-12, and 8-120). In cases of vital extirpation, fillings slightly underextended are much more comfortable to the patient than are fillings extended to the radiographic apex.

Contrary to the old suggestion of filling to the radiographic apex or slightly beyond in cases with an area of rarefaction, we have observed countless successful cases with periapical lesions filled nonsurgically to 0.5 or 2 mm short of the radiographic apex (Figs. 8-12, *B,* and 8-120). Emphasis should be on how densely and how well the entire root canal space is obturated.

Schilder[115] emphasized the distinction between overfilling and underfilling and between overextension and underextension.

In *overfilling,* the canal space is entirely obturated, with a surplus of material extruding beyond the apical foramen (Fig. 8-132). In overfilling, the apical seal is obtained and success is the usual outcome of treatment (Figs. 8-4, 8-5, 8-18, and 8-19).

In *underfilling,* the canal space is incompletely filled, leaving voids as potential areas of recontamination and infection (Fig. 8-6, *A*).

Overextension and *underextension* refer merely to the vertical extent of the root canal filling, independent of its volume.[115] An overextended filling may actually be grossly underfilled; there may be large dead spaces or voids in the pulp canal, leading to fluid percolation and ultimate failure (Fig. 8-132, *A*).

A serious effort to compact the filling material vertically, therefore, should be made to obtain a dense, homogeneous-appearing filling in its entire mass. A filling may seem dense from the buccal-lingual view but may be grossly underfilled from the mesial-distal view (Fig.

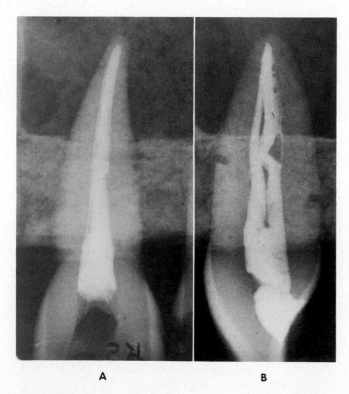

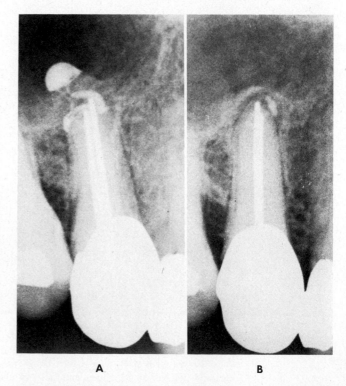

FIG. 8-133. A, Labial-lingual view of a central incisor. The canal appears well filled. **B,** Mesial-distal view. Note the gross underfilling and the large voids in the body of the filling.

FIG. 8-134. A, Maxillary premolar filled with silver cones. Note the massive excess of sealer extruded into the maxillary sinus. **B,** Nine months later, almost complete absorption of sealer.

8-133). Although the tight apical seal is of prime importance for the success of endodontic treatment, the sealing of patent accessory canals at locations other than the root apex is no less important in enhancing the chance of success toward that perfect 100% rate. An endodontic implant, used to improve the crown/root ratio, is an intentional overfilling with metal cones. Many failures observed in endodontic implants come from lack of an apical seal. This concern for an apical seal has led many clinicians to overfill the canal in an effort to obtain a tight seal or an apical "button" at the foramen (Figs. 8-132, *B,* and 8-134, *A*).

Sealers currently in use are more or less toxic when freshly mixed.[126] Gross excess of filling materials beyond the apical foramen is an *unnecessary* invasion of the attachment apparatus, resulting in needless postfilling pain and discomfort. Fortunately, tissue tolerance to commonly used filling materials is high, the excess sealer usually is absorbed, and the prognosis is for ultimate success (Figs. 8-18 and 8-132, *B* and *C*).

PATIENT INSTRUCTION AFTER CANAL OBTURATION

The patient should be advised that the tooth may be slightly tender for a few days. The discomfort may be due to sensitivity to the possible excess of filling materials pushed beyond the apical foramen. Excess sealer is usually absorbed in a few months (Fig. 8-134, *B*). Pain from temporary apical inflammation may be relieved by analgesics and frequent warm saline rinses (1 level teaspoon of salt per 8-ounce glass of very warm water). The patient is advised to hold the warm water in the affected area for 10 seconds, empty his mouth, and repeat the procedure until the entire glass of warm salt water has been used. If swelling occurs, cold compresses or an ice bag should be applied on the face over the affected area; on 10 minutes, off 20 minutes, for several hours. This intraoral warming and extraoral chilling is usually effective in relieving postendodontic swelling and discomfort. Antiinflammatory drugs such as corticosteroids (see Chapter 12) together with an antibiotic may be prescribed in severe cases. The patient should be advised not to chew unduly on the tooth until it is protected by a permanent restoration.

RECALL CHECKUP

A recall checkup for clinical evaluation of tissue repair and healing progress should be arranged before the patient is dismissed. If bone loss is extensive or the therapy was unusual or prolonged, the first recall checkup should be within 3 months; in most cases, patients are recalled in 6

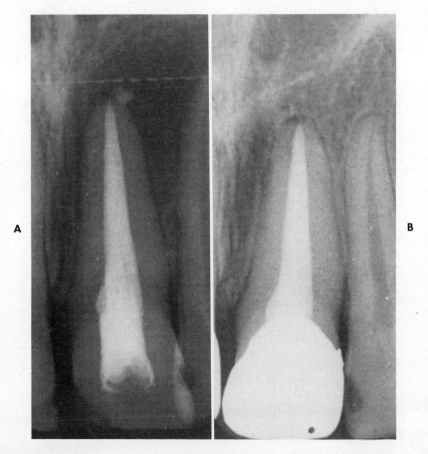

FIG. 8-135. A, Central incisor. Large chronic periapical lesion filled to the dentin-cementum junction with gutta-percha. No surgery was performed. **B,** Eighteen months later, complete healing is recognized by continuity of the periodontal ligament and lamina dura around the root apex.

months. A comparison of the new radiograph with the preceding one should show a continued regeneration of bone. Complete bone regeneration and healing require a few months to 4 years. The periapical tissue of an endodontically treated tooth without an area of rarefaction should continue to appear normal at the recall checkup. The radiograph of a successful root canal filling should show the periodontal ligament with a uniform thickness and the lamina dura continuous along the lateral surfaces of the root and around the apex (Figs. 8-9, 8-18, and 8-135). A break in the continuity of the lamina dura around the apex should be questioned as evidence of possible pathologic disturbance. The root canal filling should appear homogeneously dense and filled to the dentin-cementum junction. The tooth should be entirely comfortable to the patient and be serviceable as a useful member of the masticating apparatus.

REMOVAL OF ROOT CANAL FILLING MATERIALS

Root canal filling materials, whether pastes, cement, gutta-percha, or silver cones, may have to be removed for re-treatment or to make room for a dowel-and-core preparation.

Gutta-percha

Gutta-percha can be removed from the canal by either the Hedström file method or the solvent method.

Hedström file method

When the gutta-percha cones are loosely cemented in the canal, they can be removed quickly and efficiently by Hedström files.

As much filling as possible is removed from the cham-

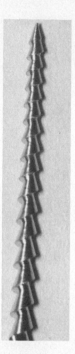

FIG. 8-137. Close-up of a Hedström file showing its cutting blades or flutes.

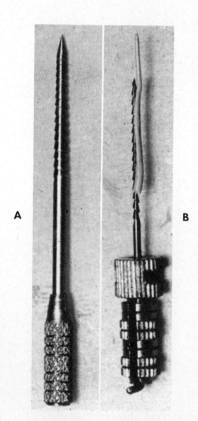

FIG. 8-136. A, Hedström file resembling a wood screw. B, Removal of a gutta-percha cone by a Hedström file. The file engages material in its flutes.

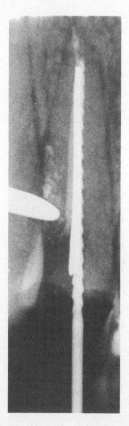

FIG. 8-138. New Hedström file inserted into the canal alongside the silver cone and advanced in a clockwise screwing motion.

ber and canal orifice with a no. 2 or 4 long-shanked round bur mounted on a miniature or pedodontic contraangle handpiece.

A new Hedström file no. 30 or larger (Figs. 8-136 and 8-137), depending on the canal size, is inserted with a clockwise rotation between the filling and canal wall until it binds in the canal (Fig. 8-138). The file is then pressed laterally against the canal wall as it is forcibly withdrawn from the canal.

Often the gutta-percha is engaged between the flutes of the file and removed in one piece (Fig. 8-136, *B*). If the first two or three attempts fail to dislodge the cone, another new Hedström file one or two sizes larger is used to engage the gutta-percha cone more positively. Usually the cone is removed after one or two further attempts.

The Hedström file method should always be tried first, especially when the gutta-percha filling protrudes beyond the apical foramen (Fig. 8-139). If a solvent is used in these cases, the apical excess of gutta-percha will likely remain in the periapical tissues or be pushed farther apically.

Solvent method

Because of its solubility in common solvents, gutta-percha can be removed by being softened with chloroform or xylol; the softened gutta-percha is then removed bit by bit with a reamer, Hedström file, or absorbent point. The solvent/file method consumes more time than the Hedström file technique and is useful when attempts to remove the gutta-percha with Hedström files are not successful. Round burs and Gates-Glidden burs are used to remove as much filling as possible before the solvent is used.

In this technique a few drops of chloroform are deposited in the pulp chamber with a syringe. The softened gutta-percha is removed bit by bit with a Hedström file or reamer. The instrument is cleaned each time by being twisted counterclockwise in a cotton roll. Fresh chloroform is added from time to time, and the process is repeated until the apical foramen is reached.

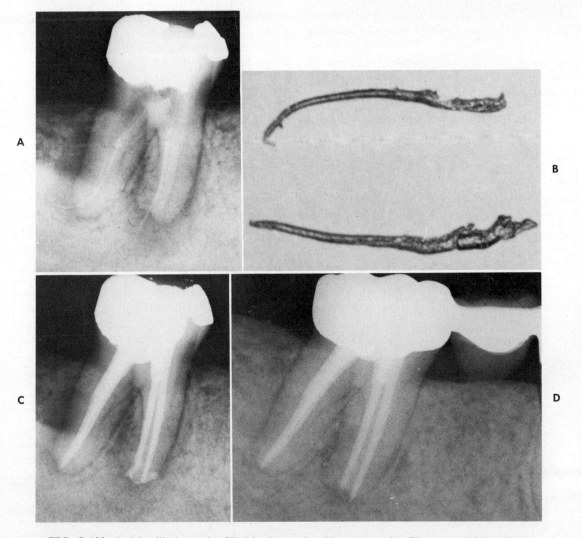

FIG. 8-139. A, Mandibular molar filled inadequately with gutta-percha. The coronal third of the filling has been drilled out with a no. 2 long-shanked round bur. Gutta-percha cones extend past the apices, yet the canals are underfilled. **B,** Gutta-percha cones removed with Hedström file technique. **C,** Canals refilled with gutta-percha. **D,** Six months later, progressive bone repair.

The procedure is performed using a rubber dam with frequent irrigations to evacuate dislodged debris.

Another way to remove the occlusal portion of gutta-percha from the canal is to use a suitable-size plugger heated red hot.

Gates-Glidden and Girdwood burs are useful in drilling out of the occlusal portion of gutta-percha to make room for a dowel-and-core-preparation.

Silver cones

Most silver cones can be removed through application of patience and proper technique; however, occasionally a tightly wedged cone will be impossible to dislodge. The access cavity should then be made larger than usual for better visibility and access.

A no. 2 long-shanked round bur, mounted on a miniature contraangle handpiece for better vision, is used to cut away the cement around the cone. Care must be taken not to nick the cone with the bur. The cement immediately adjacent to the cone is chipped off with the tip of the explorer or orifice-finder instrument.

The pulp chamber is then flooded with chloroform or xylol to soften the cement sealer. A small file or reamer is used to stir the chloroform around the cone, breaking down the cement further. The pulp chamber is dried with a blast of air and flooded again with fresh chloroform.

If the butt end of the cone extends into the pulp chamber, it may be grasped with narrow-beak pliers or splinter (Stieglitz) forceps (Fig. 8-140) and pulled out firmly. If the cone extends only slightly into the pulp chamber, it may be pried out with the blade of an excavator spoon or a silver point retriever (Fig. 8-141). Often a small file or reamer can be inserted around the side of the cone and the canal wall. With patience and perseverance, more root canal cement-sealer will be broken down and dissolved farther apically. The chamber is again flooded with chloroform.

A larger, new Hedström file may be inserted with clockwise rotation along the cone until it binds (Fig. 8-138). Because the flutes of the file are harder than silver, they will cut into the side of the cone. The file is then forcibly withdrawn from the canal, pulling or dislodging the cone from the canal. The insertion and withdrawal of the file are repeated several times, going deeper apically each time until the silver cone is dislodged and removed from the canal.

The method can also be employed to remove or dislodge broken instruments from the canal. A new file must be used each time. Excessive winding and binding of the instrument should be avoided to prevent its fracture. Frequent irrigation is done to evacuate dislodged debris. Roig-greene[108a] described the removal of foreign objects from root canals by means of a thin steel wire inserted through the lumen of a dental injection needle and tightened with small hemostat pliers.

Pastes

Most pastes are readily soluble in common solvents and are relatively simple to remove from the canal (except N-2–like paste). First, small long-shanked round burs and Girdwood burs are used and are followed by new reamers or Hedström files. The tooth length should be determined accurately by radiographs and the canal irrigated frequently to evacuate dislodged debris. If the debris is pushed beyond the apical foramen, exacerbation of an otherwise asymptomatic tooth will often result.

Cements

Zinc phosphate and silicophosphate cements (used occasionally as root canal filling materials) are difficult to remove from the canal. Small long-shanked round burs mounted on a miniature or pedodontic contraangle handpiece are used to drill the cement out slowly. Radiographs should be used frequently to verify the direction of the cut to avoid lateral root perforation.

Ultrasonic energy for the removal of cemented solid objects from canals

Ultrasonic energy, used for almost three decades to clean the external surfaces of teeth, has gained increased application in dentistry, particularly in endodontics.[38] Ultrasound waves can be employed to break and loosen the cementing bond of preformed dowels, cast posts, or silver cones from the canal, enabling the clinician to remove them with Stieglitz forceps (Figs. 8-140 and 8-143) or Hedström file (Fig. 8-138) with relative ease and without damage to the root structure.

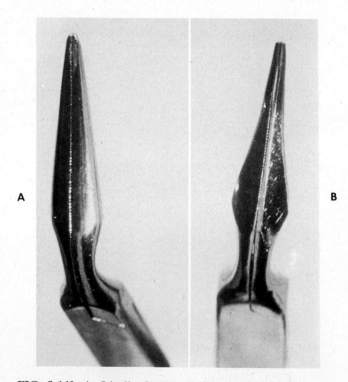

FIG. 8-140. A, Stieglitz forceps. Fine beaks are useful for handling and seating silver cones in canals and for removing broken instruments and silver cones from the canal. **B,** Forceps with beaks ground on the sides to narrow them further. This allows a deeper reach into the canal for removal of broken instruments or silver cones.

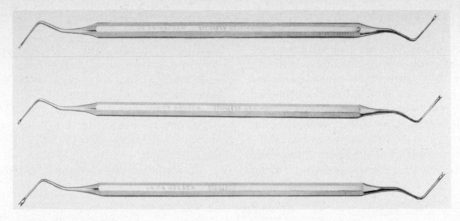

FIG. 8-141. Silver point retrievers designed by Caufield. (Courtesy Union Broach Co., Inc., Long Island City, N.Y.)

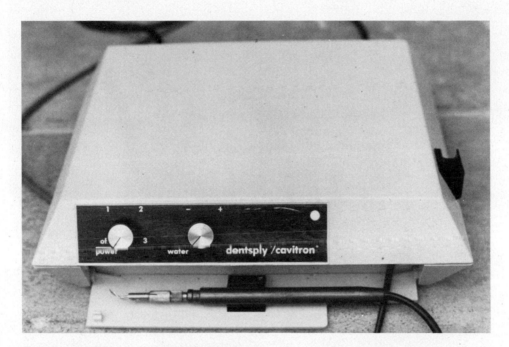

FIG. 8-142. A Cavitron unit designed for cleaning the external surfaces of teeth is used as the ultrasonic energy source to break and loosen the cement bond around cemented objects.

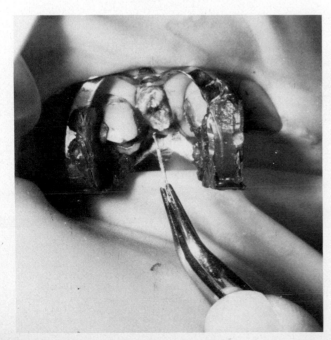

FIG. 8-143. The silver cone loosened by ultrasonic waves is removed with Stieglitz forceps. (Courtesy Dr. R. Wilcox.)

Dowels, cast posts, or silver cones that are firmly cemented into the canal space can be extremely difficult, time consuming, and often dangerous or impossible to remove. A root may be damaged by drilling or fractured by attempts to remove a tenacious post. Single-rooted teeth have been extracted accidentally by pulling strongly on an unyielding dowel.

Numerous post pullers and dowel extractors designed by dentists throughout the years have been used with varying degrees of success. The ultrasound energy method is a highly efficient and successful way to remove cemented solid objects from root canals with less damage to root structure.

A Cavitron dental unit (model 110M) adapted with a P-10 or TFI-10 insert (Fig. 8-142) may be used to provide the ultrasonic energy to break and loosen the cement bonding.

The technique requires careful chipping away of the ce-

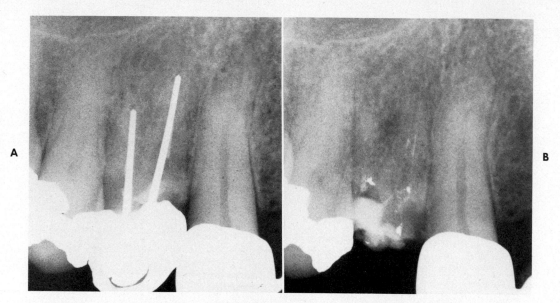

FIG. 8-144. Removal of silver cones with ultrasonic waves. **A,** Premolar with two silver cones to be removed for re-treatment, dowel reinforcement, and crown buildup. **B,** Postoperative radiograph. Silver cones removed by the ultrasonic energy, chloroform, and Stieglitz forceps. (Courtesy Dr. R. Wilcox.)

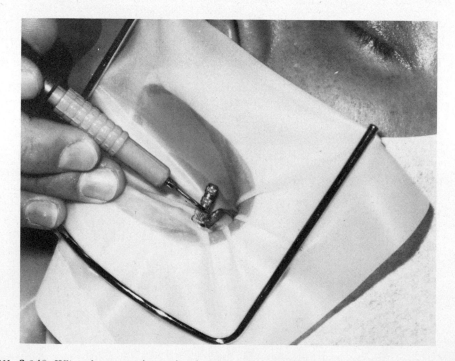

FIG. 8-145. When the access is restricted, a file may be inserted along the side of the object to be removed. The ultrasound waves are transmitted to the object when the ultrasonic probe is brought into contact with the file. (Courtesy Dr. R. Wilcox.)

ment surrounding the solid object to be removed, as described for the removal of silver cones (p. 264).

A rubber dam is used to isolate the tooth whenever possible. If the object to be removed is a silver cone, the pulp chamber is flooded with chloroform. The Cavitron is activated at setting no. 3, and the probe tip is brought into contact with the silver cone along its side. The vibration from the tip is transferred to the cone, causing the surrounding cement to shatter and loosen. The ultrasonic energy sets up shock waves in the chloroform solution and

makes the solution penetrate deeper into the canal space, exerting a faster solvent effect on the cement sealer. Also the heat generated by the ultrasound waves softens some resin cement. The loosened silver cone can be removed with minimal effort (Figs. 8-143 and 8-144).

In mandibular incisors where the access cavity may be too narrow to allow for deep penetration of the tip of the probe to reach the silver cone, a file may be inserted alongside the cone. The probe placed in contact with the file (Fig. 8-145) can transfer ultrasonic energy to the cone to facilitate its removal.

In removing a dowel cemented with insoluble cement, the ultrasonic device may be used with vacuum suction and water spray to help reduce the amount of heat generated by the ultrasound waves (Fig. 8-146). Some firmly cemented cast posts may require over 20 minutes to loosen and be removed (Fig. 8-147). Care must be taken to ensure that the tip of the probe does not come in contact with the tooth structure for a prolonged time.

Although ultrasonic energy has been used in dentistry for almost three decades, potential damage to dental supporting tissues needs to be investigated further.

SUMMARY

The aim of canal obturation is to fill the entire volume of the root canal space, including patent accessory canals and multiple foramina, completely and densely with biologically inert and compatible filling materials. Regardless of the technique used, a serious effort should be made to obtain a hermetic apical seal and contain the filling material within the confines of the root canal. An endodontic cavity preparation with a slight flare and a definite constriction or minimal opening at the dentin-cementum junc-

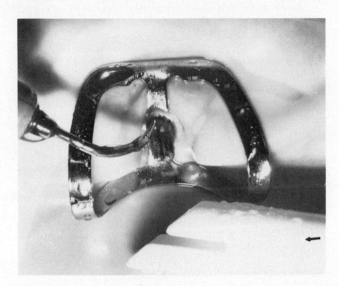

FIG. 8-146. Tip of the ultrasonic probe placed on a cemented cast dowel to be removed. Water spray is used in conjunction with vacuum suction (*arrow*) to reduce heat generated by the ultrasound waves. (Courtesy Dr. R. Wilcox.)

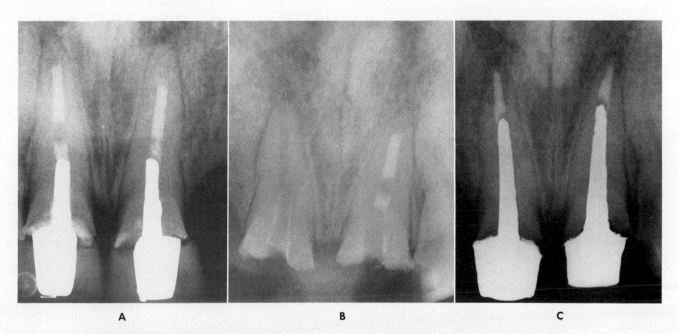

A   B   C

FIG. 8-147. Removal of cemented dowel posts with ultrasonic waves. **A,** Two cast gold posts to be removed to gain access into canals for re-treatment and construction of longer dowels on two central incisors. **B,** Dowels removed with Stieglitz forceps following application of ultrasonic energy, breaking the cement bonding. **C,** New cast gold posts cemented. (Courtesy Drs. R. Wilcox and K. Muzikar.)

tion makes it easier to obtain a three-dimensional, well-condensed gutta-percha filling with minimal apical excess. Needless invasion of the periapical space with gross excess of filling materials has no biologic justification and must be avoided.

REFERENCES

1. Allen, D.: Method of hermetically sealing smaller root canals, J. Am. Dent. Assoc. **76:**579, 1968.
2. Allison, D., Weber, C., and Walton, R.: The influence of the method of canal preparation on the quality of apical and coronal obturation, J. Endod. **5:**298, 1979.
3. Al Rafei, S.R., Sayegh, F.S., and Wright, G.: Sealing ability of a new root canal filling material. JOE, **8:**152, Apr., 1982.
4. American Dental Association, Council on Dental Therapeutics: Accepted dental therapeutics, ed. 35, Chicago, 1973-1974, The Association.
5. Antrim, D.D.: Evaluation of the cytotoxicity of root canal sealing agents on tissue culture cells in vitro. Grossman's sealer, N_2 (permanent), Rickert's selaer and Cavit, J. Endod. **2:**111, Apr. 1978.
6. Barkhordar, R.A., and Nguyen, N.T.: Paresthesia of the mental nerve after overextension with AH-26 and gutta-percha: report of case, J. Am. Dent. Assoc. **110:**202, 1985.
7. Barry, G.N., and Fried, I.L.: Sealing quality of two polycarboxylate cements used as root canal sealers, J. Endod. **1:**107, Mar. 1975.
8. Baume, L., Holz, J., and Risk, L.B.: Radicular pulpotomy for Category III pulps, parts I to III, J. Prosthet. Dent. **25:**418, 1971.
9. Bender, I.B., et al.: To culture or not to culture? Oral Surg. **18:**527, 1964.
10. Benkel, B.H., et al.: Use of a hydrophilic plastic as a root canal filling material, J. Endod. **2:**196, 1976.
11. Benner, M.D., Peters, D.D., Grover, M., and Bernier, W.: Evaluation of a new thermoplastic gutta-percha obturation technique using ^{45}Ca. J. Endod. **7:**500, 1981.
12. Biggs, J.T., Kaminiski, E.J., and Ostek, E.M.: Rat macrophage response to implanted sealer cements, J. Endod. **11:**30, 1985.
13. Block, R.M., Lewis, R.D., Sheats, J.B., and Burke, S.H.: Antibody formation to dog pulp tissue altered by N_2-type paste within the root canal, J. Endod., **8:**309, Aug. 1977.
14. Block, R.M., Lewis, R.D., Sheats, J.B., and Fawley, J.: Cell-mediated immune response to dog pulp tissue altered by Kerr (Rickert's) sealer via the root canal, J. Endod. **4:**110, Apr. 1978.
15. Block, R.M., Sheats, J.B., Lewis, R.D., and Fawley, J.: Cell-mediated response to dog pulp tissue altered by N_2 paste within the root canal, Oral Surg. **45:**131, Jan. 1978.
16. Brady, J.E., Himal, V.T., and Weir, J.C.: Periapical response to an apical plug of dentin fillings intentionally placed over root canal overcementation, J. Endod. **11:**323, Aug. 1985.
17. Brady, J.M., and del Rio, C.E.: Corrosion of endodontic silver cones in humans: a scanning electron microscope and x-ray microprobe study, J. Endod. **1:**250, 1975.
18. Bowman, G.A.: History of dentistry in Missouri, Fulton, Mo., 1983, Ovid Bell Press.
19. Brewer, D.L.: Histology of apical tissue reaction to overfill (Sargenti formula vs. gutta-percha-Grossman), J. Calif. Dent. Assoc. **3:**58, 1975.
20. Buchbinder, M.: Statistical comparison of cultured and noncultured root canal cases, J. Dent. Res. **20:**93, 1941.
21. Callahan, J.R.: Resin solution for the sealing of the dentinal tubuli and as an adjuvant in the filling of root canals, J. Allied Dent. Soc. **9:**53, 1914.
22. Carnes, E., and Skidmore, A.: Configurations and deviations of root canals of maxillary premolars, Oral Surg. **36:**880, 1973.
23. Coffae, K., and Brilliant, J.: The effect of serial preparation versus nonserial preparation on tissue removal in the root canals of extracted mandibular human molars, J. Endod. **1:**211, 1975.
24. Cohler, C.M., Newton, C.W., Patterson, S.S., and Kafrawy, A.H.: Studies of Sargenti's technique of endodontic treatment: short term response in monkeys, J. Endod. **6:**473, Mar. 1980.
25. Crane, D.L., Heuer, M.A., Kaminski, E.J., and Moser, J.B.: Biological and physical properties of an experimental root canal sealer without eugenol, J. Endod. **6:**438, Feb. 1980.
26. Czonstkowsky, M., Michanowicz, A.E., and Vasquez, J.A.: Evaluation of an injection of thermoplasticized low-temperature gutta-percha using radioactive isotopes, J. Endod. **11:**71, 1985.
27. Dow, P.R., and Ingle, J.I.: Isotope determination of root canal failure, Oral Surg. **8:**1100, 1955.
28. Eguchi, D.S., Peters, D.D., Hollinger, J., and Lorton, L.: A comparison of the area of the canal space occupied by gutta-percha following four gutta-percha techniques using Procosol sealer, J. Endod. **11:**166, 1985.
29. El Deeb, M.E., Nguyen, T.T.Q., and Jensen, J.R.: The dentinal plug: its effects on confining substances to the canal and on the apical seal, J. Endod. **9:**355, 1983.
30. Erausquin, J., and Muruzabal, M.: Response to periapical tissues in the rat molar to root canal fillings with Diaket and AH-26, Oral Surg. **21:**786, 1966.
31. Erausquin, J., and Muruzabal, M.: Tissue reactions to root canal cements in the rat molar, Oral Surg. **26:**360, Sept. 1968.
32. Evans, J.T., and Simon, J.S.: Evaluation of the apical seal produced by injected thermoplasticized gutta-percha in the absence of smear layer and root canal sealer, J. Endod. **12:**101, 1986.
33. Feldman, G., and Nyborg, H. Tissue reaction to root canal filling material. Odontol Revy **15:**33, 1964.
34. Fisher, J.: Preliminary investigation in the effectiveness of the McSpadden automated thermatic condenser. Thesis, Boston University School of Graduate Dentistry, 1980.
34a. Fogel, B.A.: A comparative study of five materials for use in filling root canal spaces, Oral Surg. **43:**284, 1977.
35. Food and Drug Administration: Memorandum to state drug officials, Washington, D.C., 1974, U.S. Government Printing Office.
36. Formaldehyde—an assessment of its health effect, National Academy of Sciences, Mar. 1980.
37. Frank, A.L.: Improvement of the crown-root ratio by endodontic endosseous implants, J. Am. Dent. Assoc. **14:**451, 1967.
38. Gaffney, J.L., et al.: Expanded use of the ultrasonic scaler, J. Endod. **5:**228, 1981.
39. Goldberg, F.: Relation between corroded silver points and endodontic failures, J. Endod. **7:**224, 1981.
40. Goldberg, F., and Gurfinkel, J.: Analysis of the use of Dycal with gutta percha points as an endodontic filling technique, Oral Surg. **47:**78, Jan. 1979.
41. Goldberg, F., and Massone, E.J.: Analysis of Hydron as an endodontic filling material. Transactions, 36th Annual Session, American Association of Endodontists, Los Angeles, 1980.
42. Goodman, A., Schilder, H., and Aldrich, W.: The thermomechanical properties of gutta-percha. IV. A thermal profile of the warm gutta-percha packing procedure, Oral Surg. **51:**544, May 1981.
43. Greenberg, M.: Filling root canals in deciduous teeth by an injection technique, Dent. Dig. **67:**574, 1961.
44. Greenberg, M.: Filling root canals by an injection technique, Dent. Dig. **69:**61, 1963.
45. Grossman, L.I.: Endodontics, ed. 9, Philadelphia, 1978, Lea & Febiger.
46. Gutiérrez, J.H., et al.: Personal communication with F. Goldberg, 1979.
47. Guttuso, J.: Histopathologic study of rat connective tissue response to endodontic materials, Oral Surg. **16:**7, 1963.
48. Hardt, N., and Kaul, A.: Untersuchungen über den Verbleib des Bleies im Wurzelkanalfüllmaterial N-2, Dtsch. Zahnaertzl. Z. **28:**580, 1973.
49. Harnden, D.G.: Tests for carcinogenicity and mutagenicity, Int. Endod. J., **14:**35, 1981.

50. Harris, G.Z., Dickey D.J., Lemon, R.R., and Luebke, R.G.: Apical seal: McSpadden vs lateral condensation, J. Endod. **6**:273, 1982.
51. The hazards of formaldehyde. Alert Sheet. U.S. Consumer Product Safety Commission (Bulletin), Mar. 1980.
52. Hendry, J.A., Jeansonne, B.G., Dummett, C.O., Jr., and Burrell, W.E.: Comparison of calcium hydroxide and zinc oxide and eugenol pulpectomies in primary teeth of dogs, Oral Surg. **54**:445, 1982.
53. Holland, G.R.: Periapical response to apical plugs of dentin and calcium hydroxide in ferret canines, J. Endod. **10**:71, Feb. 1984.
54. Holland, R., deMello, W., Nery, M.J., Bernabe, P.F.E., and deSouza, V.: Reaction of human periapical tissue to pulp extirpation and immediate root canal filling with calcium hydroxide, J. Endod. **3**:63, Feb. 1977.
55. Holland, R., deSouza, V., Nery, M.J., Bernabe, P.F.E., deMello, W., and Otoboni Filho, J.A.: Apical hard tissue deposition in adult teeth of monkeys with use of calcium hydroxide, Aust. Dent. J. **25**:189, 1980.
56. Holland, R., deSouza, V., Nery, M.J., Otoboni Filho, J.A.: Overfilling and refilling monkey's pulpless teeth, J. Can. Dent. Assoc. **6**:387, 1980.
57. Holland, R., deSouza, V., Nery, M.J., deMello, W., Bermabe, C.D., and Octoboni, J.A.: Tissue reaction following apical plugging of the root canal with infected dentin chips, Oral Surg. **49**:366, Apr. 1980.
58. Holland, R., Nery, M.J., deMello, W., deSouza, V., Bernabe, C.D., and Otoboni Filho, C.D.: Root canal treatment with calcium hydroxide. I. Effect of overfilling and refilling, Oral Surg. **47**:87, Jan. 1979.
59. Holland, R., Nery, M.J., deMello, W., deSouza, V., Bernabe, C.D., and Otoboni Filho, C.D.: Root canal treatment with calcium hydroxide. II. Effect of instrumentation beyond the apices, Oral Surg. **47**:93, Jan. 1979.
60. Holland, R., Nery, M.J., deMello, W., deSouza, V., Bernabe, C.D., and Otoboni Filho, C.D.: Root canal treatment with calcium hydroxide. III. Effect of debris and pressure filling, Oral Surg. **47**:185, Feb. 1979.
61. Ingle, J.I., and Beveridge, E.E.: Endodontics, ed. 2, Philadelphia, 1976, Lea & Febiger.
62. Ingle, J.I., and Zeldow, B.J.: An evaluation of mechanical instrumentation and negative culture in endodontic therapy, J.Am. Dent. Assoc. **57**:471, 1958.
63. Ishley D.J., and Eldeeb, M.E.: An in vitro assessment of the quality of apical seal of thermomechanically obturated canals with and without sealer, J. Endod. **9**:242, 1983.
64. Jacobson, E.L., Bery, P.F., and BeGole, E.A.: The effectiveness of apical dentin plugs in sealing endodontically treated teeth, J. Endod. **11**:289, July 1985.
65. Johnston, H.B.: The principle of diffusion applied to the Callahan method of pulp canal filling, Dent. Summ. **43**:743, 1927.
66. Jones, G.: The use of Silastic as an injectable root canal obturating material, J. Endod. **6**:552, May 1980.
67. Kapsimalis, P., and Evans, R.: Sealing properties of endodontic filling materials using radioactive isotopes, Oral Surg. **22**:386, Sept. 1966.
68. Keane, K., and Harrington, G.W.: The use of a chloroform-softened gutta-percha master cone and its effect on the apical seal, J. Endod. **10**:57, 1984.
69. Kennedy, W.A., Walker, W.A., and Gough, R.W.: Smear layer removal effects on apical leakage, J. Endod. **1**:21, 1986.
70. Kerekes, K., and Rowe, A.H.R.: Thermomechanical compaction of gutta-percha root filling, Int. Endod. J. **15**:27, 1982.
70a. Ketterl, W.: Kriterion für den Erfolg der Vitalexstirpation, Dtsch. Zahnaerztl. Z. **20**:407, 1965.
71. Krakow, A.A., and Berk, H.: Efficient endodontic procedure with the use of a pressure syringe, Dent. Clin. North Am., July 1965, p. 387.
72. Kronman, J.H., et al.: Evaluation of intracytoplasmic particles in histiocytes after endodontic therapy with a hydrophilic plastic, J. Dent. Res. **56**:795, 1977.
73. Kuttler, Y.: Microscopic investigation of root apexes, J. Am. Dent. Assoc. **50**:554, 1955.
74. Langeland, K.: Is N-2 an acceptable method of treatment? In Grossman, L.I., editor: Transactions, Fifth International Conference on Endodontics, Philadelphia, 1973, University of Pennsylvania.
75. Langeland, K., Olsson, B., and Pascon, E.A.: Biological evaluation of Hydron, J. Endod. **7**:196, 1981.
76. Lee, H., and Teigler, D.: Review of biological safety testing of Endo-Fill, research report RR-82-101, South El Monte, Calif., Apr. 1982, Lee Pharmaceuticals.
77. Leonardo, M.R., Leal, J.M., and Simoes Filho, A.P.: Pulpectomy: immediate root canal filling with calcium hydroxide, Oral Surg. **49**:441, May 1980.
78. Lewis, B.B., and Chestner, S.B.: Formaldehyde in dentistry: a review of the mutagenic and carcinogenic potential, J. Am. Dent. Assoc. **103**:429, Sept. 1981.
79. Lugassy, A.A., and Yee, F.: Root canal obturation with gutta-percha: a scanning electron microscope comparison of vertical compaction and automated thermatic condensation, J. Endod. **8**:120, 1982.
80. Lysenko, L.V.: Antiphlogistic action of eucalyptus oil azulene, Farmakol. Toksikol. **30**:341, 1967.
81. Maisto, O.A., and Erausquin, J.: Reacción de los tejidos periapicales del molar de la rata a las prastas de obturación reabsorbibles, Rev. Assoc. Odontol. Argent. **53**:12, 1965.
82. manhart, J.J.: The calcium hydroxide method of endodontic sealing. Oral Surg. **54**:219, 1982.
83. Marlin, J., et al.: Clinical use of injection-molded thermoplasticized gutta-percha for obturation of the root canal system, a preliminary report, J. Endod. **7**:277, 1981.
84. Martin, H.: Personal communication, April 1985.
84a. Martin, H.: Personal communication, April 20, 1986.
85. Maruzzela, J.C., and Sicurella, N.A.: Antibacterial activity of essential oil vapors, J. Am. Pharm. Assoc. **49**:692, 1960.
86. Mayer, A., and Ketterl, W.: Dauererfolge bei der Pulpitisbehandlung. Dtsch. Zahnaeztl. Z., **13**:883, 1958.
87. McComb, D., and Smith, D.C.: Comparison of the physical properties of polycarboxylate-based and conventional root canal sealers, J. Endod. **2**:228, Aug. 1976.
88. McElroy, D.L., and Wach, E.C.: Endodontic treatment with a zinc oxide–Canada balsam filling material, J. Am. Dent. Assoc. **56**:801, 1958.
89. Michanowicz, A.E., and Czonstkowsky, M.: Sealing properties of an injection-thermoplasticized low-temperature (70° C) gutta-percha: a preliminary study, J. Endod. **10**:563, 1984.
89a. Michanowicz, A.E., Czonstkowsky, M., and Peisco, N.: Low-temperature (70° C) injection gutta-percha: a scanning electron microscopic investigation, J. Endod. **12**:64, 1986.
90. Mohammad, A.R., Mincer, H.H., Hounis, O., Dillingham, E., and Siskin, M.: Cytotoxicity evaluation of root canal sealers by the tissue culture–agar overlay technique, Oral Surg. **45**:768, May 1978.
91. Moreno, A.: Thermomechanical softened gutta-percha technique, J. Mex. Dent. Assoc. **33**:13, Mar 1976.
92. Moreno, A.: Thermomechanically softened gutta-percha root canal filling, J. Endod. **3**:186, May 1977.
93. Morse, D.R.: The endodontic culture technique: an impractical and unnecessary procedure, Dent. Clin. North Am. **15**:793, 1971.
94. Morse, D.R., and Wilcko, J.M.: Gutta percha–eucapercha: a new look at an old technique, Gen. Dent. **26**:58, 1978.
95. Morse, D.R., Wilcko, J.M., Pullon, P.A., et al.: A comparative tissue toxicity evaluation of the liquid components of gutta-percha root canal sealers, J. Endod. **7**:545, 1981.

96. Munaco, F.S., Miller, W.A., and Everett, M.M.: A study of long-term toxicity of endodontic materials with use of an in vitro model, J. Endod. **4:**151, May 1978.

97. Murrin, J.R., Reader, A., Foreman, D.W., Beck, F.M., and Meyers, W.J.: Hydron versus gutta-percha and sealer: a study of endodontic leakage using the scanning electron microscope and energy-dispersive analysis, J. Endod. **11:**101, 1985.

98. Newton, C.W., Patterson, S.S., and kafrawy, A.H.: Studies of Sargenti's technique of endodontic treatment: six-month and one-year responses, J. Endod. **6:**509, Apr. 1980.

99. Nicholson, R.J., Nguyen, N.T., Merrill, P.W., and Casanova, F.: Tissue response to an acrylic reinforced gutta percha, J. Cal Dent. Assoc. **7:**55, Sept. 1979.

100. Nygaard-Østby, B.: Introduction to endodontics, Oslo, 1971, Scandinavian University Books.

101. Ochi, S.: Studies on the cellular response to various root canal filling materials, Bull. Exp. Biol. **14:**1, 1964.

102. Oliet, S.: Evaluation of culturing in endodontic therapy, Oral Surg. **15:**727, 1962.

103. Olsson, B., Sliwkowski, A., and Langeland, K.: Subcutaneous implantation for the biological evaluation of endodontic materials, J. Endod. **7:**355, 1981.

104. O'Neil, K.J., Pitts, D.S., and Harrington, G.W.: Evaluation of the apical seal produced by the McSpadden Compactor and by lateral condensation with a chloroform-softened primary cone, J. Endod. **9:**190, 1983.

105. Oswald, R.J., and Friedman, C.E.: Periapical response to dentin filings, Oral Surg. **49:**344, Apr. 1980.

106. Pitts, D.L., Jones, J.E., and Oswald, R.J.: A histological comparison of calcium hydroxide plugs and dentin plugs used for the control of gutta-percha root canal filling material, J. Endod. **10:**283, July 1984.

107. Rappaport, H.M., Lilly, G.E., and Kapsimalis, P.: Toxicity of endodontic filling materials, Oral Surg. **18:**785, Dec. 1964.

108. Rising, D.W., Goldman, M., and Brayton, S.M.: Histologic appraisal of three experimental root canal filling materials, J. Endod. **1:**172, May 1975.

108a. Roig-greene, J.L.: The retrieval of foreign from root canals: a simple aid, J. Endod. **9:**394, Sept. 1983.

109. Russin, T.P., Zardiachas, L.D., Reader, A., and Menke, R.A.: Apical seals obtained with laterally condensed, chloroform softened gutta percha and Grossman's sealer, J. Endod. **6:**678, 1980.

110. Saito, S.: Characteristics of glass ionomer cements and clinical application. J. Dent. Med. **10:**1, July 1979.

111. Sampeck, A.J.: The stainless steel endodontic file: its use in obturation of difficult root canals. Thesis, School of Dentistry, University of Michigan, Ann Arbor, Mich., 1961.

112. Sanders, S.H., and Dooley, R.J.: A comparative evaluation of polycarboxylate cement as a root canal sealer utilizing roughened and nonroughened silver points, Oral Surg. **37:**629, Apr. 1974.

113. Sapone, J: Endodontic abutment prosthesis, J. Prosthet. Dent. **29:**210, 1973.

114. Sargenti, A.: Endodontic course for the general practitioner, ed. 4, Brussels, 1965, European Endodontic Society.

115. Schilder, H.: Filling root canals in three dimensions, Dent. Clin. North Am., Nov. 1967, p. 723.

116. Schoeffel, C.J., Lancaster, Calif.: Personal communication, May 1982.

117. Self-study course for the thematic condensation of gutta-percha (pamphlet), Toledo, 1979, Ransom & Randolph.

118. Seltzer, S., Maggio, J., Wollard, R.R., Brough, S.O., and Barnett, A.: Tissue reactions to polycarboxylate cements, J. Endod. **2:**208, July 1976.

119. Seltzer, S., Soltanoff, W., and Smith, J.: Periapical tissue reactions to root canal instrumentation beyond the apex and root canal fillings short of and beyond the apex, Oral Surg. **36:**725, Nov., 1973.

120. Seltzer, S., et al.: A scanning electron microscope examination of silver cones removed from endodontically treated teeth. Oral Surg. **33:**589, 1972.

121. Smith, D.C.: Some observations on endodontic cements. Presented at meeting of Canadian and American Association of Endodontics, Apr. 1972.

122. Solomon, S.M., and Oliet, S.: Rejuvenation of aged (brittle) endodontic gutta percha cones, J. Endod. **5:**233, Aug. 1979.

123. Spangberg, L.: Biologic effect of root canal filling materials, Odontol. Tdskr. **77:**502, 1969.

124. Spangberg, L.: Biological effects of root canal filling materials, Odontol. Revy **20:**133, 1969.

125. Spangberg, L.: Studies on root canal medicaments, Swed. Dent. J., **64:**1, 1971.

126. Spåangberg, L., and Langeland, K.: Biologic effects of dental materials. I. Toxicity of root canal filling materials on HeLa cells in vitro, Oral Surg. **35:**402, 1973.

127. Spielman, A., Gutman, D., and Laufer, D.: Anesthesia following endodontic overfilling with AH26, Oral Surg. **52:**554, 1981.

128. Spradling, P.M., and Senia, E.S.: The relative sealing ability of paste-type filling materials, J. Endod. **8:**543, Dec. 1982.

129. Tamse, A., et al.: Paresthesia following overextension of AH26: report of two cases and review of the literature, J. Endod. **8:**88, 1982.

130. Tanzilli, J.P., Nevins, A.J., and Borden, B.B.: A histologic study comparing Hydron and gutta-percha as root canal filling materials in monkeys, J. Endod. **7:**396, 1981.

131. Torabinejad, M., Kettering, J.D., and Bakland, L.K.: Evaluation of systemic immunogical reactions to AH-26 root canal sealer, J. Endod. **5:**196, July 1979.

132. Torabinejad, M., et al.: Scanning electron microscopic study of root canal obturation using thermoplasticized gutta-percha, J. Endod. **4:**250, 1978.

133. Torneck, C.D., Smith, J.S., and Grindall, P.: Biologic effects of procedures on developing incisor teeth. II. Effect of pulp injury and oral contamination, Oral Surg. **35:**378, Mar. 1973.

134. Tronstad, L.: Tissue reactions following apical plugging of the root canal with dentin chips in monkey teeth subjected to pulpectomy, Oral Surg. **45:**297, Feb. 1978.

135. von Fraunhofer, J.A., and Branstetter, J.: The physical properties of four endodontic sealer cements, J. Endod. **8:**126, Mar. 1982.

136. Weine, F.S.: Endodontic therapy, ed. 3, St. Louis, 1982, The C.V. Mosby Co.

137. Wennberg, A.: Biological evaluation of root canal sealers using in vitro and in vivo methods, J. Endod. **6:**784, Oct. 1980.

138. Wollard, R., Brough, S., Maggio, J., and Seltzer, S.: Scanning and electron microscopic examination of root canal filling materials, J. Endod. **2:**98, Apr. 1976.

139. Wong, M., Peters, D.D., and Lorton, L.: Comparison of gutta-percha filling techniques: compaction (mechanical), vertical (warm), and lateral condensation techniques, part 1, J. Endod. **7:**151, 1981.

140. Wong, M., Peters, D.D., Lorton, L., and Bernier, W.E.: Comparison of gutta-percha filling techniques: three chloroform-gutta percha filling techniques, part 2, J. Endod. **8:**4, 1982.

141. Yates, J., and Hembree, J.: Microleakage of three root canal cements, J. Endod. **6:**591, June 1980.

142. Yee, F.S., et al.: Three dimensional obturation of the root canal using injection-molded, thermoplasticized dental gutta-percha, J. Endod. **3:**168, 1977.

143. Yee, R.D.J., Newton, C.W., and Patterson, S.S.: The effects of canal preparation and leakages characteristic of the apical dentin plug, J. Endod. **10:**308, 1984.

144. Zakariasen, K.L., and Stadem, P.S.: Microleakage associated with modified eucapercha and chlorapercha root-canal-filling techniques, Int. Endod. J. **15:**67, 1982.

145. Zeldow, B.J., and Ingle, J.I.: Correlation of the positive culture to the prognosis of endodontically treated teeth: a clinical study, J. Am. Dent. Assoc. **66:**9, 1963.

146. Zielke, D.R., Brady, J.M., and del Rio, C.E.: Corrosion of silver cones in bone: a scanning electron microscope and microprobe analysis, J. Endod. **1:**356, 1975.

147. Zmener, O., and Dominguez, F.V.: Tissue response to a glass ionomer used as an endodontic cement, Oral Surg. **56:**198, Aug. 1983.

Self-assessment questions

1. The main objective of canal obturation is to
   a. Equalize the amount of core material and sealer within the canal
   b. Obliterate the canal space in all dimensions
   c. Seal the main canal from the surrounding tissue fluids
   d. Fill the endodontic lesions in a lateral or periapical location

2. It is best to delay obturation if the tooth
   a. Is asymptomatic
   b. Is dry in the canal spaces
   c. Shows no sinus tract
   d. Has a dislodged temporary filling

3. An ideal root canal filling material should
   a. Provide sufficient shrinkage to seal the canal
   b. Seal the canal laterally and apically, conforming to canal walls
   c. Be resorbable to tissue fluids to prevent irritation
   d. Have a porous surface to support tissue growth

4. An ideal root canal sealer used with a semisolid cone will
   a. Fill irregularities between the filling and canal walls
   b. Usually be irritating to periapical tissues
   c. Be radiolucent at placement but not at final set
   d. Have little effect on the final outcome

5. Standardized gutta-percha cones are used for primary cones because such cones are
   a. Long, tapered, and soluble in chloroform
   b. Well-suited to the narrow, curved canals
   c. Similar to the diameter and taper of root canal instruments
   d. Rigid, strong, and easily placed in a root canal

6. A significant disadvantage of gutta-percha as a filling material is the
   a. Reaction between gutta-percha and periapical tissues
   b. Difficulty of preparing a post space
   c. Solubility of gutta-percha in chloroform and xylol
   d. Lack of rigidity in the smaller sizes

7. The primary gutta-percha cone must fit the canal wall tightly in the
   a. Apical third
   b. Middle third
   c. Cervical third
   d. Entire canal

8. If the radiographs show the cone to be too short, the clinician may
   a. Use a lubricant to seat the cone further
   b. Instrument the canal to a larger size and refit the cone
   c. Trim 1 mm from the end of the cone and reinsert
   d. Change to a larger cone and exert apical pressure

9. The main component of most root canal sealers is
   a. Epoxy resin
   b. Polyvinyl resin
   c. Zinc oxide–engenol
   d. Precipitated silver

10. The most widely used root canal sealer today is
    a. Rickert's sealer
    b. Wach's sealer
    c. Chloropercha
    d. Grossman-type sealer

11. Prior to obturation with gutta-percha, instrumentation must result in canal walls that are
    a. Parallel throughout their length
    b. Slightly tapered to the apical constriction
    c. Well tapered to the apical constriction
    d. Widest in the apical and midroot areas

12. The vertical condensation with warm gutta-percha technique
    a. Softens gutta-percha by heat and vertically condenses the gutta-percha mass to fill the canal in three dimensions
    b. Requires a primary cone with binding or "tugback" at the prepared canal length
    c. Utilizes pointed cold spreaders for condensation
    d. Softens the gutta-percha with a solvent, then condenses vertically with warmed blunt-ended pluggers

13. The most desirable vertical extent of a root canal filling is
    a. At the same level as the radiographic apex
    b. 0.5 mm beyond the radiographic apex
    c. 0.5 mm short of the radiographic apex
    d. 0.5 mm to 1 mm short of the radiographic apex

14. An indication for the use of silver cones as the canal filling material may be
    a. Narrow, curved canals in which enlargement beyond a no. 20 or 25 instrument is inadvisable
    b. Large canals of maxillary anterior teeth
    c. Surgical cases in which root resection is anticipated
    d. Incomplete, large, or irregular canals of young patients

9

RECORDS AND LEGAL RESPONSIBILITIES

JOSEPH SCHULTZ
EDWIN J. ZINMAN
FULTON S. YEE

Records

PURPOSES OF RECORDS

Written records are necessary in any dental practice to identify the patients; to record their status before, during, and after treatment procedures; to document their acceptance or rejection of a treatment plan; to record therapy sequence, prognoses, results, and sequelae; to measure progress at successive appointments; to document consultations and referrals; to provide for ease of transfer to another practitioner; and to manage business aspects and malpractice prophylaxis.

The records must be complete, accurate, readable, written indelibly, and dated. Although alterations are forbidden, subsequent additions may be added to expand, define, modify, or clarify so long as they are dated.[4]

The evolution of written records has resulted in a combination of the "fill in" and the "check off" types of forms.

The *fill in* or essay type allows more latitude of response to a question, possibly resulting in a more detailed description; however, it also permits oversight unless one is very conscientious in noting all clinical information (Fig. 9-1).

Certain aspects of record keeping, particularly the health history, cannot employ the essay type of response to gather all the information necessary in a reasonable amount of time. The *check off* type of format is more practical and better suited for this inquiry (Fig. 9-2). Forms with questions developed to reveal pertinent data are available to alert the clinician to medical conditions that may warrant further consideration before proceeding.

BASIC ENDODONTIC RECORDS

Although they may take many forms, the basic records necessary include patient identification, health history, radiographs, evaluation and diagnosis, consent form, and treatment record. (Business records are not discussed here.)

Patient identification

The patient is usually requested to complete a form providing information essential for identification, communication, and reference (Fig. 9-3). Name address, business

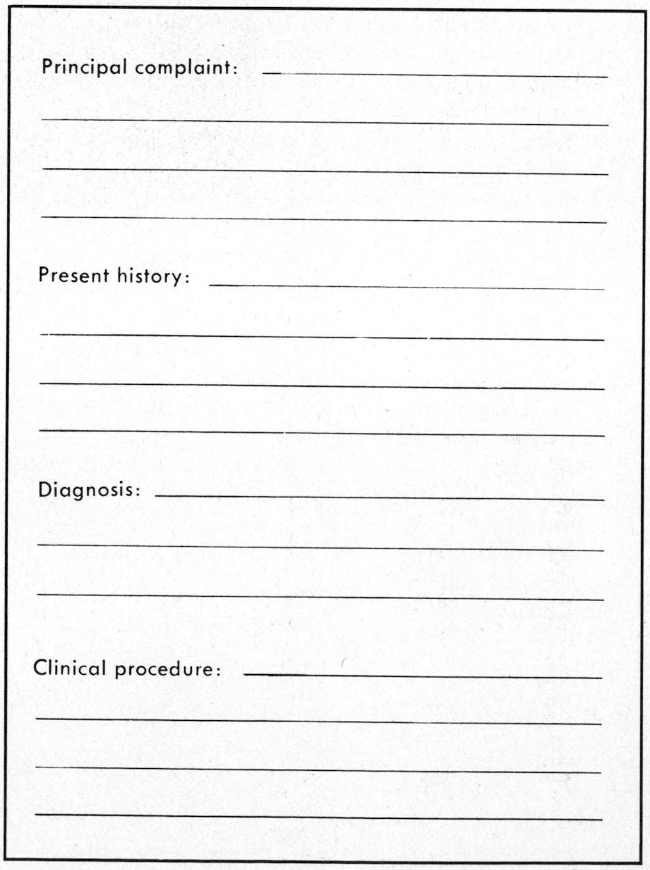
Principal complaint:
Present history:
Diagnosis:
Clinical procedure:

FIG. 9-1. "Fill-in" type of record.

Date _____

Name _____ Address _____
    Last   First   Middle   Number & Street

City _____ State _____ Zip Code _____ Home Phone _____ Business Phone _____

Date of Birth _____ Sex _____ Height _____ Weight _____ Occupation _____

Social Security No. _____ Single _____ Married _____ Name of Spouse _____

Closest Relative _____ Phone _____

If you are completing this form for another person, what is your relationship to that person? _____

Referred By: _____

In the following questions, circle yes or no, whichever applies. Your answers are for our records only and will be considered confidential.

1. Are you in good health? . . . . YES   NO

2. Has there been any change in your general health within the past year? . . . . YES   NO

3. My last physical examination was on _____

4. Are you now under the care of a physician? . . . . YES   NO

    a. If so, what is the condition being treated? _____

5. The name and address of my physician is _____
    _____
    _____
    _____

6. Have you had any serious illness or operation? . . . . YES   NO

    a. If so, what was the illness or operation? _____

7. Have you been hospitalized or had a serious illness within the past five (5) years? . . . . YES   NO

    a. If so, what was the operation? _____

8. Have you ever suffered from alcoholism or drug addiction? . . . . YES   NO

9. Do you have or have you had any of the following diseases or problems?

    a. Rheumatic fever or rheumatic heart disease . . . . YES   NO
    b. Congenital heart lesions . . . . YES   NO
    c. Cardiovascular disease (heart trouble, heart attack, coronary insufficiency, coronary occlusion,
       high blood pressure, arteriosclerosis, stroke). . . . . YES   NO
       (1) Do you have pain in chest upon exertion?. . . . . YES   NO
       (2) Are you ever short of breath after mild exercise?. . . . . YES   NO
       (3) Do your ankles swell? . . . . YES   NO
       (4) Do you get short of breath when you lie down or do you require extra pillows when you sleep? . . . . . YES   NO
       (5) Do you have a cardiac pacemaker or heart valve? . . . . YES   NO
    d. Do you have any hip or knee joint prosthesis? . . . . YES   NO
    e. Allergy . . . . YES   NO
    f. Sinus trouble . . . . YES   NO
    g. Asthma or hay fever . . . . YES   NO
    h. Hives or a skin rash . . . . YES   NO
    i. Fainting spells or seizures . . . . YES   NO
    j. Diabetes . . . . YES   NO
       (1) Do you have to urinate (pass water) more than six times a day? . . . . YES   NO
       (2) Are you thirsty much of the time? . . . . YES   NO
       (3) Does your mouth frequently become dry?. . . . . YES   NO
    k. Hepatitis, jaundice or liver disease . . . . YES   NO
    l. Arthritis . . . . YES   NO
    m. Inflammatory rheumatism (painful swollen joints) . . . . YES   NO
    n. Stomach ulcers . . . . YES   NO
    o. Kidney trouble . . . . YES   NO
    p. Tuberculosis . . . . YES   NO
    q. Do you have a persistent cough or cough up blood? . . . . YES   NO
    r. Low blood pressure . . . . YES   NO
    s. Venereal disease . . . . YES   NO
    t. AIDS or ARC . . . . YES   NO

(over)

FIG. 9-2. Health history form. (Courtesy American Dental Association.)   *Continued.*

10. Have you had abnormal bleeding associated with previous extractions, surgery, or trauma? . . . .   YES   NO

    a. Do you bruise easily? . . . .   YES   NO

    b. Have you ever required a blood transfusion? . . . .   YES   NO

       If so, explain the circumstances _____

11. Do you have any blood disorder such as anemia? . . . .   YES   NO

12. Have you had surgery or x-ray treatment for a tumor, growth, or other condition of your head or neck? . . . .   YES   NO

13. Are you taking any drug or medicine? . . . .   YES   NO

    If so, what? _____

14. Are you taking any of the following:

    a. Antibiotics or sulfa drugs . . . .   YES   NO

    b. Anticoagulants (blood thinners) . . . .   YES   NO

    c. Medicine for high blood pressure . . . .   YES   NO

    d. Cortisone (steroids) . . . .   YES   NO

    e. Tranquilizers . . . .   YES   NO

    f. Antihistamines . . . .   YES   NO

    g. Aspirin . . . .   YES   NO

    h. Insulin, tolbutamide (Orinase) or similar drug. . . . .   YES   NO

    i. Digitalis or drugs for heart trouble. . . . .   YES   NO

    j. Nitroglycerin . . . .   YES   NO

    k. Oral contraceptive or other hormonal therapy . . . .   YES   NO

    l. Other _____

15. Are you allergic or have you reacted adversely to:

    a. Local anesthetics . . . .   YES   NO

    b. Penicillin or other antibiotics . . . .   YES   NO

    c. Sulfa drugs . . . .   YES   NO

    d. Barbiturates, sedatives, or sleeping pills . . . .   YES   NO

    e. Aspirin . . . .   YES   NO

    f. Iodine . . . .   YES   NO

    g. Codeine or other narcotics . . . .   YES   NO

    h. Jewelry, wristwatches, or earings? . . . .   YES   NO

    i. Other _____

16. Have you had any serious trouble associated with any previous dental treatment? . . . .   YES   NO

    If so, explain _____

_____

17. Do you have any disease, condition, or problem not listed above that you think I should know about? . . . .   YES   NO

    If so, explain _____

_____

18. Are you employed in any situation which exposes you regularly to x-rays or other ionizing radiation? . . . .   YES   NO

19. Are you wearing contact lenses? . . . .   YES   NO

WOMEN

20. Are you pregnant? . . . .   YES   NO

21. Do you have any problems associated with your menstrual period? . . . .   YES   NO

22. Are you nursing? . . . .   YES   NO

CHIEF DENTAL COMPLAINT:

_____
SIGNATURE OF PATIENT

_____
                                                               SIGNATURE OF DENTIST

FIG. 9-2, cont'd. Health history form.

(PLEASE PRINT)   **REGISTRATION**

Date _____

Name _____ Soc. Sec. No. _____

Date of birth: _____ If a minor, parent's name: _____

Marital Status: ☐ Single   ☐ Married   ☐ Separated   ☐ Widowed   ☐ Divorced

Address _____ Phone _____

City _____ State _____ Zip Code _____

Occupation_____ Employer _____ How long? _____

Business Address _____ Phone_____

City _____ State _____ Zip Code_____

Name of spouse _____

Occupation_____ Employer _____ How long? _____

Business Address _____ Phone _____

City _____ State _____ Zip Code _____

Person responsible for account _____

Address (if different from patient's address) _____ Phone_____

City _____ State _____ Zip Code _____

Referred by: _____

Insurance Carrier _____ Group # _____ Local # _____

Name of Insured Person_____ Soc. Sec. No_____

Relationship to Patient_____
Second Insurance Carrier
(if dual coverage) _____ Group # _____ Local # _____

Name of Insured Person _____ Soc. Sec. No. _____

Relationship to Patient_____

INFORMED CONSENT

I understand Root Canal treatment is a procedure to retain a tooth which may otherwise require extraction. Although Root Canal therapy has a very high degree of clinical success, it is still a biological procedure, so it cannot be guaranteed. Occasionally, a tooth which has had Root Canal therapy may require retreatment, surgery, or even extraction.

I also understand that only the root canal treatment is to be performed at this office. The permanent (outside) restoration (filling, onlay, crown, etc.) will be done by my regular dentist.

I also acknowledge full responsibility for the payment of such services and agree to pay for them, in full, AT or BEFORE COMPLETION, unless other specific arrangements are made with the secretary.

I authorize my insurance carrier to issue the dental benefits of my plan directly to this dental office. I also authorize release of any information necessary to process dental insurance.

Signed: PATIENT, PARENT or AGENT _____

FIG. 9-3. Patient identification information. (Courtesy American Dental Association.)

address, and telephone numbers are needed to contact the patient for scheduling purposes or to inquire about treatment sequelae. Similar information about one's spouse, relative, or close friend who can be notified in an emergency is also required. In the event the patient is a minor, the parent or guardian should provide the information or be available to confirm its content. Often questions about dental insurance and financial responsibility are included to avoid any misunderstandings later.[2,4]

Health history

The patient's past and present health status should be thoroughly reviewed by the dentist before proceeding. This is to provide adequate information so dental treatment can be safely initiated (Fig. 9-2). Health questionnaires open avenues for discussion about problems of major organ systems and important biochemical mechanisms (e.g., blood coagulation). As a result of this review the dentist may suggest or insist that the patient be examined by a physician or tested by a laboratory under medical supervision to determine whether a suspected medical problem may warrant attention before endodontic therapy proceeds or whether treatment modifications should be made (e.g., drug sensitivities).[1,4]

Every health history form should require information about any current therapy, physical or psychologic, and the name of the physician. This individual may be the best one to provide advice in emergency situations. Consultation with the patient's physician may be indispensable to the patient's welfare.

These records should include general questions about the dental history and any difficulties encountered previously. A positive response should suggest further consultation.

Finally, the medical history must be updated periodically. The patient should be asked to review the original and date and sign it if conditions are unchanged. Otherwise, a new form should be completed, with the first retained for future reference.[2]

Radiographs

Radiographs are essential because they serve as additional documentation of the condition of the patient before any therapy is initiated. A panographic radiograph is not diagnostically accurate but can serve as a guide. Good periapical radiographs are essential to aid in diagnosis, to carry out endodontic therapy, to record the final result, and for follow-up comparisons at a later date.[2,3]

Evaluation and diagnosis

There should be an area on the form where the history of the current problem, clinical examination, pulp testing, and radiographic results are recorded. This information provides a basis upon which a diagnosis can be made for consultation with the patient (Fig. 9-4). If therapy is indicated, the reasons can be discussed in an organized way. At times, when other factors will affect the prognosis (e.g., strategic importance or restorability of the tooth), it will be necessary to request further evaluation before any treatment is started.

Consent form

After an endodontic treatment plan and the alternatives to endodontic treatment based on the patient's medical and dental status are presented to the patient or guardian, it is necessary to discuss thoroughly the difficulties that may be encountered with the proposed treatment *and* the problems that may ensue if the patient chooses not to undergo any dental treatment. Following this discussion it is necessary to document the acceptance or rejection of the consultation recommendations with the patient's (or guardian's) signature and date. Later changes in the proposed treatment plan should also be discussed and initialed by the patient to indicate continued acceptance and to acknowledge understanding of the risks and alternatives involved.[2,4]

Treatment record—the EndoChart (Fig. 9-4)

A chart has been devised to facilitate the recording of information pertinent to the diagnosis and treatment of the endodontic patient.

The systematic acquisition and arrangement of data from the interrogatory, clinical, and radiographic examinations will expedite the formulation of an accurate diagnosis. In addition to addressing these requirements, the EndoChart enables the clinician to record all rendered treatment in exacting detail and with minimal time and effort.

The chart is divided into several sections, which are described below with directions for their utilization.

General patient data

The name, address, and phone number(s) of the patient and referring doctor are entered here. This information is printed or typed in the corresponding space by the receptionist at the patient's initial office visit.

Appointment schedule and business record

This section is divided into two parts:
1. The first portion is completed by the attending doctor after the diagnosis and treatment plan have been formulated and presented to the patient. The tooth number and quoted fee are posted, and the treatment plan is recorded by simply circling the appropriate description. Under SPECIAL INSTRUCTIONS specific treatment requests by the referring dentist are circled. Details of planned adjunctive procedures (e.g., hemisection, root resection) may be written in the adjacent space. Along with information from the patient data section, these are used for general reference by the doctor during future treatment and by the dental secretary when scheduling appointments and establishing financial arrangements.
2. The remaining portion is completed by business personnel. Information pertaining to fiscal agreements, third party coverage, and account status are included here. Appointment data, including the day, date, and scheduled procedure, are also recorded.

• • •

Portions of the following diagnosis and treatment sections may be completed by either the doctor or the chairside assistant. To comply with medical-legal recommendations, entries made by auxiliary personnel must be reviewed, approved, and endorsed by the attending dentist.

Dental history

Under CHIEF COMPLAINT it is noted first whether the patient is symptomatic at the time of examination. Narrative facts regarding the presenting problem are then recorded in the space provided. Additional details of the chief complaint obtained during successive questioning are recorded by circling the applicable descriptive adjective within each symptom parameter. (See Chapter 2.) The pain intensity index (range, 0 to 10) or pain classification (mild +, moderate + +, or severe + + +) may be registered alongside the appropriate description. For accurate assessment of the effects of prior dental treatment pertaining to the examination site, a summary account of such procedures should be documented. All pretreatment and posttreatment symptoms are described.

Medical history

Pertinent reference information (e.g., personal physician's name, address, and phone, patient's age and date of last physical examination) are recorded. The dentist should procure a detailed medical history by completing a survey of the common diseases and disorders significant to den-

| LAST NAME | FIRST NAME | MR.
MISS
MRS. | ADDRESS | HOME
PHONE | S.F. |
| | | | | BUSINESS
PHONE | T.L. |

| REF. DR. | REF. DR. ADDRESS | REF. DR.
PHONE |

TOOTH   FEE   R——————L

TREATMENT PLAN

CONSULT   RCT: SURGERY
EET   AE PE ME $Ca(OH)_2$

SPECIAL INSTRUCTIONS
POST SPACE
PREFORMED POST/B.U.
COMP AMAL TEMP. CR.

INSURANCE S D	AMT DUE	REC'D	DATE	DAY	TIME	PRO-CEDURE	X-RAY	REMARKS:
PRE-AUTH Y N								
% COVERED								
VERIFIED								
FORM SIGNED								
PT. INFORMED								
PT. PORTION								
INS SENT								

DATE			REMARKS	SIGNATURE
MO	DAY	YR		

MIDDLE INITIAL   *FIRST NAME*   *LAST NAME*

FIG. 9-4. Appointment and business sections of endodontic records.   *Continued.*

LAST NAME	FIRST NAME	TOOTH	FEE	TREATMENT PLAN	SPECIAL INSTRUCTIONS
		R ——┼—— L		CONSULT RCT: SURGERY EET AE PE ME Ca(OH)$_2$	POST SPACE PREFORMED POST / B-U COMP AMAL TEMP. CR

DENTAL HISTORY	CHIEF COMPLAINT: symptomatic / asymptomatic

SYMPTOMS	Location	Chronology	Quality	Affected By:	Prior Tx

localized   referred
diffuse   radiating
		Inception:
		
		Clinical Course:
		
		constant momentary
		intermittent lingering
			sharp Intensity
			dull + + + + + +
			    spontaneous
			pulsating provoked
			steady reproducible
			enlarging occasional
				hot palpation
				cold manipulation
				
				biting head position
				chewing activity
				percussion time of day
					Tx: restorative Yes No
					    emergency Yes No
					    RCT Yes No
					Sx Pre-Tx: Yes No
					Sx Post-Tx: Yes No Initial:

MEDICAL HISTORY	Physician Name:	Address:	Phone:	Last Physical:	Pt. Age:

Heart Condition
angina
coronary
surgery
pacemaker
Rheumatic Fever / Murmur
Hypertension / Circulatory

Anemia / Bleeding
Diabetes / Kidney
Hepatitis / Liver
Herpes
Thyroid / Hormonal
Asthma / Respiratory
Ulcers / Digestive
Migraine / Headaches

Epilepsy / Fainting
Sinusitis / ENT
Glaucoma / Visual
Mental / Neural
Tumor / Neoplasms
Alcoholism / Addictions
Infectious Diseases
Venereal Disease

Allergies:
penicillin / antibiotics
aspirin / Tylenol
codeine / narcotics
local anesthetic
N$_2$O/O$_2$
other:

Major Medical Prob:
Females: Pregnant _____ mo.
Recent Hosp./Operation:
Current Medical TX:
Medications:
Medical Status:

Initial:

EXAMINATION	RADIOGRAPHIC		CLINICAL		DIAGNOSTIC TESTS						
Tooth	Attachment Apparatus		Tooth	Soft Tissues	Tooth No.						

WNL
caries
restoration
calcification
resorption
fracture
perforation/deviation
prior RC Tx / RCF
separated instrument
canal obstruction
post / build-up
open apex
	PDL normal
	PDL thickened
	alveolar bone, WNL
	diffuse lucency
	circumscribed lucency
	resorption
	   apical
	   lateral
	hypercementosis
	osteosclerosis
	perio:
			WNL
			discoloration
			caries
			pulp exposure
			prior access
			attrition/abrasion
			fracture
			restoration
			   amalgam
			   composite
			   inlay / onlay
			   temporary
			   crown
			   abutment
				WNL
				extra-oral swelling
				intra-oral swelling
				sinus tract
				lymphadenopathy
				TMJ
				perio:
				
				      B
				M ——┼—— D
				      L
					perio
					mobility
					percussion
					palpation
					cold
					hot
					EPT
					transillum.
					cavity
					date:						

DIAGNOSIS	PULPAL	PERIAPICAL	ETIOLOGY		PROGNOSIS		
	WNL reversible pulpitis irreversible pulpitis necrosis prior RC Tx / RCF	WNL acute apical periodontitis acute apical abscess chronic periapical inflammation phoenix abscess osteosclerosis	idiopathic trauma caries periodontal restoration orthodontic attrition / abrasion prior RC Tx developmental intentional RCT		ENDODONTIC favorable questionable poor	PERIODONTAL favorable questionable poor	RESTORATIVE favorable questionable poor

PT. CONSULT	____ Examination Findings ____ Periodontal Status ____ Fracture ____ Surgery ____ Prognosis
	____ Treatment Plan ____ Restoration ____ Discoloration ____ Recall ____ Consent Form Initial:

TREATMENT	CONS	PRE-TREATMENT	CLEANING / SHAPING	OBTURATION	SURG	Rx		REMARKS
DATE	pt. / Dr.	local / R.D. / rel oc. / O.D.	access / pulpec. / canal / test / final	G.G.B. / s. file / cotton / temp / G.P. / sealer / tech.	post / B-U / temp / I&D / retro	S. R / analg. / Ab		
mo day yr								

CANAL	REF	Elec.	X-Ray	Adj	Final	Size	Rx	MEDICATION	DOSE	DISP	INSTR.		RECALL	DATE	REMARKS
B F									x		q	h			
L P									x		q	h			
MB									x		q	h			
ML									x		q	h			
DB									x						
DL									x						

FIG. 9-4, cont'd. Diagnosis and treatment sections of endodontic records. Refer to Fig. 9-5 for explanation of abbreviations.

tistry, along with a comprehensive review of corresponding organ systems and physiologic conditions. Specific entities that have affected the patient are circled. Essential remarks regarding these entries (e.g., details of consultations with the patient's physician) should be documented in the space below. A review of the patient's medical status (including recent or current conditions, treatment, and medications) completes the health history.

Examination

After the interrogatory evaluation (dental and medical history) findings obtained from the various phases of the clinical and radiographic examinations are recorded. The lists provided within each category afford the clinician a systematic format for discerning details pertinent to a proper diagnosis. The appropriate descriptions are circled, followed by the necessary notations in the accompanying spaces. The tabular arrangement allows easy recording and comparison of diagnostic test data acquired from the same tooth on different dates, as well as from different teeth on the same date. As with entries in the dental history, a pain intensity index (0 to 10) or pain classification (mild +, moderate + +, severe + + +) should be used to document diagnostic test results whenever possible.

Diagnosis

A careful analysis of accumulated examination data should result in the determination of an accurate pulpal and periapical diagnosis. The appropriate clinical conditions are circled, as are the probably etiologic factors responsible for the presenting problem. Alternative modalities of therapy are considered and analyzed. The recommended treatment plan is circled, followed by a prognostic assessment of the intended therapeutic course.

Patient consultation

The patient should be informed of the diagnosis and treatment plan before any therapy is rendered by the attending dentist. This consultation should include an explanation of alternative treatment approaches and rationale, as well as any preexisting conditions and consequences that may affect the outcome of intended therapy. Documentation of such discussion is made by simply completing and endorsing the check list provided.

Treatment

All treatment rendered on a given date is documented by placing a check (√) within the designated procedural category. Only the most frequent treatment procedures are included for tabulation. Descriptions of occasional procedures or explanatory treatment remarks should be entered in writing. A separate dated entry should be made for each patient visit, phone communication (e.g., consultations with the patient or other doctors), and correspondence (e.g., biopsy report, treatment letters).

Individual root canal lengths are recorded by circling the corresponding anatomic designation and the method of length determination (e.g., radiograph or electronic measuring device), writing the measurement in millimeters, and indicating the reference point.

Whenever a medication is prescribed or dispensed, the date and type of drug are noted in the treatment table under ℞. The name, dosage, quantity, and instructions for use of these medications are immediately footnoted and recorded in the section below.

The intervals, dates, and results of periodic recall examinations are entered in the spaces provided.

A completed EndoChart is presented to illustrate its proper utilization (Fig. 9-5). An explanatory key listing the standard abbreviations used in the chart is also provided.

Legal responsibilities

Prophylaxis is the keystone of good dental as well as legal care. Endodontic treatment performed with the requisite standard of care not only saves treated teeth but in-

pt.	= Patient	temp	= Temporary restoration
Dr.	= Doctor	G.P.	= Gutta percha
local	= Local anesthetic	sealer	= Type of sealer used
R.D.	= Rubber dam	tech.	= Technique for canal obturation
reloc.	= Relieved occlusion	post	= Preformed stainless steel post
O.D.	= Open and drain	B-U	= Buildup of tooth
access	= Access cavity	I & D	= Incision and drainage
pulpec	= Pulpectomy	retro	= Retrograde procedure
canal	= Identify canal that has been cleaned and shaped	S/R	= Suture removal
test	= Test file	analg.	= Analgesic
final	= Final file	Ab	= Antibiotic
G.G.B.	= Gates-Glidden bur	SD	= Single insurance or dual coverage
s. file	= Serial filing	YN	= Insurance preauthorized, Yes or No
cotton	= Placed in pulp chamber between treatments	WNL	= Within normal limits

FIG. 9-5. Treatment record section used to detail progress and events.

Continued.

LAST NAME		FIRST NAME	MR. MISS MRS.	ADDRESS		HOME PHONE		S.F.
						BUSINESS PHONE		T.L.

REF. DR.		REF. DR. ADDRESS		REF. DR. PHONE

TOOTH   FEE   (CONSULT)   TREATMENT PLAN   SURGERY   SPECIAL INSTRUCTIONS

R —— L   19   EET   (RCT:)   AE PE (ME)   Ca(OH)$_2$ POST SPACE   (PREFORMED POST/B.U.)   *distal canal*   COMP (AMAL) TEMP. CR.

INSURANCE S D	AMT DUE	REC'D	DATE	DAY	TIME	PRO- CEDURE	X-RAY	REMARKS:
PRE-AUTH Y N								
% COVERED								
VERIFIED								
FORM SIGNED								
PT. INFORMED								
PT. PORTION								
INS SENT								

(side label: MIDDLE INITIAL)

DATE			REMARKS	SIGNATURE
MO	DAY	YR		
3	5	83	Filled mesial lingual canal to furcation. Recommend full veneer cast crown; Pt will call general dentist for appt.	PC

(side labels: FIRST NAME, LAST NAME)

FIG. 9-5, cont'd. For legend see previous page.

LAST NAME	FIRST NAME	TOOTH R—L 19	FEE	TREATMENT PLAN (CONSULT) (RCT) SURGERY EET AE PE (ME) Ca(OH)₂	SPECIAL INSTRUCTIONS POST SPACE (PREFORMED POST/B-U) COMP AMAL TEMP. CR

DENTAL HISTORY — CHIEF COMPLAINT: (symptomatic) asymptomatic

MOD amalgam placed on #19 three days ago by general dentist. Patient unable to locate source of pain — spontaneous; provoked by heat/cold/chewing.

SYMPTOMS	Location	Chronology	Quality	Affected By:	Prior Tx
mandibular left posterior	Inception: 3 days ago	sharp	Intensity	(hot) ++	palpation	Tx: restorative (Yes) No MOD Amalgam #19

Clinical Course:

sharp — dull
Intensity + ++ +++
(hot) ++   palpation
(cold) +++   manipulation
(pulsating) (provoked)   biting / head position
steady / reproducible   (chewing) + / activity
(spontaneous)   percussion / time of day

iocalized / referred   (constant) / momentary
(diffuse) (radiating)   intermittent / (lingering)
enlarging / (occasional)

Tx: restorative (Yes) No MOD Amalgam #19
emergency Yes (No)
RCT Yes (No)
Sx Pre-Tx: Yes (No)
Sx Post-Tx: (Yes) No   Initial: PC

MEDICAL HISTORY — Physician Name: — Address: — Phone: — Last Physical: 1-10-83 — Pt. Age: 45

Heart Condition	Anemia / Bleeding	Epilepsy / Fainting	Allergies:	Major Medical Prob:
angina	Diabetes / Kidney	Sinusitis / ENT	penicillin / antibiotics	Females: Pregnant _____ mo.
coronary	Hepatitis / Liver	Glaucoma / Visual	aspirin / Tylenol	Recent Hosp./Operation:
surgery	Herpes	Mental / Neural	codeine / narcotics	Current Medical TX:
pacemaker	Thyroid / Hormonal	Tumor / Neoplasms	local anesthetic	Medications: aspirin for toothache – ineffective
Rheumatic Fever / Murmur	(Asthma) Respiratory	Alcoholism / Addictions	N₂O/O₂	Medical Status:
Hypertension / Circulatory	Ulcers / Digestive	Infectious Diseases	other:	non-contributory
	Migraine / Headaches	Venereal Disease		

Hx childhood asthma

Initial: PC

EXAMINATION

RADIOGRAPHIC		CLINICAL		DIAGNOSTIC TESTS				

Tooth	Attachment Apparatus	Tooth	Soft Tissues	Tooth No.	18	19	20	14
WNL	PDL normal	WNL	(WNL)	perio	WNL	WNL	WNL	WNL
caries	(PDL thickened)	(discoloration)	extra-oral swelling	mobility	NO	NO	NO	1–
(restoration) pulp	(alveolar bone, WNL)	caries	intra-oral swelling	percussion	WNL	+	WNL	WNL
(calcification) chamber	diffuse lucency	pulp exposure	sinus tract	palpation	WNL	WNL	WNL	WNL
resorption	circumscribed lucency	prior access	lymphadenopathy	cold	WNL	+++	+	WNL
fracture	resorption	attrition/abrasion	TMJ	hot	WNL	++	WNL	+
perforation/deviation	apical	fracture	perio: WNL	EPT				
prior RC Tx / RCF	lateral	(restoration)		transillum.				
separated instrument	hypercementosis	(amalgam) composite		cavity				
canal obstruction	osteosclerosis	inlay / onlay		date:	³/₁/83	³/₁/83	³/₁/83	³/₁/03
post / build-up	perio:	temporary						
open apex	WNL	crown						
		abutment						

(Soft Tissues diagram) B / 1 2 / M — D / 1 1 / L

recommend RCT on #19

DIAGNOSIS

PULPAL	PERIAPICAL	ETIOLOGY		PROGNOSIS		
WNL	(WNL)	idiopathic	trauma	ENDODONTIC	PERIODONTAL	RESTORATIVE
reversible pulpitis	acute apical periodontitis	caries	periodontal	(favorable)	(favorable)	(favorable)
(irreversible pulpitis)	acute apical abscess	(restoration)	orthodontic	questionable	questionable	questionable
necrosis	chronic periapical inflammation	attrition / abrasion	prior RC Tx	poor	poor	poor
prior RC Tx / RCF	phoenix abscess	developmental	intentional RCT			
	osteosclerosis					

PT. CONSULT — ✓ Examination Findings ✓ Periodontal Status ✓ Fracture ✓ Surgery ✓ Prognosis ✓ Treatment Plan ✓ Restoration ✓ Discoloration ✓ Recall ✓ Consent Form — Initial: PC

TREATMENT

DATE	CONS	PRE-TREATMENT	CLEANING / SHAPING	OBTURATION	SURG	Rx	REMARKS
mo day yr	Pt. / Dr.	local / R.D. / rel. oc. / O.D.	access / pulpec. / canal / test / final / G.G.B. / s. file / cotton / temp	G.P. / sealer / tech. / post / B-U / temp	I&D / retro / S.R.	analg / Ab	
3 1 83	✓	reproduced pt's Sx to #19			①		
		✓ ✓ ✓	✓ MB ✓ ✓ ✓	lidocaine 2% c̄ epi 1:100,000			
			ML ✓ ✓ ✓ ✓	x2 carpules – required			
			DB ✓ ✓ ✓	intrapulpal			
			DL ✓ ✓ ✓ ✓ ✓				PC
3 5 83	✓ ✓	Pt. asymptomatic	✓ K W ✓ ✓	lido c̄ epi 1:100,000 x2			PC

filled all canals c̄ warm G-P; preformed post distal; amalgam

CANAL	REF	Elec.	X-Ray	Adj	Final	Size	Rx	MEDICATION	DOSE	DISP	INSTR.	RECALL	DATE	REMARKS
B F							①	Empirin-Cod #3	x 16	1	q 4ʰ prn	6 mos.	9/16/84	WNL – crowned
L P									x		q h	12 mos	3/2/84	WNL – asympto.
MB	MBC		✓	21.0	21.0	25			x		q h			
ML	MLC		✓	21.0	21.5	25			x		q h			
DB	BG		✓	19.5	20.0	30			x					
DL	BG		✓	20.0	20.0	35			x					

FIG. 9-5, cont'd. For legend see p. 281.

sulates the treating dentist from a lawsuit for professional negligence. Legal prophylaxis in endodontics protects the patient, by careful attention to the principles of due care, from avoidable or unnecessary risks associated with endodontic therapy.

Although varying degrees of risk are inherent in every dental procedure, failure to follow the dictates of sound dental practice increases the risk of negligently induced deleterious results. Accordingly, the keystone of the law of negligence is designed to prevent foreseeable risks of injury when reasonably possible.

STANDARD OF CARE DEFINED

Good endodontic practice as defined by the courts is the standard of care legally required to be performed by the treating dentist. The standard of care does not require perfection, ideal care, or by analogy an A + grade in endodontics. Instead the legal standard is that degree of care which a *reasonably* careful or prudent practitioner would perform under the same or similar circumstances of treatment. Therefore it is a flexible standard that accommodates individual variants in treatment. Legally acceptable due care constitutes reasonable conduct as a minimum. Additional precautionary steps that exceed the minimum floor of reasonableness and approach the ceiling of ideal care are laudable but are not legally mandated.

Standard dental practice is sometimes confused with customary practice. Custom constitutes evidence of prudent practice but not always is the equivalent. Consequently, what the majority of practitioners would do under the particular circumstances of treatment may not conform to reasonable or prudent care.[5] Common negligent customs, although widespread, are neither legal nor laudable. Jaywalking, exceeding the 55 mph speed limit, and not wearing seat belts are common examples.

Examples of negligent customary practices include failure of the majority of dentists to take diagnostic quality radiographs,[6] failure to sterilize dental instruments adequately,[7] failure to use a rubber dam in endodontics,[8] relying only on radiographs rather than a calibrated periodontal probe for diagnosing pathologic periodontal pockets,[9] and exclusive use of panoramic radiographs rather than periapicals and bite-wings for diagnosing caries or fractures.[10]

One who undertakes to render services in the practice of a profession or trade is required to possess the knowledge normally possessed by members of that profession or trade in good standing in similar communities.[11] This standard has been held also to apply to dentists in the practice of their profession.[12] There is a further duty in utilizing such knowledge—to use the care and skill ordinarily exercised in like cases by a reputable member of the profession practicing in the same or similar circumstances, and to use reasonable diligence and judgement in the exercise of such skill and application of learning.[13] This rule has been incorporated into the standard jury instruction pertaining to professional negligence of a health care provider.[14]

ORDINARY CARE EQUALS PRUDENT CARE

In lay terms ordinary is commonly understood to mean ". . . .b) lacking in excellence . . .c) being of poor or mediocre quality." However, as expressed in the context of actions for negligence, "ordinary" care has assumed a technical-legal definition somewhat different from its common meaning. *Black's Law Dictionary,* 4th edition, describes ordinary care as "that degree which persons of ordinary care and prudence are accustomed to use or employ . . . that is, reasonable care."

In adopting this distinction the courts have defined ordinary care as "that degree of care which people ordinarily prudent could be reasonably expected to exercise under circumstances of a given case."[1] It has been equated with the reasonable care and prudence exercised by ordinarily prudent persons under similar circumstances.[15]

The legal standard of ordinary care also does not contemplate what may be the average skills among all known practitioners from the best to the worst and from the most experienced to the least. "We are not permitted to aggregate into a common class the quacks, the young men who have no practice, the old ones who have dropped out of practice, the good, and the very best, and then strike an average between them."[16]

Although the standard required of a professional cannot be that of the most highly skilled practitioner, neither can it be that of the average member of the profession since those who have less than median skill may still be competent and qualify.[17] By such an illogical definition, one half of all dentists in a community would automatically fall short of the mark and be negligent as a matter of law.[18]

RELEVANCE OF CUSTOM

The standard of care that a professional must possess and exercise is peculiarly within the knowledge of experts.[19] However, there are occasions in which the conduct involved in within the common knowledge of layman; in particular, the trier of fact, such as negligence, may be determined in lieu of expert testimony.[20]

The customary practice in the community of the profession may have bearing on the determination by the trier of fact as to the standard of care required in the particular circumstances.[21] Compliance with such custom may aid the determination as to whether a standard of reasonable care was satisfied.[22]

However, the fact that conduct complies with custom does not exclude the possibility that a customary practice may be a negligent custom.[23] "What usually is done may be evidence of what ought to be done, but what ought to be done is fixed by a standard of reasonable prudence whether it is usually complied with or not."[24]

In one case[25] the evidence was undisputed that virtually no ophthamologist in the entire state routinely tested for glaucoma in patients under the age of 40 since the incidence was only 1 in 25,000 patients. Nevertheless, the Supreme Court of Washington State held the defendant ophthamologist negligent as a matter of law irrespective of the customary practice.

Moreover, compliance with a safety statute does not conclusively establish due care since regulations require only minimal care and not necessarily prudent care or what the law regards as due care.[24]

SPECIALTY CARE
Ethics

Endodontics is one of the seven recognized dental specialities by the American Dental Association.[26] Although any licensed dentist may legally practice endodontics, it is *unethical* to announce that one specializes in endodontics absent specialty training[27] or being ''grandfathered'' in endodontic practice. A general practitioner who desires to emphasize or limit his practice to endodontics is ethically permitted to advertise or list his practice only as follows:

General Practitioner—Endodontics

It is *ethically impermissible* for a general practitioner to announce his practice as ''Limited to Endodontics.''

Fraud

A nonspecialist in endodontics who misrepresents that he is an endodontist or specializes in endodontics subjects himself to the following legal liabilities:
1. Obtaining a fee by fraud or misrepresentation[28]
2. Fraudulent misrepresentation[28]

Although a dentist who refers a patient to a specialist is ordinarily insulated from any negligent act or omission performed by the specialist, the notable exception is when the general dentist refers to another dentist whom he *knows* or in the exercise of reasonable diligence *should have known* to be incompetent. Therefore, it may be argued that a fully trained specialist in endodontics possesses a greater degree of competency in diagnosing and rendering endodontic therapy, which the general dentist knew or should have known in making the referral to a nonspecialist in endodontics. Additionally, the *referring dentist* would also therefore be legally liable for fraudulent misrepresentation if, in his referral to the untrained dentist, he represented to the patient that the nonspecialist was an endodontic or root canal specialist rather than a dentist who emphasized endodontics in his general practice.

INFORMED CONSENT (Figs. 9-6 to 9-8)

The doctrine of informed consent requires that the patient be advised of the reasonably foreseeable risks of endodontic therapy, the nature of the treatment, reasonable alternatives, and the consequences of nontreatment.[29] This doctrine is premised on the legal principle that each individual has a right to do with his own body as he sees fit, regardless of preferred dental treatment, including the right to die. Thus an adult of sound mind is entitled to elect to maintain or ignore endodontic disease rather than select elective treatment once the dentist has informed the patient of the diagnosis, recommended corrective treatment or alternative therapy, and the likely risks and prognosis of treatment compared to not proceeding with recommended therapy.

Judicial intervention to compel therapy against the patient's wishes may occur only if the person is legally incompetent to make an informed and intelligent decision (e.g., a minor, a comatose or insane individual).[30]

Informed consent is a flexible standard that considers the reasonably foreseeable consequences depending upon the clinical situation present both before and during treatment. For instance, a fractured endodontic instrument left in the canal will have a foreseeable likelihood of success depending on whether the fracture occurred in the coronal, middle, or apical third of the root canal. Therefore, the dentist must advise the patient of relative risks of future failure so the patient can make an intelligent choice of either an apicoectomy, referral to an endodontist for attempt at retrieval, or watchful waiting with close observation at recall visits.

Abandonment

Once endodontic treatment is initiated, the dentist is legally obligated to complete the treatment *irrespective* of the patient paying any outstanding balance. This requirement is posited on the legal premise that any person who attempts to rescue another from harm must reasonably complete the rescue with beneficial intervention unless another rescuer (dentist) is willing to assume the undertaking.[31] Another view is that if the patient is placed in a position of danger, unless further treatment is performed, then the dentist must institute reasonable therapeutic measures to assure that adverse consequences do not result.[32]

To avoid a charge of abandonment, several prophylactic measures apply:

First, there is no legal duty to accept for treatment all patients, and a dentist may legally refuse to treat a new patient despite severe pain or infection.[32] If treatment is limited to emergency measures only, be certain that the patient is advised that only temporary emergency endodontic therapy is being provided and not complete treatment. Record on the patient's chart, for instance:

''Emergency treatment only. Endo of tooth no. _____ to be completed with another dentist.''

Also, have the patient acknowledge that treatment is limited to the existing emergency by endorsing an informed consent to emergency endodontics.

''I agree to emergency root canal therapy of my tooth and have been advised that (a) emergency treatment is for temporary relief of pain and (b) that further root canal treatment is necessary to avoid further pain, infection, fracture, abscess, or loss of tooth.''

Second, be aware that there is no legal duty to continue former patients on recalls or emergency care if former treatment is complete. Thus, endodontic completion of tooth no. 19 at a prior visit does not legally obligate the dentist to initiate endodontic therapy for tooth no. 3, whose endodontic disease began after the last treatment of tooth no. 19.

I, _____ , have been advised by Dr. _____

that I require a root canal treatment for my tooth _____ .

Dr. _____ has explained to me the method and manner of the proposed treatment, the desirability of root canal treatment compared to extractions and the consequences of not having root canal treatment including but not limited to the following:

1. Postoperative discomfort lasting a few hours to several days for which medication will be prescribed if deemed necessary by the doctor

2. Postoperative swelling of the gum area in the vicinity of the treated tooth or facial swelling, either of which may persist for several days or longer

3. Infection

4. Trismus (restricted jaw opening), which usually lasts several days but may last longer

5. Failure rate of 5-10% (If failure occurs, the treatment may have to be redone, root-end surgery may be required, or the tooth may have to be extracted.)

6. Breakage of root canal instruments during treatment, which may in the judgment of the doctor be left in the treated root canal or require surgery for removal

7. Perforation of the root canal with instruments, which may require additional surgical corrective treatment or result in premature tooth loss or extraction

8. Premature tooth loss due to progressive periodontal (gum) disease in the surrounding area

I understand that following root canal treatment my tooth will be brittle and must be protected against fracture by placement of a crown (cap) over the tooth.

I understand that I am to return in _____ months for a recall visit so that

Dr. _____ can evaluate the root canal treatment.

No warranty or guarantee of success has been or can be given in root canal treatment.

All of my questions have been answered by the doctor and I fully understand the above statements in this consent form.

Date _____

_____
signature of patient or legal guardian

FIG. 9-6. Treatment consent form.

Third, any patient may be discharged from a practice for any arbitrary reason, except racial discrimination, so long as all initiated treatment is completed.[33] Accordingly, a former patient who evokes memories of frictional rapport, who is financially irresponsible, or who arrives at your office after an absence of several years with an acute apical abscess in a different location than previous care may legally be refused treatment.

Fourth, it is not considered abandonment if a patient is given reasonable notice to seek endodontic treatment with another dentist and is willing to seek endodontic services elsewhere.[33] Thus, if there is a breakdown of rapport with the patient, do not hesitate to suggest that each of you would be better served if any remaining endodontic treatment were performed elsewhere with a different dentist.

Defective instrument

A manufacturer of an instrument is strictly liable in tort for consequential damages from a fractured instrument if it is proved to be defectively manufactured.[34] Therefore, if an instrument breaks, one should *save the unbroken end* so it can be tested for defective manufacturing. If it is

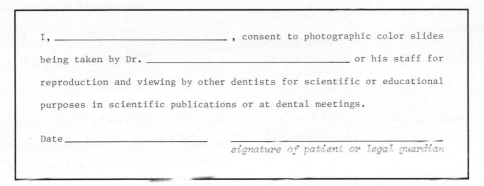

I, _____ , consent to emergency root canal therapy

to possibly save tooth _____ from extraction. Following this emergency

treatment to reduce the infection, additional root canal treatment will

be necessary. I understand that unless I have such additional treatment

by Dr. _____ or another dentist of my choice within

the next several days to _____ weeks infection will recur or continue

and the emergency root canal treatment will be ineffective in saving my

tooth.

Date _____   _____
                                    signature of patient or legal guardian

FIG. 9-7. Emergency root canal consent form.

I, _____ , consent to photographic color slides

being taken by Dr. _____ or his staff for

reproduction and viewing by other dentists for scientific or educational

purposes in scientific publications or at dental meetings.

Date _____   _____
                                    signature of patient or legal guardian

FIG. 9-8. Photography consent form.

proved to be defective, this shifts legal responsibility to the manufacturer.

Paresthesia

Endodontic surgery in the vicinity of the mental foramen carries with it the risk of injury to the mental nerve. Consequently, the patient should be advised (in lay terms) before any surgery is performed that there is a risk of temporary or permanent anesthesia or paresthesia.

Failure

A dentist is not a guarantor of success unless foolish enough to warrant saving a tooth or achieving a perfect result.[35] Endodontic failures may occur despite the best of endodontic care.[36] Therefore, the patient should be advised in advance of treatment of the inherent but relatively small risk of failure.[36] It may be adequate to advise the patient of the high statistical probability of success in endodontics so long as the clinical condition of tooth and the clinician's past success rate warrant such representation.[37] Factors to be considered in avoiding representing the national success rate of endodontics vis-a-vis a particular dentist in a given clinical situation are (1) a tooth that is periodontally ques-

tionable, and (2) a clinician known to have an unusually high endodontic failure rate.

The doctrine of informed consent protects both the dentist and the patient so there will be no surprises or patient disappointment if an adverse result manifests. Should a failure or a poor result occur, the availability of a signed informed consent form may serve as a reminder to the patient that the risk of complications was discussed in advance of treatment and that, unfortunately, the patient's endodontic treatment came out on the wrong end of the statistical curve.

Slips of the drill

A slip of the drill, like a slip of the tongue, may be unintentional but nevertheless cause harm. When a cut tongue or lip occurs, it is usually the result of operator error. To paraphrase Alexander Pope, to err is human but to forebear divine. To succeed in having a patient forebear from filing suit because of a cut lip or tongue, the clinician should follow these steps:

First, inform the patient that you are indeed sorry. This is not a legal admission of guilt but rather an admission that you are a compassionate human being.

Second, repair the injured tissue yourself or refer the patient to an oral or plastic surgeon, depending on the extent of the injury and whether a plastic revision due to scarring is likely.

Third, advise the patient that you will pay the bill for the referred treatment of the oral or plastic surgeon.

Fourth, send the oral or plastic surgeon's bill to your professional liability carrier. Most carriers will pay the claim under the medical payments provisions of the general liability policy for an "accident" rather than as a malpractice incident compensable under the professional liability policy.

Treatment of the incorrect tooth

It is not negligent to commit an error in judgment so long as it is a reasonable mistake of judgment.[38] For instance, it may be difficult to localize the source of endodontic pain, and vital pulps may on occasion be sacrificed in an attempt to diagnose the source of pain.

Nevertheless, it is unreasonable and therefore inexcusable to treat the wrong tooth because it is recorded incorrectly on the referral slip or the radiographs are mounted incorrectly or reversed.

If an unreasonable mistake of judgment occurs, then be sympathetic, waive payment for all endodontic treatment, and offer to pay the fee for the crowning of the unnecessarily treated tooth.[38] Most insurance carriers provide a "medical payments" provision in the policy for "accidents" which is broadly construed and does not count against the dentist as a malpractice incident. Stated otherwise, payment should be made under the "medical payments" portion of the general liability policy rather than the "errors or omissions" section of the professional liability policy.

Swallowing of an endodontic file

Use of a rubber dam in endodontics is mandatory.[39] Therefore, if a patient swallows a file, it is because the dentist failed to meet the standard of care (Fig. 9-9). If such incident does occur, advise the patient that you are sorry for what occurred. Refer the patient for immediate medical care to determine if it is lodged in the bronchus or stomach so that appropriate measures are taken for its removal. Finally, offer to pay for the patient's out-of-pocket medical expenses.

Overfill of a canal

A very slight overfill of a canal can occur within the standard of care (Chapter 24). Gross overfills usually indicate faulty technique. Nevertheless, so long as the overfill is not in contact with vital structures such as the mandibular nerve or sinuses, no permanent harm will likely result.[5] If, however, severe postoperative pain is foreseeable as a result of the overfill, the patient should be advised of the likelihood of postoperative discomfort due to contact of the sealing material with the surrounding tissue. Similarly, if the overfill is slight or increased postoperative pain is unlikely, the patient need not be advised since it would unnecessarily alarm him. However, a note should be made on the patient's chart regarding the overfill and

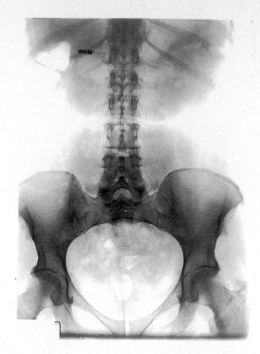

FIG. 9-9. Swallowed endodontic file demonstrates wisdom of rubber dam.

the reason for not informing the patient. Fortunately, slight overfills with inert conventional endodontic sealers (like gutta-percha) will usually repair themselves.

PROPHYLACTIC ENDODONTIC PRACTICE
Diagnosis

Competent endodontic treatment begins with adequate diagnostic procedures, as discussed in Chapters 1 and 2.

An adequate periodontal evaluation must accompany each endodontic diagnosis, which requires a diagnostic radiograph, clinical visualization and evaluation of the periodontal tissues, and probing for periodontal pockets with a calibrated periodontal probe (particularly in furcation areas).[40]

Although endodontic treatment may be successful, tooth loss may nevertheless result from progress of any residual untreated periodontitis. Consequently, a periodontal evaluation and prognostication are *mandatory* so the patient and dentist can make an informed and intelligent choice as to whether to proceed with endodontics, a combination of periodontal and endodontic techniques (Chapter 17), or extraction.

Preoperative and postoperative radiographs

It is axiomatic that the dentist should take only the number of radiographs necessary and avoid exposing the patient to unnecessary radiation. Dental societies have petitioned insurance companies to not require postoperative radiographs if therapeutically unnecessary.

A panoramic radiograph may not be as diagnostically accurate as a periapical radiograph and therefore should not be used for accurate apical measurement assessment.[10] Working films are necessary to verify apical extent of filing, canal shaping, and fill.

Posttreatment radiographs are beneficial in determining the adequacy of the endodontic seal, as discussed in Chapter 8, and are therefore recommended to assure clinical success.

Medical history

As patients live longer because of improved medical science, an adequate and updated medical history becomes increasingly important.[41] For instance, an endodontic file extended beyond the apical foramen or insertion of any endosseous implant is a potential focus of infection for subacute bacterial endocarditis, which may be avoided by the administration of prophylactic antibiotics to a patient with damaged heart valves.[42]

At the followup visit, if any treatment is necessary (e.g., apical surgery), a current medical history should be obtained. The patient is asked to review the previously signed medical history and to initial and date the prior history if there are no changes. The history should be updated for any changes in systemic health by recording the specific change differing from the prior medical history.

Record keeping

Oral, written, documentary, or circumstantial types of evidence are all equally competent and admissible evidence at trial.[43] Nevertheless, a written record is inherently more credible to a jury since there is little doubt regarding its content. Memories fade and are not as trustworthy as documented written evidence. A short pen is better than a long memory.

For example, proof of periodontal probing is best documented by probe recordings on the chart. If no pathologic pockets are detected, the fact should be recorded on the chart that all measurements are within normal limits.[44]

Abbreviations are legally acceptable as long as they are standard. Difficulties occur with abbreviations that defy credibility, such as representing a referral to a periodontist that the patient refused with the letter P* rather than a simple "referred to Dr. _____ for periodontal evaluation."

Rapport

A compassionate and concerned doctor who is able to demonstrate that the patient is cared about, as well as cared for, will abort many malpractice actions. Thus, when an iatrogenic mishap occurs, it behooves the clinician to be frank and forthright with the patient. Concealment of negligence may extend the statute of limitations, since most states with discovery statutes construe discovery as the date upon which the patient discovered the negligent cause of the injury and not merely the injury itself.[45] Furthermore, it is the belated discovery of injury from another dentist that evokes a feeling of betrayal in the patient and destroys the formerly existing rapport that would otherwise dissuade the patient from instituting litigation.

---

*An actual case of the author (EJZ) (which was settled out of court) involved this dubious abbreviation.

Peer review

If despite good rapport, candid disclosure, and an offer to pay corrective medical or surgical bills the patient is still litigious, the clinician should consider suggesting peer review.

Peer review committees award damages only for out-of-pocket losses. General damages for pain and suffering or wage loss are not permitted. Consequently, even if the committee's judgment is adverse, the damage claim will probably be less than a jury's verdict. If peer review finds for the dentist, the patient may be discouraged from proceeding further with litigation. Results of the committee's decision are not admissible at trial for either side.[46]

Insurance carriers will usually honor a peer review committee decision since a fair adjudication of the merits has been determined, judgment is less than a potential jury award, and defense costs and attorney's fees are saved.

Referral

What may appear to be a routine endodontic procedure can change if a complication such as perforation, calcified obstruction, or root fracture occurs.

If certain dental procedures are ordinarily performed by a specialist rather than a general dentist, the general dentist will be held to the higher standard of care of the specialist.[5] For example, apical surgery in the vicinity of the maxillary sinus or mental foramen is a delicate procedure for the best of dental specialists. What may appear to be a routine endodontic procedure can change if a complication such as perforation or root fracture occurs. Although it may have been prudent for the general dentist to initiate endodontic therapy, referral to a specialist may be advisable if a complication occurs that is outside the scope of the generalist's training or experience.

Endosseous implants

Endosseous implants are still regarded as experimental and are not generally accepted as a predictably reliable technique.[47] Consequently, the patient should be informed of the uncertainty of success and asked to initial an informed consent form that contains a paragraph such as the following:

I have been advised and understand that the long-term success of the implants proposed for treatment has not yet been conclusively established. No guarantee of success has been or can be given for the proposed implant.

I also understand that the following complications may result from failure of the endosseous implant:
1. Tooth loss
2. Infection
3. Sinus perforation (if applicable)
4. Temporary or permanent numbness of my lip or chin (if applicable)
5. Implant fracture
6. Surgical removal of the implant

CONCLUSION

If the dentist performs endodontics within the standards of care provided in this chapter, there should not be any concern of a successful suit for professional negligence. Suggested prophylactic measures in this chapter will avoid litigation by reducing avoidable risks associated with endodontic care. Both the patient and dentist benefit from risk reduction. It is far better and easier for the dentist to take the extra minute to *do it right* rather than subject a patient to a possible lifetime of misery.

REFERENCES

1. Keeling, D.: Malpractice claim prevention, J. Calif. Dent. Assoc. **3**(8):55, 1975.

2. Morris, W.O.: Dental litigation, ed. 2, Charlottesville, Va., 1977, The Michie Co.

3. Terezhalmy, G., and Bottomley, W.: General legal aspects of diagnostic dental radiography, Oral Surg. **48**:486, 1979.

4. Weichman, J.: Malpractice prevention and defense, J. Calif. Dent. Assoc. **3**(8):58, 1975.

5. Zinman, E.J.: Usual and customary versus prudent practice, Tenn. Dent. J. **60**:9, 1980; *Kelly v. Cunningham,* I Cal. 365 (1850); *Katz v. Hebbing,* 205 Cal. 629; 271 P. 1062; 62 A.L.R. 825 (1928); Restatement of the law of torts, ed. 2, § 245A, Comment (c); *Helling v. Carrey,* 519 P. 2d 981 (Washington) (1974); *Gates v. Jensen,* 595 P. 2d 919 (1979); Kircos, L.T., Vandre, R.H., and Lorton, L.: Exposure reduction of 96% in intraoral radiography, J. Am. Dent. Assoc. **113**:746, 1986.

6. Biedeman, R.W., Johnson, O.N., and Alcox, R.W.: A study to develop a rating system and evaluate dental radiographs submitted to a third party carrier, J. Am. Dent. Assoc. **93**:1010, 1976. (Majority of radiographs not diagnostic.)

7. Silverman, S.: Cold sterilization methods examined Dent. Surv., p. 8, Oct. 1978. See also American Dental Association, Council on Dental Therapeutics: Quaternary compounds not acceptable for disinfection of instruments and environmental surfaces in dentistry, J. Am. Dent. Assoc. **97**:855, 1978.

8. *Simpson v. Davis,* 219 Kan. 584; 549 P. 2d 950 (1976).

9. Glavind, C., and Loe, H.: Errors in the clinical assessment of periodontal destruction, J. Periodont. Res. **2**:180, 1967; Glazer, S.A.: Reliability of x-ray scores in Navy periodontal disease index, U.S. Navy Medical **60**:34, 1972; Morgulis, J.: Developing a periodontal screening evaluation, J. Calif. Dent. Assoc. **7**:59, Jan. 1979.

10. American Dental Association: Report of the Council on Dental Materials, Instruments, and Equipment, J. Am. Dent. Assoc. **94**:147, 1977; Christen, A.G., and Segreto, V.A.: Distortion and artifacts encountered in Panorex radiographs, J. Am. Dent. Assoc. **77**:1096, 1968; Mitchell, L.D., Jr.: Panoramic roentgenography, J. Am. Dent. Assoc. **66**:777, 1963; Brueggemann, I.A.: Evaluation of the Panorex unit, Oral Surg. **24**:348, 1967; Updegrave, W.G.: Panoramic dental radiography, Dent. Radiogr. Photogr. **36**:76, 1963.

11. *Agnew v. Larson,* 82 Cal. App. 2d 176, 183; 185 P. 2d 851 (1947).

12. *Keen v. Prisinyana,* 23 Cal. App. 3d 275, 279; 100 Cal. Rptr. 82 (1972).

13. *Folk v. Kilk,* 53 Cal. App. 3d 176; 126 Cal. Rptr. 172 (1975); *Bardesonno v. Michels,* 3 Cal. 3d 780; 91 Cal. Rptr. 760 (1970); 478 P. 2d 480, Am. Jur. 2d, Physicians and surgeons and other healers, 138 (1972).

14. California book of approved jury instructions, Civil, 6.00 et seq.; Witkin, B.: Summary of California law, ed. 8, Torts, §§ 514 and 516.

15. *Switzer v. Atchison, Topeka, & Santa Fe Railroad Co.,* 7 Cal. App. 2d 661, 666; 47 P. 2d 353 (1935).

16. *Scarano v. Schnoor,* 158 Cal. App. 2d 618; 323 P. 2d 178 (1958). Citing *Sims v. Weeks,* 7 Cal. App. 28, 42 (1935).

17. Restatement of the law of torts, ed. 2, § 299A, Comment (e).

18. See 61 Am. Jur. 2d, Physicians and surgeons and other healers, § 110.

19. *Sinz v. Owens,* 33 Cal. 2d 749, 753; 205 P. 2d 3; 8 A.L.R. 2d 757 (1949).

20. *Folk v. Kilk,* 53 Cal. App. 3d 176, 185 (1975).

21. *Tucker v. Lombardo,* 47 Cal. 2d 457; 303 P. 2d 1041 (1956); *Barton v. Owen,* 7 Cal. App. 2d 28; 45 P. 2d 350; 139 Cal. Rptr. 498 (1977).

22. *Cyerman v. United States Lines Co.,* 102 Cal. Rptr. 795; 498 P. 2d 1041 (1972).

23. *Kelly v. Cunningham,* 1 Cal. 365 (1850); *Katz v. Hebbing,* 205 Cal. 629; 271 P. 1062; 62 A.L.R. 825 (1928); Restatement of the law of torts, ed. 2, § 245A, Comment (c).

24. *Texas & Pacific Railway Co. v. Behymer,* 189 U.S. 468, 470; 47 L. Ed. 905; 23 S. Ct. 622 (1903).

25. *Helling v. Carrey,* 83 Wash. 2d 514; 519 P. 2d 981 (1974). But see *Meeks v. Marx,* 15 Wash. App. 571; 556 P. 2d 1158 (1976); *Gates v. Jensen,* 595 P. 2d (1979).

26. Lawyers' medical encyclopedia, § 1.17(D) (rev. ed. 1966).

27. American Dental Association: Principles of ethics and code of professional conduct, §§ 5-C and 5-D; California Dental Association, §§ 8 and 9.

28. See California business and professions code 1680 (a) and (h).

29. *Congrove v. Holmes,* 37 Ohio Misc. 95; 308 N.E. 2d 765 (1973); *Llera v. Wisner,* 557 P. 2d 805 (Mont.) (1976); *Morgenroth v. Pacific Medical Center, Inc.,* 54 Cal. App. 3d 531; 126 Cal. Rptr. 681 (1976); *Scaria v. St. Paul Fire & Marine Insurance Co.,* 68 Wis. 201; 227 N.W. 2d 647 (1975); Zinman, E.: Informed consent to periodontal surgery. Advise before you incise, J. West. Soc. Periodontol. **24**(3):101, 1976.

30. *Matter of Quinlan,* 348 A. 2d 801, 355 A. 2d 647 (1976); *Bouvier v. Superior Court* 179 CA 3d 1127 (1986); *Randolph v. Upper Manhattan Medical Group,* 501 NYS 2d 837 (1986).

31. *Lee v. Deubre* 362 S.W. 2d 900 (Tex. Civ. App., 1962); Clark v. Hoek, 219 Cal. Rptr. 845 (1985).

32. *McNamara v. Emmons,* 36 Cal. App. 2d 199; 97 P. 2d 503 (1939); *Small v. Wegner,* 267 S.W. 2d 26; 50 A.L.R. 2d 170 (Mo., 1954).

33. *Murray v. U.S.,* 329, F. 2d 270 (4 Va. Civ. App., 1964).

34. *Barker v. Lull Engineering Co.,* 20 Cal. 3d 413; 143 Cal. Rptr. 225, 573 P. 20 443 (1978); *Grimshaw v. Ford Motor Co.,* 119 Cal. Rptr. 757 (1974), Cal. Rptr. 348 (1975).

35. *Christ v. Lipsitz,* 160 Cal. Rptr. 498; 99 Cal. App. 3d 894 (1980).

36. Ingle, J., and Beveridge, E.: Endodontics, ed. 2, Philadelphia, 1976, Lea & Febiger, pp. 34 and 597; "Maloccurrence does not per se equal malpractice." Gurdin v. Dongieux, 468 So.2d 1241 (1985).

37. *Hales v. Pittman,* 118 Ariz. 305; 576 P. 22 493.

38. Witkin, B.: Summary of California law, ed. 8. Vol. 4. Torts, §514, *Fraijo v. Hartland Hospital,* 99 Cal. App. 3d 331; 160 Cal. Rptr. 246 (1979).

39. *Simpson v. Davis,* 219 Kan. 584; 549 P. 2d 950 (1976).

40. Grant, D., Stern, I., and Everett, F.: Periodontics. In the tradition of Orban and Gottlieb, St. Louis, 1979, The C.V. Mosby Co., pp. 443 to 506.

41. McCarthy, F.M.: "A new patient-administered medical history developed for dentistry," J. Am. Dent. Assoc. **111**:595, 1985.

42. Crespi, P. and Friedman, R.: "Dental examination guides for children requiring infective endocarditis prophylaxis," J. Am. Dent. Assoc. **111**:931, 1985.

43. Witkin, B.: California procedures, ed. 2, Vol. 4. Trial, §224; *Tropani v. Holzer,* 158 Cal. App. 2d 1; 321 P. 2d 803.

44. Brady, W.F., and Martinoff, J.T.: A simplified examination, diagnosis, and treatment classification of periodontal disease, J. Am. Dent. Assoc. **104**:313, 1982.

45. *Franklin v. Albert,* 411 N.E. 2d 458 (Mass.) 1980. See "Developments in the law: statutes of limitations," Harvard L. Rev. **63**:1177, 1203-05, May 1950, *Teeters v. Currey,* 518 S.W. 2d 512 (1974) (negligent sterilization operation case in which the Tennessee Supreme Court, reversing a 47-year-old time-of-negligent-act rule, shifted to the equitable "discovery doctrine"); Prosser: Torts, ed. 4, 144-145, 1971. Note, 38 Montana L. Rev. 399, 401 n.22 (1977); Annot., 80 A.L.R. 2d 368, §7(b) (1961), and Later Case Service (collecting statutes and cases); 70 A.L.R. 3d 7 (leaving foreign ob-

jects in the body); see also *Raymond v. Eli Lilly,* 412 F. Supp. 1392 (D.N.H. 1976), *aff'd,* 556 F. 2d 628 (1st Cir. 1977) (Malpractice discovery rule applied in drug products liability case involving plaintiff's blindness from use of C-Quens, an oral contraceptive); 32 A.T.L.A. L.J. 260-265 (1968) (collecting cases adopting equitable discovery rule); *Grey v. Silver Bow Cty.,* 425 P. 2d 819 (Mont. 1967) (extending discovery rule beyond "foreign-object" cases and applying it in case in which failure of defendant's hospital to use sterile techniques permitted introduction into plaintiff's body of staphylococcus infection); *Ayers v. Morgan,* 154 A. 2d 788, 792 (Pa. 1959), 25 N.A.C.C.A. L.J. 131-141 (1960) ("the man who buries a time bomb would argue futilely that he could not be held responsible for a resulting death because the explosion and death of his victim did not occur until more than a year after he had placed the bomb."); *Berry v. Branner,* 421 P. 2d 966 (Ore. 1966), 10 A.T.L.A. News L. 105 (April 1967) (a foreign-object case with

strong influential impact upon subsequent decisional law around the country, including its emphatic rejection of the defense argument that prior refusals of the legislature in a state to adopt the discovery rule by statute disables courts in that state from thereafter abandoning the time-of-the-negligent-act rule and adopting the discovery rule); note especially *Ruth v. Dight,* 453 P. 2d 631 (Wash. 1969) (a remarkable case applying the discovery rule to a case in which a sponge was left in plaintiff's body for 23 years); Sacks, Statutes of limitation and undiscovered malpractice, 16 Cleveland-Marshall, L. Rev. 65 (1967); Note, 30 Ohio St. L.J. 425 (1969).

46. California evidence code 1157.

47. American Dental Association: Report of the Council on Dental Materials, Instruments, and Equipment, J. Am. Dent. Assoc. **100:**247, 1980. The Biotes implant, classified as provisionally acceptable by the ADA Council on Dental Materials, Instruments and Equipment in 1985, is the notable exception.

Self-assessment questions

1. For dental-legal reasons the dental record should provide:
   a. Accurate legible entries dated
   b. Medical and dental condition of the patient prior to and during treatment
   c. Clear radiographic films
   d. All of the above

2. One of the following statements is false regarding the health history review:
   a. Sufficient details should be included so any dental therapy can be judged safe.
   b. A clinician may wish to suggest or insist that a patient receive medical evaluation prior to dental treatment.
   c. Any current therapy, physical or psychologic, should be included, and the patient's personal physician consulted.
   d. Problems associated with previous dental care are usually not indicated or necessary.

3. Standard of care as defined by the courts
   a. Requires absolute perfection
   b. Does not allow individual variants of treatment
   c. Equates with what a reasonably careful and prudent clinician would do under similar circumstances
   d. Is analogous to customary practice

4. One of the following statements is true:
   a. A general practitioner may ethically list his practice as "General Practitioner—Endodontics."
   b. It is ethically permissible for a general practitioner to announce his practice as "Limited to Endodontics."
   c. Without specialty training, a licensed dentist may not legally practice endodontics.
   d. A dentist referring a patient to a specialist is usually responsible for any negligent act by the specialist.

5. The doctrine of informed consent does not
   a. Require that a patient be advised of reasonably forseeable risks of treatment
   b. Require advising the patient of reasonable alternatives
   c. Give up the patient's right to do as he sees fit with his own body
   d. Require advising the patient of the consequences of nontreatment

6. Which one of the following statements is true?
   a. A dentist may legally refuse to treat a new patient despite severe pain or infection.
   b. One is legally bound to continue patients on recall or emergency care if former treatment is completed.
   c. A patient may not be discharged from a practice until all proposed treatment is completed.
   d. The patient does not need to be advised if treatment is limited to emergency procedures only.

7. Which legal responsibility is correct?
   a. When operating near the mental nerve, it is unnecessary to advise a patient of possible paresthesia.
   b. A signed informed consent form guarantees to the patient the success of treatment against failure.
   c. Treatment of the incorrect tooth is considered negligent if there is reasonable mistake in judgment.
   d. The use of a rubber dam to prevent swallowing of endodontic instruments is considered mandatory.

8. Which of the following statements is true?
   a. Endodontic diagnostic evaluation usually does not require a periodontal evaluation.
   b. Oral and written documentary testimony is equally competent admissible evidence at a trial.
   c. Peer review committees award general damages for pain and suffering.
   d. Endosseous implants are generally accepted as a predictable reliable technique.

PART TWO

THE SCIENCE OF ENDODONTICS

10

PULP STRUCTURE AND FUNCTION

HENRY O. TROWBRIDGE
SYNGCUK KIM

The dental pulp is in many ways similar to other connective tissues of the body, but its special characteristics deserve serious consideration. Even the mature pulp bears a strong resemblance to embryonic connective tissue; and yet at its periphery is a layer of highly sophisticated cells, the odontoblasts. Certain peculiarities are imposed on the pulp by the rigid mineralized tissues in which it is enclosed. For example, the ability of the pulp to increase in volume during episodes of vasodilation is quite restricted. The pulp chamber is filled with nerves, vascular tissue, fibers, ground substance, interstitial fluid, odontoblasts, fibroblasts, and other minor cellular components. Since each of these constituents is relatively incompressible, the total volume of blood within the pulp chamber cannot be increased, although reciprocal volume changes can occur between arterioles and venules. Thus, in the case of the pulp we are dealing with a low-compliance system in which careful regulation of blood flow is critically important.

No true arteries or veins enter or leave the pulp, so the circulatory system of the pulp is actually a microcirculatory system whose largest vascular components are arterioles and venules. Unlike most tissues, the pulp lacks a true collateral system and is dependent upon the relatively few arterioles entering through the root foramina and the occasional arteriole through a lateral canal. Since with age there is a gradual reduction in the luminal diameters of these foramina, the vascular system of the pulp decreases progressively.

The pulp is also a rather unique sensory organ. Being encased in a protective layer of dentin, which in turn is covered with enamel, it might be expected to be quite unresponsive to stimulation; yet, despite the low thermal conductivity of dentin, the pulp is undeniably sensitive to thermal stimuli such as ice cream and warm drinks. Later in this chapter we will consider the unusual mechanism that allows the dentin-pulp complex to function as such an exquisitely responsive sensory system.

Following tooth development the pulp retains its ability to form dentin throughout life. This enables the vital pulp partially to compensate for the loss of enamel or dentin caused by mechanical trauma or disease. How well it serves this function depends upon many factors, but the potential for regeneration and repair is as much a reality in the pulp as in other connective tissues of the body.

It is the purpose of this chapter to try to bring together what is known about the development, structure, and function of the dentin-pulp complex in the hope that this knowledge will provide a firm biologic basis for clinical decision making.

DEVELOPMENT

Embryologic studies have shown that the pulp is derived from the cephalic neural crest. Neural crest cells arise from the ectoderm along the lateral margins of the neural plate and migrate extensively. Those that travel down the sides of the head into the maxilla and mandible contribute to the formation of the tooth germs. The dental papilla, from which the mature pulp arises, develops as ectomesenchymal cells proliferate and condense adjacent to the dental lamina at the sites where teeth will develop (Fig. 10-1). It is important that we remember the migratory potential of ectomesenchymal cells, for later in this chapter we will consider the ability of pulp cells to move into areas of injury and replace destroyed odontoblasts.

During the sixth week of embryonic life, tooth formation begins as a localized proliferation of ectoderm associated with the maxillary and mandibular processes. This proliferative activity results in the formation of two horseshoe-shaped structures, one on each process, that are termed the primary dental laminae. Each primary dental lamina splits into a vestibular and a dental lamina (Fig. 10-2).

Numerous studies have indicated that the embryologic development of any tissue is promoted by interaction with

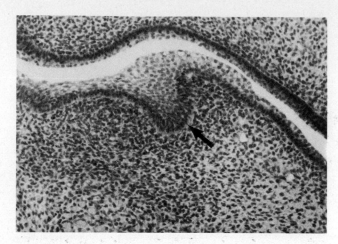

FIG. 10-1. Dental lamina *(arrow)* arising from the oral ectoderm.

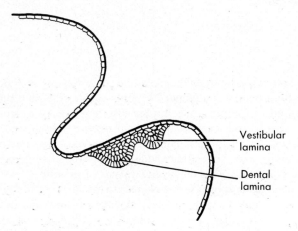

Vestibular
lamina

Dental
lamina

FIG. 10-2. Diagram showing formation of the vestibular and the dental lamina from oral ectoderm.

an adjacent tissue.* The complex epithelial-mesenchymal interactions occurring during tooth development have been extensively studied, and it is generally held that elements of the dental basement membrane direct the differentiation of ameloblasts and odontoblasts by causing these cells to change gene expression. The dental basement membrane consists of a basal lamina, which is formed by the epithelial cells, and a layer of extracellular matrix (ECM) derived from the adjacent mesenchyme. The macromolecular constituents of the ECM include glycoproteins such as laminin and fibronectin and proteoglycans such as heparin sulfate, hyaluronate, chondroitin-4-sulfate, chondroitin-6-sulfate, and collagen types I, III, and IV.[34,118,121,195-197] The composition of the basement membrane changes during tooth development, and these changes appear to modulate the successive steps in odontogenesis.[171-173] It is thought that by binding to receptors on the surface membrane of the developing ameloblasts and odontoblasts, ECM constituents such as fibronectin, laminin, and collagen influence the differentiation of these cells.

*References 82, 108, 109, 170-172, 181, and 182.

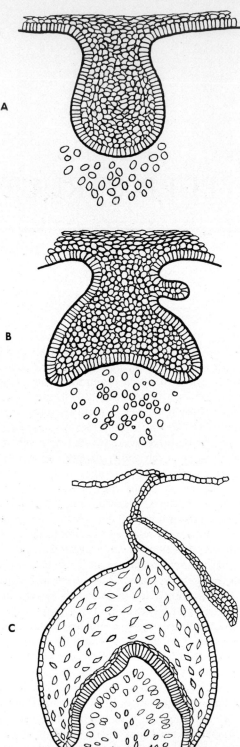

FIG. 10-3. Diagrammatic representation of, **A,** the bud, **B,** the cap, and, **C,** the bell stages of tooth development.

The initial stage of development of the dental papilla is characterized by proliferative activity beneath the dental lamina at sites corresponding to the positions of the prospective primary teeth. Even before the dental lamina begins to form the enamel organ, a capillary vascular net-

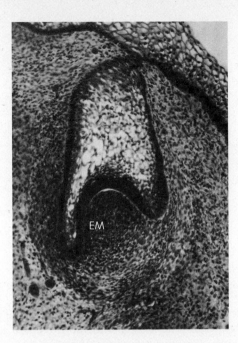

FIG. 10-4. Cap stage of tooth development. The condensed ectomesenchyme *(EM)* that will form the dental papilla lies subjacent to the concave aspect of the enamel organ.

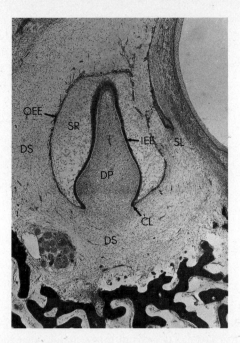

FIG. 10-5. Bell stage of tooth development showing the outer enamel epithelium *(OEE)*, stellate reticulum *(SR)*, inner enamel epithelium *(IEE)*, dental papilla *(DP)*, cervical loop *(CL)*, successional lamina *(SL)*, and dental sac *(DS)*.

work develops within the ectomesenchyme, presumably to support the increased metabolic activity of the presumptive tooth buds.[67] This primordial vascularization is thought to play a key role in odontogenic induction. Nerve fibers have also been demonstrated beneath the dental lamina prior to the appearance of the tooth buds[159]; it has been hypothesized that this early innervation influences the initiation and patterning of the tooth germs.[110]

Although formation of the tooth is a continuous process, as a matter of convenience the process has been divided into three stages: the bud, cap, and bell (Fig. 10-3). The *bud* is the initial stage of tooth development, wherein the epithelial cells of the dental lamina proliferate and produce a budlike projection into the adjacent ectomesenchyme. The *cap* stage is reached when the cells of the dental lamina have proliferated to form a concavity that produces a caplike appearance (Fig. 10-4). The outer cells of the "cap" are cuboidal and constitute the outer enamel epithelium. The cells on the inner or concave aspect of the cap are somewhat elongated and represent the inner enamel epithelium. Between the outer and inner epithelia is a network of cells termed the stellate reticulum because of the branched reticular arrangement of the cellular elements. The rim of the enamel organ (i.e., where the outer and inner enamel epithelia are joined) is termed the cervical loop. As the cells forming the loop continue to proliferate, there is further invagination of the enamel organ into the mesenchyme. The organ assumes a bell shape, and tooth development enters the *bell* stage (Fig. 10-5). During the bell stage the ectomesenchyme of the dental papilla becomes partially enclosed by the invaginating epithelium. It is also during this stage that blood vessels become established in the dental papilla.[15]

The condensed ectomesenchyme surrounding the enamel

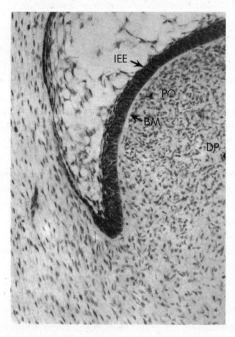

FIG. 10-6. Bell stage showing preodontoblasts *(PO)* aligned along the basement membrane *(BM)*, separating the inner enamel epithelium *(IEE)* from the dental papilla *(DP)*.

organ and dental papilla complex forms the dental sac and ultimately develops into the periodontal ligament (Fig. 10-5). As the tooth bud continues to grow, it carries a portion of the dental lamina with it. This extension is referred to as the lateral lamina. During the bell stage the lateral lamina degenerates and is invaded and replaced by mesenchymal tissue. In this way the epithelial connection between the enamel organ and the oral epithelium is severed. The

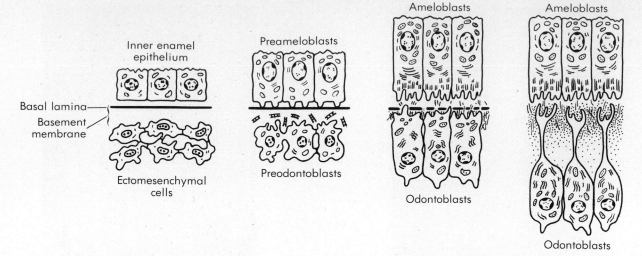

FIG. 10-7. Diagrammatic representation of the stages of odontoblast differentiation.

free end of the dental lamina associated with each of the primary teeth continues to grow and form the successional lamina (Fig. 10-5). It is from this structure that the tooth germ of the succedaneous tooth arises. As the maxillary and mandibular processes increase in length, the permanent first molar arises from posterior extensions of the dental lamina. After birth the second and third molar primordia appear as the dental laminae proliferate into the underlying mesenchyme.

Differentiation of epithelial and mesenchymal cells into ameloblasts and odontoblasts respectively occurs during the bell stage of tooth development. This differentiation is always more advanced in the apex of the "bell" (the region where the cusp tip will develop) than in the area of the cervical loop. From the loop upward toward the apex the cells appear progressively more differentiated. The preameloblasts differentiate at a faster rate than the corresponding odontoblasts so that at any given level mature ameloblasts appear before the odontoblasts have fully matured. In spite of this difference in rate of maturation, dentin matrix is formed in advance of enamel matrix.

Although it is generally held that the presence of the enamel organ is a requirement for odontoblast differentiation, in vitro culture experiments have shown that pulp cells can develop into active preodontoblasts in the absence of the inductive influences of inner enamel epithelium, suggesting that pulp ectomesenchyme has a certain capacity to autodifferentiate into odontogenic tissue.[160] This characteristic of pulp cells should be kept in mind when considering the formation of a dentinal bridge beneath a pulp exposure where no epithelium is present to provide an inductive influence.

During the bell stage of development there is still mitotic activity among the relatively immature cells of the inner enamel epithelium in the region of the cervical loop. As they commence to mature into ameloblasts, mitotic activity ceases and the cells elongate and display the characteristics of active protein synthesis (i.e., an abundance of rough endoplasmic reticulum [RER], a well-developed Golgi complex, and numerous mitochondria).

As the ameloblasts undergo differentiation, changes are taking place across the basement membrane in the adjacent dental papilla. Thanks to some excellent enlightening studies,* a comprehensive picture of dentin development has emerged. Prior to differentiation of odontoblasts, the dental papilla consists of sparsely distributed polymorphic mesenchymal cells with wide intercellular spaces (Fig. 10-6). With the onset of differentiation a single layer of cells, the presumptive odontoblasts (preodontoblasts), align themselves along the basement membrane separating the inner enamel epithelium from the dental papilla (Fig. 10-6). These cells stop dividing and elongate into short columnar cells with basally situated nuclei (Fig. 10-7). Several cytoplasmic projections from each of these cells extend toward the basal lamina. At this stage the preodontoblasts are still relatively undifferentiated.

As the preodontoblasts continue to differentiate, they become progressively more elongated and take on the ultrastructural characteristics of protein-secreting cells. Cytoplasmic processes from these cells extend through the basement membrane toward the basal lamina, and more and more collagen fibrils appear within the ECM. Large fan-shaped fiber bundles 1000 to 2000 Å in diameter, (sometimes referred to as von Korff fibers), become oriented at more or less right angles to the basal lamina. Smaller collagen fibers approximately 500 Å in diameter also accumulate, and these lie more parallel with the basal lamina. The origin of the von Korff fibers has been the subject of much debate since they were first described by Karl von Korff in 1905.[111] Several authors[12,19,112,137,142] have stated that they are derived from pulp fibroblasts and reach the region of the dentin matrix by passing peripherally between the differentiating odontoblasts. Others[192-194] believe that there are few if any collagen fibrils between the differentiating odontoblasts and that all the collagen fibrils in dentin originate from odontoblasts. Support for the latter viewpoint has been provided by studies[127,129]

---

*References 130, 147, 148, 172, 180, 186, 189, and 192.

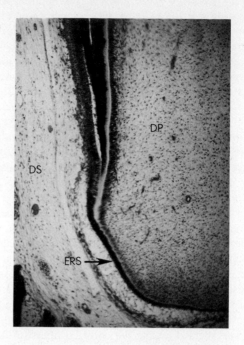

FIG. 10-8. Root development showing dental pulp *(DP)*, dental sac *(DS)*, and epithelial root sheath *(ERS)*.

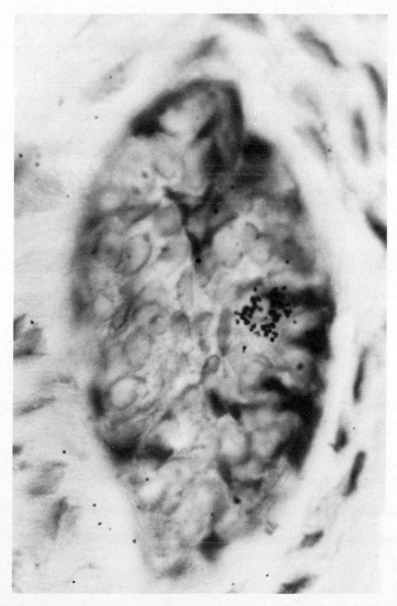

FIG. 10-9. Radioautograph of an epithelial rest cell showing ³H-thymidine labeling of the nucleus. The cell is preparing to divide. (From Trowbridge, H.O., and Shibata, F.: Periodontics **5:**109, 1967.)

demonstrating that the mantle dentin of bovine and human teeth contains no Type III collagen, a type produced by fibroblasts of the dental papilla.

Dentinogenesis first occurs in the developing tooth at sites where the cusp tips or incisal edge will be formed. It is in this region that odontoblasts reach full maturity and become tall columnar cells, at times attaining a height of 50 μm or more (Fig. 10-7). The width of these cells remains fairly constant at approximately 7 μm. Production of the first dentin matrix involves the formation, organization, and maturation of collagen fibrils and proteoglycans. As more collagen fibrils accumulate subjacent to the basal lamina, the lamina becomes discontinuous and eventually disappears. This occurs as the collagen fibers become organized and extend into the interspaces of the ameloblast processes. Concurrently the odontoblasts extend several small processes toward the ameloblasts. Some of these become interposed between the processes of ameloblasts, resulting in the formation of enamel spindles (dentinal tubules that extend into the enamel). Membrane-bound vesicles bud off from the odontoblast processes and become interspersed among the collagen fibers of the dentin matrix. These vesicles subsequently play an important role in the initiation of mineralization (to be discussed later). With the onset of dentinogenesis the dental papilla becomes the dental pulp.

As predentin matrix is formed, the odontoblasts commence to move away toward the central pulp, depositing matrix at a rate of approximately 4-8 μm per day in their wake. Within this matrix a process from each odontoblast becomes accentuated and remains to form the primary odontoblast process. It is around these processes that the dentinal tubules are formed.

Root

Root development commences after the completion of enamel formation. The cells of the inner and outer enamel epithelia, which comprise the cervical loop, begin to proliferate and form a structure known as Hertwig's epithelial root sheath (Fig. 10-8). This sheath determines the size and shape of the root or roots of the tooth. As in the formation of the crown, the cells of the inner enamel epithelium appear to influence the adjacent mesenchymal cells to differentiate into preodontoblasts and odontoblasts. As soon as the first layer of dentin matrix mineralizes, gaps appear in the root sheath, allowing mesenchymal cells from the dental sac to move into contact with the newly formed dentin. These cells then differentiate into cementoblasts and deposit cementum matrix on the root dentin.

Epithelial rests of Malassez

The epithelial root sheath does not entirely disappear with the onset of dentinogenesis. Some cells persist within the periodontal ligament and are known as epithelial rests of Malassez. Although the number of these rests gradually decreases with age, it has been shown that at least some of them retain the ability to undergo cell division[212] (Fig. 10-9). *If in later life a chronic inflammatory lesion develops within the periapical tissues as a result of pulp dis-*

ease, proliferation of the epithelial rests may produce a periapical (radicular) cyst.

Accessory canals

Occasionally during formation of the root sheath a break develops in the continuity of the sheath, producing a small gap. When this occurs, dentinogenesis does not take place opposite the defect. The result is a small "accessory" canal between the dental sac and the pulp. An accessory canal can become established anywhere along the root, thus creating a periodontal-endodontic pathway of communication and a possible portal of entry into the pulp if the periodontal tissues lose their integrity. *In periodontal disease the development of a periodontal pocket may expose an accessory canal and thus allow microorganisms or their metabolic products to gain access to the pulp.*

DENTIN

Fully matured dentin is composed of approximately 65% inorganic material by weight, nearly all of which is in the form of hydroxyapatite crystals. Collagen accounts for about 20% of dentin. Citrate, chondroitin sulfate, noncollagenous protein, lactate, and lipid account for approximately 2%. The remaining 13% consists of water. By volume, inorganic matter makes up 45% of dentin; organic molecules 33%; and water 22%. A characteristic of human dentin is the presence of tubules that occupy from 20% to 30% of the volume of intact dentin. These tubules house the major cell processes of odontoblasts. The elasticity of dentin provides flexibility for the overlying brittle enamel.

Dentin and enamel are closely bound together at the dentin-enamel junction (DEJ), and dentin joins cementum at the dentin-cementum junction (DCJ). Electron microscopy has revealed that the hydroxyapatite crystals of dentin and enamel are intermixed in the area formerly occupied by the basal lamina of the inner enamel epithelium.[93] Since the basal lamina is dissolved prior to the onset of dentinogenesis, no organic membrane separates the crystals of enamel from those of dentin. It is well known clinically that the DEJ is an area of considerable sensitivity. The reason for this is not clear, but it is thought that the branching of the dentinal tubules in the region of the DEJ plays a role.

Types of dentin

Developmental dentin is that which forms during tooth development. That formed physiologically after the root is fully developed is referred to as secondary dentin. Developmental dentin is classified as *orthodentin*, the tubular form of dentin found in the teeth of all dentate mammals. Mantle dentin is the first formed dentin and is situated immediately subjacent to the enamel or cementum. It is typified by its content of the thick fan-shaped collagen fibers deposited immediately subjacent to the basal lamina during the initial stages of dentinogenesis. Spaces between the fibers are occupied by smaller collagen fibrils lying more or less parallel with the DEJ or DCJ. The width of mantle dentin in human teeth has been estimated at 80 to 100 μm.[12,130,137]

Circumpulpal dentin is formed after the layer of mantle dentin has been deposited, and it constitutes the major part of developmental dentin. The organic matrix is composed mainly of collagen fibrils, approximately 500 Å in diameter, that are oriented at right angles to the long axis of the dentinal tubules. These fibrils are closely packed together and form an interwoven network.

Predentin is the unmineralized organic matrix of dentin situated between the layer of odontoblasts and the mineralized dentin. Its macromolecular constituents include type I collagen,[37] chondroitin-4-sulfate, chondroitin-6-sulfate, hyaluronate, dermatan sulfate, and keratin sulfate.[125] Proteoglycans, principally chondroitin sulfate, accumulate near the calcification front. Proteoglycans interact with collagen and somehow influence fibrillogenesis. In addition to proteoglycans and collagen, the odontoblast secretes phosphophoryn, a phosphoprotein involved in extracellular mineralization. This substance is unique to dentin and pulp cells and is not found in other mesenchymal cell lines.[214]

Mineralization of dentin

Mineralization of dentin matrix commences within the initial increment of mantle dentin. Hydroxyapatite crystals begin to accumulate in matrix vesicles within the predentin.[42] Presumably these vesicles bud off from the cytoplasmic processes of odontoblasts.[180] Although matrix vesicles are distributed throughout the predentin, they are most numerous near the basal lamina. The apatite crystals grow rapidly within the vesicles, and in time the vesicles rupture. The crystals thus released mix with crystals from adjoining vesicles to form advancing crystal fronts that merge to form small globules. As the globules expand, they fuse with adjacent globules until the matrix is completely mineralized.

Apparently matrix vesicles are involved only in mineralization of the initial layer of dentin. As the process of mineralization progresses, the advancing front projects along the collagen fibrils of the predentin matrix.[42] Hydroxyapatite crystals appear on the surface and within the fibrils and continue to grow as mineralization progresses, resulting in an increased mineral content of the dentin. Eventually, the crystals achieve a length of 300 to 600 Å and a width of 20 to 45 Å.[189]

Dentinal tubules

The orthodentin of mammalian teeth is characterized by the presence of tubules. Tubules form around the odontoblast processes and thus traverse the entire width of the dentin from the DEJ or DCJ to the pulp. They are slightly tapered, with the wider portion situated toward the pulp. This tapering is the result of the progressive formation of peritubular dentin, which leads to a continuous decrease in the diameter of the tubules toward the enamel.

In coronal dentin the tubules have a gentle S shape as they extend from the DEJ to the pulp. The S-shaped curvature is presumably a result of the crowding of odontoblasts as they migrate toward the center of the pulp. As they approach the pulp, the tubules converge because the

surface of the pulp chamber has a much smaller area than the surface of dentin along the DEJ.

The number and diameter of the tubules at various distances from the pulp have been determined[66] (Table 10-1). Investigators[1] found the number and diameter of dentinal tubules to be similar in rats, cats, dogs, monkeys, and humans, indicating that mammalian orthodentin has evolved amazingly constantly (Table 10-2).

Lateral tubules containing branches of the main odontoblastic processes have been demonstrated by other researchers,[100] who suggested that they form pathways for the movement of materials between the main processes and the more distant matrix. It is also possible that the direction of the branches influences the orientation of the collagen fibrils in the intertubular dentin.

Near the DEJ the dentinal tubules ramify into one or more terminal branches (Figs. 10-10 and 10-11). This is due to the fact that during the initial stage of dentinogene-

TABLE 10-1. Mean number and diameter per square millimeter of dentinal tubules at various distances from the pulp in human teeth

Distance from pulp (mm)	Number of tubules (1000/sq mm)		Tubule diameter (μm)	
	Mean	Range	Mean	Range
Pulpal wall	45	30-52	2.5	2.0-3.2
0.1-0.5	43	22-59	1.9	1.0-2.3
0.6-1.0	38	16-47	1.6	1.0-1.6
1.1-1.5	35	21-47	1.2	0.9-1.5
1.6-2.0	30	12-47	1.1	0.8-1.6
2.1-2.5	23	11-36	0.9	0.6-1.3
2.6-3.0	20	7-40	0.8	0.5-1.4
3.1-3.5	19	10-25	0.8	0.5-1.2

From Garberoglio, R., and Brännström, M.: Arch. Oral Biol. **21:**355, 1976.

TABLE 10-2. Tubule diameter, number of tubules per square millimeter, and percent area occupied by dentinal tubules in different species (mean values halfway between pulp and enamel)

Animal	Diameter (μm)	Number (per sq mm)	Percent area occupied by tubules
Rat			
Incisor	1.0	50,000	3.9
Molar	1.1	49,000	4.6
Cat	1.0	41,000	3.2
Dog	1.3	43,000	5.7
Monkey	1.1	37,000	3.5
Human			
Young	1.4	30,000	4.6
Old	1.1	29,000	2.8

From Ahlberg, K., Brännström, M., and Edwall, L.: Acta Odontol. Scand. **33:**243, 1975.

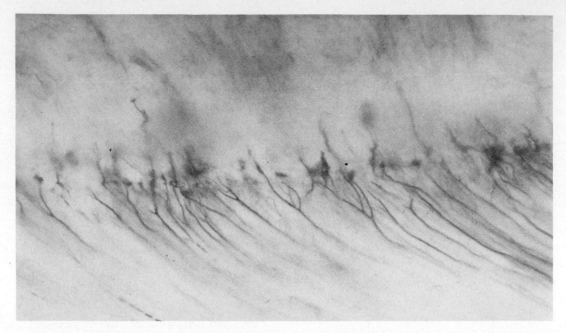

FIG. 10-10. Ground section of a tooth demonstrating branching of the dentinal tubules near the DEJ. This branching may account for the increased clinical sensitivity at the DEJ.

sis the differentiating odontoblasts extended several cytoplasmic processes toward the DEJ but, as the odontoblasts withdrew, their processes converged into one major process (see Fig. 10-7).

Peritubular dentin

Dentin lining the tubules is termed peritubular dentin, whereas that between the tubules is known as intertubular dentin (Fig. 10-12). Presumably precursors of the dentin matrix that is deposited around each odontoblast process are synthesized by the odontoblast, transported in secretory vesicles out into the process, and released by reverse pinocytosis. With the formation of peritubular dentin there is a corresponding reduction in the diameter of the process.

Peritubular dentin represents a specialized form of orthodentin not common to all mammals. Because of its lower content of collagen, peritubular dentin is more quickly dissolved in acid than is intertubular dentin.

It has also been shown that peritubular dentin is more highly mineralized and therefore harder than intertubular dentin.* Because of its hardness, peritubular dentin may provide added structural support for the intertubular dentin. The matrix of peritubular dentin also differs from that of intertubular dentin in having relatively fewer collagen fibrils and a higher proportion of sulfated proteoglycans.

Intertubular dentin

Intertubular dentin is located between the rings of peritubular dentin and constitutes the bulk of circumpulpal dentin (Fig. 10-12). Its organic matrix consists mainly of collagen fibrils having diameters of 500 to 1000 Å. These

fibrils are oriented approximately at right angles to the dentinal tubules.

Dentinal sclerosis

Partial or complete obturation of dentinal tubules may occur as a result of aging or develop in response to stimuli such as attrition of the tooth surface or dental caries.[183] When tubules become filled with mineral deposits, the dentin becomes sclerotic. Dentinal sclerosis is easily recognized in histologic ground sections because of its translucency, which is due to the homogeneity of the dentin since both matrix and tubules are mineralized. Studies using dyes, solvents, and radioactive ions[11,14,50,135] have shown that sclerosis results in decreased permeability of dentin. Thus dentinal sclerosis, by limiting the diffusion of noxious substances through the dentin, helps to shield the pulp from irritation.

One form of dentinal sclerosis is thought to represent an acceleration of peritubular dentin formation. This form appears to be a physiologic process, and in the apical third of the root it develops as a function of age.[183] Dentinal tubules can also become blocked by the precipitation of hydroxyapatite and whitlockite crystals within the tubules.[191] This type occurs in the translucent zone of carious dentin as well as in attrited dentin and has been termed "pathological sclerosis."[215] One study[61] found that, during caries, intratubular mineral deposits occurred both within the periodontoblastic space and the cytoplasm of the odontoblast process.

Interglobular dentin

The term interglobular dentin refers to organic matrix that remains unmineralized because the mineralizing globules fail to coalesce. This occurs most often in the circum-

---

*References 38, 39, 46, 56, 57, 94, 120, 207, and 215.

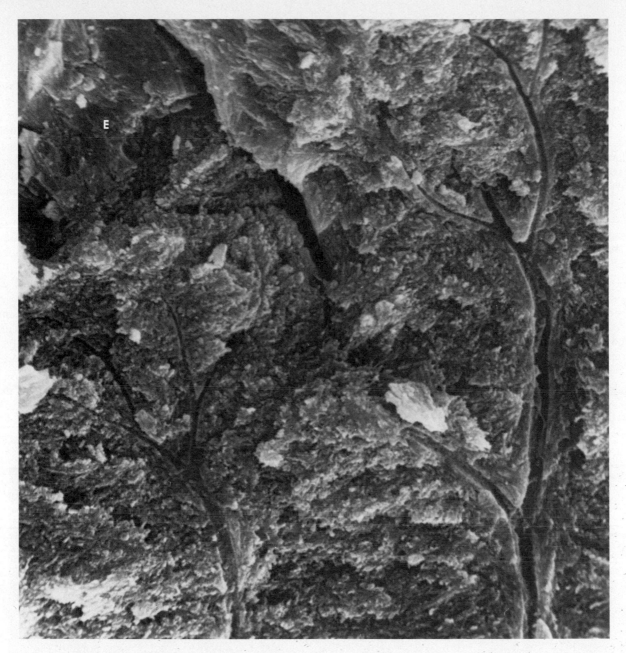

FIG. 10-11. Scanning electron micrograph of branching dentinal tubules near the DEJ. Enamel *(E)* is at the upper left. (×4800.) (Courtesy Keith W. Kelley and Charles F. Cox, School of Dentistry, University of Michigan.)

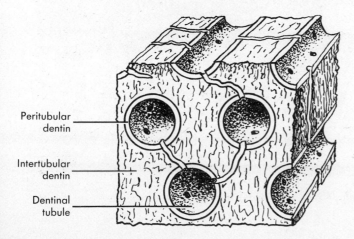

Peritubular dentin

Intertubular dentin

Dentinal tubule

FIG. 10-12. Diagram illustrating peritubular and intertubular dentin. (From Trowbridge, H.O.: Dentistry 82 **2:**22, 1982.)

pulpal dentin just below the mantle dentin where the pattern of mineralization is more likely to be globular than appositional. In certain dental anomalies (e.g., vitamin D–resistant rickets and hypophosphatasia) large areas of interglobular dentin are a characteristic feature (Fig. 10-13).

Dentinal fluid

Free fluid occupies about 22% of the total volume of dentin. This fluid is an ultrafiltrate of blood in the pulp capillaries and its composition resembles plasma in many respects. The fluid flows outward between the odontoblasts into the dentinal tubules and eventually escapes through small pores in the enamel. It has been shown that the tissue pressure of the pulp is approximately 6 mm Hg.[83] Consequently, there is a pressure gradient between the pulp and the oral cavity that accounts for the outward flow of fluid. Exposure of the tubules by tooth fracture or during cavity preparation often results in the movement of fluid to the exposed dentin surface in the form of tiny droplets. This outward movement of fluid can be accelerated by dehydrating the surface of the dentin with compressed air, dry heat, or the application of absorbent paper. The rapid flow of fluid through the tubules is thought to be a cause of dentin sensitivity. (See pp. 319-321.)

Bacterial products or other contaminants may be introduced into the dentinal fluid as a result of dental caries, restorative procedures, or growth of bacteria beneath restorations.[22,23,208] Dentinal fluid may thus serve as a sump

from which injurious agents can percolate into the pulp, producing an inflammatory response.[13]

Dentin permeability

The permeability of dentin has been well characterized* (see Pashley[153] for review). Dentinal tubules are the major channels for fluid diffusion across dentin. Since fluid permeation is proportional to tubule diameter and number, dentin permeability increases as the tubules converge on the pulp (Fig. 10-14).[151] The total tubular surface near the DEJ is approximately 1% of the total surface area of dentin,[152] whereas close to the pulp chamber the total tubular surface may be nearly 45%. Thus from a clinical standpoint it should be recognized that dentin beneath a deep cavity preparation is much more permeable than dentin underlying a shallow cavity. For the same reason peripheral dentin is stronger than dentin near the pulp.

Factors modifying dentin permeability include the presence of odontoblast processes in the tubules, the presence of collagen fibers in the tubules, and the sheath-like lamina limitans that lines the tubules. Thus the functional or physiological diameter of the tubules is only about 5 to 10% of the anatomic diameter, i.e., the diameter seen in microscopic sections.[132]

In dental caries an inflammatory reaction develops in the

---

*References 132, 151, 154-157, and 165.

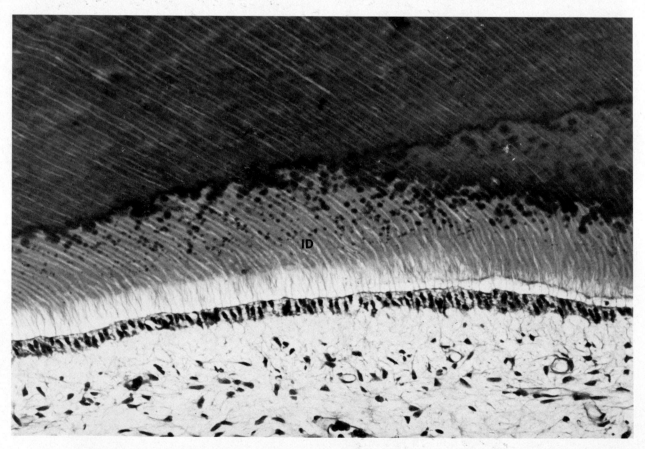

FIG. 10-13. Section showing interglobular dentin *(ID)* in a deciduous incisor from a 3-year-old boy with childhood hypophosphatasia.

pulp long before the pulp actually becomes infected.[28,166,208] This indicates that bacterial products reach the pulp in advance of the bacteria themselves. Dentinal sclerosis beneath a carious lesion reduces this permeation by obstructing the tubules, thus decreasing the concentration of irritants that are introduced into the pulp.

The cutting of dentin during cavity preparation produces microcrystalline grinding debris that coats the dentin and clogs the orifices of the dentinal tubules. This layer of debris is termed the smear layer. Because of the small size of the particles, the smear layer is capable of preventing bacteria from penetrating dentin.[133] Removal of the grinding debris by acid etching greatly increases the permeability of the dentin by decreasing the surface resistance and widening the orifices of the tubules. Consequently, the incidence of pulpal inflammation may be increased significantly if cavities are treated with an acid cleanser, unless a cavity liner or base is used.

The incidence of pulpal inflammation is increased significantly when cavities are treated with an acid cleanser (50% citric acid) as compared to controls in which the acid is omitted.[33]

In vital teeth bacteria do not readily pass through exposed dentinal tubules into the pulp. Constrictions and irregularities within the dentinal tubules are capable of arresting 99.8% of the bacteria that enter the dentin surface.[133,150] Such intratubular resistances produce a functional or physiologic tubular radius that is only about one tenth the anatomic radius.[132] In teeth from which the pulps have been removed, bacteria pass into the pulp in a relatively short time.[31] Presumably this is due to the resistance offered by the presence of dentinal fluid and odontoblast processes in the tubules of vital teeth. It is also possible that antibodies or other antimicrobial agents may be present within the dentinal fluid in response to bacterial infection of the dentin.

Since they are not motile, bacteria advance through the tubules by repeated cell division.[133] If a force such as the hydraulic pressure generated during mastication or impression taking is applied to exposed dentin, bacteria may be driven through the dentin and into the pulp.

MORPHOLOGIC ZONES OF THE PULP
Odontoblast layer

The outermost stratum of cells of the healthy pulp is the odontoblast layer (Figs. 10-15 and 10-16). This layer

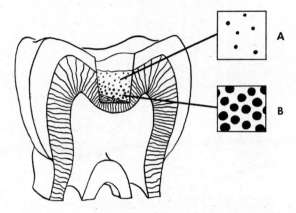

FIG. 10-14. Diagram illustrating the difference in size and number of tubules in the dentinal floor between a shallow, **A,** and a deep, **B,** cavity preparation. (From Trowbridge, H.O.: Dentistry 82 **2:**22, 1982.)

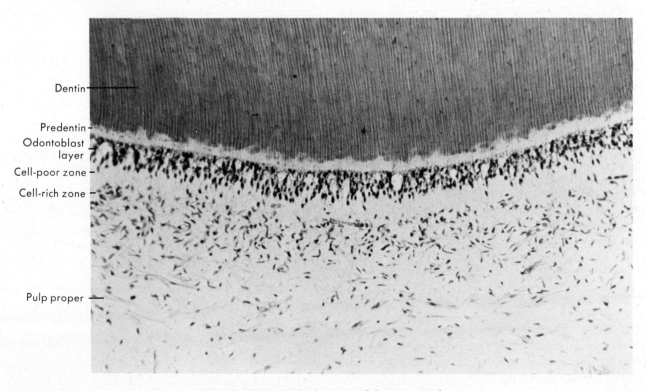

Dentin

Predentin
Odontoblast
layer
Cell-poor zone
Cell-rich zone

Pulp proper

FIG. 10-15. Morphologic zones of the mature pulp.

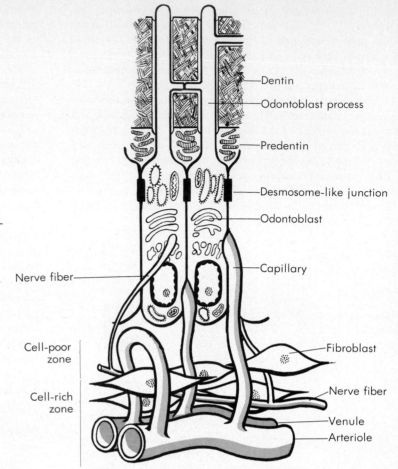

FIG. 10-16. Diagrammatic representation of the odontoblast layer and subodontoblastic region of the pulp.

Labels on figure: Dentin, Odontoblast process, Predentin, Desmosome-like junction, Odontoblast, Capillary, Nerve fiber, Fibroblast, Cell-poor zone, Cell-rich zone, Nerve fiber, Venule, Arteriole

is located immediately subjacent to the predentin. Since the odontoblast processes are embedded within the dentinal tubules, the odontoblast layer is composed principally of the cell bodies of odontoblasts. Additionally, capillaries and nerve fibers may be found among the odontoblasts.

In the coronal portion of a young pulp the odontoblasts assume a tall columnar form. The tight packing together of these tall slender cells produces the appearance of a palisade. The odontoblasts vary in height; consequently, their nuclei are not all at the same level and are aligned in a staggered array. This often produces the appearance of a layer three to five cells in thickness. Between odontoblasts there are small intercellular spaces approximately 300 to 400 Å in width.

The odontoblast layer in the coronal pulp contains more cells per unit area than in the radicular pulp. Whereas the odontoblasts of the mature coronal pulp are usually columnar (Fig. 10-17), those in the midportion of the radicular pulp are more cuboid (Fig. 10-18). Near the apical foramen the odontoblasts appear as a flattened cell layer. Since there are fewer dentinal tubules per unit area in the root than in the crown of the tooth, the odontoblast cell bodies are less crowded and are able to spread out laterally. The cell body of most of the odontoblasts borders on the predentin; the odontoblast process, however, passes on through the predentin into the dentin.

Between adjacent odontoblasts there are specialized cell-to-cell junctions.* Desmosome-like junctions provide attachment plaques that mechanically join odontoblasts in an almost continuous band near the border of the predentin.[91] Gap junctions provide a low-resistance pathway through which electrical excitation can pass rapidly from cell to cell, perhaps permitting the odontoblasts to function as a syncytium (Fig. 10-20). These cell-to-cell junctions do not form a complete and uninterupted encirclement of the odontoblasts, so fluid, plasma proteins, capillaries, and nerve fibers are able to pass between them. Gap junctions and desmosome-like junctions have been observed joining odontoblasts to fibroblasts in the subodontoblastic area.[107]

Cell-poor zone

Immediately subjacent to the odontoblast layer in the coronal pulp there is often a narrow zone approximately 40 μm in width that is relatively free of cells (Figs. 10-15 and 10-16). It is traversed by blood capillaries, unmyelinated nerve fibers, and the slender cytoplasmic processes of fibroblasts. The presence or absence of the cell-poor zone depends upon the functional status of the pulp. It may not be apparent in young pulps rapidly forming dentin or in older pulps where reparative dentin is being produced.

---

*References 80, 86, 88, 91, 107, and 170.

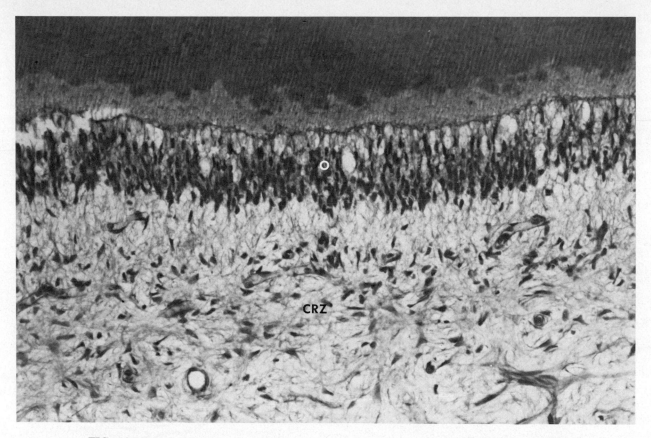

FIG. 10-17. Tall columnar odontoblasts *(O)* of the coronal pulp. Note the presence of the cell-rich zone *(CRZ)*.

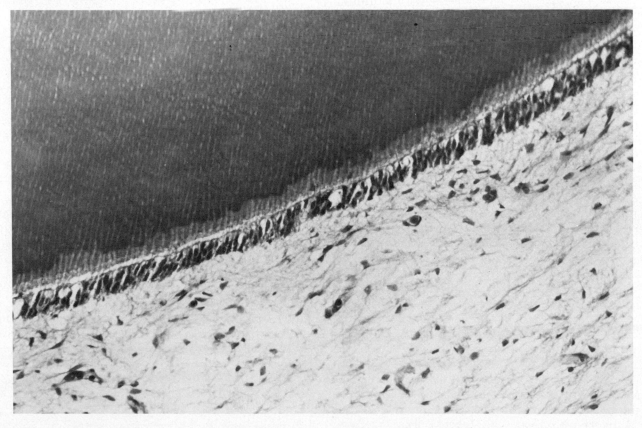

FIG. 10-18. Low columnar odontoblasts of the radicular pulp. The cell-rich zone is inconspicuous.

Cell-rich zone

Usually conspicuous in the subodontoblastic area is a stratum containing a relatively high proportion of fibroblasts compared to the more central region of the pulp (Fig. 10-15). It is much more prominent in the coronal pulp than in the radicular pulp. Besides fibroblasts, the cell-rich zone may include a variable number of macrophages, lymphocytes, or plasma cells.

On the basis of evidence obtained in rat molar teeth, it has been suggested[68] that the cell-rich zone forms as a result of peripheral migration of cells populating the central regions of the pulp, commencing at about the time of tooth eruption. Although cell division within the cell-rich zone is a rare occurrence in normal pulps, death of odontoblasts causes a great increase in the rate of mitosis.[69] Since irreversibly injured odontoblasts are replaced by cells that migrate from the cell-rich zone into the odontoblast layer,[223] this mitotic activity is probably the first step in the regeneration of the odontoblast layer. (See pp. 328-330.)

Pulp proper

The pulp proper is the central mass of the pulp (Fig. 10-15). It contains the larger blood vessels and nerve fibers. Most of the connective tissue cells in this zone are fibroblasts. These cells, together with a network of collagen fibers, are embedded within the connective tissue ground substance.

CELLS OF THE PULP
Odontoblast

Because it is responsible for dentinogenesis both during tooth development and in the mature tooth, the odontoblast is the most characteristic cell of the dentin-pulp complex. During dentinogenesis the odontoblasts form the dentinal tubules, and their presence within the tubules makes dentin a living tissue.

Dentinogenesis, osteogenesis, and cementogenesis are in many respects quite similar. Therefore it is not surprising that odontoblasts, osteoblasts, and cementoblasts have many similar characteristics. Each of these cells produces a matrix composed of collagen fibers and proteoglycans that is capable of undergoing mineralization. The ultrastructural characteristics of odontoblasts, osteoblasts, and cementoblasts are likewise similar in that each exhibits a highly ordered RER, a prominent Golgi complex, secretory granules, and numerous mitochondria. In addition, these cells are rich in RNA and their nuclei contain one or more prominent nucleoli. These are the general characteristics of protein-secreting cells.

Perhaps the most significant differences between odontoblasts, osteoblasts, and cementoblasts are their morphologic characteristics and the anatomic relationships between the cells and the structures they produce. Whereas osteoblasts and cementoblasts are polygonal to cuboidal in form, the fully developed odontoblast of the coronal pulp is a tall columnar cell. In bone and cementum the osteoblasts and cementoblasts become entrapped in the matrix as osteocytes or cementocytes respectively. The odontoblasts, on the other hand, leave behind cellular processes to form the dentinal tubules. Lateral branches between the

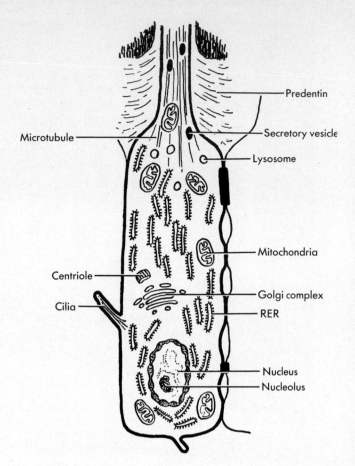

FIG. 10-19. Diagram of a fully differentiated odontoblast.

major odontoblast processes interconnect the processes through canals just as osteocytes and cementocytes are linked together through the canaliculae in bone and cementum. This provides for intercellular communication as well as circulation of fluid and metabolites through the mineralized matrix.

The ultrastructural features of the odontoblast have been the subject of numerous investigations.* The cell body of the active odontoblast has a large nucleus that may contain up to four nucleoli (Figs. 10-19 and 10-20). The nucleus is situated at the basal end of the cell and is contained within a nuclear envelope. A well-developed Golgi complex, centrally located in the supranuclear cytoplasm, consists of an assembly of smooth-walled vesicles and cisternae. Numerous mitochondria are evenly distributed throughout the cell body. RER is particularly prominent, consisting of closely stacked cisternae forming parallel arrays that are dispersed diffusely within the cytoplasm. Numerous ribosomes closely associated with the membranes of the cisternae mark the sites of protein synthesis. Within the lumen of the cisternae, filamentous material probably representing newly synthesized protein can be observed.

Apparently the odontoblast synthesizes only type I collagen and an unusual type I trimer having three alpha chains.[125] In addition to proteoglycans and collagen, the

---

*References 57, 65, 92, 94, 147, 148, 167, 168, 186, and 190.

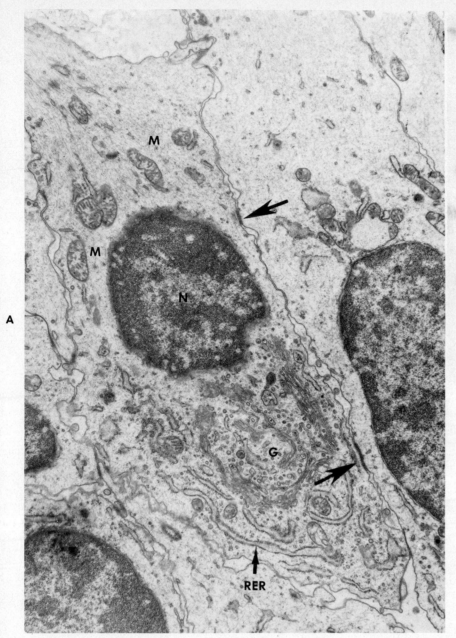

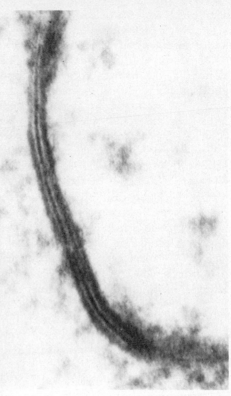

FIG. 10-20. **A,** Electron micrograph of a mouse molar odontoblast demonstrating gap junctions *(arrows)*, nucleus *(N)*, mitochondria *(M)*, Golgi complex *(G)*, and rough endoplasmic reticulum *(RER)*. **B,** High magnification of a section fixed and stained with lanthanum nitrate to demonstrate a typical gap junction. (Courtesy Dr. Charles F. Cox, School of Dentistry, University of Michigan.)

odontoblast secretes phosphophoryn, a phosphoprotein involved in extracellular mineralization. This substance is unique to dentin and is not found in any other mesenchymal cell lines.[214]

Acid phosphatase activity occurs in the Golgi complex and in lysosomes located in the cell body close to the predentin.[99] Some activity extends into the basal portion of the odontoblast process. It has been suggested that lysosomal enzymes such as acid phosphatase may be involved in digesting material that has been resorbed from the predentin matrix, possibly proteoglycans associated with mineralization.[44,99] The odontoblast also secretes alkaline phosphatase, an enzyme that is closely linked to mineralization but whose precise role is yet to be illuminated.

Two centrioles are situated in the region of the Golgi complex. One gives rise to a solitary nonmotile cilium, which may remain rudimentary or undergo further devel-

opment and extend into the interodontoblastic space.[65]

Cytoplasmic microtubules extend from the cell body into the odontoblast process. These straight structures follow a course that is parallel with the long axis of the cell and impart the impression of rigidity. Although their precise role is unknown, theories as to their functional significance suggest that they may be involved in cytoplasmic extension, transport of materials, or simply the provision of a structural framework.

In contrast to the active odontoblast, the resting or inactive odontoblast has a decreased number of organelles and may become progressively shorter. These changes can begin with the completion of root development.

Odontoblast process

Microtubules and microfilaments are the principal ultrastructural components of the odontoblast process and its lateral branches.[90] These structures have a preferential arrangement parallel with the long axis of the process. The plasma membrane of the odontoblast process closely approximates the wall of the dentinal tubule. Localized constrictions in the process occasionally produce relatively large spaces between the tubule wall and the process.[57,58,198] Such spaces may contain collagen fibrils and fine granular material which presumably represents ground substance. The peritubular dentin matrix lining the tubule is circumscribed by an electron-dense limiting membrane.[198] A space separates the limiting membrane from the plasma membrane of the odontoblast process. This space is usually narrow except in areas where, as mentioned previously, the process is constricted.

The extent to which the odontoblast process extends outward in the dentin has been a matter of considerable controversy. It has long been thought that the process is present throughout the full thickness of dentin.[7,137,161,202] However, many ultrastructural studies using scanning and transmission electron microscopy have described the process as being limited to the inner third of the dentin.[26,64,85,87,198] On the other hand, studies employing scanning electron microscopy have described the process in peripheral dentin, often extending to the DEJ.[35,71,73,101,219] One investigator[198-200] has shown that the lumen of the dentinal tubule is surrounded by an electron-dense structure, the lamina limitans, which is indistinguishable from the odontoblast process, and he has suggested that this is what others have described as being the odontoblast process. Using antibodies directed against microtubules, investigators have demonstrated immunoreactivity throughout the dentinal tubule, suggesting that the process extends throughout the entire thickness of dentin.[178,179] Obviously this problem warrants further study. Since high-speed drilling can disrupt odontoblasts, it would be of considerable clinical importance to establish conclusively the extent of the odontoblast processes in human teeth. With this knowledge the clinician would be in a better position to estimate the impact of restorative procedures on the underlying odontoblast layer.

The odontoblast is considered to be a fixed postmitotic cell in that once it has fully differentiated it apparently cannot undergo further cell division. If this is indeed the case, the life-span of the odontoblast coincides with the life-span of the viable pulp. It is conceivable, however, that cells from the cell-rich zone migrate into the odontoblast layer to replace odontoblasts that have died.

Relationship of structure to function

Isotope studies have shed a great deal of light on the functional significance of the cytoplasmic organelles of the active odontoblast.[60,167,217] In experimental animals the intraperitoneal injection of collagen precursors such as ^{3}H-proline is followed by autoradiographic labeling of the odontoblasts and predentin matrix (Fig. 10-21). Rapid incorporation of the isotope in the RER soon leads to labeling of the Golgi complex in the area where the procollagen is packed and concentrated into secretory vesicles. Labeled vesicles can then be followed along their migration pathway until they reach the base of the odontoblast process.

Here they fuse with the cell membrane and release their tropocollagen molecules into the predentin matrix by the process of reverse pinocytosis. It is now known that collagen fibrils precipitate from a solution of tropocollagen and that the aggregation of fibrils occurs on the outer surface of the odontoblast plasma membrane. Fibrils are released into the predentin and increase in thickness as they approach the calcification front. Whereas fibrils at the base of the odontoblast process are approximately 150 Å in diameter, fibrils in the region of the calcification front have attained a diameter of about 500 Å.

Similar tracer studies[216] have elucidated the pathway of synthesis, transport, and secretion of the predentin proteoglycans. The protein moiety of these molecules is synthesized by the RER of the odontoblast whereas sulfation and addition of the GAG moieties to the protein molecules takes place in the Golgi complex. Secretory vesicles then transport the proteoglycans to the base of the odontoblast process, where they are secreted into the predentin matrix. Proteoglycans, principally chondroitin sulfate, accumulate near the calcification front. The role of the proteoglycans is speculative, but mounting evidence suggests that they act as inhibitors of calcification by binding calcium. It appears that just before calcification the proteoglycans are removed, probably by lysosomal enzymes secreted by the odontoblasts.[44]

Fibroblast

Fibroblasts are the most numerous cells of the dental pulp. They produce the collagen fibers of the pulp; and since they also degrade collagen, they are also responsible for collagen turnover. Although distributed throughout the pulp, fibroblasts are particularly abundant in the cell-rich zone. The early-differentiating fibroblasts are polygonal and appear to be widely separated and evenly distributed within the ground substance.[6] Cell-to-cell contacts are established between the multiple processes that extend out from each of the cells. Many of these contacts take the form of gap junctions, which provide for electronic coupling of one cell to another. Ultrastructurally the organelles of the immature fibroblasts are generally in a rudimentary stage of development, with an inconspicuous Golgi complex, numerous free ribosomes, and sparse RER. As they mature, the cells become stellate in form and the Golgi complex enlarges, the RER proliferates, secretory vesicles appear, and the fibroblasts take on the characteristic appearance of protein-secreting cells. Along the outer surface of the cell body, collagen fibrils commence to appear. With an increase in the number of blood vessels, nerves, and fibers there is a relative decrease in the number of fibroblasts in the pulp.[6]

A colleague once remarked that the fibroblasts of the pulp are very much like Peter Pan in that they never grow up. There may be an element of truth in this statement, for these cells do seem to remain in a relatively undifferentiated modality as compared to fibroblasts of most other connective tissues.[76] This perception has been fortified by the observation of large numbers of reticulin fibers in the pulp.[130,140,161] Reticulin fibers, once believed to be precollagenous in nature and therefore the product of immature

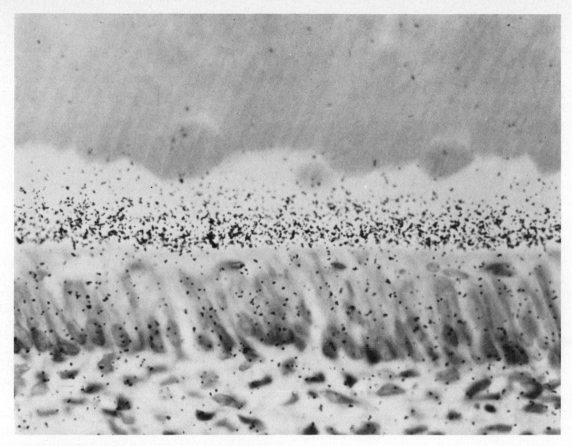

FIG. 10-21. Radioautograph demonstrating odontoblasts and predentin in a developing rat molar 1 hour after intraperitoneal injection of ^{3}H-proline.

cells, have an affinity for silver stains and are similar to the argyrophilic fibers of the pulp. However, in a careful review of the subject, Baume[12] concluded that because of distinct histochemical differences, reticulin fibers, such as those of gingiva and lymphoid organs, are not present in the pulp. He suggested that these pulpal fibers be termed argyrophilic collagen fibers. The fibers apparently acquire a GAG sheath, and it is this sheath that is impregnated by silver stains. In the young pulp the non-argyrophilic collagen fibers are sparse, but they progressively increase in number as the pulp ages.

Many experimental models have been developed to study wound healing in the pulp, particularly dentinal bridge formation following pulp exposure. One study[55] suggests that mitotic activity preceding the differentiation of replacement odontoblasts appears to occur primarily among young fibroblasts. Evidence has been presented that new odontoblasts are derived from pulpal fibroblasts that have undergone dedifferentiation and reverted to undifferentiated mesenchymal cells.[221] Through repeated cell division these cells presumably provide new cells that differentiate into odontoblasts.

Fibrocyte

The pulpal fibrocyte is recognizable by a large polymorphous nucleus surrounded by scant cytoplasm. This cell contains relatively few organelles and synthesizes little if any collagen. Although it is not commonly seen in young pulps, its number increases in older pulps which contain highly aggregated collagen fibers. Fibrocytes are thought to play a role in the maintenance of collagen fibers.

Mesenchymal cell

Undifferentiated mesenchymal cells are stem cells that can differentiate into various types of cells such as osteoblasts, skin fibroblasts, cementoblasts, etc. As mesenchymal cells mature, they become tissue-specific stem cells having the ability to differentiate into only a specific type of tissue. These cells ultimately differentiate into progenitor cells; for example, in the pulp they become odontoprogenitor cells capable of differentiating into dentin-producing cells. Thus they appear to be the only mesenchymal cells capable of producing phosphophoryn, a phosphoprotein unique to dentin matrix.[214] When the need for new odontoblasts arises following injury to the odontoblast layer, pulp fibroblasts, after repeated mitosis, differentiate into odontoblasts.[220]

Other cellular elements

Lymphocytes and plasma cells are occasionally observed in either the coronal or the radicular portion of a healthy pulp; however, they are more likely to be encountered in the subodontoblastic region of the coronal pulp. These immunologically competent cells suggest the presence of antigenic material, probably derived from the oral flora. Although it is theoretically possible for bacterial antigens from the oral cavity to reach the pulp in erupted teeth, one study[116] reported finding inflammatory cells, particularly lymphocytes and neutrophilic leukocytes, in the extravascular tissue in pulps of impacted teeth. Since plasma cells were seldom observed in the pulps of these teeth, it is possible that the lymphocytes and neutrophils were merely performing a surveillance function rather than responding to specific inflammatory stimuli.

Tissue macrophages (often referred to as histiocytes) are monocytes that have left the bloodstream and entered the tissues. They are frequently observed in the healthy pulp intimately mingled with fibroblasts, although the study just mentioned[116] seldom encountered them in the pulps of impacted teeth. These cells are avidly phagocytic and function to remove foreign particulate matter that is introduced into pulp tissue. They may accumulate such material as hemosiderin, calcium hydroxide, and particles of amalgam.

The tissue mast cell has been the subject of considerable interest, perhaps because of its dramatic role in certain inflammatory responses in which histamine is an important chemical mediator (e.g., anaphylactic reactions). While it is frequently seen in chronically inflamed pulps, until recently investigators had been unable to establish its presence in the healthy pulp.[134,222] However, it now appears that mast cells may be present in uninflamed pulps.[47]

METABOLISM

The metabolic activity of the pulp has been studied by measuring the rate of oxygen consumption and the production of carbon dioxide or lactic acid by pulp tissue in vitro.[51,52,174] Recent investigations[75] have employed the radiospirometry method.

Because of the relatively sparse cellular composition of the pulp, the rate of oxygen consumption is low in comparison to most other tissues. During active dentinogenesis, metabolic activity is much higher than following the completion of crown development.[52,174] As would be anticipated, the greatest metabolic activity is found in the region of the odontoblast layer.[51]

In addition to the usual glycolytic pathway, the bovine pulp has the ability to produce energy through a phosphogluconate (pentose phosphate) shunt type of carbohydrate metabolism,[54] suggesting that the pulp may be able to function under varying degrees of ischemia. This could explain how the pulp manages to withstand periods of vasoconstriction resulting from the use of infiltration anesthesia employing epinephrine-containing local anesthetic agents.[104]

Several commonly used dental materials (e.g., eugenol, zinc oxide–eugenol, calcium hydroxide, silver amalgam) have been shown to inhibit oxygen consumption by pulp tissue, indicating that these agents may be capable of depressing the metabolic activity of pulpal cells.[53,98] One investigation[75] found that application of orthodontic force to human premolars for 3 days resulted in a 27% reduction in respiratory activity in the pulp.

GROUND SUBSTANCE

Ground substance comprises the matrix in which connective tissue cells and fibers are embedded. Whereas the fibers and cells of the pulp have recognizable shapes, the ground substance is described as being amorphous. The cells that produce connective tissue fibers also synthesize the major constituents of ground substance.

The ground substance can be thought of as a sol (fluid colloidal system) or a gel that cannot be easily squeezed out of the connective tissue. In this respect it differs from tissue fluids that can be removed largely by drainage alone. Early in embryonic development the ground substance is quite fluid, whereas in mature connective tissue it tends to be gelatinous. The ability of connective tissue to retain water is ascribed to the GAGs, a characteristic component of the ground substance.

The principal molecular components of ground substance are often referred to as mucopolysaccharides. Since these compounds are highly acidic, they are also termed acid mucopolysaccharides. They consist of polysaccharides or glycosaminoglycans linked covalently to a protein molecule. Special histochemical stains (e.g., Alcian blue, colloidal iron) can be employed to demonstrate the presence of mucopolysaccharides in the pulp. The more up-to-date term *proteoglycan* is now frequently used in place of mucopolysaccharide.

In the dental pulp the principal proteoglycans consist of chondroitin-6-sulfate, chondroitin-4-sulfate, heparan sulfate, a hyaluronic acid,* and dermatan sulfate.[124] The proteoglycan content of pulp tissue decreases approximately 50% with tooth eruption.[126] During active dentinogenesis, chondroitin sulfate is the principal proteoglycan, particularly in the odontoblast-predentin layer, where it is involved with mineralization; but with eruption hyaluronic acid and dermatan sulfate increase and chondroitin sulfate decreases greatly.

Another component of pulpal ground substance is fibronectin, which appears to act as a mediator of cell adhesion and is found throughout the pulp.[127]

The consistency of a connective tissue such as the pulp is largely determined by the proteoglycan components of the ground substance. The long GAG chains of the proteoglycan molecules form relatively rigid coils constituting a network that holds water, thus forming a characteristic gel. Hyaluronic acid in particular has a strong affinity for water and is a major component of ground substance in tissues with a large fluid content, such as Wharton's jelly. The water content of the pulp is very high (approximately 90%), and thus the ground substance forms a cushion capable of protecting cells and vascular components of the tooth.

Ground substance also acts as a molecular sieve in that it excludes large proteins, and urea. Cell metabolites, nutrients, and wastes pass through the ground substance be-

---

*Since there is still some doubt as to whether hyaluronic acid is linked to protein, it should probably be referred to as a GAG rather than a proteoglycan.

tween cells and blood vessels. In some ways ground substance can be likened to an ion-exchange resin since the polyanionic charges of the GAGs bind cations. Additionally, osmotic pressures can be altered by excluding osmotically active molecules. Thus the proteoglycans can regulate the dispersion of interstitial matrix solutes, colloids, and water and in large measure determine the physical characteristics of the pulp.

Degradation of ground substance can occur in certain inflammatory lesions in which there is a high concentration of lysosomal enzymes. Proteolytic enzymes, hyaluronidases, and chondroitin sulfatases of lysosomal as well as bacterial origin are examples of the hydrolytic enzymes that can attack components of the ground substance. The

pathways of inflammation and infection are strongly influenced by the state of polymerization of the ground substance components.

FIBERS OF THE PULP

Two types of structural proteins are found in the pulp: collagen and elastin. However, elastin fibers are confined to the walls of arterioles and, unlike collagen, are not a part of the intercellular matrix.

A single collagen molecule, referred to as tropocollagen, consists of three polypeptide chains, designated as either α-1 or α-2 depending upon their amino acid composition and sequence. The different combinations and linkages of chains making up the tropocollagen molecule

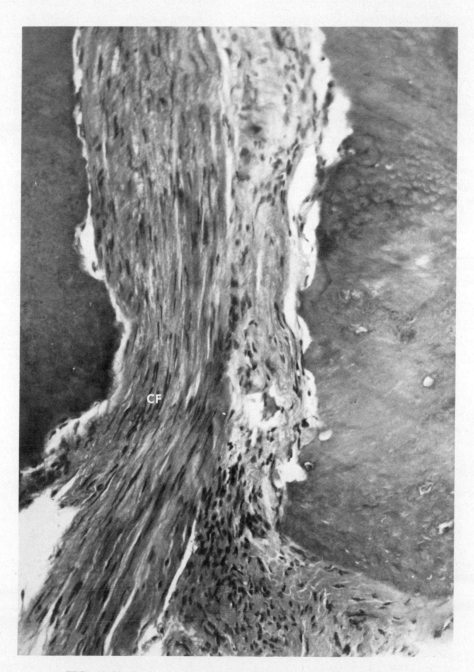

FIG. 10-22. Dense bundles of collagen fibers *(CF)* in the apical pulp.

has allowed collagen to be classified into a number of types. Type I is found in skin, tendon, bone, dentin, and pulp. Type II occurs in cartilage. Type III is found in most unmineralized connective tissues. It is a fetal form found in the dental papilla as well as the mature pulp. In the bovine pulp it comprises 45% of the total pulp collagen during all stages of development.[119] Type IV collagen is found only in basement membranes.

In collagen synthesis the protein portion of the molecule is formed by the polyribosomes of the RER of connective tissue cells. The proline and lysine residues of the polypeptide chains are hydroxylated in the cisternae of the RER, and the chains are assembled into a triple helix configuration in the smooth endoplasmic reticulum. The product of this assembly is termed procollagen, and it has a terminal unit of amino acids known as the telopeptide of the procollagen molecule. When these molecules reach the Golgi complex, they are glycosylated and packaged in secretory vesicles. The vesicles are transported to the plasma membrane and secreted via exocytosis into the extracellular milieu, thus releasing the procollagen. Here the terminal telopeptide is cleaved by a hydrolytic enzyme and the tropocollagen molecules begin aggregating to form collagen fibrils. It is believed that aggregation of tropocollagen is somehow mediated by the GAGs. The conversion of soluble collagen into insoluble fibers occurs as a result of cross linking of tropocollagen molecules.

The small collagen fibers of the pulp stain characteristically black with silver impregnation stains and are thus referred to as argyrophilic fibers. The larger collagen fibers, more often seen in older pulps, are not argyrophilic; but they can be demonstrated with special histochemical methods such as Gomori's trichrome stain or Mallory's aniline blue. At the electron microscopic level the collagen fibers of the pulp display the characteristic 640 Å crossbanding pattern of collagen.[70] Collagen fibers in the young pulp are characteristically small and irregularly oriented.[78] In older pulps larger fiber bundles are seen, particularly in the central region of the pulp. The highest concentration of collagen fibers is usually found near the apex (Fig. 10-22). Thus Torneck[206] advises that, during pulpectomy, if the pulp is engaged with a barbed broach in the region of the apex this generally affords the best opportunity to remove it intact.

INNERVATION

The pulp is a sensory organ capable of transmitting information from its sensory receptors to the central nervous system. Regardless of the nature of the sensory stimulus (i.e., thermal change, mechanical deformation, injury to the tissues), all afferent impulses from the pulp result in the sensation of pain. The innervation of the pulp includes both *afferent* neurons, which conduct sensory impulses, and *autonomic* fibers, which provide neurogenic modulation of the microcirculation and perhaps regulate dentinogenesis as well. It has been suggested[10] that some intradental nerve fibers may be capable of actually slowing dentin formation.

Nerve fibers are classified according to their function, diameter, and conduction velocity, as shown in Table 10-3. Most of the nerves of the pulp fall into two main categories, A-δ and C fibers. The principal characteristics of these fibers are summarized in Table 10-4.

During the bell stage of tooth development, "pioneer" nerve fibers enter the dental papilla following the path of blood vessels.[48] While only unmyelinated fibers are observed in the dental papilla, a proportion of these fibers are probably A fibers that have not yet become myelinated. Myelinated fibers are the last major structures to appear in the developing human dental pulp.[6] The number of nerve fibers gradually increases and some branching occurs as the fibers near the dentin, but during the bell stage very few fibers enter the predentin.

The sensory nerves of the pulp arise from the trigeminal nerve and pass into the radicular pulp in bundles via the foramen in close association with arterioles and venules (Fig. 10-23). Each of the nerves entering the pulp is invested within a Schwann cell, and the A fibers acquire their myelin sheath from these cells. With the completion of root development the myelinated fibers appear grouped

TABLE 10-3. Classification of nerve fibers

Type of fiber	Function	Diameter (μm)	Conduction velocity (m/sec)
A-α	Motor, proprioception	12-20	70-120
A-β	Pressure, touch	5-12	30-70
A-γ	Motor, to muscle spindles	3-6	15-30
A-δ	Pain, temperature, touch	1-5	6-30
B	Preganglionic autonomic	<3	3-15
C dorsal root	Pain	0.4-1.0	0.5-2
sympathetic	Postganglionic sympathetic	0.3-1.3	0.7-2.3

TABLE 10-4. Characteristics of sensory fibers

Fiber	Myelination	Location of terminals	Pain characteristics	Stimulation threshold
A-δ	Yes	Principally in region of pulp-dentin junction	Sharp, pricking	Relatively low
C	No	Probably distributed throughout pulp	Burning, aching, less bearable than A-δ fiber sensations	Relatively high, usually associated with tissue injury

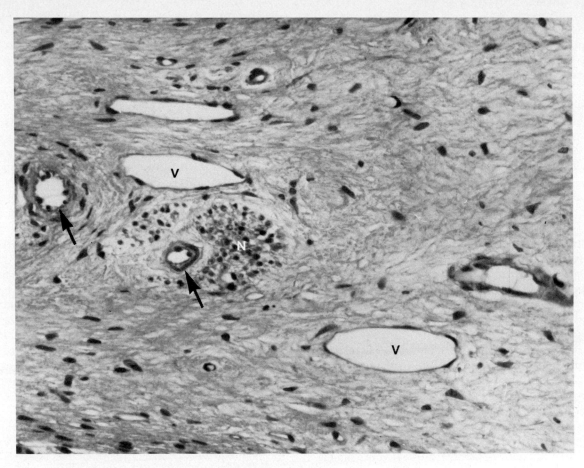

FIG. 10-23. Cross section of the apical pulp of a young human premolar demonstrating the nerve fiber bundle *(N)*, arterioles *(arrows)*, and venules *(V)*.

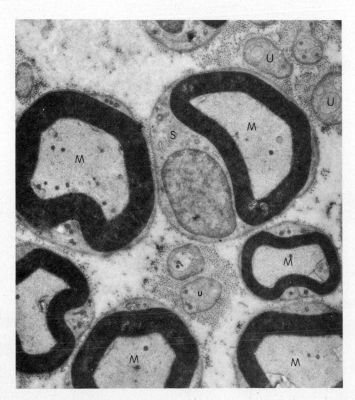

FIG. 10-24. Electron micrograph of the apical pulp of a young canine tooth showing in cross section myelinated nerve axons *(M)* within Schwann cells *(S)*. Smaller unmyelinated axons *(U)* are enclosed singly and in groups by Schwann cells. (Courtesy Dr. David C. Johnsen, School of Dentistry, Case Western Reserve University.)

in bundles in the central region of the pulp (Fig. 10-24). Most of the unmyelinated C fibers entering the pulp are located within these fiber bundles; the remainder are situated toward the periphery of the pulp.[164]

Investigators[95] found that in the human premolar the number of unmyelinated axons entering the tooth at the apex reached a maximum number shortly after tooth eruption. At this stage they observed an average of 1,800 unmyelinated axons and upwards of 400 myelinated axons, although in some teeth fewer than 100 myelinated axons were present. The number of A fibers gradually increased to upwards of 700 five years after eruption. *The relatively late appearance of A fibers in the pulp helps to explain why the electric pulp test tends to be unreliable in young teeth.*[62,63]

A quantitative study of nerve axons 1 to 2 mm above the root apex of fully developed human canine and incisor teeth has been conducted.[96] It reported a mean of 361 and 359 myelinated axons in canines and incisors respectively. The number of unmyelinated axons was much greater, with means of 2240 for canines and 1591 for incisors. Thus, approximately 80% of the nerves were unmyelinated fibers. However, some myelinated fibers may lose their sheaths before entering the apex or, in young teeth, they may not yet have acquired a sheath. Consequently, it is difficult to accurately assess the true proportion of myelinated and unmyelinated fibers entering the pulp.

The nerve bundles pass upward through the radicular pulp together with blood vessels. Once they reach the coronal pulp, they fan out beneath the cell-rich zone, branch into smaller bundles and finally ramify into a plexus of single nerve axons known as the plexus of Raschkow (Fig. 10-25). Full development of this plexus does not occur until the final stages of root formation.[49] It has been estimated that each fiber entering the pulp sends at least eight branches to the plexus of Raschkow. There is prolific branching of the fibers in the plexus, producing a tremendous overlap of receptor fields.[79] It is in the plexus that the A fibers emerge from their myelin sheaths and, while still within Schwann cells, branch repeatedly to form the subodontoblastic plexus (Fig. 10-26). Finally, terminal axons exit from their Schwann cell investiture and pass between the odontoblasts as free nerve endings (Figs. 10-27 and 10-28).

One investigator[72] studied the distribution and organization of nerve fibers in the dentin-pulp border zone of human teeth. On the basis of their location and pattern of branching, he described several types of nerve endings (Fig. 10-29). He found simple fibers that run from the subodontoblastic nerve plexus towards the odontoblast layer but do not reach the predentin. These fibers terminate in extracellular spaces in the cell-rich zone, the cell-poor zone, or the odontoblast layer. Other fibers extend into the predentin and run straight or spiral through a dentinal tubule in close association with an odontoblast process. Most of these intratubular fibers extend into the dentinal tubules for only a few microns, but a few may penetrate as far as 100 or so microns. He also observed complex fibers that reach the predentin and branch extensively (Fig. 10-30). The area covered by a single such terminal complex often reached thousands of square microns.

The anatomic relationships between the odontoblasts,

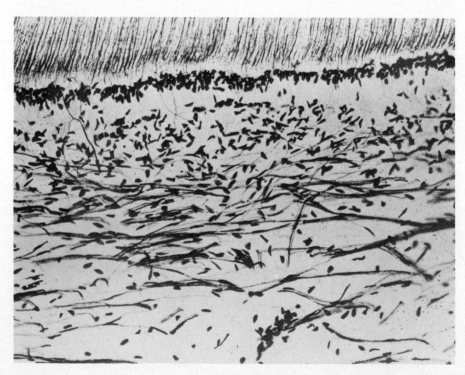

FIG. 10-25. Parietal layer of nerves (plexus of Raschkow) below the cell-rich zone. (From Avery, J.K.: J. Endod. **7:**205, 1981.)

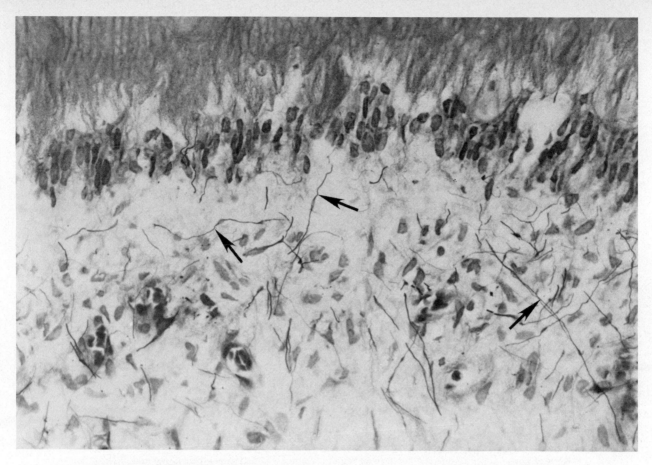

FIG. 10-26. Nerve fibers *(arrows)* in the subodontoblastic area as demonstrated by the Pearson silver impregnation method.

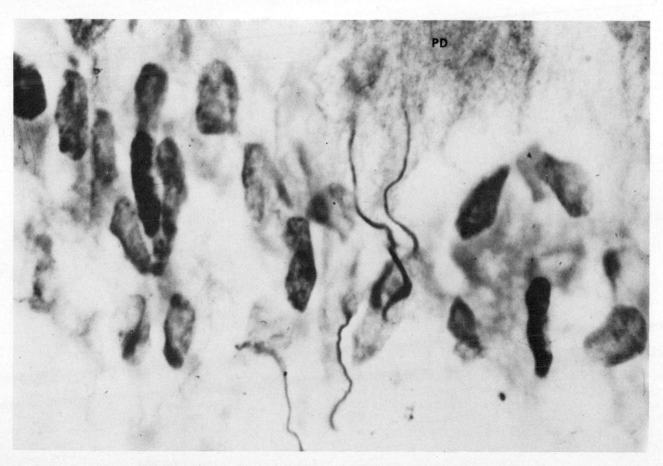

FIG. 10-27. Nerve fibers passing between odontoblasts to the predentin *(PD)*.

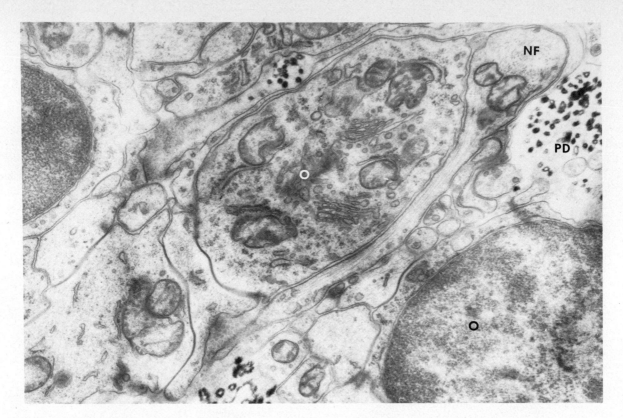

FIG. 10-28. Unmyelinated nerve fiber *(NF)* without a Schwann cell covering located between adjacent odontoblasts *(O)* overlying pulp horn of a mouse molar tooth. Predentin *(PD)* can be seen at upper right. Within the nerve there are longitudinally oriented fine neurofilaments, microvesicles, and mitochondria. (From Corpron, R.E., and Avery, J.K.: Anat. Rec. **175:**585, 1973.)

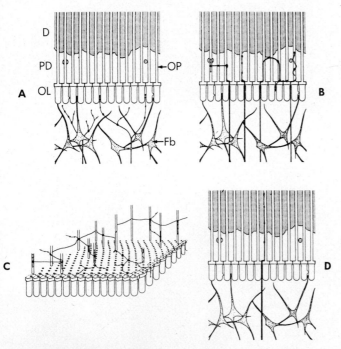

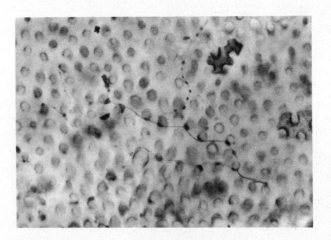

FIG. 10-29. Schematic drawing showing four types of nerve fibers in the pulpodentinal border zone. **A,** Fibers running from the subodontoblastic plexus to the odontoblast layer but not the predentin. *D,* Dentin; *PD,* predentin; *OP,* odontoblast process; *OL,* odontoblast layer; *Fb,* fibroblast. **B,** Fibers extending into dentinal tubules in the predentin. **C,** Complex fibers that branch extensively in the predentin. **D,** Intratubular fibers extending into the dentin. (Courtesy T. Gunji, Niigata University, Japan.)

FIG. 10-30. Histologic section showing a terminal branch of a complex predentinal nerve fiber. (Courtesy T. Gunji, Niigata University, Japan.)

their processes, and the intratubular nerve endings has been studied by several investigators.[5,59,86,87,169] It appears that these fibers lie in a groove or gutter along the surface of the odontoblast process.[59] Toward their terminal ends the nerve fibers twist around the process like a corkscrew. The cell membranes of the odontoblast process and the nerve fiber are closely approximated and run closely parallel for the length of their proximity.[59]

Intratubular nerve endings are most numerous in the area of the pulp horns where as many as one in four tubules contain fibers.[89,122] The number of intratubular fibers decreases in other parts of the dentin, and in root dentin only about one tubule in ten contains a fiber.[122] The functional significance of the intratubular fibers is by no means established, and there is still some question as to whether they are autonomic or sensory fibers. It has even been suggested that they may be passively trapped in the tubules during the final stage of dentin formation.[32]

Although it may be tempting to speculate that the odontoblasts and their associated nerve axons are functionally interrelated and that together they play a role in dentin sensitivity, evidence for this is lacking. If the odontoblast were acting as a receptor cell,* it would synapse with the adjacent nerve fiber. However, Byers was unable to find synaptic junctions that could functionally couple odontoblasts and nerve fibers together.[30] With regard to the membrane properties of odontoblasts, it has been reported that the membrane potential of the odontoblast is low (around -30 mv) and that the cell does not respond to electrical stimulation.[115,218] Thus, it would appear that the odontoblast does not possess the properties of an excitable cell. Furthermore, the sensitivity of dentin is not diminished following disruption of the odontoblast layer.[24,123]

The extent to which dentin is innervated has been the subject of numerous investigations. With the exception of the intratubular fibers discussed above, dentin is totally devoid of nerve fibers. This offers an explanation as to why pain-producing agents such as acetylcholine and potassium chloride do not elicit pain when applied to exposed dentin.[2] Similarly, application of topical solutions to dentin does not decrease its sensitivity.

In addition to sensory nerves, sympathetic fibers from the superior cervical ganglion appear with blood vessels at the time the vascular system is established in the dental papilla. In the adult tooth sympathetic fibers form plexuses, usually around pulpal arterioles.[4] When stimulated, these fibers cause constriction of the arterioles, resulting in a decrease in blood flow. Sympathetic fibers have also been found lying independent of blood vessels in the region of the odontoblasts. It is thought that these nerve endings may be involved in the regulation of dentin formation. One study reported finding both adrenergic and cholinergic nerve endings among the odontoblasts.[9]

Another study showed that a reduction in pulpal blood flow induced by stimulation of sympathetic fibers leading to the pulp results in depressed excitability of pulpal A fibers.[41] The excitability of C fibers is less affected than A fibers by a reduction in blood flow.[205]

Of considerable clinical interest is the evidence that nerve fibers of the pulp are relatively resistant to necrosis.[43,141] This is apparently due to the fact that nerve bundles in general are more resistant to autolysis. Even in degenerating pulps, the nerve fibers could still respond to stimulation.[43] It may be that C fibers remain excitable even after blood flow has been compromised in the diseased pulp, for C fibers are better able to maintain their functional integrity in the presence of hypoxia.[205] This may help to explain why instrumentation of the root canals of apparently nonvital teeth sometimes elicits pain.

SENSITIVITY OF DENTIN

The mechanisms underlying dentin sensitivity have been the subject of keen interest in recent years. How are stimuli relayed from the peripheral dentin to the sensory receptors located in the region of the pulp-dentin border zone? Converging evidence indicates that *movement of fluid in the dentinal tubules is the basic event in the arousal of pain* (see review by Trowbridge[209]). It now appears that pain-producing stimuli such as heat, cold, air blasts, and probing with the tip of an explorer have in common the ability to displace fluid in the tubules.[21,25,27,211] Brannstrom and his group in Stockholm[21,22,25,29] are responsible for advancing the hydrodynamic theory of dentin sensitivity. This theory helps to explain how fluid movement in the dentinal tubules is translated into electrical signals by sensory receptors located in the pulp.

In experiments on humans, brief application of heat or cold to the outer surface of premolar teeth evoked a painful response before the heat or cold could have produced temperature changes capable of activating sensory receptors in the underlying pulp.[211] The evoked pain was of very short duration, 1 or 2 seconds. The thermal diffusivity of dentin is relatively low; yet the response of the tooth to thermal stimulation is rapid, often less than a second. How can this best be explained? Evidence suggests that thermal stimulation of the tooth results in a rapid movement of fluid in the dentinal tubules that results in the deformation of the sensory nerve terminals in the underlying pulp. Heat would expand the fluid within the tubules, causing it to flow towards the pulp, whereas cold would cause the fluid to contract, producing an outward flow (Fig. 10-31). Pre-

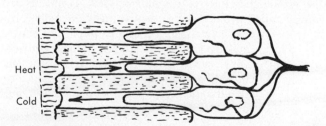

FIG. 10-31. Diagram illustrating movement of fluid in the dentinal tubules resulting from application of heat and cold to the outer surface of the tooth.

---

*A receptor cell is a non-nerve cell capable of exciting adjacent afferent nerve fibers. Synaptic junctions connect receptor cells to afferent nerves.

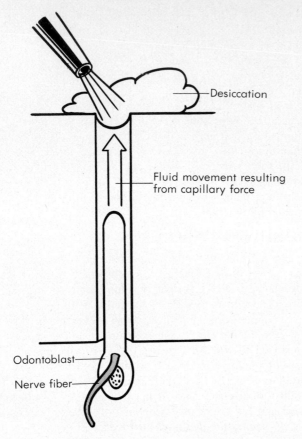

FIG. 10-32. Diagram illustrating movement of fluid in the dentinal tubules resulting from dehydrating effect of a blast of air from an air syringe.

sumably the rapid movement of fluid across the cell membrane of the sensory receptor activates the receptor. All nerve cells have membrane channels through which charged ions pass, and this current flow, if great enough, can stimulate the cell and cause it to transmit impulses to the brain. Some channels are activated by voltage, some by chemicals and some by mechanical pressure. In the case of pulpal nerve fibers that are activated by hydrodynamic forces, pressure would increase the flow of sodium and potassium ions through pressure-activated channels, thus initiating generator potentials.

The dentinal tubule is a capillary tube having an exceedingly small diameter.* Therefore, the effects of capillarity are significant, as the narrower the bore of a capillary tube, the greater the effect of capillarity. Thus, if fluid is removed from the outer end of exposed dentinal tubules by dehydrating the dentinal surface with an airblast or absorbent paper, capillary forces will produce a rapid outward movement of fluid in the tubule (Fig. 10-32). According to Brannstrom,[22] desiccation of dentin can theoretically cause dentinal fluid to flow outward at a rate of 2 to 3 mm

per second. In addition to air blasts, dehydrating solutions containing hyperosmotic concentrations of sucrose or calcium chloride can produce pain if applied to exposed dentin.[3,128]

Several investigators have shown that it is the A fibers rather than the C fibers that are activated by stimuli such as heat, cold, and air blasts applied to exposed dentin.[144] However, if heat is applied long enough to increase the temperature of the pulp-dentin border several degrees Celsius the C fibers may respond, particularly if the heat produces injury. It seems that the A fibers are only activated by a very rapid displacement of the tubular contents.[145] Slow heating of the tooth produced no response until the temperature reached 43.8° Celsius, at which time C fibers were activated, presumably because of heat-induced injury to the pulp.[145]

It has also been shown that pain-producing stimuli are more readily transmitted from the dentin surface when the exposed tubule apertures are wide and the fluid within the tubules is free to flow outward.[97] For example, other researchers found that acid treatment of exposed dentin to remove grinding debris opens the tubule orifices and makes the dentin more responsive to stimuli such as air blasts and probing.[84]

Perhaps the most difficult phenomenon to explain is pain associated with light probing of dentin. Even light pressure of an explorer tip can produce strong forces.* Presumably these forces mechanically compress the openings of the tubules and cause sufficient displacement of fluid to excite the sensory receptors in the underlying pulp. Considering the density of the tubules in which hydrodynamic forces would be generated by probing, thousands of nerve endings would be simultaneously stimulated, thus producing a cumulative effect.

Another example of the effect of strong hydraulic forces that are created within the dentinal tubules is the phenomenon of odontoblast displacement. In this reaction the cell bodies of odontoblasts are displaced upward into the dentinal tubules, presumably by a rapid movement of fluid in the tubules produced when exposed dentin is desiccated, as with the use of an air syringe or cavity-drying agents (Fig. 10-33). Such displacement results in loss of the odontoblasts since cells thus affected soon undergo autolysis and disappear from the tubules. (Displaced odontoblasts may eventually be replaced by cells that migrate from the cell-rich zone of the pulp, as discussed below.)

The hydrodynamic theory can also be applied to an understanding of the mechanism responsible for hypersensitive dentin. Hypersensitive dentin is associated with the exposure of dentin normally covered by cementum. The thin layer of cementum is frequently lost as gingival recession exposes cementum to the oral environment and cementum is subsequently worn away by brushing, flossing, or the use of toothpicks. Once exposed, the dentin may respond to the same stimuli that any exposed dentin sur-

---

*To appreciate fully the dimensions of dentin tubules, understand that the diameter of the tubules is much smaller than that of red blood cells (approximately 8 μm).

---

*A force of 10 g (0.022 lb) applied to an explorer having a tip 0.002 inch in diameter would produce a pressure of 7000 psi on the dentin.

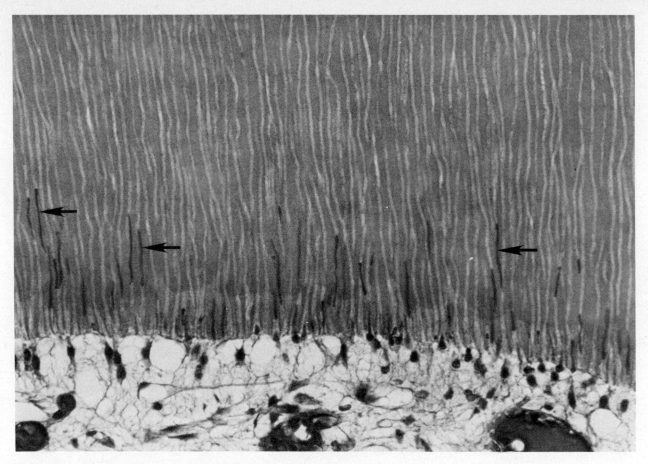

FIG. 10-33. Nuclei of odontoblasts *(arrows)* that have been displaced up into the dentinal tubules.

face responds to—mechanical pressure, dehydrating agents, etc. Although the dentin may at first be very sensitive, within a few weeks the sensitivity usually subsides. This densitization is thought to occur as a result of gradual occlusion of the tubules by mineral deposits, thus reducing the hydrodynamic forces. Additionally, the deposition of reparative dentin over the pulpal ends of the exposed tubules probably also reduces sensitivity.[210]

Painful pulpitis

From the foregoing it is apparent that pain associated with the stimulation of the A-δ fibers does not necessarily signify that the pulp is inflamed or that tissue injury has occurred. The A-δ fibers have a relatively low threshold of excitability, and painful pulpitis is more likely to be associated with nociceptive C fiber* activity. The clinician should carefully examine symptomatic teeth to rule out the possibility of hypersensitive dentin, cracked fillings, or dentinal fractures, each of which may initiate hydrodynamic forces, before establishing a diagnosis of pulpitis.

Pulpitis, or inflammation of the pulp, may be either painless or painful, but pain seems to be the exception rather than the rule. As a rule, however, the stimulation threshold of nerve fibers that mediate pain is lowered by sustained inflammation. In this case the inflamed pulp may become hypersensitive to all stimuli. Clinically it has been observed that the sensitivity of dentin is increased when the underlying pulp becomes acutely inflamed, and the tooth may be more difficult to anesthetize. Although a precise explanation for this hyperalgesia* is lacking, apparently the localized elevations in tissue pressure that accompany acute inflammation play an important role.[185,213] Hyperalgesia as a manifestation of pulp disease can be assessed clinically by means of thermal tests using agents such as ice, ethyl chloride, or carbone dioxide "snow."

How does inflammation lower the pain threshold? The answer is not clear, but pressure changes undoubtedly play an important role. Clinically we know that when the pulp chamber of an abscessed tooth is opened drainage promptly produces a reduction in the level of pain. In addition, algogenic (i.e., pain-producing) agents are known to alter the sensitivity threshold of the nociceptive fibers. The endogenous chemical mediators of inflammation such as bradykinin, 5-hydroxytryptamine (5-HT), and prostaglandins are either directly or indirectly algogenic and thus

---

*A nociceptive fiber is a pain-conducting fiber that responds to stimuli capable of injuring tissue.

---

*Hyperalgesia, lowering of the pain threshold.

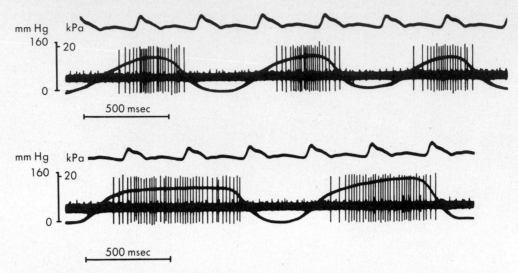

FIG. 10-34. Response of a single dog pulp nerve fiber to repeated hydrostatic pressure stimulation pulses. The lower solid wavy line of each recording indicates the stimulation pressure applied to the pulp. The upper line *(kPa)* is the femoral artery blood pressure curve recorded to indicate the relative changes in the pulse pressure and the heart cycle. (From Närhi, M.: Proc. Finn. Dent. Soc. **74**[suppl. 5]:1, 1978.)

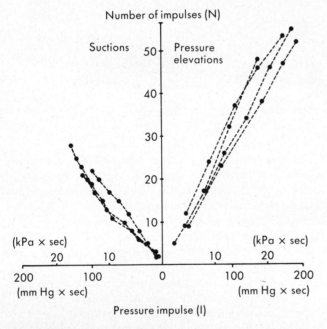

FIG. 10-35. Relationship between the number of nerve impulses *(N)* and the pressure impulse *(I)* of a small group of pulpal cat nerve fibers with three suction stimuli and four pressure elevations. The pressure impulse is labeled as both mm Hg × sec and kPa × sec. (From Närhi, M.: Proc. Finn. Dent. Soc. **74**[suppl. 5]:1, 1978.)

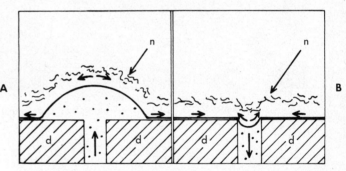

FIG. 10-36. Theoretical effect of hydrostatic pressure changes on the area of stimulation in the pulp. *d,* Dentin; *n,* nerve endings. **A,** Positive pressure. **B,** Suction. (From Närhi, M.: Proc. Finn. Dent. Soc. **74**[suppl. 5]:1, 1978.)

may be capable of affecting the excitability of sensory nerve fibers. 5-HT can increase the permeability of nerve cell membranes to sodium ions and thus alter the membrane potential, lowering the threshold of excitability.

An investigator found that application of 5-HT to the base of deep dentinal cavities consistently activated the sensory nerve fibers of the pulp in cats.[149] Vasoactive agents such as histamine and bradykinin have been shown to activate pulpal C fibers.[146] Such agents produce vasodilation and increase vascular permeability, resulting in an elevation of the interstitial pressure in the vicinity of the nerve endings. Pressure undoubtedly plays an important role in determining the stimulation threshold.

Pain associated with an inflamed or degenerating pulp may be either provoked or spontaneous. The hyperalgesic pulp may respond to stimuli that usually do not evoke pain, or the pain may be exaggerated and persist longer. On the other hand, the tooth may commence to hurt spontaneously in the absence of any external stimulus. There is not a satisfactory explanation as to why a pulp that has been inflamed but asymptomatic for weeks or months suddenly begins to ache at 3:00 in the morning. Such unprovoked pain usually manifests itself as a dull aching, poorly localized sensation that is qualitatively different from the brief, sharp, well-localized sensation associated with hydrodynamic fluid movement within the dentinal tubules. It seems reasonable to assume that spontaneous pain primarily involves nociceptive C fiber activity.

One researcher[143] has done much to elucidate the role of hydrostatic pressure changes in the activation of pulpal nerve fibers. In his experiment involving dogs and cats both positive and negative pressure changes were introduced into the pulp by means of a cannula inserted in the dentin. Using single-fiber recording techniques, he found a positive correlation between the degree of pressure change and the number of nerve impulses leaving the pulp. He theorized that the pressure changes produced local deformities in the pulp tissue, resulting in a stretching of the sensory nerve fibers (Figs. 10-34 to 10-36).

VASCULAR SUPPLY
Hemodynamics

Blood from the dental artery enters the tooth via arterioles having diameters of 100 μm or less. These vessels pass through the apical foramen or foramina in company with nerve bundles (Fig. 10-23). Smaller vessels may enter the pulp via lateral or accessory canals. The arterioles course up through the central portion of the radicular pulp and give off branches that spread laterally toward the odontoblast layer, beneath which they ramify to form a capillary plexus (Fig. 10-37). As the arterioles pass into the coronal pulp, they fan out toward the dentin, diminish in size, and give rise to a capillary network in the subodontoblastic region (Figs. 10-38 and 10-39). This network provides the odontoblasts with a rich source of metabolites.

Capillary blood flow in the coronal portion of the pulp is nearly twice that in the root portion.[105,158] Moreover, blood flow in the region of the pulp horns is greater than in other areas of the pulp.[131]

The subodontoblastic capillaries are surrounded by a basement membrane, and occasionally fenestrations (pores) are observed in their walls[163] (Figs. 10-40 and 10-41). These fenestrations are thought to provide rapid transport of fluid and metabolites from the capillaries to the adjacent odontoblasts. In addition, one study[77] observed numerous pinocytic vesicles in the capillaries of the hamster pulp and suggested that these structures might also be important in the transcapillary transport of metabolites. In young teeth, capillaries commonly extend into the odontoblast layer, thus assuring an adequate supply of nutrients for the metabolically active odontoblasts.

Blood passes from the capillary plexus first into postcapillary venules and then into progressively larger venules (Fig. 10-38). Venules in the pulp have unusually thin walls, which may facilitate the movement of fluid in or out of the vessel. The muscular coat of these venules is thin and discontinuous. The collecting venules become progressively larger as they course to the central region of the pulp. The largest venules have a diameter that may reach a maximum of 200 μm; thus they are considerably larger than the arterioles of the pulp. According to one study,[114]

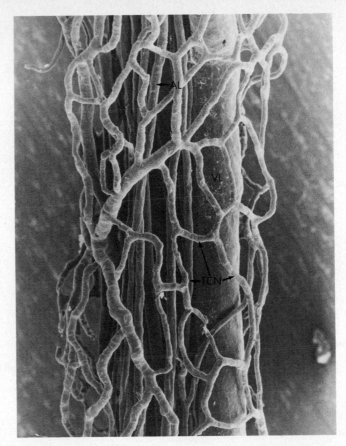

FIG. 10-37. High-power scanning electron micrograph of vascular network in the radicular pulp of a dog molar showing the configuration of the subodontoblastic terminal capillary network *(TCN)*. Venules *(VL)* and arterioles *(AL)* are indicated. (Courtesy Dr. Y. Kishi, Kanagawa Dental College, Kanagawa, Japan.)

the principal venous drainage in multirooted teeth sometimes flows down only one root canal or courses out through an accessory canal in the bifurcation or trifurcation area of the tooth.

Arteriovenous anastomoses (AVAs) may be present in both the coronal and radicular portions of the pulp, particularly in the latter.[102,114,162,188] Such vessels provide a direct communication between arterioles and venules, thus bypassing the capillary bed. The AVAs are relatively small venules, having a diameter of approximately 10 μm.[105] It is hypothesized that the AVAs play an important role in the regulation of the pulp circulation.[102,105,113] Theoretically they could provide a mechanism for shunting blood away from areas of injury where damage to the microcirculation may result in thrombosis and hemorrhage.

Among the oral tissues, the pulp has the highest volume of blood flow, but it is substantially lower than blood flow in the major visceral organs (Fig. 10-42). This reflects the fact that the respiratory rate of pulp cells is relatively low.[51] Kim reported that in young dogs blood flow in teeth with fully formed apices was approximately 40 to 50 ml/min/100 gm of pulp tissue (Fig. 10-42).

Regional blood flow distribution in the pulps of dogs has

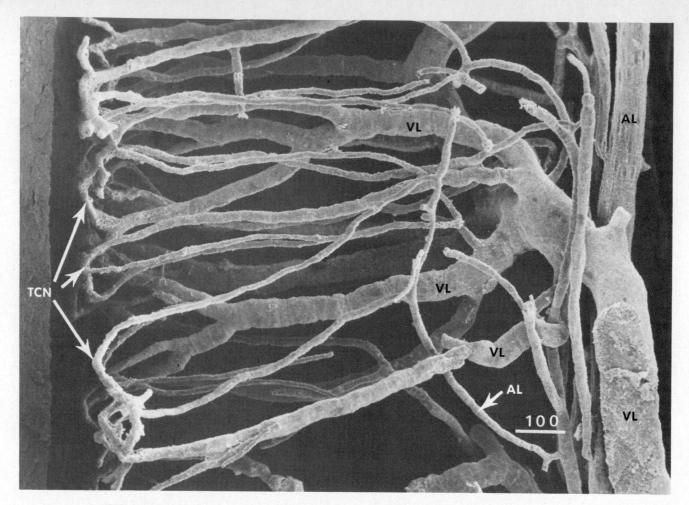

FIG. 10-38. Subodontoblastic terminal capillary network *(TCN)*, arterioles *(AL)*, and venules *(VL)* of young canine pulp. Dentin would be to the far left and the central pulp to the right. The bar is 100 μm. (From Takahashi, K., et al.: J. Endod. **8:**131, 1982.)

been studied.[102] As would be anticipated, pulpal blood flow was greater in the peripheral layer of the pulp (i.e., the subodontoblastic capillary plexus) than in the central area.

It appears that blood flow in the pulp is largely under the control of the adrenergic sympathetic system.[105] The walls of arterioles and venules are associated with smooth muscle that is innervated by unmyelinated sympathetic fibers. When stimulated, these fibers transmit impulses that cause the muscle fibers to contract, thus decreasing the diameter of the vessel (vasoconstriction). It has been shown experimentally that electrical stimulation of sympathetic fibers leading to the pulp results in a decrease in pulpal blood flow.[40,102,204] Activation of alpha-adrenergic receptors by the administration of epinephrine-containing local anesthetic solutions may result in a marked decrease in pulpal blood flow.[104] Functional evidence for cholinergic parasympathetic regulation of pulpal blood flow is lacking. However, the presence of cholinergic nerve endings among odontoblasts in mouse and monkey pulps has been reported along with the suggestion that these fibers may influence dentinogenesis.[8]

One investigation measured tissue and intravascular pressures in the pulps of cats.[204] The tissue pressure was estimated to be approximately 6 mm Hg. Pressure in the arterioles, capillaries, and venules was 43, 35, and 19 mm Hg, respectively (Fig. 10-43).

A unique feature of the pulp is that it is rigidly encased within dentin. This places it in a low compliance environment, much like the brain and bone marrow. Thus, pulp tissue has a limited ability to expand, so the total volume of blood within the pulp cannot be rapidly increased to any great extent. Evidence suggests that inflammation may increase the tissue pressure in the pulp by as much as 8 to 10 mm Hg.[213] However, the increased pressure tends to remain localized to the area of injury and does not extend to the rest of the pulp unless the inflammation is severe and persistent.[83] Presumably any sudden rise in intrapulpal pressure would be distributed equally within the area of pressure increase, including the blood vessels. Since venules have a lower intravascular pressure than capillaries or arterioles and their thin walls render them susceptible to compression, they may collapse if the intrapulpal

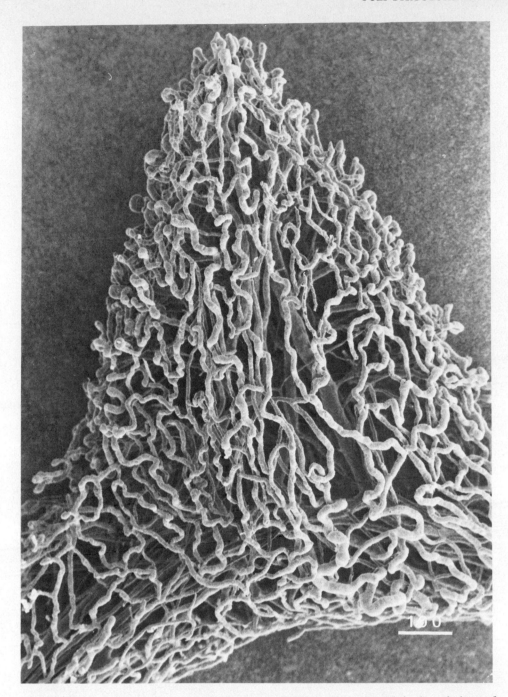

FIG. 10-39. Scanning electron micrograph of the terminal capillary network in the pulp horn of a dog molar. (Courtesy Professor K. Takahashi, Kanagawa Dental College, Kanagawa, Japan.)

pressure reaches a critical level. Thus, compression of the venules would increase vascular hindrance in the affected area of the pulp and this in turn would lead to a decrease in blood flow and tissue hypoxia. This may provide an explanation as to why injection of vasodilators such as bradykinin into an artery leading to the pulp results in a reduction rather than an increase in pulpal blood flow.[106,203]

Lymphatics

The existance of lymphatics in the pulp is still a matter of debate, since it is not easy to distinguish between venules and lymphatics by ordinary light and electron microscopic techniques. Although morphologic evidence of a lymphatic system in the pulp has been presented,[17] other researchers[138,187] have been unable to find lymphatics in the pulps of human, rabbit, guinea pig, or mouse teeth.

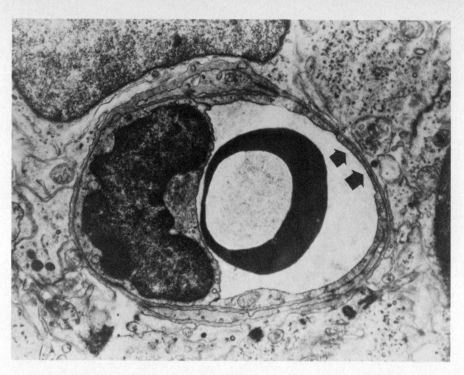

FIG. 10-40. Capillary adjacent to the predentin. Arrows show fenestrations. These 300 to 500 Å openings are bridged by the thin segment that is continuous with the endothelial cell wall. (From Avery, J.K.: J. Endod. **7**:205, 1981.)

FIG. 10-41. Part of a capillary from the subodontoblastic layer of a human pulp showing a very attenuated endothelial wall with many fenestrations *(F)*. (From Rapp, R., et al.: Arch. Oral Biol. **22**:317, 1977.)

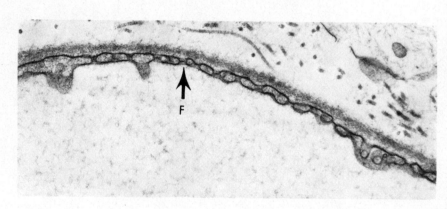

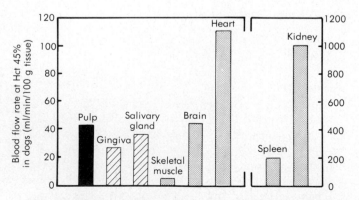

FIG. 10-42. Blood flow per 100 g tissue weight for various organs and tissues at 45% hematocrit *(Hct)* in dogs. (From Kim, S.: J. Endod. **11**:465, 1985. © by American Association of Endodontists, 1985.)

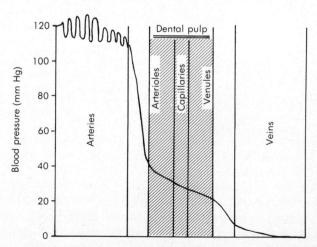

FIG. 10-43. Blood pressure fall along extrapulpal and intrapulpal blood vessels. (Modified from Heyeraas, K.J.: J. Dent. Res. **64**(spec. issue):585, 1985.)

REPAIR

The inherent healing potential of the dental pulp is well recognized. As in all other connective tissues, repair of tissue injury commences with debridement by macrophages followed by proliferation of fibroblasts, capillary buds, and the formation of collagen. Local circulation is of critical importance in wound healing and repair. An adequate supply of blood is essential to transport inflammatory elements into the area of pulpal injury and to provide the young fibroblasts with nutrients from which to synthesize collagen. Unlike most tissues, the pulp has essentially no collateral circulation; and for this reason it is theoretically more vulnerable than most other tissues. Thus, in the case of severe injury, healing would be impaired in teeth with a limited blood supply. It is well recognized that the highly cellular pulp of a young tooth, with a wide open apical foramen and rich blood supply, has a much better healing potential than does an older tooth, with a narrow foramen and a restricted blood supply.

Dentin that is produced in response to the injury of primary odontoblasts has been known by a number of different names:

Irregular secondary dentin
Irritation dentin
Reaction dentin
Defense dentin
Replacement dentin
Adventitious dentin
Atypical dentin
Tertiary dentin
Reparative dentin

Although attempts have been made to reach accord on a single term, several of these terms are still in popular use. That most commonly applied to irregularly formed dentin

is *reparative* dentin, presumably because it so frequently forms in response to injury and appears to be a component of the reparative process. It must be recognized, however, that this type of dentin has also been observed in the pulps of normal unerupted teeth without any obvious injury.[116]

It will be recalled that secondary dentin is deposited circumpulpally at a very slow rate throughout the life of the vital tooth. In contrast, the formation of reparative dentin

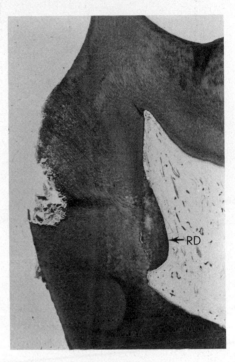

FIG. 10-44. Reparative dentin *(RD)* deposited in response to a carious lesion in the dentin. (From Trowbridge, H.O.: J. Endod. 7:52, 1981.)

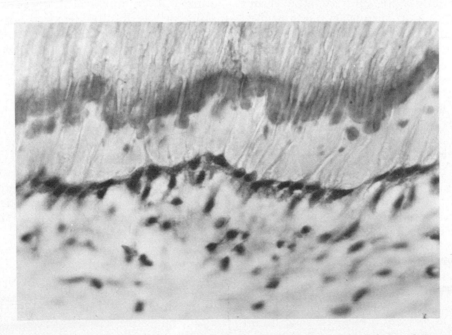

FIG. 10-45. Layer of cells forming reparative dentin. Note the decreased tubularity of reparative dentin as compared to the developmental dentin above.

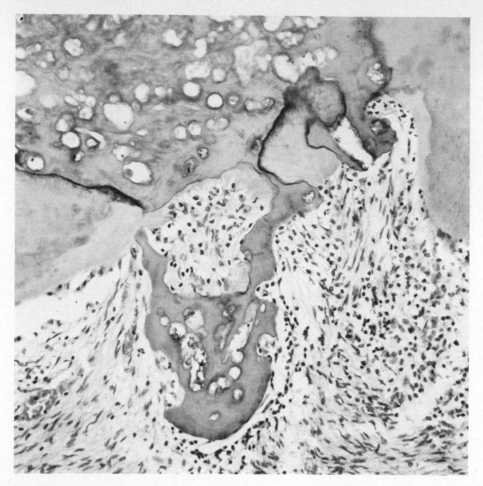

FIG. 10-46. Swiss cheese type of reparative dentin. Note the numerous areas of soft tissue inclusion and infiltration of inflammatory cells in the pulp.

occurs at the pulpal surface of primary or secondary dentin at sites corresponding to areas of irritation. For example, when a carious lesion has invaded dentin, the pulp usually responds by depositing a layer of reparative dentin over the dentinal tubules of the primary or secondary dentin which communicate with the carious lesion (Fig. 10-44). Similarly, when occlusal wear removes the overlying enamel and exposes the dentin to the oral environment, reparative dentin is deposited over the exposed tubules. In general, the amount of reparative dentin formed in response to caries or attrition of the tooth surface is proportional to the amount of primary dentin that is destroyed. Thus the formation of reparative dentin allows the pulp to retreat behind a barrier of mineralized tissue.

Compared to primary dentin, reparative dentin is less tubular and the tubules tend to be more irregular with larger lumina. In some cases no tubules are formed. The cells that form reparative dentin are not as columnar as the primary odontoblsts of the coronal pulp and are often cuboidal (Fig. 10-45). The quality of reparative dentin (i.e., the extent to which it resembles primary dentin) is quite variable. If irritation to the pulp is relatively mild, as in the case of a superficial carious lesion, the reparative dentin formed may resemble primary dentin in terms of tubularity and degree of mineralization. On the other hand, re-

parative dentin deposited in response to a deep carious lesion may be relatively atubular and poorly mineralized with many areas of interglobular dentin. The degree of irregularity of reparative dentin is probably determined by factors such as the amount of inflammation present, the extent of cellular injury, and the state of differentiation of the replacement odontoblasts.

The poorest quality of reparative dentin is usually observed in association with marked pulpal inflammation. In fact, the dentin may be so poorly organized that areas of soft tissue are entrapped within the dentinal matrix. In histologic sections these areas of soft tissue entrapment impart a Swiss cheese appearance to the dentin (Fig. 10-46). As the entrapped soft tissue degenerates, products of tissue degeneration further contribute to the inflammatory stimuli assailing the pulp.

It has been reported[36] that trauma caused by cavity preparation which is too mild to result in the loss of primary odontoblasts does not lead to reparative dentin formation, even if the cavity preparation is relatively deep. This evidence would suggest that reparative dentin is formed principally by replacement cells.[136] Regeneration of the odontoblast layer has been the subject of numerous studies. For many years it has been recognized that destruction of primary odontoblasts is soon followed by increased mitotic

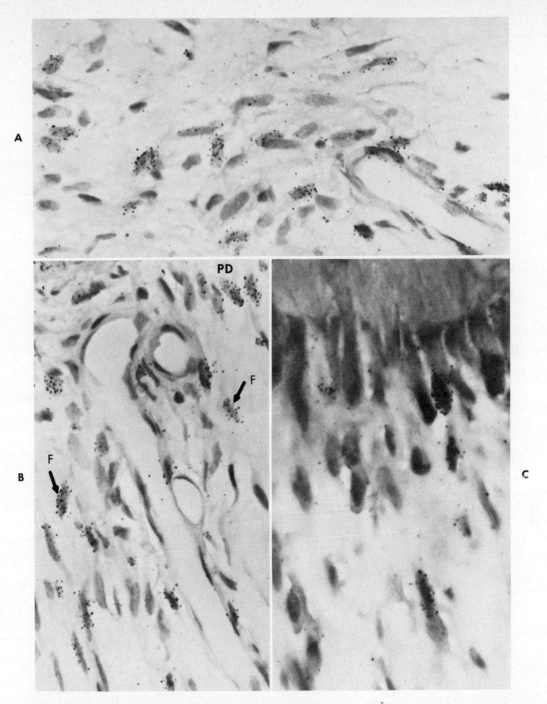

FIG. 10-47. Autoradiographs from dog molars illustrating uptake of ^{3}H-thymidine by pulp cells preparing to undergo cell division following pulpotomy and pulp capping with calcium hydroxide. **A,** Two days after pulp capping. Fibroblasts, endothelial cells, and pericytes beneath the exposure site are labeled. **B,** By the fourth day preodontoblasts adjacent to the predentin *(PD)* as well as fibroblasts *(F)* are labeled, which suggests that differentiation of preodontoblasts occurred within 2 days. **C,** Six days after pulp capping, new odontoblasts are labeled and tubular dentin is being formed. (Tritiated thymidine was injected 2 days after the pulp capping procedure in **B** and **C**.) (From Yamamura, T., et al.: Bull. Tokyo Dent. Coll. **21:**181, 1980.)

activity within the subjacent cell-rich zone. However, the origin of the replacement cells has been a matter of speculation. Odontoblasts can be replaced by differentiation of pulpal fibroblasts into functioning odontoblasts.[55] Other investigators[221] have studied dentin bridge formation in the teeth of dogs and found that pulpal fibroblasts appeared to undergo dedifferentiation and revert to undifferentiated mesenchymal cells (Figs. 10-47 and 10-48). These cells divided and the new cells then redifferentiated in a new direction to become odontoblasts. Recalling the migratory potential of ectomesenchymal cells from which the pulpal fibroblasts are derived, it is not difficult to envision the differentiating odontoblasts moving from the subodonto-blastic zone into the area of injury to constitute a new odontoblast layer.

Baume[12] has suggested that the formation of atubular "fibrodentine" results in the secondary induction of odontoblast differentiation, provided a capillary plexus develops beneath the fibrodentin. This is consistent with the observation made by other researchers[221] that the newly formed dentin bridge is composed first of a thin layer of atubular dentin upon which a relatively thick layer of tu-bular dentin is deposited. The fibrodentin* was lined by cells resembling undifferentiated mesenchymal cells, whereas the tubular dentin was associated with cells closely resembling odontoblasts.

Still other researchers[184] studied reparative dentin formed in response to relatively traumatic experimental Class V cavity preparations in human teeth. They found

---

*Actually the term osteodentin was used rather than fibrodentin.

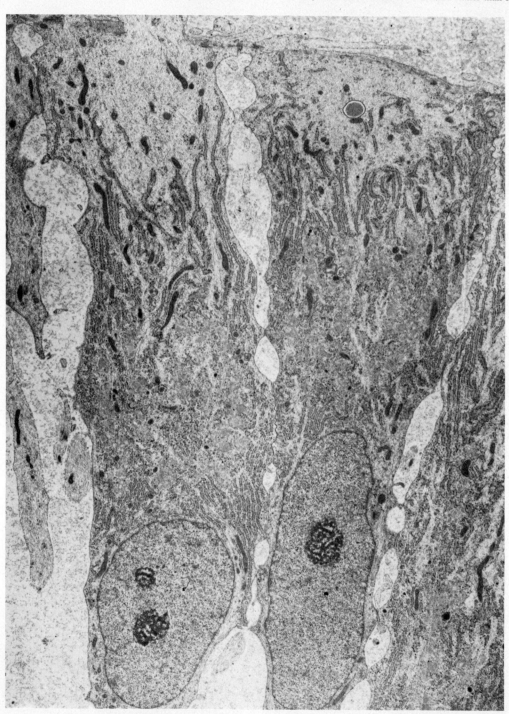

FIG. 10-48. Electron micrograph of new odontoblasts corresponding to the labeled odontoblasts depicted in Fig. 14-45, *C*. (From Yamamura, T., et al.: Bull. Tokyo Dent. Coll. **21**:181, 1980.)

that seldom was reparative dentin formed until about the thirtieth postoperative day, although in one case dentin formation was observed on day 19. The rate of formation was 3.5 μm per day for the first 3 weeks after the onset of dentin formation. Then it decreased markedly. By postoperative day 132, dentin formation had nearly ceased. Assuming that most of the odontoblasts were destroyed during cavity preparation, as was likely in this experiment, it is probable that the lag phase between cavity preparation and the onset of reparative dentin formation represented the time required for the proliferation and differentiation of new replacement odontoblasts.

Does reparative dentin protect the pulp or is it simply a form of scar tissue? To serve a protective function, it would have to provide a relatively impermeable barrier that would exclude irritants from the pulp and compensate for the loss of developmental dentin. The junction between developmental and reparative dentin has been studied.[176] This study found, in addition to a dramatic reduction in the number of tubules, that the walls of the tubules along the junction were thickened and often occluded with material similar to peritubular matrix. Furthermore, others[135] have reported that the junction is less permeable to dyes than is normal developmental dentin. These observations would indicate that the junctional zone between develop-

mental and reparative dentin is an area of relatively low permeability.

One group studied the effect of gold foil placement on human pulps and found that this was better tolerated in teeth in which reparative dentin had previously been deposited beneath the cavity than in teeth that were lacking such a deposit. It would thus appear that reparative dentin can protect the pulp, but it must be emphasized that this is not always the case. It is well known that reparative dentin can be deposited in a pulp that is irreversibly inflamed and that its presence does not necessarily signify a favorable prognosis (Fig. 10-46). The quality of the dentin formed, and hence its ability to protect the pulp, to a large extent reflects the environment of the cells producing the matrix.

Periodontally diseased teeth have smaller root canal diameters than do teeth that are periodontally healthy.[117] The root canals of such teeth are narrowed by the deposition of large quantities of reparative dentin along the dentinal walls.[177] The decrease in root canal diameter with increasing age, in the absence of periodontal disease, is more likely to be the result of secondary dentin formation.

In one study, it was shown in a rat model that scaling and root planing frequently result in reparative dentin formation along the pulpal wall opposite the instrumented root surface.[81]

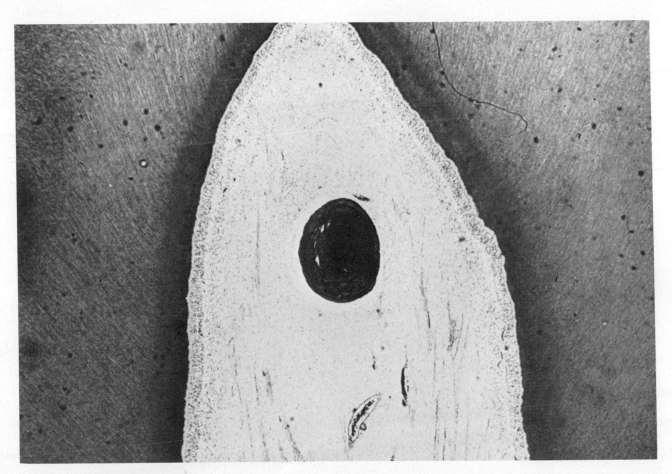

FIG. 10-49. Pulp stone with a smooth surface and concentric laminations in the pulp of a newly erupted premolar extracted in the course of orthodontic treatment.

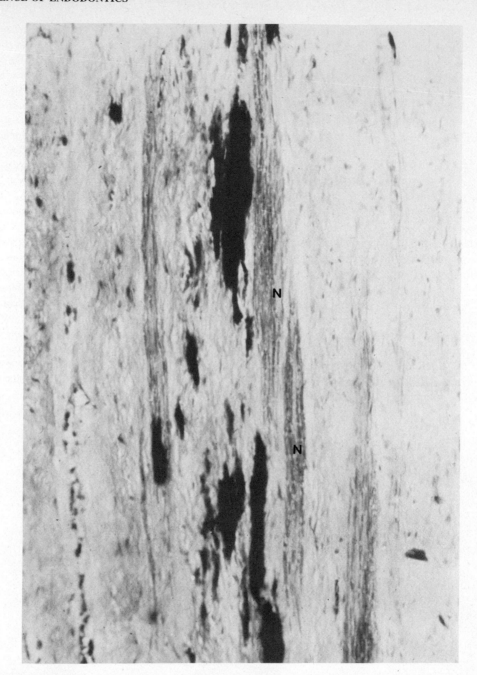

FIG. 10-50. Diffuse calcification in a radicular pulp. The calcification appears to be associated with nerve trunks *(N)*.

Fibrosis

Not uncommonly the cellular elements of the pulp are largely replaced by fibrous connective tissue. It appears that in some cases the pulp responds to noxious stimuli by accumulating large fiber bundles of collagen rather than by elaborating reparative dentin. However, fibrosis and reparative dentin formation often go hand in hand, indicating that both are expressions of a reparative potential.

PULPAL CALCIFICATIONS

Calcification of pulp tissue, generally regarded as a pathologic condition, is a very common occurrence. In the coronal pulp calcification usually takes the form of discrete pulp stones (Fig. 10-49), whereas in the radicular pulp calcification tends to be diffuse (Fig. 10-50).

Pulp stones range in size from small microscopic particles to accretions that occupy almost the entire pulp chamber (Fig. 10-51). Histologically two types of pulp stones are recognized: those that are round or ovoid with smooth surfaces and concentric laminations (Fig. 10-49) and those that assume no particular shape, lack laminations, and have rough surfaces (Fig. 10-52). Both types have an organic matrix composed principally of collagen fibrils in which hydroxyapatite crystals are embedded. The lami-

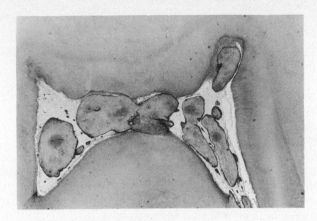

FIG. 10-51. Pulp stones occupying much of the pulp chamber.

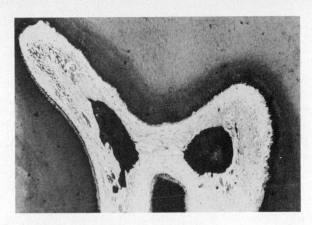

FIG. 10-52. Rough surface form of pulp stones. Note the hyalinized appearance of collagen fibers in the pulp.

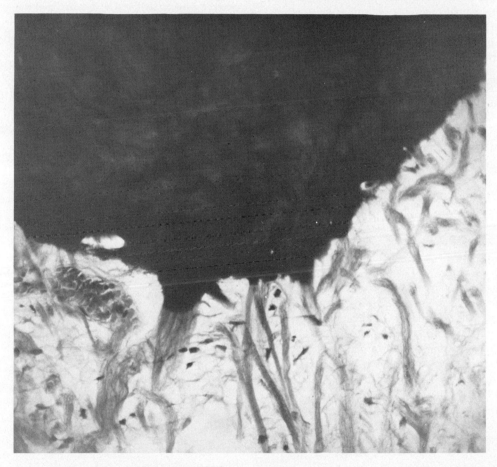

FIG. 10-53. High-power view of a pulp stone from Fig. 10-52 showing the relationship of mineralization fronts to collagen fibers.

nated stones appear to grow in size by the addition of collagen fibrils to their surface, whereas the unlaminated stones develop via the mineralization of preformed collagen fiber bundles. In the latter type the mineralization front seems to extend out along the coarse fibers, making the surface of the stones appear fuzzy (Fig. 10-53). Often these coarse fiber bundles appear to have undergone hyalinization, thus resembling old scar tissue.

Pulp stones that form around epithelial cells (remants of Hertwigs epithelial root sheath) are termed denticles.[139] Presumably the epithelial remnants induce adjacent mesenchymal cells to differentiate into odontoblasts. Characteristically these pulp stones are found near the root apex and contain dentinal tubules.

The cause of pulpal calcification is largely unknown. Calcification may occur around a nidus of degenerating cells, blood thrombi, or collagen fibers. Many authors believe this represents a form of dystrophic calcification. In this type calcium is deposited in tissues where degenerative changes are occurring. When cells degenerate, calcium phosphate crystals may be deposited within the cell, initially within the mitochondria, because of the increased membrane permeability to calcium that results from a failure to maintain active transport systems within the cell membranes. Thus degenerating cells serving as a nidus may initiate calcification of a tissue. In the absence of obvious tissue degeneration the cause of pulpal calcification is enigmatic. It is often difficult to assign the term dystrophic calcification to pulp stones since they so often occur in apparently healthy pulps. For example, pulpal calcifications have been reported in teeth that have not erupted,[116] suggesting that functional stress need not be present for calcification to occur. However, a positive relationship between pulpal calcification and pulpal pathology is recognized, particularly where there has been long-standing chronic irritation, as with dental caries.[74,175]

Although soft tissue collagen does not usually calcify, it is not at all uncommon to find calcification occurring in old hyalinized scar tissue in the skin. This may be due to the increase in the extent of cross linking between collagen molecules, since increased cross linkage is thought to enhance the tendency for collagen fibers to calcify. There may thus be a relationship between pathologic alterations in collagen molecules within the pulp and pulpal calcification.

Diffuse calcification is most often found in the perivascular adventitia and vascular walls within the radicular pulp. This form of pulpal calcification increases with age and seems to accompany the decrease in vascularity and innervation that are thought to represent age changes in the pulp.

Calcification replaces the cellular components of the pulp and may possibly embarrass the blood supply, although concrete evidence for this is lacking. Pain has frequently been attributed to the presence of pulp stones; but because calcification so often occurs in pathologically involved pulps, it is difficult to establish a cause-and-effect relationship, particularly since pulp stones are so frequently observed in teeth lacking a history of pain. (Perhaps their greatest endodontic significance is that they may hinder root canal instrumentation.) Investigators[18] have described the effect of calcification on the aging pulp.

AGE CHANGES

Continued formation of secondary dentin throughout life gradually reduces the size of the pulp chamber and root canals. In addition, certain regressive changes in the pulp appear to be related to the aging process. There is a gradual decrease in cellularity as well as a concomitant increase in the amount of collagen, particularly in the radicular pulp.[20] The odontoblasts decrease in size and number and may disappear altogether in certain areas of the pulp, particularly on the pulpal floor over the bifurcation or trifurcation areas of multirooted teeth.

Decrease in size of the pulp is thought to be related to

a reduction in the number of nerves and blood vessels.[16,18] Fibrosis appears to occur in relation to the pathways of degenerated vessels or nerves, and the thick collagen fibers may serve as foci for pulpal calcification.[18]

There is also evidence that aging results in an increase in the resistance of pulp tissue to the action of proteolytic enzymes[224] as well as hyaluronidase and sialidase,[20] suggesting an alteration of both collagen and proteoglycans in the pulps of older teeth.

The main changes in dentin associated with aging are the increase in peritubular dentin, dentinal sclerosis, and the number of dead tracts.* Dentinal sclerosis produces a gradual decrease in dentinal permeability as the dentinal tubules become progressively reduced in diameter.

ACKNOWLEDGMENTS

We are deeply indebted to the following individuals whose research, advice, technical assistance, and moral support have so greatly assisted and guided us in the development of this chapter:

James K. Avery, D.D.S., Ph.D., Professor of Oral Biology, University of Michigan.

Louis J. Baume, D.D.S., Professor of Dentistry, University of Geneva, Switzerland.

I.B. Bender, D.D.S., Emeritus Professor of Endodontics, University of Pennsylvania.

Martin Brännström, Odont. Dr., Professor of Histopathology, Karolinska Institute, Stockholm, Sweden.

Charles F. Cox, M.S., Instructor in Oral Histology, University of Michigan.

Robert Emling, D. Ed., Director of Admissions, School of Dental Medicine, University of Pennsylvania.

Patricia Jenks, Sonoma California.

David H. Pashley, D.D.S., Ph.D., Professor of Oral Biology, Medical College of Georgia.

REFERENCES

1. Ahlberg, K., Brännström, M., and Edwall, L.: The diameter and number of dentinal tubules in rat, cat, dog and monkey. A comparative scanning electronic microscopic study, Acta. Odontol. Scand. **33**:243, 1975.
2. Anderson, D.J., Curwen, M.P., and Howard, L.V.: The sensitivity of human dentin. J. Dent. Res. **37**:669, 1958.
3. Anderson, D.J., Matthews, B., and Goretta, C.: Fluid flow through human dentine, Arch. Oral Biol. **12**:209, 1967.
4. Anneroth, G., and Nordenberg, K.A.: Adrenergic vasoconstrictor innervation in the human dental pulp. Acta Odontol. Scand. **26**:89, 1968.
5. Arwill, T.: Studies on the ultrastructure of dental tissues. II. The predentin-pulpal border zone, Odontol. Rev. **18**:191, 1967.
6. Avery, J.K.: Structural elements of the young normal human pulp, Oral Surg. **32**:113, 1971.
7. Avery, J.K.: Dentin. In Bhaskar, S.N., editor: Orban's oral histology and embryology, ed. 9, St. Louis, 1980, The C.V. Mosby Co.
8. Avery, J.K.: Repair potential of the pulp, J. Endod. **7**:205, 1981.
9. Avery, J.K., Cox, C.F., and Chiego, D.J., Jr.: Presence and location of adrenergic nerve endings in the dental pulps of mouse molars, Anat. Rec. **198**:59, 1980.

---

*The term dead tract refers to a group of dentinal tubules in which odontoblast processes are absent. Dead tracts are easily recognized in ground sections as the empty tubules refract transmitted light and the tract appears black in contrast to the light color of normal dentin.

10. Avery, J.K., Cox, C.F., and Corpron, R.E.: The effects of combined nerve resection and cavity preparation and restoration on response dentine formation in rabbit incisors, Arch. Oral Biol. **19**:539, 1974.

11. Barber, D., and Massler, M.: Permeability of active and arrested carious lesions to dyes and radioactive isotopes, J. Dent. Child. **31**:26, 1964.

12. Baume, L.J.: The biology of pulp and dentine. In Myers, H.M., editor: Monographs in oral science, Vol. 8, Basel, 1980, S. Karger AG.

13. Bergenholtz, G.: Effect of bacterial products on inflammatory reactions in the dental pulp, Scand. J. Dent. Res. **85**:122, 1977.

14. Berggren, H.: The reaction of the translucent zone of dentine to dyes and radioisotopes, Acta Odontol. Scand. **23**:197, 1965.

15. Bernick, S.: Vascular supply to the developing teeth of rats, Anat. Rec. **137**:141, 1960.

16. Bernick, S.: Effect of aging on the nerve supply to human teeth, J. Dent. Res. **46**:694, 1967.

17. Bernick, S.: Lympatic vessels of the human dental pulp, J. Dent. Res. **56**:70, 1977.

18. Bernick, S., and Nedelman, C.: Effect of aging on the human pulp, J. Endod. **1**:88, 1975.

19. Bevelander, G.: The development and structure of the fiber system of dentin, Anat. Rec. **81**:79, 1941.

20. Bhussry, B.R.: Modification of the dental pulp organ during development and aging. In Finn, S.B., editor: Biology of the dental pulp organ: a symposium, Birmingham 1968, University of Alabama Press.

21. Brännström, M.: The transmission and control of dentinal pain. In Grossman, L.J., editor: Mechanisms and control of pain, New York, 1979, Masson Publishing USA, Inc.

22. Brännström, M.: Dentin and pulp in restorative dentistry, Nacka, Sweden, 1981, Dental Therapeutics AB.

23. Brännström, M: Communication between the oral cavity and the dental pulp associated with restorative treatment Oper. Dent. **9**:57, 1984.

24. Brännström, M., and Åström, A.: A study of the mechanism of pain elicited from the dentin, J. Dent. Res. **43**:619, 1964.

25. Brännström, M., and Åström, A.: The hydrodynamics of the dentine: its possible relationship to dentinal pain, Int. Dent. J. **22**:219, 1972.

26. Brännström, M., and Garberoglio, R.: The dentinal tubules and the odontoblast processes, Acta Odontol. Scand. **30**:291, 1972.

27. Brännström, M., and Johnston, G: Movements of the dentine and pulp liquids on application of thermal stimuli. An in vitro study, Acta Odontol. Scand. **28**:59, 1970.

28. Brännström, M., and Lind, P.O.: Pulpal response to early dental caries, J. Dent. Res. **44**:1045, 1965.

29. Brännström, M., Lindën, L.-A., and Åström, A.: The hydrodynamics of the dental tubule and of pulp fluid. A discussion of its significance in relation to dentinal sensitivity, Caries Res. **1**:310, 1967.

30. Byers, M.R.: Large and small trigeminal nerve endings and their association with odontoblasts in rat molar dentin and pulp. In Bonica, J.J., Liebeskind, J.C., and Able-Fessard, D.G., editors: Advances in pain research and therapy, Vol. 3, New York, 1979, Raven Press.

31. Chirnside, I.M.: Bacterial invasion of nonvital dentin, J. Dent. Res. **40**:134, 1961.

32. Corpron, R.E., and Avery, J.K.: The ultrastructure of intradental nerves in developing mouse molars, Anat. Rec. **175**:585, 1973.

33. Cotton, W.R., and Siegel, R.L.: Human pulpal response to citric acid cavity cleanser, J. Am. Dent. Assoc. **96**:639, 1978.

34. Cournil, I., et al.: Immunohistochemical localization of proteoglycans. I. Light microscopic distribution of procollagen I, III, and IV antigenicity in the rat incisor tooth by the indirect peroxydase-antiperoxydase method. Histochem. Cytochem. **27**:1059, 1979.

35. Crooks, P.V., O'Reilly, C.B., and Owens, P.D.A.: Microscopy of the dentine of enamel-free areas of rat molar teeth, Arch. Oral Biol. **28**:167, 1983.

36. Diamond, R.D., Stanley, H.R., and Swerdlow, H.: Reparative dentin formation resulting from cavity preparation, J. Prosthet. Dent. **16**:1127, 1966.

37. Dodd, C.M.,and Carmichael, D.J.: The collagenous matrix of bovine predentin, Biochem. Biophys. Acta **577**:117, 1979.

38. Dreyfuss, F., Frank, R.M., and Gutmann, B.: La sclérose dentinaire, Bull. Groupe Int. Recherch. Scientific. Stomatol. **7**:207, 1964.

39. Eda, S., and Takuma, S.: Microstructure of the peritubular matrix in horse dentin, Bull. Tokyo Dent. Coll. **6**:1, 1965.

40. Edwall, L., and Kindlová, M.: The effect of sympathetic nerve stimulation on the rate of disappearance of tracers from various oral tissues, Acta Odontol. Scand. **29**:387, 1971.

41. Edwall, L., and Scott, D. Jr.: Influence of changes in microcirculation on the excitability of the sensory unit in the tooth of the cat, Acta Physiol. Scand. **82**:555, 1971.

42. Eisenmann, D.R., and Glick, P.L. Ultrastructure of initial crystal formation in dentin, J. Ultrastruct. Res. **41**:18, 1972.

43. England, M.C., Pellis, E.G., and Michanowicz, A.E.: Histopathologic study of the effect of pulpal disease upon nerve fibers of the human dental pulp, Oral Surg. **38**:783, 1974.

44. Engström, C., Linde, A., and Persliden, B.: Acid hydrolases in the odontoblast-predentin region of dentiongenically active teeth, Scand. J. Dent. Res. **84**:76, 1976.

45. Engström, C., and Röckert, H.O.E.: Effects of local anestetics on aerobic and anaerobic metabolism of the dental pulp, Swed. Dent. J. **4**:119, 1980.

46. Ericsson, S.G.: Quantitative microradiography of cementum and abraded dentine, Acta Radiol. (Supply. 246), 1965.

47. Farnoush, A.: Mast cells in human dental pulp, J. Endod. **10**:250, 1984.

48. Fearnhead, R.W.: The neurohistology of human dentine, Proc. Roy. Soc. Med. **54**:877, 1961.

49. Fearnhead, R.W.: Innervation of dental tissues. In Miles, A.E.W., editor: Structure and chemical organization of teeth, Vol. 1, New York, 1967, Academic Press, Inc.

50. Fish, E.W.: Experimental investigation of the enamel, dentine, and dental pulp, London, 1932, John Bale Sons & Danielson, Ltd.

51. Fisher, A.K.: Respiratory variations within the normal dental pulp, J., Dent. Res. **46**:424, 1967.

52. Fisher, A.K., et al.: The influence of the stage of tooth development on the oxygen quotient of normal bovine dental pulp, J. Dent. Res. **38**:208, 1959.

53. Fisher, A.K., et al.: Effects of dental drugs and materials on the rate of oxygen consumption in bovine dental pulp, J. Dent. Res. **36**:447, 1957.

54. Fisher, A.K., and Walters, V.E.: Anaerobic glycolysis in bovine dental pulp, J. Dent. Res. **47**:717, 1968.

55. Fitzgerald, M.: Cellular dynamics of dentinal bridge repair using 3H-thymidine, J. Dent. Res. **58**:(D):2198, 1979.

56. Frank, R.M.: Electron microscopy of undecalcified sections of human adult dentine, Arch. Oral Biol. **1**:29, 1959.

57. Frank, R.M.: Etude au microscope électronique de l'odontoblaste et du canalicule dentinaire humain, Arch. Oral Biol. **11**:179, 1966.

58. Frank, R.M.: Ultrastructure of human dentine. In Fleisch, H., Blackwood, H.J.J., and Owen, M., editors: Third European Symposium on Calcified Tissues, New York, 1966, Springer-Verlag New York, Inc.

59. Frank, R.M.: Ultrastructural relationship between the odontoblast, its process and the nerve fibre. In Symons, N.B.B., editor: Dentine and pulp, Dundee, 1968, University of Dundee.

60. Frank, R.M.: Etude autographradiographique de la dentinogenèse en microscopie électronique à l'aide de la proline tritiée chez le chat, Arch. Oral Biol. **15**:583, 1970.

61. Frank, R.M., and Voegel, J.C.: Ultrastructure of the human odontoblast process and its mineralization during dental caries, Caries Res. **14:**367, 1980.

62. Fulling, H.-J., and Andreasen, J.O.: Influence of maturation status and tooth type of permanent teeth upon electrometric and thermal pulp testing, Scand. J. Dent. Res. **84:**286, 1976.

63. Fuss, Z., et al.: Assessment of reliability of electrical and thermal pulp testing agents. J. Endod. **12:**301, 1986.

64. Garant, P.R.: The organization of microtubules within rat odontoblast processes revealed by perfusion fixation with gluteraldehyde, Arch. Oral Biol. **17:**1047, 1972.

65. Garant, P.R., Szabo, G., and Nalbandian, J.: The fine structure of the mouse odontoblast, Arch. Oral Biol. **13:**857, 1968.

66. Garberoglio, R., and Brännström, M.: Scanning electron microscopical investigation of human dentinal tubules, Arch. Oral Biol. **21:**355, 1976.

67. Gaunt, W.A.: The vascular supply to the dental lamina during early development, Acta Anat. **37:**232, 1959.

68. Gotjamanos, T.: Cellular organization in the subodontoblastic zone of the dental pulp. 2. Period and mode of development of the cell-rich layer in rat molar pulps, Arch. Oral Biol. **14:**1011, 1969.

69. Gotjamanos, T.: Mitotic activity in the subodontoblastic cell-rich layer of adult rat molar pulps, Arch. Oral Biol. **15:**905, 1970.

70. Griffin, C.J., and Harris, R.: Ultrastructure of collagen fibrils and fibroblasts of the developing human dental pulp, Arch. Oral Biol. **11:**659, 1966.

71. Grossman, E.S., and Austin, J.C.: Scanning electron microscope observations on the tubule content of freeze-fractured peripheral vervet monkey dentine (Ceropithecus pygerythrus), Arch. Oral Biol. **28:**279, 1983.

72. Gunji, T.: Morphological research on the sensitivity of dentin, Arch. Histol. Jap. **45:**45, 1982.

73. Gunji, T., and Kobayashi, S.: Distribution and organization of odontoblast processes in human dentin, Arch. Histol. Jap. **46:**213, 1983.

74. Hall, D.C.: Pulpal calcifications—a pathological process? In Symons, N.B.B., editor: Dentine and pulp, Dundee, 1968, University of Dundee.

75. Hamersky, P.A., Weimer, A.D., and Taintor, J.F.: The effect of orthodontic force application on the pulpal tissue respiration rate in the human premolar, Am. J. Orthod. **77:**368, 1980.

76. Han, S.S.: The fine structure of cells and intercellular substances of the dental pulp. In Finn, S.B., editor: Biology of the dental pulp organ, Birmingham, 1968, University of Alabama Press.

77. Han, S.S., and Avery, J.K.: The ultrastructure of capillaries and arterioles of the hamster dental pulp, Anat. Rec. **145:**549, 1963.

78. Harris, R.: Histogenesis of fibroblasts in the human dental pulp, Arch. Oral Biol. **12:**459, 1967.

79. Harris, R., and Griffin, C.J.: Fine structure of nerve endings in the human dental pulp. Arch. Oral Biol. **13:**773, 1968.

80. Hasty, D.L.: Freeze-fracture studies of neonatal mouse incisors, Anat. Rec. **205:**405, 1983.

81. Hattler, A.B., and Listgarten, M.A.: Pulpal response to root planing in a rat model, J. Endod. **10:**471, 1984.

82. Hay, E.D., and Meier, S.: Tissue interaction in development. In Shaw, J.H., Sweeney, E.A., Cappuccino, C.C. and Meller, S.M., editors: Textbook of oral biology, Philadelphia, 1978, W.B. Saunders Co.

83. Heyeraas, K.J.: Pulpal, microvascular, and tissue pressure, J. Dent. Res. **64:**(Spec. Iss.):585, 1985.

84. Hirvonen, T., and Närhi, M.: The excitability of dog pulp nerves in relation to the condition of dentine surface, J. Endod. **10:**294, 1984.

85. Holland, G.R. The dentinal tubule and odontoblast process in the cat, J. Anat. **120:**169, 1975.

86. Holland, G.R.: Membrane junctions on cat odontoblasts, Arch. Oral Biol. **20:**551, 1975.

87. Holland, G.R.: The extent of the odontoblast process in the cat, J. Anat. **121:**133, 1976.

88. Holland, G.R.: Lanthanum hydroxide labelling of gap junctions in the odontoblast layer, Anat. Rec. **186:**121, 1976.

89. Holland, G.R.: The incidence of dentinal tubules containing more than one process in the cuspal dentin of cat canine teeth, Anat. Rec. **200:**437, 1981.

90. Holland, G.R.: The odontoblast process: form and function, J. Dent. Res. **64**(Spec. Iss.):499, 1985.

91. Iguchi, Y., et al.: Intercellular junctions in odontoblasts of the rat incisor studied with freeze-fracture, Arch. Oral Biol. **29:**487, 1984.

92. Jessen, H.: The ultrastructure of odontoblasts in perfusion fixed, demineralized incisors of adult rats, Acta Odontol. Scand. **25:**491, 1967.

93. Johansen, E.: Ultrastructure of dentine. In Miles, A.E.W., editor: Structural and chemical organization of the teeth, Vol. 2, New York, 1967, Academic Press, Inc.

94. Johansen, E., and Parks, H.F.: Electron microscopic observations on sound human dentine, Arch. Oral Biol. **7:**185, 1962.

95. Johnsen, D.C., Harshbarger, J., and Rymer, H.D.: Quantitative assessment of neural development in human premolars, Anat. Rec. **205:**421, 1983.

96. Johnsen, D., and Johns, S.: Quantitation of nerve fibers in the primary and permanent canine and incisor teeth in man, Arch. Oral Biol. **23:**825, 1978.

97. Johnson, G., and Brännström, M.: The sensitivity of dentin. Changes in relation to conditions at exposed tubule aperatures, Acta Odontol. Scand. **32:**29, 1974.

98. Jones, P.A., Taintor, J.F., and Adams, A.B.: Comparative dental material cytoxoicity measured by depression of rat incisor pulp respiration, J. Endod. **5:**48, 1979.

99. Katchburian, E., and Holt, S.J.: Ultrastructural studies on lysosomes and acid phosphatase in odontoblasts. In Symons, N.B.B., editor: Dentine and pulp, Dundee, 1968, University of Dundee.

100. Kaye, H., and Herold, R.C.: Structure of human dentine. I. Phase contrast, polarization, interference, and bright field microscopic observations on the lateral branch system, Arch. Oral Biol. **11:**355, 1966.

101. Kelley, K.W., Bergenholtz, G., and Cox, C.F.: The extent of the odontoblast process in rhesus monkeys (Macaca mulatta) as observed by scanning electron microscopy, Arch. Oral Biol. **26:**893, 1981.

102. Kim, S.: Regulation of blood flow of the dental pulp: macrocirculation and microcirculation studies, Doctoral thesis, Columbia University, 1981.

103. Kim, S.: Microcirculation of the dental pulp in health and disease, J. Endod. **11:**465, 1985.

104. Kim, S. et al.: Effects of local anesthetics on pulpal blood flow in dogs, J. Dent. Res. **63:**650, 1984.

105. Kim, S., Schuessler, G., and Chien, S.: Measurement of blood flow in the dental pulp of dogs with the 133xenon washout method, Arch. Oral Biol. **28:**501, 1983.

106. Kim, S., et al.: Effects of bradykinin on pulpal blood flow in dogs, J. Dent. Res. **61:**293, 1982.

107. Koling, A., Rask-Andersen, H., and Bagger-Sjöbäck, D.: Membrane junctions on odontoblasts. A freeze-fracture study, Acta Odontol. Scand. **39:**355, 1981.

108. Kollar, E.J., and Baird, G.R.: Tissue interactions in embryonic mouse tooth germs. 1. Reorganization of the dental epithelium during tooth-germ reconstruction, J. Embryol. Exp. Morphol. **24:**159, 1970.

109. Kollar, E.J., and Baird, G.R.: Tissue interactions in embryonic mouse tooth germs. 2. The inductive role of the dental papilla, J. Embryol. Exp. Morphol. **24:**173, 1970.

110. Kollar, E.J., and Lumsden, A.G.S.: Tooth morphogenesis: The role of the innervation during induction and pattern formation, J. Biol. Buccale **7:**49, 1979.

111. von Korff, K.: Die Entwicklung der Zahnbeingrundsubstanz der Saugetiere, Arch. Mikrosckp. Anat. **67:**1, 1905.

112. von Korff, K.: Zur Histologie und Histogenese des Bindegewebes, besonders der Knochen-und Dentingrundsubstanz, Ergeb. Anat. Entwickl. **17:**251, 1909.

113. Kramer, I.R.H.: The vascular architecture of the human dental pulp, Arch. Oral Biol. **2**:177, 1960.

114. Kramer, I.R.H.: The distribution of blood vessels in the human dental pulp. In Finn, S.B. editor: Biology of the dental pulp organ, Birmingham, 1968, University of Alabama Press.

115. Kroeger, D.C., Gonzales, F., and Krivoy, W.: Transmembrane potentials of cultured mouse dental pulp cells, Proc. Soc. Exptl. Med. **108**:134, 1961.

116. Langeland, K., and Langeland, L.K.: Histologic study of 155 impacted teeth, Odontol. Tidskr. **73**:527, 1965.

117. Lantelme, R.L., Handleman, S.L., and Herbison, R.J.: Dentin formation in periodontally diseased teeth, J. Dent. Res. **55**:48, 1976.

118. Lau, E.C., and Ruch, J.V.: Glycosaminoglycans in embryonic mouse teeth and the dissociated dental constituents, Differentiation **23**:234, 1983.

119. Lechner, J.H., and Kalnitsky, G.: The presence of large amounts of type III collagen in bovine dental pulp and its significance with regard to the mechanism of dentinogenesis, Arch. Oral Biol. **26**:265, 1981.

120. Lefèvre, R., Frank, R.M., and Voegel, J.C.: The study of human dentine with secondary ion microscopy and electron diffraction, Calcif. Tiss. Res. **19**:251, 1976.

121. Lesot, H., Osman, M., and Ruch, J.V.: Immunofluorescent localization of collagens, fibronectin and laminin during terminal differentiation of odontoblasts, Dev. Biol. **82**:371, 1981.

122. Lilja, J.: Innervation of different parts of the predentin and dentin in young human premolars, Acta Odontol. Scand. **37**:339, 1979.

123. Lilja, J., Noredenvall, K.-J., and Brännström, M.: Dentin sensitivity, odontoblasts and nerves under desiccated or infected experimental cavities, Swed. Dent. J. **6**:93, 1982.

124. Linde, A.: Glycosaminoglycans (mucopolysaccharides) of the porcine dental pulp, Arch. Oral Biol. **15**:1035, 1970.

125. Linde, A.: Glycosaminoglycans of the odontoblast-predentin layer in dentinogenically active porcine teeth, Calcif. Tissue Res. **12**:281, 1973.

126. Linde, A.: A study of the dental pulp glycosaminoglycans from permanent human teeth and rat and rabbit incisors, Arch. Oral Biol. **18**:49, 1973.

127. Linde, A.: The extracellular matrix of the dental pulp and dentin, J. Dent. Res. **64**(Spec. Iss.):523, 1985.

128. Lindén, L.A., and Brännström, M.: Fluid movements in dentine and pulp, Odontol. Rev. **18**:227, 1967.

129. Magloire, H., et al.: Distribution of type III collagen in the pulp parenchyma of the human developing tooth. Light and electron microscope immunotyping, Histochemistry **74**:319, 1982.

130. Martens, P.: Human dentinogenesis with special regard to the formation of peritubular crown dentin and zones in fetal deciduous and unabraded permanent teeth. A morphologic, microradiographic, and histochemic study, Odontol. Tidskr. **76**:5, 1968.

131. Meyer, M.W., and Path, M.G.: Blood flow in the dental pulp of dogs determined by hydrogen polarography and radioactive microsphere methods, Arch. Oral Biol. **24**:601, 1979.

132. Michelich, V., Pashley, D.H., and Whitford, G.M.: Dentin permeability: a comparison of functional versus anatomical tubular radii, J. Dent. Res. **57**:1019, 1978.

133. Michelich, V.J., Schuster, G.S., and Pashley, D.H.: Bacterial penetration of human dentin in vivo, J. Dent. Res. **59**;1398, 1980.

134. Miller, G.S., et al.: Histologic identification of mast cells in human dental pulp, Oral Surg. **46**:559, 1978.

135. Miller, W.A., and Massler, M.: Permeability and staining of active and arrested lesions in dentine, Br. Dent. J. **112**:187, 1962.

136. Mjör, I.A.: Dentin-predentin complex and its permeability: pathology and treatment overview. J. Dent. Res. **64**(Spec. Iss.):621, 1985.

137. Mjör, I.A., and Pindborg, J.J.: Histology of the human tooth, Copenhagen, 1973, Einar Munksgaard.

138. Mori, K.: Identification of lymphatic vessels after intra-arterial injection of dyes and other substances, Microvasc. Res. **1**:268, 1969.

139. Moss-Salentijn, L., and Klyvert, M.H.: Epithelially induced denticles in the pulps of recently erupted, noncarious human premolars, J. Endod. **9**:554, 1983.

140. Mowry, R.W.: The histochemical detection and identification of complex carbohydrates in human connective tissues. In Finn, S.B., editor: Biology of the dental pulp organ, Birmingham, 1968, University of Alabama Press.

141. Mullaney, T.P., Howell, R.M., and Petrich, J.D.: Resistance of nerve fibers to pulpal necrosis, Oral Surg. **30**:690, 1970.

142. Mummary, J.H.: Microscopic anatomy of the teeth. Oxford, 1919, Oxford University Press.

143. Nähri, M.: Activation of dental pulp nerves of the cat and the dog with hydrostatic pressure, Proc. Finn. Dent. Soc. **74**(Suppl. 5):1, 1978.

144. Närhi, M.V.O., Hirvonen, T.J., and Hakumäki, M.O.K.: Activation of intradental nerves in the dog to some stimuli applied to the dentine. Arch. Oral Biol. **27**:1053, 1982.

145. Närhi, M., et al.: Activation of heat-sensitive nerve fibers in the dental pulp of the cat, Pain **14**:317, 1982.

146. Närhi, M., et al.: Functional differences in intradental A- and C-nerve units in the cat, Pain Suppl. **2**:S242 (abstract), 1984.

147. Nylen, M.U., and Scott, D.B.: An electron microscopic study of the early stages of dentinogenesis, USPHS Publication No. 613, Washington, D.C., 1958, Government Printing Office.

148. Nylen, M.U., and Scott, D.B.: Electron microscopic studies of dentinogenesis, J. Indiana Dent. Assoc. **39**:406, 1960.

149. Olgart, L.: Influence of pharmacologic agents on blood flow and sensory nerves in the pulp. Grossman, L.I., editor: The mechanism and control of pain, New York, 1979, Masson Publishing USA, Inc.

150. Olgart, L., Brännström, M., and Johnson, G.: Invasion of bacteria into dentinal tubules. Experiments in vivo and in vitro, Acta Odontol. Scand. **32**:61, 1974.

151. Outhwaite, W.C., Livingston, M.J., and Pashley, D.H.: Effects of changes in surface area, thickness, temperature, and post-extraction time on human dentine permeability, Arch. Oral Biol. **21**:599, 1976.

152. Pashley, D.J.: Dentin conditions and disease. In Lazzari, G., editor: CRC handbook of experimental dentistry, Boca Ratan, FL, 1893, CRC Press.

153. Pashley, D.H.: Dentin-predentin complex and its permeability: physiologic overview, J. Dent. Res. **64**(Spec. Iss.):613, 1985.

154. Pashley, D.H., et al.: Comparison of in vitro and in vivo dog dentin permeability, J. Dent. Res. **60**:763, 1981.

155. Pashley, D.H., and Livingston, M.J.: Effect of molecular size on permeability coefficients in human dentine, Arch. Oral Biol. **23**:391, 1978.

156. Pashley, D.H., Livingston, M.J., and Greenhill, J.D.: Regional resistances to fluid flow in human dentine, in vitro, Arch. Oral Biol. **23**:807, 1978.

157. Pashley, D.H., Nelson, P., and Pashley, E.: In vivo fluid movement across dentine, in the dog, Arch. Oral Biol. **26**:707, 1981.

158. Path, M.G., and Meyer, M.W.: Heterogeneity of blood flow in the canine tooth of the dog, Arch. Oral Biol. **25**:83, 1980.

159. Pearson, A.A.: The early innervation of the developing deciduous teeth, J. Anat. **123**:563, 1977.

160. Pourtois, M.: Étude de la différenciation des odontoblastes en culture in vitro, Arch. Biol. (Liege) **77**:107, 1966.

161. Provenza, D.V.: Oral histology. Inheritance and development, Philadelphia, 1964, J.B. Lippincott Co.

162. Provenza, D.V.: Comparative morphology of the pulp vascular system. In Finn, S.B. editor: Biology of the dental pulp organ: a symposium. Birminghan, 1968, University of Alabama Press.

163. Rapp, R., et al.: Ultrastructure of fenestrated capillaries in human dental pulps, Arch. Oral Biol. **22**:317, 1977.

164. Reader, A., and Foreman, D.W.: An ultrastructural qualitative investigation of human intradental innervation, J. Endod. **7**:161, 1981.

165. Reeder, O.W., et al.: Dentin permeability: determinants of hydraulic conductance, J. Dent. Res. **57**:187, 1978.

166. Reeves, R., and Stanley, H.R.: The relationship of bacterial penetration and pulpal pathosis in carious teeth, Oral Surg. **22:**59, 1966.

167. Reith, E.J.: Collagen formation in developing molar teeth of rats, J. Ultrastruct. Res. **21:**383, 1968.

168. Reith, E.J.: Ultrastructural aspects of dentinogenesis. In Symons, N.B.B., editor: Dentine and pulp, Dundee, 1968, University of Dundee.

169. Roane, J.B., et al.: An ultrastructural study of dentinal innervation in the adult human tooth, Oral Surg. **35:**94, 1973.

170. Ruch, J.V.: Odontoblast differentiation and the formation of the odontoblast layer. J. Dent. Res. **64**(Spec. Iss.):489, 1985.

171. Ruch, J.V., and Karcher-Djuricic, V.: On odontogenic tissue interactions. In Slavkin, H.C., and Greulich, R.C. editors: Extracellular matrix influences on gene expression, New York, 1975, Academic Press, Inc.

172. Ruch, J.V., Karcher-Djuricic, V., and Thiebold, J.: Cell division and cytodifferentiation of odontoblasts, Differentiation **5:**165, 1976.

173. Ruch, J.V.,. et al.: Facts and hypotheses concerning the control of odontoblast differentiation, Differentiation **21:**7, 1982.

174. Sasaki, S.: Studies on the respiration of the dog tooth germ, J. Biochem. **46:**269, 1959.

175. Sayegh, F.S., and Reed, A.J.: Calcification in the dental pulp, Oral Surg. **25:**873, 1968.

176. Scott, J.N., and Weber, D.F.: Microscopy of the junctional region between human coronal primary and secondary dentin, J. Morphol. **154:**133, 1977.

177. Seltzer, S., Bender, I.B., and Ziontz, M.: The interrelationship of pulp and periodontal disease, Oral Surg. **16:**1474, 1963.

178. Sigal, M.J., et al.: The odontoblast process extends to the dentinoenamel junction: An immunocytochemical study of rat dentine, J. Histochem. Cytochem. **32:**872, 1984.

179. Sigal, M.J., et al.: A combined scanning electron microscopy and immunofluorescence study demonstrating that the odontoblast process extends to the dentinoenamel junction in human teeth, Anat. Rec. **210:**453, 1984.

180. Sisca, R.F., and Provenza, D.V.: Initial dentin formation in human deciduous teeth. An electron microscopic study, Cacif. Tiss. Res. **9:**1, 1972.

181. Slavkin, H.C.: The nature and nurture of epithelial-mesenchymal interactions during tooth morphogenesis, J. Biol. Buccale **6:**189, 1978.

182. Slavkin, H.C., et al.: editors: Epithelial derived basal lamina regulation of mesenchymal cell differentiation. In Weber, R., and Burger, M.: Proceedings of the International Society of Developmental Biologists, New York, 1982, A.R. Liss.

183. Stanley, H.R., et al.: The detection and prevalance of reactive and physiologic sclerotic dentin, reparative dentin and dead tracts beneath various types of dental lesions according to tooth surface and age, J. Oral Pathol. **12:**257, 1983.

184. Stanley, H.R., White, C.L., and McCray, L.: The rate of tertiary (reparative) dentin formation in the human tooth, Oral Surg. **21:**180, 1966.

185. Stenvik, A., Iverson, J., and Mjör, I.A.: Tissue pressure and histology of normal and inflamed tooth pulps in Macaque monkeys, Arch. Oral Biol. **17:**1501, 1972.

186. Symons, N.B.B.: The microanatomy and histochemistry of dentinogenesis. In Miles, A.E.W., editor: Structural and chemical organization of the teeth, Vol. 1, New York, 1967, Academic Press, Inc.

187. Takada, T.: The structures of the vessels in the dental pulp studied by light and electron microscopy, with special reference to presence or absence of lymphatic vessels and fine structure of venules (Japanese), Kaibogaku Zasshi **48:**118, 1973.

188. Takahashi, K., Kishi, Y., and Kim, S.: A scanning electron microscope study of the blood vessels of dog pulp using corrosion resin casts, J. Endod. **8:**131, 1982.

189. Takuma, S: Ultrastructure of dentinogenesis. In Miles, A.E.W., editor: Structure and chemical organization of the teeth, Vol. 1, New York, 1967, Academic Press, Inc.

190. Takuma, S., and Nagai, N.: Ultrastructure of rat odontoblasts in various stages of their development and maturation, Arch. Oral Biol. **16:**993, 1971.

191. Takuma, S., et al.: Electron microscopy of carious lesions in human dentin, Bull. Tokyo Dent. Coll. **8:**143,1967.

192. Ten Cate, A.R.: A fine structural study of coronal and root dentinogenesis in the mouse: observations on the so-called "von Korff fibers" and their contribution to mantle dentin. J. Anat. **125:**183, 1977.

193. Ten Cate, A.R.: Oral histology: development, structure, and function, ed. 2, St. Louis, 1985, The C.V. Mosby Co.

194. Ten Cate, A.R., et al.: The non-fibrous nature of the von Korff fibers in developing dentine. A light and electron microscopic study, Anat. Rec. **168:**491, 1970.

195. Thesleff, I., et al.: Changes in the distribution of type IV collagen, laminin proteoglycan and fibronectin during mouse tooth development, Dev. Biol. **81:**182, 1981.

196. Thesleff, I., Lehtonen, E., and Saxon, L.: Basement membrane formation in transfilter tooth culture and its relations to odontoblast differentiation, Differentiation **10:**71, 1978.

197. Thesleff, I., et al.: Changes in the matrix proteins, fibronectin and collagen during differentiation of mouse tooth germs, Dev. Biol. **70:**116, 1979.

198. Thomas, H.F.: The extent of the odontoblast process in human dentin, J. Dent. Res. **58**(D):2207, 1979.

199. Thomas, H.F.: The lamina limitans of human dentinal tubules, J. Dent. Res. **63:**1064, 1984.

200. Thomas, H.F., and Payne, R.C.: The ultrastructure of dentinal tubules from erupted human premolar teeth, J. Dent. Res. **62:**532, 1983.

201. Thomas J.J., Stanley, H.R., and Gilmore, H.W.: Effects of gold foil condensation on human dental pulp, J. Am. Dent. Assoc. **78:**788, 1969.

202. Tomes, J.: On the presence of the fibrils of soft tissue in the dentinal tubules, Philos. Trans. **146:**515, 1856.

203. Tönder, K.J.H.: Effect of vasodilating drugs on external carotid and pulpal blood flow in dogs: "stealing" of dental perfusion pressure, Acta Physiol. Scand. **97:**75, 1976.

204. Tönder, K.J.H., and Naess, G.: Nervous control of blood flow in the dental pulp in dogs, Acta Physiol. Scand. **104:**13, 1978.

205. Torebjörk, H.E., and Hanin, R.G.: Perceptual changes accompanying controlled preferential blocking of A and C fiber responses in intact human skin nerves, Exp. Brain Res. **16:**321, 1973.

206. Torneck, C.D.: Dentin-pulp complex. In Ten Cate, A.R.: Oral histology: development, structure, and function, ed. 2, St. Louis, 1985, The C.V. Mosby Co.

207. Tronstad, L.: Quantitative microradiography of intact and worn human coronal dentine, Arch. Oral Biol. **18:**533, 1973.

208. Trowbridge, H.O.: Pathogenesis of pulpitis resulting from dental caries, J. Endod. **7:**52, 1981.

209. Trowbridge, H.O.: Intradental sensory units: physiological and clinical aspects, J. Endod. **11:**489, 1985.

210. Trowbridge, H.O.: Mechanisms of pain induction in hypersensitive teeth. In Rowe, N.H., editor: Hypersensitive dentin: origin and management, Ann Arbor, 1985, University of Michigan.

211. Trowbridge, H.O., et al.: Sensory response to thermal stimulation in human teeth, J. Endod. **6:**405, 1980.

212. Trowbridge, H.O., and Shibata, F.: Mitotic activity in epithelial rests of Malassez, Periodontics **5:**109, 1967.

213. Van Hassel, H.J.: Physiology of the human dental pulp, Oral Surg. **32:**126, 1971.

214. Veis, A., Tsay, T.-G., and Kanwar, Y.: The preparation of antibodies to dentin phosphophoryns. In Ruch, J.V., and Belcourt, A.B., editors: Tooth morphogenesis and differentiation, Paris, 1984, Inserm Symposia Series. (In press.)

215. Weber, D.F.: Human dentine sclerosis: a microradiographic study, Arch. Oral Biol. **19**:163, 1974.
216. Weinstock, A., Weinstock, M., and Leblond, C.P.: Autoradiographic detection of 3H-fucose incorporation into glycoprotein by odontoblasts and its deposition at the site of the calcification front in dentin, Calcif. Tiss. Res. **8**:181, 1972.
217. Weinstock, M., and Leblond, C.P.: Synthesis, migration and release of precursor collagen by odontoblasts as visualized by radioautography after 3H-proline administration, J. Cell Biol. **60**:92, 1974.
218. Winter, H.F., Bishop, J.G., and Dorman, H.L.: Transmembrane potentials of odontoblasts, J. Dent. Res. **42**:594, 1963.
219. Yamada, T., et al.: The extent of the odontoblast process in normal and carious human dentin, J. Dent. Res. **62**:798, 1983.
220. Yamamura, T.: Differentiation of pulpal cells and inductive influences of various matrices with reference to pulpal wound healing, J. Dent. Res. **64**(Spec. Iss.):530, 1985.
221. Yamamura, T., et al.: Differentiation and induction of undifferentiated mesenchymal cells in tooth and periodontal tissue during wound healing and regeneration, Bull. Tokyo Dent. Coll. **21**:181, 1980.
222. Zachrisson, B.U.: Mast cells in human dental pulp, Arch. Oral Biol. **16**:555, 1971.
223. Zander, H.A.: The physiology of the dental pulp, Queensland Dent. J. **6**:33, 1953.
224. Zerlotti, E.: Histochemical study of the connective tissue of the dental pulp, Arch. Oral Biol. **9**:149, 1964.

Self-assessment questions

1. Root development begins
   a. Prior to enamel formation
   b. Simultaneous with enamel formation
   c. After completion of enamel formation
   d. Prior to Hertwig's epithelial root sheath formation
2. A characteristic of human dentin is the presence of
   a. Tubules that occupy 20% to 30% of intact dentin
   b. von Korff fibers in the predentin layer
   c. Mineralized predentin adjacent to dentin
   d. Presence of odontoblasts in the dentinal tubules
3. In dental caries an inflammatory reaction develops in the pulp prior to actual pulp infection because
   a. Sclerotic dentin precedes the caries process
   b. Bacterial products reach the pulp before the bacteria
   c. Dentin permeability is less near the pulp space
   d. Peripheral dentin is much more permeable
4. Although similar in function, the odontoblast differs from the osteoblast and cementoblast in
   a. Morphologic characteristics
   b. Ultrastructures
   c. Matrix production
   d. Being a protein-secreting cell
5. The extent to which the odontoblast process extends outward in dentin
   a. Has been shown conclusively in recent years
   b. Is variable depending on the vitality of the pulp
   c. Depends on continued mitotic activity of the odontoblast
   d. Will affect the impact of restorative procedures on the pulp
6. Fibroblasts
   a. Are the least numerous cells of the pulp
   b. Produce and degrade collagen fibers of the pulp
   c. Increase in numbers as blood vessels, nerves, and fibers increase
   d. Undergo active differentiation in the pulp as do fibroblasts of other connective tissues
7. The pathways of pulpal inflammation and infection are strongly influenced by
   a. The two structural proteins in the pulp: collagen and elastin
   b. Dental materials that depress pulpal metabolic activity
   c. The state of polymerization of the ground substance components in the pulp
   d. Osmotic pressures as regulated by proteoglycans
8. Regardless of the nature of the sensory stimulus, all afferent impulses from the pulp result in the sensation of
   a. Proprioception
   b. Pain
   c. Heat
   d. Touch
9. The nerve fibers of the pulp tissue are
   a. Unmyelinated C fibers
   b. Relatively resistant to necrosis
   c. Primarily from the facial nerve
   d. Evenly distributed throughout the pulp
10. Fluid movement in dentinal tubules is known as the
    a. Hydrodynamic theory
    b. Osmotic pressure
    c. Mechanical deformation theory
    d. Hydraulic theory
11. Painful pulpitis associated with an inflamed or degenerating pulp
    a. Is caused by a decrease of intrapulpal pressure
    b. Results from a reduction of nerve cell permeability
    c. Is associated with stimulation of A fibers
    d. Is most likely due to nociceptive C fiber activity
12. Capillaries are found throughout the pulp, and are most dense in the
    a. Pulp horns
    b. Central pulp
    c. Subodontoblastic region
    d. Radicular area
13. A healthy dental pulp responds to an injury by
    a. An effective collateral circulation to transport inflammatory elements to the area
    b. Deposition of well-mineralized and highly tubular reparative dentin
    c. Initiation of an inflammatory response, followed by partial and complete pulp necrosis
    d. The formation of reparative dentin at the pulpal surface corresponding to areas of irritation
14. Pulpal calcifications
    a. May compromise the pulpal blood supply
    b. Are of no significance in root canal therapy
    c. Usually have an inorganic matrix of collagen
    d. Are not associated with age, attrition, or pathology

11

PATHOLOGY

JAMES H.S. SIMON

The study of pulpal and periapical disease provides the clinician with a scientific basis for diagnosis and treatment and a means of evaluating both the success or failure of each. Our concern here will be mainly with the microscopic progression of disease, which the clinician must have in mind when confronted with the clinical realities of endodontic practice.

In the past, many attempts were made to correlate a set of clinical findings with a specific microscopic picture of the pulp. Investigators[19,60,63] have now shown the futility of this approach. Since it is generally agreed that no reliable correlation exists, the microscopic and clinical findings are usually divided into separate classifications. Thus, after the clinical findings have been gathered, the clinician is faced with the uncertainty of the histologic status of the pulp. However, with the following basic understanding of the disease processes, one should be able to arrive at a reasonably accurate decision as to whether the pulp requires treatment and, if so, if it is amenable to preventive therapy or requires endodontic treatment. This is what is important to the clinician. Furthermore, once endodontic therapy has been rendered, the clinician should be able to predict and evaluate the results of treatment.

AGING

To understand pulp pathology, one must have a thorough knowledge of what is considered normal as described in Chapter 10. Although aging may not strictly be considered a pathologic process, several factors merit consideration here because of their effects on the disease processes. When confronted with a diagnostic problem, the clinician must take into account the patient's age and the underlying changes.

By merely surviving, pulp tissue is subject to retrogressive or atrophic changes, on which other reactions may be superimposed:

1. Because of the elaboration of reparative dentin, the size and volume of pulp tissue are reduced. Thus there is

a smaller area in which pathologic processes may take place.

2. The cellular components are usually decreased, and

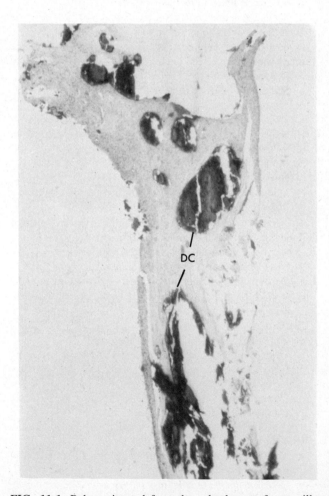

FIG. 11-1. Pulp extirpated from the palatal root of a maxillary molar. Note the numerous dystrophic calcifications *(DC)*. These were not visible on the radiograph.

there is a corresponding increase in the number and thickness of collagen fibers. Zach[90] has reported a diminution in the number and size of odontoblasts.

3. The vascular and nerve supplies also decrease in number and quality. This may explain in part the decrease in sensitivity and metabolic rate in older teeth.[8-10] Any tissue that has a reduced blood supply is hampered in its ability to respond to injury.

4. With increasing age, there is an increase in incidence of pulp stones and dystrophic calcifications. The diffuse foci of calcification are more prevalent in the apical areas of the pulp (Fig. 10-48). Most of these calcifications have been described as being perivascular and perineural.[57] Other calcifications have been classified as either true or false. True denticles consist of dentin with evidence of tubules and odontoblasts. The false denticles are composed of concentric layers of calcification around a nidus of necrotic cells or a thrombus in blood vessels. Although the cause of these calcifications is unknown, they may aggravate or impede an inflammatory reaction within the pulp (Fig. 11-1). Thus, in the interpretation of a pulpal response in an older tooth, these underlying changes must be considered in determining the pulp's healing capacity.

INFLAMMATION

The basic disease process that is involved in pulp and periapical disease is infection. Many definitions of inflammation exist but none is precise.* Menkin defined inflammation as the complex vascular, lymphatic, and local tissue reaction of a higher organism to an irritant.[35] Because infection is the reaction to a viable (i.e., microorganisms) irritant, *the terms inflammation and infection are not interchangeable.* This distinction is important. A patient can have an inflammatory response without having an infection. However, the converse is not valid. In any event inflammation is basically a vascular phenomenon.

Vascular changes

The initial vascular change in inflammation is a transient contraction of the microcirculation that possesses muscle tissue: the arterioles, metarterioles, and precapillary sphincters. This contraction is followed almost immediately by dilation of the vessels (Figs. 11-2 and 11-3). Because of the dilation the blood flow slows, and the white blood cells that usually flow in the center of the vessel drop to the periphery and stick to the endothelial wall. This is termed margination (Fig. 11-4). The arteriole dilation leads to an increase of the pressure in the microcirculation and also leakage of fluid though the endothelial venule walls. Although platelets try to plug these gaps, fluid (plasma) leaks into the extravascular tissue. Because of this plasma leakage the tissue pressure increases until it equals the leaking pressure. At this point the leaking slows down. The precapillary sphincters, however, allow more blood than is normal to flow into the capillaries and ven-

*References 17, 54, 56, 59, 84, 88.

ules, which forces more plasma protein into the tissues. All this results in edema.

In general the leakage may be of a histamine type in the venules, where the contraction of the endothelial cells opens the fenestrations in the wall and allows fluid to pass through, or leakage may occur by direct injury to the vessel wall. This lasts for a longer time than the histamine type.

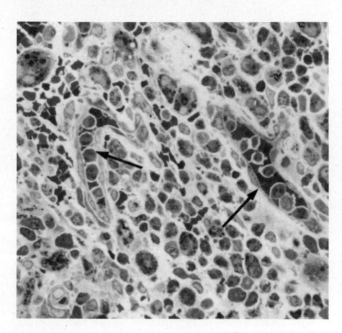

FIG. 11-2. Photomicrograph of an area of inflammation with two capillaries showing white and red cells flowing through the vessels *(arrows).* (×400.)

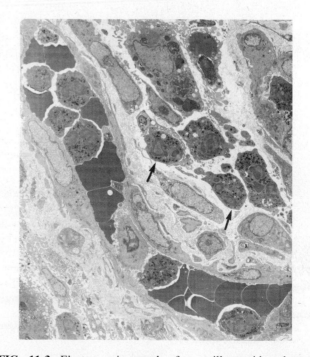

FIG. 11-3. Electron micrograph of a capillary with polymorphonuclear leukocytes and erythrocytes inside. Note PMN's in the extravascular tissue *(arrows).* (×3,450.)

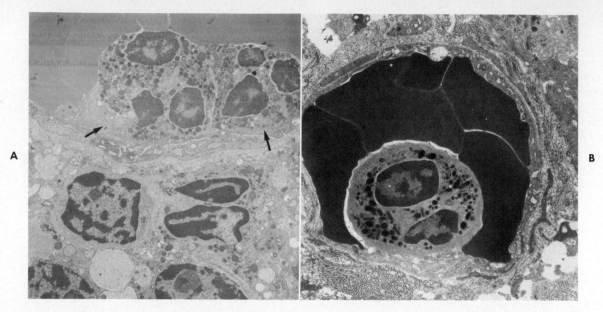

FIG. 11-4. A, Electron micrograph of a portion of a large vessel showing margination of two leukocytes *(arrows)*. (×11,000.) **B,** Smaller vessel with PMN about to squeeze through the wall.

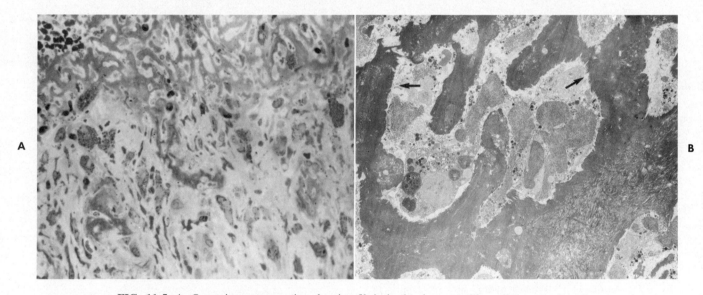

FIG. 11-5. A, One-micrometer section showing fibrin in the tissues walling off the resection. **B,** Ultrastructural picture of fibrin in the tissue *(arrows)*.

As the vessel walls become more permeable large plasma protein molecules pass into the tissue. For example, fibrinogen is converted to fibrin in the tissues and acts as a meshwork to wall off the reaction (Fig. 11-5). The white blood cells that now line the endothelial wall of the vessels squeeze through the gaps into the tissue by ameboid movement. This movement is called diapedesis. It is a tight movement through the gaps with no fluid leakage around the cells.

Acute inflammation

In acute inflammation the first cells to go through the vessel wall are the polymorphonuclear leukocytes (PMNs) followed by the monocytes. When the monocyte migrates into the tissue, it is now termed a macrophage (Fig. 11-6).

The neutrophils survive for hours whereas the monocytes last for days to months. The neutrophil is characterized by its lobulated nucleus and its many cytoplasmic granules whereas the macrophage has a single large nucleus. In addition many heterogeneous dense granules and pinocytic vesicles are present in the cytoplasm.

Phagocytosis. In the inflammatory process both cell types function as phagocytes. The process of phagocytosis involves three stages:

1. Attachment—to be phagocytized, bacteria or an antigen is coated or opsonized with IgG, IgM, or C3b from the complement system.
2. Ingestion—after attachment the bacteria are taken into the cell. Pseudopods from the cell fuse around the particle, forming a phagosome. At the same

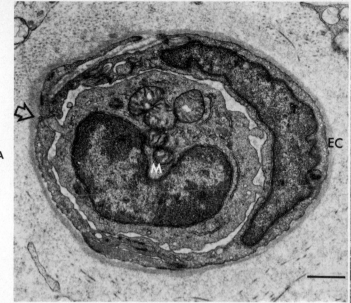 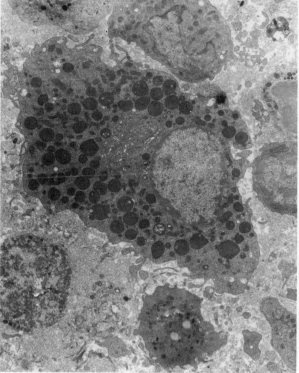

FIG. 11-6. **A,** Monocyte *(M)* in a capillary with three psueodo-pods extended. (×12,900.) One pseudopod *(upper left)* is beginning to squeeze through the intercellular gap *(arrow)*. Note the prominent endothelial cells *(EC)*. **B,** Electron micrograph of a macrophage now out in the tissue.

time, cytoplasmic granules converge on the phagosome, fuse with it, and then degranulate or discharge onto the bacteria.

3. Breakdown of the bacteria or antigen—the bacteria are killed or degraded by:
   a. Lysosomal hydrolytic enzymes
   b. An acid pH in the vacuole
   c. Cationic proteins
   d. Lactoferrin
   e. Superoxide anion
   f. Hydrogen peroxide

Thus the process of phagocytosis includes coating, ingesting, and then destroying the bacteria.

Mediators. These vascular and cellular changes are directed by nerves and to a large extent certain chemicals that are called mediators of inflammation. The mediators may be exogenous (such as from bacterial products) or endogenous. The endogenous mediators come from the plasma or are released from the tissues. Mediators released from plasma are:
1. Kinin system
2. Complement system
3. Clotting system

Mediators released from tissue are:
1. Vasoactive amines (histamines from mast cells, basophils, and platelets). These are released in response to:
   a. Physical injury (i.e., trauma)
   b. Chemicals (i.e., neutrophilic lysosomal cationic protein)
   c. IgE sensitized cells
   d. Exposure to C3a and C5a
2. Acidic lipids (i.e., SRS-A and prostaglandins)

3. Lysosomal components
   a. Cationic proteins
   b. Acid proteases
   c. Neutral proteases
4. Lymphocyte products (i.e., lymphokines from T cells)
5. Other

The PMN's macrophages, and effects of the mediators result in the microscopic picture and chain of events for acute inflammation (Fig. 11-7). Thus we can now account for the five original signs of inflammation.
1. Redness—results from the increased dilation of the vessels and some from hemorrhage.
2. Swelling—results from the escape of fluid into the tissues, causing edema.
3. Pain—the accumulation of fluid in the tissues, causing increased pressure on nerve endings.
4. Heat—the increased blood supply causes the warm or hot feeling of the tissues.
5. Loss of function—this is the result of the acute inflammatory process with tissue destruction. Hemostasis leads to reduction in oxygen exchange and enzymes result in necrosis.

Healing. When the bacteria or antigen is destroyed, healing may take place. If the tissue returns to its original state, it is called regeneration. If the original tissue is replaced with dense fibrous connective tissue, it is called a scar.

The two cell types involved in healing are (1) the macrophages that clean up the debris in the area and (2) the fibroblasts that repair the damage. Because this process requires a great deal of oxygen, capillary buds and lymphatics must also be present. If a scar is formed, myofibro-

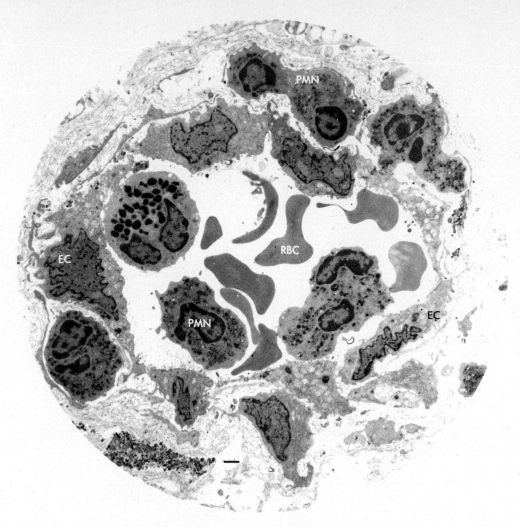

FIG. 11-7. Small venule showing margination of PMNs in the lumen. (×4400.) Other PMNs have already migrated into the interstitial tissue. Red blood cells *(RBC)* are also visible in the lumen, and the endothelial cells *(EC)* are prominent.

blasts that contain actin predominate. Since they act like smooth muscle and can contract, the typical appearance is of wavy collagen.

Chronic inflammation

If the acute process does not heal but continues, then the reaction becomes chronic. The predominant cell types are the lymphocytes and plasma cells. The purpose of the immune system is to neutralize, inactivate, or destroy a stimulus (antigen or bacteria). This is accomplished by:

1. Direct neutralization by antibody binding to the stimulus (antigen) and/or destruction of the stimulus by sensitized lymphocytes.
2. Activation of biochemical and cellular mediator systems that can destroy the antigen.

People are either immunocompetent or immunodeficient. Immunocompetence is the abiltity to generate an immune response that can overcome many diseases and infections. Immunodeficient people cannot make this response and are thus afflicted with many inflammatory and infectious diseases. This specific response to an anti-

gen or immunogen is determined genetically so that each person differs in their response to various antigens. This has been referred to as "host resistance."

Development of lymphocytes. Cell development begins shortly after conception in the yolk sac. Hemopoietic stem cells form that are to become the red blood cells (erythrocytes), granulocytes, macrophages, and lymphocytes. As fetal development progresses, these cells move to the spleen and liver and then on to the bone marrow. The immature lymphocytes go in two different directions:

1. One group of stem cells migrates to the thymus gland, where they mature and become T cells (thymus-dependent lymphocytes). The T cells are concerned with cell-mediated immunity and form a subpopulation for each of the following functions:
   a. Killer T cells
   b. Effector T cells
   c. Helper T cells—help the B cells to produce antibody
   d. Suppressor T cells—turn off the response and prevent autoimmune reactions

Effector T cells are specifically reactive lymphocytes derived from progenitor recognition T cells. Following immunogen stimulation these T cells become lymphoblasts and then multiply by clonal expansion. They do not become plasma cells and do not have RER or make antibodies like plasma cells. However, they do have abundant ribosomes. As an effector cell, this T cell with antigen produces activity in the cytoplasm. As a result, active biochemical and biologic mediators (called lymphokines) are released.

2. The other group remains in the bone marrow and matures to form the B cells (bone marrow derived or bursa equivalent lymphocytes). The B cells give rise to antibody forming plasma cells.

Both groups then migrate to the peripheral lymphatic tissues: the lymph, blood, lymph nodes, spleen, Peyer's patches, appendix, and tonsils. While both cell types look identical microscopically, they can be differentiated. B cells can be identified by detecting the immunoglobulin and complement receptors on the cell membrane by using immunofluorescent techniques, T cells have the ability to form rosette clusters when exposed to sheep red blood cells.

Recognition. Each T cell and B cell has specific recognition sites on its membrane surfaces that can chemically recognize and react with specific antigens. Only a few cells of the total number have a specific site for a specific antigen. Thus, after the cell is stimulated, it rapidly reproduces by clonal expansion to produce enough cells for the specific antigen.

Stimulation also triggers the differentiation of the B cells to form into a blast cell, which then becomes a plasma cell (Fig. 11-8). For this process helper T cells and macrophages (to hold the antigen on the cell surface) are necessary. The life span of a plasma cell is approximately 12 hours.

Antigens (immunogens). Immunogens are any biologic or chemical macromolecule that can react with an antibody or cell product of the immune response. Antigens are usually:

1. Nonself or foreign
2. Macromolecules
3. Proteins, carbohydrates, glycoprotein, or nucleic acids

Fats are *not* immunogenic.

Each lymphocyte is specific for its receptor sites; therefore, it will not bind two different antigens to its surface. The antibody only reacts with six amino acids. This area of the antigen with the amino acids is called the antigenic determinant. There are two types of molecular determinants within an antigen:

1. Haptenic determinants—these are small molecules that by themselves cannot stimulate antibody formation. These must be attached to a carrier molecule to initiate antibodies. (A hapten cannot stimulate a B cell to produce antibody, but once this antibody is made the hapten can cause a reaction.)
2. Carrier determinants—these are less exposed, much larger than haptens, and within the molecular framework or alongside.

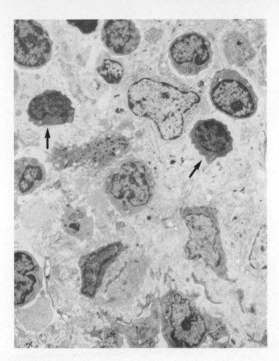

FIG. 11-8. Electron micrograph of numerous lymphocytes *(arrows)* in the lymphoblast stage transforming into plasma cells. Note the presence of a macrophage. (×5,240.)

In general, B cells mainly react with haptens and T cells with carrier determinants.

Antibodies. Antibodies are immunoglobulins that are proteins synthesized by plasma cells. The plasma cell can secrete five classes of immunoglobulin molecules: IgG, IgA, IgM, IgE, and IgD (Fig. 11-9). Each type is produced by a specific lymphocyte that cannot produce more than one type.

The function of the immunoglobulins may be summarized as follows:

IgG—activates complement in the tissues or circulation. Its highest concentration is in the serum. IgG passes the placental barrier.

IgM—activates complement in the tissues and circulation. IgM is the most efficient fixer of complement.

IgE—binds to cell membranes of mast cells and basophils in the Fc region. After reacting with an immunogen at the cell membrane surface, vasoactive factors are released from the mast cell or basophil that cause edema and swelling.

IgA—binds along epithelial surfaces in body secretions and blocks antigen entry across mucous membranes. It may also activate the alternate pathway of complement. Its highest concentration is in saliva.

IgD—functions as a surface molecule (receptor) on cell membranes of maturing B lymphocytes.

For further information, the reader is referred to Chapter 12.

Complement. Complement has nine components (C1-C9) with many subunits. It is produced by the liver and macrophages but is present in an inactive form. Therefore, to exert its activity it must be activated.

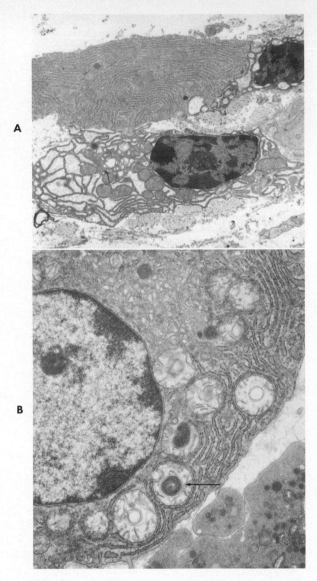

FIG. 11-9. A, Electron micrograph of two plasma cells, one with normal RER and the other with very dilated RER. This dilation is thought to indicate immunoglobulin production and synthesis. (×3,450.) **B,** High-power electron micrograph of part of a plasma cell showing the RER with ribosomes on the surface and myelin figures in the Golgi apparatus *(arrow).* (×23,700.)

There are two pathways for the activation of the complement cascade:

1. Classic pathway—triggered by an antigen/antibody reaction in order C1-C4-C2-C3-C5-C6-C7-C8-C9-. It can be activated by IgG and IgM.
2. Properdin or alternate pathway—the non immune pathway that is triggered by cell surfaces and plant and bacterial carbohydrates but *not* by antigen/antibody reactions. This system is activated by C3-C5-C6-C7-C8-C9. It can be activated by a variety of substances, including IgA, lysosomal enzymes, gram-positive bacterial cell wall, and endotoxin.

In the complement systems C1 is the recognition unit, C2 to C4 is the activation unit, and C5 to C9 is the membrane attack unit.

C1—binds with the antigen/antibody complex and triggers the entire sequence.

C2 and C2a—activate the kinin system that causes endothelial cells to contract and thus increases vascular permeability.

C3a and C5a—are chemotactic for PMNs and monocytes. They also have an anaphylatoxic effect, that is, they interact with specific receptors on the surface of mast cells and basophils that result in:

1. Degranulation and release of histamine
2. Production of SRS-A and intermediate substances of prostaglandin
3. Release of enzymes to form bradykinin

All of these increase vascular permeability.

C3b—becomes bound to cell membranes and has a role in phagocytosis and immune adherence reactions.

C5b—binds to cell membranes.

C5b,6,7—are also chemotactic for PMNs, which release enzymes that destroy cell tissue.

C8 & C9—result in cell lysis.

Since the alternate pathway begins at C3, these reactions are lacking C2a, which activates the kinin system. Thus there are two forms of complement-mediated injury:

1. Cytotoxic. It occurs at the cell membrane and results in phagocytic destruction and cell lysis due to an antigen/antibody complex. The attack cells are sensitized by IgG reacting with antigens on their cell surfaces, and the killer T cells disintegrate the target cell.
2. Immune complex injury. This occurs following the localization of immune complexes in the tissues. It can be in reaction to antigens from bacteria, bacterial fragments, viruses, foreign protein, drugs, etc. These complexes are mediated by IgG or IgM and activate complement through the classic pathway. This attracts PMNs that release lysosomal enzymes that cause tissue destruction and necrosis (Fig. 14-9). These enzymes degrade ground substance, collagen, elastic tissue, carbohydrates, nucleic acids, and other tissue proteins. The Arthus reaction is the prototype of the complement-dependent reaction.

Immunopathologies. The immunopathologies are divided into two broad groups:

1. Immediate-type hypersensitivities—reactions that occur within 24 hours and are caused by antibodies in the serum.
   a. Anaphylaxis—may be local or systemic, but the sensitizing antibody is always IgE. This fixes along mast cell and basophil membranes to trigger release of granules that cause vascular permeability and smooth muscle contraction. The substances are: histamine, serotonin, SRS-A, ECF, and enzymes that catalyze the formation of bradykinin.
   b. Immune complex disease—the sensitizing antibody is IgG and IgM and activates complement by the classic pathway. An example of this is the Arthus phenomenon that occurs between the basement membrane and endothelial cells of the vasculature, leading to localized necrosis.

2. Delayed hypersensitivities—reactions that occur in 24 to 96 hours and are mediated by T cells.
   a. Contact dermatitis—caused by fat-soluble allergens that penetrate the skin and combine with skin proteins. They act as haptens.
   b. Infectious allergies—reactions mediated by effector T cells but also require helper T cells and macrophages. The effector T cells produce the lymphokines that attract and activate macrophages, which release enzymes that destroy the antigen and self. These reactions are caused by infectious agents (i.e., tuberculosis).

Evidence indicates that *all of these processes take place in pulp and periapical inflammatory reactions*. Thus, in the following descriptions, all these reactions may be occurring.

Pulpal pathophysiology

The inflammatory process in the pulp is basically the same as elsewhere in the body connective tissue. However, several factors combine to somewhat alter the response:

1. The pulp is unique insofar as it is connective tissue that is almost totally surrounded by hard tissue—the dentin walls. This limits the area for tissue expansion, thus restricting the pulp's ability to tolerate edema.
2. A factor limiting the pulp's capacity for healing is the almost total lack of collateral circulation. There are a few major vessels that supply the pulp through the apical foramen and small vessels that enter through lateral or accessory canals, but this system does not compare favorably with collateral circulation in other connective tissue. This factor, in combination with factor 1, appears to severely limit the ability of the pulp to cope with necrotic tissue and debris.
3. The pulp is the only organ that can produce reparative dentin to protect itself from injury.

During the inflammatory process the role of tissue pressure becomes critical.[88] When the inflammatory exudate leaves the vessels because of an increase in hydrostatic pressure, there is a corresponding rise in the interstitial pressure. Since the fluid is not compressible and there is little room for edema, the pressure rise may cause a local collapse of the venous portion of the microcirculation. Because this interrupts the blood transport system, local tissue hypoxia and anoxia can occur, which in turn may lead to localized necrosis. The necrotic tissue releases more breakdown products, increasing the interstitial concentration of osmotically active small protein molecules. This aids in pulling more fluid from the vessels, possibly resulting in increased pressure. These products also increase permeability of adjacent vessels, leading to further spread of inflammation. If pus is formed, resulting in microabscess, the process is predictably irreversible. Total necrosis of the pulp may then result from the continued spread of local inflammation. The end result of the inflammatory process is a necrotic pulp devoid of viable tissue.

Etiologic factors

The etiologic factors involved in inflammation of the pulp can be grouped into four general categories: bacterial, iatrogenic, traumatic, and idiopathic.

Bacterial factor

Bacteria and their products are the most common cause of endodontic disease.[27,81,82,85] In work on both conventional and gnotobiotic rats, researchers[25] graphically showed the importance of bacteria—specifically that exposed pulps would degenerate and become totally necrotic with abscess formation *only* if bacteria were present. In the germ-free rats not only was there no infection but healing of soft and hard tissue occurred.[27]

Pulpal response to caries. The pulpal response to caries is inflammatory because the dentinal tubules are permeable. Many biologically active substances (bacterial enzymes, bacterial peptides, endodotoxins, polysaccharides, antibodies, immune complexes, complement proteins, and products of tissue destruction) are able to go through the tubules. However, this is not a one-way street. A study[50] has shown that serum proteins are able to go from the pulp outward.

The first response of dentin to decay is sclerosis. The matrix and tubules calcify with a deposition that resembles peritubular dentin. The purpose of the sclerosis is to reduce dentin permeability. Needle-shaped crystals may also attempt to block the tubules. If the carious lesion is more severe, the odontoblasts and their processes are quickly destroyed, leaving dead tracts that are highly permeable. If the odontoblasts are not destroyed, then reparative dentin may be formed at the pulpal end.

According to Trowbridge,[82] the carious lesion in dentin has four zones:

1. Outer zone of destruction—bacteria and debris are present and the tubules are destroyed.
2. Zone of infection—the tubules are still recognizable and may contain bacteria.
3. Zone of demineralization—there is a loss of peritubular dentin and a decrease in crystal size. The previously sclerosed tubules are now reopened and permeable.
4. Zone of sclerosis—the tubules are trying to wall off the advancing lesion.

If this lesion is mild and advances slowly, reparative dentin may be formed to wall off the lesion and the pulp tissue remains uninflamed (Fig. 11-10). However, this reparative dentin is less tubular and more irregular and has larger lumina than does primary dentin. It may also be atubular, be poorly calcified, and have interglobular dentin, which may not be sufficient to prevent noxious substances from irritating the pulp.

If the carious lesion is more severe or is not removed, pulpal changes take place.[3-7,21,45] Since caries is a chronic disease, the first changes are thought to be chronic. It is an immune response composed of lymphocytes, plasma cells, and macrophages. A study has shown lymphocytes in the pulp when the carious lesion is still confined to enamel.[13]

Odontoblastic changes. With an increase of dentin permeability the immunogens may reach the pulp. Injury to the odontoblasts releases enzymes and the vascular changes of inflammation are set in motion (Figs. 11-11 and 11-12). This initial chronic inflammatory response is believed to be either an immune complex–mediated type of hypersensitivity or a delayed type of hypersensitivity. If the lesion is removed and treated, these pulpal changes may be reversible and healing may occur.

Abscess formation. When the bacteria penetrate the primary or reparative dentin, neutrophils are drawn to the area by chemotaxis. The neutrophils play a role in phagocytosis but also destroy pulp tissue. Eventually the PMNs result in suppuration that may be diffuse or small discrete areas that form microabscesses. Few bacteria are found because they have been engulfed by the PMNs and macrophages. The fibroblasts attempt to wall off the whole reaction. Once this reaction occurs in the pulp, it is thought to be irreversible and will ultimately result in necrosis of the pulp (Fig. 11-13).

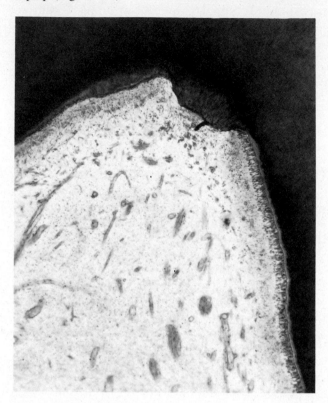

FIG. 11-11. Pulp horn demonstrating reparative dentin formation and engorged vessels (early transitional stage).

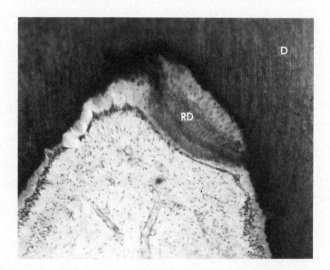

FIG. 11-10. High-power view of a pulp horn exhibiting reparative dentin formation in response to early caries with no apparent inflammatory cell infiltrate. *RD*, Reparative dentin; *D*, dentin.

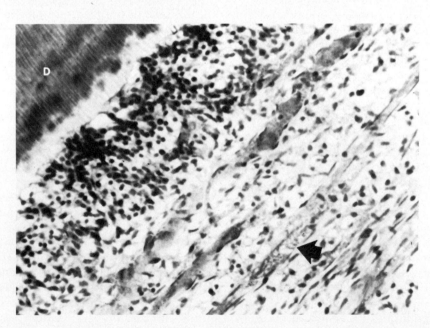

FIG. 11-12. Early inflammation. Disruption of the odontoblasts and infiltration of the subodontoblastic area by inflammatory cells are evident. Note the engorged vessels *(arrow)*. *D*, Dentin.

Hyperplastic pulpitis. Once a carious exposure of the pulp has occurred, a surface ulceration is formed. On occasion this may elicit a proliferative reaction that forms a hyperplastic pulpitis. The tissue grows out of the carious opening and may eventually be covered by epithelium from the surrounding mucosa (Fig. 11-14). This can also occur in teeth with traumatic pulp exposure.

Iatrogenic factors

The second most common cause of endodontic disease occurs as a result of attempts to correct the ravages of dental disease. The effects of operative procedures resulting in excessive heat or drying, or both, are described in Chapter 14. Pulpal changes have also been reported in response to impression techniques whereby bacteria were forced through the dentinal tubules into the pulp. Many materials and chemicals used in dentistry have been found to cause irritation in the pulp.

Pulpal response to operative procedures and chemicals. In assessing the pulpal response to operative procedures, many variables must be taken into account (see Chapter 14). However, the pulp responds with inflammatory reactions that may or may not be reversible. A prominent researcher claims[77] the single most important factor in determining pulpal response to a stimulus is the amount of dentin remaining between the base of the stimulus and the pulp.[71] For cavity preparations the minimal distance remaining between the base of the preparation and the pulp is 2 mm.

The combination for operative procedures that produce minimal pulpal changes was high speed (50,000 to 300,000 rpm), temperature control, and a light load. Since Stanley found that the less the pulpal response, the greater the chance for complete healing, the above combination was judged best.[71]

After an injury, reparative dentin does not begin to form until the twentieth day. Then reparative dentin is formed at the rate of about 1 μm per day. When using high speed with water-cooled temperature control, the greater the distance the bottom of the cavity preparation is from the pulp, the less the chance of reparative dentin being formed.

Another factor to consider in cavity or crown preparations is the pressure of condensation. Pressure condensation in excess of 8 ounces can cause a prominent inflammatory response, whereas no more than 4 ounces appears biologically acceptable.

If heat becomes excessive because of inadequate coolants, no water spray, or toxic materials, then the pulp may respond with coagulation necrosis and intrapulpal abscess formation. This extends past the cut dentinal tubules and produces a burn lesion that may lead to total pulp necrosis. As opposed to caries, the initial response to operative procedures and materials is usually acute inflammation, which may or may not lead to healing. Furthermore, this is not an immune response. Thus, in the treatment of disease, further disease can be created.

Traumatic factors

The different responses to trauma, as described in Chapter 15, appear to be particularly dependent on the severity of the trauma. For example, relatively light trauma from occlusion may cause little or no effect. However, heavier trauma from occlusion may have a significant pulpal effect. One paper[27] reported a case of pulpal necrosis, apparently the result of bruxism.[24]

The response to trauma from blows or accidents can be varied. Some pulps apparently heal with no adverse ef-

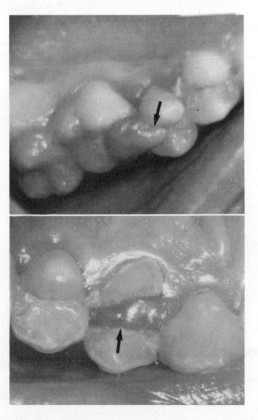

FIG. 11-14. Two clinical examples of hyperplastic pulpitis. The hyperplastic pulp tissue has grown out of the lesion instead of becoming necrotic *(arrows)*.

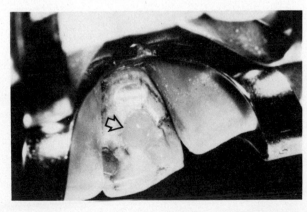

FIG. 11-13. Lingual view of a maxillary anterior tooth that responded to endodontic testing procedures in the higher range. When the pulp chamber was opened, several drops of pus exuded followed by hemorrhage *(arrow)*. Vital pulp tissue was found in the apical portion of the canal.

fects, whereas others become necrotic. There appears to be a middle ground (i.e., some teeth respond to trauma by increased pulpal calcification). This may be so extensive that radiographically the entire canal appears calcified. Fig. 11-15 shows two different responses to the same

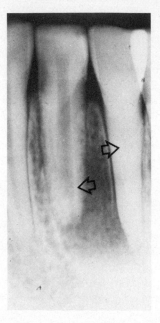

FIG. 11-15. Diverse responses to trauma: calcification *(right)*, necrosis *(left)*.

trauma. One tooth became necrotic, and the other responded with increased calcification.

Trauma causing a cracked or fractured tooth secondarily provides a pathway for the oral flora to reach the pulp. Once the pulp is exposed to the oral environment, inflammation is a predictable complication (Fig. 11-16). These cracked teeth can result in bizarre clinical symptoms as described in Chapter 1, making diagnosis very difficult.

Pulpal response to trauma. If the trauma is sufficient, there is direct vascular damage and hemorrhage that leads to inflammation and tissue destruction. This usually results in either healing or total necrosis of the pulp. An accurate prognosis is not predictable. Studies on intact teeth with necrotic pulps and a history of trauma state that many of these teeth are positive for bacteria. Their presence has been explained by anachoresis, i.e., the process of bacteria lodging in an area of previously damaged tissue. The acute and chronic inflammatory response is not an immunologic process until bacteria are present in the tissues.

A very different histologic picture of the pulp occurs if the apical blood supply is severed by sudden trauma. One investigator has described this as ischemic infarction.[72] The occlusion of the apical vessels leads to ischemia, the capillary walls are damaged, and red blood cells hemorrhage into the tissues. The hemoglobin is eventually converted to a homogeneous granular debris that replaces the pulp tissue. Eventually no cellular detail is visible, only the uniform red material remains. Since the blood supply

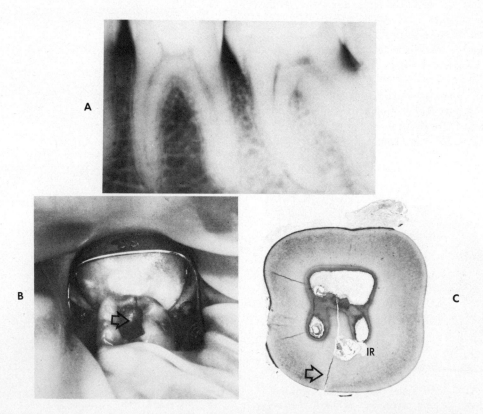

FIG. 11-16. A, Preoperative view. Occlusal and buccal restoration but otherwise unremarkable. **B,** The tooth has been isolated and the occlusal alloy removed. The crack *(arrow)*, running in a mesial-distal plane, is now visible. **C,** Cross section of a different tooth showing the extent of a crack *(arrow)*. Note the partial pulpitis and the internal resorption *(IR)*.

has been severed, inflammatory cells cannot get to the tissues. Thus the nerves, vessels, and fibroblasts degenerate with no inflammatory response. In some cases all that remains is a collagen "skeleton." These are the cases that do not respond to pulp testing procedures, but upon extirpating the pulp a nonbleeding material that has the form of a pulp is removed. Clinically these have been referred to as a "fibrotic" pulp. If bacteria are present, there is no blood supply to provide a response. However, the cellular products and debris do diffuse out the apex of this tooth and lead to periapical inflammation and a radiolucency on the radiograph.

Idiopathic factors

Pulpal changes also occur for reasons that are as yet unknown (i.e., are idiopathic). A common example is internal resorption (Fig. 11-17). Although trauma has been implicated to an extent in internal resorption, this does not explain the whole phenomenon.[43] These teeth are frequently asymptomatic and are discovered on routine dental radiographs, as described in Chapter 16. Microscopically, macrophages and multinucleated giant cells are found close to the resorbing dentin. The tissue replacing the lost dentin usually is chronically inflamed. If the pulp has become necrotic, the resorption stops because vital tissue is necessary for the resorptive process. Endodontic therapy

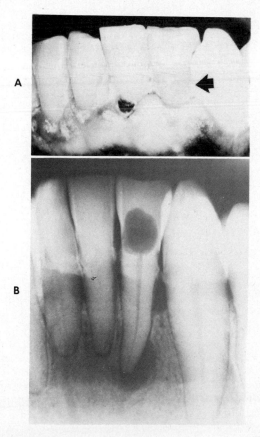

FIG. 11-17. A, Discoloration *(arrow)* of the gingival half of crown of the mandibular left lateral incisor. Internal resorption was immediately suspected. **B,** The clinical impression of internal resorption is confirmed. This case led to chronic apical periodontitis.

will arrest the internal resorptive process. However, if the lesion perforates externally, then the prognosis becomes more guarded. Also a periapical radiolucency may be associated with internal resorption, signifying pulpal necrosis as a sequela to the reaction (Fig. 11-17).

Classification. Because no reliable correlation has been demonstrated between the clinical status and the histologic status of the pulp, many classifications have been based on one or the other finding.[19,30,61-63] The most difficult aspect to accept is that *there is no correlation between the severity of pain and the extent of pulpal involvement.*[36,45] The critical decision for the clinician is whether to treat the pulp endodontically or attempt preventive measures. Once the decision is made to institute endodontic therapy, the precise histologic state of the pulp is academic because the treatment is total extirpation. However, in the early stages of pulpal pathology the pulp passes from a reversible to an irreversible pulpitis. This diagnosis is not always an easy one to make because the dividing line can be very obscure.

Reversible and irreversible pulpitis. To decide whether a pulpitis is reversible or irreversible, we depend on test results, clinical symptoms, and clinical judgment as described in Chapter 1. The patient's history of pain and the presence or absence of spontaneous pain are of critical importance. By this we mean pain that is not brought on by specific stimulus (i.e., heat or cold).

For example, a patient who has had a restoration replaced 1 month before now appears with a complaint of pain. After a period of quiescence the pain is coming and going at no specific time. During the past year there have been several episodes of spontaneous pain. Irreversible pulpitis is immediately suspected. Thermal tests may be valuable at this stage, because pain usually lingers after thermal stimuli are applied and withdrawn. The pulp tester may show a higher reading on adjacent and contralateral teeth.

On the one hand, if the pain is elicited only by thermal stimulation and goes away immediately when the stimulus is removed, reversible pulpitis is suspected. No history of previous pain would add to this diagnosis. However, if a more acute or prolonged sensation exists, irreversible pulpitis is usually diagnosed.

Seltzer[60] believes that the most definitive factor in irreversible pulpitis is the presence of an intrapulpal abscess. This diagnosis is based on a history of previous pain (moderate to severe), no response to pulp tests, or vitalometer tests differing markedly from those on control teeth. In addition, the presence of spontaneous severe pain or a prolonged response after thermal testing usually indicates irreversible pulpitis. In the presence of two or more findings, irreversible pulpitis if fairly easy to diagnose. The real diagnostic challenge is the gray area preceding this stage. Mistakes in diagnosis can be made; however, good clinical judgment and understanding of the basic pathologic processes keep these to a minimum.

Seltzer[60] summed up the entire spectrum of pulpal histopathology by the following classification:

Atrophic pulp
Transitional stage

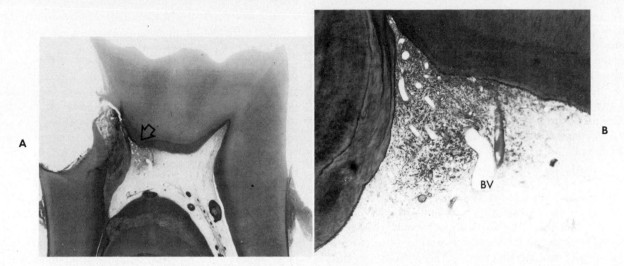

FIG. 11-18. A, Low-power view of the beginning inflammatory response to caries *(arrow)* in the pulp horn of a mandibular molar. The remainder of the pulp shows no inflammatory infiltrate. Calcifications and reparative dentin on the chamber floor are evident in the remaining pulp tissue. **B,** Higher-power view of the pulp horn area showing the inflammatory infiltrate and dilated blood vessels *(BV)*.

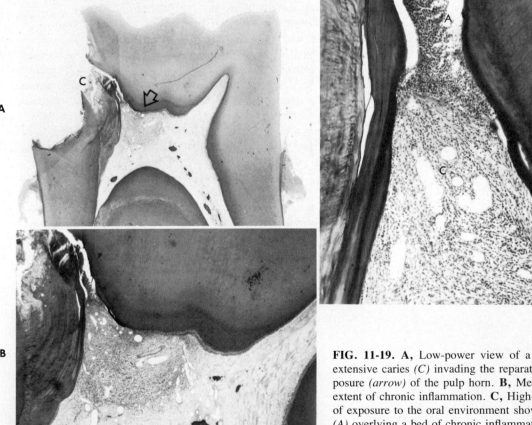

FIG. 11-19. A, Low-power view of a mandibular molar with extensive caries *(C)* invading the reparative dentin. Note the exposure *(arrow)* of the pulp horn. **B,** Medium-power view of the extent of chronic inflammation. **C,** High-power view at the point of exposure to the oral environment showing acute inflammation *(A)* overlying a bed of chronic inflammation *(C)*.

Acute partial pulpitis
Chronic partial pulpitis
Chronic partial pulpitis with liquefaction necrosis
Total pulp necrosis

Each of these stages can be seen as a step in the spectrum of the inflammatory process. The stages are fixed and static only in microscopic tissue sections (Figs. 11-18 to 11-22). In vivo the inflammatory process is dynamic and ever changing.

Periapical extension of pulpal inflammation

Periapical inflammation begins *before* the pulp is totally necrotic. Bacterial products, mediators of inflammation, and deteriorating pulp tissue leak past the apex and evoke a chronic inflammatory response from the vessels in the periodontal ligament. This explains why it is possible to

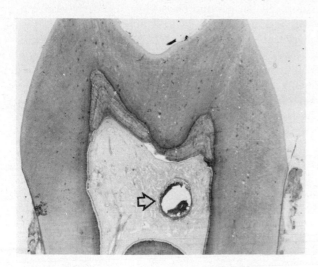

FIG. 11-20. Microabscess *(arrow)* in the depth of reparative dentin of the pulp horns.

have a periapical radiolucency and still have some vital tissue remaining in the root canal. The vascular response is the same as in the pulp except that it is aided by the collateral circulation of the periodontal ligament and the rapid resorbability of bone as compared to dentin. The inflammatory response may be acute, chronic, or mixed depending on the time that the lesion is seen.[14] The progression of the inflammatory response may be classified into several microscopic descriptions, but it is all part of the inflammatory response.*

Chronic inflammation (granuloma)

Chronic apical inflammation is a relatively low-grade, long-standing response to canal irritants. Clinically this lesion is usually asymptomatic and is detected by an apical radiolucency on the radiograph. Microscopically the lesion is characterized by a predominance of lymphocytes, plasma cells, and macrophages surrounded by a relatively uninflamed fibrous capsule made up of collagen, fibroblasts, and capillary buds (Fig. 11-23). In the inflammatory area large amorphous circles with very pale staining may be seen. These are Russell bodies that are thought to be associated with plasma cells. Cords or strands of proliferating epithelium may or may not be present. This lesion is usually not purely chronic in nature, as some PMNs may be seen scattered in the lesion.

Suppurative inflammation (granuloma with fistulation)

An apical lesion that has established drainage through a sinus tract is termed suppurative inflammation. Clinically, the patient may complain of a "gumboil" or a bad taste in the mouth. Pus may be expressed through the opening

---

*References 55, 56, 66, 69, 79, 88.

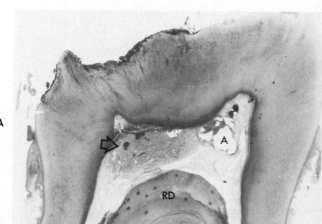
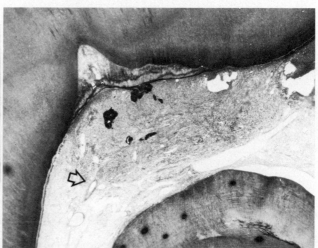

FIG. 11-21. Extensive inflammatory infiltrate *(arrow)* involving almost the entire pulp chamber. Note the reparative dentin *(RD)* on the chamber floor and the possible intrapulpal abscess *(A)*. **B,** Higher-power view showing the inflammatory infiltrate beginning to penetrate the radicular pulp *(arrow)*.

by gentle pressure. A radiograph should be taken with a gutta-percha probe inserted into the tract to determine the cause of the lesion. Microscopically the tract may be filled with PMNs or pus. Chronic inflammatory cells may line the periphery and in later stages epithelium may be present.

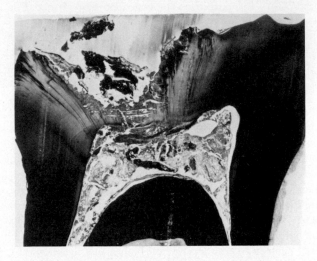

FIG. 11-22. Total pulpal necrosis of the pulp chamber with impaction of food debris.

Acute inflammation

Acute apical inflammation is a very painful response that occurs before alveolar bone is resorbed. PMNs and edema rapidly fill the periodontal ligament between the tooth and bone. Because the fluid is not compressible, any external pressure on the tooth forces the fluid against nerve endings, resulting in exquisite pain. The pain will continue until the bone begins to resorb and space is created to accommodate the edema fluid. The patient will also complain of the tooth feeling elevated in the socket, but no lesion is demonstrable on the radiograph.

Acute apical abscess

An acute apical abscess may result when large numbers of bacteria get past the apex and overwhelm the body defenses. The inflammatory response is acute with the dominating cell the polymorphonuclear leukocyte resulting in pus formation (Fig. 11-24). An abscess is defined as a localized collection of pus. All tissue in the local area is destroyed in this highly acidic environment. Clinically, swelling to various degrees is present along with pain and a feeling that the tooth is elevated in the socket. An elevated temperature and malaise are additional symptoms. The body tries to handle the abscess by turning it into a

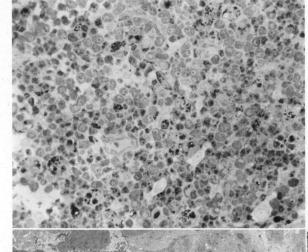

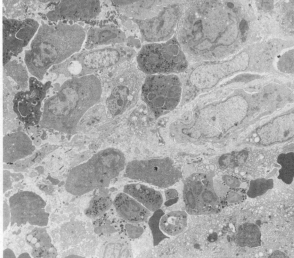

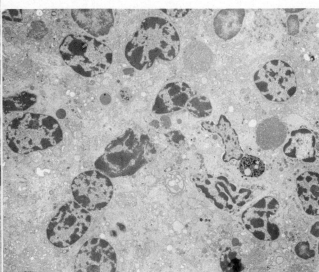

FIG. 11-23. A, One-micrometer section stained with toliudine blue showing both acute and chronic cells in a granuloma. (×400.) **B,** Electron micrograph showing predominantly PMNs, plasma cells, and fibroblasts. **C,** Electron micrograph of tissue destruction in inflammation. Cells have lost their cytoplasmic membrane, granules are free in the tissue, and edema is present. The nuclei show clumping of chromatin and are losing their membranes. (×3,000.)

chronic lesion and establishing drainage through fistulation to an outer or external surface. However, if the abscess spreads along facial planes to form a cellulitis, serious infection such as Ludwig's angina and cavernous sinus thrombosis may result. Microscopically pus is composed of dead cells, debris, and PMNs. Macrophages are also present.

If a radiolucency is present, this acute inflammatory response superimposed on a preexisting chronic lesion is termed a *phoenix abscess*. It is an acute exacerbation of a previously existing chronic inflammation.

Foreign body reaction

A foreign body response may occur to many types of substances. The reaction can be acute or chronic. What usually distinguishes these lesions microscopically is the presence of multinucleated giant cells surrounding a foreign material (Fig. 11-25). If the material is soluble in the

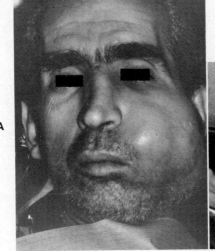
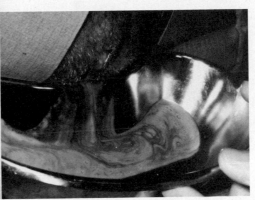

FIG. 11-24. A, Clinical photgraph of an acute apical abscess. B, Pus and blood draining externally into a basin from the incised abscess.

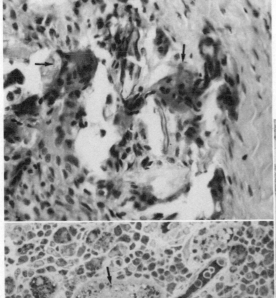
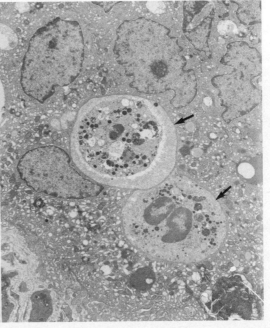

FIG. 11-25. A, Photomicrograph of a foreign body reaction at the apex of a tooth. Note giant cells and foreign material (arrows). (×400.) B, Photomicrograph of 1-mm section of a different patient showing a large multinucleated giant cell (arrow). (×400.) C, Electron micrograph of a part of the same cell showing many nuclei and two ingested PMNs (arrows). (×11,000.)

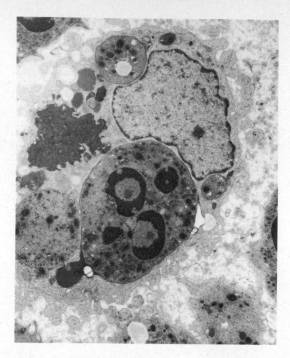

FIG. 11-26. Electron micrograph of a macrophage that has engulfed a polymorphonuclear leukocyte. This is possibly the beginning of giant cell formation. ($\times 11,000$.)

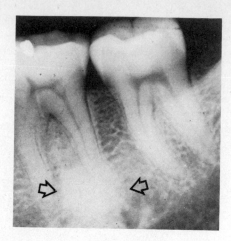

FIG. 11-27. Increased radiopacity *(arrows)* and trabeculation around the distal root of the mandibular first molar.

materials used to prepare the histologic section, then the giant cells will appear to be surrounding a space. Usually the giant cells are surrounded by a chronic inflammatory infiltrate. The giant cells are thought to be formed by the joining together of many macrophages into one cell, but retaining many nuclei (Fig. 11-26). This giant phagocytic cell is capable of engulfing the PMNs that have to ingest the foreign body. These lesions may or may not be symptomatic, depending on what stage the clinician happens to see the patient.

Osteosclerosis or condensing osteitis

The inflammatory response is modified depending on the quality, duration, and virulence of the irritant. A very low-grade, subclinical response may lead to an increase in the bone density rather than resorption. This lesion may be clinically asymptomatic and radiographically shows increased bone density and trabeculation (Fig. 11-27). Microscopically dense bone with growth lines is prevalent with a mild chronic inflammatory infiltrate in the marrow spaces. Not much is known about this lesion, but if it is associated with a necrotic pulp, endodontic therapy may lead to healing.

Osteomyelitis

Osteomyelitis, as described in Chapter 12, may be a serious progression of periapical infection that results in a diffuse spread through the medullary spaces and necrosis of varying amounts of bone. Acute osteomyelitis may be localized or spread throughout large areas of bone. The patient usually has severe pain, an elevated temperature, and swollen lymph nodes. The teeth are loose and sore but

in the early stages no swelling or radiographic changes are detectable. Microscopically the medullary spaces are filled with neutrophils predominantly that may or may not have formed pus. The osteoblasts are destroyed and bone resorption has begun.

If untreated the acute form may progress to chronic or arise directly from a dental infection.[53] Chronic suppurative osteomyelitis is clinically the same as acute except that the symptoms are milder and diffuse bone resorption is evident on radiographs. Osteomyelitis is a very serious extension of periapical disease and must be treated promptly and properly (Fig. 11-28).

Role of epithelium

One of the normal components of the lateral and apical periodontal ligament is the epithelial rests of Malassez. The term *rests* is misleading in that it has been shown to be a fishnet-like, three-dimensional, interconnected network of epithelial cells. In many periapical lesions, epithelium is not present and therefore is presumed to have been destroyed.[64] If the rests remain, their first response to stimulus from the pulp canal is to proliferate. To wall off the irritants coming out of the apex, the epithelium is surrounded by chronic inflammation and is termed an epitheliated granuloma (Fig. 11-29, *A*). If the source of irritation continues, the epithelium continues to proliferate and wall off the irritants. The microscopic picture is termed a "bay" cyst (Fig. 11-29, *B*). This is a chronic inflammatory lesion that has epithelium lining the lumen, but the lumen has a direct communication with the root canal system. It is not a true cyst, because a cyst is a three-dimensional, epithelial-lined cavity with no connection between the lumen and the canal system.

When periapical lesions are studied in relation to the root canal, true epithelial lined cavities are found.[68] These are termed "true" cysts (Fig. 11-29, *C*). Confusion has occurred when lesions are studied only on curetted biopsy material. Since the tooth is not attached to the lesion, orientation to the apex is lost. Thus, the criterion used for diagnosis of a cyst is "a strip of epithelium that appears to be lining a cavity." It is readily apparent that curetting

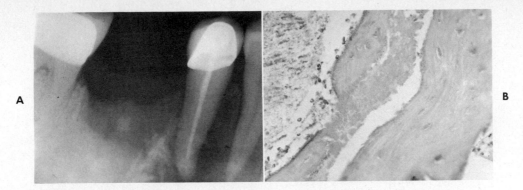

FIG. 11-28. **A,** Radiograph of chronic osteomyelitis showing extensive bone destruction in the mandible. **B,** Histologic section of necrotic bone with bacterial colonies.

both a "bay" cyst and a "true" cyst could give the same microscopic appearance and prevent differentiation. A "bay" cyst could be sectioned in such a way that it could resemble or give the false appearance of a "true" cyst.

This distinction between a "bay" and a "true" cyst is important from the standpoint of healing. Endodontists state that they heal some cysts with nonsurgical root canal treatment, whereas surgeons state that cysts have to be surgically excised.* It may be that "true" cysts have to be surgically removed, but "bay" cysts that communicate with the root canal may heal with nonsurgical root canal therapy. Since root canal therapy can directly affect the lumen of the "bay" cyst, the environmental change may bring about resolution of the lesion. *The "true" cyst, however, no longer has anything to do with the root canal system; thus root canal therapy may have no effect on the "true" cyst.* This would explain the discrepancy between the endodontic and surgical opinions on the treatment of cysts.

Healing

Part of the progression of periapical inflammation may lead to scar formation. This occurs when the tissue that was originally present is replaced with dense fibrous connective tissue after the irritant has been destroyed. This may also occur after surgical intervention takes place where both the buccal and the lingual cortical plates have been lost. Radiographically this shows as a radiolucency but does not require treatment. To all intents and purposes this lesion has healed. Microscopically there is an abundance of dense collagen bundles with some fibroblasts. In earlier stages macrophages may be present with more fibroblasts and capillary buds (Fig. 11-30).

Immunologic aspects

In describing the microscopic pictures of inflammation it is apparent that the cells involved in immunologic reactions are present in periapical lesions.† In addition, C3 complement fragment and immunoglobulins IgM, IgG,

IgE, and IgA have been found in these lesions. Thus the canal irritants (bacteria, bacterial products, and tissue breakdown products) are capable of sensitizing the host and causing immune reactions.

The response of the periapical tissues to noxious products from the root canal system is inflammatory. These are not separate diseases but rather different aspects of the inflammatory response that are static only under the microscope. Acute and chronic reactions can go back and forth and quite often are not only present in different parts of the same section, but they also may be seen mixed together.

Immune complex disease

In this immediate-type hypersensitivity the sensitizing antibodies are IgG and IgM (also see Chapter 12). Complement is activated by the classic pathway. Thus to produce an Arthus reaction immune complexes, the complement system, and PMNs are required. All ingredients have been found in periapical lesions. Thus the antigen-antibody complexes activate complement by the classic pathway, which is chemotactic for PMNs. Since the antigen continues from the root canal, this process becomes chronic and leads to the microscopic picture seen in chronic inflammation (granuloma).

Anaphylaxis

The other type of immediate hypersensitivity, anaphylaxis, may also occur at the apex of teeth. The sensitizing antibody is IgE, which has also been found in periapical lesions along with mast cells and IgE-containing plasma cells (also see Chapter 12). Thus it is assumed that anaphylactic reactions can occur at the apex.

Infectious allergies

These delayed hypersensitivity reactions are mediated by effector T cells with the aid of helper T cells and macrophages (also see Chapter 12). Antibody is not required. The interaction of the antigen and the previously sensitized lymphocytes stimulates the production of lymphokines. These result in enhanced macrophage activity that phagocytizes and digest foreign debris. Other effects (lymphotoxin) are cell lysis and bone resorption. The results of this response seem compatible with periapical lesions.

---

*References 10-12, 29, 31, 32, 39-41, 64, 66, 75.
†References 16, 18, 20, 26, 28, 33, 34, 37, 38, 42, 46, 47, 70, 73, 76, 78-80, 89.

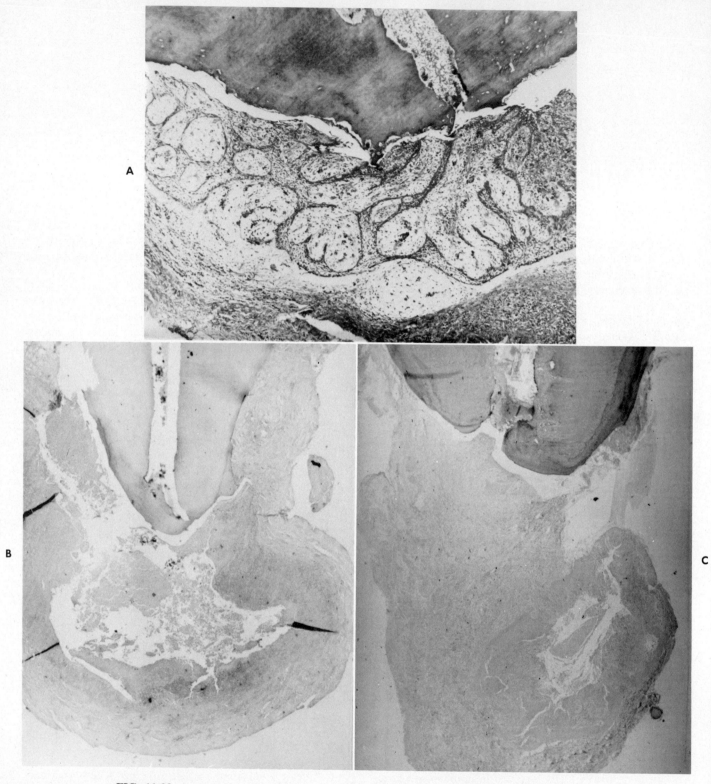

FIG. 11-29. A, Chronic apical periodontitis with proliferating cords of epithelium. **B,** Low-power photomicrograph of a bay cyst or apical periodontal pocket. The root canal opens directly into the lumen of this epithelium-lined lesion. **C,** Low-power photomicrograph of a true cyst. This is a cavity completely lined with epithelium and does *not* communicate with the root canal system.

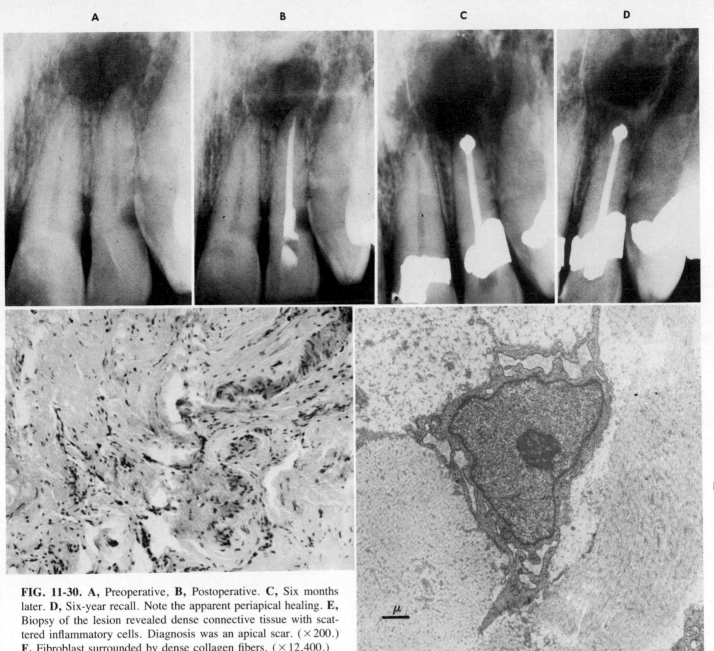

FIG. 11-30. A, Preoperative, **B,** Postoperative. **C,** Six months later. **D,** Six-year recall. Note the apparent periapical healing. **E,** Biopsy of the lesion revealed dense connective tissue with scattered inflammatory cells. Diagnosis was an apical scar. ($\times 200$.) **F,** Fibroblast surrounded by dense collagen fibers. ($\times 12,400$.)

PERIAPICAL DISEASE OF NONPULPAL ORIGIN

Not all radiolucencies or radiopacities in the apical region are the result of pulpal disease. In addition to inflammatory lesions, other pathologic conditions can and do occur, quite often resembling endodontic lesions to the extent that the unwary diagnostician may be fooled. They may be reactive, neoplastic, or developmental. The reader is referred to a textbook on pathology to cover all these lesions, several notable examples will be presented here.

Inflammatory diseases (e.g., radiation necrosis, osteomyelitis), as discussed earlier, may be associated with a tooth.

Reactive lesions (e.g., central giant cell granuloma) may occur (Fig. 11-31). Although there is controversy concern-

ing this disease, it is a benign process characterized microscopically by giant cells in a fibrous tissue stroma with many proliferating fibroblasts and small capillaries.[53] Diagnosis is established by clinical, microscopic, and laboratory value determination. (Hyperparathyroidism can show similar lesions.) The central giant cell granuloma may appear at the apex of a tooth and simulate endodontic disease. It must therefore be on any periapical differential diagnosis list.

There is also a gray area represented by the so-called fibro-osseous lesions (e.g., periapical osseous dysplasia [cementoma]) (Fig. 11-32). Histologically the cementoma consists of fibroblasts, collagen, and a few blood vessels. It may progress through three stages, each increasing in

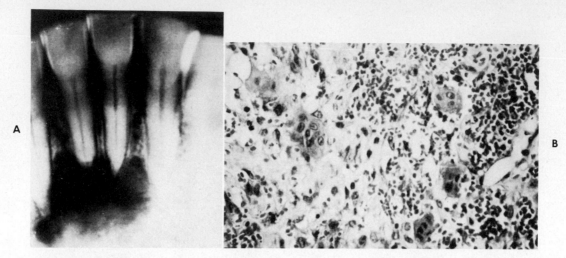

FIG. 11-31. **A,** Diffuse apical radiolucency. All teeth responded to testing procedures within normal limits. **B,** Biopsy of the lesion revealed multinucleated giant cells in a fibrous tissue stroma. Diagnosis was giant cell granuloma. (Courtesy Drs. Albert M. Abrams and Raymond J. Melrose.)

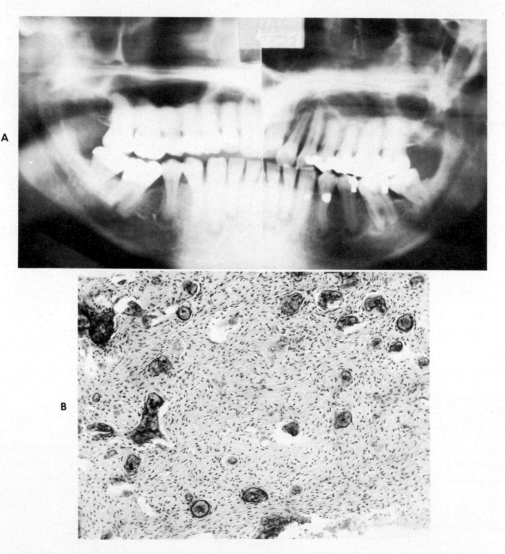

FIG. 11-32. **A,** Multiple periapical radiolucent areas. The patient was totally without symptoms. **B,** Biopsy of apical tissue from the mandibular left first premolar revealed numerous calcifications within a cellular fibrous connective tissue stroma. There was no inflammatory infiltrate. Diagnosis was periapical osseous dysplasia.

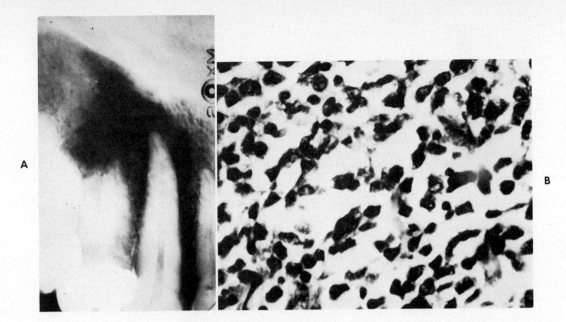

FIG. 11-33. **A,** Diffuse radiolucent area approximating the maxillary canine. **B,** High-power view revealing dense lymphocytic infiltrate. Diagnosis was malignant lymphoma. (Courtesy Drs. Albert M. Abrams and Raymond J. Melrose.)

the amount of calcification. The case presented in Fig. 11-32 showed multiple radiolucencies; if only one periapical radiograph had been exposed, the radiolucencies might have been mistaken for disease of pulpal origin. All the involved teeth responded within normal limits to endodontic testing procedures.

Malignant tumors (e.g., malignant lymphoma) can also occur at the apex of the tooth (Fig. 11-33). In this particular case the only complaints by the patient may be numbness and tingling sensations over the apex of the canine. These symptoms can be indicative of perineural invasion by tumor cells. Therefore, although these symptoms can occur for other reasons, a malignancy must be ruled out first.

Developmental processes (e.g., primordial cysts) may also mimic periapical disease of pulpal origin.

In summary, although most of the radiolucencies in the apical region are of pulpal origin, the clinician must be vigilant for the case that is something else. For this reason, endodontic testing procedures should not be ignored or underestimated in the diagnosis.

ACKNOWLEDGMENT

A special acknowledgement is in order to Sol Bernick, M.D., Department of Anatomy, School of Medicine, University of Southern California, for providing much of the histologic material on pulpal disorders. (The transmission electron microscopic work displayed in this chapter was done by Sant S. Sekhon, Ph.D., and Nora L. Tong, M.A., of the Veterans Administration Medical Center, Long Beach, CA.)

REFERENCES

1. Andreason, J.O., and Hjorting-Hansen, E.: Replantation of teeth. I. Radiographic and clinical study of 110 human teeth replanted after accidental loss, Acta Odontol. Scand. **24:**287,1966.
2. Andreason, J.O., and Hjorting-Hansen, E.: Replantation of teeth. II. Histological study of 22 replanted anterior teeth in humans, Acta Odontol. Scand. **24:**287, 1966.
3. Avery, J.: Repair potential of the pulp, J. Endod. **7:**205, 1981.
4. Avery, J.K.: Symposium on pulpal response to dental caries, J. Endod. **7**(1):6, 1981.
5. Baume, L.J.: Diagnosis of diseases of the pulp, Oral Surg. **29:**102, 1970.
6. Bender, I.B.: Pulp biology conference: A discussion, J. Endod. **4**(2):37, 1978.
7. Bergenholtz, G.: Inflammatory response of the dental pulp to bacterial irritation, J. Endod. **7.**100, 1981.
8. Bernick, S.: Age changes in the blood supply to human teeth, J. Dent. Res. **46:**544, 1967.
9. Bernick, S.: Effect of aging on the nerve supply to human teeth, J. Dent. Res. **45:**694, 1967.
10. Bhaskar, S.N.: Periapical lesions—types, incidence, and clinical features, Oral Surg. **21:**657, 1966.
11. Bhaskar, S.N.: Nonsurgical resolution of radicular cysts, Oral Surg. **38:**458, 1972.
12. Block, R.M., et al.: A histopathologic, histobacteriologic, and radiographic study of periapical endodontic surgical specimens, Oral Surg. **42**(5):656, 1976.
13. Brännström, M., and Lind, P.O.: Pulpal response to early dental caries, J. Dent. Res. **44:**1045, 1965.
14. Brynolf, I.: A histologic and roentgenologic study of the periapical region of human upper incisors, Odont. Rev. **18**(Supp. II):1, 1976.
15. Cohen, M.: Pathways of inflammatory cellular exudate through radicular cyst epithelium: SCM study, J. Oral Pathol. **8:**369, 1979.
16. Dwyer, T.G., and Torabinejad, M.: Radiographic and histologic evaluation of the effect of endotoxin on the periapical tissues of the cat, J. Endod. **7:**31, 1981.
17. Eisen, H.N.: Immunology, ed. 2, New York, 1980, Harper & Row, Publishers.
18. Eleazer, P.D., Farber, P.A., and Seltzer, S.: Lack of lymphocyte stimulation by root canal products, J. Endod. **1:**388, 1975.
19. Garfunkel, A., Sela, J., and Ulmansky, M.: Dental pulp pathosis; clinicopathologic correlations based on 109 cases, Oral Surg. **35:**110, 1973.
20. Greening, A.B., and Schonfeld, S.E.: Apical lesions contain elevated immunoglobulin G levels, J. Endod. **6:**867, 1980.
21. Grossman, L.I.: Origin of microorganisms in traumatized pulpless sound teeth, J. Dent. Res. **26:**551, 1967.
22. Honjo, H., et al.: Localization of plasma proteins in the human dental pulp, J. Dent. Res. **49:**888, 1970.

23. Howell, F.V., de la Rosa, V.M., and Abrams, A.M.: Cytologic evaluation of cystic lesions of the jaw: a new diagnostic technique, J.S.C. Dent. Assoc. **36**:161, 1968.
24. Ingle, J.I.: Alveolar osteoporosis and pulpal death associated with compulsive bruxism, Oral Surg. **13**:1371, 1960.
25. Kakehashi, S., Stanley, H.R., and Fitzgerald, R.J.: The effects of surgical exposure of dental pulps in germ-free and conventional laboratory rats, Oral Surg. **20**:340, 1965.
26. Kettering, J.D., and Torabinejad, M.: Concentrations of immune complexes, IgG, IgM, IgE, and C3 in patients with acute apical abscesses, J. Endod. **10**:417, 1984.
27. Korzen, B.H., Krakow, A.A., and Green, D.B.: Pulpal and periapical tissue responses in conventional and monoinfected gnotobiotic rats, Oral Surg. **37**:782, 1974.
28. Kuntz, D.D., et al.: Localization of immunoglobulins and the third component of complement in dental periapical lesions, J. Endod. **3**:68, 1977.
29. Lalonde, E.R., and Luebke, R.G.: The frequency and distribution of periapical cysts and granulomas, Oral Surg. **25**:861, 1968.
30. Langeland, K.: Management of the inflamed pulp associated with deep carious lesions, J. Endod. **7**:169, 1981.
31. Langeland, K., Block, R.M., and Grossman, L.I.: A histopathologic and histobacteriologic study of 35 periapical endodontic surgical specimens, J. Endod. **3**:8, 1977.
32. Langeland, K., Rodrigues, H., and Dowden, W.: Periodontal disease, bacteria and pulpal histopathology, Oral Surg. **37**:257, 1974.
33. Malmstrom, M.: Immunoglobulin classes of IgG, IgM, IgA and complement components C3 in dental periapical lesions of patients with rheumatoid disease, Scand. J. Rheumatol. **4**:57, 1975.
34. Mathiesen, A.: Preservation and demonstration of mast cells in human periapical granulomas and radicular cysts, Scand. J. Dent. Res. **81**:218, 1973.
35. Menkin, V.: Dynamics of inflammation, New York, 1940, Macmillan Publishing Co., Inc.
36. Mitchell, D., and Tarpley, R.: Painful pulpitis, Oral Surg. **13**:1360, 1960.
37. Morse, D.R., Lasater, D.R., and White, D.: Presence of immunoglobulin producing cells in periapical lesions, J. Endod. **1**:338, 1975.
38. Morse, D.R., Lasater, D.R., and White, D.: Presence of immunoglobulin-producing cells in periapical lesions, J. Endod. **1**(10):338, 1975.
39. Morse, D.R., Patnick, J.W., and Schoeterle, G.R.: Electrophoretic differentiation of radicular cysts and granulomas, Oral Surg. **35**:249, 1973.
40. Mortenson, H.: Periapical granulomas of cysts, Scand. J. Dent. Res. **78**:241, 1970.
41. Mortensen, H., Winther, J.E., and Birn, H.: Periapical granulomas and cysts: an investigation of 1600 cases, Scand. J. Dent. Res. **78**:141, 1971.
42. Morton, T.H., Clagett, J.A., and Yavorsky, J.D.: Role of immune complexes in human periapical periodontitis, J. Endod. **3**:261, 1977.
43. Mount, G.J.: Idiopathic internal resorption, Oral Surg. **33**:801, 1972.
44. Mullaney, T.P., Howell, R.M., and Petrich, J.D.: Resistance of nerve fibers to pulpal necrosis, Oral Surg. **30**:690, 1970.
45. Mumford, J.M.: Relationship between the pain-perception threshold of human teeth and their histological condition of the pulp, J. Dent. Res. **44**:1167, 1965.
46. Naidorf, I.J.: Immunoglobulins in periapical granulomas: a preliminary report, J. Endod. **1**:15, 1975.
47. Nisengard, R.J.: The role of immunology in periodontal disease, J. Periodontol. **48**:505, 1977.
48. Norton, L.A., Proffit, W.R., and Moore, R.R.: In vitro bone growth inhibition in the presence of histamine and endotoxins, J. Periodontol. **41**:153, 1970.
49. Nyborg, H., and Tullin, B.: Healing processes after vital extirpation, Odontol. Tidskr. **73**:430, 1965.
50. Okamura, K., et al.: Serum proteins and secretory component in human carious dentin, J. Dent. Res. **58**:1127, 1979.
51. Patterson, S.S., Shafer, W.G., and Healey, H.J.: Periapical lesions associated with endodontically treated teeth, J. Am. Dent. Assoc. **68**:191, 1964.
52. Quint, J.H., Lehrman, M., and Loveman, C.E.: Reparative giant-cell granuloma, Oral Surg. **17**:142, 1964.
53. Roane, J.B., and Marshall, F.J.: Osteomyelitis: a complication of pulpless teeth, Oral Surg. **34**:257, 1972.
54. Roitt, I., Brostoff, J., and Male, D.: Immunology, London, 1985, Gower Medical Publishing.
55. Rowe, A.H.R., and Binnie, W.H.: Correlation between radiological and histological inflammatory changes following root canal treatment, J. Br. Endod. Soc. **7**:57, 1974.
56. Ryan, G.B., and Majno, G.: Inflammation, Kalamazoo, MI, 1977, The Upjohn Company.
57. Sayegh, F.S., and Reed, A.J.: Calcification in the dental pulp, Oral Surg. **25**:873, 1968.
58. Schein, B., and Schilder, H.: Endotoxin content in endodontically involved teeth, J. Endod. **1**:19, 1975.
59. Sell, S.: Immunology, immunopathology and immunity, ed. 2, New York, 1975, Harper & Row, Publishers.
60. Seltzer, S.: Classification of pulpal pathosis, Oral Surg. **34**:269, 1972.
61. Seltzer, S., and Bender, I.B.: The Dental Pulp, ed. 3, Philadelphia, 1985, J.B. Lippincott Co.
62. Seltzer, S., Bender, I.B., and Nazimov, H.: Differential diagnosis of pulp conditions, Oral Surg. **19**(3):383, 1965.
63. Seltzer, S., Bender, I.B., and Ziontz, M.: The dynamics of pulp inflammation: correlations between diagnostic data and actual histologic findings in the pulp: I and II, Oral Surg. **16**:846, 969, 1963.
64. Seltzer, S., Soltanoff, W., and Bender, I.B.: Epithelial proliferation in periapical lesions, Oral Surg. **27**:111, 1969.
65. Seltzer, S., et al.: Biologic aspects of endodontics: III. Periapical tissue reactions to root canal instrumentation, Oral Surg. **26**:694, 1968.
66. Seltzer, S., Soltanoff, W., and Smith, J.: Biologic aspects of endodontics. V. Periapical tissue reactions to root canal instrumentation beyond the apex and root canal fillings short of and beyond the apex, Oral Surg. **36**:725, 1973.
67. Shear, M.: Cholesterol in dental cysts, Oral Surg. **16**:1465, 1963.
68. Simon, J.H.S.: Incidence of periapical cysts in relation to the root canal, J. Endod. **6**:845, 1980.
69. Sinai, I., et al.: Biologic aspects of endodontics. II. Periapical tissue reactions to pulp extirpation, Oral Surg. **23**:664, 1967.
70. Stabholz, A., and McArthur, W.P.: Cellular immune response of patients with periapical pathosis to necrotic dental pulp antigens determined by release of LIF, J. Endod. **4**:282, 1978.
71. Stanley, H.R.: Human pulp response to operative procedures, Gainesville, 1976, University of Florida.
72. Stanley, H.R., et al.: Ischemic infarction of the pulp: sequential degenerative changes of the pulp after traumatic injury, J. Endod. **4**:325, 1978.
73. Stuart, W.W., et al.: Humoral response to endodontic cements, J. Endod. **5**:214, 1979.
74. Ten Cate, A.R.: The epithelial cell rests of Malassez and the genesis of the dental cyst, Oral Surg. **34**:957, 1972.
75. Toller, P.: Origin and growth of cysts of the jaws, Ann. R. Coll. Surg. Engl. **40**:306, 1967.
76. Torabinejad, M., and Bakland, L.K.: Immunopathogenesis of chronic periapical lesions, Oral Surg. **46**:685, 1978.
77. Torabinejad, M., and Bakland, L.K.: Prostaglandins: their possible role in the pathogenesis of pulpal and periapical disease, Part I, J. Endod. **6**:733, 1980; Part II, J. Endod. **6**:769, 1980.
78. Torabinejad, M., and Kettering, J.D.: Detection of immune complexes in human dental periapical lesions by anticomplement immunofluorescence technique, Oral Surg. **48**:256, 1979.
79. Torabinejad, M., and Kettering, J.D.: Identification and relative concentration of B and T lymphocytes in human chronic periapical lesions, J. Endod. **11**:122, 1985.

80. Torabinejad, M., Kettering, J.D., and Bakland, L.K.: Localization of IgE immunoglobulin in human dental periapical lesions by the peroxidase-antiperoxidase method, Arch. Oral Biol. **26**:677, 1981.
81. Torneck, C.D.: A report of studies into changes in the fine structure of the dental pulp in human caries pulpitis, J. Endod. **7**:8, 1981.
82. Trowbridge, H., and Daniels, T.: Abnormal immune response to infection of the dental pulp, Oral Surg. **43**:902, 1977.
83. Trowbridge, H.O.: Pathogenesis of pulpitis resulting from dental caries, J. Endod. **7**:52, 1981.
84. Trowbridge, H., and Daniels, T.: Abnormal immune response to infection of the dental pulp, Oral Surg. **43**:902, 1977.
85. Trowbridge, H.O., and Emling, R.C.: Inflammation, a review of the process, Bristol, 1978, Distribution Systems Inc.
86. Tucker, E.S.: I: Basic concepts of immunology. II: Mechanisms of immunologic tissue injury, Chicago, 1978, American Society of Clinical Pathologists.
87. Van Hassel, H.J.: Physiology of the human dental pulp, Oral Surg. **32**:126, 1971.
88. Van Hassel, H.J.: Inflammation, Atlanta, 1978, American Association of Endodontists.
89. Wesselink, P.R., Thoden van Velzen, S.K., and Makkes, P.C.: Release of endotoxin in an experimental model simulating the dental root canal, Oral Surg. **45**(5):789, 1978.
90. Zach, L.: Pulp liability and repair; effect of restorative procedures, Oral Surg. **33**:111, 1972.
91. Zweifach, B.W.: Microcirculatory aspects of tissue injury, Ann. N.Y. Acad. Sci. **116**:831, 1964.

Self-assessment questions

1. The aging process affects the pulp tissue in which way?
   a. Decreases the size and volume of pulp tissue
   b. Increases the cellular component at the expense of the fiber component
   c. Increases the vascular supply with a decrease in fiber component
   d. Decreases the vascular supply at the expense of the fibrous component
2. After the initial microcirculatory changes of inflammation, what cells are first to arrive at the area of irritated tissue?
   a. Macrophages
   b. Lymphocytes
   c. Polymorphonuclear neutrophils (PMNs)
   d. Monocytes
3. What is the function of fibrin in the inflammatory process?
   a. Acts as a meshwork to wall off the reaction
   b. Increases vascular permeability
   c. Releases antibody
   d. Hemostatic effect on PMNs
4. What is the most probable effect of a microabscess on vital pulp tissue?
   a. Insignificant; pulp tissue will remain vital and healthy
   b. Cyclic breakdown of tissue damage with a spreading area of destruction
   c. Formation of a calcific bridge of repair, resulting in the maintenance of pulp vitality
   d. Pulp necrosis resulting from strangulation of the blood supply
5. Chronic inflammation demonstrates a predominance of what cell type?
   a. Monocytes
   b. Polymorphonuclear leukocytes (PMNs)
   c. Lymphocytes
   d. Fibroblasts
6. How does the inflammatory process in the pulp differ from the inflammatory process elsewhere in the body?
   a. The pulp is surrounded by hard tissue, limiting tissue expansion.
   b. The pulp is devoid of reparative cells.
   c. The pulp has a well-established collateral circulation system.
   d. The pulp readily copes with necrotic tissue and debris.
7. What effect does edema have on pulp physiology?
   a. It has no effect on blood transport system.
   b. Fluid is compressed within the vessels, limiting intercellular pressure.
   c. There is a decrease in interstitial pressure due to increased vascularity.
   d. Localized tissue necrosis results from hypoxia and anoxia.
8. Which statement is false?
   a. Periapical inflammation is an extension of the pulpal inflammatory process.
   b. Periapical inflammation involves a poor vascular network; therefore, the ability to heal at the apex is decreased.
   c. Initial periapical inflammation is difficult to detect radiographically.
   d. It is possible to have some vital pulp tissue as well as an apical radiolucency with the same tooth.
9. Chronic suppurative apical periodontitis is characterized by
   a. Acute inflammatory cells lining a draining sinus tract.
   b. A lesion with established drainage through a sinus tract
   c. A patient in severe to moderate pain
   d. The presence of swelling and/or cellulitis
10. Acute apical periodontitis is characterized by
    a. A histologic predominance of PMNs and edema
    b. A chief complaint of lingering pain to sweets
    c. No discomfort to percussion
    d. A draining sinus tract
11. An acute apical abscess is characterized by
    a. Pus formation
    b. Varying degrees of swelling
    c. Varying degrees of pain
    d. All of the above
12. Periapical osteosclerosis is characterized by
    a. Host resistance to pulpal irritation
    b. A decrease of bone density
    c. Acute inflammation
    d. Expansion of the cortical plates of bone
13. What type of healing may be expected when both the buccal and the lingual cortical plates are involved?
    a. Ankylosis
    b. Scar tissue
    c. Normal regeneration of bone
    d. Osteosclerosis
14. Nonpulpal periapical pathosis
    a. Includes the giant cell granuloma
    b. Includes the possibility of a malignant tumor
    c. Includes the fibro-osseous lesion cementoma
    d. All of the above

12

MICROBIOLOGY AND PHARMACOLOGY

DONALD R. MORSE

In this chapter the microbiologic and pharmacologic aspects of endodontics are discussed. Included within the microbiologic section are the following concepts: (1) the endodontic flora, (2) pulpal pathways, (3) host-parasite interaction (including microbial virulence factors and host resistance factors), (4) oral pathways of infection including bloodstream pathways, (5) immunologic considerations, (6) detection of microbes, and (7) local antimicrobial agents. Antibiotics simultaneously ends the microbiologic section and begins the pharmacologic section. After antibiotics, the other drugs covered are: (1) analgesics, (2) sedatives and antianxiety agents, (3) anti-inflammatory agents, and (4) nutrients.

ENDODONTIC FLORA

Various media and techniques have been used in numerous studies on the pulpal and periapical microbial flora. The numbers and types of microorganisms isolated in these studies have varied according to the following factors[148,150,153,213,245]:

1. Types of media used. All media, including transport media,[88a] inhibit some microbes. However, some researchers[43] found that a high recovery of bacteria occurs if the transport medium is fluid thioglycollate, U.S.P.

2. Whether phase and dark-field microscopy were used. These methods are necessary for spirochete identification.

3. Whether gram-stained smears were used. Many species seen on smears fail to grow under culture conditions.

4. Whether identification of microbes in tissue sections was done. Although it is not usual, microbes may present in periapical tissues. For example, in recent studies, colonies of actinomyces and streptococci were found in periapical granulomas and occasionally microbes were found in periapical macrophages.* In two recent studies [15a,130a] microbes (especially obligate anaerobes) were found in periapical "areas" (usually associated with necrotic tissue and abscess cavities).

5. Relative conditions of aerobiosis or anaerobiosis. (As the result of recent techniques using obligate anaerobic techniques, many more microbes have been isolated from root canals.)

6. Environmental and nutritional conditions such as temperature, humidity, pH, osmotic pressure, oxygen tension, and nutrients of the media. Most microbes grow best under conditions simulating in vivo situations. Anaerobes are most fastidious.[214]

7. Methods of isolation: (a) the number of absorbent points used (more points may mean more inoculum); (b) the depth of penetration of the points (results depend on the location of microbes. In a recent study, it was found that obligate anaerobes predominated in the apical part of the root canal system[74]); (c) the use of wet or dry points (usually wet points pick up a greater inoculum); (d) whether strict aseptic conditions were used (e.g., contamination can result from a permeable temporary seal, saliva, or an improper rubber dam seal or from air, hand, and breath contamination); (e) whether students or experienced clinicians did the isolation (students may have more contaminants); (f) the number of days for the incubation (some anaerobic species grow only after 1 to 2 weeks)[74]; (g) whether isolation is via the root canal or the alveolar mucosa (with the latter method there is a greater chance of contamination); (h) whether the tooth is intact (closed case, usually one or a few species) or is open to the oral cavity (open case, usually a mixed flora).

8. Timing of the culture. Culturing at the conclusion of the visit may detect a reduced microbial flora; culturing before or after cleaning and shaping of the root canal system alters the type of microbes isolated. These changes are because of the mechanical removal of some microbes and the chemical destruction of others that follow irrigation and the use of medicaments. In a recent study, it was shown that mechanical instrumentation greatly reduced the number of bacteria from the beginning of the visit to the end of the same visit.[74] In some dental schools, it was taught to have a separate visit to take a root canal culture. Because of leakage of temporary seals, it would be almost impossible to have a negative culture provided that sensitive culture media were used.[150] In other dental schools, the culture was taken at the conclusion of the instrumentation visit. If instrumentation and irrigation were thorough, those cases would invariably have had temporary negative cultures.[40] However, there still could have been microbes remaining behind. It has been shown that in long-standing root canal infections, the microbes invade

---

*References 86, 128, 161, 172, 214, 237.

364

the dentinal tubules and accessory canals and are protected from routine instrumentation and irrigation, which is mainly effective on the surface layers of the root canal walls.[12]

9. Width of the canal. A narrow canal may not be penetrable, although it may be infected; also there may be microbes present periapically that cannot be sampled. In a recent study, investigators[154] found a statistically significantly higher incidence of failures in cases with periapical lesions when the canals had apical calcifications and couldn't be penetrated as compared to cases when instrumentation went into the periapical lesion.

10. Whether the patient is receiving antibiotics systemically. Antibiotics may cause destruction of some root canal microbes and allow overgrowth of others. For example, investigators[86] reported a case in which a patient was being treated for a bladder infection with the antibiotic combination Bactrim DS. As a result, an acute exacerbation developed in an upper central incisor with an overgrowth of *Streptococcus faecalis*.

11. Host resistance. With a vigorous host response, only phagocytes may be detected in a particular sample. A later sample may show growth.

12. Presence of systemic disease or a bacteremia. It is possible to detect in the root canal system the microbes found in diseases like tuberculosis, actinomycosis, and leprosy (hematogenous spread). Normally these species are not isolated. It is also possible for microbes to lodge in the pulp from a secondary site following a transient bacteremia (anachoresis).

13. Type of teeth in the sample. Differences in numbers and types of flora may result from (a) vital as opposed to pulpless [necrotic] cases, (b) teeth with periapical radiolucencies as compared to teeth without radiolucencies and (c) original cases as compared to re-treatment cases. For example, in vital-inflamed cases, most of the pulp is usually sterile and any microbes found may result from oral contamination[198] These type cases could safely be treated in one visit. Teeth with periapical radiolucencies appear to always have infected root canals with a high incidence of obligate anaerobes and especially *bacteroides* species.[41,213] Obligate anaerobes in conjunction with α-hemolytic and nonhemolytic streptococci predominate in long-standing cases.[210] *Streptococcus faecalis* has been found in some persistent infection cases and in some re-treatment cases[150]; *Actinomyces israeli* has also been found in some failure cases.[214] However, other investigators have failed to implicate any specific microbes in persistent endodontic infections.[41]

14. Patient habits. It is possible for nonindigenous microbes to be found in the oral cavity or in the root canal system solely by chance. If a sample were taken at a different time, the indigenous flora may destroy the transients and the latter might not be detected.

Despite the influence of these factors on the variety of microorganisms detected, most studies conducted through the 1960s[148,150,153,213,245] have shown that the predominant microbial group found was the facultative anaerobic α-hemolytic streptococci. Other microbes frequently isolated were enterococci, diptheroids, micrococci, staphylococci, lactobacilli, enteric bacteria, and *Candida, Neisseria,* and *Veillonella* species. These microorganisms were isolated using standard aerobic culture techniques with media such as brain-heart infusion broth, thioglycollate broth, and trypticase-soy broth with agar. When the techniques of isolation and culturing were varied, the types and numbers of recoverable microbes also varied. For example, the use of phase and dark-field microscopy resulted in the isolation of significant numbers of spirochetes and fusobacteria.[148,220a] In contradistinction, the use of a lactose-fuchsin broth yielded an increased recovery of coliform and *Candida* species.[153]

A major breakthrough was achieved in the 1970s with the major improvement of obligate anaerobic techniques for use in both isolation and growth of microbes.[148] These techniques using prereduced media and roll tubes were first developed for medical microbiology but were soon adapted for use in endodontic microbiology. A literature search revealed that at least 22 endodontic studies* used these obligate anaerobic techniques. The consensus from the studies was that *obligate anaerobes are routinely found in pulpal-periapical disease,* have clinical importance, and may be the predominant species. Investigators who did not use strict anaerobic techniques found, as was the case previously, that α-hemolytic streptococci were predominant.

Researchers[16,168] found that *obligate anaerobes predominate in pulpal-periapical disease.* According to a monkey research study,[74] staphylococci, neisseria, lactobacilli, and fungi are rarely found in root canals with necrotic pulp tissue. In early stages of pulpal infection, facultative anaerobic streptococci and staphylococci are found. One group[90-92] found that microbes such as *Streptococcus salivarius* and *Staphylococcus epidermidis* can be contaminants. However, by the time periapical "areas" are formed, the root canals have been found to always be infected and the flora almost always consists of obligate anaerobes including *Bacteroides* species, fusobacteria and some gram-positive rods.[41,74,213,214] It appears that deep within the root canal after a sufficient time period, an anaerobic milieu develops and there are sufficient nutrients available for growth from necrotic pulp tissue and serum.[74] In an earlier human study,[25] a higher incidence of root canal infection was found in teeth with periapical lesions as compared to teeth without periapical lesions. Sundqvist examined human teeth and found that gram-positive facultative anaerobes are the most significant microbes in developing pulpitis.[214] He also found that in teeth with necrotic pulps and periapical lesions, the flora is almost exclusively obligate anaerobic. One study[210] found that in cases without periapical radiolucencies, there was only a 28% incidence of positive bacteriologic cultures. In a recent series of studies on flare-ups from asymptomatic teeth with necrotic pulps and associated periapical radiolucencies, it was found that teeth with very large periapical lesions had the greatest incidence of flare-ups. Others found that the larger the periapical lesion, the greater the number of obligate anaerobic strains present.[213] These flare-ups are of the type that Ingle[115] has called "phoenix abscess." In that same series of studies on flare-ups, it was[155] found that the second most frequent incidence of flare-ups occurred with teeth with small periapical lesions. These cases had initial flare-ups and may have been cases of "acute apical abscess."[94] Although the cases were not examined microbiologically, because of the recent development of the periapical lesion, these flare-ups may have shown more facultative anaerobic than obligate anaerobic species.

---

*Available from author on request.

ROOT CANAL MICROBES

1. α-Hemolytic streptococci (viridans streptococci, greening streptococci)
   a. *S. mitis*
   b. *S. salivarius*
   c. *S. mutans*[121,208]
   d. *S. sanguis*
   e. *S. milleri*[40]
   f. *S. mitior*
   g. *S. morbillorum*
   h. *S. intermedius*

2. Enterococci (Lancefield Group D antigenic-type streptococci)
   a. *S. faecalis*
   b. *S. liquefaciens*
   c. *S. zymogenes*
   d. *S. faecium*

3. *Staphylococci*
   a. *S. epidermidis (albus)*[90]
   b. *S. citreus* (rarely found)
   c. *S. aureus* (rarely found)[242]

4. *Corynebacterium* species (diphtheroids)
   a. *C. xerose*
   b. *C. hofmannii (C. pseudodiphtheriticum)*

5. *Lactobacillus* species
   a. *L. casei*
   b. *L. acidophilus*
   c. *L. fermenti*
   d. Anaerobic lactobacilli (e.g., *L. catinaforme*)

6. *Candida* species
   a. *C. albicans*
   b. *C. krusei*
   c. *C. mortifera*
   d. *C. guilliermondi*

7. Gram-negative cocci
   a. *Neisseria* species *(N. catarrhalis [Branhammella catarrhalis], N. flava, N. sicca)*
   b. *Veillonella* species *(V. alcalescens, V. parvula)*

8. Obligate anaerobic gram-positive cocci
   a. *Peptostreptococcus* species *(P. intermedius, P. anaerobius, P. micros)*
   b. *Peptococcus* species, *(P. morbillorum, P. variabilis, P. magnus)*

9. β-Hemolytic streptococci (predominantly the Lancefield Groups H and K)

10. Micrococci

11. Gram-negative, non-spore-forming, facultative anaerobic rods (the Enterobacteriaceae, or enteric bacteria, and related groups)
    a. *Aerobacter aerogenes*
    b. *Escherichia coli*
    c. *Klebsiella pneumoniae* (Friedländer's bacillus)
    d. *Proteus vulgaris*
    e. *Salmonella typhosa* (typhoid bacillus)
    f. *Alcaligenes faecalis*
    g. *Pseudomonas aeruginosa (Pseudomonas pyocyanea)*
    h. *Haemophilus influenzae* (Pfeiffer's bacillus)

ROOT CANAL MICROBES—cont'd

    i. *Mima polymorpha*
    j. *Campylobacter sputcrum*[218]
    k. *Eikenella corrodens*[63,88]
    l. *Enterobacter agglomerans*

12. *Pneumococcus (Diplococcus pneumoniae)*

13. *Actinomyces* species[34,161,237]
    a. *A. israelii*
    b. *A. bovis*
    c. *A. viscosus*
    d. *A. naeslundii*
    e. *A. odontolyticus*
    f. *A. propionicus (Arachnia propionicus)*
    g. *Streptobacillus monoiliformis*
    h. *Bacterionema matruchotii*

14. *Norcardia asteroides*

15. *Bacillus* species
    a. *B. subtilis*
    b. *B. cereus*

16. Gram-negative, non-spore-forming, obligate anaerobic rods
    a. *Bacteroides* species *(B. fragilis, B. asaccharolyticus, B. endodontalis, B. gingivalis* [found in some spreading infections], *B. intermedius* [found in some localized infections], *B. melaninogenicus,*[213,218] *B. oralis, B. ruminicola, B. fragilis, B. disastonics)*
    b. *Fusobacterium* species *(F. fusiforme, F. varium, F. nucleatum, F. necrophorum)*
    c. *Leptotrichia buccalis*
    d. *Selenomonas* sputigena
    e. *Actinobacillus actinomycetemcomitans* (A.A.; rarely found)[214]
    f. *Wolinella* (formerly known as *Vibrio sputorum, V. succinogenes,* and *Bacteroides corrodens)*[218]
       (1) *W. succinogenes*
       (2) *W. recta* (commonly found)
    g. *Capnocytophaga*[87] (formerly *B. ochraceus)*

17. Gram-positive, nonmotile, non-spore-forming rods
    a. *Propionibacterium acnes*
    b. *Propionibacterium avidum*
    c. *Bifidobacterium dentium*
    d. *Bifidobacterium adolescentis*
    e. *Eubacterium alactolyticum*
    f. *Eubacterium lentum*

18. Spirochetes
    a. *Borrelia vincentii*
    b. *Treponema microdentium*
    c. *Treponema macrodentium*

19. *Mycobacterium* species
    a. *Mycobacterium tuberculosis* (tubercle bacillus)
    b. *Mycobacterium leprae* (leprosy bacillus)

20. *Mycoplasma salivarium*

21. Yeasts
    a. *Saccharomyces* species
    b. *Cryptococcus* species

Sundqvist stated that there are over 500 species of microbes in the oral cavity, but only a small percentage are regularly found in root canals.[214] He further stated that the root canal flora is a selection of the periodontal pocket microbial flora, which is, in turn, a partial selection of the oral cavity flora. Therefore the current concept is that obligate anaerobes are the most clinically important and especially in periapical lesion cases. A list of identifiable root canal microbes is presented on pp. 364 and 365.

There have also been investigations into the possibility that viruses are present in endodontic diseases, but none have been identified.[201] As can be seen in the list of endodontic microbial flora, many microorganisms either singly or in combination may be involved in endodontic diseases. Until 1976, no correlations had been shown between any specific root canal microbe and any endodontic disease or clinical manifestation. However, in that year Sundqvist[213] did an exhaustive bacteriologic study of necrotic pulps and found *Bacteroides melaninogenicus* in samples from all teeth with acute periapical inflammation (tenderness, swelling, and exudation) but not in teeth without those symptoms. *B. melaninogenicus* always was present with some other species *(Peptostreptococcus anaerobius, Peptostreptococcus micros,* and *Campylobacter sputorum).*

Other studies have failed to confirm Sundqvist's findings. However, the techniques and samples were different. As did Sundqvist, Matusow[139] studied intact teeth (no carious or traumatic pulpal exposures); but he did not employ a strict anaerobic method of detection and culturing. In Matusow's examination of the ''acute pulpal-alveolar cellulitis syndrome,'' he found the predominant microbial group to be streptococci, with a complete absence of *Bactercides melaninogenicus.* Others[91,92] partially corroborated Sundqvist's findings. They examined pulps from both traumatized teeth (as did Sundqvist) and cariously involved teeth. Using a specially developed anaerobic culture technique, they found that *Bacteroides melaninogenicus* was significantly related to pain, sinus tract formation, and foul odor. They also suggested relationships between that microorganism and the presence of apical sensitivity and local swelling. Unlike Sundqvist, however, they did not find 100% correlation between pain and periapical radiolucencies with the presence of *Bacteroides melaninogenicus.* Other investigators[16,168] also investigated the pulps of traumatized and cariously involved teeth using strict obligate anaerobic methods. These workers found no correlation between root canal microorganisms and the presence of pulpal-periapical signs and symptoms. Although it is tempting to hypothesize cause-and-effect relationships between specific microbes and endodontic manifestations, the evidence does not support that contention. Nevertheless, *Bacteroides melaninogenicus* does appear to be of importance in symptomatic cases. However, endodontic infections are invariably mixed infections.[96,213] Oral microbes usually interact synergistically in the development of oral infections and *B. melaninogenicus* appears to be a key component. Experimentally induced periapical lesions rarely occur with pure cultures of single microbes. Mixed infection is almost always necessary to induce

periapical lesions. In a recent study using dark-field microscopy[233a] it was found that endodontic abscesses could be differentiated from periodontal abscesses. There were significantly more cocci in the endodontic lesions and significantly more spirochetes in the peridontal lesions.

PULPAL PATHWAYS

Microbes and microbial products may reach the pulp through several pathways:

1. Through a carious lesion either directly or via dentinal tubules[198]
2. Through a cavity preparation, either when the pulp is directly exposed or via dentinal tubules
3. As a result of periodontal disease, from a pocket or furca involvement, via lateral canals or dentinal tubules (Fig. 17-19), or form apical blood vessels or lymphatics by apical extension of a periodontal pocket.[109] In a recent study, similar anaerobic microbes were found in deep pockets and the pulps of the same teeth.[126]
4. Through enamel lamellae and dead tracts in dentin
5. From an adjoining periapical lesion, via apical or lateral canals[109,126]
6. As a result of anachoresis. Microbes present in the bloodstream (bacteremia) can lodge in a traumatized or inflamed pulp. Under restorations the pulp shows various gradations of inflammation. It is not known how severe the inflammation has to be in order to attract microbes. However, clinically it is a common observation that pulps become necrotic and infected beneath sound restorations that had been inserted years previously.[198]
7. From heat and pressure (e.g. compound copper band impressions) through dentinal tubules[198]
8. By abrasion, erosion, attrition, fracture, or developmental anomalies such as a dens-in-dente or a palatogingival groove[64,143,147]

The most common pathway is direct extension from caries and cavity preparations.[198] Nevertheless, many endodontists observe that most of their patients do not have carious lesions that have invaded the pulp. Rather the teeth have sound restorations that had been placed months or years previously. The most likely scenario for these cases is the following: The combination of caries, operative procedures, insertion of the restoration, the chemical irritation from the restoration, and leakage of the restoration causes cumulative pulpal damage. This results in varying degrees of pulpal inflammation.[198] Once the inflammation reaches a sufficient intensity, microbes are attracted (anachoresis).[60,62] This then leads to chronic pulpitis and/or necrosis with the necessity for endodontic intervention. In regard to caries, regardless of the type, most studies have shown that the deeper layers are sterile.[198] Hence, with good case selection, indirect pulp capping (Chapter 22) is a feasible procedure.

HOST-PARASITE INTERACTION

The results of host-parasite interaction depend on microbial virulence factors and host resistance factors.

Microbial virulence factors

Microbial virulence factors are substances that are inherent in or produced by microorganisms; they give microorganisms the capability of causing tissue damage. If clinical disease is produced, the microbes are considered pathogenic. Microbes associated with pulp and periapical

ROOT CANAL MICROBIAL VIRULENCE FACTORS

1. Coagulase—formed by staphylococci, coliforms and *Pseudomonas* species.

2. Collogenase[92,125]—formed by *Bacteroides,* eubacteria, bifidobacteria, peptostreptococci, peptococci, and streptococci.

3. Deoxyribonuclease (streptodornase)—formed by streptococci.

4. Leukocidin[125]—formed by streptococci and staphylococci. *Bacteroides* species may impair functioning of PMNs and prevent phagocytosis by degrading immunoglobulins and C_3.[90]

5. Hemolysin—formed by streptococci and staphylococci.

6. Necrotoxin—formed by staphylococci. A.A. inhibits fibroblast reproduction, inhibits epithelial and endothelial cells, destroys PMNs, inhibits lymphocytes, and has collagenase activity.[100]

7. Gelatinase[125]—formed by *Bacteroides,* bifidobacteria, propionibacteria, peptostreptococci, peptococci, *Actinomyces, Veillonella,* staphylococci, and streptococci species.

8. Capsules[90]—formed by *Bacteroides* and pneumococci species.

9. Anti-opsonins (factors that depress phagocytosis by PMNs)[223]—formed by *Bacteroides,* coliforms, staphylococci, and mycobacteria species.

10. Carotenoid pigments[223] (quench singlet O_2, which enables microbes to survive the PMNs "respiratory burst")—formed by *Staphylococcus aureus.*

11. Plasmids that confer resistance to complement-mediated lysis—formed by *Staphylococcus aureus.*

12. Factors that inhibit chemotaxis—formed by *Bacteroides melaninogenicus.*[90]

13. Factors that induce chemotaxis—the pathogenicity of pyogenic bacteria may depend on their extreme ability to attract PMNs, which then break down and release damaging lysosomal enzymes.[215]

14. Kinases (fibrinolysins)—formed by streptococci (streptokinase), staphylococci (staphylokinase), and *Bacteroides melaninogenicus.*

15. Lecithinase[90]—formed by *Bacteroides melaninogenicus.*

16. Proteases—formed by streptococci, fusobacteria, *Bacteroides,* and gram-negative cocci species. *S. sanguis* produces a protease that degrades IgA.

17. Sulfatases—formed by fusobacteria species.

18. β-Glucuronidase[125]—formed by streptococci.

19. Chondroitin sulfatase[125]—formed by diphtheroids, streptococci, staphylococci, lactobacilli, *Bacteroides,* bifidobacteria, propionibacteria, peptostreptococci, and fusobacteria species.

20. Hyaluronidase (spreading factor)[125]—formed by streptococci, staphylococci, diphtheroids, pneumococci, clostridia, *Bacteroides,* fusobacteria, eubacteria, bifidobacteria, propionibacteria, and peptostreptococci species.

21. Edema-producing factor—formed by pneumococci.

22. Catalase (inactivates the PMNs' H_2O_2 to H_2O and O_2)—formed by many facultative anaerobes.

Continued.

23. Exotoxins—formed by clostridia species, which are very rarely found in root canals.

24. Endotoxins[65,125,173,191,194]—particularly damaging and have the following properties: chemotactic for PMNs; cause blood platelet damage; cause the degranulation of mast cells with the release of histamine; activates the Hageman factor (initiates blood clotting and leads to the production of bradykinin, a potent pain-producing mediator); activates macrophages; decreases cellular respiration; activates the complement cascade; stimulates and attracts osteoclasts; stimulates bone resorption; induces leukopenia; induces hypoglycemia; causes elevated fever; leads to hypotension; can induce shock; causes impaired perfusion of essential organs; activates localized and generalized Schwartzman reaction (a nonspecific inflammatory response); induces the hypersensitivity Arthus reaction; and can lead to death. The administration of 0.1 μg/kg body weight of an endotoxin had, in human volunteers, a marked deleterious effect on lymphocyte distribution and function.[78] Schein and Schilder[191] found that significant concentrations of endotoxin were recovered from endodontically involved teeth, especially those with periapical "areas." Schonfeld et al.[194] found endotoxin in 75% of periapical granulomas.

25. Peptidoglycans[39]—derived from the cell wall of grampositive bacteria. They produce similar, but less potent, effects as endotoxins.

26. Plasmids that confer resistance to antibiotics (e.g., penicillinase)—formed by *Staphylococcus aureus*.

27. Resistance to intracellular destruction[223]—mycobacteria and corynebacteria can be engulfed by macrophages but can replicate within them in an environment free of host antibody, hence the normal immune response is ineffective.

28. Glutathione peroxidase (breaks down H_2O_2 and reduces the antimicrobial hypothiocyanite ion and sulfenyl derivatives)—formed by some facultative anaerobes.

29. Immunosuppressive factors[223]—formed by *Wolinella (Vibrio)* and mycobacteria species.

30. Cyclical antigenic variation[223]—destruction of many of the bacteria (e.g., *Campylobacter* species) by a local immune response leaves a residual portion of the microbes that possess antigens differing from the original population. These persisters can multiply and may later be eliminated by a second immune response, leaving a residual population with a third type of antigen. This process can be repeated and because of a poor memory response by IgA, these microbes can reutilize antigens without stimulating a strong immune response.

31. Various odorous microbial breakdown products—include indole, skatole, various amines, ammonia, and antigens.[147] Experimental evidence has shown that the primary cause of oral malodor is putrefaction of sulfurcontaining proteinaceous substrates by predominantly gram-negative oral microbes.[225] Griffee et al.[92] found a strong corellation between foul odor and the presence of *Bacteroides melaninogenicus*. Therefore even though sterile breakdown of the host's own cells can produce malodor (discussed shortly), if an endodontically involved tooth emits a strong odor, it is most likely caused by gram-negative anaerobic microbes.

BENEFICIAL HOST RESISTANCE FACTORS

1. Platelet factors[223] including β-lysins (active against gram-positive microbes); plakin (active against gram-positive microbes); and basic polyamines, polypeptides, and proteins (active against gram-positive microbes).

2. Serum factors[29,113,223] including antibodies (IgG, IgM—active against bacteria; IgA—active against viruses; IgE—active against helminths); complement (active against gram-positive microbes; with lysozyme, active against gram-negative microbes; also active against viruses and protozoa); transferrin (an iron-binding protein that is active against gram-positive and gram-negative microbes); haptoglobin[67] (a hemoglobin-binding protein that appears to prevent bacteria from using hemoglobin iron as a nutrient); opsonins (γ-globulins that facilitate phagocytosis by binding to foreign particles); tuftsin (a tetrapeptide that activates phagocytes into higher rates of foreign particle ingestion); and the acidic pH during inflammation that can also destroy microorganisms.

3. Leukocytic factors[76,143,238] including lysozyme (hydrolyzes glycosidic linkages between the N-acetyl-muramic acid and N-acetyl glucosamine of the bacterial cell wall peptidoglycan of gram-positive bacteria, thereby destroying them; in conjunction with complement, it destroys gram-negative bacteria); leukin (a basic protein that is active against gram-positive bacteria); phagocytin (a basic protein that is active against gram-positive bacteria); lactoferrin[8] (an iron-binding protein that is active against gram-positive and gram-negative bacteria; myeloperoxidase-halide ion-H_2O_2 system[76,143,234,238] (the "respiratory burst") (it occurs within the phagolysosome but it can be released extracellularly; peptidoglycan is the preferred substrate for the system.)

$$O_2 \rightarrow \overset{*}{O_2} \xrightarrow[\text{dismutase}]{\text{Superoxide}} H_2O_2^* \xrightarrow{\text{Myeloperoxidase}} HOCl^{-*} + \text{Amino acids}$$

Superoxide ion — Supercoxide ion

O_2^1* / Chloride ion Cl^- — Hypochlorite ion

$OH^{\cdot}*$ Singlet oxygen   Hydroxyl radical — Chloramine*

$NH_3 \quad CO_2 \quad Cl^- \quad$ Aldehyde*

4. Macrophage factors[223] including lysosomal enzymes and proteins (similar to PMNs); "respiratory burst" (less intense than PMNs, no myeloperoxidase but has catalase); fibronectin[235] (which binds to several species of bacteria and may promote the uptake of bacteria by phagocytic cells, i.e., acts an opsonin); interferon (antiviral); lymphocyte-activating factor; and leukotrienes (chemotactic for PMNs, promotes collagen formation by fibroblasts, and stimulates the release of acute phase proteins from the liver.

5. Phagocytosis—in early stages, PMNs dominate; in later stages, macrophages dominate.

6. Lymphocyte factors[223] including lymphotoxin (a lymphokine released by T cells that destroys cells); macrophage activating factor (a lymphokine released by T cells that causes macrophages to become much more bactericidal [e.g., allows them to destroy intracellular parasites such as mycobacteria and corynbacteria]); interferon (released by T cells and is antiviral). The B cells form plasma cells, which are precursors of the serum antibodies.

7. Salivary factors including lysozyme; antibodies (primarily IgA); flow of saliva (physically removes microbes that are then swallowed or expectorated); antibiotic factors released by normal microbial flora (destroys invading microbes [e.g., peroxides released by streptococci and lactic acid released by lactobacilli]); anaerobic conditions (can destroy facultative anaerobic microbes; blockage of sites or niches by normal microbial flora (invaders have no available niches); and lactoperoxidase-thiocyanate-H_2O_2 system[1,80,81,175,221] (somewhat similar to myeloperoxidase system in PMNs; antimicrobial action depends in part on its penetration into cells; it is more effective against gram-positive than gram-negative bacteria). Small cationic proteins, mucins, lactoferrin and complement are also found in saliva and have antimicrobial activity.[81]

8. Gastric acid—HCl from the stomach rapidly destroys swallowed oral microbes.

9. Fever[26,127,134]—with elevated body temperatures, there is an enhanced destruction of gram-negative but not gram-positive microbes. The thermal alteration of the gram-negative cell wall might be partially responsible. In an animal experiment, all of the individuals were infected with a gram-negative species.[26] Half were given aspirin; they did not develop a fever and they subsequently died. The other half were not given aspirin; they developed a fever and survived (something to consider when we usually try to reduce elevated body temperatures).

---

*Believed to have antimicrobial activity. Methionine sulfoxide is another product of the system that is believed to have antimicrobial activity. Hypochlorite is believed to chlorinate the bacterial cell wall and lead to the degradation of the amino acid content of the wall. This system is active against gram-positive and gram-negative bacteria, viruses, and protozoa. Collagenases, lipases, and ribonucleases are more important in destroying dead, than living, microbes. There are also antimicrobial cationic proteins derived from lipids.[66]

DELETERIOUS HOST RESISTANCE FACTORS

1. Lysosomal enzymes and "respiratory burst" factors[113]

2. Acidic polysaccharides and nucleic acids

3. Prostaglandins, collagenase, fibrinolysin, proteases, complement, and corticosteroids

4. Histamine and other vasoactive amines (result of Type I hypersensitivity)[223,229]

5. Lymphotoxin (result of Type IV hypersensitivity)[223,229]

6. Metabolic breakdown products including indole, skatole, various amines, ammonia, and antigens[147]

REGULATING HOST RESISTANCE FACTORS

1. Inhibitors of inflammatory enzymes[46,223] including antiproteases such as alpha$_1$-antitrypsin and alpha$_2$-macroglobulin (block proteases that are released from lysosomes of PMNs); plasma carboxypeptidase (inactivates C_{5a}, C_{3a}, and bradykinin); inhibitors of the complement cascade; and eosinophilic enzymes (can destroy the major inflammatory mediators).

2. Acute phase proteins[46,223] including C-reactive protein (activates the complement system, suppresses the immune response, and may prevent the production of autoantibodies to proteins released by damaged cells); ceruloplasmin; and ferritin (helps limit injury and promotes repair).

3. Under conditions of stress endogenous corticosteroids are elevated,[148,151,152] but even under normal conditions they are produced. As corticosteroids inhibit the inflammatory and immune responses, their activity would also tend to regulate an overreactive inflammatory and immune response.

---

disease are relatively avirulent; however, some of them produce factors with the potential of causing tissue damage. In vitro examples of virulence may not necessarily correlate with in vivo tissue destruction. Microbes may be virulent and yet not pathogenic. The outcome of the host-parasite interrelationship is what decides whether infectious disease will result.

Studies do not show any correlation between the number and type of virulence factors produced by root canal isolates and the size or type of radiographic periapical lesions.[29] However, it is possible that certain combinations of microbial products interact with the host to produce a pathologic state.[125] Substances related to virulence may be exotoxins, capsules, endotoxins, enzymes, metabolic end products, or antigenic components.[135]

In a recent study, investigators found that bacterial cell wall components and products can induce pulpal and peri-

apical disease.[208] Viable bacteria were not essential. Root canal microbial virulence factors are given on p. 368.

Host resistance factors

The reactions of the host to the presence of microbes or their products may be beneficial or detrimental. There are certain substances produced during the inflammatory reaction that may be more deleterious than the microbial factors themselves. These are given on this page. On the beneficial side are various factors and conditions that are important for host resistance. These are given on p. 369. There are also regulating factors that moderate the inflammatory and immune responses. These are given on this page.

ORAL PATHWAYS OF INFECTION

Once infection occurs in the pulp, there are several possible pathways of infection.[147] They are:

1. It can remain in the pulp and stimulate the formation of either a granuloma (lateral or periapical), a radicular cyst, or condensing osteitis (see Chapter 11).

2. It can perforate through the root apex and temporarily overwhelm the host defensive cells and form either an acute apical abscess (if no previous periapical lesion was present) or an acute exacerbation of a periapical granuloma (i.e., phoenix abscess) or a radicular cyst (see Chapter 1).

3. It can perforate through the root apex and penetrate the nasal fossa and form a nasal abscess or penetrate the maxillary sinus and form a maxillary sinusitis.

4. It can have recurrent flare-ups and form a chronic apical abscess and then create a path through the alveolar mucosa or skin. This path is called either a sinus tract (if it is lined by granulomatous tissue) or a fistula (if it is lined by epithelium).[197] Sinus tracts are more frequent. These pathways can drain: (a) through the labial (or buccal) or palatal (or lingual) mucosa into the oral cavity; (b) into the gingival sulcus (or periodontal pocket); (c) into the furcation region of molars; and (d) through the skin of the face. The last is more likely to occur in long-standing, untreated cases. In the oral cavity, at the site of the intermittent discharge of the "pus" (liquefied microbial cellular, and tissue breakdown products), a proliferation of granulomatous tissue can form that is known as a parulis (stoma, "gumboil") (see Chapter 18).

5. Finally, the infection can drain into the blood circulatory system and the lymphatics. This will now be discussed.

Microorganisms in the bloodstream

All of the following serious, and sometimes fatal, conditions are dependent upon the presence of microorganisms in the bloodstream: bacteremia, septicemia, septic shock, anachoresis, cellulitis, Ludwig's angina, actinomycosis, orbital cellulitis, osteomyelitis, cavernous sinus thrombosis, brain abscess, mediastinitis, hemiplegia, paresthesia, surgical emphysema, air embolism, and focal disease. Before the advent of antibiotics, these conditions were not unusual sequelae to pulpally induced periapical pathosis. Because of the introduction of antibiotics and improved patient education, a great reduction occurred in these untoward complications. However, recently, primarily because of the fear of inducing serious hypersensitivity reactions, many dentists have decreased their usage of appropriate antibiotics for endodontically related periapical pathosis. As a result, there has been an upsurge in these life-threatening complications (as determined by a review of the recent literature). Let us now consider these serious conditions.

Microbes and their products can be released into the bloodstream and lymphatics from a periapical site. The main pathway of bacteria into the bloodstream from a primary site (e.g., the apex) is indirect via the lymphatics.[23] The clinical result of bacteria in the bloodstream depends on the virulence of the microbes and the resistance of the host. The various terms used in describing microbes in the bloodstream are bacteremia (bacteria), septicemia (bacteria and toxins), toxemia (toxins), pyemia (pus), and viremia (viruses).

Bacteremia

Bacteria can be released into the bloodstream in the normal person following various dental procedures, such as extraction, periodontal treatment, and endodontic therapy. Bacteremia can also result from the simple act of chewing and toothbrushing. Although any oral microbe may be involved in bacteremia, the α-hemolytic streptococci had formerly been found most frequently. Recently, with the use of strict anaerobic methods, obligate anaerobes such as *Bacteroides melaninogenicus* have been isolated with increasing frequency.[155] One of the greatest dangers with organisms such as *Bacteroides* is that they have a strong tendency to invade veins. A danger in infections of this type is septic embolization. The small infarctions that result from emboli are a fertile breeding ground for microbes and metastatic abscess formation is common.[13]

In patients with a history of rheumatic fever who have a heart murmur or mitral valve prolapse,[35] heart valve damage is present. Bacteria in the bloodstream can lodge in damaged heart valves and lead to the serious and sometimes fatal disease infective endocarditis (previously called subacute bacterial endocarditis).[35,142] Patients with no obvious predisposing factors for infective endocarditis have recently shown an increased incidence of this potentially fatal disease.[130,195] There are now more older individuals and the elderly have an increased incidence of primary endocarditis.[224] From 50% to 80% of narcotic-associated infective endocarditis occurs in individuals with no known preexisting heart disease.[118]

In the healthy person, the bacteria are disposed of within 10 minutes by the body's blood-clearing mechanisms (primarily antibodies and phagocytosis).[17,21] In patients whose defense mechanisms are impaired (suppressed immune system) by drugs (e.g., alcohol, corticosteroids, other immunosuppressants, stimulants, hallucinogens, narcotics), disease, dehydration, vitamin deficiencies, malnutrition, lack of sleep, and debilitation, the normal blood-clearing mechanisms are diminished or inoperative. Microbes can then multiply in the bloodstream, and the results can be serious or fatal diseases.[147] With many of these patients, there are no overt signs and symptoms and the history is frequently negative. For example, it is estimated that in the United States, almost 5% of the population has diabetes mellitus and that about 50% of these people have the disease undiagnosed.[241] Poorly controlled, or uncontrolled, diabetics often have exacerbations of infections.[116] Poorly controlled diabetics have abnormalities in red blood cells and vascular disease which may hamper good wound healing on the basis of poor oxygen delivery to the wound area. They also have decreased PMNs response to stress, decreased leukocyte adherence, and abnormalities in PMN migration, chemotaxis, phagocytosis, and bacterial killing.[101] For example, a case was recently reported[101] of a poorly controlled diabetic patient who developed a life-threatening deep space neck infection from a routine periodontal abscess of the lower left central incisor following extraction and *nonuse* of antibiotics. This is an important, medically and legally relevant case, which could also have occurred under similar situations following endodontic therapy and nonuse of antibiotics.

Alcoholics are also often undiagnosed. They have an impaired immune system and can also have serious exacerbations.[176] Stress, which is uncommonly evaluated in the dental office, can result in high levels of circulating corticosteroids, which can allow for a rapid spread of infection.[151] The 1985 recommendations of the American Heart Association state that "periapical infections may induce bacteremia even in the absence of dental procedures."[55] Bender further stated: "On occasion, these quiescent lesions may change spontaneously into acute abscesses ('phoenix' abscess) in the absence of dental instrumentation."[22] Hence dentists should be aware of the possibility of serious reactions in patients with pulpally induced periapical pathosis, especially if there is suspicion of drug and alcohol intake, undetected serious disease (such as diabetes), and stress.

In a patient who has received a transplant or artificial valves, there is a dual problem. First, this individual would be receiving immunosuppressive drugs, which seriously affect resistance to infection. Second, microbes can adhere more readily to artificial valves or sites of transplant attachment and multiply.

Various dental procedures differ in their ability to cause bacteremias. According to Bender et al.[21] the incidence of bacteremia was least following nonsurgical endodontic therapy (Table 12-1). Bacteremias following extraction varied from 51.5% (single extractions) to 93.4% (multiple extractions, heavy trauma). It can be seen from this table that *nonsurgical endodontic therapy, within the confines of the root canals, is the least likely dental procedure (of those tested) to cause bacteremia*. Judging by the negative results after 10 minutes, one finds that even vigorous *endodontic overinstrumentation is less detrimental than extraction or periodontal therapy*. These results were confirmed in two studies in which anaerobic as well as aerobic techniques were used.[17]

Regardless of the results, special-risk patients, such as (1) those receiving immunosuppressants, (2) those with artificial valves or transplants, (3) those with a history of rheumatic fever or mitral valve prolapse, and (4) those whose resistance is impaired, should all be premedicated with antibiotics during endodontic therapy. Because of poor resistance and impaired clearing mechanisms, even a slight bacteremia can prove devastating to these patients.

TABLE 12-1. Incidence of bacteremia in dental procedures

Procedure	Number of cases	Immediately after extraction (No.)	(%)	10 minutes after extraction (No.)	(%)
Incidence of bacteremia in exodontic manipulation					
Multiple extraction	93	79	84.9	41	44.0
Heavy trauma	61	57	93.4	30	49.2
Mild trauma	32	22	68.7	11	34.3
Single extraction	33	17	51.5	8	24.2
		Immediately after manipulation (No.)	(%)	10 minutes after manipulation (No.)	(%)
Incidence of bacteremia in periodontic manipulation					
Gingivectomy	12	10	83.3	3	25.0
Deep scaling	15	8	53.3	2	13.3
Light scaling	20	6	30.0	1	5.0
Incidence of bacteremia following endodontic manipulation					
Group A (within root canal)	50	0	0.0	0	0.0
Group B (beyond root canal)	48	15	31.2	0	0.0
TOTAL	98	15	15.3	0	0.0

*Modified from Bender, I.B., et al.: Oral Surg. **16**:466, 1963.

The need for antibiotic premedication in patients with joint and hip replacements has not been definitiely established.[133] Although many orthopedic surgeons want their patients protected with antibiotics during dental procedures, there is no consensus on drugs, dosage, or the duration of protection. It is suggested that consultation with the physician be done before routinely prescribing any antibiotics for these patients. (For a discussion on specific drug and dosage, see ''Antibiotics,'' p. 383.)

Septicemia

Septicemia is a serious, life-threatening bloodstream invasion by microbes and their noxious products. It generally occurs when resistance is impaired and/or infection is overwhelming. It is associated with severe signs and symptoms.[147]

In one case,[129] the patient was a 13-year-old apparently healthy girl who presented with a history of intermittent pain associated with the upper left central incisor. The pulp was necrotic and there was a periapical lesion present. The author stated that he probably instrumented beyond the apex and then a small amount of pus emerged from the canal. The tooth was left open for drainage and the patient was given an appointment to return in 3 days provided that no problems occurred sooner. Antibiotics were not prescribed because there was no evidence of local spread or systemic involvement. The next day, the patient felt sick and although her left lip and cheek became swollen, she did not return to seek immediate treatment as advised. By nightfall, she had become pyrexic and delerious. The patient was admitted to a hospital, drowsy, with a high fever, uncharacteristically aggressive, and dissociated in time and place. Her pulse rate was 156. The diagnosis was septicemic meningitis. The patient was given massive penicillin therapy and fortunately she recovered by the seventh day. The endodontic therapy was then completed uneventfully. The author hypothesized that apparently inadvertent instrumentation beyond the apex or blockage of the root canal opening led to spread of infection deep into the periapical tissues.

From the results of the studies by other investigators,[155,239] it appears that blockage of the root canal opening is a more likely etiologic factor than instrumentation beyond the apex in a case with an endodontically originated periapical radiolucency.

In a study[157] on the electrophoretic differentiation of radicular cysts and granulomas, it was found that in about 25% of the cases of periapical granulomas, liquefaction necrosis (pus) was found and it only drained through the root canal(s) when instrumentation was extended into the approximate center of the lesions. The investigators also observed that about 50% of the radicular cysts only drained through the root canals when overinstrumentation was done. Therefore in many cases of periapical lesions, overextension of small files (''overinstrumentation'') was essential to ensure drainage. This is apparently important. Seltzer,[197] in his description of periapical granulomas, stated: ''may produce violent symptoms resulting from further formation of liquefaction necrosis. The pus, confined and unable to be evacuated, may produce pressure on nerve endings resulting in severe pain and swelling. Once the pus has been evacuated, symptoms subside, and the status quo is reestablished.''

Bender[20] in his description of healing of periapical cysts as the result of instrumentation into the lesion stated, ''Once the inflammation (created by the overinstrumentation) subsides, the excess fluid is drained or resorbed by the adjacent cells and the fibroblasts begin to proliferate. As the fibroblasts mature, they elaborate collagen. The subsequent increase in collagen deposition begins to squeeze down on the rich capillary network within the granulomatous tissue, with ultimate shutting off of the blood supply to the cells. This type of action is similar to that which is observed when granulation tissue becomes converted into scar tissue in the process of healing. As more collagen is deposited, the starved epithelial cells become entrapped, undergo degeneration, and are removed by macrophages.''

Bender[20] gave further support to the concept of overextension of small files in periapical radiolucency cases when he stated: ''The instrument is inserted to break the wall of the cyst or abscess in order to establish drainage and reduce the pressure. It would be better to insert the instrument at least one half the distance into the region of rarefaction to make certain that it traverses the center of the granuloma or cyst. The cystic cavity is usually found in the center of the granuloma. . . . If the instrument goes through the lesion, drainage is established more often."

However, others,[129] are of the opinion that overinstrumentation in these type cases spreads infection and causes clinical flare-ups. Grossman[93] stated that overinstrumentation could cause "an endodontic emergency." Several investigators[13] believe that overinstrumentation could result in an "exacerbation."[13,30,163] "Instrumentation beyond the apex will push these toxic products out into the periapical tissues, as demonstrated by Ingle,[115] and aggravate the tissue disintegration, compounding the damaging effect of the mechanical irritation. Clinically, this is known as a flare-up of iatrogenic etiology."[30] However, there is no clinical evidence that instrumentation into asymptomatic periapical radiolucencies will cause "a flare-up of iatrogenic etiology."[30] In fact, it is more likely that, rather than induce infectious flare-ups, overextension of small files in these quiescent periapical lesions may remove microbes and their inflammatory products and/or bring them into a region where body defenses are high. That is the periapical granulomatous region, a site with a high concentration of blood vessels, lymphatics, and host defensive cells (i.e., lymphocytes, plasma cells, macrophages, giant cells, and polymorphonuclear leukocytes.[197] Since microbes can lodge in dentinal tubules and later cause problems,[187,202] it appears to be more logical to thoroughly instrument necrotic pulp cases to dislodge those microbes (easier to do by going beyond the apex and then file occlusally). As mentioned previously, in long-standing root canal infections (as occurs with periapical "area" cases), the microbes invade the dentinal tubules and accessory canals[187,202] and are protected from routine instrumentation and irrigation, which is mainly effective on the surface layers of the root canal walls.[12] In the healthy individual, if microbes are inadvertently pushed beyond the apex, they are rapidly destroyed.

It has been observed that in symptomless teeth with necrotic pulps and associated periapical rarefactions, there was a trend toward fewer flare-ups when instrumentation was more complete.[13] Instrumentation short of the apex (two-thirds the way up the root canal) resulted in flare-ups in 14.3% of the cases. Instrumentation to the radiographic apex (which is in reality often slight overinstrumentation) resulted in flare-ups 10% of the time. One investigator observed that flare-ups occurred more than twice as frequently when complete instrumentation was not done as compared to when it was done.[192] Support has been given to the concept that overinstrumentation is not important in inducing flare-ups in these cases.[213] Investigators did three studies on asymptomatic teeth with necrotic pulps and associated periapical radiolucencies.[155] They were done in three different practices at three different time periods. In the first study, pre–flare-up antibiotics were *not* used and instrumentation was done to the radiographic apex (time period was 1963 to 1970). In that study, the incidence of flare-ups (unscheduled emergency appointments necessitated by pain and swelling combined or swelling alone) was 19.6%. In the second study, the patients were given a prescription for an antibiotic to be taken at the first sign of swelling and instrumentation was done to the approximate center of the periapical lesion (time period was 1978 to 1983). In that study, the incidence of flare-ups was 4.3%. In the third study, antibiotic usage was mandatory and instrumentation was again into the approximate center of the periapical lesions and the cases were completed in one visit (time period, 1983 to 1985). In that study, the flare-up incidence was only 1.5% and the cases were mild and easily controlled. Although the antibiotic usage was a primary consideration (discussed further in the Antibiotics section), it did appear that the overinstrumentation may help in the reduction of the flare-ups.

There is extensive resorption of dentin and cementum in the apices of teeth with periapical areas of pathosis of endodontic origin. In addition, the granulomatous tissue invades the root canal from the periapical region and is found several millimeters coronally from the apex. Overinstrumentation facilitates the removal of necrotic dentin and cementum and possibly the breakdown of granulomatous tissue. Granulomatous tissue apparently must first be broken down and then resorbed before repair can take place. In teeth with periapical granulomas and radicular cysts, the pulp tissue, the dentin, the cementum, and some of the epithelium become altered as the result of the chronic inflammation. These altered tissues, along with root canal microbes, are antigenically foreign to the host.[149,229] Antigenically foreign material can induce a hypersensitivity reaction, either immediate or delayed (discussed further later), which may be a component of the flare-up reactions. By overinstrumentation, these altered foreign materials can either be withdrawn through the access opening or be forced into the periapex where there is an active drainage system. Therefore, for these various reasons, the hypothesis[129] that overinstrumentation was partly responsible for the septicemia may not be valid. A second hypothesis on the cause of the septicemia—blockage of the root canal opening after leaving the tooth open to drain—appears to be one of the reasons for the serious sequelae to periapical disease. It has been the clinical experience of many endodontists that when a tooth is left open to drain, there is a high likelihood that the opening would become occluded with food or debris. This would then allow the oral microbes that entered the root canal from the oral cavity to multiply in a relatively protected environment. For this reason, it is suggested that a tooth should only be left open for drainage when there is unremitting purulent discharge that is not relieved by thorough instrumentation and irrigation.

It also appears from the other studies that the use of prophylactic antibiotics in pulpally induced periapical lesion cases may have prevented this severe septicemia (discussed further in the section on antibiotics).[137,155]

Septic shock

Septic shock has been related to alcoholism.[176] In alcohol-induced bone marrow depression, there is a lack of healthy and vigorous PMNs, and alcoholics have a decreased ability to clear bacteria from the bloodstream. These patients become prone to septic shock, which is often fatal. Septic shock is secondary to the release of endotoxin, which has been found in high concentrations in teeth with necrotic pulps and associated periapical "areas."[191,194] In a recent case report,[176] an alcoholism-related case of odontogenic septic shock was presented. Since many patients drink alcoholic beverages, and some are unrecognized alcoholics, this serious sequela must be considered when cases of endodontically related periapical pathosis are present.

Anachoresis

Anachoresis denotes the localization of blood-borne microbes or their products to an inflamed area. This process has been demonstrated experimentally in animals[3,60,62,149] and indirectly in humans.[153] It could account for cases of infected pulps and periapical areas in (1) traumatized teeth that have had no previous pulpal exposures or restorations and (2) teeth with sound restorations with underlying pulp inflammation. One study[62] showed that anachoresis does not occur to stagnant tissue fluid of instrumented but unfilled root canals. It has been hypothesized that pulpal blood circulation (as would be found in traumatized inflamed pulps or beneath sound restorations) is essential for anachoresis to take place. In another study[3] investigators found that bacteria can spread from periapical granulomas to primarily noninfected but pulpectomized roots. Additionally, it has been shown[60] that anachoresis would occur in instrumented, unfilled root canals if overinstrumentation was done and bleeding occurred within the root canals.

Cellulitis

Cellulitis secondary to pulpally induced periapical pathosis is not unusual in clinical practice. A cellulitis is an acute inflammation of the alveolar and loose connective tissues and is a diffuse, spreading type of inflammation. There are two principal types: superficial and deep. The superficial type is where the exudate courses between the superficial fascia and the superficial layer of the deep cervical fascia.[147] These infectious processes look very serious but generally can be readily controlled by antibiotics and drainage. Examples of superficial cellulitis are involvements of the canine space, the buccal space, and the mental space. In the deep cellulitis, the exudate travels beneath the superficial layer of the deep cervical fascia, below muscle attachments, and between fascial sheets.[147] These infectious processes look serious and are potentially dangerous; they require more vigorous antibiotic, drainage, and supportive measures. For example, investigators[132] reported a near fatal case in which the obligate anaerobes peptococci and *Bacteroides* were found. Examples of deep cellulitis are involvement of the submental space, the sublingual space, the submaxillary (submandibular) space, the infratemporal space, the temporal space, the superficial masticator space, the deep masticator space, and the lateral pharyngeal space. With severe infectious disease and lowered patient resistance, more posterior spaces can become involved including the retropharyngeal space, the "danger" space, and the prevertebral space. These complications are potentially fatal. Cellulitis is the clinical manifestation of what is commonly called a flareup. Let us briefly consider the possible ways that a flareup may occur.

1. As a result of the access preparation, oxygen enters the root canal system, which may facilitate facultative anaerobes to multiply and interact with obligate anaerobes to produce inflammatory and edematous substances.[160]

2. It was postulated in 1905 that overinstrumentation can force necrotic debris and microbes through the apex, which could then temporarily overwhelm the host defensive cells and produce severe inflammation.[37] However, bacteremias are reduced to 0% within 10 minutes, even following overinstrumentation.[21]

3. *Bacteroides melaninogenicus* has been implicated in flareup cases.[90,92,213] The trauma from endodontic instrumentation

may indirectly result in the proliferation of this species and its synergistic interaction with other microbes.[90]

4. Microbial products such as endotoxin[191,194] and enzymes[125] can be forced into the periapex. Many gram-negative microbes found in root canals of periapical "area" cases produce endotoxin.[92,191,194] As mentioned in the section on microbial virulence factors endotoxin is dangerous and has been found in high concentration in necrotic pulps and associated periapical lesions.[65,173,191,194] Microbial cell wall components (in addition to endotoxin), enzymes,[125,226] toxins, and antigens may serve as etiologic agents in the initiation of flareups by causing inflammatory edema.

5. Impaired resistance and stress can allow microbes to multiply and disseminate.[151]

6. Hypersensitivity reactions to the microbes and their products may be a component of the flareup reactions[199] (see Immunologic Considerations).

7. Occasionally, foreign bodies can induce flareups. Flareups have been observed related to the extrusion of paper points or cotton fibers into the periapex.

8. Seltzer[197] stated that: "Excessive bleeding causes a pericementitis inasmuch as the extravasated blood causes compression of the tissue and inflammatory changes—pooled blood is an excellent culture medium for the growth of microorganisms."

9. Finally, regardless of etiology (e.g., microbes, foreign bodies), there is a release of inflammatory precursors and mediators such as Hageman factor, plasmin, histamine, serotonin, prostaglandins, leukotrienes, kinins, complement, lysosomal enzymes, lymphokines, platelet-activating factor, and cyclic GMP. These are pain- and edema-producing, thereby contributing to the flareup.[199,226]

Microbes are the primary etiologic factor of flareups; the principal method of managing and preventing cellulitis is the use of appropriate antibiotics (primarily penicillin V and erythromycin).

Even cases that are not serious (e.g., superficial cellulitis such as buccal space) can cause patients grief. The reason is frequently they had no previous discomfort (generally their first awareness of an endodontic problem was when the dentist told them they had a periapical lesion). Even when they are forewarned about possible flareups, many patients become distressed because of the pain and facial distortion.

Recently, the American Association of Endodontists has made a definitive effort to improve the negative image the public has about endodontics.[193] Nevertheless, patients who develop flareups from teeth that were symptomless before treatment tend to have a negative image of endodontics. If those flareups could be minimized or prevented, with proper antibiotic prophylaxis, this would help improve the image of endodontics.

Ludwig's angina

One of the most serious types of cellulitis is the fulminating bilateral involvement of the submaxillary, sublingual, submental, lateral pharyngeal, and retropharyngeal spaces known as Ludwig's angina. The tongue is enlarged and displaced superiorly and posteriorly against the soft palate, leading to respiratory difficulties. The floor of the mouth is boardlike in consistency. Rapid spread of infection can occur through the fascial spaces into the cranium or mediastinum.[147] Other possible complications are meningitis, septicemia, pneumonitis, and death.[112] Before the advent of antibiotics, Ludwig's angina had a mortality of 54%. Since the introduction of penicillin, the rate has been reduced to 4%.[4]

Actinomycosis

Actinomycosis is a suppurative infectious disease caused by various strains of *Actinomyces* microbes (e.g., *A. israeli, A. bovis, A. viscosus, A. naeslundii*) acting synergistically with streptococci and staphylococci.[24,147] Trauma, including endodontic instrumentation and more frequently extraction, is believed to be a precondition for the onset of the disease.[122] The primary site of the cervicofacial variety in the oral cavity is the mandible, where multiple external skin sinus tracts are often found. In the last few years, several cases have been reported of actinomycosis of the pulp and periapex of varying degrees of severity.[24,34,161,237] If untreated or inadequately treated, actinomycosis can be a serious disease. Fortunately, it is amenable to penicillin V therapy, but the antibiotic therapy must be prolonged.[122]

Orbital cellulitis

Orbital cellulitis is an inflammatory condition of the eye orbit. It can be a sequela to pulpal-periapical pathosis. Orbital cellulitis can lead to orbital abscess, optic neuritis, abducens nerve paralysis, cavernous sinus thrombosis, blindness, and death.[117]

Three recent periapical lesion–originating cases in apparently healthy individuals have been reported. One[211] was a case that originated from a carious lower left second premolar with a necrotic pulp and associated periapical radiolucency. The outcome was unilateral blindness. Another[117] discussed a serious case of orbital cellulitis in a 14-year-old boy who had a toothache and swelling for 4 days originating from a cariously involved upper first molar with a mesiobuccal periapical lesion. Another report[38] presented four cases of orbital cellulitis and reviewed several others. Of the four cases, one, which occurred in a previously healthy 12-year-old boy, was fatal. There was no evidence that antibiotics were used at the time of the extraction of the upper right first molar. Two weeks later, the boy died.

Osteomyelitis

Osteomyelitis is an inflammation of bone that begins in the marrow spaces, then involves the associated periosteum, and finally becomes enmeshed in the cortical plates of bone.[147] Ischemia results and various parts of the calcified tissues become necrotic and are sequestered. Osteomyelitis can occur as the result of direct medullary spread from the apex of an acute or chronically involved periapical "area" case. The mandible is affected much more commonly than the maxilla, possibly because of the inferior blood supply of the mandible. Several serious cases have been reported.[9,174,184,205,236] Once osteomyelitis is established, resolution is much more difficult. That is why it is even more important to prevent the disease by the use of prophylactic antibiotics (see section on antibiotics).

Cavernous sinus thrombosis (thrombophlebitis)

A thrombophlebitis of the cavernous sinus may be caused by direct extension of infectious processes from adjoining veins (e.g., the facial vein, the internal jugular vein, or the pterygoid plexus).[27] However, the most common is from the maxillary and mandibular third molars via the pterygoid plexus.

Cavernous sinus thrombosis is a dangerous condition that causes impairment of cerebral vascular drainage. Although it is much less frequent since the advent of antibiotics, it can still follow severe periapical pathosis in debilitated persons. Septic emboli can occur from the breaking off of the thrombi and their passage through the bloodstream and may result in lung abscesses and cerebral abscesses, among other possibilities. Even today, cavernous sinus thrombosis is a serious condition and recovery can still produce residual brain damage. Treatment consists of massive antibiotic therapy and surgical drainage.

Brain abscess

There are numerous case reports regarding the severity of brain abscess.[11,49,121,182] Brain abscess can result from pulpal-periapical disease. Clinically, there is generally a latent period of several days or weeks following the endodontic treatment or tooth extraction before the clinical manifestations of brain abscess occur.[110] The encapsulation of a brain abscess begins within a week of infection and usually requires 4 to 6 weeks for completion.[141]

Mediastinitis

Mediastinitis is a serious and usually fatal[71] complication of pulpally induced periapical pathosis. The clinical manifestations are chest pain, persistent fever, dyspnea, and radiographic indication of a widened mediastinum.[147]

Hemiplegia

Hemiplegia is paralysis of one lateral half of the body. Before the advent of antibiotics, neurologic complications such as this were not unusual and they were frequently fatal.[104]

Paresthesia (dysesthesia)

From a life-threatening viewpoint, paresthesia is a less severe neurologic complication than is hemiplegia. Nevertheless, it is a very disturbing symptom and has precipitated many malpractice suits. Paresthesia is defined as "a morbid, abnormal, or perverted sensation such as burning, prickling, numbness, or itching; it can include any deviation from normal sensation."[82] Although inferior alveolar nerve paresthesia is usually related to trauma from periapical surgery (frequent) and overinstrumentation (rare) and pressure and chemical irritation from overfilling (common, especially with paraformaldehyde-containing root canal pastes), it can also occur from microbial infection.[7,84,217]

Also related to neuronal damage by microorganisms, investigators[178,185] found that in patients with idiopathic trigeminal neuralgia and atypical facial neuralgia, jawbone cavities from extracted teeth sites contained mixed polymicrobial aerobic and anaerobic species. Their treatment consisted of curettage of the jawbone cavities along with the use of antibiotics. Resolution was the usual outcome.

Surgical emphysema and air embolism

Surgical emphysema is the introduction of air into the subcutaneous tissues resulting in marked edema with (usually) noticeable swelling and discoloration.[147] It most often occurs rapidly following procedures such as (1) the use of the air turbine handpiece during oral surgery, (2) directing compressed air from the air syringe into the root canal, and (3) using hydrogen peroxide vigorously as a root canal irrigant.[75] Quite often, microbes are forced in along with the air and then the situation can become serious. If the air (with the associated microbes) dislodges into a blood vessel, this is called an air embolism. It is very serious (and potentially fatal) if it occurs in the lungs or brain.[179] If a dentist inadvertently blows compressed air into a root canal, antibiotics should be given immediately (preferably penicillin) and the patient should be kept under close observation. However, it is a cardinal principle in endodontics to *never use compressed air in a root canal*. There have been several case reports strongly suggesting cause and effect between various ailments and root canal etiology.[171,196,200]

Focal disease

Focal disease (focal infection) is a secondary disease resulting from blood-borne infection that originated at a primary site.[147] The primary site is called a focus of infection. In the previous discussion of bacteremias it was stated that bacteria can lodge and colonize in damaged heart valves, producing the serious disease infective endocarditis. This is the *only* definitely authenticated example of focal disease from an oral microbial focus of infection.

Eye, ear, and nasal infections can occur as a result of direct extension of severe periapical pathosis and conceivably can occur as a result of hematogenous spread of microbes or their products. Extensive investigations[149] have been conducted of eye conditions that apparently were related to oral foci of infection. Therefore, if a patient has periapical disease with concomitant eye, ear, or nasal disorders, there is a *possibility* of focal disease. However, if the symptoms persist in the eye, ear, or nasal region after the return to normalcy of the dental condition, then the patient should be referred to the appropriate physician for consultation.

Although it has never been proved, oral microbes (e.g., α-hemolytic streptococci) may sensitize tissues at a secondary site, such as joint tissues. The sensitized tissue antigens may then evoke an autoimmune-type response, and a secondary disease could result. This could occur even though the original inciting microbes were destroyed. A similar autoimmune mechanism has been proposed for the development of rheumatic fever. In spite of the fact that the concept of focal disease is not currently popular, there are indications that *secondary disease from an oral focus can occur*.

IMMUNOLOGIC CONSIDERATIONS*

The interaction of microbes or other foreign antigens with the host can result in an immunologic response. Such a response may be favorable (protective or prophylactic), resulting in the destruction of the microbes or other foreign antigens, or it may be deleterious, resulting in an immediate or delayed hypersensitivity reaction (allergic response). The reaction may also be a combination of favorable and unfavorable responses. There are two types of lymphocytes: B cells and T cells. B cells lead to plasma cells, which then form antibodies. B cell protective responses involve interaction of antigen with antibodies and complement (antigen-antibody complexes or immune complexes). This leads to the removal and destruction of the antigens (microbes, toxins, or microbial products) by phagocytes. There is a minimum of damage to host tissue cells. Antigens are substances that are foreign to the host and stimulate the production of serum antibodies or a delayed hypersensitivity (cellular) reaction. Antibodies are humoral (serum) and are of five classes: IgG, IgM, IgE, IgA, and IgD.

IgG is the principal antibody involved in the protective reaction against microbes and their products. IgM is also involved in the protective reaction and is a larger molecule, usually formed in response to large microbes. IgA—found in urine, colostrum, respiratory and gastrointestinal tract secretions, tears, and saliva—is involved in antiviral action in those areas. IgA prevents the adherence of bacteria and viruses to epithelial surfaces.

The function of IgD is not definitely known.

Studies[149] however, have shown that IgD is on the surface of B lymphocytes (antibody producers) and may be involved in switching the lymphocyte from IgM to IgG production. IgD may also be involved in the prevention of immunologic tolerance (no immunologic response). IgE is active against parasitic worm (helminth) infections. Complement is a complex system involved with IgG and IgM. It aids in phagocytosis and can cause lysis of cells, including microbes.

T-cell protective responses are related to the four types of T cells.

1. T-inducer lymphocytes produce lymphokines. These substances recruit inflammatory cells to the site and activate and maintain them.
2. T-helper lymphocytes stimulate B lymphocytes to differentiate into mature antibody-secreting plasma cells. The T-helper lymphocytes also stimulate T-lymphocyte precursors to become the third type of T cells, the T-cytotoxic lymphocytes.
3. T-cytotoxic lymphocytes lyse cells infected by nonself antigen (primary viruses).
4. T-suppressor lymphocytes reduce antibody production by plasma cells and turn off T-lymphocyte precursors so that they do not become T-cytotoxic lymphocytes. (In essence, they prevent "overkill.")

It appears that the main protective response for the T cells, by themselves, is for the destruction of tumor cells.

The deleterious hypersensitivity responses involve both B and

---

*References 58, 149, 223, 229.

T cells and are of four types. Type I (immediate hypersensitivity) involves the binding of IgE to the surface of mast cells with the subsequent release of vasoactive substances from the mast cells including histamine, serotonin, kinins, and leukotrienes. Massive accumulation is found of eosinophils, which secrete enzymes that neutralize the agents released by mast cells (prevents overreaction). Clinical manifestations of Type I hypersensitivity are anaphylaxis, respiratory allergy (e.g., hay fever, rhinitis, asthma), and food allergy (results in diarrhea). Type II hypersensitivity (cytotoxic hypersensitivity) involves the destruction of host cells (such as erythrocytes) through the action of antibodies (generally IgM) and complement and by cytotoxic cells such as activated T cells, macrophages, and PMNs. The destruction of erythrocytes occurs when transfusion to another individual is done. The transfused erythrocytes are eliminated by the action of antibodies, complement, and macrophages (clinical example is erythroblastosis fetalis). Type III hypersensitivity (immune-complex, Arthus phenomenon) involves the formation of antigen-antibody (IgG) complexes (immune complexes) with the activation of complement. The destructive effect is related to the release of lysosomal enzymes from PMNs that are attracted to the site by two complement factors. Type IV hypersensitivity (delayed hypersensitivity, cell-mediated hypersensitivity) involves T lymphocytes and is a late reaction occurring 24 hours or more after the initial contact.

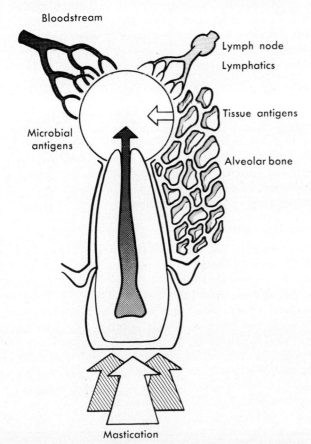

FIG. 12-1. Proposed immunologic mechanism for periapical disease. *Bloodstream,* Antibodies may become stimulated by released antigen. *Lymph node,* Lymphocytes may become stimulated by released antigen. *Alveolar bone* may allow for prolonged retention of antigen at the site. *Mastication* may allow for repeated release of antigen at intervals into the lymphatics or bloodstream.

Various lymphokines are released and adjoining cells are destroyed (destruction results from release of the lymphokine, lymphotoxin, and vasoactive factors from mast cells). There is also a monocyte infiltration. Clinical examples of Type IV hypersensitivity are contact dermatitis of the skin from formaldehyde; poison ivy, oak, and sumac; the granulomatous response to virus and bacteria such as tuberculosis; and transplant rejection. Related to endodontics, one of the released lymphokines is osteoclast-activating factor, which could partially account for periapical bone destruction.

The allergic (hypersensitivity) responses may be to (1) microbial antigens, (2) altered host tissue antigens (autoimmunity), (3) both microbial and tissue antigens (microbially incited autoimmunity, as proposed for rheumatic fever), (4) intracanal medicaments, irrigants, and (5) root canal filling materials.

There have been various investigations into the immunologic factors in pulpal-periapical diseases and evidence has been given of types I, II, III, and IV hypersensitivities.* Most of these investigations have been on periapical lesions. Therefore the following hypothetical immunologic mechanism for periapical disease is proposed (Fig. 12-1). Because the periapical area is surrounded by alveolar bone, there may be prolonged reduction of antigen at the inoculation site. This site is exposed to the pressure and irritation produced by mastication, which could allow for the release of small amounts of antigen into the lymphatics or bloodstream. The repeated release of antigen could stimulate circulating antibodies as well as lymphocytes in the regional lymph nodes. If the products of tissue breakdown in the chronic periapical area were rendered antigenically active (as the result of exposure of a hidden site or interaction with a microbial antigen), it is probable that antibodies to these active antigens would be produced regularly. These antibodies might cross-react with the altered tissue components, and an autoimmune response could result. Therefore the immunologic response in periapical tissues is probably a combination of protective (antigen destroyed) and allergic reactions.

Several studies[228-230] found that in cases of chronic periapical lesions, immune complexes are formed between the root canal antigens and periapical antibodies. These immune complexes basically remain localized and "it appears that chronic periapical lesions cannot act as a focus to cause systemic diseases via immune complexes." Other investigators, in contrast, found that patients with acute apical abscesses[124] had statistically significantly higher levels of circulating immune complexes and other immune components. "These immune complexes have the potential in certain individuals to cause systemic diseases." Therefore although the method of systemic involvement of root canal antigens is not known, systemic reactions from pulpal-periapical disease remains a distinct possibility.

The various possible components involved in periapical reactions (pain, swelling, and bone destruction) (Fig. 12-2) may be summarized as follows:

---

*References 29, 31, 32, 58, 124, 148, 149, 167, 226-230.

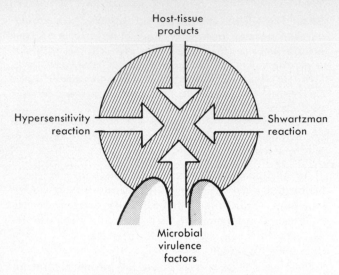

Host-tissue products

Hypersensitivity reaction

Shwartzman reaction

Microbial virulence factors

FIG. 12-2. Periapical destruction.

1. *Microbial virulence factors* (e.g., collagenase, hyaluronidase, streptokinase). After endodontic therapy is completed, irritating factors released from filling materials (e.g., corrosion products from silver cones) can replace microbial factors as irritants.

2. *Host tissue products* (e.g., histamine, bradykinin, prostaglandins).

3. *Hypersensitivity reactions.* The antigens involved in periapical disease may be bacterial products, host tissue products, or even intracanal medicaments. Low-molecular-weight chemicals such as intracanal medicaments can act as haptens and induce a hypersensitivity response. Rabbit and dog dental pulps are made antigenically active by treatments with the use of eight different sealer components including formaldehyde.[31,32,167] The clinician should consider the possibility that root canal sealer components interact with host proteins to make antigenically active substances that could induce an allergic reaction.[108] Patients can develop Type I hypersensitivity reactions to the penicillin component of the polyantibiotic root canal dressing. Other substances used in endodontic therapy have been shown to act as haptens: phenol and camphor (both in camphorated parachlorophenol, CMCP), iodine compounds, eugenol, balsam of Peru (in some root canal cements), creosote, urea, benzalkonium chloride (Zephiran), sodium hypochlorite, H_2O_2 (the latter four are irrigants), EDTA (calcium-chelating agent), and local anesthetics occasionally utilized for intrapulpal anesthesia or irrigation.[31,32] Gutta-percha may also act as a hapten.[149] Considering these various possibilities, one should use the least inflammatory drugs for irrigation, intracanal medication, and obturation.

One investigator[227] believes that activated epithelial cell rests in the periapical region can acquire antigenic properties and the resulting immunologic reactions may destroy the proliferating epithelial cells and thus facilitate the formation of a periapical cyst. He lists four possible ways of epithelium becoming antigenic: (1) epithelial cells ingest antigenic material from root canals, (2) there is antigenic cross-reactivity between root canal antigens and proliferating cell rests, (3) immunologic responses within the proliferating epithelium can be directed against the metabolic products of these proliferating epithelial cells, and (4) the aged epithelial cell rests have altered antigens and an autoimmune response occurs.

4. *Shwartzman reaction.* This is a reaction that is related to the presence of endotoxin. It is a nonimmunologic phenomenon causing local tissue destruction. The destruction results from the release of lysosomal enzymes from PMNs. Endotoxin (released in gram-negative microbes) has other effects including stimulating bone resorption, attracting osteoclasts, and acting as an antigen and complement activator.

DETECTION OF MICROBES

To detect microbes, a root canal exudate and fluid from a draining sinus tract or a fluctuant lesion can be used for the following tests: Gram stain, microbial culture tests, antibiotic sensitivity tests, and phase microscopy.

Gram stain

Gram stain examination shows the presence or absence of microbes (gram-positive or gram-negative), epithelial cells, erythrocytes, and PMNs. Because endodontic disease processes can contain practically any strain of oral microbes, the Gram stain and culture tests are not specific in the diagnosis of any endodontic symptom or disease. Gram staining also does not separate live from dead microbes. However, it does give some indication of the microbial flora involved in the particular condition. One advantage of the Gram stain is that it gives some insight into the host response. Detection of large numbers of PMNs and few or no organisms indicates a favorable host reaction. The presence of many microbes with the absence of PMNs indicates salivary contamination. However, it could also be a sign of immune deficiency.

Microbial cultures tests

It is believed that microbial culture tests are not useful for determining when to obturate a root canal system but may have some role in diagnosis. Even in diagnosis, a sole culture medium should not be used. The most commonly available culture media, such as brain-heart infusion broth, trypticase soy broth with agar, glucose ascites medium, and thioglycolate broth, do not permit good growth of all the possible microbes that might be present. The usual result of culturing in these media is an overgrowth of gram-positive cocci. Another problem is that some obligate anaerobic strains do not grow in these media, even when the culture tubes are incubated anaerobically. Many infectious diseases (probably including endodontic diseases) and most blood infections are caused by obligate anaerobes. Methods are now available to aid in the detection of obligate anaerobes from root canals. However, in present these methods are not readily available in most commercial laboratories. Hence the clinician who is interested in determining endodontic infection must depend on the not-too-reliable culture media currently available. The recent development of simplified chairside techniques may make culturing more practical.[44,91,189] Nevertheless, the determination of microbes in vivo has significance only if a specific endodontic pathogen (or combination of pathogens) is found or if some rare or unusual microbe is uncovered (e.g., actinomyces species, *Mycobacterium tuberculosis*).

For the following reasons a culture test is *not* advocated as an aid in determining when to obturate a root canal:[147,148,150]

1. There are many causes for a false-positive culture: failure in sterilization of the operating field, and instruments; rubber dam leaks; use of unsterile paper points and cotton tube plugs; forcing of microbes apically; air, breath, and hand contamination; root fractures; infected maxillary sinus; patent sinus tract; periodontal disease with exposure of lateral canals; and incomplete seal of temporary restoration.

2. A false-negative culture can occur with the following: incomplete penetration of a paper point; use of a paper point that is too narrow; a relatively dry canal; undetectable microbes (hidden in dentinal tubules, accessory or lateral canals, or cementum lacunae); culturing at the termination of the visit; phagocytes in the sample; dormant microbes in the sample; presence of antimicrobial materials in the canal; insufficient incubation time; only visual determination for growth; failure to consider culture reversal (negative culture at the obturation visit becoming positive after the obturation visit); and use of a single culture medium that fails to allow for growth of obligate anaerobic microbes and other hard-to-culture species.

3. No positive correlation exists between any root canal microbe (or microbial product) and any endodontic disease or clinical manifestation. Thus there is no definite need to totally eradicate any particular microbe as there is in a systemic disease (e.g., actinomycosis). However, there is an indication that *Bacteroides melaninogenicus*, in combination with other microbes, may be correlated with the presence of endodontic flare-ups.[92,213]

4. A culture test does not reveal the microbial virulence, the microbial population, or the host's resistance. The host's response is of major importance in determining when to obturate a root canal system.

5. An untoward host response (pain, swelling, fluid exudation) may result from an allergic reaction to the host's own tissue products as well as from microorganisms or their products. Therefore, if the response of the host is considered as one of the major determinants of when to obturate, the original cause is not relevant as long as the host's response becomes normal. (The indications for canal obturation are described in Chapter 8.)

6. All the findings* except one[172] have shown that microbes remaining in accessory and lateral canals, dentinal tubules, and cementum lacunae either remain inactive or die off (probably as the result of lack of nutrients).

7. The outcome of clinical studies of success and failure relative to positive and negative culture findings is inconclusive.[148]

8. The biggest danger in the use of the culture is the dentist's reliance on the culture results to the exclusion of other indices of readiness for obturation (e.g., dry canal and asymptomatic). Since temporary seals are porous[147,148] and most intracanal medicaments are inactive after 48 hours,[145] if proper culturing techniques are done (including strict anaerobic culturing and phase microscopy), positive cultures would be the rule rather than the

exception. If there are no complicating factors (e.g., pain, swelling, inadequate time), it appears to be more logical and biologically compatible to treat cases in one visit whenever possible. In that manner, there would be no problem with porous seals, ineffective intracanal medicaments, and unreliable microbiologic culturing. If the root canal is well obturated, any remaining microbes would tend to die (see 6, above).

However, cultures have some value[278]—to check aseptic technique (a good teaching tool for dental students)[28] and to show that microbes are important in the development of endodontic diseases. Clinicians are not at fault if they want to use the culture test as *one* indicator for determining when to fill a root canal system, provided they realize the potential for error in the technique and they do not needlessly prolong the treatment.

The clinician must realize that the *most important* consideration is the host's resistance. A tooth should *never* be extracted because of a persisting positive culture when the host resistance factors are normal (e.g., pain, exudation, swelling, and tenderness all absent).

Antibiotic sensitivity testing

Some clinicians have advocated the taking of a culture during an endodontic patient's first visit.[160] They state that the culture should then be incubated and sent to a microbiologic laboratory for identification and antibiotic sensitivity testing. Their rationale is that if acute symptoms develop the dentist will have available a specific effective antibiotic. The fallacies in this reasoning and some shortcomings of antibiotic sensitivity testing are as follows.

1. Microbial detection using only a single culture medium is difficult, and the species detected may not be the one causing the disease.

2. Microbes that are present at the first visit may differ from the microbes that may cause acute symptoms at a subsequent visit.

3. Detection of obligate anaerobes is difficult because most microbiologic laboratories in dental schools do not have the necessary equipment. In addition, antibiotic sensitivity testing is more exacting for obligate anaerobes than it is for aerobes and facultative anaerobes. However, several techniques[91] may be helpful in this regard.[44,91,189]

Another major problem is that most clinical laboratories have been reluctant to perform routine anaerobic antibiotic susceptibility testing because of (1) the technical difficulties of obtaining pure cultures of microbial isolates (as discussed previously) and (2) the lack of standardized methods of analysis.[59] An additional problem is that many anaerobic infections are caused by a mixed anaerobic flora (as occurs in endodontic infections). It is impossible to isolate and test all the species present in a reasonable time period. Also, as will be discussed shortly, the empirical use of penicillin V and erythromycin (to a lesser extent) has been effective against oral anaerobes.[2,73] Therefore there has been little need for *routine* antibiotic susceptibility testing.

4. Cellulitis may be the result of hypersensitivity (allergic) reaction. Because antibiotic sensitivity testing does not consider microbial virulence, it may be that the microbes are only ''innocent bystanders'' and not causally related to the disease process.

5. Interpretations must consider the clinical dose range, which

---

*References 6, 14, 57, 138, 187, 197.

may be altered by the allergenicity, toxicity, and routes of administration of the antibiotic and the age, weight, and systemic condition of the patient.

Nevertheless, there are rare times (e.g., in severe unresponsive cellulitis) when it is important for the clinician to try to determine which microbes are present so that an effective antibiotic can be prescribed. Hence, even with its shortcomings, antibiotic sensitivity testing may be needed if fluid can be aspirated and culturing can be done anaerobically.

Phase microscopy

The phase microscope is a special optical microscope that allows for visualization of living, unstained microorganisms. It can be used for demonstrating living root canal microorganisms to the patient when the clinician is discussing the importance of techniques (e.g., cleaning and shaping) for removing microbes.

LOCAL ANTIMICROBIAL AGENTS

Local antimicrobial action can occur in five ways: (1) mechanical instrumentation of the root canal system, (2) canal irrigation (physical dislodgement of microbes and antiseptic action of a drug), (3) intracanal medication (antiseptic action of a drug), (4) canal obturation (entombs the microbes; cements and fillings also have antimicrobial action), and (5) periodontal curettage (in endodontic-periodontal cases of periodontal origin).

Mechanical instrumentation of the root canal system

During pulpectomy and instrumentation, there is a gross removal of microbes.[95] Subsequent studies have shown that some microbes may remain behind in dentinal tubules.[187,202] However, if the root canal is well obturated, these microbes usually die or remain dormant.

Irrigation

In vital cases, *sodium hypochlorite at high concentrations is not advocated,* because it is a pulp tissue solvent[162] and could irritate tissue in lateral canals. In vitro findings have shown that *5.25% sodium hypochlorite (usual clinical concentration) is more destructive to vital tissues than to microbes whereas 0.5% sodium hypochlorite dissolves necrotic tissue but not vital tissue.*[207] Hence, a 0.5% to 1.0% concentration of sodium hypochlorite is recommended for vital cases. In necrotic cases, where there is a probability of dead tissue in lateral and accessory canals, irrigation with higher concentrations of sodium hypochlorite, which is a good necrotic tissue solvent,[162] is suggested. It is also recommended in those types of cases because of its antimicrobial effect. One study[40] reported that 0.5% sodium hypochlorite was more effective than saline as an antimicrobial agent. However, it did show that instrumentation and irrigation with saline could temporarily render root canals sterile 50% of the time. They also found *no* significant antimicrobial difference between 0.5% and 5.0% sodium hypochlorite. These same investigators also reported that the combined use of EDTA and 5.0% sodium hypochlorite was the most effective antimicrobially. It has

also been shown that ultrasonics along with sodium hypochlorite irrigation increased the effectiveness of the irrigant in debris removal.[146] Cavitation, which occurs from ultrasonic therapy, can destroy bacteria.

Care must be taken that no sodium hypochlorite solution is forcibly expressed beyond the apical foramen, because pain and swelling will result.[19] Hydrogen peroxide (3%) alone and in combination with sodium hypochlorite (5%) has also been used effectively for irrigation. However, forceful expression of hydrogen peroxide can result in pain and emphysema.[123] One study has shown that the combination technique is no more effective than sodium hypochlorite used alone.[216] It was also found that a combination of Gly-Oxide (10% urea peroxide in an anhydrous glycerol base) and 5.25% sodium hypochlorite was no more effective than the hypochlorite alone in destroying *Bacteroides melaninogenicus.*[76] Saline was totally ineffective against this species. Investigators also found that 5.25% sodium hypochlorite was the most effective irrigant against *Bacteroides melaninogenicus.* As emphasized in this chapter, this anaerobe is a dangerous root canal pathogen. Nevertheless, Grossman[94] has stated that merely opening the tooth and introducing atmospheric oxygen is sufficient to destroy obligate anaerobes; however, Foley, et al. found that atmospheric oxygen was totally ineffective against *Bacteroides melaninogenicus.* When properly used, 5.25% sodium hypochlorite causes no more pain than does saline and is the most effective irrigant for chemical-mechanical removal of pulpal and dentinal debris.[103] In support of this, others[39] found that sodium hypochlorite effectively detoxified bacterial endotoxins. Chlorhexidine has been investigated as an antibacterial root canal irrigant.[181] Although it was must more effective than saline, it was *less* effective than 2.5% sodium hypochlorite. Considering all the evidence, it appears that sodium hypochlorite is the irrigant of choice but the optimum concentration has not yet been definitely established.

Intracanal medication

In pulpless cases the main use of a medicament is to help destroy microbes; it may also be used for anodyne effect and for fluid removal. Although periapical healing may be faster after the use of polyantibiotic root canal paste, results of a controlled study showed no difference in healing between cases treated with polyantibiotics and those treated with nonspecific intracanal medications.[212]

PBSC (a polyantibiotic) was withdrawn from clinical use by the action of the Food and Drug Administration.[114] It is not advocated because of the allergy-inducing possibilities of the penicillin component. Formocresol is highly irritating and must be used cautiously in the canal in a diluted (1:50) and almost dry form. Propylene glycol has been shown to be effective in diluting formocresol.[222]

Formocresol may also act as a hapten because of the formalin content and, therefore, may cause deleterious hypersensitivity reactions.[206] Beechwood creosote has been shown to be less irritating than formocresol but formocresol had greater bactericidal activity.[136] Camphorated monochlorophenol (CMCP) has been shown to be less irritating than formocresol.[220] Other studies[240] indicate that glutaraldehyde is effective but much less toxic than formaldehyde. In a recent in vitro study,[177] a new medicament, dimethylsubermidate, fixed tissue as well or better than formalin and was less antigenic than formalin or glutaraldehyde. In vitro studies[52,148,207] have shown 2% iodine-potassium iodide to be the most tissue-tolerant drug combination that is still antimicrobial, although the iodine component can also act as a hapten, a possibility that must be considered for allergic persons. Another iodine mixture that has been suggested as having potential as a root canal medicament is a povidone-iodine mixture.[45] It is reported to have low toxicity and a wide antimicrobial spectrum. It was shown to be less irritating than both CMCP and eugenol and greater antimicrobial activity than eugenol and cresatin. One study[243] reported that dequalinium acetate is an effective irrigant and intracanal medicament with low tissue toxicity. Calcium hydroxide ($Ca[OH]_2$) has antimicrobial activity and recently has been evaluated as an intracanal medicament. In one study,[209] it was found not to be as effective as CMCP. In two more recent comprehensive studies,[42,190] calcium hydroxide was shown to be a better and longer lasting antimicrobial medicament than either 2% iodine-potassium iodide or CMCP. Hence, *calcium hydroxide may prove to be the intracanal medicament of choice for pulpless cases.*

In vital cases when treatment is completed in one visit, no intracanal medicaments are used. In vital cases completed in multiple vitis, a sedative-type dressing such as eugenol or metacresylacetate (Cresatin) may be used.[15,222] Corticosteroids are also used clinically for intracanal sedation. In a recent controlled double-blind study,[159] it was shown that the intracanal use of the corticosteroid solution Decadron (dexamethasone, 4 mg/ml) as an irrigant and intracanal medicament was statistically significantly better than a placebo in the control of postoperative pain in the first 24 hours following instrumentation of vital-inflamed cases. In contrast, another report[135] states that no medicaments, including Cresatin and eugenol, were better than a dry cotton pellet in reducing interappointment pain.

Another possible problem with intracanal medicaments is their short-lived antibacterial activity. Part of the rationale for the use of intracanal medicaments is that their use might prevent reinfection of the canal via coronal or periapical leakage and reduce the risk of microbial proliferation within the canal. One recent report[145] found that 90% to 95% of CMCP is lost within 24 hours, but others found that calcium hydroxide maintained its antimicrobial activity for weeks.[214] An experimental method for the controlled release of intracanal medicaments has been devised that hopefully will overcome the problem of rapid inactivation of medicaments.[232]

Obturation

Some cements (e.g., paraformaldehyde-containing pastes) have antimicrobial effects, but tissue destruction usually results as well. Silver cones and amalgam are supposed to have an oligodynamic effect (antimicrobial action from the heavy metal ions). In these also, tissue destruction may result. The obturation process itself can cause entrapment of microbes. A recent study showed that these microbes die following obturation.[61]

Periodontal curettage

There are cases of the endodontic-periodontal syndrome in which open lateral canals or dentinal tubules feed microbes and their products into the pulp (Chapter 17). Apparently periodontal therapy, including curettage and surgical procedures, can decrease the ingress of these microbes into the pulp.

ANTIBIOTICS

If swelling is minor in degree and limited in scope and if it can be relieved by root canal or soft tissue drainage, antibiotics are not necessary. However, even in these limited cases, if the swelling recurs or if the drainage procedures are not effective within 24 hours, then antibiotics should be used to prevent the serious complications that were discussed earlier.

Patients with cellulitis and osteomyelitis must be treated with antibiotics. Patients with the following conditions should be protected with antibiotics during treatment[147]: rheumatic or congenital heart disease, heart prosthesis, organ transplant, Addison's disease, Cushing's disease (or conditions treated with corticosteroids), asplenic[219] immunologloglobulin or T-cell deficiency diseases,[219] uncontrolled or poorly controlled diabetes,[101] valvular prosthesis or grafts, total hip replacements, uremia, leukemia, granulocytopenia, hypothyroidism, multiple myeloma, Paget's disease, conditions treated with immunosuppressive drugs, radiation, and antimetabolites, and malnutrition. Earlier a discussion was given of the impaired resistance of diabetics. Leukemic patients have neutropenia, impaired migration and decreased killing ability of PMNs, reduced level of immunoglobulins,[89] and impairment of T-cell immune responses. Patients with implanted vascular autografts generally do not need antibiotic prophylaxis, but in patients with implanted synthetic vascular grafts, antibiotic prophylaxis is mandatory.[131] Whether to use antibiotics for routine periapical surgery is debatable. However, a recent study[70] indicates that routine surgery results in a marked impairment of PMNs to kill microbes. In addition, the stress related to surgery and the increased protein catabolism temporarily impairs the immune response. Hence, it may be beneficial to prophylactically use antibiotics before periapical surgery.

Systemic administration of antibiotics is usually recommended when a traumatically avulsed tooth is replanted, in order to prevent the deleterious effects from microbial contamination. In a recent study,[99a] it was also shown that systemic antibiotic administration at the time of replantation results in a dramatic reduction of inflammatory root resorption.

The clinician must use antibiotics for manipulative endodontic procedures on patients with true heart murmurs. This is because oral microbes can be dispersed into the bloodstream and attack damaged heart valves. Infective endocarditis can result and is serious and difficult to treat. For these patients, penicillin should be used before each visit but it is preferable to do the case in one visit. If penicillin allergy exists, erythromycin is indicated.

The following treatment schedule is recommended by the Committee on Rheumatic Fever and Infective Endocarditis of the American Heart Association in consultation with the Council on Dental Therapeutics of the American Dental Association.[55]

1. Standard regimen. Penicillin V, 2 g 1 hour before the procedure, and then 1 g 6 hours later. For patients unable to take oral antibiotics, 2 million units of aqueous penicillin G is given intravenously or intramuscularly 30 to 60 minutes before the procedure, then 1 million units 6 hours later.

2. Standard regimen for patients allergic to penicillin. Erythromycin, 1 g 1 hour before the procedure, and then 500 mg 6 hours later. For those who cannot tolerate either penicillin or erythromycin, an oral cephalosporin may be useful in the same dosage schedule as erythromycin. However, data are lacking on this regimen. Tetracyclines are not recommended.

3. Patients taking oral penicillin for secondary prevention of rheumatic fever or for other purposes. Erythromycin, following dosage schedule given in 2, or vancomycin 1 g intravenously slowly over 1 hour, starting 1 hour before the procedure.

4. Patients with prosthetic heart valves and others with highest risk of endocarditis. Ampicillin 1 to 2 g plus gentamycin 1.5 mg/kg, both intramuscularly or intravenously ½ hour before the procedure, followed by either 1 g oral penicillin V six hours later or a repeat of the parenteral regimen 8 hours later.

In all these cases, the clinician should first verify that the patient took the appropriate antibiotics. There is no evidence that patients who have had coronary artery bypass surgery are at risk for infective endocarditis. Although they are at low risk for endocarditis, dentists may choose to use prophylactic antibiotics for patients with cardiac pacemakers.

With endodontically related infections, penicillins G and V or phenethicillin potassium (if taken orally) are the drugs of choice if no allergy exists. As mentioned previously, oral microbes usually interact synergistically in the development of oral infections and penicillin inhibits this synergistic activity by killing the penicillin-sensitive microbes and rendering the penicillin-resistant microbes nonpathogenic[96] Even though penicillin does not appear to affect the cell wall of gram-negative microbes such as *Bacteroides melaninogenicus,* it may still render them ineffective by its destruction of gram-positive species on which the gram-negatives are dependent. One possible way is related to the finding that certain gram-positive microbes provide vitamin K to the *Bacteroides* as an essential metabolite. When the gram-positive strains are destroyed by penicillin, the *Bacteroides* no longer are provided with the vitamin K and therefore perish.[92] Almost all of the recent studies have shown that penicillin V remains the preferred antibiotic to treat outpatient odontogenic infections.* Penicillin V has low direct tissue toxicity but the highest allergy-inducing potential of all the endodontically useful antibiotics[83] (discussed further in the latter part of this section). If it cannot be used, erythromycin is the next choice. Other antibiotics that may be useful are clindamycin hydrochloride hydrate (Cleocin) and the cephalosporins (Keflex, Duricef). Evidence exists, however, that serious

or even fatal reactions can occur from the use of clindamycin. Therefore it should be used only if no other antibiotics are effective. Tetracyclines and lincomycin (Lincocin) are rarely indicated.

The penicillins and cephalosporins are bactericidal. They act selectively to inhibit the formation of bacterial cell walls.[119] The resultant action causes (1) the development of protoplasts (bacteria without cell walls) that can rupture easily or (2) direct lysis of the bacteria. There is probably a difference in the chemical nature of the wall in gram-positive and gram-negative bacteria, accounting for the fact that gram-positive bacteria are attacked more readily. It is preferable to use a bactericidal agent rather than a bacteriostatic agent. This is especially true for patients who have a decreased ability to fight infection, such as diabetics and those taking immunosuppressant drugs. Another advantage of penicillin is that it has a narrow spectrum, which decreases the chance of superinfection (which causes gastrointestinal distress) and reduces the possibility of the development of resistant microbes.[204]

Erythromycin, lincomycin, clindamycin, and the tetracyclines all inhibit bacterial protein synthesis. Because the direct death of the microbes does not occur (as is the case with penicillin), it is necessary for host defensive cells to aid in the destruction of the microbes.

The bacteria may recover if alternate enzymatic pathways are developed for protein synthesis. In addition, if the host's resistance is sufficiently reduced or the antibiotic dose is not adequate, the microbes can recover. There is also a good chance that resistant strains will develop if therapy is insufficient. Erythromycin is effective, but is not as effective as penicillin against penicillin-sensitive microbes. Nonetheless, an investigation[140] found erythromycin to be the antibiotic of choice for the "acute pulpal-alveolar cellulitis" syndrome. One form of erythromycin, ERYC, is in the form of pellets. It is purported to give better absorption and cause fewer gastrointestinal side effects than other forms of erythromycin.

Lincomycin may cause severe gastrointestinal distress, and clindamycin can cause serious or fatal reactions. One advantage of clindamycin is its low incidence of hypersensitivity reactions. Neither lincomycin nor clindamycin is as effective as penicillin against penicillin-sensitive organisms. Cephalosporins may show cross allergenicity with penicillin; consequently they are not indicated for patients allergic to penicillin. The cephalosporins have a wider spectrum that does penicillin and are bactericidal, but they are also more toxic than penicillin.

Broad-spectrum antibiotics, including ampicillin (a semisynthetic penicillin) and the tetracyclines, are less useful since endodontic infectious diseases are generally caused by gram-positive microbes, which are usually susceptible to penicillin. Penicillin and erythromycin (in high doses) are bactericidal whereas the tetracyclines are only bacteriostatic. Other disadvantages of the tetracyclines are as follows:[72,111,164]

1. Their use can lead to overgrowth of nonsusceptible microbes.

---

*References 48, 96, 105, 120, 165, 166, 169, 204, 243.

2. There is a high incidence of adverse drug interactions between the tetracyclines and various other drugs.
3. Tooth discoloration (photosensitivity) can occur if drugs are given during the developmental period of the involved teeth.
4. There are more side effects than with penicillin or erythromycin.

Although ampicillin has a broader spectrum than penicillin V, it is apparently less effective against the usual gram-positive microbes found in pulpal-periapical disease. Recently, it has been shown that metronidazole (Flagyl) is an effective and relatively nontoxic antimicrobial agent for the treatment of anaerobic infections of the jaws.[48,105] Metranidazole is bactericidal and does not show cross-allergenicity with penicillin, erythromycin, and clindamycin since it is chemically unrelated to them. Hence, it can be used for patients allergic to the other antibiotics. Metronidazole may cause an intolerance to alcohol; therefore, they should not be mixed.[48]

Antibiotics, used therapeutically, should usually be given for approximately 5 days in order to eliminate the microbes. Therapy of 2 weeks or longer can lead to allergic reactions, drug toxicity, and superinfections from resistant organisms and therefore should be avoided.

Antibiotic sensitivity testing is fallible, but it does have its indications. For example, if after 36 to 48 hours the original antibiotic is apparently not effective in patients with cellulitis, then antibiotic sensitivity testing should be done by aspirating fluid (if present). However, as discussed previously anaerobes are usually involved in cellulitis cases and they are difficult to culture and test for antibiotic sensitivity. Also, quite frequently the swelling is firm and diffuse and if an incision is made, only blood is withdrawn. Therefore one is faced with making an empiric choice for another antibiotic. The three main possible etiologic factors of the cellulitis are penicillinase-producing microbes, gram-negative microbes, and obligate anaerobic microbes. Penicillinase-producing microbes are more likely to be found in the confined atmosphere of a hospital, where resistant strains can rapidly emerge and facultative organisms such as *Staphylococcus aureus* are more likely. In that case, the semisynthetic penicillinase-resistant penicillins (e.g., Unipen) should be tried. These drugs should not be used as the sole antibiotic because they are not as effective as penicillins G and V or phenethicillin potassium (Syncillin) against most oral microbes. Most oral infections appear to be of the gram-positive, synergistic gram-negative variety (susceptible to penicillin V); but if penicillin V is not producing results, the assumption can be made that gram-negative microbes are predominantly involved. In addition, if the cellulitis is not superficial, then it is likely that obligate anaerobes are involved (prevalent in deep space infections). Considering that many pathogenic obligate anaerobes are also gram-negative (e.g., *Bacteroides melaninogenicus),* in this situation one should choose an antibiotic that is effective against gram-negative anaerobes. Such an antibiotic is clindamycin. Since the possible toxic responses to clindamycin usually occur after prolonged use (2 weeks or longer), a desirable dosage is

300 mg q. 6 h. until the cellulitis is gone (generally within 3 days) and then 150 mg q. 6 h. for another 4 days (to eliminate persisters). If gram-positive anaerobes are involved, clindamycin is also effective against most of them. Nevertheless, because of its possible serious adverse effects, clindamycin should only be used if none of the other antibiotics is effective. Another antibiotic effective against obligate anaerobes is metronidazole (Table 12-2).

As discussed before, because of the decreased usage of antibiotics by dentists for fear of inducing serious hypersensitivity reactions and inducing resistant strains of microbes, there has occurred what appears to be an alarming increase in serious life-threatening infectious diseases secondary to pulpal-periapical diseases. Many of the patients did not show any clinical signs of impaired resistance and their medical histories were noncontributory. In addition, several of the life-threatening sequelae to pulpal-induced periapical pathosis occurred in individuals who, when first seen by the dentist, had either no untoward signs and symptoms or minimal negative clinical manifestations. As was discussed previously,[41,213] researchers,[41] found that in every instance in which a necrotic pulp with a periapical lesion was present, the root canal was infected with obligate anaerobes. The aforementioned life-threatening infections were almost always caused by some combination of obligate anaerobic microbes. Since penicillin V and erythromycin are usually effective against these microbes, it seems to make good sense to use either of the antibiotics as a prophylactic measure to prevent these serious sequelae. (The use of antibiotics for asymptomatic teeth with necrotic pulps and associated periapical lesions is not prophylaxis in the strict sense since researchers have not demonstrated that these cases are always infected with the dangerous obligate anaerobes.[41] Hence, treatment is really of an existing infection before it has had an opportunity to exacerbate.) However, in terms of risk vs. benefit, the risk of flare-up is substantially reduced with prophylactic administration of antibiotics for nonvital cases.[155]

When penicillin V or erythromycin is used prophylactically, serious sequela have not occurred. The rationale for antibiotic prophylaxis is that the antibiotic would attack the microbes during the period of contamination before colonization had occurred, or if colonization had occurred, before actual invasion had begun (i.e., while the microbes are limited to the root canal).

It has been shown that the antibiotic prophylactic regimen can prevent serious sequelae from pulpal-periapical pathosis; let us consider the possible objections. First, hypersensitivity reactions are examined. The major disadvantage of penicillin is its high hypersensitivity-inducing ability.[83] With the increased use of penicillin in clinical medicine and dentistry, veterinary medicine, industry, and agriculture, many patients have been exposed to penicillin without their prior knowledge.[5] This partly accounts for allergic reactions in patients having their first clinical exposure to penicillin. Nevertheless, oral penicillin is much safer in regard to inducing hypersensitivity reactions than is injectable penicillin.

Now, let us consider the development of resistant strains

TABLE 12-2. Useful antibiotics

	Use	Usual dosage*
Penicillin V	Antibiotic of choice if no allergy exists	One tablet (500 mg) every 6 hr
Erythromycin stearate or base (ERYC)†	Antibiotic of choice if penicillin allergy exists	One capsule or tablet (500 mg) every 6 hr
Penicillinase-resistant penicillins (Staphcillin, Prostaphlin, Unipen)	Penicillinase producers are detected and are sensitive to these antibiotics	One tablet (500 mg) every 6 hr
Ampicillin (Penbritin, Omnipen, Polycillin)	Gram-negative microbes are detected and are sensitive to these antibiotics	One capsule (500 mg) every 6 hr
Cephalexin monohydrate (Keflex)	Broader spectrum than penicillin; not affected by penicillinase but affected by cephaloridase; more side reactions than penicillin, cannot be used for patients with penicillin allergy	Two tablets (500 mg) every 6 hr
Cefadroxil (Duricef, Ultracef) Cephradine (Anspor, Velosef)		One capsule (500 mg) twice a day or one tablet (1 g) once daily
Clindamycin (Cleocin)‡		Two tablets (total of 300 mg) every 6 hr for first 3 days (or until swelling is markedly decreased); then one tablet (150 mg) every 6 hr for the next 2 days
Metronidazole (Flagyl)	Penicillin and erythromycin have not been effective for a cellulitis case (apparently anaerobic) that is not improving	Two tablets (total of 500 mg) every 6 hr for first 3 days or until swelling is markedly decreased); then one tablet every 6 hr for 4 days

*For patients with cellulitis and no signs of toxemia (high fever, disorientation) the adult dosage should be at least 500 mg every 6 hours for 2 to 3 days followd by 250 mg every 6 hours for another 4 to 5 days. For cellulitis plus signs of toxemia, IV or IM injections of massive doses and hospitalization may be required.

†The stearate or base form is recommended because an infrequent side effect of the estolate form is cholestatic hepatitis.[161]

‡Be aware of the possibility of pseudomembranous colitis (see text).

of microbes from antibiotic usage. It is true that microbes are becoming resistant to antibiotics at an increasing rate.[48] Nevertheless, it appears from this vantage point to be more important to use the antibiotics that are most effective at the time (i.e., penicillin V with gram-positive synergistic anaerobic infections of the pulp and periapex). In the event resistant strains develop in the future, newer antibiotics are continually being produced that can deal with most of these emerging resistant strains.

There is one other advantage for the prophylactic use of antibiotics in periapical "area" cases; that is, the reduction of pain.

In a recent study in which antibiotics were used,[155] it was observed that although the patients were given narcotic analgesic prescriptions, in many of the cases the prescriptions were not used. Apparently, the antibiotics effectively controlled much of the pain while simultaneously preventing the swelling. The swelling is most likely controlled by antimicrobial action. The destruction or inhibition of the microbes would subsequently prevent the release of their inflammatory and exudate-producing substances. With the inactivation of the microbial irritants, the host's own inflammatory substances would soon stop being produced. This would then allow the lymphatic system to drain the exudate. The end result would be an absence or diminution of swelling. Concerning the pain inhibition, it appears that swelling causes pressure on nerve endings. Microbial and host defensive cells also produce pain-inciting inflammatory substances. When

the swelling is reduced as a result of the antibiotic's activity, the pressure on the nerve endings should subsequently be decreased with an alleviation of the pain. With the inhibition or destruction of the microbes, the release of pain-producing substances by the microbes and host cells would soon cease. This, in turn, would result in minimizing or avoiding pain.

Therefore it appears that the prophylactic use of antibiotics for asymptomatic teeth with necrotic pulps and associated periapical lesions imposes much less risk to the patient in terms of allergy and bacterial resistance than the risk of serious sequelae such as septicemia, Ludwig's angina, cavernous sinus thrombosis, and brain abscess.

When failures occur and periapical lesions develop or fail to heal, except in the case of radicular cysts, where the lesion is self-perpetuating either on an irritant or immunologic basis,[157,158,227] the primary etiologic factor is microbes. The primary cause of failures is incomplete obturation.[115] In essence, there are voids in the root canal system and it is not tissue fluids that causes the periapical breakdown as several investigators[77,85,170,231] who have debunked the "hollow tube" theory have shown. It is microbes. Where do they come from? Two studies[60,62] have shown that anachoresis does not occur to necrotic tissue; vital-inflamed tissue is essential. Where does the vital-inflamed tissue come from in obturated root canals? There

TABLE 12-3. Useful analgesics

	Ingredients	Degree of pain*	Usual dosage†
Aspirin (acetylsalicylic acid)		Mild to moderate	300 to 600 mg every 3 to 4 hr
Darvocet-N	Proproxyphene napsylate (50 mg) and acetaminophen (325 mg)	Mild to moderate	Two tablets every 4 hr
Darvon (32 mg propoxyphene hydrochloride)		Mild to moderate	One capsule every 4 hr
Tylenol (acetaminophen)		Mild to moderate	One or two tablets (325 to 650 mg) every 3 to 4 hr
Ponstel (mefenamic acid)		Mild to moderate	Two tablets (500 mg) to begin with; then one tablet every 6 hr
Motrin	Ibuprofen (400, 600, 800 mg)	Moderate to severe	One tablet every 4 to 8 hr depending on dosage form
Dolobid	Diflunisal/MSD (500 mg)	Moderate to severe	Two tablets to begin with; then one tablet every 12 hr (some patients may require one every 8 hr)
Suprol	Suprofen	Moderate to severe	One tablet every 4 to 6 hr
Anaprox	Naproxen (275 mg)	Moderate to severe	Two tablets to begin with; then one tablet every 6 to 8 hr
Codeine alone and in other combinations		Moderate to severe	30 mg every 4 hr
Vicodin	Hydrocodone bitartrate (5 mg) and acetaminophen (500 mg)	Moderate to severe	One tablet every 6 hr
Synalgos-DC	Dihydrocodeine (16 mg), aspirin (356.4 mg), caffeine (30 mg)	Moderate to severe	One or two capsules every 4 hr
Talwin (pentazocine hydrochloride)		Moderate to severe	One tablet (50 mg) every 3 to 4 hr
Percodan	Oxycodone hydrochloride (4.5 mg), oxycodone terephthalate (0.38 mg), aspirin (325 mg)	Severe	One tablet every 6 hr
Demerol (meperidine hydrochloride)		Severe	One tablet (50 mg) every 4 hr

*Author's opinion.
†For a 150-pound adult.

are two sources.[197] The first is pulp tissue remnants that have not been removed before the obturation. They can be either in accessory canals, lateral canals, secondary canals, or primary canals. The second is granulomatous tissue (in the case of periapical lesions), which invades the root canal and fills in any voids in the root canal system. This tissue has an abundant blood supply and is protected inside the solid walls of dentin. Therefore anachoresis can occur to this tissue as well. One may ask: "What about the microbes that could have been left behind in the dentinal tubules or the root canal system?" This has been discussed previously when it was shown that several studies revealed that remaining microbes either become entombed, inert, or die following obturation and they have no effect on success rate.* Therefore a logical conclusion is that it is essential to have a well-obturated root canal system with a material that may be initially antimicrobial but that becomes inert in a relatively short time (unlike corroding silver cones, which are a continuous irritant, and are most likely the primary nonmicrobial source of periapical breakdown). Even nonendodontic failures from endodontic

cases have a strong microbiologic etiologic component. When failures result from cases in which there is gross occlusal leakage because of a poor or absent coronal restoration, the microbes travel from the oral cavity along obturation defects (no seal is perfect) in the primary or lateral canals. When failures result from fractures, microbes travel along the fracture lines. When failures result from post preparations, defects are created in the obturation along which microbes and/or their products travel. Finally, when failures result from post perforations, microbes travel along the perforations.

OTHER TYPICAL SYSTEMIC DRUGS AND SUPPLEMENTS USED IN ENDODONTICS

The following categories of drugs and supplements are discussed in this section: analgesics, sedatives and antianxiety agents, antiinflammatory agents, and nutritional supplements. For each category, certain information is given: indications, side effects, contraindications, and dosages. *When writing prescriptions, the clinician should include "label as such" on the prescription. This precaution will ensure that the bottle will have the name of the drug labeled.* In cases of allergic reactions, drug interactions, and drug toxicity, labeling is very important.

*References 6, 14, 57, 61, 138, 187, 197.

Analgesics

Analgesics are drugs given for pain relief. They may be used before, during, or after treatment. A summary chart showing useful analgesics is given in Table 12-3.

The placebo effect should be considered when dispensing or prescribing analgesics. It has been suggested that placebo analgesia may be mediated by endorphins (naturally occurring morphine like pain-reducing substances).[71] Hence, the clinician should prescribe and dispense with enthusiasm to maximize the potential placebo effect.

The two major types of analgesics are nonnarcotics and narcotics.[33,111] The nonnarcotics act principally at the peripheral nerve endings by inhibiting the synthesis of prostaglandins. They do not produce addiction or tolerance and their toxicity is much less than that of the narcotics. However, they may be effective only for mild to moderate pain. The narcotics act within the central nervous system and do cause addiction and produce tolerance. However, they produce potent analgesia and varying degrees of sedation and euphoria. Because of the different sites of activity and the different mechanisms of action, a combination of nonnarcotic and narcotic analgesics is generally very effective for endodontic pain.

Mild to moderate pain

Nonnarcotic drugs (aspirin, propoxyphene formulations, acetaminophen, mefenamic acid) are used to treat patients with mild to moderate pain.

Aspirin (acetylsalicylic acid). Aspirin remains the most widely used analgesic. It is contraindicated for patients receiving corticosteroids or anticoagulants; those with gout, gastric ulcer, or asthma; or those allergic to it. A rare series of reactions to aspirin —including the triad of chronic rhinitis, nasal polyposis, and asthma—comprise aspirin idiosyncrasy. Dentists should avoid aspirin use in patients with a history of any of the triad symptoms.

A typical dose is one or two tablets (300 to 600 mg) every 3 to 4 hours. Common aspirin compounds include Anacin (aspirin 400 mg and caffeine 32 mg), Bufferin (aspirin 324 mg, aluminum glycinate 49 mg, and magnesium carbonate 97 mg), Ecotrin (an enteric-coated aspirin tablet designed to minimize the gastrointestinal irritation of aspirin [this has not been proved]), Excedrin (acetaminophen 250 mg, aspirin 250 mg, and caffeine 65 mg), and Empirin Compound (aspirin 325 mg). There is no definite proof that these preparations are more effective than aspirin alone. However, caffeine is included in some preparations to establish a sense of well-being, and the aluminum and magnesium compounds are included in Bufferin to minimize the irritating gastric effects of aspirin; this has not been proved.[49]

Propoxyphene formulations. These products (Darvon, Darvon Compound-32, Darvon Compound-65, Darvon-N with A.S.A., Darvocet-N) are all preparations made up or composed of one or more of the following: propoxyphene hydrochloride, propoxyphene napsylate, aspirin, and acetaminophen. Plain Darvon can be prescribed for patients with aspirin allergies. The most popular formulation has

been Darvon Compound-65. Studies reported by the Lilly Company,[69] however, have shown that it may be no more effective than aspirin, although the evidence is inconclusive.

Darvon was formerly thought to be nonaddictive, but recent findings[111] have indicated that people can become habituated to it. Darvon-N 100 with A.S.A. was made to prevent addicts from "mainlining" (injecting the propoxyphene into their veins). A combination of these drugs (excluding aspirin) is Darvocet-N, devised to give the advantages of acetaminophen and of Darvon. This formulation is especially desirable for patients in whom aspirin is contraindicated. Side effects are dizziness, euphoria, gastrointestinal disturbances, and occasional sedation and skin rash. An average dose is one capsule every 4 to 6 hours for Darvon Compound-65 and Darvon-N with A.S.A. Two tablets of Darvocet-N should be given every 4 hours. Propoxyphene can cause dizziness and euphoria; therefore patients should be warned about driving a motor vehicle.

Acetaminophen (N-acetyl-*p*-aminophenol). Acetaminophen (e.g., Phenaphen) is the active breakdown product of phenacetin. Acetaminophen is useful in patients with aspirin allergies or who are taking uricosuric drugs for gout treatment. Unlike aspirin, it does not affect the action of anticoagulants or cause gastrointestinal bleeding.[111] It is not indicated for long-term use in patient with kidney or liver diseases.

Formulations containing acetaminophen are Tylenol (acetaminophen 325 mg), Nebs (acetaminophen 325 mg), Valadol (acetaminophen 325 mg), Phenaphen (acetaminophen 325 mg), Empracet (acetaminophen 300 mg), Anacin 3 (acetaminophen 500 mg), Percogesic (acetaminophen 325 mg and phenytoxamine citrate 30 mg), Trigesic (acetaminophen 125 mg, aspirin 230 mg, and caffeine 30 mg), and the aforementioned Darvocet-N. Usual dosage is one to two tablets (325 mg) every 3 to 4 hours. Trigesic and Excedrin contain aspirin; therefore they are contraindicated for any person who cannot take aspirin. Unlike aspirin and the nonsteroidal antiinflammatories (discussed shortly), acetaminophen has little, if any, antiinflammatory activity.[111] Since pulpal and periapical pain are related to inflammation, if there are no contraindications, aspirin and the nonsteroidal antiinflammatories are preferable to control endodontically related pain.

Mefenamic acid. The common preparation is Ponstel Kapseals (mefenamic acid 250 mg).

This drug is useful for patients with aspirin allergies. It should not be given to the following patients: (1) those with intestinal ulcers, asthma, abnormal kidney function, or gastrointestinal inflammations, (2) children under 14 years of age, and (3) women in the childbearing age (or who are pregnant). Side effects include headache, dizziness, drowsiness, nausea, and nervousness. The usual dose is two tablets (500 mg) at the onset, followed by one tablet (250 mg) every 6 hours. Ponstel should not be used for more than 1 week. Patients should be cautioned against operating a motor vehicle when taking Ponstel because of the possible side effects.[49]

Tryptophan. In a recent controlled double-blind study,[203] it was shown that tryptophan was significantly better than a placebo in the control of postoperative endodontic pain in the first 24 hours following the initiation of treatment. All types of cases were involved (i.e., anterior, posterior, vital-inflamed, and necrotic teeth with and without periapical "areas"). The finding of the effectiveness of tryptophan for pain relief is important for two reasons: (1) Generally, the most intense and highest frequency of endodontic pain occurs in the first 24 hours following initial treatment. It was during this time period that tryptophan was most effective. (2) Tryptophan is an essential amino acid with minimal side effects as compared to other analgesics. Further studies should be done to either corroborate or dispute these interesting findings.

Moderate to severe pain

Nonsteroidal antiinflammatories. The antiinflammatories have recently been introduced in dentistry for patients with moderate to severe pain. The principal preparations are Motrin (ibuprofen* 400, 600, 800 mg), Dolobid (diflusinal/MSD 500 mg), Anaprox (naproxen 275 mg), and Meclomen (meclofenamate 100, 200 mg).[188] A few of these have been shown in some studies[56,68] to outperform codeine in relieving dental pain. Clinical experience suggests that the drugs may be as effective as 30 mg of codeine. Their main advantages over narcotics are that they are neither addictive nor habit forming and they are well tolerated. Their most frequent side effect is mild gastrointestinal disturbance (generally less frequent and severe than aspirin).[111]

Nonnarcotics. The principal drug in this category is the benzomorphan pentazocine.

Pentazocine hydrochloride. Talwin, a benzomorphan, is reported to be as effective in a 50 mg dose as 60 mg of codeine and is useful in patients with codeine allergy. Its onset is more rapid and its action slightly shorter than those of codeine. It is contraindicated in patients with asthma and other lung diseases, cranial injuries, or cyanosis and in children under 12 years of age (not enough clinical trials have been conducted with children). Previously it was thought to be nonaddictive, but there have been reported cases of dependence.[97] The usual dosage is 50 mg every 3 to 4 hours. For severe pain, 100 mg can be used. Because of possible side effects patients should be cautioned against driving.

Narcotics. These drugs are indicated for severe to extreme pain and cause a degree of sedation. The effective range is from codeine, hydrocodone bitartrate (Vicodin), and oxycodone hydrochloride (Percodan) for severe pain to meperidine hydrochloride (Demerol) for more intense pain.[98]

The narcotics should not be prescribed for patients with respiratory tract diseases and hypotension unless a medical clearance is obtained. Patients should be cautioned against operating a motor vehicle while under the influence of narcotics because of the depressant effects of the drugs. Narcotics should not be given to patients with cerebral diseases, lesions, and injuries.

Codeine. Alone, combined with aspirin, or as a constituent of proprietary compounds, codeine is the most frequently prescribed analgesic in dentistry for relief of severe pain. When all the narcotics are compared, codeine is the least addictive analgesic. Its side effects include constipation, nausea, sedation, and respiratory depression.

Persons may be allergic to codeine, but *usually it is the safest of the strong analgesics.* Commonly used forms and dosages include the following: one tablet codeine phosphate (30 mg) with two tablets aspirin (600 mg) every 4 hours; one capsule Phenaphen with ½ gr codeine phosphate (32.4 mg) every 4 hours; one tablet Empirin Compound no. 3 (30 mg codeine) every 4 hours; one tablet Tylenol with ½ gr codeine (30 mg) every 4 hours; one capsule Fiorinal no. 3 with codeine (30 mg codeine, 50 mg butalbital, 40 mg caffeine, 325 mg aspirin) every 4 to 6 hours, and one capsule Percogesic with codeine (codeine 32.4 mg). Tylenol and Phenaphen are useful in patients with aspirin allergy. Fiorinal and Percogesic contain a sedative used to control the anxiety that often accompanies pain (anxiety lowers the pain threshold).[49]

Hydrocodone preparations. Two compounds containing hydrocodone have been marketed: Vicodin and Synalgos-DC.[49,98]

Vicodin is a formulation for moderate to moderately severe pain. It contains hydrocodone bitartrate (5 mg), a semisynthetic analogue of codeine that purportedly has six times the potency of codeine, and acetaminophen, which is present in almost twice the dose found in most codeine-acetaminophen combinations. Vicodin is rapid acting (within 30 minutes) and long lasting. The usual adult dose is one tablet every 6 hours. It should not be administered to children. The drug has addiction potential. Vicodin can be prescribed by phone in most states and may prove to be an effective analgesic for endodontically induced pain.

The other, somewhat similar, codeine-type preparation that has been used effectively in endodontics is Synalgos-DC. This product contains dihydrocodeine (16 mg) in combination with aspirin (356.4 mg) and caffeine (30 mg). Its usual dosage is two capsules every 4 hours.

Severe pain

The two principal drugs in this category are Percodan and Demerol.

Oxycodone preparations. The complete formula of Percodan is oxycodone hydrochloride (4.5 mg), oxycodone terephthalate (0.38 mg), and aspirin (325 mg). The analgesic effect is comparable to that of codeine, but Percodan apparently has a longer duration. Its addiction potential is greater than that of codeine. Percodan should not be prescribed for patients who are allergic to any of the components. The usual dosage is one tablet every 6 hours.

For pain of less intensity or for children under 12, Percodan-Demi can be prescribed. It contains approximately

---

*Ibuprofen in a 200 mg formulation (Advil, Nuprin) is sold over the counter and is useful for mild to moderate pain.

TABLE 12-4. Sedatives and antianxiety agents

Agent	Category	Usual dosage*
Secobarbital (Seconal)	Sedative	50 mg night before appointment; 50 mg 30 min before appointment
Pentobarbital (Nembutal)	Sedative	30 mg night before appointment; 60 mg 30 min before appointment
Chloral hydrate (Noctec)†	Sedative	500 mg (in syrup) 30 min before appointment
Ethinamate (Valmid)	Sedative	One of two tablets (500 mg to 1 gr) night before appointment; one tablet 30 min before appointment
Diazepam (Valium)	Antianxiety	One tablet (5 mg) at night; one tablet on arising; one tablet 2 hours before appointment
Hydroxyzine hydrochloride (Atarax, Vistaril)	Antianxiety	50 mg night before appointment; 50 mg 30 min before appointment
Meprobamate (Equanil, Miltown)	Antianxiety	One tablet (400 mg) four times/day starting the night before appointment

*For 150-pound adult.
†Must never be given to a patient who is taking an anticoagulant. Hemorrhage can result from drug interactions.[36]

half the average adult dose. For people who cannot take aspirin, a formulation with acetaminophen is available. Known as Percocet-5 (5 mg oxycodone hydrochloride and 325 mg acetaminophen), it has been shown to be effective in relieving moderate to severe dental pain.[54] A similar analgesic combination is found in Tylox.

Meperidine hydrochloride. Demerol is a stronger analgesic than codeine, hydrocodone, or oxycodone. It also induces sedation. It is also more addicting than codeine. The average dose is one 50 mg tablet every 4 hours. For intense pain 100 mg can be prescribed. For children under 16, a 25 mg dose is recommended. The oral route is not as effective as the parenteral route.

Sedatives and antianxiety agents (Table 12-4)

Sedatives and antianxiety drugs are useful for premedication and "comedication" of the apprehensive patient. They do not have an analgesic effect. However, an anxious patient will experience less pain if some form of sedation is used with the analgesic. The resulting relaxation may potentiate the effect of the analgesic.[50] There are three categories: barbiturates, nonbarbiturate sedatives, and the antianxiety agents (meprobamate, phenothiazines, diazepines, and hydroxyzine). Sedatives affect the cortical centers. Antianxiety agents selectively depress the subcortical regions and are less likely to cause a decrease in mental alertness; they may also arrest aggressive actions.

The most popular antianxiety agents are the benzodiazepines. They offer certain advantages over the sedatives. They have fewer adverse reactions; the development of tolerance is less; they have many fewer drug interactions; and unlike the sedatives, mortality from drug overdose is almost unknown when the drugs are taken by themselves. Dependence may occur from long-term use (has been reported with diazepam) but withdrawal is less severe than with barbiturates. All of the benzodiazepines begin to take effect within 30 minutes after oral administration. A typical benzodiazepine is Valium (diazepam 5 mg). If there is need to help the patient have a good night's sleep prior to the endodontic procedures, two benzodiazepines are effective hypnotics. They are (1) Dalmane (flurazepam), 30 mg taken before retiring, and (2) Restoril (temazepam), 15 to 30 mg taken before retiring.

Alcohol and other CNS depressants should not be mixed with any of the benzodiazepines because of severe depressive interactive effects. Use of these agents is contraindicated in pregnant patients, as they may cause fetal damage. Patients who take antianxiety agents must be cautioned against driving because these drugs may cause drowsiness or lethargy.

Patients who take sedatives must not be allowed to drive. The clinician may want to give an extremely fearful patient a hypnotic dose the night before an endodontic visit.

Antiinflammatory agents (Table 12-5)

To control postsurgical swelling in endodontic therapy, antiinflammatory drugs have been and are currently being used. Yet a great deal of controversy surrounds their efficacy or need.[11,98] One may question the usefulness of interfering with inflammation because it is the normal reaction to injury and initiates repair. Nevertheless, for esthetic and functional reasons, limiting postsurgical swelling may be useful. When infection is present or suspected, an antibiotic must also be given. In addition, as endodontically related pain is invariably keyed to inflammation, it may be prudent to try to control inflammation. The nonsteroidal antiinflammatories and aspirin (see Analgesics, p. 387) have both analgesic and antiinflammatory action and should prove useful for endodontic inflammations.

Of the corticosteroids, dexamethasone (Decadron) has the highest antiinflammatory potential (over 30 times as potent as cortisone).[11] As discussed before, Decadron is effective for pain relief.

Nutritional supplements

To aid in repair, the patient should be given sufficient proteins, minerals, vitamins A, C, and B complex, and fluid (about 2.5 liters of water daily). It has been shown that stress depletes the vitamin C level in the blood,[180] and most patients experience stress before, during, or after surgery. Stress has also been found to be common before endodontic therapy.[148] In a study,[182] high daily dosages of vitamin C (500 to 3000 mg) were shown to accelerate wound healing significantly in patients judged to be not deficient in that vitamin. Furthermore, studies indicate that

TABLE 12-5. Antiinflammatory agents

Agent	Category	Usual dosage*
Aspirin (acetylsalicylic acid)	Analgesic	300 to 600 mg every 3 to 4 hr for few days
Ibuprofen (Motrin)	Analgesic	400 mg every 4 hr for few days
Diflunisal/MSD (Dolobid)	Analgesic	500 mg every 12 hr for few days
Naproxen (Anaprox)	Analgesic	275 mg; 2 tablets to start; then 1 every 6 to 8 hr
Dexamethasone (Decadron)	Corticosteroid	Two tablets (0.75 mg) twice a day for 2 days; then one tablet twice a day for 2 days; finally one tablet once a day for 2 days

*For a 150-pound adult.

vitamin C has antimicrobial activity.[183] Therefore a good practice is to give these individuals vitamin C presurgically and preendodontically and for a few days postsurgically and postendodontically (500 mg twice a day, preferably in a sustained- or slow-release capsule).

Since vitamin C is important for bone matrix formation, it is especially important in periapical lesion cases, as Seltzer[197] has stated: "It seems logical, therefore, that following endodontic treatment, especially of teeth with areas of rarefaction, the patient's diet should be supplemented with a daily intake of 300 mg vitamin C and larger quantities of protein to help promote healing of the bony tissue."

REFERENCES

1. Adams, M., and Carlsson, J.: Lactoperoxidase and thiocyanate protect bacteria from hydrogen peroxide, Infect. Immun. **35:**20, 1982.
2. Allard, U., Dornbusch, K., and Erik-Nord, C.: Susceptibility of bacteria isolated from oral infections to nine antibiotics in vitro, Swed. Dent. J. **2:**1, 1978.
3. Allard, U., et al.: Experimental infections with *Staphylococcus aureus, Streptococcus sanguis, Pseudomonas aeruginosa,* and *Bacteroides fragilis* in the jaws of dogs, Oral Surg. **48:**454, 1979.
4. Allen, D., Loughnan, T.E., and Ord, R.A.: A re-evaluation of the role of tracheostomy in Ludwig's angina, J. Oral Maxillofac. Surg. **43:**436, 1985.
5. Altman, L.C., and Tomkins, L.S.: Toxic and allergic manifestations of antimicrobials, Postgrad. Med. **64:**157, 1978.
6. Andreasen, J.O., and Rud, J.: A histobacteriologic study of dental and periapical structures after endodontic surgery, Int. J. Oral Surg. **1:**272, 1972.
7. Antrum, D.D.: Paresthesia of the inferior alveolar nerve caused by periapical pathology, J. Endod. **4:**220, 1978.
8. Arnold, R.R., et al.: Bactericidal activity of human lactoferrin: differentiation from the stasis of iron deprivation, Infect. Immun. **35:**792, 1982.
9. Austin, G., Deasy, M., and Walsh, R.F.: Osteomyelitis associated with routine endodontic and periodontal therapy: a case report, J. Oral Med. **33:**120, 1978.
10. Baddour, H.M., Durst, N.L., and Tilson, H.B.: Frontal lobe abscess of dental origin: report of case, Oral Surg. **47:**303, 1979.
11. Bahn, S.L.: Glucocorticosteroids in dentistry, J. Am. Dent. Assoc. **105:**476, 1982.
12. Baker, N.A., et al.: Scanning electron microscopic study of the efficacy of various irrigating solutions, J. Endod. **1:**127, 1975.
13. Balaban, F.S., Skidmore, A.E., and Griffin, J.A.: Acute exacerbations following initial treatment of necrotic pulps, J. Endod. **10:**78, 1984.
14. Barker, B.C.W., and Lockett, B.C.: Concerning the fate of bacteria following the filling of infected root canals. Aust. Dent. J. **17:**98, 1972.
15. Barnett, F., et al.: Tissue response to anodyne medicaments, Oral Surg. **58:**605, 1984.
15a. Barnett, F., et al.: Anaerobic bacteria in periapical lesions of human teeth (abstract 29), J. Endod. **12:**131, 1986.
16. Baum, R.H., et al.: Persistence of bacteria in infected root canals, Abstracts of the American Society of Microbiologists, no. B52, 77th annual meeting, 1977.
17. Baumgartner, J.C., Heggers, J.P., and Harrison, J.W.: Incidence of bacteremias related to endodontic procedures. II. Surgical endodontics, J. Endod. **3:**399, 1977.
18. Baumgartner, J.C., and Plack, W.F., III: Dental treatment and management of a patient with a prosthetic heart valve, J. Am. Dent. Assoc. **104:**181, 1982.
19. Becker, G.L., Cohen, S., and Borer, R.: The sequelae of accidentally injecting sodium hypochlorite beyond the root apex, Oral Surg. **38:**633, 1974.
20. Bender, I.B.: A commentary on General Bhaskar's hypothesis, Oral Surg. **34:**469, 1972.
21. Bender, I.B., et al.: Dental procedures in patients with rheumatic heart disease, Oral Surg. **16:**466, 1963.
22. Bender, I.B.: Recommendations questioned, J. Am. Dent. Assoc. **110:**874, 1985.
23. Bennett, I.L., Jr., and Beeson, P.B.: Bacteremia: a consideration of some experimental and clinical aspects, Yale J. Biol. Med. **26:**241, 1954.
24. Benoliel, R., and Asquith, J.: Actinomycosis of the jaws, Int. J. Oral Surg. **14:**195, 1985.
25. Bergenholtz, G.: Micro-organisms from necrotic pulp of traumatized teeth, Odont. Rev. **25:**347, 1974.
26. Bernheim, H.A., and Kluger, M.J.: Fever: effect of drug-induced antipyresis on survival, Science **193:**237, 1976.
27. Bhaskar, S.: Synopsis of oral pathology, ed. 7, St. Louis, 1986, The C.V. Mosby Co.
28. Biesterfeld, R.C., James, G.A., and Taintor, J.F.: Endodontic culturing—an educational aid, Dent. Manag. **19:**41, 1979.
29. Blechman, H.: Infections of pulp and periapical tissues. In Nolte, W.A., editor: Oral microbiology, ed. 4, St. Louis, 1982, The C.V. Mosby Co.
30. Block, R.M., et al.: A histopathologic, histobacteriologic, and radiographic study of periapical endodontic surgical specimens, Oral Surg. **42:**656, 1976.
31. Block, R.M., et al.: Cell-mediated immune response to dog pulp tissue altered by formocresol within the root canal, J. Endod. **3:**424, 1977.
32. Block, R.M., et al.: Antibody formation and cell-mediated immunity to dog pulp tissue altered by either endodontic sealers via the root canal, Int. Endod. J. **15:**105, 1982.
33. Bloomquist, D.S.: Pain control in endodontics, Dent. Clin. North Am. **23:**543, 1979.
34. Borssén, E., and Sundqvist, G.: Actinomyces of infected dental root canals, Oral Surg. **51:**643, 1981.

35. Brackett, S.E.: Infective endocarditis and mitral valve prolapse—the unsuspected risk, Oral Surg. **54**:273, 1982.

36. Brown, A.A.: Sedatives, hypnotics, and anxiolytics, Ont. Dent. **54**(2):14, 1977.

37. Buckley, J.P.: The chemistry of pulp decomposition, with a rational treatment for this condition and its sequelae, Dent. Cosmos **47**:223, 1905.

38. Bullock, J.D., and Fleishman, J.A.: The spread of odontogenic infections to the orbit: diagnosis and management, J. Oral Maxillofac. Surg. **43**:749, 1985.

39. Buttler, T.K., and Crawford, J.J.: The detoxifying effect of varying concentrations of sodium hypochlorite on endotoxins, J. Endod. **8**:59, 1982.

40. Byström, A., and Sundqvist, G.: Bacteriologic evaluation of the efficacy of mechanical root canal instrumentation in endodontic therapy, Scand. J. Dent. Res. **89**:321, 1981.

41. Byström, A., and Sundqvist, G.: The antibacterial action of sodium hypochlorite and EDTA in 60 cases of endodontic therapy, Int. Endod. J. **18**:35, 1985.

42. Byström, A., Claesson, R., and Sundqvist, G.: The antibacterial effect of camphorated paramonochlorophenol, camphorated phenol and calcium hydroxide in the treatment of infected root canals, Endod. Dent. Traumatol. **1**:170, 1985.

43. Carlsson, J., and Sundqvist, G.: Evaluation of methods of transport and cultivation of bacterial specimens from infected dental root canals, Oral Surg. **49**:451, 1980.

44. Carlsson, J., Frölander, R.F., and Sundqvist, G.: Oxygen tolerance of anaerobic bacteria isolated from necrotic dental pulps, Acta Odont. Scand. **35**:139, 1977.

45. Cartwright, J.W., Jr., and Todd, M.J.: A comparison of endodontic medications, Gen. Dent. **30**:334, 1982.

46. Cejka, J.: Laboratory consultant: what is the mechanism of the acute-phase response? Clin. Chem. News **11**(10):12, 1985.

47. Churton, M.C., and Greer, N.D.: Intracranial abscess secondary to dental infection, N. Z. Dent. J. **76**:58, 1980.

48. Ciancio, S.G.: Drugs in dentistry: antibiotics, Dent. Manag. **24**(9):48, 1984.

49. Ciancio, S.G.: Drugs in dentistry: analgesics, Dent. Manag. **24**(4):64, 1984.

50. Ciancio, S.G.: Drugs in dentistry: agents for anxiety disorders, Dent. Manag. **25**(6):66, 1985.

51. Cogan, M.I.C.: Necrotizing mediastinitis secondary to descending cervical cellulitis, Oral Surg. **44**:7, 1977.

52. Collet, R., et al.: The biocompatibility of some root canal medicaments and irrigants, Int. Endod. J. **14**:115, 1981.

53. Conover, M.A., Kaban, L.B., and Mulliken, J.B.: Antibiotic prophylaxis for major maxillocraniofacial surgery, J. Oral Maxillofac. Surg. **43**:865, 1985.

54. Cooper, S.A., et al.: Evaluation of oxycodone and acetaminophen in treatment of postoperative dental pain, Oral. Surg. **50**:496, 1980.

55. Council on Dental Therapeutics: Prevention of bacterial endocarditis: a committee report of the American Heart Association, J. Am. Dent. Assoc. **110**:98, 1985.

56. Crossley, H.L., Bergman, S.A., and Wynn, R.L.: Nonsteroidal anti-inflammatory agents in relieving dental pain: a review, J. Am. Dent. Assoc. **106**:61, 1983.

57. Cvek, M., Hollender, L., and Nord, C.E.: Treatment of non-vital permanent incisors with calcium hydroxide. VI. A clinical, microbiological and radiological evaluation of treatment in one sitting of teeth with mature or immature root, Odont. Rev. **27**:93, 1976.

58. Cymerman, J.J., et al.: Human T lymphocyte subpopulations in chronic periapical lesions, J. Endod. **10**:9, 1984.

59. Dalton, H.P.: State of the art of antimicrobial agent susceptibility testing: a clinical microbiologist's view, Am. Soc. Microb. News **48**:513, 1982.

60. Delivanis, P.D., and Fan, V.S.C.: The localization of blood-borne bacteria in instrumented unfilled and overinstrumented canals, J. Endod. **10**:521, 1984.

61. Delivanis, P.D., Mattison, G.D., and Mendel, R.W.: The survivability of F_{43} strain of *Streptococcus sanguis* in root canals filled with gutta-percha and Procosol cement, J. Endod. **9**:407, 1983.

62. Delivanis, P.D., Snowden, R.B., and Doyle, R.J.: Localization of blood-borne bacteria in instrumented unfilled root canals, Oral Surg. **52**:430, 1981.

63. DeMello, F.J., and Leonard, M.S.: *Eikenella corrodens:* a new pathogen, Oral Surg. **47**:401, 1979.

64. DeSmit, A., and Demaut, L.: Nonsurgical endodontic treatment of invaginated teeth, J. Endod. **8**:506, 1982.

65. Dwyer, T.G., and Torabinejad, M.: Radiographic and histologic evaluation of the effect of endotoxin on the periapical tissues of the cat, J. Endod. **7**:31, 1981.

66. Dye, E.S., and Kapral, F.A.: Partial characterization of a bactericidal system in staphyloccal abscesses, Infect. Immun. **30**:198, 1980.

67. Eaton, J.W., Brandt, P., and Malloney, J.R.: Haptoglobin: a natural bacteriostat, Science **215**:691, 1982.

68. Editorial: New drugs beat codeine in relieving postoperative pain, Med. World News **20**(21):14, 1981.

69. Eli Lilly & Co. Newsletter, May 19, 1972.

70. El-Maullem, H., and Fletcher, J.: Effects of surgery on neutrophil granulocyte function, Infect. Immun. **32**:38, 1981.

71. Epstein, J.B.: Understanding placebos in dentistry, J. Am. Dent. Assoc. **109**:71, 1984.

72. Epstein, S., and Scopp, I.W.: Antibiotics and the intraoral abscess, J. Periodontol. **48**:236, 1977.

73. Ernest, M.A., Conte, M.V., and Keudell, K.C.: Antibiotic sensitivity patterns of facultative and obligate anaerobic bacteria from pulp canals, J. Endod. **3**:106, 1977.

74. Fabricus, L.: Oral bacteria and apical periodontitis: an experimental study in monkey (thesis), Department of Oral Microbiology, University of Göteborg, Göteborg, Sweden, 1982.

75. Falomo, O.O.: Surgical emphysema following root canal therapy, Oral Surg. **58**:101, 1984.

76. Foley, D.B., et al.: Effectiveness of selected irrigants in the elimination of *Bacteroides melaninogenicus* from the root canal system: an in vitro study, J. Endod. **9**:236, 1983.

77. Friend, L.A., and Browne, R.M.: Tissue reactions to some root filling materials, Br. Dent. J. **125**:291, 1968.

78. Gale, R.P., Opelz, G., and Golde, D.W.: The effect of endotoxin on circulating lymphocytes in normal man, Br. J. Haem. **36**:49, 1977.

79. Geisler, P.J., et al.: Isolation of anaerobes in Ludwig's angina, J. Oral Surg. **37**:60, 1979.

80. Germaine, G.R., and Tellefson, L.M.: Effect of human saliva on glucose uptake by *Streptococcus mutans* and other oral microorganisms, Infect. Immun. **31**:598, 1981.

81. Gilbert, D.B., Germaine, G.R., and Jensen, J.R.: Inactivation by saliva and serum of the antimicrobial activity of some commonly used root canal sealer cements, J. Endod. **4**:100, 1978.

82. Gilbert, B.O., and Dickerson, A.W.II: Paresthesia of the mental nerve after an acute exacerbation of chronic apical periodontitis, J. Am. Dent. Assoc. **103**:588, 1981.

83. Glauda, N.M., Henefer, E.P., and Super, S.: Nonfatal anaphylaxis caused by oral penicillin: report of case, J. Am. Dent. Assoc. **90**:159, 1975.

84. Goldberg, M.H., and Galbreath, D.A., Late onset of mandibular and lingual dysesthesia secondary to postextraction infection, Oral Surg. **58**:269, 1984.

85. Goldman, M., and Pearson, A.H.: A preliminary investigation of the "hollow tube" theory in endodontics, J. Oral Therap. Pharmacol. **6**:618, 1965.

86. Goldstein, J., and McKinney, R.: Development of a periapical infection in the presence of antibiotic therapy, J. Endod. **7**:89, 1981.

87. Goodman, A.D., and Munson, P.A.: *Capnocytophaga* found in root canal system of a nonvital tooth, Oral Surg. **53**:622, 1982.

88. Goodman, A.D.: *Eikenella corrodens* isolated in oral infections of dental origin, Oral Surg. **44:**128, 1977.

88a. Goodman, A.D.: Isolation of anaerobic bacteria from the root canal systems of necrotic teeth by the use of a transport system, Oral Surg. **43:**766, 1977.

89. Greenberg, M.S., et al.: The oral flora as a source of septicemia in patients with acute leukemia, Oral Surg. **53:**32, 1982.

90. Griffee, M.B., et al.: *Bacteriodes melaninogenicus* and dental infections: some questions and some answers, Oral Surg. **54:**486, 1982.

91. Griffee, M.B., et al.: Comparison of bacterial growth in an improperly but commonly used medium versus reduced thioglycolate with the use of an anaerobic sampling technique, Oral Surg. **52:**433, 1981.

92. Griffee, M.B., et al.: The relationship of *Bacteroides melaninogenicus* to symptoms associated with pulpal necrosis, Oral Surg. **50:**457, 1980.

93. Grossman, L.I.: Endodontic emergencies, Oral Surg. **43:**948, 1977.

94. Grossman, L.I.: Endodontic practice, ed. 10, Philadelphia, 1981, Lea & Febiger.

95. Grossman, L.I.: Endodontic treatment of pulpless teeth, J. Am. Dent. Assoc. **61:**671, 1960.

96. Guralnick, W.: Odontogenic infections, Br. Dent. J. **156:**440, 1984.

97. Gurney, B.F.: Chemotherapy: non-narcotic analgesics. I. Pentazocine, Dent. Dig. **77:**598, 1971.

98. Gurney, B.F.: Clinical pharmacology in endodontics and intracanal medicaments, Dent. Clin. North Am. **18:**257, 1974.

99. Hall, W.E.: Antibiotics: basic management principles, AAOMS Surg. Update **1:**2, 1985.

99a. Hammarström, L., et al.: Replantation of teeth and antibiotic treatment, Endod. Dent. Traumatol. **2:**51, 1986.

100. Hammond, B.: Mechanisms of cytotoxicity and tissue destruction Presented at the 8th International Conference on Endodontics, Philadelphia, September, 1985.

101. Harrison, G.A., Schultz, T.A., and Schaberg, S.J.: Deep neck infection complicated by diabetes mellitus: report of a case, Oral Surg. **55:**133, 1985.

102. Harrison, J.W., Baumgartner, J.C., and Svec, T.A.: Incidence of pain associated with clinical factors during and after root canal therapy. Part 2. Postobturation pain, J. Endod. **9:**434, 1983.

103. Harrison, J.W., Baumgartner, J.C., and Zielke, D.R.: Analysis of interappointment pain associated with the combined use of endodontic irrigants and medicaments, J. Endod. **7:**272, 1981.

104. Haymaker, W.: Fatal infections of the central nervous system and meninges after tooth extraction with analysis of 28 cases, Am. J. Orthodont. Oral Surg. **31:**117, 1945.

105. Head, T.W., et al.: A comparative study of the effectiveness of metronidazole and penicillin V in eliminating anaerobes from postextraction bacteremias, Oral Surg. **58:**152, 1984.

106. Heidke, T.W.: Successful treatment of Ludwig's angina, Dent. Surv. **52**(19):52, 1976.

107. Henig, E.F., et al.: Brain abscess following dental infection, Oral Surg. **45:**955, 1978.

108. Hensten-Pettersen, A., Orstavik, D., and Wennberg, A.: Allergic potential of root canal sealers, Endod. Dent. Traumatol. **1:**61, 1985.

109. Hildebrand, C.N., and Morse, D.R.: Periodontic-endodontic interrelationships, Dent. Clin. North Am. **24:**797, 1980.

110. Hollin, S.A., Hayashi, H., and Gross, S.W.: Intracranial abscesses of odontogenic origin, Oral Surg. **23:**277, 1967.

111. Holroyd, S.: Clinical pharmacology in dental practice, ed. 2, St. Louis, 1983, The C.V. Mosby Co.

112. Hought, R.T., et al.: Ludwig's angina: Report of two cases and review of the literature from 1945 to January 1979, J. Oral Surg. **38:**849, 1980.

113. Iacono, V.J., et al.: Selective antibacterial properties of lysozyme for oral microorganisms, Infect. Immun. **29:**623, 1980.

114. Ineffective drugs, FDA Papers **5:**13, 1971.

115. Ingle, J.I.: Endodontics, Philadelphia, 1965, Lea & Febiger.

116. Isselbacher, K.J., et al.: Harrison's principles of internal medicine, ed. 9, New York, 1980, McGraw-Hill Book Co.

117. Janakarajah, N., and Sukumaran, K.: Orbital cellulitis of dental origin: case report and review of the literature, Br. J. Oral Maxillofac. Surg. **23:**140, 1985.

118. Jaspers, M.T., and Little, J.W.: Infective endocarditis: a review and update, Oral Surg. **57:**606, 1984.

119. Jawetz, E., Melnick, J.L., and Adelberg, E.A.: Review of medical microbiology, ed. 10, Los Altos, Calif., 1972, Lange Medical Publications.

120. Johnson, W.T.: Managing odontogenic infections, Am. Fam. Physician **29**(5): 167, 1984.

121. Kantz, W.E., and Henry, C.A.: Incidence of *Streptococcus mutans* in root canals, J. Dent. Res. **52:**1163, 1973.

122. Kanya, K.J.: Cervico-facial actinomycosis (a case report), J. Oral Med. **40:**166, 1985.

123. Kaufman, A.Y.: Facial emphysema caused by hydrogen peroxide irrigation: report of case, J. Endod. **7:**470, 1981.

124. Kettering, J.D., and Torabinejad, M.: Concentrations of immune complexes, IgG, IgM, IgE, and C_3 in patients with acute apical abscesses, J. Endod. **10:**417, 1984.

125. Keudell, K., and Conte, M.: Enzymes of microbial isolates from infected pulp chambers—a preliminary report, J. Endod. **2:**217, 1976.

126. Kiplioti, A., et al.: Microbiological findings of infected root canals and adjacent periodontal pockets in teeth with advanced periodontitis, Oral Surg. **58:**213, 1984.

127. Kluger, M.J., and Rothenburg, B.A.: Fever and reduced iron: their interaction as a host defense response to bacterial infection, Science **203:**374, 1979.

128. Langeland, K., Block, R.M., and Grossman, L.I.: A histopathologic and histobacteriologic study of 35 periapical endodontic surgical specimens, J. Endod. **3:**8, 1977.

129. Lee, G.T.R.: Septicaemia as a complication of endodontic treatment, J. Dent. **12:**241, 1984.

130. Lerner, P.I., and Weinstein, L.: Infective endocarditis in the antibiotic era, N. Engl. J. Med. **274:**199, 1966.

130a. Lin, L.M., et al.: Histopathologic and histobacteriologic study of endodontic failure (abstract 38), J. Endod. **12:**133, 1986.

131. Lindemann, R.A., and Henson, J.L.: The dental management of patients with vascular grafts placed in the treatment of arterial occlusive disease, J. Am. Dent. Assoc. **104:**625, 1982.

132. Linkous, C.M., and Welch, J.T.: Massive facial infection of odontogenic origin: report of case, J. Oral Surg. **33:**209, 1975.

133. Little, J.W.: The need for antibiotic coverage for dental treatment of patients with joint replacements, Oral Surg. **55:**20, 1983.

134. Mackowiak, P.A., and Marling-Cason, M.: Hyperthermic enhancement of serum antimicrobial activity: mechanism by which fever might exert a beneficial effect on the outcome of gram-negative sepsis, Infect. Immun. **39:**38, 1983.

135. Maddox, D.L., Walton, R.E., and Davis, C.O.: Incidence of post-treatment endodontic pain related to medicaments and other factors. J. Endod. **3:**447, 1977.

136. Marquez-Aviles, J.R., and Miller, J.: Bactericidal and irritant properties for endodontics, Br. Dent. J. **149:**105, 1980.

137. Mata, E., et al.: Prophylactic use of penicillin V in teeth with necrotic pulps and asymptomatic periapical radiolucencies, Oral Surg. **60:**201, 1985.

138. Matsumiya, S., and Kitamura, H.: Histo-pathological and histobacteriological studies of the relation between the condition of sterilization of the interior of the root canal and the healing process of periapical tissues in experimentally infected root canal treatment, Bull. Tokyo Dent. Coll. **1:**1, 1960.

139. Matusow, R.J.: Acute pulpal-alveolar cellulitis syndrome. I. Clinical study of bacterial isolates from pulps and exudates of intact teeth, with description of a specific culture technique, Oral Surg. **48:**70, 1979.

140. Matusow, R.J.: Acute pulpal-alveolar cellulitis syndrome. II. Clinical assessment of antibiotic effectiveness against microbes isolated from intact teeth, Oral Surg. **52:**187, 1981.

141. McCann, V.J., et al.: Intracranial abscesses, Med. J. Aust.**1:**75, 1979.

142. McGowan, D.A.: Endodontics and infective endocarditis, Int. Endod. J. **15:**127, 1982.

143. Meister, F., et al.: Successful treatment of a radicular lingual groove: case report, J. Endod. **9:**561, 1983.

144. Melcher, A.: Repair of granulomatous lesions, Presented at Temple University School of Dentistry, March, 1972.

145. Messer, H.H., and Chen, R.S.: The duration of effectiveness of root canal medicaments, J. Endod. **10:**240, 1984.

146. Moorer, W.R., and Wesselink, P.R.: Factors promoting the tissue dissolving capability of sodium hypochlorite, Int. Endod. J. **15:**187, 1982.

147. Morse, D.R.: Clinical endodontology: a comprehensive guide to diagnosis, treatment and prevention, Springfield, IL, 1974, Charles C Thomas Publisher.

148. Morse, D.R.: Endodontic microbiology in the 1970s, Int. Endod. J. **14:**69, 1981.

149. Morse, D.R.: Immunologic aspects of pulpal-periapical diseases. Oral Surg. **43:**436, 1977.

150. Morse, D.R.: The endodontic culture technique: an impractical and unnecessary procedure. Dent. Clin. North Am. **15:**793, 1971.

151. Morse, D.R., and Furst, M.L.: Stress and relaxation: application to dentistry, Springfield, IL, 1978, Charles C Thomas, Publisher.

152. Morse, D.R., and Furst, M.L.: Stress and the oral cavity. In Selye, H., editor: Selye's guide to stress research, vol. 2, New York, 1983, Van Nostrand Reinhold Co.

153. Morse, D.R., and Hoffman, H.: The presence of coliforms in root canals: preliminary findings, Israel J. Dent. Med. **21:**79, 1972.

154. Morse, D.R., et al.: A radiographic evaluation of the guttapercha-eucapercha endodontic obturation method: a one-year follow-up study, Oral Surg. **55:**607; **56:**89, 190, 1983.

155. Morse, D.R., et al.: Asymptomatic teeth with necrotic pulps and associated periapical radiolucencies: relationship of flare-ups to endodontic instrumentation, antibiotic usage and stress in three separate practices at three different time periods. Int. J. Psychosom. **33**(1):3, 1986.

156. Morse, D.R., et al.: Stress, meditation and saliva: a study of separate salivary gland secretions in endodontic patients, J. Oral Med. **38:**150, 1983.

157. Morse, D.R., Patnik, J.W., and Schacterle, G.R.: Electrophoretic differentiation of radicular cysts and granulomas, Oral Surg. **35:**249, 1973.

158. Morse, D.R., Wolfson, E., and Schacterle, G.R.: Nonsurgical repair of electrophoretically diagnosed radicular cysts, J. Endod. **1:**158, 1975.

159. Moskow, A., et al.: Intracanal use of a corticosteroid solution as an endodontic anodyne, Oral Surg. **58:**600, 1984.

160. Naidorf, I.J.: Endodontic flare-ups: bacteriological and immunological mechanisms, J. Endod. **11:**462, 1985.

161. Nair, P.N.R., and Schroeder, H.E.: Periapical actinomycosis, J. Endod. **10:**567, 1984.

162. Nakamura, H., et al.: The solvent action of sodium hypochlorite on bovine tendon collagen, bovine pulp, and bovine gingiva, Oral Surg. **60:**322, 1985.

163. Natkin, E.: Treatment of endodontic emergencies, Dent. Clin. North Am. **18:**243, 1974.

164. Neidle, E.A., Kroeger, D.C., and Yagiela, J.A.: Pharmacology and therapeutics for dentistry, St. Louis, 1980, The C.V. Mosby Co.

165. Nelson, C.I., and Hutton, C.E.: Biosis, antibiosis, and how to select an antibiotic, Compend. Contin. Ed. Dent. **5:**815, 1984.

166. Neu, H.C.: Anaerobes in endodontic abscesses show need for more than penicillin, Infect. Dis., vol. 16, 1984.

167. Nishida, O., et al.: Investigation of homologous antibodies to an extract of rabbit dental pulp. Arch. Oral Biol. **16:**733, 1971.

168. Pakman, L.M., et al.: Root canal infections: symptoms versus bacterial isolates, Abst. Am. Soc. Microbiol., no. C-38, 80th Annual meeting, 1980.

169. Pecuch, J.F.: Odontogenic infections, Dent. Clin. North Am. **26:**129, 1982.

170. Phillips, J.M.: Rat connective tissue response to hollow polyethylene tube implants, J. Can. Dent. Assoc. **33:**59, 1967.

171. Pickney, L.E., Currarino, G., and Highgenboten, C.L.: Osteomyelitis of the cervical spine following dental extraction, Radiology **135:**335, 1980.

172. Pitt Ford, T.R.: The effects on the periapical tissues of bacterial contamination of the filled root canal, Int. Endod. J. **15:**16, 1982.

173. Pitts, D.L., Williams, B.L., and Morton, T.H., Jr.: Investigation of the role of endotoxin in periapical inflamation, J. Endod. **8:**10, 1982.

174. Price, J.D.: Bone sequestration following root canal therapy: a case report, Int. Endod. J. **18:**55, 1985.

175. Purdy, M.A., et al.: Effect of growth phase and cell envelope structure on susceptibility of *Salmonella typhimurium* to the lactoperoxidase-thiocyanate-hydrogen peroxide system, Infect. Immun. **39:**1187, 1983.

176. Quinn, P., and Guernsey, L.H.: The presentation and complications of odontogenic septic shock, Oral Surg. **59:**336, 1985.

177. Ranly, D.M., and Lazzari, E.P.: A biochemical study of two bifunctional reagents as alternatives to formocresol, J. Dent. Res. **62:**1054, 1983.

178. Ratner, E.J., et al.: Jawbone cavities and trigeminal and atypical facial neuralgias, Oral Surg. **48:**3, 1979.

179. Rickles, N.H., and Joshi, B.A.: Death from air embolism during root canal therapy, J. Am. Dent. Assoc. **67:**397, 1963.

180. Riccitelli, M.L.: Vitamin C: a review and reassessment of pharmacological and therapeutic uses, Conn. Med. **39:**609, 1975.

181. Ringel, A.M., et al.: In vivo evaluation of chlorhexidine gluconate solution and sodium hypochlorite solution as root canal irrigants, J. Endod. **8:**200, 1982.

182. Ringsdorf, W.M., Jr., and Cheraskin, E.: Vitamin C and human wound healing, Oral Surg. **53:**231, 1982.

183. Ringsdorf, W.M. Jr., Cheraskin, E., and Medford, F.H.: Vitamin C and antibiotics, J. Oral Med. **35**(1):14, 1980.

184. Roane, J.B., and Marshall, F.J.: Osteomyelitis: a complication of pulpless teeth, Oral Surg. **34:**257, 1972.

185. Roberts, A.M., and Person, P.: Etiology and treatment of idiopathic trigeminal and atypical facial neuralgia, Oral Surg. **48:**298, 1979.

186. Roberts, P.: The effect of dietary zinc sulfate supplements on the healing of extraction wounds, Chron. Omaha Dist. Dent. Soc. **26:**127, 1973.

187. Rowe, A.H.R. and Binnie, W.H.: The incidence and location of microorganisms following endodontic treatment, Br. Dent. J. **142:**91, 1977.

188. Rowe, N.H., Aseltine L.F., and Turner, J.L.: Control of pain with meclofenamate sodium following removal of an impacted molar, Oral Surg. **59:**446, 1985.

189. Rysz, T.J.: A comparison of culture media and methods of specimen collection, abst. 13, AAE Annual Meeting, J. Endod. **10:**121, 1984.

190. Safavi, K.E., et al.: A comparison of antimicrobial effects of calcium hydroxide and iodine-potassium iodide, J. Endod. **11:**454, 1985.

191. Schein, B., and Schilder, A.: Endotoxin content in endodontically involved teeth, J. Endod. **1:**19, 1975.

192. Schilder, H.: Cleaning and shaping the root canal, Dent. Clin. North Am. **18:**269, 1974.

193. Schilder, H.: Public awareness, J. Endod. **11:**317, 1985.

194. Schonfeld, S.E., et al.: Endotoxic activity in periapical lesions, Oral Surg. **53:**82, 1982.

195. Scopp, I.W., and Orvieto, L.D.: Gingival degerming by povidone-iodine irrigation: bacteria reduction in extraction procedures, J. Am. Dent. Assoc. **83:**1294, 1971.

196. Sela, M., and Sharav, Y.: The dental focal infection as an origin for uveitis, Isr. J. Dent. Med. **24**:31, 1975.

197. Seltzer, S.: Endodontology: biologic considerations in endodontic procedures, New York, 1971, McGraw-Hill Book Co.

198. Seltzer, S., and Bender, I.B.: The dental pulp: biologic considerations in dental procedures, ed. 3, Philadelphia, 1984, J.B. Lippincott Co.

199. Seltzer, S., and Naidorf, I.J.: Flare-ups in endodontics: 1. Etiological factors, J. Endod. **11**:472, 1985.

200. Shepherd, J.P.: Osteomyelitis of the tibia following dento-alveolar abscess: a case report, Br. Dent. J. **145**:267, 1978.

201. Shindell, E.: Studies on the possible presence of a virus in subacute and chronic periapical granulomas, Oral Surg. **15**:1382, 1962.

202. Shovelton, D.S.: The presence and distribution of microorganisms within non-vital teeth, Br. Dent. J. **117**:101, 1964.

203. Shpeen, S.E., Morse, D.R., and Furst, M.L.: The effect of tryptophan on postoperative endodontic pain, Oral Surg. **58**:446, 1984.

204. Siegel, I.A.: Pharmacology of antibiotics used in dentistry, Int. Dent. J. **31**:133, 1981.

205. Silberman, M., Maloney, P.L., and Doku, H.C.: Mandibular osteomyelitis in the patient with chronic alcoholism: etiology, management, and statistical correlation, Oral Surg. **38**:530, 1974.

206. Simon, M., VanMullem, P.J., and Lamers, A.C.: Allergic skin reactions provided by a root canal disinfectant with reduced formaldehyde concentration, Int. Endod. J. **17**:199, 1984.

207. Spångberg, L., Rutberg, M., and Rydinge, E.: Biologic effects of endodontic antimicrobial agents, J. Endod. **5**:166, 1979.

208. Stabholz, A., and Sela, M.N.: The role of oral microorganisms in the pathogenesis of periapical pathosis. 1. Effect of *Streptococcus mutans* and its cellular constituents on the dental pulp and periapical tissue of cats, J. Endod. **9**:171, 1983.

209. Stevens, R.H., and Grossman, L.I.: Evaluation of the antimicrobial potential of calcium hydroxide as an intracanal medicament, J. Endod. **9**:372, 1983.

210. Stobberingh, E.E., and Eggink, C.O.: The value of the bacteriological culture in endodontics.II. The bacteriological flora of endodontic specimens, Int. Endod. J. **15**:87, 1982.

211. Stone, A., and Stratigos, G.T.: Mandibular odontogenic infection with serious complications, Oral Surg. **47**:395, 1979.

212. Strindberg, L.Z.: Lokal användning av antibiotika vid konserverande rotbehandling. En jämförande klinisk, bacteriologisk och röntgenologisk undersökning, Sven. Tandlak. Tidskr. **56**:639, 1963.

213. Sundqvist, G.: Bacteriological studies of necrotic dental pulps, Umeå University Odontological Dissertations, no. 7, 1976.

214. Sundqvist, G.: Microbial etiology of pulpal and periodontal diseases. Presented at the 8th International Conference on Endodontics, September, 1985, Philadelphia.

215. Sundqvist, G., and Johansson, E.: Neutrophilic chemotax is induced by anaerobic bacteria isolated from necrotic dental pulps, Scand. J. Dent. Res. **88**:113, 1980.

216. Svec, T.A., and Harrison, J.W.: The effect of effervescence on debridement of the apical region of root canals in single-rooted teeth, J. Endod. **7**:335, 1981.

217. Szmigrelski, S., et al.: Injury of myelin sheaths in isolated rabbit vagus nerves by alpha toxin of Staphylococcus aureus, Toxicol. **17**:363, 1979.

218. Tanner, A.C.R., Visconti, R.A., Holdeman, L.V., et al.: Similarity of *Wolinella recta* strains isolated from periodontal pockets and root canals, J. Endod. **8**:294, 1982.

219. Terezhalmy, G.T., and Hall, E.H.: The asplenic patient: A consideration for antimicrobial prophylaxis, Oral Surg. **57**:114, 1984.

220. The, S.D., Maltha, J.C., and Plasschaert, A.J.M.: Reactions of guinea pig subcutaneous connective tissue to direct or long distance exposure to parachlorophenol-or formalin-containing endodontic drugs, J. Endod. **7**:22, 1981.

220a. Thilo, B.E., Bachni, P., and Holy, J.: Dark-field observation of the bacterial distribution in root canals following pulp necrosis, J. Endod. **12**:202, 1986.

221. Thomas, E.L.: Inhibition of *Streptococcus mutans* by the lactoperoxidase antimicrobial system, Infect. Immun. **39**:767, 1983.

222. Thomas, P.A., Bhat, K.S., and Kotian, K.M.: Antibacterial properties of dilute formocresol and eugenol and propylene glycol, Oral Surg. **49**:166, 1980.

223. Tizard, I.R.: Immunology: an introduction, Philadelphia, 1984, W.B. Saunders Co.

224. Tomsect, R., and Skryska, C.: Reappraising clinical features of bacterial endocarditis, Postgrad. Med. **42**:462, 1967.

225. Tonzetich, J.: Production and origin of oral malodor: a review of mechanisms and methods of analysis. J. Periodontol. **48**:13, 1977.

226. Torabinejad, M.: Mediators of pulpal and periapical inflammation. Presented at the 8th International Conference on Endodontics, September, 1985, Philadelphia.

227. Torabinejad, M.: The role of immunological reactions in apical cyst formation and the fate of epithelial cells after root canal therapy: a theory, Int. J. Oral Surg. **12**:14, 1983.

228. Torabinejad, M., and Kettering, J.D.: Identification and relative concentration of B and T lymphocytes in human chronic periapical lesions, J. Endod. **11**:122, 1985.

229. Torabinejad, M., Eby, W.C., and Naidorf, I.J.: Inflammatory and immunological aspects of the pathogenesis of human periapical lesions, J. Endod. **11**:479, 1985.

230. Torabinejad, M., et al.: Quantitation of circulating immune complexes, immunoglobulins G and M, and C_3 complement component in patients with large periapical lesions, Oral Surg. **55**:186, 1983.

231. Torneck, C.D.: Reaction of rat connective tissue to polyethylene tube implants, Oral Surg. **21**:379, 1966.

232. Tronstad, L., et al.: Controlled release of medicaments in endodontic therapy, Endod. Dent. Traumatol. **1**:130, 1985.

233. Trope, M., and Grossman, L.I.: Root canal culturing survey: Single visit endodontics, J. Endod. **11**:511, 1985.

233a. Trope, H., Rosenberg, E., and Tronstad, L.: Dark field microscopy as a diagnostic aid in differentiating endodontic and periodontal abscesses. Presented at the 43rd Annual Session of the American Association of Endodontists, Boston, April 16-20, 1986.

234. Tsan, M-F: Mycloperoxidase-mediated oxidation of methionine and amino acid decarboxylation, Infect. Immun. **36**:136, 1982.

235. Van DeWater, L., Destree, A.T., and Hynes, R.O.: Fibronectin binds to some bacteria but does not promote their uptake by phagocytic cells, Science **220**:204, 1983.

236. Walker, D.G.: Severe infection of the mandible, Proc. Roy. Soc. Med. **40**:309, 1947.

237. Weir, J.C., and Buck, W.H.: Periapical actinomycosis: report of a case and review of the literature, Oral Surg. **54**:336, 1982.

238. Weiss, S.J., Lampert, M.B., and Test, S.T.: Long-lived oxidants generated by human neutrophils: characterization and bioactivity, Science **222**:625, 1983.

239. Weisz, G.: A clinical study using automated instrumentation in root canal therapy, Int. Endod. J. **18**:203, 1985.

240. Wemes, J.C., Jansen, H.W.B., Purdell-Lewis, D., and Boering, G.: Histologic evaluation of the effect of formocresol and glutaraldehyde on the periapical tissues after endodontic treatment, Oral Surg. **54**:329, 1982.

241. Wheat, L.J.: Infection and diabetes mellitus, Diabetes Care **3**:187, 1980.

242. Wyman, T.P., Dowden, W.E., and Langeland, K.: *Staphylococcus aureus* isolation from a clinically nonexposed root canal, J. Endod. **4**:122, 1978.

243. Young, E.W., et al.: Evaluation of treatment provided patients hospitalized with orofacial odontogenic infections: a retrospective study, Oral Surg. **59**:28, 1985.

244. Zach, A., and Kaufman, Y.: Quantatitive evaluation of the influence of dequalinum acetate and sodium hypochlorite on human dentition, Oral Surg. **55**:524, 1983.

245. Zavistoski, J., et al.: Quantitative bacteriology of endodontic infections, Oral Surg. **49**:171, 1980.

Self-assessment questions

1. It has been found that the microbial flora of necrotic pulps with associated periapical areas consists mostly of
   a. Gram-positive facultative anaerobes
   b. Obligate anaerobic organisms
   c. Staphylocci and lactobacilli
   d. Facultative anaerobic streptococci
2. The most common pathway for microbes and microbial products to reach the pulp is
   a. Directly through a carious lesion
   b. Apical extension of periodontal disease
   c. Pulpal inflammation and anachoresis
   d. From adjoining necrotic pulps and periapical lesions
3. The outcome of a microbial pulp infection will depend on the
   a. Virulence of the microbes
   b. Products of the microbes
   c. Resistance of the host
   d. Host-parasite interrelationship
4. The author suggests that instrumentation into quiescent periapical lesions may
   a. Remove microbes and their inflammatory products
   b. Destroy blood vessels, lymphatics and host defensive cells
   c. Cause a flare-up of iatrogenic etiology
   d. Cause a considerable delay in healing
5. A cellulitis between the superficial fascia and the superficial layer of the deep cervical fascia requires treatment that includes
   a. Vigorous antibiotic and supportive measures
   b. Endotoxins and drainage
   c. Antibiotics and drainage
   d. Rest, fluids and supportive measures
6. In order to control the incidence of post-treatment flare-ups of previously asymptomatic periapical "areas," the author recommends
   a. Proplylactic systemic antibiotic coverage
   b. Instrumentation within the root canal spaces
   c. Antibiotic coverage if symptoms develop
   d. The use of antibiotic sensitivity testing
7. The American Heart Association recommendation for use of oral penicillin for premedication is
   a. 4 tablets (250 mg) 1 hour before procedure then 1 tablet (250 mg) every 6 hours for one week
   b. 2 gm 30 minutes before procedure, then 500 mg every 6 hours for eight doses
   c. 2 gm 1 hour before the procedure and 1 gm 6 hours later
   d. 250 mg every 6 hours the day before the procedure, the day of the procedure, and three days following the procedure

8. IgG is the principal antibody that
   a. Prevents adherence of bacteria and viruses to epithelial surfaces
   b. Provides a protective reaction against microbes and their products
   c. Is active against parasitic worm infections
   d. Prevents immunological tolerence (no immunological response)
9. Periapical bone destruction may be a Type IV (delayed) hypersensitivity due to the
   a. Destruction of host cells by antibodies
   b. Formation of antigen-antibody complexes
   c. Production of lysosomal enzymes
   d. Release of osteoclast-activating factor
10. A drug such as penicillin may induce an immediate or delayed hypersensitivity response because its breakdown products may act as a
   a. Complete antigen
   b. IgE antibody
   c. Hapten
   d. Tissue protein
11. A false-negative culture may occur due to
   a. A rubber dam leak near the involved tooth
   b. Incomplete penetration of the paper point
   c. The use of unsterile paper points
   d. Periodontal disease with exposed lateral canals
12. The concentration of sodium hypochlorite that causes the least vital tissue destruction is
   a. 0.5%
   b. 1.0%
   c. 2.25%
   d. 5.25%
13. According to recent studies, the intracanal medicament with the longer-lasting antimicrobial effect is
   a. Cresatin
   b. CaOH
   c. 2% iodine-potassium iodide
   d. CMCP
14. Which of the following is not a basic principle in the management of infected necrotic pulps with associated periapical areas
   a. Determine and remove the cause by intracanal procedures
   b. Arrest and eradicate the organisms by chemotherapy
   c. Evacuate pus and maintain drainage
   d. Provide adequate irritation to periapical area to form granulomatous tissue

13

INSTRUMENTS AND MATERIALS

MICHAEL A. HEUER
LEO J. MISERENDINO

The purpose of this chapter is to provide information on the biologic effects and physical properties of the more popular instruments and materials that either have been or are currently being used within root canals. Presumably one may then select instruments and materials best suited to one's professional skills and to the particular clinical problem with which one is faced

The armamentarium of endodontics has grown in complexity over the last 20 years as increasing numbers of clinicians have applied their talents to the resolution of recurrent clinical situations. The technical skills required in endodontics invariably lead to a high degree of personalized artistry in their execution. Hence the development of a body of literature frequently partisan toward a particular instrument, material, or technique is certainly evident

In addition to personal, subjective influences, the literature dealing with endodontic instruments and material reflects prevailing concepts of endodontic pratice in vogue at the time. *This occurs despite the nearly universal conviction that cleaning, shaping, and sealing the root canal system lie at the heart of the clinical practice of endodontics.* For example, when the attention of the profession was centered on countering the concept that pulpless teeth were "foci of infection," emphasis was placed on instrumentation techniques directed toward "disinfection" of the root canal and toward root canal filling materials with a strong and persistent potential for antisepsis. Later, endodontic techniques subtly shifted toward minimization of instrumentation trauma to the periodontal ligament and toward the use of materials better tolerated by pulpal and periapical tissues. Until recently neither endodontic instruments nor materials were investigated as merely instruments or materials apart from clinical techniques.

Changes in emphasis from one mode of instrumentation, material, or root canal filling technique to another do not imply that either the instruments or the materials used in endodontics have been radically altered in the last 50 years. On the contrary, most of the instruments and mate-

rials employed clinically today have been used for several decades, and clinical success with them has been significant. Usually emphasis has been placed on clinical reports and investigations directed toward the improvement or modification of longstanding clinical practices. This has often resulted in involved and convoluted rationalizations for the continued use of these practices rather than in the development of entirely new concepts, instruments, or materials. Seemingly radical instruments, materials, or techniques in endodontics have been, for the most part, technologic improvements on existing models rather than new inventions

ENDODONTIC INSTRUMENTS

The principal investigations of endodontic instrument designs and physical characteristics were initiated in the 1950s at the University of Michigan. Ralph F. Sommer, a prominent clinician and teacher and Chairman of the Endodontic Department, was an ardent advocate of the use of silver cones as a root canal filling material. This was predicated on the hypothesis that the natural structure of the apex was conical and the apex could be readily and accurately prepared to provide a seat for a prefabricated silver cone to be cemented in place, thereby sealing the root canal.

Because the University of Michigan initiated one of the pioneer programs in advanced education in endodontics, several interrelated investigations were conducted by a succession of graduate students to establish a firm scientific foundation for the highly successful clinical technique being taught. Apical stricture and its relationship to the sizing of root canal instruments were investigated. The relationship of silver cones to root canal preparations made by endodontic files was examined. Problems in precisely fitting prefabricated silver cones to prepared root canals were encountered, and several proposals to overcome these were offered.

Meanwhile, Ingle and Levine[82] on the faculty of the

University of Washington, advocated standardization of the endodontic instrument armamentarium.

The Michigan group also began to evaluate the feasibility of using the endodontic file *itself*, rather than a silver cone, to seal the root canal, thus eliminating problems with matching sizes. To determine whether stainless steel files (thought at the time to be suitable for implantation in tissue) were comparable in physical and working characteristics to the commonly used carbon steel files, investigators had to determine their properties. This was done by analyzing the physical and structural characteristics of standardized files and reamers in 1959. These investigations and others that followed were the first in which endodontic instruments were studied as entities apart from their use in clinical situations.[35-37] Pressure was brought to bear on manufacturers of root canal instuments to maintain closer instrument tolerances, quality control, and standardization of products.

Attempts to develop techniques whereby root canals could be routinely prepared to receive accurately a solid-core filling point may not have been successful in accomplishing that end, but they did stimulate interest in studies of endodontic instruments and instrumentation. Researchers at The University of Pennsylvania investigated the efficiency of files and reamers in prepared simulated root canals.[129] Some studied the deterioration of endodontic reamers during root canal preparation; others conducted investigations of instrument fractures as encounterd in clinical practice. Proponents of rigid-core root canal filling techniques were hard pressed to substantiate their hypotheses. Conflicting studies supported or rejected the premise that accurate geometric preparations of the root canal sytems are possible

The relationship of the instrumentation technique to the root canal filling procedure remains controversial to this day. Standardization has come to mean standardization of the endodontic instruments and materials themselves rather than the canal preparation or filling. In a search for more simplistic and efficient methods of endodontic instrumentation, engine-driven instruments have been reintroduced and new studies to evaluate their potential are being objectively reported. The dichotomy of opinion regarding techniques of instrumentation persists in the semantics of endodontics. Proponents of instrumentation systems leading to geometric root canal shapes suitable for rigid-core filling techniques speak in terms of root canal preparation, whereas opponents of this philosophy speak only in terms of cleaning and shaping. Often, sweeping statements have been made regarding the shape of the root canal following instrumentation. In general, these statements are based on neither investigation nor observation but on predetermined notions of what a particular filling technique or material requires to satisfy real or hypothetical biologic considerations. The claims are many; the facts are few; and the criteria of success or failure remain inconsistently defined.

TYPES OF ENDODONTIC INSTRUMENTS AVAILABLE

The instruments used in endodontics have been grouped, according to use, by the International Standards Organization (I.S.O.) and the Fédération Dentaire Internationale (F.D.I.) through a Joint Working Group on Root Canal Instruments.[5]

Group I: endodontic instruments, hand use only. Included are K-type (Kerr) and H-type (Hedström) files, K-type reamers, R-type rasps (rattail files), barbed broaches, probes (smooth broaches), applicators, filling condensers (pluggers), and filling spreaders (Fig. 13-1).

Group II: endodontic instruments, engine driven; two-part shaft and operative head. Included are instruments having shafts designed for use only in a straight handpiece, a contraangle handpiece, or specially designed endodontic contraangle handpieces. The operative head is identical either with the root canal files, reamers, rasps, or barbed broaches of Group I or with the specially designed root canal instruments such as B-2 or quarter-turn reamers or Lentulo paste carriers (Fig. 13-2).

Group III: endodontic instruments, engine driven; one-part shaft and operative head. Included are B-1, G-type

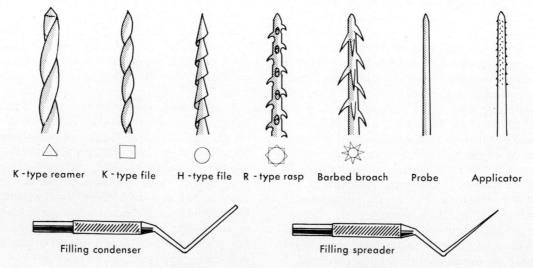

K-type reamer   K-type file   H-type file   R-type rasp   Barbed broach   Probe   Applicator

Filling condenser   Filling spreader

FIG. 13-1. Group I: endodontic instruments for hand use only.

(Gates-Glidden), P-type (Peeso), A-type, D-type, O-type, Ko-type, T-type, and M-type reamers as well as the root facer (Fig. 13-3).

Group IV: endodontic points. Included are absorbent (paper) points and filling points.

The foregoing classification and terminology for endodontic instruments were adopted by the Joint Working Group on Root Canal Instruments in 1973 for presentation to the I.S.O. member countries (including the United States) and the F.D.I. Commission on Dental Materials, Instruments, Equipment, and Therapeutics. In addition to classifying the various types of root canal instruments, the Task Group on Terminology was able to arrive at descriptive definitions for these instruments as well as a symbol code to be used for quick identification of the most commonly used types.

Rasps, broaches, and applicators

R-type rasps, broaches, applicators, and probes are historically the oldest form of endodontic instrument, dating well back to the nineteenth century (Chapter 25). The probe is a light, slender, fairly flexible, smooth or edged, metal hand instrument usually pointed and tapered; it is used for exploring root canals. Probes are generally made of soft iron wire. Rasps, broaches, and applicators are manufactured from soft iron wire by the placement of a series of incisions along the shaft and the subsequent elevation of the edge of the incision to create a cutting prominence with a barbed or rough surface. The depth and angle of cut in the shaft are the principal determinants of the instrument type (Fig. 13-4).

R-type endodontic rasps are hand-operated, tapered, and pointed instruments on which the cutting prominences are distinct points. The incisive cuts of the manufacturing tool

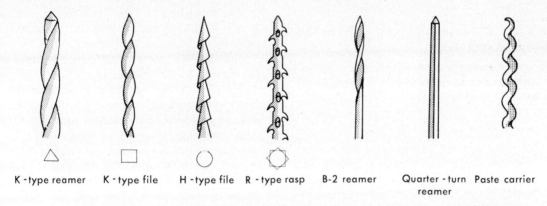

K-type reamer   K-type file   H-type file   R-type rasp   B-2 reamer   Quarter-turn reamer   Paste carrier

FIG. 13-2. Group II: engine-driven endodontic instruments, two-part shaft and operative head.

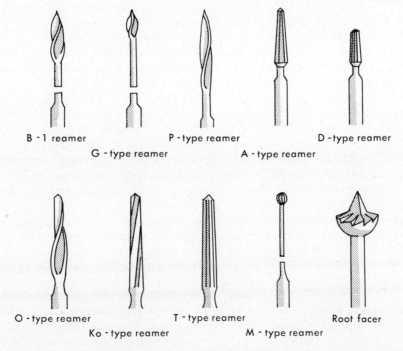

B-1 reamer

G-type reamer

P-type reamer

A-type reamer

D-type reamer

O-type reamer

Ko-type reamer

T-type reamer

M-type reamer

Root facer

FIG. 13-3. Group III: engine-driven endodontic instruments, one-part shaft and operative head.

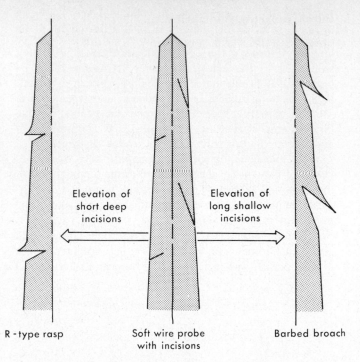

Elevation of
short deep
incisions

Elevation of
long shallow
incisions

R -type rasp

Soft wire probe
with incisions

Barbed broach

FIG. 13-4. Endodontic barbed broaches and rasps. The soft wire probe can be converted into an R-type rasp or a barbed broach, depending on the depth and angle of the cut.

are shallow and nearly perpendicular to the soft iron shaft. As a consequence the cutting prominences produced are a series of ovoid or semicircular elevations along the operative head of the instrument. Rasps are used to enlarge the root canal by abrasive action on the dentinal surfaces. The term rattail file was previously applied to this instrument . The identification symbol for R-type rasps is an eight-pointed polyhedron.

Endodontic broaches are thin, flexible usually tapered and pointed, metal hand instruments with sharp projections curving backward and obliquely. The incisive cuts of the manufacturing tool are a series of sharply pointed barbs along the operative head of the tool. Broaches are used in engaging and removing the pulp and other substances intact from the root canal or pulp chamber. Their identification symbol is an eight-pointed star.

Endodontic applicators are light, slender, tapering, fairly flexible, pointed instruments that are circular in cross section; the working head is rough to aid in holding cotton fibers or liquids for application into root canals. They are similar to some root canal probes except for the rough surfaces of their working portion. The incisive cuts of the manufacturing tool are shallow, and the elevation of the special portion of the cut (in the manner of root canal rasp or broach) is slight.

Rasps, broaches, applicators, and probes are of limited usefulness in modern endodontic practices in the United States. Usually of these four types of instruments, only the broaches (and, at best, a limited selection of these) will be found in the armamentarium of the endodontist.

Files and reamers

K-type endodontic files and reamers were developed shortly after the turn of the century by the Kerr Manufacturing Company to meet the need for more effective cutting instruments in root canals. They are manufactured from carbon steel wire and stainless steel wire onto which is machined either a three- or a four-sided, tapered, pyramidal blank. The blank portion is then twisted to introduce a series of spirals into what will become the operating head of the instrument (Fig. 13-5). By this method the manufacturing process for a file is identical to that for a reamer. The blank portion of the wire can be a square, a rhombus, or an equilateral triangle in cross section.

A blank twisted to produce from one quarter to over a half of a spiral per millimeter of length, depending on size, produces an instrument with from 1.97 to 0.88 cutting flutes per millimeter of operating head; this is designated a file. A blank so twisted as to produce from less than a quarter to less than a tenth of a spiral per millimeter of length, depending on size, produces an instrument having from 0.80 to 0.28 cutting flute per millimeter of operating head; this is designated a reamer.

Although the essential difference between K-type files and reamers is the number of spirals or cutting flutes per unit of length, the tendency (particularly in wire sizes larger than 0.30 mm diameter) is for files to be twisted from square-cross section blanks and reamers to be twisted from triangular-cross section blanks. Most, if not all, K-type instruments are twisted from blanks that are of square cross section in wire sizes smaller than 0.30 mm diameter. Thus files are usually manufactured from blanks that are square in cross section throughout their range of sizes; this is not true of reamers. Recently a line of endodontic files manufactured from blanks that are rhomboid or diamond shaped in cross section has been introduced. These instruments are purported to have features that are intermediate between those of the usual square-blank files and those of the triangular-blank reamers.

The relationship of cross-sectional shape to instrument identification is responsible for much confusion in the empirical literature of these types of endodontic instruments. The selection of blank shape is a manufacturer's prerogative and varies by company for both files and reamers.

K-type reamers are hand- or power-operated (Groups I and II), usually tapered and pointed, metal instruments with spiral cutting edges, sometimes serrated; they are used to enlarge root canals by a rotary cutting action. The identification symbol for K-type reamers is an equilateral triangle.

K-type files are hand-operated (Group I), tapered and pointed, metal instruments with tight spiral cutting edges so arranged that cutting occurs on either a pushing or a pulling stroke. They are used to enlarge the root canal by a rotary cutting or abrasive action. The identification symbol for K-type files is a square.

H-type (Hedström) files are made by machine grinding the flutes of the file into the metal stock of the operating head of the instrument so as to form a series of intersecting

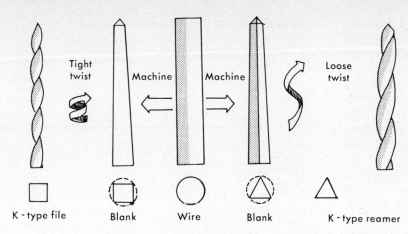

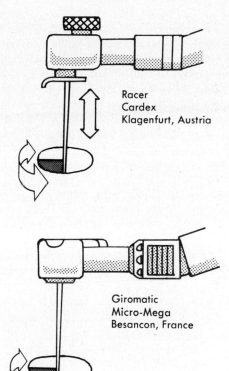

FIG. 13-5. K-type endodontic files and reamers.

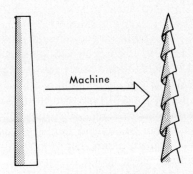

FIG. 13-6. H-type endodontic files.

FIG. 13-7. Endodontic contraangle handpieces.

cones successively larger from the tip toward the handle (Fig. 13-6). These instruments are similar in design to buttress threaded screws. The helical angle of the usual H-type instrument is close to 90 degrees, or nearly perpendicular to the instrument's central axis. New forms of H-type files with helical angles significantly less than 90 degrees have been developed. They possess increased potential for cutting by rotary as well as withdrawal movement, a feature not normally associated with H-type instruments. The H-type files are tapered and pointed metal instruments, hand or power operated (Groups I and II), with spiral cutting edges arranged so the cutting occurs principally on the pulling stroke. They are used to enlarge the root canal by either a cutting or an abrasive action. The identification symbol for H-type files is a circle.

Condensers and spreaders

Endodontic filling condensers and spreaders generally have long handles of stainless steel or chromiumplated brass much like those on similar instruments used in operative dentistry; short-handled condensers and spreaders, however, are relatively recent and are used principally as "finger pluggers" (Luks). The operating head of the condenser can be either uniangular or bayonet style (Fig. 13-1).

Condensers (pluggers) are smooth, flat-ended and slightly tapered, metal instruments used to condense filling material vertically in a root canal. Spreaders are smooth, pointed, and tapered metal instruments for laterally condensing filling material in a canal.

Engine-driven instruments

Although, historically, engine-driven endodontic instruments have not been extensively advocated in the United States (principally because of the hazards of root perforation or instrument breakage), a number of types have been developed. Introduction of the Giromatic and Racer engine-driven contraangle handpieces, specifically designed for endodontic use, has rekindled interest, long smoldering, in engine-driven instrumentation. The Giromatic handpiece operates by rotary reciprocal action through a 90-degree arc, whereas the principal action of the Racer handpiece is by vertical oscillation within the root canal (Fig. 13-7).

Instruments that are adaptable to slow-speed contraangles and operate in the usual 360-degree rotary fashion are also available. Two that are designed especially for engine operation are the B-2 and quarter-turn reamers. Both belong to Group II, because the shaft and operating head are two pieces (Fig. 13-2). The B-2 reamer has a cylindrical working head with two cutting edges forming a spiral. Its cross-sectional shape is a rectangle, and its working head and shank are similar to those of the more familiar K-type reamers. The quarter-turn reamer is a power-operated, tapered, and pointed metal instrument designed for use in special endodontic handpieces. It possesses four straight side-cutting edges and is used to enlarge or widen the root canal by cutting axial walls. This reamer is similar in shape to the blank of a K-type file before the twisting procedure.

The Lentulo paste carrier is a power-operated small spiral instrument used in conveying filling material or medicaments into the root canal (Fig. 13-2).

The McSpadden compactor is a specially designed instrument, not unlike the H-type file, in which the spiraling is reversed. The effect of this is to direct material apically rather than occlusally when the instrument is rotated clockwise. It is used in gutta-percha root canal filling techniques in which the frictional heat generated softens the gutta-percha and the apically directed spiral molds it into the root canal system.

The various endodontic instruments comprising Group II and the types of shafts available for them are shown in Table 13-1. Numerous engine-driven instruments are made with the shaft and operative head as one piece, similar to most dental burs. With the exception of the root facer (Fig. 13-3), all of these Group II instruments are termed reamers.

The G-type reamer is more familiarly known as the Gates-Glidden drill. It has a short, flame-shaped head with side-cutting blades spiraling slightly with a wide rake angle. It usually has a short noncutting guide at the tip to minimize its potential for perforating the root surface. The head is connected to the shank by a long thin neck. The instrument can also be obtained without the short noncutting guide at the tip.

The B-1 reamer is similar to the G-type reamer with the exception that the working head of the B-1 reamer is generally about twice as long.

The O-type reamer has a fairly long, tapered head consisting of three spiraling blades that end in a plane angle, giving the instrument a blunt tip. The head is connected to the shank by a short neck.

The P-type reamer is more familiarly known as the Peeso drill. It has a long, narrow, tapering head with side-cutting, slightly spiraling, blades that have a wide rake angle. The head is connected to the shank by a short thick neck. The instrument can be obtained with or without a noncutting guide at the tip.

A-type and D-type reamers are similar in design. The A-type reamer has a long, tapered, pyramid-shaped, pointed head that is square in cross section with four

TABLE 13-1. Group II endodontic instruments

Instrument	Type of shaft used		
	Contraangle handpiece	Straight handpiece	Giromatic or Racer contraangle handpiece only
K-type reamer	X	X	—
B-2 reamer	X	X	—
H-type file	—	—	X
R-type rasp	—	—	X
Barbed broach	—	—	X
Quarter-turn reamer	—	—	X
Lentulo paste carrier	X	X	—

straight side-cutting blades and straight grooves between the edges. The head is connected to the shank by a short, narrow neck. The D-type reamer has a heavier, shorter neck with a shorter pyramidal point.

Ko-type, T-type, and M-type reamers are orifice enlargers intended for either straight or contraangle handpieces. The Ko-type reamer has a head similar to but longer than a tapered and pointed-fissure bur without a crosscut. Its eight side-cutting blades spiral slightly. The head is connected to the shank by a short neck. The T-type reamer has 12 to 16 straight side-cutting blades and a slightly shorter head length. The M-type reamer has an entirely round head with six to eight cutting blades. The neck is extremely long and somewhat flexible.

The root facer is a power-operated rotating instrument used in facing the exposed root surface of a crownless tooth. It has a thin wheel-shaped end-cutting and/or side-cutting head in whose center is a cylindrical truncated cone or pointed projection with smooth surfaces that enters the root canal.

Although they are not endodontic instruments in the strictest sense of the word, absorbent points and root canal filling points have been considered part of the Group IV armamentarium under the developing international standards. Root canal absorbent points are slender cones made of paper or other absorbent material; they are used for drying the canal, for conveying medicaments into the canal, and for obtaining canal cultures. Root canal filling points are smaller, slender cones of solid material; they are used for canal obturation and will be considered more fully in the discussion of root canal materials.

INSTRUMENT STANDARDIZATION

In 1962, at the annual session of the American Association of Endodontists, the research committee of the Association met with several representatives of the manufacturers and suppliers of root canal instruments to discuss standardization of the endodontic armamentarium. Out of these discussions was formed a working committee on endodontic instruments and materials under the auspices of the North American Section of the International Associa-

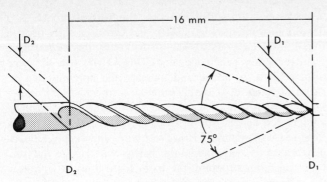

Terminology = D_1 expressed in hundredths of a mm
Diameters D_2 = D_1 plus 0.32 mm
Taper = 0.02 mm per mm
Tip angle = 75° ± 15° included angle
Tolerance = ± 0.02 mm
Length blade (D_1 to D_2) = 16.0 mm

FIG. 13-8. Standardized endodontic instruments.

TABLE 13-2. Terminology and color coding of endodontic instruments

Size	D_1 (mm)	D_2 (mm)	Color	Abbreviation
10	0.10	0.42	Purple	Pur
15	0.15	0.47	White	Wh
20	0.20	0.52	Yellow	Yel
25	0.25	0.57	Red	Red
30	0.30	0.62	Bluc	Blu
35	0.35	0.67	Green	Grn
40	0.40	0.72	Black	Blk
45	0.45	0.77	White	Wh
50	0.50	0.82	Yellow	Yel
55	0.55	0.87	Red	Red
60	0.60	0.92	Blue	Blu
70	0.70	1.02	Green	Grn
80	0.80	1.12	Black	Blk
90	0.90	1.22	White	Wh
100	1.00	1.32	Yellow	Yel
110	1.10	1.42	Red	Red
120	1.20	1.52	Blue	Blu
130	1.30	1.62	Green	Grn
140	1.40	1.72	Black	Blk
150	1.50	1.82	White	Wh

tion for Dental Research. In 1964 this group consolidated its efforts with those of the National Bureau of Standards, the National Institute of Dental Research, and the American Dental Association. The following year the American Association of Endodontists adopted the terminology and nomenclature of the proposed standardized instrument systems as the officially recognized system of the Association. In response to numerous developments in standardization of dental materials and devices on a worldwide basis, the responsibility for standard development was transferred to the American National Standards Institute (A.N.S.I.) and its Committee Z-156 (Dentistry), later to be designated Committee MD-156 (Medical Devices), with the Council on Dental Materials, Instruments, and Equipment of the American Dental Association acting as secretariat for the United States.[3]

Under the joint auspices of the F.D.I. and the I.S.O., whose memberships consist of several national standards of institutes, the development of worldwide standards for endodontic instruments is guided by (Technical Committee) TC-106 JWG-1 (Joint Working Group) and its task groups on terminology, dimensions and measuring systems, physical properties, and quality control.[5]

The F.D.I./I.S.O. TC-106 JWG-1 continues to progress in the development of international standards for endodontic instruments, and its efforts are well coordinated at many levels.

Both the American national standard (specification no. 28)[4] and the developing international standard contain several departures from the original concept of instrument uniformity as proposed by Ingle and Levine[82] (Fig. 13-8), most notably in the location of the measurements D_1 and D_2 and in the 0.02 mm increase in the differential (from 0.30 to 0.32 mm) between D_1 and D_2. In the new standards the shape and dimensions of the tip of the instrument are accounted for; they were not accounted for in the original (Ingle and Levine) proposal. The terminology remains

as proposed and a color-coding identification system has been added (Table 13-2).

The American national standard (no. 28) is for K-type reamers and files and does not include H-type files; nor does it include rasps, broaches, probes, applicators, condensors, or spreaders. All of these are included in Group I of the developing international specification. A separate specification (no. 58) for H-type (Hedström) instruments has been developed and was adopted by the Council on Dental Materials, Instruments, and Equipment of the A.D.A. and A.N.S.I. in 1981.[6] A subcommittee is continuing work on a specification for barbed broaches and instruments of this generic type (specification no. 63).

The files and reamers of the American national standard are made of stainless steel because carbon steel K-type instruments have been discontinued by most manufacturers. The specification calls for detailed dimensions and tolerances for the diameters, taper, tip, and length of the spiral cutting section of the instrument. Specific procedures for the measurement of dimensions are noted. Unlike the international standard, as yet to be adopted, the American specification includes physical tests of the instruments, detailing the equipment and procedures to record acceptable limits of resistance to fracture by twisting, stiffness, and corrosion resistance. Requirements as well as color coding are also included in the American specification.

The American standard calls for an included angle of 75 degrees, with a tolerance of ±15 degrees, to define the tip. The lengths of the tips of H-type files cannot be greater than twice the D_1 diameter. The development of the international standard has led to the adoption of automated testing and recording equipment for the measurement of physical tests analogous to those of the American standard. Evidence seems to indicate that although some progress has been made in the standardization of the endodontic armamentarium much work remains to be done.[87,97]

USE OF ENDODONTIC INSTRUMENTS

The most common endodontic instruments are shown in Fig. 13-9; they are the barbed broach, the K-type reamer, and the K-type file.

Barbed broaches are used primarily for the removal of intact pulp tissue. The instrument is introduced slowly into the root canal until gentle contact with the canal walls is made. It is rotated 360 degrees in either a clockwise or a counterclockwise manner to entangle the pulpal tissue in the protruding barbs. It is then withdrawn directly from the root canal. If successful, the entire pulp comes with it.

If the vital pulp is so inflamed that the gel-sol state of the ground substance has been altered by edema or the collagenous fibrous network has been destroyed, it probably cannot be removed intact by a barbed broach. The instrument will only lacerate the already hemorrhagic tissues. Unless a necrotic pulp maintains a high degree of cellular or fibrous integrity, it will not lend itself to removal by the barbed broach.

Because of these biologic realities and the design of the broach, this instrument has limited use in clinical practice. Occasionally it will effectively retrieve a paper point or cotton dressing inadvertently lodged in the canal.

Because of its soft wire core, the barbed broach is a flexible instrument (Fig. 13-10) and can be readily broken if not used cautiously. The incisions in the core (these form the barbs when elevated) (Fig. 13-4) extend some distance into the metal and increase the potential for instrument fracture. If the instrument is forced deeply into a tapering narrow root canal, the tips of the barbs will be compressed against the instrument shaft and will create a false sense of security. However, when the deeply embedded broach is withdrawn, the barbs will engage the surrounding tooth structure; the more force used to withdraw the instrument, the deeper the barbs will dig into the predentinal surfaces. If enough force is applied, the barbs will (1) bend back on themselves, allowing the instrument to be withdrawn (rare), (2) break off in the walls of the root canal (more common), or (3) tear at the base of the incision that produced them, resulting in a fracture of the instrument (most common). To avoid these hazards, the clinician must have a fine tactile sense; the use of a heavy-handled "broach holder" is *not* recommended. Rather, barbed broaches without handles or with light short handles are preferred.

Barbed broaches have been used in engine-driven contraangle handpieces designed for endodontics (Table 13-1) without significant incidents of instrument fracture.[76] They were selected for use in the Giromatic rotary reciprocal handpieces primarily because of their flexibility. Investigations have revealed that they are ineffective as root canal–cleaning instruments when used in endodontic contraangle handpieces because the rotary action of the instrument compresses the barbs against the core of the instrument and burnishes them in place after a very few minutes

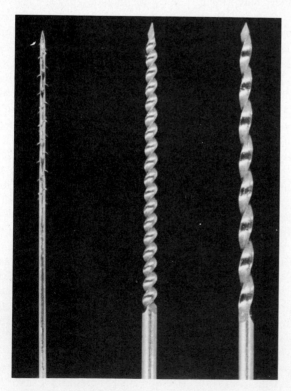

FIG. 13-9. Endodontic instruments: barbed broach, K-type file, and K-type reamer.

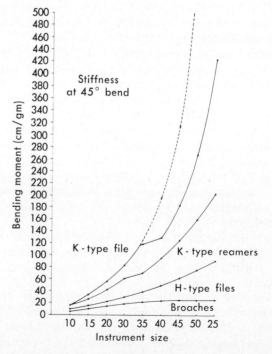

FIG. 13-10. Flexibility of endodontic instruments. The displacement of the curves for K instruments to the right indicates the change in blade shape from four sided to three sided.

at the 1000 to 1800 rpm normally used.[96,118] In effect, the barbed broach becomes a smooth root canal probe in a short time and exerts little if any cleaning action.

R-type rasps, being similar in design to barbed broaches (Fig. 13-4) but with shallower and more rounded protrusions, have also been utilized in engine-driven contraangle handpieces designed for endodontics; results have been slightly better than with broaches as far as cleaning effectiveness is concerned.[57] They produce rough-walled preparations in comparison to the other types of root canal instruments, as might be anticipated by their design. For rasping or honing a root canal, they have been superceded by H-type files in most techniques.

Endodontic applicators and probes (Fig. 13-1) are seldom used in routine practice. If it is necessary to swab a root canal by means of cotton fibers on a metal instrument, a fine-barbed broach can easily serve as an applicator. In place of root canal probes, once used extensively for the exploration of a root canal before instrumentation, the smallest-size K-type file is usually the instrument of choice in modern practice.

Endodontic files and reamers are by far the most frequently used root canal instruments in modern practice. The principal instruments are the K-type (more common) or H-type files. K-type reamers are less useful.

More is known about K-type files and reamers than about other types of instruments in endodontics, not only because of their widespread acceptance but also because of the impetus given to instrument investigation by the development of national and international standards. K-type root canal instruments are, size for size, stiffer and stronger than comparable types of instruments[75] (Fig. 13-10). This is mostly because of their mode of manufacture (Fig. 13-5), wherein the grain structure of the fabricating wire is preserved and the entire bulk of metal in the working portion of the instrument makes up the blade with its cutting edges. The ductility of the instrument, whether of carbon steel or stainless steel, varies according to the work hardening induced during drawing and fabrication.

Work hardening is a function of size, shape, and tightness of twist. For a given amount of twist, the larger instrument of the same shape will be more work hardened because of greater strains at its outer surfaces and edges. Similarly a square-shafted instrument with greater bulk at the outer extremities will have more work hardening than a triangular shafted instrument. The tighter the twist, the more work hardening will be induced. A reamer has about half the number of twists of a file the same size and as a consequence has about half the work hardening. A no. 60 file is three times larger than a no. 20 file, has approximately three fourths the number of twists, and is subjected to about two and one half times more work hardening. Stainless steel is more ductile than carbon steel, but this means little as far as reamers are concerned; for clinical purposes stainless steel is more significant in files.

The shape of the shaft of the instrument can be important in clinical practice. The triangular shaft requires a one-third rotation of the instrument to complete a cutting circle of the root canal wall, whereas the square shaft re-

quires but a quarter turn to accomplish the same end. An instrument having a triangular shaft gives a deeper cut with thicker cutting chips than does an instrument having a square shaft because of the triangular shaft's smaller contact angle with the root canal wall.[155] An instrument having a diamond-shaped or rhomboid shaft combines two acute edge angles and two obtuse edge angles, thus increasing the cutting efficiency of a four-sided instrument. When the blade engages the root canal wall in either instance, a large amount of compression/distortion occurs in the dentin, resulting in cracks that grow as tangents to the orbit of movement of the instrument's edge. When the cracks extend to certain distances, a chip of the surface 0.005 to 0.01 mm deep and 1 to 4 mm long will break away. Whether a K-type file or reamer is being used, the net result is the same if a cutting circle is completed.[72]

Because of differences in bulk, instrument ductility, and contact angle with the root canal wall between the square-shafted file and the triangular-shafted file, the clinical feel of the instrument and its consequences can be significant. Note that the curve for K-type files in Fig. 13-10 abruptly changes between sizes 30 and 35, as does the curve for K-type reamers between sizes 25 and 30. This is because of a shift that some manufacturers make from square shafts in smaller instruments to triangular shafts in larger instruments. If the K-type files continued to be made of square shafts, the curve for stiffness would go on as indicated by the dotted line. If this change of instrument shaft shape is not perceived and compensation made, the clinician is likely to experience an increase in instrument breakage by assuming a naturally increasing progression of applied forces during instrumentation.[98]

Three K-type files, one with a square shaft, one with a

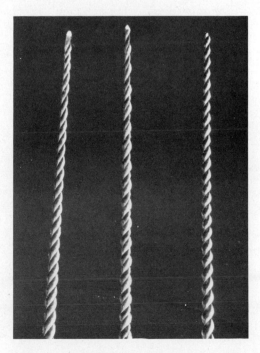

FIG. 13-11. K-type endodontic files. *Left to right,* Square, rhomboid, and triangular shafts.

rhomboid shaft, and one with a triangular shaft, are shown in Fig. 13-11. The irregular appearance of the file with the rhomboid shaft is due to the alternating low-profile obtuse angles with high-profile acute angles of the shaft as it is twisted to form a working blade.

A root canal preparation that is round in cross section can be made only by the rotary action of a K-type file.[170] In relatively straight root canals this can be accomplished 80% of the time at the apical 1 mm level. In severely curved canals it can be accomplished approximately 33% of the time at the same level.[146] Neither K-type files nor K-type reamers will produce any significant deviation from circular canal preparations when used with a reaming action; however, files used with a filing action will produce significant deviations from circular preparations. Aside from being slightly more flexible and less susceptible to fracture, K-type reamers offer no advanges over K-type files.

A comparison of the common square-shafted files to triangular-shafted reamers is given in Table 13-3. The triangular- or rhomboid-shafted files are similar to reamers despite the increased effectiveness of the newer designs.[171,174] The carrier effect is the ability of an instru-ment to carry or withdraw debris from the root canal. For most instrumentation the K-type file has replaced the K-type reamer as the instrument of choice.

Too deep a bite of the cutting edge of a K-type file or reamer into the root canal wall during rotary movement of the instrument can lock the instrument into the tooth. If continued torque is applied in a clockwise cutting motion, the spirals will first elongate and then twist on themselves as the elastic limits of the metal are exceeded. Endodontic instruments with uneven spacing of the spirals or flutes of their working blades are subjected to these forces and are liable to fracture. If irreversible instrument stress is detected, the instrument should be discarded. Two types of fracture of K-type instruments have been observed.[94] The first is a splintering of the instrument as continued clockwise torque is applied (Fig. 13-12, *A*); the second is a sudden clean break of the instrument, usually seen when counterclockwise torque is applied to a locked instrument (Fig. 13-12, *B*). The minimum values for torque as required by the American specification are shown in Fig. 13-13. These are values for a clockwise instrument fracture and are significantly higher than those for a counterclockwise instrument fracture.

Many methods for removing fractured root canal instruments have been reported in the literature—from wrapping broaches with cotton to entangle and remove a loose fragment, isolating with burs and removing the tip with splinter forceps, and working rasps or files alongside the fragment before honing it out, to using trepan burs, ultrasonic vibration, and the Masserann Extractor (a hollow tube with an internally locking stylus) to remove the fragment.[54] No known method is either totally effective or totally without hazards. Often the fragment can be bypassed and sealed in the tooth by being incorporated into the root canal filling. If it is occluding the apical foramen, the instrument frag-

TABLE 13-3. Comparison of common K-type endodontic files and reamers

Feature	Reamers	Files
Helical angle of edge	Small	Large
Carrier effect	Poor	Good
Ration of spiral numbers	Few	Many
Tactile sense inside canal	Rough	Smooth
Cutting mode	Clockwise turn only	Clockwise turn with pull, or pull only

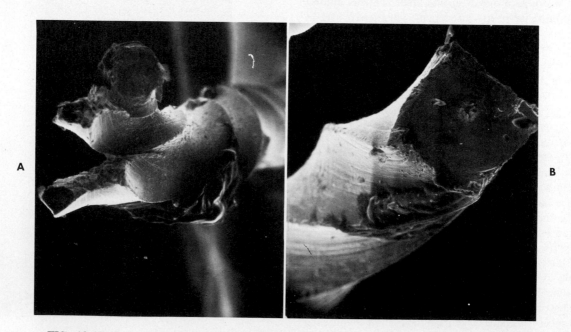

FIG. 13-12. Fracture of a K-type file by, **A,** clockwise torque ($\times 100$) and, **B,** counterclockwise torque ($\times 200$).

ment can actually serve as the apical seal when sealer is forced onto or around it. The condition of the tooth at the time of instrument fracture and the location of the fragment are significant to the prognosis of the case. When instruments are broken during the removal of vital intact pulps, the prognosis is better than when breakages occur in teeth with chronic periapical lesions and necrotic pulps. Instrument fragments tightly bound at the apical foramen afford a better clinical prognosis than do fragments located elsewhere (assuming they cannot be incorporated into the root canal filling).

Apicoectomies and retrograde root canal closure should be considered where indicated (Chapter 18). The clinician must keep in mind that many teeth with accidentally or intentionally broken instruments occluding the apical foramen have proved to be as clinically successful as have teeth in which routine root canal procedures under more usual circumstances have been performed.[39]

K-type files and reamers have not been used as engine-driven instruments because they are generally too stiff to negotiate any but large and straight canals.

The potential for tooth fracture as well as the hazards of root canal perforation due to the stiffness of these instruments are very real dangers with rotary engine-driven handpieces. To overcome the lack of flexibility found in the usual K-type instruments, a quarter-turn reamer has been developed for use with endodontic contraangle handpieces (Fig. 13-2). This instrument lacks the spiraling and resulting work hardening of the K-type instruments and closely resembles the blank from which K-type instruments are fabricated. No reports of the effectiveness of this instrument are obtainable as yet.

The H-type file, more commonly known as the Hedström file, is frequently used in endodontic practice for flaring of the canal from the apical region to the occlusal or incisal orifice. The design of the H-type file is such that the bulk of metal in the working blade supporting the cutting surfaces does not extend to the edges of the instrument but occurs as a central core of metal (Fig. 13-6). This relationship between the overall size of the instrument and its inherent strength and flexibility can be deceptive, because the instrument is only as strong or as flexible as the central core of metal from which the cutting edges protrude. When placed in contact with a root canal wall, the cutting edges contact the wall at angles approaching 90 degrees and when the instrument is withdrawn exert an effective honing action. Newly introduced H-type files such as the Unifile, designed by Burns and McSpadden, have cutting edges that contact root canal walls at angles significantly less than 90 degrees (Fig. 13-14). Although this feature does reduce somewhat the effectiveness of the instrument used as a file, it also increases the effectiveness of the instrument used as a reamer. Thus Unifiles are useful not only for honing but for rotary cutting as well.

A comparison of the common H-type instrument with a near 90-degree helical angle to a square-shafted K-type instrument is given in Table 13-4, which illustrates the extremes of the instrument types. If H-type instruments of the Unifile design were compared to K-type instruments with triangular or rhomboid shafts, the features of each type would overlap in several instances. What should be firmly kept in mind is that the designation H-type or K-type is a generic classification based upon manufacturing process and does not apply to any single design or line of instruments.

To use root canal files for maximal effectiveness, Shoji[55,156] recommends the K-type file for preparation of the circular apical retention form and the H-type file for cleaning and shaping the coronal half of the root canal

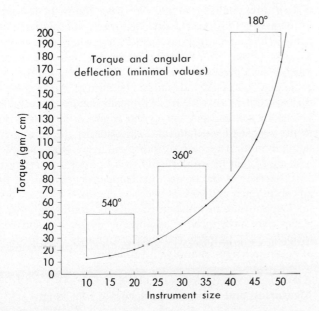

FIG. 13-13. K-type endodontic files and reamers under torque; minimum accepted standard, clockwise rotation only.

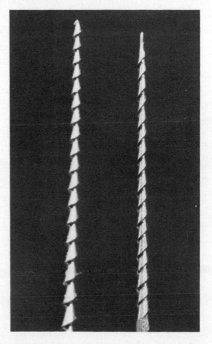

FIG. 13-14. H-type root canal files. Hedström *(left)*, Burns Unifile *(right)*.

TABLE 13-4. Comparison of common K-type and H-type (Hedström) endodontic files

Feature	K	H
Mode of use	Clockwise turn with pull, or pull only	Pull only
Rake angle of edge	45 degrees	90 degrees
Cutting efficiency	Average to good	Excellent
Carrier effect	Good	Good
Shaping of nonround canal	Average	Good
Resistance to fracture	Average to good	Poor
Cross section of prepared canal	Circular	Variable

system. The sequence as adopted by many similarly inclined clinicians would be to clean and shape the canal by means of serial filing and recapitulation using K-type files with rotary twists of a quarter turn or more followed by withdrawal strokes, thereby creating a conical preparation to the apical foramen, and then following through with H-type files to create a flare for accessibility from the apical third of the canal to the occlusal or incisal orifice.

In investigations of the thoroughness of dentinal wall preparation by means of root canal instruments,[57] the K-type files produced the cleanest and smoothest surfaces. Surfaces produced by H-type files, although clean, were not as smooth. No engine-driven instrument has been demonstrated to be as effective as the hand-operated K- or H-type file.[119,141] H-type files have been used in endodontic contraangle handpieces where it was thought their feasibility and design would be well suited; but because they cut only on withdrawal, they proved to be ineffective when rotary forces of a reciprocating nature were applied. Rapid vertical strokes only revealed the deceptive vulnerability of these files to fracture without demonstrating their full potential when forced into narrow canals. Nygaard-Østby recommended modification of the basic H-type file by blunting or removal of the sharp tip of the instrument, and this modified file has some merit when used in the recommended manner. The modification of the basic H-type file by reduction of the helical angle of the shaft spiral has been noted previously.

Single-part engine-driven instruments

The various single-part engine-driven root canal instruments of Group III (Fig. 13-3) are primarily used in the coronal third or orifice of a canal; they are not well adapted to use in the deeper middle and apical thirds of the canal. All of these, including the root facer, have special purposes for which they were designed.

The principal ones seen in American endodontics are the G-type reamer (Gates-Glidden drill) and the P-type (Peeso) reamer. Both instruments have had a long and checkered history in endodontics but currently are enjoying a revival; they are being recommended by some clinicians for finishing and enlarging the orifice and coronal third of a root canal *following* serial filing and flaring with files.[1] However, the improper use of either instrument to enlarge an uninstrumented root canal or to prepare the root for a post-

core retainer is fraught with dangers of root perforation. Preferably the canal should be enlarged with hand instruments, whether it contains pulpal debris or root canal filling material, and the engine-driven reamers of Group III should be considered as auxiliary instruments to taper the preparation only. In many instances long tapered diamond stones can be used in this manner, with little if any danger of removing excessive tooth structure or of perforating the root.

As stated earlier, there has been a revival of interest in engine-driven root canal instruments since the introduction of the Giromatic contraangle handpiece in 1964. The mechanical principle of reciprocating rotary motion and its application to the use of endodontic instruments have been known for many years. Agricultural workers are familiar with the difficulty of forcing posts directly into the earth as opposed to working them in with back-and-forth rotary motions. The endodontic contraangle handpieces produce this action mechanically. The Racer instrument also moves the instrument vertically with short pushing-pulling action. Aware of the dangers of pushing debris beyond the confines of the root canal by the injudicious use of apically directed strokes of root canal instruments, most clinicians have been cautious in adopting the Racer instrument. The Giromatic instrument and similar types have received more attention in spite of data from several sources indicating that barbed broaches, "Giromatic files" (R-type rasps), and H-type (Hedström) files, when used with these contraangles, are *significantly less successful* in cleaning canals than are conventional hand-operated instruments.

The effectiveness of special designed engine-driven reamers remains to be proved. Claims for operating efficiency are often made for engine-driven instruments in comparison to the "time-consuming" use of hand-operated root canal instruments; but in a study comparing the Giromatic instrument with broaches to hand-operated H-type files in 41 canals,[76] no significant differences in operating time could be found. Nor have claims of lessened incidences of instrument breakage been substantiated by comparative investigations, particulary when the ineffectiveness of the instruments used in the endodontic contraangle handpieces is considered. The contraangle for root canal exploration has advantages because of the fact that a fine instrument placed in a Giromatic handpiece can negotiate curved and fine canals, no doubt, in large part due to the sustained mechanical application of the rolling-rotating motion. This ease of root canal negotiation, coupled with significant losses of tactile sensation, creates the principal hazards of the device; inadvertent penetration of the apical foramen and lack of accurate control over the working length of the instrument. Endodontic contraangle handpieces may have merit if appropriate instrument and contraangle sizes, properly designed instruments, and methods of accurate length control can be achieved.

AIDS TO INSTRUMENTATION
Measuring and maintaining accurate root length

Determining and remaining within the confines of the working length of the root canal during instrumentation are a recurrent problem in endodontics. Several devices are available to help solve the problem. Historically the method of choice for the determination of the working length of a tooth in endodontics has been to take a radiograph of the tooth with a radiopaque instrument extending into the canal to the apical constriction as determined by digital-tactile sense. The measuring instrument is either bent or collared in such a fashion as to provide a mark or stop at an occlusal or incisal reference point, which will then be detectable on the radiograph. By measuring the length of the radiographic images of both the tooth and the measuring instrument, as well as the actual length of the instrument, the clinician can determine the actual length of the tooth by a mathematical formula.

Actual length of tooth =

$$\frac{\text{Actual instrument length} \times \text{Radiographic tooth length}}{\text{Radiographic instrument length}}$$

This principle can be used with measuring probes[22,24] having specially designed occlusal stops for ready reference both intraorally and on the radiograph.

Ingle and Tanter[83] recommended the following procedure: Measure on a preoperative radiograph the approximate working length of the canal by placing rubber occlusal stop on the shaft of a file used as an explorer; place the file in the canal, and expose a radiograph; on the exposed film, measure the distance between the tip of the instrument and the apical foramen; then determine the working length by making appropriate adjustments of the rubber stop on the instrument shaft. Other authors have recommended luting a metal pin of known length to the surface of the tooth parallel with its long axis before taking a preoperative radiograph. By means of a specially designed transparent BW gauge, through which the length of the pin and the length of the pulp canal are measured, compensation for radiographic distortion is made and the working length of the tooth determined.[16]

The method of determining the working length of a root canal as proposed in 1962 by Sunada[161] (see Fig 13-15) does not require radiographs. Sunada's work was based on the experimental studies of iontophoresis by Suzuki in 1942; in these studies the electrical resistance between the mucous membrane of the oral cavity and the periodontium was considered to be constant. Electrical resistance between the oral mucous membrane and the periodontal ligament supposedly would also register a constant reading when a measuring probe reached the periodontium via the pulp canal. This resistance to the passage of an electric current when a metal instrument introduced into the root canal reaches the apical area has been found to be consistent and equal to approximately 6.5 Ω. Several electronic devices based upon this principle are currently available. (See Fig. 7-26.) Some use dials or gauges to indicate the electrical resistance relationships of the oral mucosa and the periodontal ligament at the tooth apex; others use audible tones or signals.

Evaluations of the various means and devices used for determining root length indicate that the radiographic methods may still be consistently the most accurate.[22,132] The use of the BW gauge causes great variations in mea-

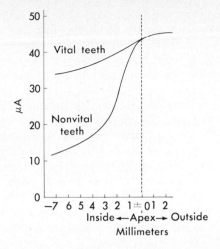

FIG. 13-15. Electrical resistance of teeth. (From Sunada, I.: J. Dent. Res. **41**:375, 1962.)

surements, as does use of the actual length-radiographic length formulas, particularly when the measuring probes are not placed close to the apical foramen.[147] There are indications that just the digital-tactile sense of the experienced clinician (without radiographic references) may detect the apical constriction and produce an accurate determination of the working length 60% or more of the time.

Clinical reports on the accuracy of electronic locators of the apical foramen are conflicting. Some indicate a rather high degree of accuracy (from 83% to 89%) whereas others report the level of accuracy to be less than 50%. Radiographic determination of the location of the apical foramen would appear to be no more accurate in most instances.[32] Although there appears to be merit in the use of nonradiographic devices to determine working lengths in endodontic therapy, the lack of a permanent record for comparisons and the time and technical factors involved have not led to their widespread adoption.

The recent introduction of the NeoSono-D (digital) has substantially reduced the time and technical problems associated with electronically determining the location of the apical foramen. (For further discussion of this device see Chapter 7.)

To control the working length of an instrument while it is being used once the working length has been determined, several varieties of instrument markers or stops are available. The simplest and perhaps most common are little pieces of rubber dam made with an ordinary paper punch or clippings from rubber bands of various sizes and colors. Small multicolored markers made of nylon or soft plastic are available commercially from several sources. These rubber or plastic markers are placed around the instrument shaft by passing the instrument through them. Also available commercially are tubular instrument stops made of plastic that clip onto the base of the instrument handle after the working blade has been passed through them. These in effect extend the length of the handle while reducing the length of the instrument shaft, thus providing a positive marking or stop. One type has a fine tubular extension that ensheathes the instrument shaft and acts as a stop at the floor of the pulp chamber. These plastic stops are available in a variety of colors, lengths, and sizes. The Kruegar stop is a sliding metal clip that fastens onto a long-handled instrument and projects forward over the instrument shaft, which passes through it. Working lengths can be adjusted by sliding the clip along the instrument handle.

Another system uses the Unigauge test handle. Endodontic instruments (K-type reamers, K-type and H-type files, and R-type rasps) are *unmounted,* and a short portion of the terminal end of the shaft is bent at a right angle to fit a specially designed adjustable handle. Unigauge test handles can be obtained in either the long or the short design. By means of a knurled locking nut on the forward portion of the handle in combination with a slotted posterior portion of the handle, the length of the working blade is adjustable from 20 to 28 mm.

Irrigation

Irrigation during instrumentation is not only desirable but imperative. In current endodontic practice, sodium hypochlorite is generally recognized as the irrigant of choice. However, a commerical disodium ethylenediaminetetraacetate (EDTA) preparation containing cetyl trimethylammonium bromide, sodium hydroxide solution, and distilled water (REDTA) is the most effective agent discovered to date for chemically cleaning the walls of a root canal.[110] Both agents appear to be less caustic than sodium hypochlorite and—except for dissolving pulp tissue and microorganisms—equal to it in every respect. Other types of EDTA solutions and lubricating gels or pastes are often recommended because of their chelating effects.

Scanning electron microscopic investigations[9] indicate that the particular irrigating solution or lubricating agent used may not be as important in removing root canal debris as is the *volume* of the irrigating agent. Since the removal of debris seems to be a function of the *quantity* of irrigant used rather than the *type* of solution, physiologic saline may well suffice in many instances and is certainly less toxic to viable tissues. However, other histologic and electron microscopic investigations show NaOCl to be essential for removing organic components associated with root canal cleaning and shaping; and solutions of EDTA are essential for removal of the inorganic debris produced.[62,120,162,173]

Several technical problems are associated with endodontic irrigation: getting sufficient volume of the solution to the working area of the instrument, particularly in fine or tortuous root canal systems; aspirating the expended fluid and debris from the tooth and operating field; and preventing the extrusion of either irrigating solution or debris beyond the apical confines of the tooth.[141,154]

Devices have been developed to assist the clinician in overcoming these problems. The endodontic irrigating syringe is the simplest approach. It consists of a disposable 3 ml syringe with a specially designed disposable irrigating needle. The needle is blunted and slit for 4 to 5 mm along one side from the tip toward the hub to provide an escape for fluids should the needle inadvertently bind in a canal. Patented needles with an occluded tip and a series of per-

forations along their sides have been developed especially for endodontics.[60,62] However, the hydraulic pressure necessary to force liquid through the minute perforations of these needles may well render the design impractical for clinical use.[91]

Several syringes have been either proposed or marketed for use with endodontic irrigation needles. They provide for aspiration of irrigating solution as well as deposition of the solution within the tooth, and they range from simple adaptations of tubing connected to saliva ejectors (for aspiration) to sophisticated patented devices that inject and aspirate as the clinician wishes.

Severe injuries have been caused by the inadvertent injection of irrigating solutions into periapical tissues during endodontic procedures.[11,18,74,172] Air embolism has also been reported as a consequence of syringes blowing compressed air into the open root canals of teeth.[138] The possibility of a resulting fatal reaction has been demonstrated in dogs. The severity of the reaction due to the irrigating solution's being forced beyond the confines of the apical foramen is dependent on the volume injected, the toxicity of the solution itself, and the location of the periapical tissues. In experimental situations [169] instrumentation of teeth flooded with irrigating solution by larger instruments (size 45 and above) has been shown to increase the potential for extruding debris and irrigant beyond the apical foramen. Selection of the type of irrigating solution to use, the device for using it, and the safest method for a particular clinical procedure involving irrigants should be made with these hazards firmly in mind.

Root canal filling devices

As stated previously, condensers and spreaders are available in a variety of sizes and handle designs. Several types of pliers, cutters, and forceps are available to meet the needs of silver point and gutta-percha filling techniques. For details of these the reader is referred to any of the general catalogs of instruments available from endodontic supply houses.

Paste root canal fillings and sealers present somewhat different clinical problems, and instruments have been designed specifically for use with them. The most commonly used instrument is the root canal paste carrier, or Lentulo spiral (Fig. 13-2). Mounted in either a straight or a contraangle handpiece, it is dipped into paste and rotated slowly into a root canal, at first to the length of the prepared root and then, with additional amounts of paste, to successively more occlusal levels until the canal is filled. Filling a root canal by this method does *not* produce a densely compacted root canal filling, and much reliance is placed on the adherence of the paste to the walls of the canal. The pastes used with the paste carrier to fill a canal often contain very radiopaque additives to give the *illusion* of a filling much denser than it actually is.

The paste carrier has also been recommended for the placement of root canal sealers into a prepared tooth before cementation of cones of silver or gutta-percha.

Pastes or sealers are mixed to a readily flowable consistency if they are to be used with the paste carrier. Thicker mixes of zinc oxide–eugenol paste are recommended for obturation of the root canal system in surgical cases or for primary teeth, where the consequences of extruding filler beyond the apical foramen are not as serious. Jiffy tubes have been found by most clinicians to be less than satisfactory. Disposable syringes designed for use with elastic impression materials do not allow for the extrusion of mixes of the desired consistency. Disposable 1 ml tuberculin syringes that, because of their size and construction, allow thick mixers to be expelled from modified 1 ½-inch, 18-gauge disposable needles or from plastic- or rubber-based injection tips cemented to the syringe do have some merit.[84] The thicker the root canal paste, the more dense and stable the ultimate root canal filling will be.

In selected cases the Pulpdent pressure syringe[66,67] (Fig. 8-103) has been adapted for use in the permanent dentition, particularly in cases involving immature roots, fine and tortuous root canals, and retrograde root canal fillings. The device consists of an internally threaded octagon-shaped syringe barrel; one end is machined to receive blunt-tipped needles with threaded hubs, and the other end contains a screw-type plunger with a knurled handle. Filling paste or sealer is placed in the hub of a needle selected to suit the size of the root canal to be obturated; that is, a 30-gauge needle corresponds to root canal instrument sizes 15 to 30, a 25-gauge needle to a size 50 instrument, and an 18-gauge needle to approximately 100 to 110. Seven sizes of needles (from 30 to 19 gauge) are available for the device. The paste-laden needle is screwed onto the syringe barrel, forcing some material into the barrel itself. Additional paste can be added by repeating the procedure of filling the needle hub and screwing it onto the syringe barrel. The screw-type plunger is inserted into the open end of the syringe barrel and turned clockwise until the compression forces created cause paste to appear at the needle tip. The handle of the plunger has four lines on it, indicating the distance of a quarter turn of the screw. By careful manipulation of the plunger, predetermined lengths of paste can be extruded from the needle tip. An accessory wrench is supplied; this not only assists in tightly screwing the needle in place but can also be used as a handle for the device when its closed end is slipped over the syringe barrel, with the bend of the wrench directed away from the operating field and the patient.

The Pulpdent syringe has been shown to be most effective for the purposes for which it was intended.[14] Pastes as thick as those used for temporary coronal restorations can be used with it, provided the mesh size of the zinc oxide or other base particles allows for flow through narrow apertures.

A mechanical compactor for gutta-percha also has been developed by McSpadden. This instrument, which resembles an H-type file with a reversal of the direction of its spiral, fits into a contraangle handpiece (Fig. 13-16). When rotated in a root canal in which a gutta-percha cone has been placed with a minimal amount of cement, it generates frictional heat sufficient to render the gutta-percha soft. The shape and direction of the instrument spiral puddle the softened material and force it apically, producing

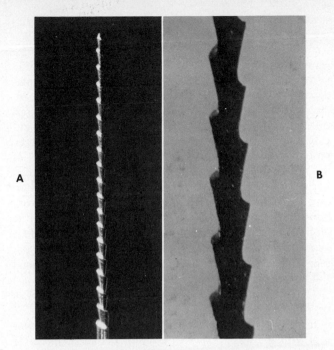

FIG. 13-16. A, McSpadden compactor. B, Longitudinal section of the compactor.

adaptation to irregular root canal surfaces. The device is effective in sealing certain types of root canal systems where there is minimal hazard of extrusion of material beyond the apex (p. 251).

ENDODONTIC MATERIALS

Modern concepts of root canal filling date to 1840. Since that time many materials have been used for filling the root canal. A partial list would include gold foil, gold foil with a shellacked surface, tricalcium phosphate with eugenol, zinc oxide and hydrochloric acid, pulverized animal charcoal with iodoform, orangewood points dipped into Black's 1-2-3 solution, iodoform and phenol paste, oxychloride of zinc and mineral wood, tin foil, lead foil with a paste of phenol and iodol, wood points soaked in bichloride of mercury (1:200), red cedar dipped into paraffin, equal parts of zinc oxide and iodoform in a paste with creosote, cotton points saturated with cinnamon oil or Campho-Phenique, thymol iodide and paraffin mixed under low heat, phenl salicylate and balsam in conical shapes, copper amalgam, zinc oxide-eugenol paste, dog dentin, ivory dust, and human dentin. The most widely used canal filling material until the middle of the twentieth century, however, was gutta-percha in solid forms or in a multitude of solvents.

Despite widespread usage, no scientific studies on the physical properties of gutta-percha were available until the exhaustive report in 1918 by Price and Miller. These authors were concerned principally with the physical changes observed in gutta-percha when heated, and they concluded that a contraction of 1% to 2% occurred if the material was heated to 75° C at the time of canal insertion. They suggested that solvents such as chloroform, eucalyptol, or rosin-chloroform mixtures were better than heat for inducing plasticity in gutta-percha, although it was noted that teeth filled with combinations of solvents and gutta-percha showed significant losses of volume and loss of adhesion to the root canal wall when the solvent evaporated; shrinkage took place toward the center of the material mass. Although the introductions of rosin-chloroform preparations by Callahan and eucapercha (gutta-percha dissolved in eucalyptol) by Buckley were designed to reduce shrinkage problems, the ultimate result was the same regardless of the solvent used, according to Price and Miller. Price and Miller also noted that a skin formed on the surface of chloropercha compounds, especially the rosin-chloroform combinations; under this surface skin the liquid retained all its original fluidity because of vapor control by the surface membrane film. Therefore, many months will elapse before these mixtures will obtain maximum contraction and solidification into honeycombed masses.

The modern era of root canal filling materials began with a series of studies reported by Dixon and Rickert[47,48] in the 1930s. Their presentation of the ''hollow tube'' concept in 1931 was followed by tissue-tolerance studies of dental materials in 1933 and histologic verification of the results of root canal therapy in experimental animals in 1938. It was through these investigations that Rickert's formula root canal sealer was developed and tested. The hollow-tube concept remained unchallenged until the late 1960s,[25,63,166,167] when evaluation of the efficacy of root canal fillings by the use of radioisotopes and newer fluorescing dyes rekindled interest in root canal sealing investigations.

Although the methods of evaluating the biocompatibility of endodontic filling materials have technically improved with the development of introasseous and cell culture techniques, as well as with refinements of the subcutaneous and intramuscular implantation techniques used by Dixon and Rickert, there are still many who believe the basic premises of Dixon and Rickert remain valid. Surprisingly few investigations of the physical properties of endodontic filling materials have appeared in the literature in the half century since Price and Miller. In 1955 McElroy[112] noted that few of the numerous clinical claims for root canal filling materials were supported by clinical evidence and that very little data existed concerning the physical properties of endodontic materials. Since then several investigations of the physical properties of root canal filling materials have appeared and at least two treatises[4,34] have been published as chapters in dental materials texts.

The methods most frequently used to seal root canals are described in Chapter 8.

Although many authors using dye or radioisotope penetration studies have evaluated the efficacy of root canal fillings, few reports are more extensive than the one by Marshall and Massler.[103] These authors used four different root canal sealers with three gutta-percha and two silver point techniques and evaluated them by means of six different radioisotopes to measure leakage about the root canal filling from within and without the root canal. In all instances where silver cones were used to seal the root canal without a root canal sealer, complete penetration of isotopes occurred; by contrast, a gutta-percha cone without sealing of the root canal resulted in complete penetration of isotopes only half the time and partial penetration the other half. A gutta-percha cone with a sealer provided the best seal, showing less penetration than a silver cone with a sealer. Condensation of accessory cones was *not* used. Apical compaction of gutta-percha segments without sealer was not as successful as techniques using sealers. Although minor differences existed between the zinc oxide-eugenol based root canal sealers (Kerr, Grossman's, and Wach's), these sealers were all superior to chloropercha as cementing agents in this study. Unlike previous dye studies, the use of an occlusal seal did not affect the results of radioisotope penetration from the exterior of the tooth.

In another fluorescent dye investigation of the sealing properties of some root canal filling materials. Messing[114] summed up the situation by concluding that a good seal is possible with any conventional method of root canal filling provided careful technique is followed. The same conclusion applies with rare exception to most of the materials used in root canal filling.

ROOT CANAL FILLING MATERIALS
Gutta-percha

Gutta-percha, the purified coagulated exudate from ''mazer wood trees'' indigenous to the islands of the Malay archipelago, has been used in dentistry since the nineteenth century. Every conceivable use for such a ''plastic'' (trinkets, substitutes for cloth, instruments, tools, and even entire structures such as boats) has been made. (See Chapter 25).

Since gutta-percha deforms when warmed, its use resulted in the softening of garments, shoes, and structures with heat. At first, gutta-percha as a pure substance was found to be useless in dentistry; but the discovery that its innate hardness could be altered by the addition of zinc oxide, zinc sulfate, alumina, whiting, precipitated chalk, lime, or silex in various combinations increased its potential as a restorative material. Attempts to use the polymer with various inert fillers (the original composite) as a permanent restorative material proved futile by the middle of the nineteenth century, but its use in temporary restorations continued unabated for over 100 years. As a root canal filling material, it has been reported from as early as 1865.

Before the addition of waxes, fillers, and opacifiers, gutta-percha is a reddish tinged, gray translucent material, rigid and solid at ordinary temperatures. It becomes pliable at 25° to 30° C and is a soft mass at 60°; it melts, partially decomposing, at 100° C.

Chloroform, carbon disulfide, and benzene are the best solvents for gutta-percha, as they are for most hydrocarbons. Exposed to light and air, gutta-percha changes crystalline form and may oxidize, becoming a brittle resinous material. Ozone and sulfur cause similar reactions. Gutta-percha is 60° crystalline at ordinary temperatures; the remainder of the mass is amorphous. It exhibits a property common to polymers—viscoelasticity—being elastic and viscous simultaneously.

Our understanding of polymers is relatively recent. Nat-

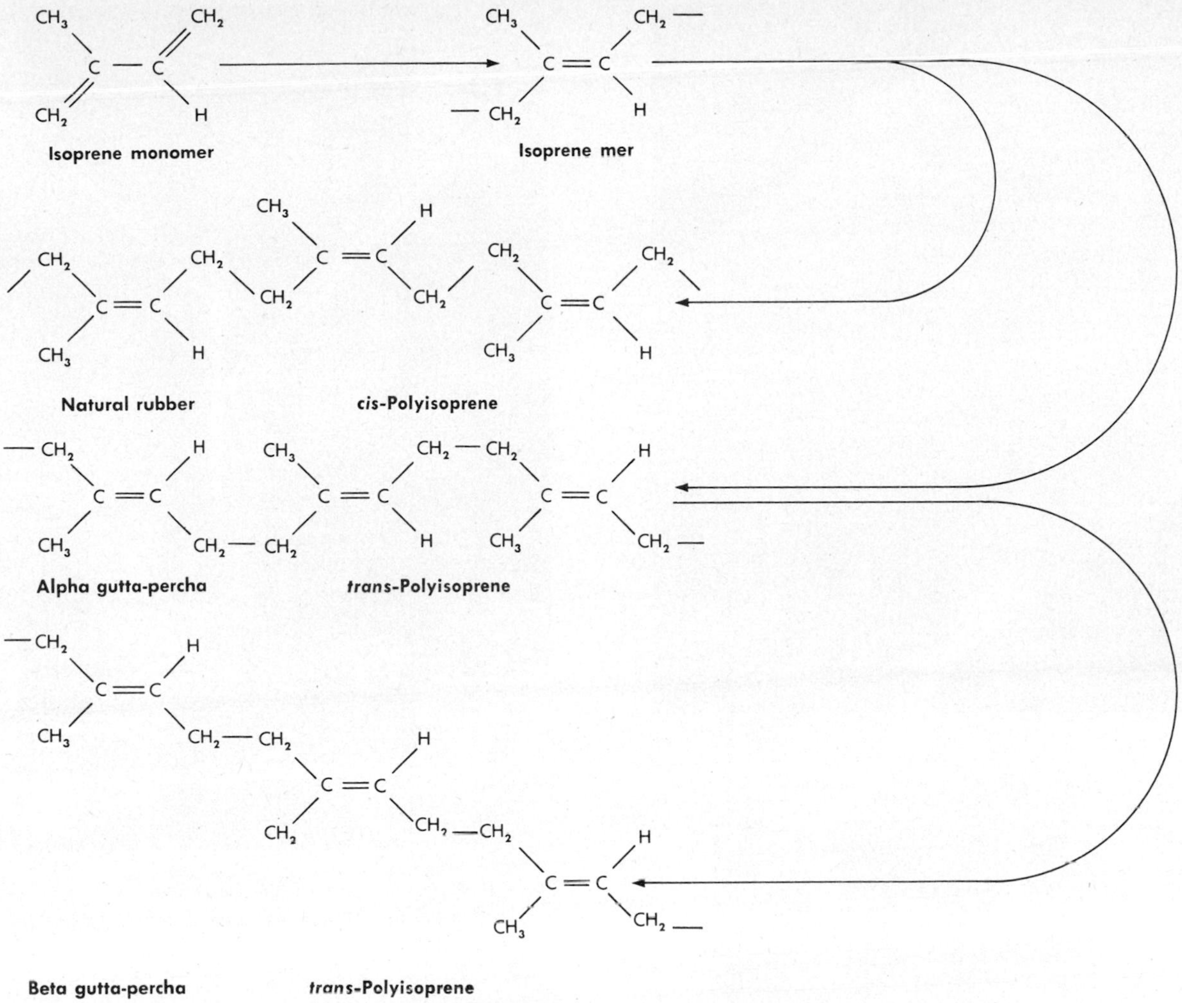

FIG. 13-17. Molecular chemistry of gutta-percha.[65]

ural rubber and gutta-percha represent an interesting example of isomerism. Both are high-molecular weight polymers structured from the same basic building unit or isoprene monomer (Fig. 13-17). Natural rubber, *cis*-polyisoprene, exists with its CH_2 groups (the chain forming the links of the individual isoprene units) on the same side of the double bond; gutta-percha, *trans*-polyisoprene, exists with its chain of CH_2 groups on the opposite sides of the double bond. The *trans* form of polyisoprene is more linear and crystallizes more readily; consequently gutta-percha is harder, more brittle, and less elastic than natural rubber. Two crystalline forms of *trans*-polyisoprene exist, differing only in single-bond configuration and molecular repeat distance.

If the naturally occurring *alpha* crystalline gutta-percha is heated above 65° C, it becomes amorphous and melts. If the amorphous material is cooled extremely slowly (0.5° C or less per hours), the alpha form will recrystallize. Routine cooling of the amorphous melted material, however, results in crystallization of the *beta* form; this occurs in most commercial gutta-percha, which becomes more amorphous when reheated at lower temperatures than does the naturally occurring material.

The reversion of the *beta* crystalline form to the naturally occurring alpha crystalline form, which is more brittle, is, according to investigators,[130,158] the primary reason why the gutta-percha cones used in endodontics become brittle with age. Gutta-percha aging can be delayed by storage under frozen or refrigerated conditions or can be reversed by tempering the brittle cones in hot tap water for a few minutes.

This complex admixture of alpha and beta crystalline forms, crystalline and amorphous states in the same mass, as well as the purity, molecular weight, compounding, and mechanical history of the batch, all affect the temperature-related volume changes and the related physical properties of gutta-percha.[145] Manufacturers of dental gutta-percha, through either trade secrecy or scientific ignorance, refuse to divulge information regarding the nature and source of their base material or the procedures involved in the processing. As a consequence, investigations of the composite used in dentistry are neither uniform nor comparable.[85]

Gutta-percha points used as root canal filling materials have been reported to contain 17% gutta-percha, 79% zinc oxide, and 4% zinc silicate; or else 15% gutta-percha, 75% zinc oxide, and 10% waxes, coloring agents, antiox-

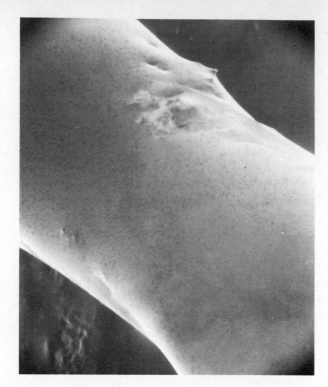

FIG. 13-18. Gutta-percha point. (×110.)

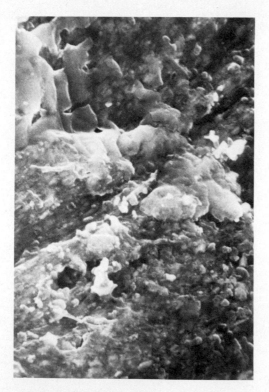

FIG. 13-19. Gutta-percha point. (×3000.)

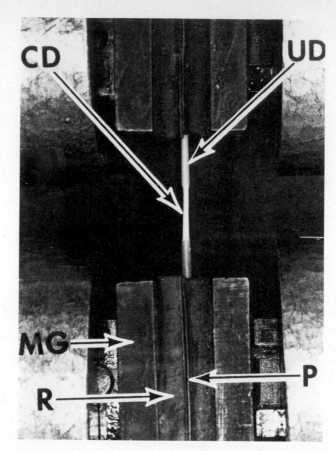

FIG. 13-20. Gutta-percha point deformed under tension.[56] *UD*, Undeformed point; *CD*, deformed point under stress; *MG, R,* and P, clamping apparatus.

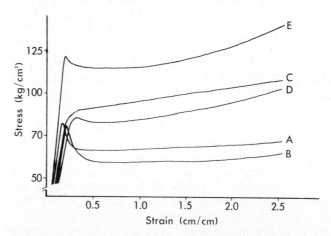

FIG. 13-21. Tensile stress-strain curves for five brands of gutta-percha.[56]

idation agents, and opacifiers.[56] Chemical analysis of five currently used brands of endodontic points has revealed a content of gutta-percha from 18.9% to 21.8%, zinc oxide from 56.1% to 75.3%, heavy metal sulfates from 1.5% to 17.3%, waxes and resins from 1% to 4.1%. The ration of gutta-percha and organic waxes and resins to zinc oxide

and heavy metal sulfates appears to be fairly constant despite variations in the specifics of either the organic or the inorganic components of the material. In spite of the secrecy surrounding the composition of the material, it is reasonable to assume that gutta-percha endodontic points are composed of approximately 20% gutta-percha, 16% filler, 11% radiopacifier, and 3% plasticizer. The appearance of the material under scanning electron microscope examination corroborates the chemical analysis. At 110×

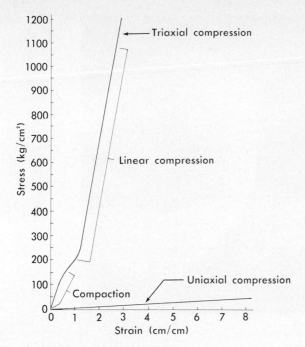

FIG. 13-22. Comparison stress-strain curves for gutta-percha.[144]

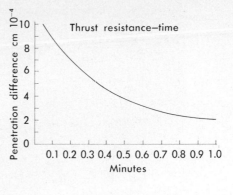

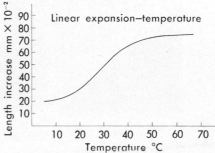

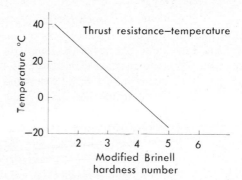

FIG. 13-23. Physical properties of gutta-percha.[71]

(Fig. 13-18) an amorphous irregular surface is seen wherein the speckled effect is probably zinc oxide particles on the surface along with waxes acting as plasticizers and antioxidants. At 3000× (Fig. 13-19) fine particles of zinc oxide (barium sulfate) are seen embedded in an amorphous and crystalline gutta-percha matrix.

Deformation of gutta-percha endodontic points under tension (Fig. 13-20) and plots of the resultant stress-strain curves (Fig. 13-21) reveal the elastic and plastic characteristics of the material.[56] The mechanical properties demonstrated correspond to those of a typical viscoelastic, partially crystalline, material. This is a substance that is extremely strain-rate sensitive, demonstrating a linear relationship between load and elongation up to the yield point, followed by a precipitous decrease in load tolerance. Comparison of these stress-strain data with the composition of the material reveals an inverse relationship between the zinc oxide concentration and the percentage elongation, possibly indicating that zinc oxide acts like a vulcanizing agent as well as simply an extender of filler.

Testing of compounded dental gutta-percha by the application of compression loads reveals some of the same characteristics (Fig. 13-22). Unrestrained flow in uniaxial testing prevents the development of stress levels sufficient to produce any molecular compression. Compressibility values obtained for dental gutta-percha in triaxial testing have proved to be less than those of water, which, for all practical purposes, is considered to be incompressible.[144] Below these levels of pressure, there is compaction of the material due to consolidation and the collapse of internal voids, as could be predicted from high-powered scanning electron microscope examinations. Contrary to empirical clinical claims, no molecular "springback" can be expected to assist in sealing the dentin–gutta-percha interface

by condensation techniques advocated for gutta-percha root canal fillings.

Several other parameters of the physical properties of gutta-percha have been reported.[71] Penetration of a gutta-percha sample by the thrust of a modified Gilmore needle apparatus (Fig. 13-23) shows a continuous distortion of the material with constant pressure over a period of time. The resistance of the material to penetration by a modified Gilmore needle is affected by the temperature of the material; there is a uniform rate of increase in resistance as well as in hardness and/or stiffness with decreasing temperature. Gutta-percha also undergoes linear expansion with alterations of temperature (Fig. 13-23). A gutta-percha point cooled to 15° C undergoes three fourths of its expansion by the time it reaches body temperature (37° C). Attempts to utilize the increased stiffness and subsequent expansion of gutta-percha by freezing gutta-percha root canal points with ethyl chloride spray have not been widely adopted because retention of these properties by the frozen point in room temperatures of 27° C has been found to be approximately 3 seconds.[71] Carrying heating instruments into a

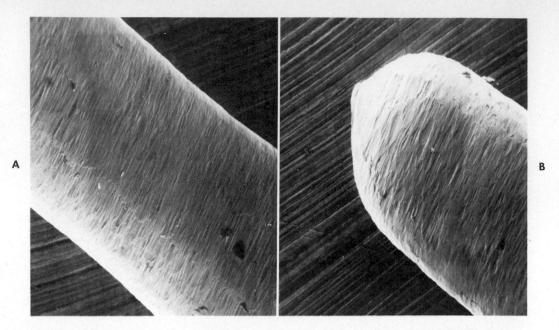

FIG. 13-24. A, Silver point (Star). (×110.) **B,** Silver point tip (Star). (×110).

root canal partially filled with gutta-percha in order to make use of these temperature-related properties probably does have some immediate effect; but the long-term result is inconclusive, with an increase in temperature of 4° C or less at the apex of simulated root canals by the time warm gutta-percha condensation techniques have been completed. Because gutta-percha remains solid at temperatures 10° C (or more) higher than body temperature, alterations of temperature within the root canal during root canal filling are most likely insignificant in clinical practice.[78] Thermoplasticized injection-molded gutta-percha has been advocated as a root canal filling—the ultimate in temperature-altered use of the material[183] (Fig. 8-90).

Alteration of gutta-percha by chemical solvents has had a long history in endodontic therapy. The effectiveness of solvent techniques in duplicating the intricate internal anatomy of a root canal system is evident; however, the material loses dimensional stability as the solvent is lost from the mixture.[93,112] The stiffer the gutta-percha point, the less compactible it is; and the more fluid the gutta-percha paste, the higher the shrinkage potential it has following evaporation of the solvent. At some future date gutta-percha points may be manufactured and marketed with varying chemical compositions and hence differing mechanical properties.

Silver cones

As root canal filling materials, metals have had a long history—equal to that of gutta-percha. Gold and lead were used as early as 1757 for filling the root canals of extracted teeth prior to replantation. In the nineteenth century, gold wire and gold foil were common root canal filling materials. Tinfoil, lead wire and cones, silver and copper amalgam, and gold-tin alloys have been recommended at one time or another.

Aside from its availability and physical properties, one of the reasons silver was selected in preference to other metals was undoubtedly its bactericidal effect, referred to as its oligodynamic property. The term *oligodynamic* dates from the 1980s and refers to the toxic effect on living cells of exceeding small quantities of a substance in solution. In the 1920s and 1930s silver, with its oligodynamic property, was widely recommended. The mechanism of oligodynamic activity was thought to be related to the surface area of soluble silver salts. The bactericidal effects were due to the affinity of silver ions for sulfhydryl enzymes, which ultimately caused protein denaturation.

As used in endodontics, silver is manufactured into tapering points designed to match the form of the canal after cleaning and shaping. Root canal sealers are needed to cement silver cones. Three common brands of silver points are shown in Figs. 13-24 to 13-26. Note that the surface texture and physical shape of silver points vary considerably by manufacturer. The relatively smooth but imprecise surface and tip shown in Fig. 13-24 can be contrasted with the machined and regular surface of those shown in Fig. 13-25 and with the cruder configurations shown in Fig. 13-26. Preciseness of shape affects accuracy of fit, and surface texture affects both cement adherence and corrosive potential.[164]

Despite manufacturing differences, the chemical composition of these brands is similar; and potentiostatic investigation shows no significant differences in their corrosion behavior in 0.9% NaCl, Ringer's solution, or serum. The silver content of these points ranges from 99.8% to 99.9%; nickel and copper are the elements next highest in concentration, 0.04% to 0.15% and 0.02% to 0.08% respectively. The hardness values for silver points average 112 Knoop hardness, corresponding to a region of Knoop values expected for cold-worked samples of commercial-

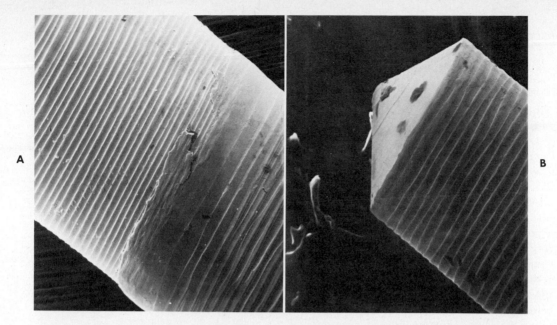

FIG. 13-25. A, Silver point (Kerr). (×110.) **B,** Silver point tip (Kerr). (×110.)

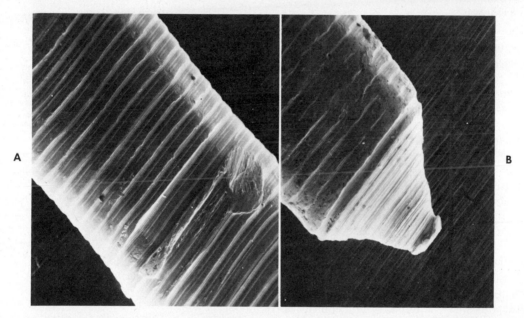

FIG. 13-26. A, Silver point (Premier). (×110.) **B,** Silver point tip (Premier). (×110.)

grade silver (99.9%). The tensile strength values determined for endodontic silver points (44,491 to 65,194 psi) fall in the range of values expected for cold-worked silver. The mechanical data available indicate that the degree of cold working associated with silver points probably lies in the range of 20% to 50%. Values for percent of elongation, proportional limit, and modulus of elasticity have been determined but are suspect because of induced experimental errors.

The salts formed by the corrosion of silver cones are silver chloride and silver carbonate or silver oxide. Sealers will protect a silver point extended into tissue for a short period of time, until the sealer is absorbed. Eugenol USP,

a common ingredient of sealers, is noncorrosive to silver. Corrosion of a silver point can be limited by sealing the point entirely within the root canal so it is surrounded and protected by sealer.

Most investigators[47,51,53] of the cytotoxicity of silver have concluded that, even though diffuse granular pigmentation is present in the tissue surrounding the implant and the implant itself shows signs of corrosion, the material is generally well tolerated. Cell culture studies have shown a similar tissue tolerance, but this could be anticipated because of the low solubility of silver in these techniques.[159] Tissue toxicity of the corrosion products of silver points was reported by Seltzer et al.[151] and investigations of the relationship of silver corrosion to tissue toxicity have followed.[21] Gutta-percha, by comparison, has been well established as a material with a very low cytotoxicity. Gutta-percha, including the paste forms once the solvent has dissipated,[90,159] is the least tissue-toxic material used in endodontics.[51,100,105,159]

In almost all clinical situations, core materials are used with a root canal sealer or cement. The bond between the sealer and the core material is nonadhesive.[23,90] The core-sealer root canal filling techniques therefore involve two interfaces: between the core and the sealer, and between the sealer and the dentin. One of the objectives of obturation techniques is to maximize the amount of core material to achieve dimensional stability by minimizing the amount of sealer. The critical relationship of core material to sealer has been demonstrated on several occasions wherein the adherence of sealing material to the tooth structure was at variance with the adherence to the core.[10,23,142] Investigations of the physical and chemical properties of root canal sealers and cements are therefore of prime importance to our understanding the technical endodontics.

ROOT CANAL SEALER-CEMENTS
Eugenol sealer-cements

Several types of sealers have been formulated for use in endodontics. The most common in current usage are based on zinc oxide–eugenol formulations. These include Kerr sealer (Rickert's formula), ProcoSol sealer (Grossman's formula), and Wach's paste (Table 13-5). They are the most widely used sealers and are manufactured and distributed throughout the United States.

Rickert's formula was developed in 1931 as an alternative to the chloropercha and eucapercha sealers of the period.[48] Gutta-percha–based sealers (chloropercha, eucapercha) lack dimensional stability after setting; Rickert's formula was developed to eliminate this problem. Several versions of Rickert's formula have been reported, and the range of ingredients in the powder component has varied slightly.

Because the relatively rapid setting time of Rickert's formula (Kerr sealer) caused some clinical hardships, Grossman's formula appeared in 1936, with the purpose of overcoming these problems. The formulas did not differ in essentials; both used precipitated silver. However, the use of precipitated silver for radiopacity was criticized[68]; a revision of Grossman's formula was marketed for many years as ProcoSol nonstaining root canal cement. Grossman's formula was again revised by the addition of sodium borate to the powder component and by the elimination of all ingredients except eugenol from the liquid component.[70] This is essentially how the material is formulated today, whereas the Kerr sealer (Rickert's formula) remains largely unchanged since its introduction nearly 45 years ago.

Kerr sealer and ProcoSol sealer enjoy the most widespread popularity of the zinc oxide–type root canal sealers. Wach's paste, a variant of a zinc oxide–eugenol formula, was originally compounded in 1925 but did not receive widespread adoption until its publication and reintroduc-

TABLE 13-5. Zinc oxide–eugenol sealers

Sealer	Content	Percent
Kerr sealer (Rickert, 1931)		
Powder	Zinc oxide	34.0-41.2
	Silver (precipitated-molecular)	25.0-30.0
	Oleoresins (white resin)	30.0-16.0
	Thymol iodide	11.0-12.8
Liquid	Oil of cloves	78.0-80.0
	Canada balsam	20.0-22.0
ProcoSol radiopaque silver cement (Grossman, 1936)		
Powder	Zinc oxide USP	45.0
	Silver(precipitated)	17.0
	Hydrogenated resin	36.0
	Magnesium oxide	2.0
Liquid	Eugenol	90.0
	Canada balsam	10.0
ProcoSol nonstaining cement (Grossman, 1958)		
Powder	Zinc oxide (reagent)	40.0
	Staybelite resin	27.0
	Bismuth subcarbonate	15.0
	Barium sulfate	15.0
Liquid	Eugenol	80.0
	Sweet oil of almond	20.0
Grossman's sealer (Grossman, 1974)		
Powder	Zinc oxide (reagent)	42.0
	Staybelite resin	27.0
	Bismuth subcarbonate	15.0
	Barium sulfate	15.0
	Sodium borate (anhydrous)	1.0
Liquid	Eugenol	100.0
Tubliseal (Kerr, 1961)		
Base	Zinc oxide	59.0-57.4
	Oleoresins	18.5-21.25
	Bismuth trioxide	7.5
	Thymol iodide	5.0-3.75
	Oils and waxes	10.0-10.1
Catalyst	Eugenol	
	Polymerized resin	
	Annidalin	
Wach's paste (Wach, 1925-1955)		
Powder	Zinc oxide	61.0-61.4
	Calcium phosphate tribasic	12.0-12.2
	Bismuth subnitrate	21.0-21.4
	Bismuth subiodide	2.0-1.9
	Magnesium oxide (heavy)	4.0-3.1
Liquid	Canada balsam	74.0-76.9
	Oil of clove USP	22.0-23.1
	Eucalyptol	2.0
	Beechwood creosote	2.0

tion circa 1955. It now is marketed under several commercial brand names with minor variations in formulation. Tubliseal, introduced by the Kerr Manufacturing Company in 1961 as an alternative to Rickert's formula, is a two-paste system as opposed to the powder-liquid systems of the other zinc oxide types. The exact formula is a trade secret, but its approximation is given in Table 13-5.

Zinc oxide–eugenol sets by a combination of chemical and physical processes, yielding a hardened mass of zinc oxide embedded in a matrix of long, sheathlike crystals of

TABLE 13-6. Sealers without eugenol

Sealer	Content	Percent
Kloroperka N-() (Nygaard-Østby, 1939)		
Powder	Canada balsam	19.6
	Rosin	11.8
	Gutta-percha	19.6
	Zinc oxide	49.0
Liquid	Chloroform	100.0
Diaket (Schmitt, 1951)		
Powder	Zinc oxide	98.0
	Bismuth phosphate	2.0
Liquid	2,2′-Dihydroxy-5,5′-dichlorodi- phenylmethane	
	Propionylacetophenone	
	Triethanolamine	
	Caproic acid	
	Copolymers of vinyl acetate, vinyl chloride, and vinyl isobutyl ether	
AH-26 (Schroeder, 1957)		
Powder	Silver powder	10.0
Liquid	Bismuth oxide	60.0
	Hexamethylene tetramine	25.0
	Titanium oxide	5.0
	bis-Phenol diglycidyl either	100.0
Chloropercla (Moyco)		
	Gutta-percha composition	9.0
	Chloroform	91.0

zinc eugenolate ($[C_{10}H_{11}O_2]_2Zn$). Excess eugenol is invariably present and is absorbed by both zinc oxide and the eugenolate. The presence of water, the particle size of zinc oxide, the pH, and the additives are all important factors in the setting reaction.[33,55,124] During the setting reaction a current sorption of eugenol takes place. Hardening of the mixture is due to the zinc eugenolate formation; the unreacted eugenol remains trapped and tends to weaken the mass.[157]

The method of preparation of the zinc oxide is closely related to the setting time of a zinc oxide–eugenol mixture. Increases in temperature or humidity decrease setting time. The longer and more vigorously the mixture is spatulated, the shorter the setting time. Setting time can be increased by decreasing the particle size of the zinc oxide. Free eugenol usually remains after the setting of zinc oxide–eugenol cements, including root canal sealers, and the comparative hardness of fresh dentin exposed to zinc oxide–eugenol sealers is increased in direct proportion to the amount of free eugenol available.[19] The significance of free eugenol is most apparent in increased cytotoxicity rather than through alteration of the physical properties of dentin.

Noneugenol sealer-cements

Table 13-6 gives the formulas of the most popular root canal sealers other than the zinc oxide–eugenol types. Kloroperka N-Ø was introduced circa 1939 from Norway and is similar to several empirical and domestic formulas dating from the early 1900s. Chloropercha (Moyco) is a direct

descendant, relatively unaltered, of materials in use for nearly a century. Diaket is an organic polyketone compound introduced in Europe by Schmitt (1951). It enjoyed some popularity in the United States following favorable reports concerning its superior strength and physical properties. The material consists of a very fine powder and a thick viscous liquid. The resin resulting from the mixing of the components of the sealer is very tacky in texture, adheres readily to tooth structure, and is often difficult to manipulate. As a polyvinyl resin, Diaket is essentially a keto complex in which basic salts and metal oxides react with neutral organic agents, forming polyketones, which in turn unite with metallic substances in the material to form cyclic complexes that are insoluble in water but soluble in organic solvents or chloroform. Used commercially as an industrial adhesive and insulator, AH-26, introduced in Europe by Schroeder (1957), is an epoxy-type resin for use in endodontic therapy. The addition of a hardener, hexamethylene tetramine, makes the cured resin chemically and biologically inert. Several proponents have demonstrated the favorable properties of AH-26 as an endodontic sealer.

At the Third International Conference on Endodontics, held in Philadelphia in 1963, Grossman[69] expressed the opinion that the development of simpler, more accurate, and more certain root canal filling materials would be the next significant breakthrough in endodontics. At the same symposium Buoncore indicated that polyethylenes, polypropylenes, nylons, and Teflon were unsuitable for endodontic usage because, in addition to requiring cure conditions of unacceptable times, temperatures, and pressures, nothing bonds to them; nor do they bond to other material. Vinyls require highly toxic solvents and root canal cements currently available would not adhere to them. Buoncore believed that injectable root canal fillings would be the path of the future. Recently Silastic materials and the hydrophilic acrylic resin Hydron had shown promise in this manner whereas the polycarboxylate sealer-cements in conjunction with cores had proved rather a disappointment.[10,139,142]

Crane et al.[38] reported on a zinc oxide root canal sealer that does not contain eugenol and that is analogous to periodontal packs without eugenol currently on the market. This sealer appears to possess physical and biologic properties making it favorable for use in endodontics.

Therapeutic sealer-cements

Table 13-7 gives the formulas of a group of root canal cements for which therapeutic properties are claimed. These materials usually are used without core materials; hence they are introduced into the root canal by means of either a Lentulo spiral or some type of injection device. The claim is made, particularly for the formulas containing either paraformaldehyde or iodoform (as well as other powerful and toxic antiseptics, that failures of the materials to provide a compact root canal filling are compensated by their prolonged or permanent therapeutic properties. Riebler's paste is the most extreme example of this type of agent, whereas Mynol cement and iodoform paste are somewhat similar in their composition and usage as cements or as sealers with core materials. Endomethasone and N-2 (Sargenti, 1970) are similar insofar as they contain, besides paraformaldehyde, corticosteroids in an attempt to alleviate the severe postoperative complications not infrequently seen with these types of materials. Both these materials contain lead as an oxide, which by increas-

TABLE 13-7. Medicated cements

Sealer	Content	Percent
Riebler's paste (Riebler)		
Powder	Zinc oxide	
	Formaldehyde (polymerized)	
	Barium sulfate	
	Phenol	
Liquid	Formaldehyde	
	Sulfuric acid	
	Ammonia	
	Glycerin	
Mynol cement		
Powder	Zinc oxide	
	Iodoform	
	Rosin	
	Bismuth subnitrate	
Liquid	Eugenol	
	Creosote	
	Thymol	
Iodoform paste (Wolkhoff, 1928)		
Powder	Iodoform	
Liquid	Parachlorophenol	45.0
	Camphor	49.0
	Menthol	6.0
Endomethasone		
Powder	Zinc oxide	
	Lead oxide	
	Bismuth subnitrate	
	Dexamethasone	
	Hydrocortisone	
	Thymol iodide	
	Paraformaldehyde	
Liquid	Eugenol	
N-2 (Sargenti, 1970)		
Powder	Zinc oxide	69.0-62.0
	Lead tetroxide	12.0-11.0
	Paraformaldehyde	6.5
	Bismuth subcarbonate	5.0-9.0
	Bismuth subnitrate	2.0-4.0
	Titanium dioxide	2.0-3.0
	Barium sulfate	2.0-3.0
	Phenylmercuric borate	0.1
	Hydrocortisone	1.2
	Prednisolone	0.2
Liquid	Eugenol	92.0-100
	Geraniol (perfume)	8.0
Calcium hydroxide paste (Laws, 1962)		
Powder	Calcium hydroxide	
Liquid	Propylene glycol	
Calcium hydroxide paste (Frank, 1962)		
Powder	Calcium hydroxide USP	
Liquid	Camphorated parachlorophenol USP	

ing radiopacity not only gives the illusion of the material's compactness once inserted but also, at least in the case of N-2, may contribute to the extreme hardness and slow solubility of the final set. Apparently lead oxide reacts and binds with eugenol in a more permanent manner than does zinc oxide. Some current formulations of N-2 contain neither corticosteroids nor lead tetroxide but still continue the use of paraformaldehyde.

Paraformaldehyde-containing root canal cements have had a long and intermittent history in dentistry. In current practice they may well have a place in temporary pulpotomy procedures, but they are *not* indicated for use in total pulpectomy procedures or in the treatment of necrotic pulp canals in the permanent dentition. Paraformaldehyde-containing pastes may be *clinically* successful in vital pulpotomy and pulpectomy procedures, but their limitations must be recognized. Formaldehyde causes necrosis of vital tissue. This is the basis of fixing tissues with formalin for histologic examination. Since tissue fixation with formaldehyde is a slow low-grade process, pain is seldom a problem (unless the material is injected forcibly beyond the apical foramen) and "clinical success" may *appear* to have been achieved. The consequences of accidentally extruding these materials beyond the confines of the tooth are often severe, as even their proponents recognize. Iodoform is somewhat less toxic; but it presents a similar hazard even though it does not achieve its antibacterial activity by cell fixation, as does paraformaldehyde.

The inclusion of heavy metal ions (e.g., mercury or lead) is potentially dangerous in root canal sealers because these ions are disseminated throughout the body, posing particular problems for target organs remote from the teeth.[31,133] Corticosteroids used in conjunction with these materials to suppress clincial symptoms may, additionally, pose hazards that are as yet unsuspected.

Calcium hydroxide pastes have also been formulated for use as root canal filling materials.[95] These serve as therapeutic temporary or interim root canal fillings when continued root development or osseous repair prior to final canal obturation is desired. Pastes of calcium hydroxide and sterile water are often used in vital pulpotomy procedures for much the same reasons.

Nontherapeutic filling pastes

Although at one time or another most of the sealer-cements recommended for core and cement root canal filling systems have been used independently as root canal filling pastes, few have been adopted for widespread use in clinical practice. Heavy thick mixes of PCA cement, a variant of Wach's paste, are recommended for use with the pressure syringe as a root canal filling material. Chloropercha techniques, in which gutta-percha is dissolved in chloroform or chloroform-rosin solution in situ within the root canal, have historically been a widely used means of obturation. The use of therapeutic sealer-cements to seal root canal systems has just been noted. What all these systems have in common is the elimination of one of the interfaces inherent in core and sealer-cement techniques. With core and sealer-cement techniques there must be a bond between the sealer-cement and the dentin as one interface and between the sealer-cement and the core as the other interface, whereas with the paste filling techniques referred to here there is only a single interface between the filling material and the dentin. The theoretical attractiveness of this single interface approach should be apparent. The one nontherapeutic material specifically designed for root canal filling by injection of a self-polymerizing resin system is the hydrophilic acrylic resin Hydron.[12]

Hydrophilic polymers have been used for contact lenses and surgical implants and as a coating for surgical sutures. Hydron, poly-2-hydroxyethylmethacrylate, a hydrophilic gel with barium sulfate added for radiopacity, was introduced as a root canal filling material in 1978. When injected into a root canal by a specially designed device, it polymerizes in situ, depending upon the remaining moisture in the root canal available for its polymerization and expansion. Initial reports of the system held great promise; but closer investigations[61,88,92] have raised serious doubts as to its stability in the root canal once polymerized, its lack of homogenity as a filling material, its ability to seal a root canal system, its tissue tolerance prior to and shortly after polymerization, and the reproducibility of acceptable clinical results with it.

PHYSICAL PROPERTIES OF ENDODONTIC MATERIALS

The evaluation of an endodontic material for safety, efficacy, and appropriateness can be done in three ways. These are, in ascending order of importance, assessments of its *physical properties,* its *biologic properties,* and ultimately its *clinical usefulness.* A well-conceived regimen for the development of a new endodontic material would most likely call for physical testing of the material to ascertain whether these parameters were suitable for endodontics; this would be followed by biologic testing to ascertain whether the material was compatible with living tissue and finally by clinical testing to determine its efficacy and safety under conditions in which it was to be used. Unfortunately, endodontic research has been concentrated primarily on the biologic properties of endodontic materials, with scant attention to their physical properties or the relationship of these with the observed biologic reactions. Well-designed and admittedly difficult to control clinical studies are even rarer than studies of the physical properties of endodontic materials.

The Committee on Dental Materials, Instruments, and Equipment of the American National Standards Institute (A.N.S.I.MD-156) and its Council counterpart in the American Dental Association have recently adopted a specification (no. 57) for endodontic filling materials.[6] Although the endodontic literature is replete with references to the requirements of the ideal root canal filling material (see Chapter 8), these listings have not been defined in the form of scientifically observable physical properties. From an overview of the endodontic literature dealing with root canal filling points, sealer-cements, and filling pastes, a consensus of what physical properties are of primary importance can be derived. These properties are addressed in

Specification no. 57 as well as in a series of specifications for endodontic filling materials under development by I.S.O. working groups.

Specification no. 57 classifies endodontic filling materials as follows:

Type I. Core (standardized) and auxiliary (conventional) points to be used with sealer cements
  Class 1. Metallic
  Class 2. Polymeric
Type II. Sealer-cements to be used with core materials
  Class 1. Powder and liquid nonpolymerizing
  Class 2. Paste and paste nonpolymerizing
  Class 3. Polymer resin systems
Type III. Filling materials to be used without either core materials or sealer cements
  Class 1. Powder and liquid nonpolymerizing
  Class 2. Paste and paste nonpolymerizing
  Class 3. Metal amalgams
  Class 4. Polymers

Endodontic filling materials of all types must meet certain general requirements. Metals or alloys should be pure and free of inclusions and other extraneous matter, with no evidence of tarnishing or corrosion when examined without magnification. Polymeric materials should be constituted from quality materials and free of impurities and inclusions with the uniform distribution of additives throughout.

The components of these materials should be free of extraneous materials and manufactured according to high standards. The components as well as the mixed or combined materials should be nontoxic in use and such that, when mixed or combined in accordance with the manufacturer's instructions, they will set to the requisite condition within a suitable time. The materials and components also should comply with the relevant sections of American National Standards Institute-American Dental Association Document no. 41 ("Recommended standard practices for the biological evaluation of dental materials")[7]

Type I materials (core and auxiliary points) are expected to conform to certain design, workmanship, and color requirements.[59] These are given in Table 13-8 and Fig. 13-27, for core points, and Table 13-9 and Fig. 13-28, for auxiliary points. The nominal length of Type 1 materials must not be less than 30 ± 2.0 mm, with diameter tolerances of ± 0.02 mm for Class 1 (metallic) points and ± 0.05 mm for Class 2 (polymeric) points including gutta-percha. Type 1 materials are color coded either individually or by unit packs, as are correspondingly sized instruments. After sterilization by methods recommended by the manufacturer, core and auxiliary points should still comply with the physical and mechanical properties called for in Specification no. 57, and neither the components as supplied nor the materials of Type 11 and Type 111 should sustain or enhance the growth of microorganisms.

All the types of endodontic materials covered in the specification must exhibit suitable radiopacity.[17] Since dentin or cortical bone has a demonstrated radiopacity

TABLE 13-8. Identification and dimensions of endodontic core (standardized) points

Size designation	Projected diameter at tip (mm)	Diameter D_1 (1 mm from tip) (mm)	Diameter D_3 (3 mm from tip) (mm)	Diameter D_{16} (16 mm from tip) (mm)
10	0.10	0.12	0.16	0.42
15	0.15	0.17	0.21	0.47
20	0.20	0.22	0.26	0.52
25	0.25	0.27	0.31	0.57
30	0.30	0.32	0.36	0.62
35	0.35	0.37	0.41	0.67
40	0.40	0.42	0.46	0.72
45	0.45	0.47	0.51	0.77
50	0.50	0.52	0.56	0.82
55	0.55	0.57	0.61	0.87
60	0.60	0.62	0.66	0.92
70	0.70	0.72	0.76	1.02
80	0.80	0.82	0.86	1.12
90	0.90	0.92	0.96	1.22
100	1.00	1.02	1.06	1.32
110	1.10	1.12	1.16	1.42
120	1.20	1.22	1.26	1.52
130	1.30	1.32	1.36	1.62
140	1.40	1.42	1.46	1.72

Notes:

All dimensions must be measured to an accuracy of 0.005 mm.

A tolerance of ± 0.02 mm for Class 1 core points and ± 0.05 mm for Class 2 core points applies to D_1, D_3, and D_{16}.

Taper proportion is 0.02 mm per millimeter of uniform taper.

Overall length is not less than 30 ± 2.0 mm unless otherwise specified.

TABLE 13-9. Identification and dimensions of endodontic auxiliary (conventional) points

Normal size designation	Diameter D_3 (3 mm from tip) (mm)	Diameter D_{16} (16 mm from tip) (mm)
XF (Extra-Fine)	0.20	0.45
FF (Fine-Fine)	0.24	0.56
MF (Medium-Fine)	0.27	0.68
F (Fine)	0.31	0.80
FM (Fine-Medium)	0.35	0.88
M (Medium)	0.40	1.10
ML (Medium-Large)	0.43	1.25
L (Large)	0.49	1.55
XL (Extra-Large)	0.52	1.60

Notes:

All dimensions must be measured to an accuracy of 0.005 mm.

A tolerance of ± 0.05 mm applies to D_3 and D_{16}.

Taper proportion is variable dependent upon nominal size but is uniform.

Overall length is not less than 30 ± 2.0 mm unless otherwise specified.

equivalent to 1100 aluminum alloy, endodontic materials must be more radiopaque than this. A 2 mm differential in the thickness of aluminum has been shown to produce a reasonable differential of radiopacity when applied to clinical endodontics, and most if not all commercially available materials meet this criterion.

Specification no. 57 sets out requirements for the physical properties of Type II and Type III endodontic materials (sealer-cements and filling pastes). The tests to be utilized have been standardized and call for administration at a temperature of 23 ± 2° C and 50% ± 5% relative humidity after the materials or components have been preconditioned for at least 24 hours prior to testing. Setting time, dimensional stability, and solubility and disintegration tests are conducted at a temperature of 37 ± 1° C and a relative humidity of not less than 95% in addition to bench testing at room temperature and humidity.

The physical characteristics of the materials with which the specifications is concerned are as follows:

1. *Working time.* This is determined only for materials whose fabrication requires less than ½ hour. Starting 210 ± 5 seconds after the commencement of mixing, 0.5 ± 0.02 ml of material is placed between two glass plates, the upper plate is weighted to a total of 120 g, and the time it takes for a disc to form that is 10% smaller than one formed after 10 minutes is recorded. Sufficient working time is important for endodontic materials and is a property related to but independent of setting time. The working time of the material is required to be within ± 10% of that claimed by the manufacturer.

2. *Flow.* This is determined in much the same manner as working time. Ten minutes after the commencement of mixing, the weighted cover glass is removed and the average major and minor diameters of the compressed disc of material are recorded. If these diameters do not agree to within 1 mm, the test is repeated. When tested by this method, the material should show a disc diameter of at least 25 mm. The flow of root canal sealers has been reported from (a) testing by displacement in glass tubes, (b) recording unimpeded flow down tilted glass surfaces and (c) rheologic studies capable of producing sophisticated data.[111,168,179,184] None of these methods is as practical or as simple as that called for in the specifications.

3. *Film thickness.* This is determined by a method similar to

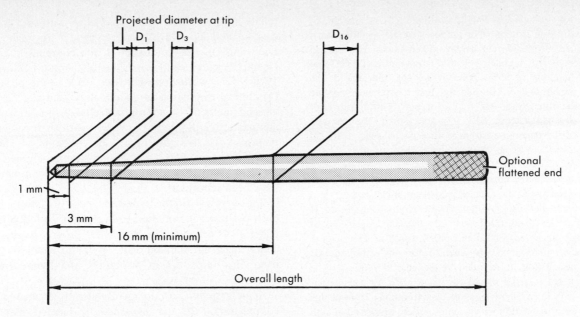

FIG. 13-27. Diagrammatic representation of core (standardized) points. Diameters: D_1, D_3, and D_{16} for each nominal size designation (see Table 13-8) Taper proportions: 0.02 mm per 1 mm D_{16} = Projected diameter at tip + 0.32 (Table 13-8) Overall lengths: Not less than 30 mm ± 2.0 mm unless otherwise specified.

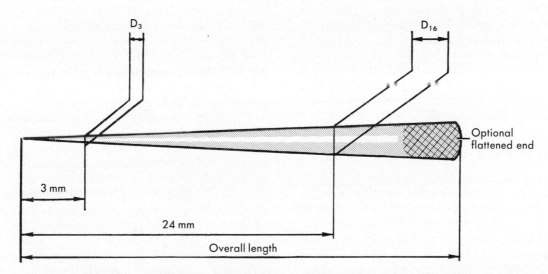

FIG. 13-28. Diagrammatic representation of auxiliary (conventional) points. Diameters: D_3 and D_{16} (see Table 13-9) Taper proportions: Variable according to nominal size Overall lengths: Not less than 30 mm ± 2.0 mm unless otherwise specified.

that described for the determination of working time and flow. In the case of film thickness the material fills the entire area between the glass plates and is placed under a force of 15 kg. After 10 minutes from the commencement of mixing, the thickness of the plates and the interposed sealer-cement film is measured to the nearest 5 mm. The film thickness compares favorably with that provided by the better luting cements in restorative dentistry. Film thickness measurements reported by others[62] seem to show this requirement to be appropriate.

4. *Setting time.* This is determined by means of a Gilmore needle with a mass of 100 ± 0.5 g having a flat end 2.0 ± 0.1 mm in diameter. A mold with the material in it is placed under the vertically descending needle after 150 ± 10 seconds have elasped from the commencement of mixing. The test is conducted at 37° C and 95% humidity. The setting time must be within ± 10% of that claimed by the manufacturer. Setting times of from 12 minutes to infinity have been reported under conditions similar to those called for in the specification. For this very reason the developing ISO standards classify root canal materials into setting and nonsetting types. As yet there appears to be no consensus as to what, if any, the ideal range for setting time should be for a root canal filling material; and clinical requirements may well be such that no definitive answer to this question can be given.[15,78,111,178]

5. *Dimensional stability*. This is an important characteristic of a root canal filling material. For purposes of the specification it is determined by placing the freshly mixed material in a mold and transferring it to a chamber with a temperature of 37° C and a relative humidity of 95%. When it has set, the ends of the specimen are ground or polished flat and the thickness of the specimen measured to an accuracy of 1 μm. Thirty days after storage in distilled water at 37° C it is remeasured. The maximal shrinkage of the material as a linear dimensional change should not exceed 1.0%. Various methods have been reported for the measurement of dimensionl stability in endodontic filling materials; all emphasize the importance that shrinkage of these materials can be relative to the maintenance of an apical seal.[15,178]

6. *Solubility and disintegration*. These physical properties of endodontic sealers in distilled water are measured by means of prepared specimens suspended in bottles stored at 37° C for 1 week. The net mass of the specimens before and after storage, and after desiccation, is recorded to the nearest 0.001 g. The solubility of the material should not exceed 3% by weight, nor should the specimens show signs of disintegration. Tests of this type have been reported in which samples were immersed in both water and dilute acetic acid.[78,111] The appropriateness of the test incorporated is well established by these tests as well as by histologic and clinical evidence.

Specification no. 57 does not call for the testing of either the compressive or the tensile strengths of root canal filling materials. It is questionable whether this information is truly applicable to the clinical circumstances in which these materials are used and whether performance requirements for strength would add to the safe or effective use of these materials. Because it is reported for cementing agents used in restorative dentistry, it has been investigated in endodontic studies as well.

BIOLOGIC PROPERTIES OF ENDODONTIC FILLING MATERIALS

The toxicity of endodontic filling materials has been of concern to dentistry for many decades, since the materials are placed in direct apposition to the connective tissues of either the pulp or the periapex when they are used clinically. These concerns for the biocompatibility of dental materials have consumed a great deal of time and effort on the part of endodontic researchers and have been extended to all types of materials used in dentistry. Until recently no standard protocol existed for the biologic evaluation of dental materials; then in 1971 the Council on Dental Materials and Devices of the American Dental Association approved for circulation and use in an interim period (from 1972 until 1975) recommended standard practices for toxicity tests of dental materials as developed by a subcommittee of the American National Standards Institute.

A.N.S.I./A.D.A. Document no. 41 ("Recommended practices for biological evaluation of dental materials") contains procedures for the use of endodontic materials. Under the document Type III, Class 2, materials are designated as root canal filling materials for which cytotoxicity, hemolysis, Ames, cell transformation, subcutaneous implantation, sensitization, and endodontic usage tests are described.

Protocols for the clinical evaluation of endodontic ma-

terials have also been published as a result of a workshop cosponsored by the American Dental Association, the Food and Drug Administration, the National Institute for Dental Research, and the National Institutes of Health in 1978.[77] The workshop addressed itself to the problems of (1) clinical evaluation of endodontic materials, (2) materials and methods of appropriate clinical research, and (3) administrative problems associated with such endeavors. It presented the thoughts of a wide spectrum of clinicians, teachers, researchers, and administrators applied to this problem. As yet no studies utilizing its recommendations have been reported.

An overview of the types of toxicity studies that have been proposed for or used in evaluating endodontic filling materials is presented in Fig. 13-29. In vivo evaluations of dental materials include acute systemic reactions, contact irritations, implantation responses, and long-duration responses.

Acute systemic reactions are generally evaluated by oral administration of the hardened or reacted material by stomach tube to at least 10 small animals. Dosage levels are 1 mg of the material per kilogram of body weight of the animal. The material is suspended or dissolved in a suitable vehicle. Observations for death or toxic effects are made daily for at least 2 weeks, at which time all surviving animals are sacrificed. If fewer than 50% of the animals have died, the material is generally considered acceptable. The systemic injection of freshly mixed materials to determine the minimum lethal dosage and the 50% lethal dosage level for therapeutic agents is the second category involved when tests for acute systemic reactions are being conducted. To date, however, there have been no reports in the literature of endodontic filling materials tested for acute systemic reactions.

Contact irritation testing as applied to dental materials usually involves the evaluation of mucous membrane irritations. This is done by holding the material in contact with the oral mucous membranes or gingival tissues of at least 10 animals of appropriate species and size for 2 weeks and then taking color photographs and biopsies of the exposed areas. The use of control materials as well as test materials is necessary. The testing of liquids, such as root canal medicaments and freshly mixed filling materials, has also been done by dropping the substances into the eyes of the rabbits.

There have been no reports in the endodontic literature of contact irritation studies done for endodontic filling materials, with the exception of one using rabbits' eyes. *Implantation responses* have been preferred as the method of evaluating endodontic filling materials. Freshly mixed materials are invariably irritating to tissues. However, as the material sets, the components of the material are bound into masses that often show a high degree of biocompatibility.[13]

In vivo studies of *long-duration responses* to endodontic filling materials have not been conducted. The incidence of cellular metaplasia or tumor production associated with these materials, which are evaluated over periods of time in excess of 1 or 2 years, in unknown. The immunologic consequences of the use of these materials is also un-

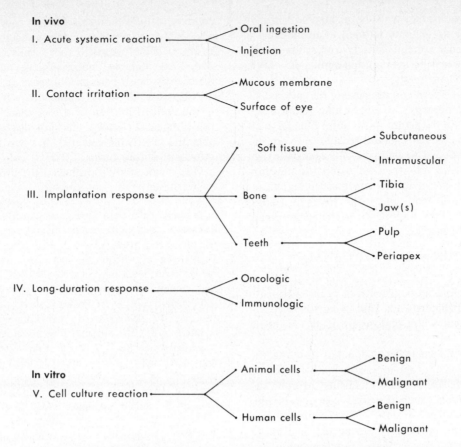

FIG. 13-29. Types of toxicity studies for endodontic materials.

known. Not only do several of the materials contain protein complexes that may well be capable of initiating antigen-antibody responses, some even produce tissue necrosis and fixation (e.g., paraformaldehyde) and may be capable of autoimmune reactions.[20] The immunocompetence of the pulp and periodontal ligament has been established, but the effects of endodontic filling materials on them have not.

The in vitro use of cell cultures has been developed as a means of evaluating the cytotoxicity of root canal filling materials.[159] The most commonly used human cells have been HeLa cells. As a screening mechanism, cell culture reactions are extremely sensitive.

From the foregoing mass of seemingly disjointed data some general conclusions can be drawn:

1. All endodontic filling materials are cytotoxic when freshly mixed; the degree of cytotoxicity is directly related to the ingredients contained in the material. For example, eugenol, eucalyptol, chloroform, iodoform, paraformaldehyde, and acids are all very tissue toxic (as reflected in the evaluations of materials containing them). This apparently is true for such materials as freshly mixed dental amalgams as well.

2. The sooner and more completely an endodontic filling material sets or becomes chemically stable, the higher will be its biocompatibility. Not only do endodontic sealers with a large eugenol content (resulting in the continuous presence of free eugenol) have retarded setting times, but the leaking of eugenol into tissues effects a long-term tissue irritation. N-2 and some of the other "therapeutic cements" are deceptive because their initial inflammatory response appears to be delayed due to the rapid setting of the material, the addition of antiinflammatory agents, or the fixation of tissues; however, there is a steadily increasing tissue reaction as the "therapeutic" agents leak out; the viable tissue responses to the fixed tissues then appear. The more inert the material becomes, the more biocompatible it is. Encapsulation by extensive layers of connective tissue is not a measure of biocompatibility but is indicative of the body's need to wall off a continuing low-grade irritant.

3. The more biodegradable the material is, the higher its biocompatibility. Biodegradable materials have not been extensively explored in endodontics and need further investigation. Materials that can effectively seal the root canal system and yet be completely absorbed and replaced by the tissues of the body so as to create a viable material-soft tissue interface while maintaining a seal may have an important place in the future of endodontics. Therapeutic cements that are absorbable are more biocompatible than are those that are not, even though both types as presently compounded have relatively high degrees of tissue irritation when compared to inert filling materials.

4. The more effective the filling material is in sealing the root canal system and maintaining that seal, the more biocompatible it is likely to be. A material with a very low

degree of tissue toxicity may well be unsuitable for endodontics because of its inability to seal, or to maintain a seal, of the root canal system. This is true of the gutta-percha–based root canal pastes and apparently of Silastic materials as well.[133]

By being aware of information regarding the physical as well as the biologic properties of endodontic filling materials, and hopefully in the future meaningful clinical evaluations, responsible clinicians should be able to select materials that are best suited to their patients and their own needs. The progressing programs of standards development nationally and internationally are making significant contributions toward this end, and more clinicians need to be aware of them and their importance to the advancement of dental science and practice.

INSTRUMENTATION AND ROOT CANAL FILLING

The intimate relationship between root canal instrumentation (cleaning and shaping) and root canal filling lies at the very heart of endodontic philosophy in the twentieth century.

One of the most fundamental precepts has been that the unfilled root canal system functions as a hollow tube and that even in the absence of microorganisms, necrotic debris, or toxic materials, such unsealed spaces will ultimately result in periapical disease. The mechanism was postulated by Rickert and Dixon[137] to be the invasion of the unsealed space by tissue fluids, the stagnation and breakdown of these fluids, and the subsequent release of toxins creating periapical inflammatory responses. This conception of the root canal system underlies much endodontic philosophy even today.

During his research (1959-1960) on the tissue toxicity of intracanal root canal medications using polyethylene tube implants, Torneck[166,167] discovered that tissue breakdown at the open tube ends was *not* a common finding. Pursuing the matter over a period of some years, he reported (1966-1967) that the experimental evidence for the "hollow tube" theory was apparently in error and that the entire concept deserved reexamination.

Other authors[63] conducted experiments of their own, and their results supported Torneck's conclusions: (1) there is circulation in and out of implanted tubes; (2) there is no evidence of inflammation at the open ends of implanted tubes; and (3) the ingrowth of tissue in open tubes of short length and large diameter as well as the invagination of tissue into tubes with small diameter and one end sealed does occur. It was also shown that the least favorable prognosis for repair occurred when the lumen of an implanted tube was filled with tissue debris and microorganisms.

Still other authors[25] showed that fibrous tissue will fill the lumen of a tube 5 mm long with a 0.5 mm bore implanted in tissue after having been filled with isotonic saline if the tube is open at both ends but will not fill the lumen of a similar tube sealed at one end. The absence of inflammatory changes in either case, as well as in the instance of tubes filled with absorbable cement, was in direct contrast to the reports of Rickert and Dixon. We can be reasonably certain that in the absence of microorganisms or tissue debris, unfilled root canals or root canals filled with biodegradable and resorbable materials will not of themselves cause periapical disease.

Nygaard-Østby[126] recommended a blood clot be created in the unfilled portion of a root canal as an aid to apical tissue repair. In effect, this provided a natural biodegradable and resorbable material that was replaced by the ingrowth of fibrous tissue.

One major study[46] evaluated the effects of underfilling or overfilling with gutta-percha:

In *Group I* the teeth were grossly overfilled with gutta-percha and sealer extended beyond the tooth apex; all such cases showed pathologic responses.

In *Group II,* wherein the root canals were filled to the apex but sealer extruded beyond the tooth, 60% of the cases showed mild chronic inflammation, and 40% evidence of bone loss and subsequent repair. These findings support the evidence of Seltzer et al.[148-150,152] gathered over a period of years.

In *Group III,* the so-called ideal situation, in which the tooth was filled to the working length of the instrumentation (within 1 mm of the apex) and no filling material extruded beyond the tooth, 25% of the cases showed moderate inflammation with evidence of repair, 10% showed necrotic tissue in branching root canals with marked inflammation and focal necrosis of the periodontium, and 65% showed normal, intact periapical tissues. This tends to support the autopsy findings obtained from humans as reported by Brynolf.[26]

In *Group IV,* in which the teeth were instrumented to within 1 mm of the apex but filled short of this by 3 mm or more, all cases showed chronic inflammation, 50% of which involved focal necrosis. This supports the contention of Dixon and Rickert[48] and the clinical view of many endodontists.

In *Group V,* in which the teeth were instrumented to, or slightly beyond, the apex but filled short of the apex by 3 mm or more, there was healing in every case, not only in the periodontium but in the unfilled canal space as well. In this group 25% of the cases showed plugs of dentin covered with new cementum, 25% demonstrated bone deposition, and 50% revealed the formation of a new attachment apparatus including bone, ligament, and secondary cementum within the root canal space. No residual inflammation of the periodontium was found in any of the cases reported in Group V. This corroborates the findings of Nygaard-Østby and other skeptics of the "hollow tube" theory.

The findings in Group V are not at all unusual, although most of the available evidence seems to support the contention that the least amount of soft tissue irritation is produced during root canal instrumentation when the root canal files or reamers are kept within the confines of the root canal itself. The long-term effects of the level of instrumentation, the influence of injury from root canal cleaning and shaping, the material used to seal the root canal system, and the efficacy of that seal are all factors not yet thoroughly examined.

It is not out of the ordinary that the procedure apparently producing the most inflammatory response within acceptable limits also produces the most profound resolution of the overall problem; and this may be the case with root canal instrumentation, provided insult is not added to injury by injections or the use of filling materials with poor biocompatibility.

In conclusion, it should be obvious to the reader that clinicians have not been able either to define clearly the objectives of endodontic therapy in concise terms or to determine with clarity what they expect their instruments to do, their devices to assist in doing, and their materials to accomplish. When these objectives are determined, careful evaluations of existing instruments, devices, and materials can and should be done to assist in our selection of them and in the development of new tools or materials. A great deal needs to be done and is being done by many dedicated clinicians, researchers, and teachers; hopefully the next generation will see more progress than has been witnessed by all those who have gone before.

RECENT DEVELOPMENTS IN ENDODONTIC INSTRUMENTS, MATERIALS, AND DEVICES

The technical demands and level of precision required for successful performance of endodontic procedures have traditionally been achieved by careful manipulation of hand instruments within the root canal space and by strict adherence to the biologic and surgical principles essential for disinfection and healing. The highly successful and predictable outcome of endodontic treatment afforded by adherence to traditional methods and principles has perhaps contributed to the tendency among most to view with skepticism or reject radical changes in methodology. As increasing numbers of patients have become aware of the advantages of endodontic treatment and the many benefits derived through preservation of the natural dentition, the demand for endodontic services has increased dramatically over the past two decades.[00] Concurrently, increasing numbers of clinicians have sought to develop the skills and techniques necessary to provide this valuable service to their patients, through formalized advanced and continuing educational programs.

Equally aware of the rise in patient demand for root canal therapy and cognizant of the growing number of clinicians prepared to provide endodontic services, dental manufacturers have realized an expanding market in the field of endodontics. Consequently, a number of new products have been introduced aimed at reducing operating time and fatigue and intended to facilitate a more efficient and efficacious means of providing endodontic treatment. Although most of these products may be regarded as new to endodontics, many represent merely an application of materials or devices already in use in other facets of dentistry and industry, adapted for endodontic purposes. The recent development of mechanized or automated systems may also be interpreted as being the result of the profession's preference for instruments aimed at improving the speed or efficiency of treatment, with a somewhat lesser emphasis on the precision or accuracy of endodontic procedures. Viewed from a historical prospective, this tendency may reflect a shift in direction away from the earlier objectives of instrument standardization and toward greater performance of instruments. It may be too early to predict whether or not this tendency will have a significant effect upon the outcome or clinical success previously experienced with endodontic treatment.

While the literature appears to reflect disparity of opinion with regard to the safety and efficacy of specific products, and dominated by preferences among individuals, the consensus regarding the basic aims and objectives of endodontic treatment remains essentially unchanged. The ultimate goal of endodontic instrumentation techniques and procedures continues to be centered around the established biologic and surgical principles of asepsis, debridement, and provision of an environment conducive for healing and repair. While differences in philosophy between various groups may be inferred by their predilection for terms such as "chemomechanical" vs "biomechanical" preparation, essentially these apparent differences only reflect minor variations in methodology rather than in concept.

Recognizing then that these new developments represent the logical sequelae of a changing technology rather than a radical departure from conventional endodontic principles we have attempted to include them in this discussion in order to evaluate their usefulness as either alternatives or supplements to instruments, materials, and devices previously employed in endodontics.

Endodontic instrument design
Hand-operated instruments

Modifications or departures from K-type, H-type, or R-type files have been made, apparently intended to alleviate some of the clinical difficulties encountered in instrumentation procedures such as ledging or perforation of the root canal wall, or to aid in the penetration and enlargement of severely curved or constricted canals. Generally these modifications have consisted of either (1) changes in the cross-sectional design (Fig. 13-30), (2) changes in the depth or angle of the cutting edges of the flutes, or (3) changes in the design of the tip of the instruments.

The effect of minute variations in design have been reported to have a significant effect on an instrument's physical and mechanical properties such as cutting efficiency,[8,123] torsional strength, and flexibility,[49,89] as measured in laboratory comparisons. Others have presented clinical evidence in support of their theories that specific design modifications related to instruments govern their clinical performance and an operator's ability to successfully achieve the objectives of endodontic procedures.[140]

A recent addition to the endodontic armamentarium is an unclassified hand instrument, called the Pathfinder, designed specifically to negotiate highly calcified root canals. This instrument, developed by the Kerr Manufacturing Company, is similar in appearance to the K-type file but possesses a narrower taper to uniformly distribute the axial stress along the instrument shaft, thus reducing the tendency to bend at the tip. The instrument handle is color-coded orange to differentiate it from standardized sizes.

Modifications of the cross-sectional design of K-type files from square (Fig. 13-31) to triangular or rhombus (diamond shaped) (Fig. 13-32) has resulted in significantly

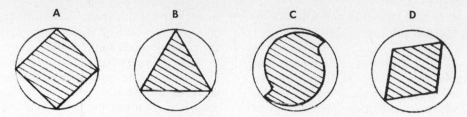

FIG. 13-30. Cross-sectional design of instruments: (a) square, (b) triangular, (c) S-shaped, (d) rhombic. Differences in bulk for these variations in cross-sectional design affect the flexibility of the instrument and other physical properties.

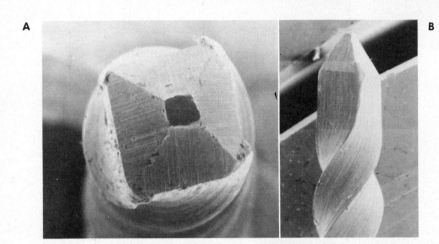

FIG. 13-31. Kerr, K-file. **A,** (×100.), top view. **B,** (×25), side view.

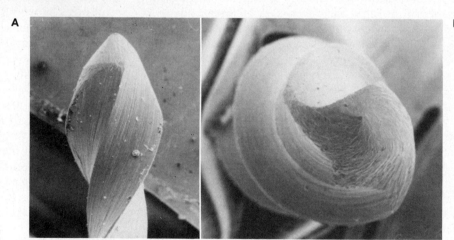

FIG. 13-32. Kerr, K-flex. **A,** (×100), top view. **B,** (×50), side view.

greater flexibility, especially in the larger diameter instruments (Fig. 13-32).[49,89] The alternating flute depth resulting from the rhombic cross-sectional design may also be responsible for the apparent increase in debris removal from constricted canals, facilitated by a decrease in instrument bulk along the shaft.[116,123] Similarly, a 37.5% decrease in cross-sectional surface area is produced by a change from square to triangular design for the same size instrument (Fig. 13-33).[123,140]

Other cross-sectional variations of K-type and H-type geometry have been produced by milling or grinding, rather than by twisting the wire shaft. Two examples of such instruments are the Unifile and the S-file. These instruments possess a S-shaped cross-section and flutes with

geometric shapes not achievable by twisting as with the K-type instruments (Fig. 13-34). These varieties of instruments by definition belong to the H-type classification. While both of these instruments display cutting efficiency similar to the H-type variety because of their positive rake angle, they are somewhat stiffer and stronger since the depth of the flutes is less, leaving greater bulk in the shaft. The S-file, of Swedish design, like the Unifile and H-type instruments is ground or machined from a solid piece of stainless steel wire, which produces very sharp cutting edges. The Unifile and S-file differ from the conventional H-type design in that a double cutting edge (S-shape) is observed in cross-section. The Unifile differs from the S-file in that the angle of the flutes varies along the instru-

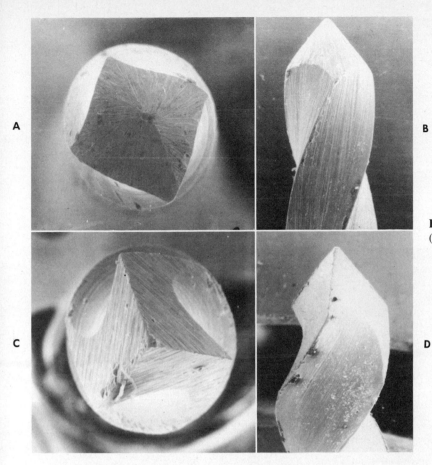

FIG. 13-33. A and **B,** Micro-Mega (×100). **C** and **D,** Triocut (×50).

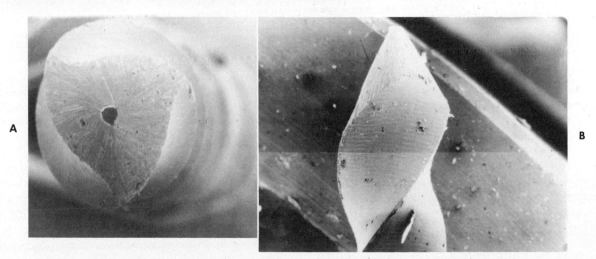

FIG. 13-34. A, Union Broach (×100), top view. **B,** Flex-R (×25), side view.

ment shaft. With the S-file, the angle of the flutes remains uniform, while the pitch and depth of the flutes increases from the tip to the handle. The S-file also possesses a 90 degree cutting tip, designed to provide a positive apical seat for the purpose of obturation. For both of these instruments depth control is facilitated by a millimeter scale etched into the shaft between the cutting region and the handle.

The S-file displays unique features that could enable it to be used as a "universal instrument" for the preparation of straight and curved canals, without the necessity of other instruments (Fig. 13-35). The manufacturers of this instrument maintain that its unique flute design provides improved cutting efficiency whether used in filing motion as with H-type files or in reaming motion as with K-type files and reamers. Laboratory comparisons of the cutting efficiency of the S-file to other instrument designs tend to substantiate these claims. Most recently, attention has

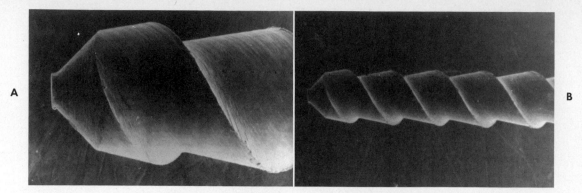

FIG. 13-35. Maillefer. **A,** (×100), top view. **B,** (×50), side view.

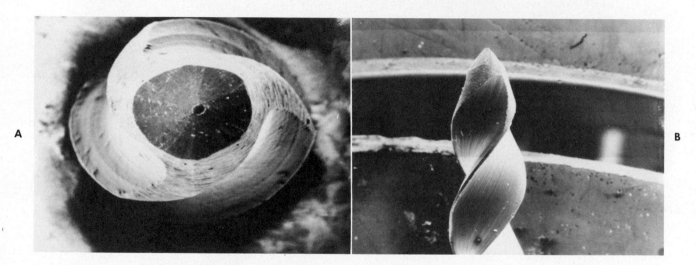

FIG. 13-36. A, Vereinigte (×100), top view. **B,** Dental Werke (×50), side view.

shifted from flute design to the design of the tip of endodontic instruments. Early investigators of the effect of instrumentation procedures on the shape of the prepared root canal have observed that the removal of cutting edges from the tip of the instrument could prevent the occurrence of ledging and perforation of curved roots.[117,175,176] More recent investigations further support the opinion that the tips of endodontic instruments possess potentially active cutting surfaces.[140]

The Flex-R file, developed by the Union Broach Corp., is one example of an instrument with a noncutting tip design. According to Roane,[140] its designer, the tendency for transportation during instrumentation of curved canals is inherent in the design of K-type files. Transportation or ledging commonly occurs at the outer curvature of the apical canal wall as a result of unbalanced forces and the presence of cutting edges on the tips of these (K-type) instruments. It is reasonable to assume that the energy stored by bending an instrument shaft creates a restoring force proportional to the inherent flexibility of the metal and the degree of curvature or bending. It is also plausible that when the sum of these forces is concentrated at the tip of the instrument, cutting of the outer dentin wall will occur more readily if cutting edges are prominent at the tip. According to the manufacturer,* the Flex-R file also differs from conventional designs in that the fluted edges are milled rather than twisted. This process allows control of instrument flexibility and cutting efficiency and influences torsional strength. By precise milling, the manufacturer is able to vary the depth and angle of the cutting edge, which determines not only sharpness but also the cross-sectional area. The variation in cross-sectional area for different sizes of instruments can provide increased stiffness and torsional strength in smaller sizes or provide increased flexibility in larger sizes with minimal reduction in torsional strength.

Examples of instruments with noncutting tips are illustrated in Fig. 13-36. Potentially, these instruments may be of benefit in specific clinical applications. The Endosonic Diamond, Rispi, and Shaper files represent a new variety of endodontic instruments, as described here.

Ultrasonic and sonic instrument systems

A new generation of instrumentation has recently evolved based on the vibrational action of energized in-

---

*Union Broach Corp., Long Island City, NY.

TABLE 13-10. Vibratory instruments

Size/length (mm)	Cavi-Endo		Enac			Endostar	Sonic 3000			
	21	25	21	25	30	25	19	21	22	25
10							r	r	r	r
15		k	k	*	*	k	r	r&k	r	r&k
20		k	*	*	*	k	r	r&k	r	r&k
25	k	d	*	*	*		r	r&k	r	r&k
30			k	*	*		r	r&k	r	r&k
35		d	*	*	*	k	r	r&k	r	r&k
40			k	*	*		r	r&k	r	r&k
45		d	*	*	*					
50			*	*	*					

k, K-file; r, R-file; d, diamond file; *, holders available for use with k-type files from other sources; blank, not available

struments within the root canal. Generally, two categories of devices have been developed, based on the frequency of vibration imparted to the instruments and source of power. The ultrasonic systems that generate vibration above the audible range of perception are powered by means of electric currents passing through an arrangement of lamillar metal plates. Alternating attractive and repulsive forces between the plates affect the mechanical vibratory movements, which are then transferred to the instrument. Sonic systems produce vibrations within the audible frequency range by means of compressed air, which activates a rotor-shaft assembly as a source of vibration.

Sonic and ultrasonic instrumentation differs from rotary or hand procedures since the cutting of dentin is facilitated by a mechanical device that imparts a sinusoidal motion to the instrument by the transfer of vibrational energy along the shaft. The term *ultrasonic instrumentation* has been used to describe these types of systems.[81] The first use of ultrasonics in root canal therapy and root resection has been credited to Richman.[136] The phrase "endosonic ultrasonic synergistic system" has also been applied to describe the combined effects of ultrasound on instrumentation and irrigation achieved with these devices.[43]

The Cavi-Endo ultrasonic unit was the first system of its type commercially available in the United States. Its development resulted from the extensive research performed at the Naval Research Center in Bethesda by Drs. Howard Martin and Walter Cunningham. Their original intention was to introduce ultrasonics to the root canal for the purpose of sterilization by sonication of bacteria.[105] More recently introduced, the Enac ultrasonic unit features detachable accessories to be used for removal of cemented castings and for the softening and condensation of gutta-percha. Interchangeable instrument holders are also provided with this system for varying the angle of the instrument to the handle assembly for easier insertion. The Endostar-5* and Endosonic 3000† are two sonic endodontic handpieces, similar to sonic air-driven scalers, that have

been modified for use as vibratory endodontic instrumentation devices.

Length control during instrumentation differs between the various systems. Both the Cavi-Endo and Enac ultrasonic units employ a section of plastic tubing as a movable marker or gauge around the instrument shaft for visual reference. Endodontic rubber stoppers should not be used since they interfere with the flow of irrigant down the instrument shaft. Length control with the sonic systems is provided by means of a metal guide bar that limits the depth of instrument insertion, thus mechanically preventing overinstrumentation.

Another major difference between these systems is in the method of irrigation and the type of irrigant employed. Both sonic and ultrasonic systems allow the clinician to adjust the rate or level of irrigation. The ultrasonic systems, however, permit the use of either an inert sterile or chemically active irrigant selected by the clinician. Irrigation with the sonic units is limited to filtered tap water as delivered through the dental unit cooling system. Other physical differences related to the number of sizes, lengths, and types of instruments available for use with the various systems are illustrated in Table 13-10.

Instruments provided for use in these systems have for the most part been modifications of either the K-type or R-type hand instruments (Table 13-10). The Endosonic Diamond file, on the other hand, has been designed specifically for use as an energized vibrational instrument and represents a considerable departure from previous types of instruments (Fig. 13-37). Diamond particles bonded to a metal shaft provide the cutting edges for dentin removal. Cutting of dentin by abrasion occurs from contact of the instrument with the canal wall by vibrational movement imparted by the mechanical device and by manual filing movement. Use of the Endosonic Diamond file, however, is limited to coronal enlargement within the straight portion of canals since it is relatively inflexible as compared to other types of instruments.

Greater cutting efficiency as reported by the developers of this system[106,109] might be expected because of automated debris removal from the cutting surface of the instrument. By combining the effects of irrigation with in-

*Syntex Dental Products, Inc., Valley Forge, PA.
†Medidenta International Inc., Woodside, NY.

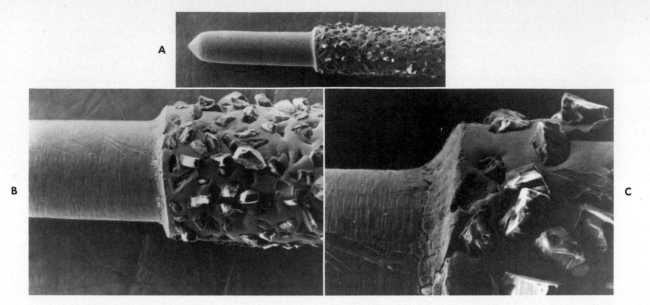

FIG. 13-37. Endosonic diamond file. **A,** ×30; **B,** ×100; **C,** ×300. Diamond particles embedded in the instrument shaft, cut by abrasive action on the dentinal canal wall.

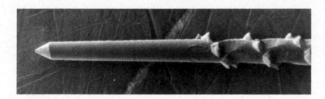

FIG. 13-38. Rispi, R-type File (×30.) Raised cutting edges cut by abrasion of dentin.

strumentation, dentin chips and debris are removed simultaneously with cutting procedures. Before this, instrumentation, irrigation, and removal of debris from the canal and instrument surfaces would necessarily be performed as separate manipulations.

Vibratory instruments belonging to the R-type (rat-tail) category are typified by the Rispi and, with some modification, the Shaper files (Figs. 13-38 and 13-39). Like the barbed broach or rasp-type hand instruments, cutting edges are created along the instrument shaft by a series of incisions that become elevated during the manufacturing process to form a roughened surface. The mechanism of cutting, like that of the diamond file, is by abrasion rather than by cutting per se. Both the ultrasonic diamond file and the sonic R-type instruments display a greatly improved cutting efficiency over the K-type designs when employed in these systems or when compared to hand instrumentation. These three instruments are also characterized by a noncutting tip design.

The recommended technique for the use of these types of instruments is by circumferential filing. The effect of instrumentation procedures on the shape of the root canal preparation has been reported with various results.[29,160,180] The ability of ultrasonic instrumentation techniques to maintain the original canal curvature appears to be similar

to hand instrumentation for smaller sizes (no. 15) files,[29] but the occurrence of ledging and tendency toward perforation has been reported for larger sizes of files.[160,180]

The customary tactile sense experienced in hand instrumentation is greatly altered with the energized systems, and since a greater cutting efficiency is claimed for these devices, caution must be exercised in their use to avoid perforations.[91] Although the biological effects of overinstrumentation on the periapical tissues has not been reported, some manufacturers have elected to include instruments with a noncutting tip, presumably to avoid this potential complication.

Since rotational movement of the instrument within the canal is limited with these systems, current specifications no. 28 and no. 57 for K-type and H-type endodontic instruments regarding torsional strength do not appear to be appropriate for these types of instruments. However, the vibrational force subjects these instruments to stresses not encountered with hand instrumentation. Although the incidence of instrument failure in clinical use has not been reported to be greater than with other types of instruments, the potential for fatigue failures is very high for instruments of this variety.

Vibrational energy absorbed by the instrument can induce fractures at points of high stress concentration such as (1) surface cracks or areas of corrosion, (2) sharp indentations and irregularities of design, (3) internal defects within the metal (voids and impurities), and (4) at points of flexure where the instrument becomes work hardened due to bending movements encountered in these types of systems. Fig. 13-40 illustrates two types of failures occurring with these types of instruments under experimental conditions. Fig. 13-40, *A,* illustrates a typical fatigue failure of the instrument as evidenced by two distinct surfaces at the fracture site. The area marked *A* has a rough, torn

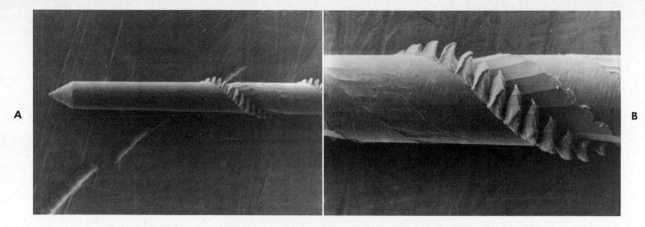

FIG. 13-39. Shaper file. **A,** $\times 30$; **B,** $\times 100$. Unique design of the spiralled cutting edges provide a roughened surface for abrasive cutting of dentin.

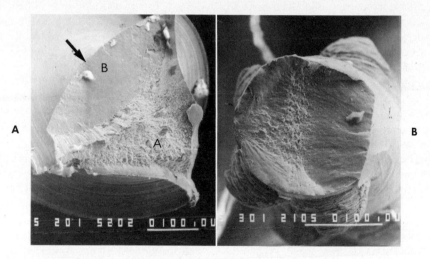

FIG. 13-40. A, Fatigue failure ($\times 100$). **B,** Brittle failure ($\times 100$).

appearance and depicts plastic deformation. Area *B* has a smooth, beachlike appearance with concentric crescent-shaped lines spreading toward the area of plastic deformation. Note that the crescent-shaped area (B) spreads out from the instrument surface (arrow). The nucleus or nuclei mark the origin, and the concentric crescent-shaped lines represent spreading of the crack under cyclic loading. Propagation of the crack in the direction of the arrow reduces the cross-sectional area progressively until the instrument is weakened sufficiently to cause brittle fracture. Fig. 13-40, *B,* on the other hand illustrates a nonfatigue, brittle fracture in which instrument failure was attributed to excessive tensile loading forces.

In light of these observations it may be advised to develop different safety standards for these types of instruments to include a minimum value for fatigue life expectancy so that the clinician may intelligently discard files before failure. Manufacturers' recommendations must be followed with regard to file usage to avoid breakage until further information becomes available.

Evaluation. While a great number of statements have been made regarding the superiority of these devices over hand instrumentation, thus far clinical and laboratory comparisons have resulted in a disparity of conclusions regarding their usefulness. In addition to their intended use as root canal preparation and irrigation devices, it has been suggested that they may also aid in the removal of foreign objects, cemented posts, silver cones, or other filling materials from the root canal.[113,160]

The clinical performance of some of these systems has been investigated by a number of independent researchers; however, the scope and extent of these investigations have been somewhat limited. Much confusion also exists related to the safety and effectiveness of these systems since many of the early reports were performed with either prototype or laboratory models and do not necessarily apply to the systems presently available. More inclusive and comprehensive research is therefore needed to objectively evaluate the actual commercial models, which are relatively new to the marketplace.

The clinical usefulness of the Cavi-Endo ultrasonic unit has been evaluated by investigators.[160] In a 10-month clinical study they examined its performance in a variety of procedures such as canal preparation, pathfinding, and removal of obstructions. As a result of their investigations, they considered the unit to be "a valuable tool with a multiplicity of uses."

Other researchers also found the Cavi-Endo unit helpful in the removal of foreign objects from the root canal. They were able to retrieve separated instruments with less loss of tooth structure than by other methods.[113]

One of the reported advantages of ultrasonic instrumentation has been a reduced incidence of postoperative pain,[108] which has been attributed to a superior debris-removing ability from canal irregularities[43] and reduction of material extruded from root apices.[42] The effect of temperature on the tissue solvent ability and antimicrobial effectiveness of sodium hypochlorite has been investigated by a number of sources.[2,40,41,134] Ultrasonic vibration apparently is able to enhance debridement and disinfection as a result of the warming action of the instrument on the irrigant solution by the generation of frictional heat. The enhanced tissue solvent action and antimicrobial effect experienced with ultrasound and sodium hypochlorite irrigation has been attributed to mechanical agitation and the increased chemical activity of the irrigant.[42,107] Cameron also demonstrated that ultrasonic irrigation with EDTA following instrumentation procedures could effectively remove the smear layer from the dentinal surface.[27] Investigations employing adaptations of the Cavitron and prototype models of the present Cavi-Endo unit found ultrasonic irrigation to be highly successful in the removal of debris and dentinal fillings.[42] Other investigations performed with either the Cavi-Endo unit or experimental systems are not in agreement with these reports. Scanning electron microscopic comparisons of root canals prepared by hand or by ultrasonic instrumentation with irrigation were made by investigators.[44] They found no difference in the appearance of canals prepared by either method. Tauber et al. in a magnifying lens comparison found no difference in debridement between ultrasonics, hand instrumentation, and ultrasonics with hand instrumentation.[163] Other investigators, in a quantitative comparison of ultrasonic, hand instrumentation, and a combination of ultrasonic and hand instrumentation, found the combined technique to be the most effective.[64] One study histologically compared the ability of the Endostar-5, the Micro Mega 3000, the Cavi-Endo unit, and hand instruments to clean extracted human teeth and monkey teeth in vivo.[91] They observed that none of the instrumentation systems examined demonstrated total debridement of the canals and concluded from their findings that root canal anatomy was the factor influencing the efficacy of debridement.[91] Another study, using an experimental ultrasonic system, also observed that neither an ultrasound stepback technique nor a stepback serial preparation technique with irrigation would consistently clean the canals and the isthmuses of the mesial roots of mandibular molars at all levels. While the ultrasonic stepback technique was judged to be better in some areas, differences were also observed in operator technique as well.[64]

One many conclude from these investigations that the effectiveness of ultrasonic irrigation and instrumentation procedures on debris removal would depend on the type of system used,* and may be influenced by operator technique[64] as well as by variations in root canal anatomy.[91]

Although it may be desirable to rely on a more extensive account of the safety and efficacy of these systems, based on the reports presently available it is reasonable to conclude that they may offer some advantages in the performance of routine and less prosaic endodontic procedures. Whether or not these systems are to be employed to replace or as adjuncts to previous forms of instruments is at the discretion of the individual clinician. An adequate level of caution and care should be exercised in the performance of endodontic procedures, regardless of the type of instruments or instrument systems selected. The safety and effectiveness of endodontic treatment will ultimately depend on an individual's clinical skills and familiarity with the instrument employed, as well as his knowledge and understanding of the principles of endodontics.

Obturation devices, instruments, and materials

Obturation of the root canal space would necessarily involve the introduction of a suitable, biologically compatible filling material to prevent the egress of microorganisms or toxic products into the vital periapical tissues. A discussion of instruments or devices intended for use in the process of obturation will therefore require some mention of the filling materials themselves. In an effort to provide guidelines and establish minimum standards for the various types of filling materials manufactured and used in endodontics, the Committee on Dental Materials, Instruments, and Equipment of the American National Standards Institute and corresponding council of the American Dental Association have adopted specification no. 57 for endodontic filling materials. This specification sets the requirements for the physical, dimensional, and biologic properties of both filling materials and sealer cements to be used in root canal obturation (see pp. 421-424).

Instruments and devices for sealing the root canal

The most recent developments related to endodontic filling instruments and devices have been those directed toward facilitating the placement of either semisolid or plasticized gutta-percha into the root canal space. The desirability for injectable materials or materials that have the ability to accurately conform to the anatomic irregularities of the root canal system is evidenced by the introduction of a number of synthetic polymers as endodontic filling materials over the past few years.[12,86,182] Other attempts to utilize the thermoplastic properties of gutta-percha to produce root canal fillings that form a homogeneous mass and seal the canal in three dimensions may also have been the impetus for the development of delivery systems and devices for this same purpose.[143] Irrespective

---

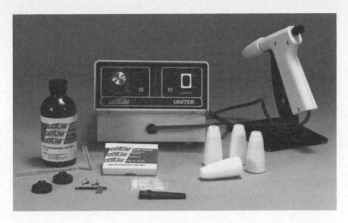

FIG. 13-41. Obtura System (Unitek Corp.) for thermoplastic injection of gutta-percha.

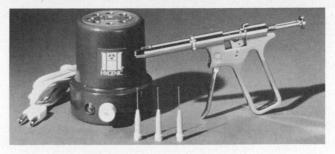

FIG. 13-42. Ultrafil System (Hygenic Corp.) for thermoplastic injection of gutta-percha.

of the factors influencing their development, devices intended for the placement of thermoplasticized or injection molded gutta-percha have recently become available.

Two systems have recently become commercially available. The Obtura* (Fig. 13-41) consists of a pistol-like delivery unit for introduction of the plasticized gutta-percha into the root canal through either 20- or 23-gauge silver injection tips. The delivery unit is connected by an electrical cord to a control unit that adjusts the temperature of the heating element within the delivery unit, thus regulating the viscosity of the extruded gutta-percha. The maximum internal temperature of the heating element with this system is 204° C. The temperature of the gutta-percha material as expressed is 160° C and has a reported working time of 3 to 5 minutes within the root canal. Gutta-percha pellets loaded into a chamber in the delivery unit become softened sufficiently within approximately 2 minutes to be extruded through the silver applicator tips by means of a ratchet plunger mechanism. It is recommended that once placed in the chamber, the gutta-percha should be injected within 15 minutes, the best results being achieved within 4 minutes. Disposable polystyrene cones are used to insulate the delivery unit adjacent to the applicator tip. A special bending tool is provided with the system for preshaping the silver applicator tips for easier insertion into areas of difficult access. The applicator tips are reusable and may be resterilized by glass bead sterilization.

The Ultrafil† system (Fig. 13-42) for delivery of thermoplasticized gutta-percha has been recently introduced. This system differs from that offered by Unitek in that the temperature of the gutta-percha as extruded is 70° C and thus it has been termed the "low-temperature" injection system. Other major differences are that the Ultrafil system consists entirely of three separate components; (1) preloaded gutta-percha filled canules with 22-gauge stainless steel needles, (2) a heating/holding unit, and (3) an autoclavable injection syringe. The preloaded canules are in-

dividually packaged and are disposable after use. The stainless steel needles may be preshaped for easier insertion before tempering in the heating unit, which holds up to four canules for storage. The proper temperature for injection is achieved within 15 minutes and the canules may be held within the heated unit for up to 4 hours. Filling or obturation is performed by inserting the prewarmed canules into the injection syringe and slowly squeezing the ratchet mechanism to express the plasticized material.

The manufacturers of the Obtura advocate the use of sealer cements to lubricate the root canal walls for better flow of the gutta-percha material. Specialized preparation techniques may also be required to allow placement of the injection tip or needle to within 3 to 6 mm of the apex. Filling may be accomplished by either passive injection of the material into the canal or with vertical condensation by hand instruments once placed. Reportedly a single canal may be obturated easily within 30 seconds.

The quality of the apical seal and adaptation of the filling produced by thermoplastic injection-molding techniques has been evaluated by the developers of these systems and other investigators. In a scanning electron micrographic comparison of thermoplastic injection of gutta-percha to conventional techniques, Torabinejad et al. found that the adaptation of gutta-percha to the dentin wall surface of the root canal was comparable to that achieved with the traditional methods.[165] Leakage as measured by both dye penetration and with radioisotope tracers has indicated that sealing by thermoplastic injection-molding of gutta-percha with sealer cement is as effective as obturation by other conventional methods.[45,115] Other investigators have found the quality of the apical seal to be acceptable; however, they additionally reported a high occurrence of overfills when the apices were intentionally overinstrumented or when vertical condensation was used. The incidence of overfilling was reduced from 75% to 12.5% when passive injection was used without vertical condensation.[50] The clinical success of injection-molded thermoplasticized gutta-percha obturation following biomechanical instrumentation was evaluated for 125 cases based on clinical and radiographic findings by investigators.[102] They reported an average success rate of 97% over a 12-month period for cases presenting either with or without periapical radiolucent areas.

The results of these studies suggest that thermoplastic

*Unitek Corp., Monrovia, CA.
†Hygenic Corp., Akron, OH.

injection-molding of gutta-percha for obturation of the root canal appears to produce fillings that compare favorably with other methods in both clinical and laboratory tests. Systems designed for the delivery of warm, semisolid gutta-percha may be beneficial as time-saving devices capable of achieving the objectives desired in endodontic obturation procedures.

Hand instruments for sealing the root canal

To those familiar with the history and development of endodontic instruments, the adoption of specifications 28, 57, and 58 may represent some of the most significant advancements toward achieving the objectives of endodontic treatment. The effects of dimensional uniformity between brands of instruments and solid core filling materials have simplified and improved the profession's ability to effectively cleanse, prepare, and seal the complex anatomic system of the root canal. Recently, the standardization of endodontic auxiliary (conventional) gutta-percha cone sizes would also represent further advancement along these lines. However, the advantage of dimensional uniformity in filling materials can be realized only if filling instruments are similarly standardized to conform in both sizing and dimension. In a recent survey of endodontic hand and finger spreaders,[115a] it was found that instrument nomenclature (spreader size) provided no indication of a corresponding auxiliary cone size for most brands tested. Designations of instruments such as "D-11" or "D-11-T" provide no information as to the appropriate auxiliary cone size to be used and thereby necessitate a trial and error method for selection of a suitably sized filling. In addition, instruments with the same nominal size designation were found to differ markedly in diameter and taper between brands. It would seem logical that instruments intended to prepare a space for the placement of a filling material having a uniform taper and dimension should likewise be dimensioned and sized to facilitate that placement.

Of the five major brands examined, only two were found to have instruments whose nomenclature and dimensions correspond to the nomenclature and dimensional requirements prescribed in specification 57 for endodontic filling materials. Finger spreaders produced by one source* were determined to correspond in both size designation and dimension to auxiliary cone sizes. Hand spreaders with standardized sizing and dimensions were also observed to correspond to that of standardized gutta-percha cones as produced by another company.† It is hoped that other manufacturers will similarly take the initiative to further the advancements achieved through standardization of endodontic instruments and materials and reduce the ambiguity in sizing for both spreaders and pluggers as it presently exists.

Endodontic sealer-cements

The biologic activity of calcium hydroxide in both vital pulp therapy and endodontic procedures has been documented extensively throughout the literature. A number of calcium hydroxide preparations have also been tested experimentally as root canal filling materials or sealer-cements in leakage and histologic studies.[58,80,154] Recently two commercial preparations have become available as endodontic sealer-cements to be used in conjunction with core filling materials. "CRCS," termed the calciobiotic root canal sealer, represents the first of the calcium hydroxide based sealers.† Sealapex,* another calcium hydroxide base preparation, appeared shortly afterward. The two differ in that CRCS consists of a powder-liquid combination, whereas Sealapex is in the form of a two tube/two paste preparation. Both may be classified as biologically active type sealers intended to promote periapical healing, with calcium hydroxide as the active ingredient. Holland and de Souza have reported the ability of Sealapex and calcium hydroxide filling material to induce apical closure by cementum deposition in histologic studies with both primates and dogs.[79] Other unpublished data tend to support their findings.[181]

REFERENCES

1. Abou-Rass, M., and Jastrab, R.J.: The use of rotary instruments as ancillary aids to root canal preparation of molars, J. Endod. **8:**78, 1982.
2. Abou-Rass, M., and Oglesby, S.W.: The effects of temperature, concentration and tissue type on the solvent ability of sodium hypochlorite, J. Endod. **7:**376, 1981.
3. American Dental Association, Council on Dental Materials and Devices: New American Dental Association, specification no. 28 for endodontic files and reamers, J. Am. Dent. Assoc. **93:**813, 1976.
4. American Dental Association, Council on Dental Materials, Instruments, and Equipment: Revised American Dental Association specification no. 28 for endodontic files and reamers, J. Am. Dent. Assoc. **104:**506, 1982.
5. American National Standards Institute: Meeting of the ISO Committee TC-106 (Dentistry), Chicago, 1974, American Dental Association.
6. American National Standards Institute: Meeting of the ISO Committee MD-156 (Dental Materials, Instruments, and Equipment), Chicago, 1982, American Dental Association.
7. American National Standards Institute/American Dental Association Document no. 41, J. Am. Dent. Assoc. **99:**697, 1979.
8. Anderson, J., Corcoran, J., and Craig, R.: Cutting ability of square versus rhombus cross-sectional endodontic files, J. Endod. **11:**212, 1985.
9. Baker, N.A., et al.: Scanning electron microscope study of the efficacy of various irrigating solutions, J. Endod. **1:**127, 1975.
10. Barry, G.N., Heyman, R.A., and Fried, I.L.: Sealing quality of instruments cemented in root canals with polycarboxylate cements, J. Endod. **1:**112, 1975.
11. Becker, G.L., Cohen, S., and Borer, R.: The sequelae of accidently injecting sodium hypochlorite beyond the root apex, Oral Surg. **38:**633, 1974.
12. Benkel, B.H., et al.: Use of a hydrophilic plastic as a root canal filling material, J. Endod. **2:**196, 1976.
13. Benner, M.D., et al.: Evaluation of a new thermoplasticized gutta-percha obturation technique using ^{45}Ca, J. Endod. **7:**500, 1981.
14. Berk, H., and Krakow, A.: Efficient endodontic procedures with the use of the pressure syringe, Dent. Clin. North Am., p. 387, July 1965.
15. Bernatti, O., Stolf, W.C., and Ruhnke, L.A.: Verification of the consistency, setting times, and dimensional changes of root canal filling materials, Oral Surg. **46:**107, 1978.

---

*Kerr Manufacturing Division, Sybron Corp., Romulus, MI.
†Hygienic Corp., Akron, OH.

16. Best, E.J., et al.: A new method of tooth length determination for endodontic practice, Dent. Dig. **66:**450, 1960.

17. Beyer-Olsen, E.M., and Orstavik, D.: Radiopacity of root canal sealers, Oral Surg. **51:**320, 1981.

18. Bhat, K.S.: Tissue emphysema caused by hydrogen peroxide, Oral Surg. **38:**304, 1974.

19. Biven, G.M., Bapna, R.J., and Heuer, M.A.: Effect of eugenol and eugenol-containing root canal sealers on the microhardness of human dentin, J. Dent. Res. **51:**1602, 1972.

20. Block, R.M., et al.: Cell moderated immune response to dog pulp tissue altered by N_2 paste within the root canal, Oral Surg. **45:**131, 1978.

21. Brady, J.M., and del Rio, C.E.: Corrosion of endodontic silver cones in humans: a scanning electron microscope and x-ray microprobe study, J. Endod. **1:**205, 1975.

22. Bramante, C.M., and Berbert, A.: A critical evaluation of some methods of determining root canal length, Oral Surg. **37:**463, 1974.

23. Brayton, S.M., Davis, S.R., and Goldman, M.: Gutta percha root canal fillings: an in vitro analysis. I, Oral Surg. **35:**226, 1973.

24. Bregman, R.C.: A mathematical method of determining the length of a tooth for root canal treatment and filling, J. Can. Dent. Assoc. **16:**305, 1950.

25. Browne, R.M., and Friend, L.A.: An investigation into the irritant properties of some root filling materials, Arch. Oral Biol. **13:**1355, 1968.

26. Brynolf, I.: A histological and roentgenological study of the periapical region of human incisors, Odontol. Rev. **18**(suppl.):11, 1967.

27. Cameron, J.A.: The use of ultrasound in the cleaning of root canals: a clinical report, J. Endod. **8:**472, 1982.

28. Canadian Dental Association, Council for Dental Materials and Devices: Status report, root canal sealing materials, J. Can. Dent. Assoc. **43:**538, 1977.

29. Chenail, B., and Teplitsky, P.: Endosonics in curved root canals, J. Endod. **11:**369, 1985.

30. Chivian, N.: Endodontics: an overview. Dent. Clin. North Am. **28:**057, 1984.

31. Chong, R., and Senzer, J.: Systemic distribution of 210 PbO from root canal fillings, J. Endod. **2:**381, 1976.

32. Chunn, C.B., Zardiakas, L.P., and Menke, R.A.: *In vivo* root canal length determination using the Forameter, J. Endod. **7:**515, 1981.

33. Copeland, H.I., Brauer, G.M., and Forziati, A.: The setting mechanism of zinc oxide and eugenol mixtures, J. Dent. Res. **34:**740, 1955.

34. Craig, R.G., editor: Dental materials; a problem oriented approach, St. Louis, 1986, The C.V. Mosby Co.

35. Craig, R.G., McIlwain, E.D., and Peyton, F.A.: Bending and torsion properties of endodontic instruments, Oral Surg. **25:**239, 1968.

36. Craig, R.G., and Peyton, F.A.: Physical properties of carbon steel root canal files and reamers, Oral Surg. **15:**213, 1962.

37. Craig, R.G., and Peyton, F.A.: Physical properties of stainless steel endodontic files and reamers, Oral Surg. **16:**206, 1963.

38. Crane, D.L., et al.: Biological and physical properties of an experimental root canal sealer without eugenol, J. Endod. **6:**438, 1980.

39. Crump, M.C., and Natkin, E.: Relationshp of broken root canal instruments to endodontic case prognosis: a clinical investigation, J. Am. Dent. Assoc. **80:**1341, 1970.

40. Cunningham, W.T., and Balekjian, A.Y.: Effect of temperature on collagen-dissolving ability of sodium hypochlorite endodontic irrigant, Oral Surg. **49:**175, 1980.

41. Cunningham, W.T., and Joseph S.W.: Effect of temperature on the bacteriocidal action of sodium hypochlorite endodontic irrigant, Oral Surg. **50:**569, 1980.

42. Cunningham, W.T., and Martin, H.: A scanning electron microscope evaluation of root canal debridement with the endosonic synergistic system, Oral Surg. **53:**527, 1982.

43. Cunningham, W.T., Martin, H., and Forrest, W.: Evaluation of root canal debridement by the endosonic ultrasonic synergistic system, Oral Surg. **53:**401, 1982.

44. Cymerman, J.J., Jerome, L.A., and Moodnick, R.M.: A scanning electron microscope study of comparing the efficacy of hand instrumentation of the root canal, J. Endod. **9:**327, 1983.

45. Czonstkowsky, M., Michanowicz, A., and Vasquez, J.: Evaluation of an injection of thermoplasticized low-temperature gutta-percha using radioactive isotopes, J. Endod. **11:**71, 1985.

46. Davis, M.S., Joseph, S.W., and Bucher, J.F.: Periapical and intracanal healing following incomplete root canal fillings in dogs, Oral Surg. **31:**662, 1971.

47. Dixon, C.M., and Rickert, U.G.: Tissue tolerance to foreign materials, Am. Dent. Assoc. J. **20:**1458, 1933.

48. Dixon, C.M., and Rickert, U.G.: Histologic verification of results of root canal therapy in experimental animals, Am. Dent. Assoc. J. **25:**1781, 1938.

49. Dolan, D.W., and Craig, R.G.: Bending and torsion of endodontic files with rhombus cross sections, J. Endod. **8:**260, 1982.

50. El Deeb, M.: The sealing ability of injection-molded thermoplasticized gutta-percha, J. Endod. **11:**84-86, 1985.

51. Feldman, G., and Nyborg, H.: Tissue reactions to root filling materials. I. Comparison between gutta percha and silver amalgam implanted in rabbits, Odontol. Rev. **13:**1, 1962.

52. Feldman, G., and Nyborg, H.: Tissue reactions to filling materials. II. A comparison of implants of silver and root filling material AH 26 in rabbits, Odontol. Rev. **15:**33, 1964.

53. Feldman, G., Nyborg, H., and Conrado, C.A.: Tissue reactions to root filling materials. III. A comparison between implants of root filling material N_2 and silver in jaws of rabbits, Odontol. Rev. **18:**387, 1967.

54. Feldman, G., et al.: Retrieving broken endodontic instruments, J. Am. Dent. Assoc. **88:**588, 1974.

55. Fragola, A., et al.: The effect of varying particle size of the components of Grossman's cement, J. Endod. **5:**366, 1979.

56. Friedman, C.E., et al.: The chemical composition and mechanical properties of gutta-percha endodontic filling materials, J. Endod. **3:**304, 1977.

57. Fromme, H.G., and Reidel, H.: Treatment of dental root canals and the marginal contact between filling material and tooth, studied by SEM, J. Br. Endod. Soc. **6:**17, 1972.

58. Goldberg, F., and Garfinkel, J.: Analysis of the use of Dycal with gutta-percha points as an endodontic filling technique, Oral Surg. **47:**78, 1979.

59. Goldberg, F., Garfinkel, J., and Spielberg, C.: Microscopic study of standardized gutta-percha points, Oral Surg. **47:**275, 1979.

60. Goldman, L.B., et al.: Scanning electron microscope study of a new irrigation method in endodontic treatment, Oral Surg. **48:**79, 1979.

61. Goldman, L.B., et al.: Adoption and porosity of poly-HEMA in a model system using two microorganisms, J. Endod. **6:**683, 1980.

62. Goldman, M., et al.: New method of irrigation during endodontic treatment, J. Endod. **2:**257, 1976.

63. Goldman, M., and Pearson, A.H.: A preliminary investigation of the "hollow tube" theory in endodontics: studies with neotetrazolium, J. Oral Ther. Pharmacol. **1:**618, 1965.

64. Goodman, A., et al.: An in vitro comparison of the efficacy of the step-back technique versus a step-back ultrasonic technique in human mandibular molars, J. Endod. **11:**249, 1985.

65. Goodman, A., Schilder, H., and Aldrich, W.: The thermomechanical properties of gutta percha. II. The history and molecular chemistry of gutta percha, Oral Surg. **37:**954, 1974.

66. Greenberg, M.: Filling root canals of deciduous teeth by an injection technique, Dent. Dig. **67:**574, 1961.

67. Greenberg, M.: Filling root canals by an injection technique, Dent. Dig. **69:**61, 1963.

68. Grossman, L.I.: An improved root canal cement, J. Am. Dent. Assoc. **56:**381, 1958.

69. Grossman, L.I.: Present status of plastic root canal filling materials, Transactions, Third International Conference on Endodontics, Philadelphia, 1963, University of Pennsylvania.

70. Grossman, L.I.: Endodontic practice, ed. 10, Philadelphia, 1981, Lea & Febiger.

71. Gurncy, B.F., Best, E.J., and Gervasio, G.: Physical measurements of gutta percha, Oral Surg. 32:260, 1971.

72. Gutiérrez, J.H., and Garcia, J.: Microscopic and macroscopic investigation on results of mechanical preparations of root canals, Oral Surg. 25:108, 1968.

73. Gutiérrez, J.H., Gigoux, C., and Sanhueza, J.: Physical and chemical deterioration of endodontic reamers during mechanical preparation, Oral Surg. 28:394, 1969.

74. Harris, W.E.: Unusual endodontic complication: report of a case, J. Am. Dent. Assoc. 83:358, 1971.

75. Harty, F.J., and Stock, C.J.R.: A comparison of the flexibility of Giromatic and hand-operated instruments in endodontics, J. Br. Endod. Soc. 7:64, 1974.

76. Harty, F.J., and Stock, C.J.R.: The Giromatic system compared with hand instrumentation in endodontics, Br. Dent. J. 137:239, 1974.

77. Heuer, M.A.: Clinical evaluation of endodontic materials, J. Endod. 7:105, 1981.

78. Higginbotham, T.L.: a comparative study of the physical properties of five commonly used root canal sealers, Oral Surg. 24:89, 1967.

79. Holland, R., and de Souza, V.: Ability of a new calcium hydroxide root canal filling material to induce hard tissue formation, J. Endod. 11:535, 1985.

80. Holland, R., et al.: Reaction of the human periapical tissue to pulp extirpation and immediate root canal filling with calcium hydroxide, J. Endod. 3:63, 1977.

81. Horton, J.E., Tarpley, T.M., and Jacoway, J.R.: Clinical applications of ultrasonic instrumentation in the surgical removal of bone, Oral Surg. 51:236, 1981.

82. Ingle, J.I., and Levine, M.: The need for uniformity of endodontic instruments, equipment, and filling materials, Transactions, Second International Conference of Endodontics, Philadelphia, 1958, University of Pennsylvania.

83. Ingle, J.E., and Tanter, J.F.: Endodontics, ed. 2, Philadelphia, 1976, Lea & Febiger.

84. Ireland, J.F., and Dolce, J.L.: Modification of technique for injection obturation, J. Endod. 1:156, 1975.

85. Johansson, B.I.: A methodological study of the mechanical properties of endodontic gutta-percha points, J. Endod. 6:781, 1980.

86. Jones, G.: The use of Silastic as an injectable root canal obturating material, J. Endod. 6:552, 1980.

87. Kerekes, K.: Evaluation of standardized root canal instruments and obturating points, J. Endod. 5:145, 1979.

88. Kronman, J.H., et al.: Microscopic evaluation of poly-HEMA root canal filling material, Oral Surg. 48:175, 1979.

89. Krupp, J., Brantley, W., and Gerstein, H.: An investigation of the torsional and bending properties of seven brands of endodontic files, J. Endod. 10:372, 1984.

90. Langeland, K.: Root canal sealants and pastes, Dent. Clin. North Am. 18:309, 1974.

91. Langeland, K., Liao, K., and Pascon, E.A.: Work-saving devices in endodontics: efficacy of sonic and ultrasonic techniques, J. Endod. 11:499, 1985.

92. Langeland, K., Olsson, B., and Pascon, E.A.: Biological evaluation of Hydron, J. Endod. 7:196, 1982.

93. Larder, T.C., Prescott, A.J., and Brayton, S.M.: Gutta-percha; a comparative study of three methods of obturation, J. Endod. 2:289, 1976.

94. Lautenschlager, W.P., et al.: Brittle and ductile torsional failures of endodontic instruments, J. Endod. 3:175, 1977.

95. Laws, A.J.: Calcium hydroxide as a possible root filling material, N.Z. Dent. J. 58:199, 1962.

96. Laws, A.J.: Preparation of root canals—an evaluation of mechanical aids, N.Z. Dent. J. 64:156, 1968.

97. Lentine, F.N.: A study of torsional deflection of endodontic files and reamers, J. Endod. 5:181, 1979.

98. Lilley, J.D., and Smith, D.C.: An investigation of the fracture of root canal reamers, Br. Dent. J. 120:364, 1966.

99. Luks, S.: Analysis of root canal instruments, J. Am. Dent. Assoc. 58:85, 1959.

100. Marcotte, L.R., Dowson, J., and Rowe, N.H.: Apical healing with retrofilling materials, amalgam and gutta percha, J. Endod. 1:63, 1975.

101. Marlin, J., and Schilder, H.: Physical properties of gutta-percha when subjected to heat and vertical condensation, Oral Surg. 36:872, 1973.

102. Marlin, J., et al.: Clinical use of injection-molded thermoplasticized gutta-percha for obturation of the root canal system, J. Endod. 7:277, 1981.

103. Marshall, F.J., and Massler, M.: The sealing of pulpless teeth evaluated with radioisotopes, J. Dent. Med. 16:172, 1961.

104. Marshall, F.J., Massler, M., and Dute, H.L.: Effects of endodontic treatments on permeability of root dentine, Oral Surg. 13:208, 1960.

105. Martin, H.: Ultrasonic disinfection of the root canal, Oral Surg. 42:92, 1976.

106. Martin, H., and Cunningham, W.T.: The effect of endosonic and hand manipulation on the amount of root canal material extruded, Oral Surg. 53:611, 1982.

107. Martin, H., and Cunningham, W.T.: An evaluation of postoperative pain incidence following endosonic and conventional root canal therapy, Oral Surg. 54:74, 1982.

108. Martin, H., Cunningham, W.T., and Norris, J.P.: A quantitative comparison of the ability of diamond and K-type files to remove dentin, Oral Surg. 50:566, 1980.

109. Martin, H., et al.: Ultrasonic vs. hand filing of dentin: a quantitative study, Oral Surg. 49:79, 1980.

110. McComb, D., and Smith, D.C.: A preliminary scanning electron microscopic study of root canals after endodontic procedures, J. Endod. 1:238, 1975.

111. McComb, D., and Smith, D.C.: Comparison of physical properties of polycarboxylate-based and conventional root canal sealers, J. Endod. 2:228, 1976.

112. McElroy, D.L.: Physical properties of root canal filling materials, J. Am. Dent. Assoc. 50:433, 1955.

113. Meidinger, D., and Kabes, B.: Foreign object removal utilizing the Cavi-Endo ultrasonic instrument, J. Endod. 11:301, 1985.

114. Messing, J.J.: An investigation of the sealing properties of some root filling materials, J. Br. Endod. Soc. 4:18, 1970.

115. Michanowicz, A., and Czonstkowsky, M.: Sealing properties of an injection-thermoplasticized low-temperature (70° C) gutta-percha: a preliminary study, J. Endod. 10:563, 1984.

115a. Miserendino, L.J.: Report submitted to ADA/ANSI Committee on Endodontists Instruments and Materials at the 42nd annual meeting of the American Association of Endodontics, San Diego, Cal, 1985.

116. Miserendino, L.J., et al.: Cutting efficiency of endodontic instruments, Part 1. A quantitative comparison of the tip and fluted regions, J. Endod. 11:435, 1985.

117. Miserendino, L.J., et al.: Cutting efficiency of endodontic instruments, Part 2. An analysis of the design of the tip, J. Endod. 12:8, 1986.

118. Molven, O.: Engine- and hand-operated root canal exploration, Odontol. Tidskr. 76:61, 1968.

119. Molven, O.: A comparison of the dentin removing ability of five root canal instruments, Scand. J. Dent. Res. 78:500, 1970.

120. Moodnik, R.M., et al.: Efficacy of biomechanical instrumentation: a scanning electron microscope study, J. Endod. 2:261, 1976.

121. Moser, J.B., and Heuer, M.A.: Forces and efficacy in endodontic irrigation systems, Oral Surg. 53:425, 1982.

122. Naidorf, I.J.: Clinical microbiology in endodontics, Dent. Clin. North Am. **18:**329, 1974.

123. Newman, J.G., Brantley, W.A., and Gerstein, H.: A study of the cutting efficiency of seven brands of endodontic files in linear motion, J. Endod. **9:**316, 1983.

124. Norman, R.D., et al.: The effect of particle size on the physical properties of zinc oxide eugenol mixtures, J. Dent. Res. **43:**252, 1964.

125. Nyborg, H., and Halling, A.: Amputation instruments for partial pulpal extirpation. II. A comparison between the efficiency of the Antaeos root canal reamer and the Hedström file with cut tip, Odontol. Tidskr. **71:**277, 1963.

126. Nygaard-Østby, B.: Pulp and root canal treatment, Int. Dent. J. **13:**23, 1963.

127. Nygaard-Østby, B., and Hjortdal, O.: Tissue formation in the root canal following pulp removal, Scand. J. Dent. Res. **79:**333, 1971.

128. O'Connell, D.T., and Brayton, S.M.: Evaluation of root canal preparation with two automated endodontic handpieces, Oral Surg. **39:**298, 1975.

129. Oliet, S., and Sorin, S.M.: Cutting efficiency of endodontic reamers, Oral Surg. **36:**243, 1973.

130. Oliet, S., and Sorin, S.M.: Effect of aging on the mechanical properties of hand-rolled gutta percha endodontic cones, Oral Surg. **43:**954, 1977.

131. Olsson, B., Slikowski, A., and Langeland, K.: Intraosseous implantation for biological evaluation of endodontic materials, J. Endod. **7:**253, 1981.

132. O'Neill, L.J.: A clinical evaluation of electronic root canal measurement, Oral Surg. **38:**469, 1974.

133. Oswald, R.J., and Cohen, S.A.: Systemic distribution of lead from root canal fillings, J. Endod. **1:**59, 1975.

134. Raphael, D., et al.: The effect of temperature on the bacteriocidal efficiency of sodium hypochlorite, J. Endod. **7:**330, 1981.

135. Rappaport, H.M., Lilly, G.E., and Kapsimalis, P.: Toxicity of endodontic filling materials, Oral Surg. **18:**785, 1964.

136. Richman, M.J.: The use of ultrasonics in root canal therapy and root resection, J. Dent. Med. **12:**12, 1957.

137. Rickert, U.G., and Dixon, C.M.: The controlling of root surgery, Transactions, Eighth International Dental Congress, sect. IIIa, Paris, 1931.

138. Rickles, N.H., and Joshi, B.A.: Death from air embolism during root canal therapy, J. Am. Dent. Assoc. **67:**397, 1963.

139. Rising, D.W., Goldman, M., and Brayton, S.M.: Histologic appraisal of three experimental root canal filling materials, J. Endod. **1:**172, 1975.

140. Roane, J., Sabala, C., and Duncanson, M.: The balanced force concept for instrumentation of curved canals, J. Endod. **11:**203, 1985.

141. Salzgeber, R.M., and Brilliant, J.D.: An in vivo evaluation of the penetration of an irrigating solution in root canals, J. Endod. **3:**394, 1977.

142. Sanders, S.H., and Dooley, R.J.: A comparative evaluation of polycarboxylate cement as a root canal sealer utilizing roughened and nonroughened silver points, Oral Surg. **37:**629, 1974.

143. Schilder, H.: Filling root canals in three dimensions, Dent. Clin. North Am. **11:**723, 1967.

144. Schilder, H., Goodman, A., and Aldrich, W.: The thermomechanical properties of gutta-percha. I. The compressibility of gutta-percha, Oral Surg. **37:**946, 1974.

145. Schilder, H., Goodman, A., and Aldrich, W.: The thermomechanical properties of gutta-percha. III. Determination of phase transition temperatures for gutta-percha, Oral Surg. **38:**109, 1974.

146. Schneider, S.W.: A comparison of canal preparations in straight and curved root canals, Oral Surg. **32:**271, 1971.

147. Seidberg, B.H., et al.: Clinical investigation of measuring working lengths of root canals with an electronic device and with digital-tactile sense, J. Am. Dent. Assoc. **90:**379, 1975.

148. Seltzer, S., et al.: Biologic aspects of endodontics, Oral Surg. **22:**375, 1966.

149. Seltzer, S., et al.: Biologic aspects of endodontics. III. Periapical tissue reactions to root canal instrumentation, Oral Surg. **26:**534, 694, 1968.

150. Seltzer, S., et al.: Biologic aspects of endodontics. IV. Periapical tissue reactions to root filled teeth whose canals had been instrumented short of their apices, Oral Surg. **28:**724, 1969.

151. Seltzer, S., et al.: A scanning electron microscope examination of silver cones removed from endodontically treated teeth, Oral Surg. **33:**589, 1972.

152. Seltzer, S., Soltanoff, W., and Smith, J.: Biologic aspects of endodontics. V. Periapical tissue reactions to root canal instrumentation beyond the apex and root canal fillings short of and beyond the apex, Oral Surg. **36:**725, 1973.

153. Senia, E.S., Marshall, F.J., and Rosen, S.: The solvent action of sodium hypochlorite on pulp tissue of extracted teeth, Oral Surg. **31:**96, 1971.

154. Shiveley, J., et al.: An in vitro autoradiographic study comparing the apical seal of uncatalyzed dycal to Grossman's sealer, J. Endod. **11:**62, 1985.

155. Shoji, Y.: Studies on the mechanism of the mechanical enlargement of root canals, Nihon Univ. Sch. Dent. J. **70:**71, 1965.

156. Shoji, Y.: Systematic endodontics. Berlin, 1973, Buch- und Zeitschriften-Verlag.

157. Smith, D.C.: The setting of zinc oxide–eugenol mixtures, Br. Dent. J. **105:**313, 1958.

158. Sorin, S.M., Oliet, S., and Pearlstein, F.: Rejuvenation of aged (brittle) endodontic gutta percha cones, J. Endod. **5:**233, 1979.

159. Spångberg, L., and Langeland, K.: Biologic effects of dental materials. 1. Toxicity of root canal filling materials on HeLa cells in vitro, Oral Surg. **35:**402, 1973.

160. Stamos, D.G., et al.: Endosonics: clinical impressions, J. Endod. **11:**181, 1985.

161. Sundada, I.: New method for measuring the length of the root canal, J. Dent. Res. **41:**375, 1962.

162. Svec, T.A., and Harrison, J.W.: Chemomechanical removal of pulpal and dentinal debris with sodium hypochlorite and hydrogen peroxide vs. normal saline solution, J. Endod. **3:**49, 1977.

163. Tauber, R., et al.: A magnifying lens comparative evaluation of conventional and ultrasonically energized filing, J. Endod. **9:**269, 1983.

164. Tayler, R.L., et al.: Characterization of endodontic silver points, IADR Abstr. **54:**520, 1975.

165. Torabinejad, M., et al.: Scanning electron microscopic study of root canal obturation using thermoplasticized gutta-percha, J. Endod. **4:**245, 1978.

166. Torneck, C.D.: Reaction of rat connective tissue to polyethylene tube implants. I, Oral Surg. **21:**379, 1966.

167. Torneck, C.D.: Reaction of rat connective tissue to polyethylene tube implants. II, Oral Surg. **24:**674, 1967.

168. Urich, J., Moser, J.B., and Heuer, M.A.: Rheology of selected root canal sealer cements, J. Endod. **4:**373, 1978.

169. Vande Visse, J.E., and Brilliant, J.D.: Effect of irrigation on the production of extruded material at the root apex during instrumentation, J. Endod. **1:**243, 1975.

170. Vessey, R.A.: The effect of filing versus reaming on the shape of the prepared root canal, Oral Surg. **27:**543, 1969.

171. Villalobos, R.L., Moser, J.B., and Heuer, M.A.: A method to determine the cutting efficiency of root canal instruments in rotary motion. J. Endod. **6:**667, 1980.

172. Walker, J.E.: Emphysema of soft tissues complicating endodontic treatment using hydrogen peroxide; a case report, Br. J. Oral Surg **13:**98, July 1975.

173. Walton, R.E.: Histologic evaluation of different methods of enlarging the pulp canal space, J. Endod. **2:**304, 1976.

174. Webber, J., Moser, J.B., and Heuer, M.A.: A method to determine the cutting efficiency of root canal instruments in linear motion. J. Endod. **6:**829, 1980.

175. Weine, F.S., Kelly, R.F., and Brag, K.: Effect of preparation with endodontic handpieces on original canal shape, J. Endod. **2:**298, 1976.

176. Weine, F.S., Kelly, R.F., and Lio, P.S.: The effect of preparation procedures on canal shape and apical foramen shape, J. Endod. **8:**255, 1975.
177. Weiner, B.H., and Schilder, H.: A comparative study of important physical properties of various root canal sealers. I. Evaluation of setting times, Oral Surg. **32:**768, 1971.
178. Weiner, B.H., and Schilder, H.: A comparative study of important physical properties of various root canal sealers. II. Evaluation of dimensional changes, Oral Surg. **32:**928, 1971.
179. Weisman, M.I.: A study of the flow rate of ten root canal sealers, Oral Surg. **29:**255, 1970.
180. Weller, N.R., Brady, J.M., and Bernier, W.E.: Efficacy of ultrasonic cleaning, J. Endod. **6:**740, 1980.
181. Wilcko, W.M.: Comparative study of two endodontic sealers in rats (master's thesis), West Virginia University, Morgantown, WV, 1982.
182. Yee, F.S., Lugassy, A.A., and Peterson, J.N.: Filling of root canals with adhesive materials, J. Endod. **1:**145, 1975.
183. Yee, F.S., et al.: Three-dimensional obturation of the root canal using injection-molded, thermoplasticized, dental gutta-percha, J. Endod. **3:**168, 1977.
184. Young, A.R., et al.: Working and setting times of root canal sealers via oscillating rheometer (Abstract 1152), J. Dent. Res. **61:**306, 1982.

Self-assessment questions

1. The endodontic broach is a flexible hand instrument with sharply pointed barbs used to
   a. Remove the roof of the pulp chamber
   b. Engage and remove pulp tissue from the pulp spaces
   c. Smooth dentin of the canal walls
   d. Establish an apical seat near the root apex
2. The essential difference between K-type files and K-type reamers is
   a. The number of spirals or cutting flutes per unit of length
   b. All files are twisted from square cross section blanks
   c. All reamers are twisted from triangular cross section blanks
   d. The K-type files may be hand or power operated
3. The working portion of an endodontic (root canal) spreader is
   a. Smooth, flat-ended, and slightly tapered
   b. Smooth, flat-ended, and uniform width
   c. Smooth, pointed, and uniform width
   d. Smooth, pointed, and uniform width
4. In order to complete a cutting circle of the canal wall, the triangular shaft instrument requires
   a. One-fourth turn
   b. One-third turn
   c. One-half turn
   d. One full turn
5. Significant deviations from circular canal preparations will occur when using a
   a. K-type reamer with a reaming action
   b. K-type reamer with a filing action
   c. K-type file with a filing action
   d. K-type file with a reaming action
6. An important factor to evaluate regarding an instrument fragment lodged in a canal is its
   a. Length
   b. Diameter
   c. Location
   d. Flexibility
7. The popular use of the Hedström file is
   a. To flare the canal from the apical region to the orifice
   b. To establish a circular canal in the apical third
   c. To prepare the canal for a post restoration
   d. For rotary cutting of the canal wall
8. The engine-driven reamers of Group III are recommended by the author for
   a. Removing pulp remnants and debris
   b. Instrumentation of middle and apical portion of the canal
   c. Final finishing and burnishing of entire canal walls
   d. Finishing and enlarging the orifice and coronal third of the canal
9. A criticism of the use of endodontic contra-angle handpieces is
   a. An increase in instrumentation time
   b. The loss of tactile sensation
   c. The reduced effectiveness in shaping canal walls
   d. An inability to negotiate root canals rapidly
10. Some investigations have indicated that the most important aspect of irrigation is the
    a. Volume of irrigant used
    b. Chelating action of the solution
    c. Lumen of the irrigating needle
    d. Aspiration of the solution
11. Which statement regarding gutta-percha is true?
    a. Gutta-percha endodontic points are composed of approximately 20% gutta-percha.
    b. Molecular springback properties assist in sealing the dentin gutta-percha interface.
    c. Gutta-percha is dimensionally stable when used with a chemical solvent.
    d. Gutta-percha aging is hastened by refrigeration.
12. Which statement regarding silver cones is true?
    a. Silver content is approximately 70%.
    b. Surface texture has no affect on cement sealer adherence.
    c. Silver cones are the least toxic materials in endodontics.
    d. Silver cones have corrosion properties capable of cytotoxicity.
13. The significance of free eugenol in root canal sealer-cements is an increase in
    a. Dimensional stability
    b. Setting time
    c. Cytotoxicity
    d. Strength
14. Paraformaldehyde containing root canal cements may be used in
    a. Temporary pulpotomy procedures
    b. Tooth pulpectomy procedures
    c. Treatment of necrotic pulps
    d. Root canal fillings

14

PULPAL REACTION TO CARIES AND DENTAL PROCEDURES

SYNGCUK KIM
HENRY O. TROWBRIDGE

At the dental centenary celebration held in Baltimore in 1940, Bodecker commented on the current state of dentistry: "Operative procedures in the reconstruction of teeth have always been governed by engineering principles."[102] While this is still true today, 46 years later, many other basic concepts of restorative dentistry have been changed drastically since then. One fundamental change in dental treatment in the past 40 years has been preservation of dentition and the pulp. Unfortunately, however, greater dental preservation all too often results in damage to the pulp. Of the various forms of dental treatment, operative procedures by far are the most frequent cause of pulpal injury. It is accepted that trauma to the pulp cannot always be avoided, particularly when the tooth requires extensive restoration. Nonetheless, the competent clinician, by recognizing the hazards associated with each step of the restorative process, can often minimize if not prevent trauma and thus preserve the vitality of the tooth.

In the past, pulpal responses to various dental procedures and materials have been discussed almost exclusively from a histologic perspective. Fortunately, active physiologic investigations in the last decade have shed new light on the dynamic changes in the pulp in response to dental procedures and materials. It is the purpose of this chapter to discuss new knowledge together with the old to understand pulpal responses to caries and to various restorative procedures and materials.

DENTAL CARIES

Dental caries is a localized, progressive destruction of tooth structure and the most common cause of pulp disease. It is now generally accepted that for caries to develop, specific bacteria must become established on the tooth surface. Products of bacterial metabolism, notably

organic acids and proteolytic enzymes, cause the destruction of enamel and dentin. Bacterial metabolites are also capable of eliciting an inflammatory reaction. Eventually, extensive invasion of the dentin results in bacterial infection of the pulp. Basic reactions that tend to protect the pulp against caries involve (1) a decrease in the permeability of the dentin, (2) the formation of new dentin, and (3) inflammatory and immunologic reactions.

Inward diffusion of toxic substances from carious lesions occurs mainly through the dentinal tubules. Therefore, the extent to which toxins permeate the tubules and reach the pulp is of critical importance in determining the extent of pulpal injury. *The most common response to caries is dentin sclerosis.* In this reaction the dentinal tubules become partially or completely filled with mineral deposits consisting of apatite as well as whitlockite crystals.[28,100] Researchers[88] reported finding dentin sclerosis at the periphery of carious lesions in 95.4% of 154 teeth examined. Studies using dyes, solvents, and radioactive ions have shown that dentin sclerosis has the effect of decreasing the permeability of dentin, thus shielding the pulp from irritation.[4, 9, 26, 56] Evidence suggests that, in order for sclerosis to occur, vital odontoblast processes must be present within the tubules.[11,38]

The ability of the pulp to produce reparative dentin beneath a carious lesion is another mechanism for limiting the diffusion of toxic substances to the pulp (see Fig. 10-44). Researchers[88] reported the presence of reparative dentin in 63.6% of teeth with carious lesions and found that it often occurred in combination with dentin sclerosis. The characteristics of reparative dentin have already been discussed (see Chapter 10). In general, the amount of reparative dentin formed is proportional to the amount of primary dentin destroyed. The rate of carious attack also seems to be an influencing factor, since more dentin is formed in response to slowly progressing chronic caries than to rapidly advancing acute caries. For this reason,

Supported in part by NIDR grants DEO-5605 and DEO-0121.

441

carious exposure of the pulp is likely to occur earlier in acute caries than in chronic caries.

Research has shown that along the border zone between primary and reparative dentin, the walls of dentinal tubules are thickened and the tubules are frequently occluded with material resembling peritubular dentin.[77] Thus the border zone appears to be considerably less permeable than ordinary dentin and may serve as a barrier to the ingress of bacteria and their products.

The formation of a dead tract in dentin is yet another reaction that may occur in response to caries. Unlike dentin sclerosis and the formation of reparative dentin, this response is not considered to be a defense reaction. A dead tract is an area in dentin within which the dentinal tubules are devoid of odontoblast processes. The origin of these tracts in dental caries is uncertain, but most authorities are of the opinion that they are formed as a result of the early death of odontoblasts. Dead tracts are most often observed in young teeth affected by rapidly progressing lesions. Because dentinal tubules of dead tracts are patent, they are highly permeable,[80] and therefore they are a potential threat to the integrity of the pulp. Fortunately the healthy pulp responds to the presence of a dead tract by depositing a layer of reparative dentin over its surface, thus sealing it off.[26]

Dentin is demineralized by organic acids (principally lactic acid) that are products of bacterial fermentation. These acids also play a role in degrading the organic matrix of enamel and dentin. While very few oral bacteria possess collagenases, the collagenous matrix of dentin can be degraded by bacterial proteases if the collagen is first denatured by acid.

There is some controversy as to when caries first elicits an inflammatory response in the underlying pulp. One study observed an accumulation of chronic inflammatory cells in the pulp beneath enamel caries that had not yet invaded dentin.[16] Another study,[54] on the other hand, did not observe pulpal inflammation until the caries had penetrated beyond the enamel. There is general agreement that by the time caries has invaded the dentin some changes are occurring in the pulp. These changes represent a response to the diffusion of soluble irritants and inflammatory stimuli into the pulp. Such substances include bacterial toxins, bacterial enzymes, antigens, chemotaxins, organic acids, and products of tissue destruction. Substances also pass outward from the pulp to the carious lesion. Researchers reported finding plasma proteins, immunoglobulins, and complement proteins in carious dentin.[1,2,63-65] It is conceivable that some of these factors are capable of inhibiting bacterial activity in the lesion.

Unfortunately, diagnosis of the extent of pulpal inflammation beneath a carious lesion is difficult. Many factors play a role in determining the nature of the caries process, so the individuality of each carious lesion should be recognized. The response of the pulp may vary depending on whether the caries process is progressing rapidly or slowly or is completely inactive (arrested caries). Moreover, caries tends to be an intermittent process with periods of rapid activity alternating with periods of quiescence.[54] The rate of attack may be influenced by any or all of the following:

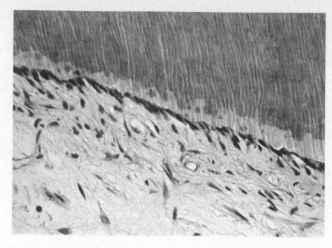

FIG. 14-1. Low cuboidal odontoblasts beneath a carious lesion. Compare the appearance of these cells with normal odontoblasts in Fig. 10-17.

Age of the host
Composition of the tooth
Nature of the bacterial flora of the lesion
Salivary flow
Buffering capacity of the saliva
Antibacterial substances in the saliva
Oral hygiene
Cariogenicity of the diet and frequency with which acidogenic food is ingested
Caries-inhibiting factors in the diet

Early morphologic evidence of a pulpal reaction to caries is found in the underlying odontoblast layer. Even before the appearance of inflammatory changes in the pulp there is an overall reduction in the number and size of odontoblast cell bodies.[93] Although normally tall, columnar cells, odontoblasts affected by caries appear flat to cuboidal in shape (Fig. 14-1). Electron microscopic examination of odontoblasts beneath carious lesions has revealed signs of cellular injury in the form of vacuolization, ballooning degeneration of mitochondria, and reduction in the number and size of other cytoplasmic organelles, particularly the endoplasmic reticulum.[53] These findings are in accord with biochemical studies[42,43] in which a reduction in the metabolic activity of odontoblasts was noted.

Concomitant with changes in the odontoblastic layer, a hyperchromatic line (calciotraumatic response) may develop along the pulpal margin of the dentin (Fig. 14-2). Formation of this line is thought to represent a disturbance in the normal equilibrium of the odontoblasts.[49] It may also delineate the point at which the primary odontoblasts succumbed to the caries process and were replaced by odontoprogenitor cells arising from the cell-rich zone. In either event, as new dentin is formed the hyperchromatic line persists and becomes permanently embedded in the dentin.

Dental caries is a protracted process and lesions progress over a period of months or years. One investigator found that the average time from the stage of incipient caries to clinically detectable caries in children is 18 ± 6 months.[68] Consequently, it is not surprising that pulpal inflammation

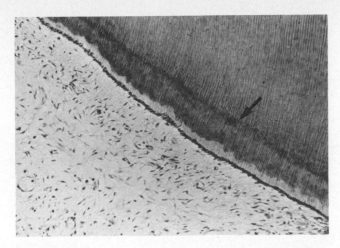

FIG. 14-2. Hyperchromatic line *(arrow)* in dentin beneath a carious lesion. (From Trowbridge, H.: J. Endod. **7**:52, 1981. © by American Association of Endodontists, 1981.)

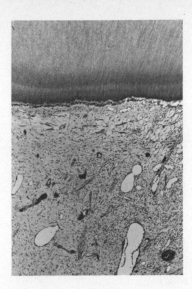

FIG. 14-3. Chronic inflammatory response evoked by a carious lesion in the overlying dentin.

evoked by carious lesions begins insidiously as a low-grade, chronic response rather than an acute reaction (Fig. 14-3). The initial inflammatory cell infiltrate consists principally of lymphocytes, plasma cells, and macrophages.[19] Within this infiltrate are immunologically competent cells responding to antigenic substances diffusing into the pulp from the carious lesion.[92] Additionally, there is a proliferation of small blood vessels and fibroblasts and the deposition of collagen fibers. This pattern of inflammation is regarded as an inflammatory-reparative process. It is well to remember that not all injuries result in permanent damage. Should the carious lesion be eliminated or become arrested, connective tissue repair would ensue.

The extent of pulpal inflammation beneath a carious lesion depends on the depth of bacterial invasion as well as the degree to which dentin permeability has been reduced by dentinal sclerosis and reparative dentin formation. In a study involving 46 carious teeth, investigators found that if the distance between the invading bacteria and the pulp (including the thickness of reparative dentin) averaged 1.1 mm or more, the inflammatory response was negligible.[76] When the lesions reached to within 0.5 mm of the pulp, there was a significant increase in the extent of inflammation, but it was not until the reparative dentin that had formed beneath the lesion was invaded by bacteria that the pulp became acutely inflamed.

As bacteria converge on the pulp, the characteristic features of acute inflammation become manifest. These include vascular and cellular responses in the form of vasodilation, increased vascular permeability, and the accumulation of leukocytes. Neutrophils migrate from blood vessels to the site of injury in response to certain split products of complement that are strongly chemotactic. These products are formed when complement is activated in the presence of antigen-antibody complexes.

Pulpal abscess

Carious exposure of the pulp results in progressive mobilization of neutrophils and eventually to suppuration, which may be diffuse or localized in the form of an abscess. The exudate associated with this reaction is called pus. Pus is formed when neutrophils release their lysosomal enzymes and the surrounding tissue is digested (a process known as liquefactive necrosis). The digested tissue has a greater osmotic pressure than the surrounding tissue, and this pressure differential is one of the reasons why abscesses are often painful and why drainage provides relief.

Few bacteria are found in an abscess, because bacteria entering the lesion are promptly destroyed by the antibacterial products of neutrophils. In addition, many bacteria cannot tolerate the low pH resulting from the release of lactic acid from neutrophils. However, as the size of the exposure enlarges and an ever-increasing number of bacteria enter the pulp, the defending forces are overwhelmed. It must be remembered that the pulp has a finite blood supply. Therefore when the demand for inflammatory elements exceeds the ability of the blood to transport them to the site of bacterial penetration, the bacteria become too numerous for the defenders and are able to proliferate without constraint. This ultimately leads to pulp necrosis.

Chronic ulcerative pulpitis

In some cases an accumulation of neutrophils may produce surface destruction (ulceration) of the pulp rather than an abscess. This is apt to occur when drainage is established through a pathway of decomposed dentin. The ulcer represents a local excavation of the surface of the pulp resulting from liquefactive necrosis of tissue. Because drainage prevents the build-up of pressure, the lesion tends to remain localized and asymptomatic. The base of the ulcer consists of necrotic debris and a dense accumulation of neutrophils. Granulation tissue infiltrated with chronic inflammatory cells is found within the deeper layers of the lesion. Eventually a space is created between the area of suppuration and the wall of the pulp chamber, giving the lesion the appearance of an ulcer (Fig. 14-4).

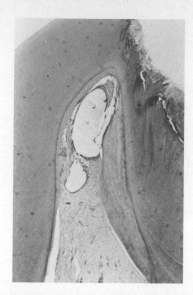

FIG. 14-4. Chronic ulcerative pulpitis.

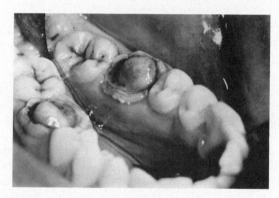

FIG. 14-5. Hyperplastic pulpitis (pulp polyp) in a lower first permanent molar (Courtesy Dr. A. Stabholz, Jerusalem.)

Hyperplastic pulpitis

Hyperplastic pulpitis occurs almost exclusively in primary and immature permanent teeth with open apices. It develops in response to carious exposure of the pulp when the exposure enlarges to form a gaping cavity in the roof of the pulp chamber. This opening provides a pathway for drainage of the inflammatory exudate. Once drainage is established, acute inflammation subsides and chronic inflammatory tissue proliferates through the opening created by the exposure form a "pulp polyp" (Fig. 14-5). Presumably the young pulp does not become necrotic following exposure because its natural defenses and rich supply of blood allow it to resist bacterial infection. Clinically the lesion has the appearance of a fleshy mass that may cover most of what remains of the crown of the tooth.

EFFECTS OF LOCAL ANESTHETICS ON THE PULP

The purpose of adding a vasoconstrictor to local anesthetics is to potentiate and prolong the anesthetic effect by reducing blood flow in the area in which the anesthetic is

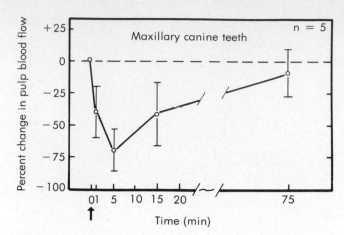

FIG. 14-6. Effects of infiltration anesthesia (2% lidocaine with 1:100,000 epinephrine) on pulpal blood flow in the maxillary canine teeth of dogs. There is a drastic decrease in pulpal blood flow soon after the injection. The arrow indicates the time of injection. The bar depicts S.D. (From Kim, S.: J. Dent. Res. 63[5]:650, 1984.)

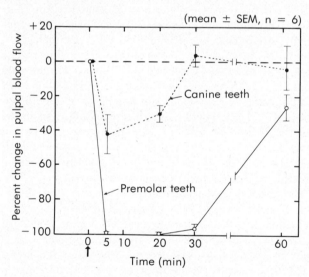

FIG. 14-7. Effects of ligamental injection (2% lidocaine with 1:100,000 epinephrine) on pulpal blood flow in the mandibular canine and premolar teeth of dogs. The injection was given at the mesial and distal sulcus of the premolar teeth. The injection caused total cessation of pulpal blood flow, which lasted about 30 minutes in the premolar teeth. The arrow indicates the time of injection. (From Kim, S.: J. Endod. 12[10]:486, 1986. © by American Association of Endodontists, 1986.)

administered. Although this enhances anesthesia, a recent study has shown that an anesthetic such as 2% lidocaine with epinephrine 1:100,000 is capable of significantly decreasing pulpal blood flow.[48] This reduction in blood flow may place the pulp in jeopardy for reasons explained later. Both infiltration and mandibular block injections cause a significant decrease in pulpal blood flow, although the flow reduction lasts a relatively short time (Fig. 14-6). With the ligamental injection, pulpal blood flow ceases completely for about 30 minutes when 2% lidocaine with 1:100,000 epinephrine is used (Fig. 14-7). With a higher concentra-

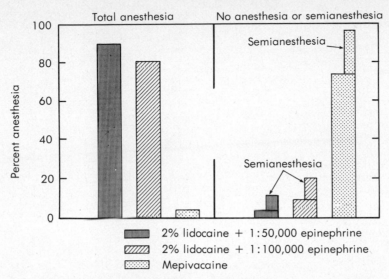

FIG. 14-8. Ligamental injection was effective in obtaining anesthesia in about 90% of cases with 2% lidocaine with 1:50,000 epinephrine and in about 80% of cases with 2% lidocaine with 1:100,000 epinephrine. The injection with mepivacaine (Carbocaine) practically failed to achieve anesthesia. The criteria for total anesthesia is no pain to pulp extirpation and canal instrumentation; semianesthesia is characterized by discomfort as a file approaches the apex.

tion of epinephrine the cessation of pulp flow lasts even longer. There is a direct relationship between the length of the flow cessation and the concentration of the vasoconstrictor used.[47] Because the rate of oxygen consumption in the pulp is relatively low, the healthy pulp can probably withstand a period of reduced blood flow. Researchers reported that pulpal blood flow and sensory nerve activity returned to normal levels after 3 hours of total cessation of blood flow.[66] Recently, it has been demonstrated that little histologic change takes place in the pulp following ligamental injection of an anesthetic solution containing a vasoconstrictor.[51] However, a prolonged reduction in oxygen transport could interfere with cellular metabolism and alter the response of the pulp to injury. Irreversible pulpal injury is particularly apt to occur when dental procedures such as full crown preparation are performed immediately following a ligamental injection. At least four documented cases have occurred in which the mandibular anterior teeth were devitalized as a result of crown preparation following ligamental injection.[47] Presumably irreversible pulp damage resulting from tooth preparation is caused by the release of substantial amounts of vasoactive agents, such as substance P, into the extracellular compartment of the underlying pulp.[67] Under normal circumstances these vasoactive substances are quickly removed from the pulp by the bloodstream. However, when blood flow is drastically decreased or completely arrested, the removal of vasoactive substances from the pulp is greatly delayed. Accumulation of these substances as well as other metabolic waste products may thus result in permanent damage to the pulp. One investigator has shown that the concentration of substances diffusing across the dentin into the pulp depends in part on the rate of removal via the pulpal circulation.[69] Thus a significant reduction in blood flow during a restorative procedure could lead to an increase in the

concentration of irritants accumulating within the pulp. *Therefore, whenever possible, it is advisable to use vasoconstrictor-free local anesthetics for restorative procedures on vital teeth.* Since the addition of epinephrine at a concentration of 1:100,000 to local anesthetics appears to provide adequate vasoconstriction, stronger concentrations should be avoided during routine restorative procedures.

For dental treatments where clinicians need not be concerned about the vitality of the pulp, such as endodontic therapy and extractions, the use of a vasoconstrictor-containing local anesthetic is recommended. When used with an epinephrine-containing anesthetic, the ligamental injection is effective in obtaining anesthesia (Fig. 14-8). Over 80% of the problem teeth were successfully anesthetized with epinephrine 1:100,000 containing anesthetic. Endodontists have found the ligamental injection to be an important tool to obtain profound anesthesia when treating so-called hot mandibular molars.

CAVITY AND CROWN PREPARATION

"Cooking the pulp in its own juice" is how Bodecker described tooth preparation without proper coolant.[79] As shown in Fig. 14-9, pulpal responses to cavity and crown preparation depend on many factors. These include thermal injury, especially frictional heat; transsection of the odontoblastic processes; vibration; desiccation of dentin; pulp exposure; smear layer; remaining dentin thickness; and agents for cavity cleansing, drying, sterilization, and acid etching.

Thermal injury

Cutting of dentin with a rotating bur or stone produces a considerable amount of frictional heat. The amount of heat produced is determined by speed of rotation, size and shape of the cutting instrument, length of time the instru-

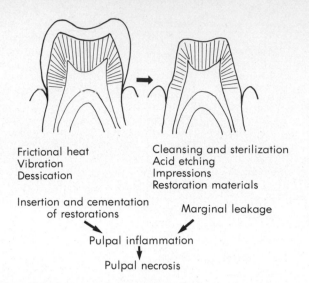

Frictional heat
Vibration
Dessication

Cleansing and sterilization
Acid etching
Impressions
Restoration materials

Insertion and cementation
of restorations

Marginal leakage

Pulpal inflammation

Pulpal necrosis

FIG. 14-9. Schematic illustration on factors that might cause pulpal reaction.

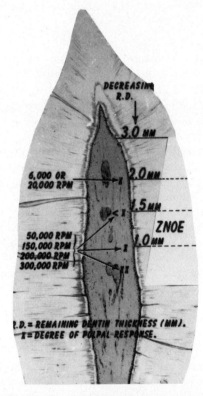

FIG. 14-10. With adequate water coolant, the same cutting tools, and a comparable remaining dentin thickness, the intensity of the pulpal response with high-speed techniques (decreasing force) is considerably less traumatic than with lower-speed techniques (increasing force). (From Stanley, H.R., and Swerdlow, H.: J. Prosthet. Dent. **14**:365, 1964.)

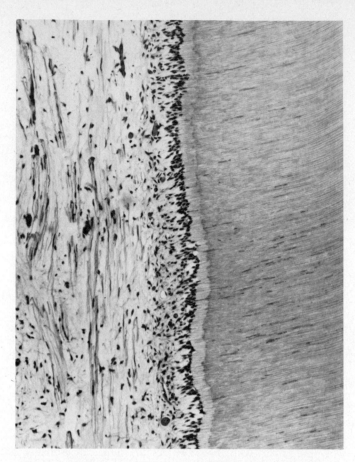

FIG. 14-11. Two-day specimen, high speed with air-water spray. The superficial layers lack infiltrating inflammatory cells. Some odontoblast displacement is present. Pulp architecture is generally intact. (From Swerdlow, H., and Stanley, H.R.: J. Prosthet. Dent. **9**:121, 1959.)

ment is in contact with the dentin, and amount of pressure exerted on the handpiece. If high temperatures are produced in deep cavities by continuous cutting without proper cooling, the underlying pulp may be severely damaged.[85] According to one investigator,[102] the production of

heat within the pulp is the most severe stress that restorative procedures impart to the pulp. If damage is extensive and the cell-rich zone of the pulp is destroyed, reparative dentin may not form.[62]

The thermal conductivity of dentin is relatively low. Therefore heat generated during the cutting of a shallow cavity preparation is much less likely to injure the pulp than a deep cavity preparation. One study found that temperatures and stresses developed during dry cutting of dentin were sufficiently high to be detrimental to tooth structure.[20] These investigators found that the greatest potential for damage was within a 1- to 2-mm radius of the dentin being cut.

The importance of the use of water-air spray during cavity preparation has been well established. For example, more than 15 years ago it was reported that high-speed cutting with an adequate coolant caused cooling of the pulp to subambient level.[102] Without a coolant the pulpal temperature rose to a critical level, 11° F above the ambient temperature. The same is true in the case of slow-speed cutting (11,000 rpm). The reaction of the pulp to cavity preparation with and without a water spray has been studied histologically (Figs. 14-10 to 14-12).[86] When water-air spray was used, there was a negligible response, providing the remaining dentin thickness was greater than 1 mm (Fig. 14-10). However, when the same procedure was performed without using a water spray, severe damage was found underneath the cutting site (Fig. 14-13). Recently a physiologic investigation[46] revealed that a full crown preparation without water spray in dog canine teeth leaving 1 mm remaining dentin resulted in a drastic reduction in pulpal blood flow. The flow was further reduced 1 hour after the completion of the crown preparation, suggesting irreversible damage. In a similar experiment utilizing a water spray we observed only minor changes in pulpal blood flow (Fig. 14-14).

Other researchers[62] investigated the effects of heat on the pulps of anesthetized young premolar teeth scheduled for orthodontic extraction. Class V cavities were prepared in the teeth, leaving an average of 0.5 mm remaining dentin thickness. Subsequently, a constant heat of 150° C was applied to the surface of the exposed dentin for 30 seconds. Following this procedure the teeth remained asymptomatic for a month, following which the teeth were extracted. Histologic examination of the pulps revealed varying degrees of pathosis, which included development of a homogenized collagenous zone along the dentin wall, disappearance of the "cell-rich" zone, and generalized cellular degeneration. Localized abscesses were observed in some of the teeth.

"Blushing" of teeth during or after cavity or crown preparation has been attributed to frictional heat. Characteristically the coronal dentin develops a pinkish hue very soon after the dentin is cut. This pinkish hue represents vascular stasis in the subodontoblastic capillary plexus blood flow. Under favorable conditions this reaction is reversible and the pulp survives. However, a dark purplish color indicates thrombosis, and this is associated with a poorer prognosis. Histologically, the pulp tissue adjacent to the blushed dentinal surface is engorged with extravasated red blood cells, presumably due to the rupture of capillaries in the subodontoblastic plexus.[58] The incidence of dentinal blushing is greatest beneath full crown preparations in teeth that were anesthetized by ligamental injection using 2% lidocaine plus 1:100,000 epinephrine.[47] In such cases, the cessation of pulpal blood flow following ligamental injection may be a contributing factor. Tooth preparation may lead to the release of various vasoactive substances such as Substance P, and accumulation of such agents as a result of cessation of pulpal blood flow following ligamental injection may cause the tooth to "blush."

Transsection of the Odontoblastic Processes

The length of the odontoblast process in fully formed teeth is still a matter of controversy. For many years it was believed that the process is confined to the inner third of the dentin. However, recent scanning electron microscopic studies have provided evidence suggesting that many of the processes extend all the way from the odontoblast layer to the dentinoenamel junction.[45] In any event, amputation of the distal segment of odontoblast processes is often a consequence of cavity or crown preparation. Histologic in-

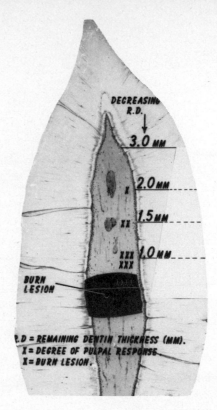

FIG. 14-12. Without adequate water coolant, larger cutting tools (e.g., a no. 37 diamond point) will create typical burn lesions within the pulp when the remaining dentin thickness becomes less than 1.5 mm. (From Stanley, H.R., and Swerdlow, H.: J. Prosthet. Dent. **14**:365, 1964.)

vestigation would indicate that amputation of a portion of the process does not invariably lead to death of the odontoblast. We know from numerous cytologic studies involving microsurgery that amputation of a cellular process is quickly followed by repair of the cell membrane. However, it would appear that amputation of the odontoblast process close to the cell body results in irreversible injury.[78]

It is not always possible to determine the exact cause of death when odontoblasts disappear following a restorative procedure, since these cells may be subjected to a variety of insults. Frictional heat, vibration, amputation of processes, displacement due to desiccation, exposure to bacterial toxins, and other chemical irritants may each play a role in the demise of odontoblasts.

Vibratory phenomena

Surprisingly little is known about the vibratory agitation that may be produced by high-speed cutting procedures. One study[34] demonstrated violent disturbances in the pulp chambers of teeth beneath the point of application of the bur as well as at other points remote from the cavity preparation. According to the observations, the shock waves produced by vibration were particularly pronounced when the cutting speed was reduced; therefore, stalling of the bur by increased digital pressure on the handpiece should be avoided. Obviously this problem deserves further study.

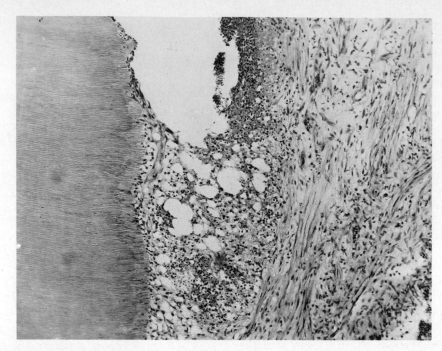

FIG. 14-13. Burn lesion with necrosis and an expanding abscess formation in a 10-day specimen. Cavity prepared dry at 20,000 rpm with remaining dentin thickness is 0.23 mm. (From Swerdlow, H., and Stanley, H.R.: J. Am. Dent. Assoc. **56:**317, 1958.)

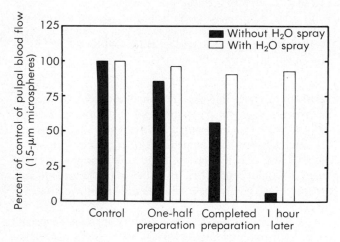

FIG. 14-14. Effects of crown preparation, in dogs, with and without water-air spray (at 350,000 rpm) on pulpal blood flow. The tooth preparation without water spray caused a substantial decrease in pulpal blood flow, whereas that with water spray caused insignificant changes in the flow.

Desiccation of dentin

When the surface of freshly cut dentin is dried with a jet of air, there is a rapid outward movement of fluid through the dentinal tubules as a result of the activation of capillary forces within.[15] According to the hydrodynamic theory of dentin sensitivity, this movement of fluid results in stimulation of the sensory nerve of the pulp. Fluid movement is also capable of drawing odontoblasts up into the tubules. These "displaced" odontoblasts soon die and disappear as they undergo autolysis. However, desiccation

of dentin by cutting procedures or with a blast of air does not injure the pulp.[12,15] While one might expect that death of odontoblasts would evoke an inflammatory response, probably too few cells are involved to evoke a significant reaction. Moreover, since death occurs within the dentinal tubules, dentinal fluid would dilute the products of cellular degeneration that might otherwise initiate an inflammatory response. Ultimately, odontoblasts that have been destroyed as a result of desiccation are replaced by new odontoblasts that arise from the cell-rich zone of the pulp, and in 1 to 3 months reparative dentin is formed.[12]

Pulp exposure

Exposure of the pulp during cavity preparation occurs most often in the process of removing carious dentin. Accidental mechanical exposure may result during the placement of pins or retention points in dentin. In both types of exposure, injury to the pulp appears to be due primarily to bacterial contamination. Investigators demonstrated that surgical exposure of the pulps of germ-free rats was followed by complete healing with no appreciable inflammatory reaction.[41,99] Another investigator has shown that pulps exposed during the removal of carious dentin become infected by bacteria that are carried into the pulp by dentin chips harboring microorganisms.[21] It is safe to state that carious exposure results in much more bacterial contamination than mechanical exposure.

Smear layer

The smear layer is an amorphous, relatively smooth layer of microcrystalline debris whose featureless surface cannot be seen with the naked eye.[70] Although the smear layer may interfere with the adaptation of restorative materials to dentin, it may not be desirable to remove the entire layer, since its removal greatly increases dentin permeability. By removing most of the layer but leaving plugs of grinding debris in the apertures of the dentinal tubules, dentin permeability is not increased, yet the walls of the cavity are relatively clean. Whether or not the smear layer should be removed is a matter of controversy. One view is that microorganisms present in the smear layer may irritate the pulp. Initially few bacteria are present in the smear layer, but if conditions for growth are favorable these will multiply, particularly if a gap between the restorative material and the dentinal wall permits the ingress of saliva.[14] Brännström believes that most restorative materials do not adhere to the dentinal wall.[14] Consequently, contraction gaps form between such materials and the adjacent tooth structure, and these gaps are invaded by bacteria either from the smear layer or from the oral cavity. As a result, bacterial metabolites diffuse through the dentinal tubules and injure the pulp.

Remaining dentin thickness

As discussed in Chapter 10, dentin permeability increases almost logarithmically with increasing cavity depth due to the difference in size and number of dentinal tubules. In short, permeability of the dentin is of great importance in determining the degree of pulpal injury resulting from restorative procedures and materials. Stanley[86] found that the distance between the floor of the cavity preparation and the pulp (i.e., the remaining dentin thickness) greatly influences the pulpal response to restorative procedures and materials. He suggested that a remaining dentin thickness of 2 mm would protect the pulp from the effects of most restorative procedures, provided that all other operative precautions are observed.

Agents for cavity cleansing, drying, sterilization, and acid etching

Cleansing agents are used to reduce microorganisms on the cut surface of dentin and to remove the smear layer that remains on the dentin after cavity preparation. It is believed that if this superficial smear layer were removed, a liner or cement would adapt better to the cut surface of dentin. Cleansing agents contain either an acid or a chelating agent such as ethylenediamine-tetra-acetic acid (EDTA). In one study it was found that the incidence of pulpal inflammation increased significantly when cavities were treated with an acid cleansing agent (50% citric acid) before being filled as compared with controls where the cleanser was omitted.[22] Another study[87] reported that Epoxylite Cavity Cleaner intensified and prolonged the severity of pulpal reactions when used in conjunction with a composite resin filling material. It has also been demonstrated that by removing the smear layer and enlarging the orifices of the dentinal tubules, acid cleansing agents greatly increase the permeability of dentin, thus enhancing penetration of the dentin by irritating substances.[72] It follows that if bacteria grow beneath a restoration, the toxins they produce will more readily diffuse through dentin that

has been cleansed with acid. Another product, Cavilax, was developed to eliminte residual eugenol after removal of temporary fillings. The ingredients are 50% methylethyl ketone and 50% ethyl acetone. Investigators[23] found that use of this cleanser resulted in only a very mild pulpal response and some odontoblast displacement.

Drying agents: Cavity drying agents generally contain organic solvents such as ether and acetone. Solvent-containing drying agents should not be used in very deep cavities, since these agents are capable of damaging odontoblast processes and cells of the pulp. Apparently when used in shallow to moderately deep cavities they produce no significant pulpal inflammation, but because of their desiccating effect, they are apt to cause odontoblast displacement.

Cavity sterilization: At one time cavity-sterilizing agents such as phenol, silver nitrate, and their germicidal agents were used routinely. However, it became obvious that agents capable of efficiently destroying bacteria are also highly irritating to pulp tissue, and today such caustic agents are seldom used. Recently, disinfectants such as benzalkonium chloride, chlorhexidine, and 9-aminoacridine have been employed to reduce the risk of bacterial contamination beneath restorations. One researcher[15] advocates the use of a cavity cleanser that contains a low concentration of EDTA (0.2%) to remove the superficial smear layer and benzalkonium chloride to disinfect the walls of the cavity.

Acid etching: While acid etching of cavity walls is cleansing, acid etching is specifically designed to enhance the adhesion of restorative materials. In the case of dentin, however, the ability of acid etching to improve long-term adhesion has been questioned.[35] Acid cleansers applied to dentin have been shown to widen the openings of the dentinal tubules, increase dentin permeability, and enhance bacterial penetration of the dentin.[98] One study showed that in deep cavities, pretreatment of the dentin with 50% citric or 50% phosphoric acid for 60 seconds is capable of significantly increasing the response of the pulp to restorative materials.[87] Results of a recent physiologic investigation have shown that acid etching a small Class V cavity having a remaining dentin thickness of 1.5 mm has little effect on pulpal blood flow.[84] Thus direct effect of the acid on the pulpal microvascular vessels appears to be negligible, possibly due to a rapid buffering of the acid by the dentinal fluid. However, it is possible that in very deep cavities acid etching may contribute to pulpal injury.

TAKING OF IMPRESSIONS

Heated modeling compound has been reported to produce significant injury to the pulp when applied to cavity or full crown preparations. Presumably this is due to the combination of heat and pressure exerted on the pulp.[79] Investigators demonstrated intrapulpal temperatures of up to 52° C during impression taking with modeling compound in copper bands.[31] Other investigators[103] have shown that an intrapulpal temperature increase of this magnitude may result in severe pulpal injury. Another[52] also observed vascular and odontoblastic changes. Crown

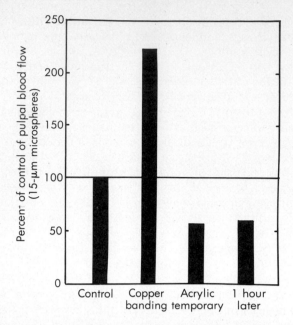

FIG. 14-15. Effects of impression taking using modeling compound with copper banding on pulpal blood flow in dogs.

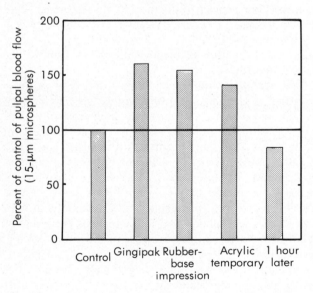

FIG. 14-16. Effects of impression taking using rubber base material on pulpal blood flow in dogs.

preparation and impression taking with modeling compound caused an arteriolar dilation and formation of an irregular odontoblastic layer. A drastic increase in pulpal blood flow was seen immediately after heated modeling compound was placed on crown preparations in canine teeth in dogs.[47] Pulpal blood flow then decreased significantly when acrylic temporary material contacted the prepared tooth surface (Fig. 14-15). The use of modeling compound with a copper band poses two hazards to the pulp: heat generation and hydraulic force, since the copper band tightly fits the prepared tooth. Thus Lindholm's observation on the irregular odontoblastic layer and our observation on the changes in pulpal blood flow suggest that this impression technique may damage the pulp.

In contrast, histologists have found that *rubber-base and hydrocolloid impression materials are well tolerated by the pulp.*[50] Recent physiologic evidence supports this finding. Pulpal blood flow changed insignificantly when an impression was taken with a rubber-based material (Fig. 14-16).

INSERTION OR CEMENTATION OF RESTORATIONS

Strong hydraulic forces may be exerted on the pulp during cementation of crowns and inlays, as the cement is driven toward the pulp, thus compressing the fluid in the dentinal tubules. In extreme cases this may actually cause a separation of the odontoblast layer from the dentin. This will not occur if the exposed dentin is first covered by a liner or base. In addition to hydraulic forces, chemical effects of cementing materials seem to occur. There is experimental evidence that cementation of a crown with zinc phosphate cement causes inflammatory reactions in the pulp. In view of other reports[73] that chemical ions of the luting agent have no effect on the pulp. Obviously, there is a need for additional research in this area.

RESTORATIVE MATERIALS

How do restorative materials evoke a response in the underlying pulp? For many years it was believed that toxic ingredients in the materials were responsible for pulpal injury. However, pulpal injury associated with the use of these materials could not be correlated with their cytotoxic properties. Thus irritating materials such as zinc oxide–eugenol (ZOE) produced a very mild pulpal response when placed in cavities, whereas less toxic materials such as composite resins and amalgam produced a much stronger pulp response. Besides chemical toxicity, some of the properties of materials that might be capable of producing injury include:
1. Acidity (hydrogen ion concentration)
2. Absorption of water during setting
3. Heat evolved during setting
4. Poor marginal adaptation resulting in bacterial contamination

Investigators[73] found that the pulpal response beneath a material is not associated with the material's hydrogen ion concentration. The acid percent in restorative materials is probably neutralized by the dentin and dentinal fluid.[19] As the superficial dentin is demineralized, phosphate ions are liberated, thus producing a buffering effect. However, placement of an acidic material such as zinc phosphate at luting consistency in a deep cavity may have a toxic effect on the pulp since the diffusion barrier is extremely thin. In a study conducted in our laboratory, zinc phosphate cement of luting consistency placed on a deep (0.5 mm remaining dentin layer) and large Class V cavity on canine tooth caused a moderate decrease in pulpal blood flow as measured with the 15 μm microsphere method. After the cement had hardened for about 30 minutes blood flow had again increased, suggesting that the cement had a temporary and transitory effect on the pulpal circulation (Fig. 14-17). The changes in pulpal blood flow may have been due to chemical and/or exothermal effects of the cement. One

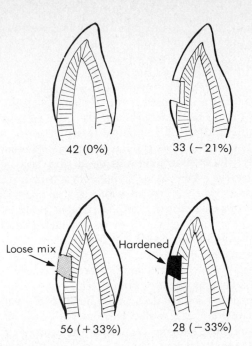

FIG. 14-17. Effects of zinc phosphate cement on pulpal blood flow (ml/min/100 g). A cement of luting consistency was placed in a deep and large Class V in the canine teeth of dogs and pulpal blood flow was measured. A 33% increase was observed initially, but the hardened cement caused a decrease in pulpal blood flow.

study found that of all materials studied, zinc phosphate cement was associated with the greatest temperature rise — an increase of 2.14° C.[73] This amount of temperature increase, however, is not sufficient to produce tissue injury.[102] In a microcirculatory study using hamster cheek pouch, a drop of zinc phosphate liquid caused stasis, followed by hemolysis, resulting in total cessation of blood flow in the vessels that were in contact with the liquid. Thus there seems to be a real possibility of pulpal damage if the pulp is in close contact with the liquid portion of the cement. Absorption of water during the setting of a material can also be ruled out as a cause of pulpal injury. Compared with the removal of fluid from dentin by an airstream during cavity preparation (which produces no inflammatory response in the pulp), absorption of water by a material is insignificant. Researchers[73] found no relationship between the hydrophilic properties of materials and their effect on the pulp.

This brings us to bacterial contamination. It has long been recognized that, in general, dental materials do not adapt to tooth structure well enough to provide a hermetic seal. Thus it has been acknowledged that bacteria may penetrate the gap between the restored material and the cavity wall. Presumably, bacteria growing beneath restorations create toxic products that can diffuse through the dentinal tubules and evoke an inflammatory reaction in the underlying pulp. Converging evidence suggests that *products of bacterial metabolism are the major cause of pulpal injury resulting from the insertion of restorations*. Let us briefly review some of that evidence. One investigator

showed that materials such as composite resins, zinc phosphate, and silicate cements produced only a localized tissue reaction when placed directly on exposed pulps in germ-free animals.[99] The same procedure in conventional animals resulted in total pulp necrosis. Employing bacterial staining methods, researchers[19] demonstrated that the growth of bacteria under restorations was correlated with the degree of inflammation of the adjacent pulp tissue. They also found that bacteria did not grow when the margins of restorations were surface-sealed with ZOE. When bacterial growth was thus inhibited, pulpal inflammation was negligible. Similar studies[8] showed that colonies of bacteria become established under restorative materials that do not provide an adequate marginal seal. Of the materials they tested—Dispersalloy amalgam,* Concise composite resin,† Hygienic gutta percha,‡ MQ silicate cements,§ and ZOE—only ZOE consistently prevented bacteria from becoming established beneath the restoration.

In vitro and in vivo studies on marginal adaptation of restorative materials have often yielded conflicting results. Obviously it is difficult to duplicate clinical conditions in the laboratory. Two important factors affecting marginal adaptation are temperature changes and masticatory forces. Nelson et al.[59] were the first to study the opening and closing of the margin of restorations that were subjected to temperature changes. If a material was a different coefficient of thermal expansion than tooth structure, temperature change is likely to produce gaps between the material and the cavity wall. Another investigator[75] demonstrated a marked effect of functional mastication on marginal adaptation of composite restorations. He found gap formation along 71% of the restorations in teeth that were in functional occlusion, whereas leakage occurred in only 28% of teeth with no antagonist.

As yet no permanent filling material has been shown to consistently provide a perfect marginal seal, so leakage and bacterial contamination are always a threat to the integrity of the pulp. Consequently, an adequate cavity liner or cement base should be employed to seal the dentinal tubules before inserting restorative materials. Despite these findings, it must be acknowledged that pulps frequently remain healthy under restorations that leak. Factors that determine whether bacterial growth beneath a restoration will injure the pulp probably include pathogenicity of the microorganisms, permeability of the underlying dentin (i.e., degree of sclerosis, number of tubules, thickness of dentin), and the ability of the irritated pulpal to produce reparative dentin.

Since there is convincing evidence that bacterial growth beneath restorations is the primary cause of pulpal injury, the antibacterial properties of filling materials may be of considerable importance. Not all materials have been stud-

---

*Johnson & Johnson Products Co., East Windsor, NJ.
†3M Co., St. Paul, MN.
‡The Hygienic Corp., Akron, OH.
§White Dental Products, Philadelphia, PA.

ied, but there is evidence that ZOE, calcium hydroxide, and polycarboxylate cement have some ability to inhibit bacterial growth. Zinc phosphate cement, the restorative resins, and silicate cements lack antibacterial ingredients, and it is these materials that are most often associated with injury to the pulp.

Zinc oxide–eugenol (ZOE)

ZOE is used for a variety of purposes in dentistry. In addition to being a popular temporary filling material, it is used for provisional and permanent cementation of inlays, crowns, and bridges, as a pulp capping agent, and as a cement base. Eugenol, a phenol derivative, is known to be toxic, and it is capable of producing thrombosis of blood vessels when applied directly to pulp tissue.[74] It also has anesthetic properties and is used as an anodyne in relieving the symptoms of painful pulpitis. This presumably results from its ability to block the transmission of action potentials in nerve fibers.[96] Experimentally, ZOE has been shown to suppress nerve excitability in the pulp when applied to the base of a deep cavity.[94] This effect is only obtained when a fairly thin mix of ZOE, e.g., powder-to-liquid ratio 2:1 w/w, is used. Presumably it is the free eugenol in the cement that is responsible for the anesthetic effect. ZOE has two important properties that explain why it is such an effective base material: (1) it adapts very closely to dentin, thus providing a good marginal seal, and (2) its antibacterial properties inhibit bacterial growth on cavity walls. However, because eugenol is injurious to cells, some authorities question whether ZOE should be used in very deep cavity preparations where there is a risk of pulp exposure.

Zinc phosphate cement

One study[36] found that, when a liner was omitted, severe pulpal reactions (principally abscess formation) occurred in all teeth in which deep Class V cavities were restored with zinc phosphate cement. The pulpal response was attributed to the phosphoric acid contained in the cement. In retrospect, however, it is likely that irritation to the pulp was due primarily to marginal leakage rather than to acidity.[18] Because of its high modulus of elasticity, zinc phosphate is the cement base of choice for amalgam restorations. This results from the fact that it is better able to resist the stresses of mastication than other cements.[25]

Silicate cements

Silicate cement restorations are very damaging to the pulp if not used with a liner or base. While many investigators have attributed the injurious effects to the low pH of silicate cement, it seems likely that microleakage resulting in the growth of bacteria on the walls of the cavity beneath silicate cement fillings is responsible for pulpal injury.

Zinc polycarboxylate cements

Polycarboxylate cement is well tolerated by the pulp, being roughly equivalent to ZOE cements in this respect.[36] This may be due to its ability to adapt well to dentin. Ad-

ditionally, it has been reported that this cement has bactericidal qualities.[5]

Restorative resins

The original unfilled resins were associated with severe marginal leakage, caused by dimensional changes that resulted from a high coefficient of thermal expansion. This in turn resulted in marked pulpal injury. The development of sulfinic acid catalyst systems and the nonpressure insertion techniques have improved the performance of resins considerably. The epoxide resins with a benzoyl peroxide catalyst that are 75% filled with glass or quartz (the so-called composite resins) represent another group of resins. These have much more favorable polymerization characteristics and a lower coefficient of thermal expansion than the original unfilled resins. The marginal seal has been further improved by acid etching of beveled enamel and the use of a bonding agent or primer. This reduces the risk of microbial invasion but does not eliminate bacteria that may be present on cavity walls. However, it has been shown that the initial marginal seal tends to deteriorate as the etched composite restoration ages.[40] Furthermore, one study showed that functional mastication is capable of producing gaps that result in increased leakage.[75] Many investigators[19,82] have shown that unlined composite resins are harmful to the pulp, primarily because of bacterial contamination beneath the restoration. Thus the use of a cavity liner is strongly recommended. Since copal varnish is not compatible with the restorative resins, the use of a polystyrene liner has been advocated.[17] Bases containing calcium hydroxide have also been shown to provide good protection against bacteria.

Glass-ionomer cement restorations

Studies on glass-ionomer cements indicate that they are well tolerated by the pulp.[44,61] However, researchers[3] have shown that leakage may occur around ionomer cement fillings, so this material should be used in conjunction with a liner or base. There have been reports of postcementation tooth sensitivity following the use of glass-ionomer cements to cement gold castings, but the cause of this sensitivity has not been determined.

Dental amalgam

Dental amalgam, first used for the restoration of carious teeth in the sixteenth century, is still the most popular restorative material in dentistry. Unvarnished amalgam restorations leak severely when they are first inserted, but within a period of 12 weeks a marginal seal develops that resists dye penetration beyond the dentinoenamel junction.[37] One investigator[33] found that pulp responses to unlined amalgams (Sybraloy,* Dispersalloy,† Tytin,‡ and Spheraloy*) consisted of slight to moderate inflammation. The inflammation tended to diminsh with time, and within

---

*Kerr Mfg. Co., Romulus, MI.
†Johnson & Johnson, East Windsor, NJ.
‡S.S. White Dental Products, Philadelphia, PA.

a few weeks reparative dentin was deposited. Another investigator[74] theorized that the high mercury content of amalgam may exert a cytotoxic effect on the pulp, as he found that mercury penetrates into the dentin and pulp beneath an amalgam restoration. He has also reported that rubbing the bottom of the cavity with a calcium hydroxide/water mixture protects the pulp from the irritating effects of amalgam. Bacteria were found beneath unlined amalgams, while the pulps of teeth in which a ZOE liner was used exhibited a milder response and no bacteria was present. In vitro bacterial tests indicated that amalgam has no inhibitory effect on bacterial growth.

It is well known that insertion of amalgam restorations may result in postoperative thermal sensitivity, even when amalgam is placed in a shallow cavity. Brännström[13] is of the opinion that such sensitivity results from expansion or contraction of fluid that occupies the gap between the amalgam and the cavity wall. This fluid is in communication with fluid in the subjacent dentinal tubules, so variations in temperature would cause axial movement of fluid in the tubules. According to the hydrodynamic theory of dentin sensitivity, this fluid movement would stimulate nerve fibers in the underlying pulp, thus evoking pain.[94] The use of a cavity varnish or base is recommended in order to seal the dentinal tubules and prevent this form of postoperative discomfort.

Cavity varnish

The effectiveness of cavity varnish in providing protection for the pulp is highly controversial. One study[27] has called attention to the fact that in vivo surfaces are wet and therefore the application of liners or varnishes may not result in an impervious coating. Even the application of two or three coats of varnish may not prevent gaps from occurring in the lining. Furthermore, other investigators[17] have reported that a double layer of Copalite did not prevent bacterial leakage and growth of bacteria on the cavity walls. Nonetheless, several reports indicate that varnish can act as a barrier to the toxic effects of restorations.[24,29,83,101] One study[60] assessed the ability of several commercial varnishes to decrease microleakage beneath a high-copper spherical alloy restorative material and found Copalite to be the most effective.

HEAT OF POLISHING

One study reported temperature increases in the pulp of over 20° C when amalgam restorations were polished continuously with prophylactic cups.[30] This is sufficient to cause severe pulpal injury. They found that polishing appliances made of rubber created higher temperatures than cup brushes. Continuous polishing using high speeds of rotation was associated with greater heat than intermittent polishing using low speeds.

POSTOPERATIVE SENSITIVITY

Postoperative discomfort, though usually transient, indicates that the restorative procedure has inflicted trauma on the tooth and/or supporting structures. Severe persistent pain almost certainly signifies that pulpal inflammation has resulted in hyperalgesia. Researchers[81] examined 40 patients who had received dental treatment involving insertion of amalgam and composite restorations. They found that 78% of the patients experienced some degree of postoperative discomfort. Sensitivity to cold was the most frequent complaint, whereas sensitivity to heat occurred much less often. Another study[39] found that there was a positive correlation between heat sensitivity and pulpal inflammation. The significance of sensitivity to cold has not been fully established. Since the response occurs very soon after stimuli such as ice, cold water, and cold air come into contact with the tooth, it is believed that pain is caused by the stimulation of sensory nerve fibers of the pulp by hydrodynamic forces.[95] Because these fibers have a relatively low excitability threshold, they will respond to low-level stimuli that do not necessarily produce tissue injury. However, the presence of hyperalgesia associated with inflammation produce an exaggerated response to cold. Sensitivity that develops soon after a restoration is placed may also be due to poor marginal adaptation, resulting in leakage of saliva under the filling.

CURRENT THINKING ON THE CAUSE OF PULPAL REACTION TO RESTORATION

In the past, pulp reactions to dental procedures was thought to be due to mechanical insults, such as frictional heat, and generally this is true. The reaction to dental materials, on the other hand, has been attributed to chemical effects, such as acidity of the restorative materials. Although the chemical effects cannot be entirely discounted, especially in a deep cavity where only a very thin layer of dentin remains, in current thinking *pulpal injury is primarily due to microleakage through gaps between the filling material and the walls of the cavity.* It is believed that bacteria growing in these gaps elaborate products that diffuse through the dentinal tubules and irritate the pulp. It must be recognized that all permanent filling materials may allow these gaps to form! It is a miracle that all restored teeth do not show some degree of pulpal inflammation. On the other hand, it is not surprising that many teeth that have been restored require endodontic therapy. One study[8] reported that the quantity of bacterial toxins filtered from the base of a Class V cavity depends on the type of restorative material used. The greatest amount of leakage occurred with silicate cements, followed by composite resins and amalgam fillings. Little or no leakage occured when zinc oxide–eugenol was used. Even full crown restorations have been found to leak.

It is impossible to examine pulpal reactions without understanding structural and functional properties of the dentin. Pulp reactions begin when irritants make contact with the surface of the dentin. As the dentin thickness decreases, the danger of pulpal reaction increases dramatically. A simple physiologic law of diffusion states that the rate of diffusion of substances depends on two factors: (1) concentration gradient of the substances and (2) the surface area available for diffusion. Of importance in determining the extent of pulp reactions is the surface area of dentin available for diffusion. Because the dentinal tubules vary in

TABLE 14-1. Surface area of dentin available for diffusion at various distances from the pulp

Distance from pulp	Number of tubules (million/cm^2)		Tubular radius (cm × 10^4)		Area of surface (Ap) (%)*	
(mm)	mean	range	mean	range	mean	range
0.1-0.5	4.5	3.0-5.2	1.25	2.0-3.2	22.1	9-42
0.6-1.0	4.3	2.2-5.9	0.95	1.0-2.3	12.2	2-25
1.1-1.5	3.8	1.6-4.7	0.80	1.0-1.6	7.6	1-9.0
1.6-2.0	3.5	2.1-4.7	0.60	0.9-1.5	4.0	1-8.0
2.1-2.5	3.0	1.2-4.7	0.55	0.8-1.6	2.9	1-9.0
2.6-3.0	2.3	1.1-3.6	0.45	0.6-1.3	1.5	0.3-6
3.1-3.5	2.0	0.7-4.0	0.40	0.5-1.4	1.1	0.1-6
	1.9	1.0-2.5	0.40	0.5-1.2	1.0	0.2-3

Modified from Garberoglio and Brännström (1976); from Pashley, D.H.: Operative Dent. (Suppl.) **3**:13, 1984.
*Ap = nr^2, where n is the number of tubules/cm^2; Ap represents the percentage of the total area of the physical surface available for diffusion.

diameter and density across the thickness of the dentin, the surface area (i.e., product of tubular area and density) available for diffusion varies one region of the dentin to the other. Table 14-1 demonstrates the available dentinal surface for diffusion at various distance from the pulp. For example, the diffusible surface area is 1% of the total dentin surface area at the dentinoenamel junction, whereas it is 22% at the pulp. Thus the harmful effects of an insult increases significantly as the thickness of dentin over the pulp decreases.

The natural defense mechanisms of the tooth should be recognized. In some situations the dentinal tubules may become blocked by hydroxyapatite and other crystals, a condition known as dentin sclerosis. Another reaction resulting in a decrease in dentin permeability is reparative dentin formation.

The smear layer also influences the permeability of dentin and thus protects the pulp by hindering the diffusion of toxic substances through the tubules. According to one investigation, the smear layer accounts for 86% of the total resistance to flow fluid.[70] Thus acid etching, which removes the smear layer, greatly increases permeability by increasing the diffusable surface area (Fig. 14-18). The question arises of what to do with the smear layer. Should it be removed or be left alone? Some authorities are of the opinion that it should be removed, since the smear layer may harbor bacteria. On the other hand, the presence of a smear layer constitutes a physical barrier to bacterial penetration of the dentinal tubules.[55,98] However, another investigator demonstrated that the presence of the smear layer cannot prevent diffusion of bacterial products, although it effectively blocks actual bacterial invasion.[6] It has been shown that bacterial products reaching the pulp are capable of evoking an inflammatory response.[7] It follows that the best way to solve the problem is to remove the smear layer and replace it with a "sterile, nontoxic" artificial smear layer. Research in the field has yielded some agents that look promising, two of which are potassium oxalate[32] and 5% ferric oxalate.[10]

Since at the present time there is no material that can bond chemically to dentin and thus prevent leakage, the

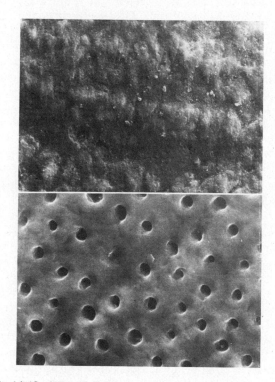

FIG. 14-18. SEM photomicrographs of smear layer intact and smear layer removed. Notice the patent dentinal tubules. (Courtesy Dr. D.H. Pashley.)

use of a cavity liner to seal dentin is highly recommended. According to one investigator, there are three possible routes for microleakage: (1) within or via the smear layer (2) between the smear layer and the cavity varnish or cement, and (3) between the cavity varnish or cement and the restorative material (Fig. 14-19).[70]

Compensatory pulpal reaction to outside insults

Mechanisms exist by which the pulp is able to ward off insults. The ability of the pulp to deposit reparative dentin beneath a restoration is an excellent example. In addition, the vascular system is able to respond to mechanical insults. For example, it has been shown that deep drilling

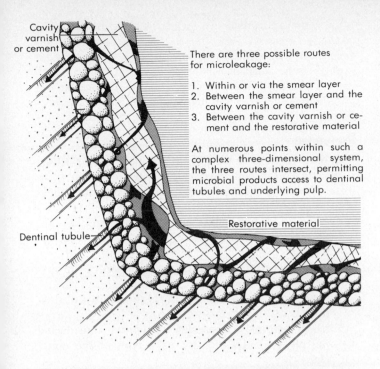

Cavity varnish or cement

Dentinal tubule

There are three possible routes for microleakage:

1. Within or via the smear layer
2. Between the smear layer and the cavity varnish or cement
3. Between the cavity varnish or cement and the restorative material

At numerous points within such a complex three-dimensional system, the three routes intersect, permitting microbial products access to dentinal tubules and underlying pulp.

Restorative material

FIG. 14-19. Schematic representation of the interface of dentin and restorative material in a typical cavity. The granular constituents of the smear layer have been exaggerated out of their normal proportion for emphasis. Three theoretical routes for microleakage are indicated by arrows. (Reprinted with permission from Pashley, D.H., et al.: Arch. Oral Biol. **23**:391, 1978. Copyright 1978, Pergamon Press, Ltd.)

without proper water coolant causes a profound decrease in pulpal blood flow in the area of injury. Blood is shunted away from the area by an abrupt increase in the flow of blood through arteriovenous anastomoses (AVAs) or U-turn loops located in the root canal (Fig. 14-20). It is possible that opening of the previously closed AVAs occurs as pulpal tissue pressure increases to critical levels. The opening of the AVAs is a compensatory mechanism of the pulp to maintain blood flow within physiologically normal limits (Fig. 14-20).

It should be remembered that the pulp is a very resilient tissue and that it has a great potential for healing. It is only when all compensatory mechanisms fail that the pulp becomes necrotic. Fig. 14-21 depicts the current thinking on the pathophysiologic mechanisms involved in pulp necrosis. Since the pulp is rigidly encased in mineralized tissues, it is protected from most forms of trauma to which the tooth is exposed. Nevertheless, insults such as dental caries and restorative procedures are capable of producing localized inflammatory lesions in the pulp. The tissue adjacent to the inflammatory lesion may show no sign of inflammation and physiologic analysis may reveal no abnormalities. Thus investigators found that pulpal tissue pressure near a site of localized inflammation was almost normal.[91] This indicates that tissue pressure changes do not spread rapidly. Similar findings have been reported by another researcher.[97] Local insults cause inflammation by

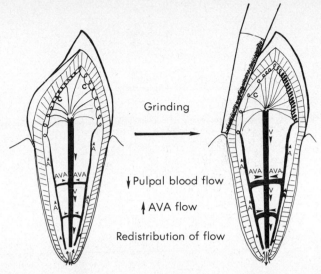

Grinding

↓ Pulpal blood flow

↑ AVA flow

Redistribution of flow

FIG. 14-20. Schematic representation of the changes in pulpal blood flow distribution in response to dry preparation. Notice that there is an increase in flow through the arteriovenous anastomoses.

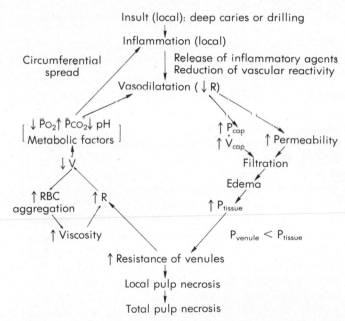

Insult (local): deep caries or drilling

Inflammation (local)

Circumferential spread

Release of inflammatory agents
Reduction of vascular reactivity

Vasodilatation ($\downarrow$ R)

$\left[\begin{array}{c} \downarrow Po_2 \uparrow Pco_2 \downarrow pH \\ \text{Metabolic factors} \end{array} \right]$

$\uparrow P_{cap}$
$\uparrow V_{cap}$

$\uparrow$ Permeability

Filtration

Edema

$\downarrow$ V

$\uparrow$ RBC aggregation $\uparrow$ R

$\uparrow P_{tissue}$

$\uparrow$ Viscosity

$P_{venule} < P_{tissue}$

$\uparrow$ Resistance of venules

Local pulp necrosis

Total pulp necrosis

FIG. 14-21. Pathophysiologic mechanism of pulp inflammation and necrosis. This hypothetical mechanism is constructed from the results of many structural and functional investigations.

triggering the release of various inflammatory mediators and reducing vascular reactivity. These mediators produce vasodilation and decrease the flow resistance in the resistance vessels. Vasodilation and decreased flow resistance cause an increase in both intravascular pressure and blood flow in the capillaries, which in turn precipitate an increase in vascular permeability, favoring filtration of serum proteins and fluid from the vessels. As a result, the tissue becomes edematous. This results in an increase in the tissue pressure. Since the pulp is encased in mineralized tis-

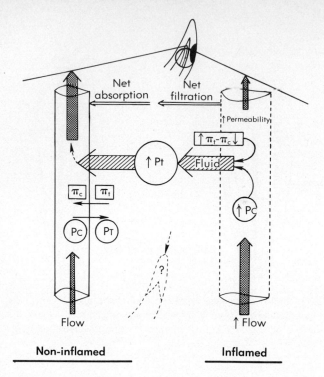

FIG. 14-22. Schematic representation of the compensatory mechanism of the pulp during inflammation. PC and PT, Hydrostatic pressure of capillary and tissue, respectively. π_c and π_t, Osmotic pressure of capillary and tissue, respectively.

sue, it is in a low compliance environment. As the tissue pressure increases it may exceed that of the venules, in which case the venules will be compressed, thus producing an increase in flow resistance. This in turn results in a decrease in blood flow since the venous drainage is impeded. The sluggish flow of blood flow causes the red blood cells to aggregate, resulting in an elevation of blood viscosity. This vicious cycle leads to even greater problems by producing hypoxia and thus suppressing cellular metabolism in the affected area of the pulp. The stagnation of blood flow not only causes rheologic changes (i.e., RBC aggregation and increased blood viscosity), it also causes an increase in carbon dioxide and a decrease in pH levels in the blood. The increase in PCO_2 results from impaired removal of waste products from the tissue. These changes in local metabolism lead to vasodilation in the adjacent area and the gradual spread of inflammation. The spread of inflammation is circumferential as was demonstrated in an elegant experiment by Van Hassel.[97] Thus, total pulp necrosis is the gradual accumulation of local necroses.

It has been shown that the pulp has tremendous healing potential. This raises the question as to how the pulp recovers from the adverse effects of localized inflammation. Although the exact physiologic mechanisms are not yet known, recent research findings suggest the following: First, as the tissue pressure increases as a result of an increase in blood flow, the arteriovenous anastomoses (AVAs) or the U-turn loop vessels open and shunt the blood before it reaches the inflamed region of the coronal

of the pulp. This prevents a further increase in blood flow and tissue pressure. Also, the increase in tissue pressure pushes macromolecules back into the bloodstream via the venules in the adjacent healthy region (Fig. 14-22). Once the macromolecules and accompanying fluid leave the extracellular tissue space through the venule, the tissue pressure decreases and normal blood flow is restored.

Prevention

In order to preserve the integrity of the pulp, the dentist should observe ertain precautions while rendering treatment. The following is a list of do's and don'ts that should prevent or minimize injury to the pulp.

> **Cutting procedures: use light, intermittent cutting, an efficient cooling system, and high speeds of rotation.**
>
> **Avoid desiccating the dentin: do not overdry the cavity preparation.**
>
> **Do not apply irritating chemicals to freshly cut dentin.**
>
> **Choose restorative materials carefully, considering the physical and biologic properties of the material.**
>
> **Do not use caustic cavity sterilizing agents.**
>
> **Assume that all restorative materials will leak. Use a cavity liner or base to seal the openings of exposed dentinal tubules.**
>
> **Do not use excessive force when inserting a restoration.**
>
> **Employ polishing procedures that do not subject the pulp to excessive heat.**
>
> **Establish a patient recall system that ensures periodic evaluation of the status of pulps that have been exposed to injury.**

REFERENCES

1. Ackermans, F., Klein, J.P., and Frank, R.M.: Ultrastructural localization of immunoglobulins in carious humane dentine, Arch. Oral Biol. **26**:879, 1981.
2. Ackermans, F., Klein, J.P., and Frank, R.M.: Ultrastructural localization of *Streptococcus mutans* and *Streptococcus sanguis* antigens in carious human dentine, J. Biol. Buccale **9**:203, 1981.
3. Alperstein, K.S., Graver, H.T., and Herold, R.C.B.: Marginal leakage of glass-ionomer cement restorations, J. Prosthet. Dent. **50**:803, 1983.
4. Barber, D., and Massler, M.: Permeability of active and arrested carious lesions to dyes and radioactive isotopes, J. Dent. Child. **31**:26, 1964.
5. Beagrie, G.S., and Smith, D.C.: Development of a germicidal polycarboxylate cement. J. Can. Dent. Assoc. **44**:409, 1978.
6. Bergenholtz, G.: Effect of bacterial products on inflammatory reactions in the dental pulp, Scand. J. Dent. Res. **85**:122, 1977.
7. Bergenholtz, G., and Reit, C.: Reactions of the dental pulp to microbial provocation of calcium hydroxide treated dentin, Scand. J. Dent. Res. **88**:187, 1980.
8. Bergenholtz, G., et al.: Bacterial leakage around dental restorations: its effect on the dental pulp, J. Oral Path. **11**:439, 1982.
9. Berggren, H.: The reaction of the translucent zone to dyes and radio-isotopes, Acta Odontol. Scand. **23**:197, 1965.
10. Bowen, R.L., Cobb, E.N., and Rapson, J.E.: Adhesive bonding of various materials to hard tooth tissues: improvement in bond strength to dentin, J. Dent. Res. **61**:1070, 1982.
11. Bradford, E.W.: The dentine, a barrier to caries, Br. Dent. J. **109**:387, 1960.

12. Brännström, M.: The effect of dentin desiccation and aspirated odontoblasts on the pulp, J. Prosthet. Dent. **20**:165,1968.

13. Brännström, M.: A new approach to insulation, Dent. Pract. **19**:417, 1969.

14. Brännström, M.: Dentin and pulp in restorative dentistry, London, 1982, Wolfe Medical Publications Ltd.

15. Brännström, M.: Communication between the oral cavity and the dental pulp associated with restorative treatment, Operative Dent. **9**:57, 1984.

16. Brännström, M., and Lind, P.O.: Pulpal response to early dental caries, J. Dent. Res. **44**:1045, 1965.

17. Brännström, M., et al.: Protective effect of polystyrene liners for composite resin restorations, J. Prosthet. Dent. **49**:331, 1983.

18. Brännström, M., and Nyborg, H.: Pulpal reaction to polycarboxylate and zinc phosphate cements used with inlays in deep cavity preparations, J. Am. Dent. Assoc. **94**:308, 1977.

19. Brännström, M., Vojinovic, O., and Nordenvall, K.J.: Bacterial and pulpal reactions under silicate cement restorations, J. Prosthet. Dent. **41**:290, 1979.

20. Brown, W.S., Christensen, D.O., and Lloyd, B.A.: Numerical and experimental evaluation of energy inputs, temperature gradients, and thermal stresses during restorative procedures, J. Am. Dent. Assoc. **96**:451, 1978.

21. Cotton, W.R.: Bacterial contamination as a factor in healing of pulp exposures, Oral Surg. **38**:441, 1974.

22. Cotton, W.R., and Siegel, R.L.: Human pulpal response to citric acid cavity cleaner, J. Am. Dent. Assoc. **96**:639, 1978.

23. Eames, W.B., Hedrix, K., and Mohler,H.C.: Pulpal response in rhesus monkeys to cementation agents and cleaners, J. Am. Dent. Assoc. **98**:40, 1979.

24. Edwards, D.L.: The response of the human dental pulp to the use of a cavity varnish beneath amalgam fillings, Br. Dent. J. **145**:39, 1978.

25. Farah, J.W., Hood, J.A., and Craig, R.G.: Effects of cement base on the stresses in amalgam restorations, J. Dent. Res. **54**:10, 1975.

26. Fish, E.W.: An experimental investigation of the enamel, dentine and dental pulp, London, 1933, John Dale Sons, and Danielson, Ltd.

27. Frank, R.M.: Reactions of dentin and pulp to drugs and restorative materials, J. Dent. Res. **54**:176, 1975, 1975.

28. Frank R.M., and Voegel, J.C.: Ultrastructure of the human odontoblast process and its mineralization during dental caries, Caries Res. **14**:367, 1980.

29. Going, R.E., and Massler, M.: Influence of cavity liners under amalgam restorations or penetration by radioactive isotopes, J. Prosthet. Dent. **2**:298, 1961.

30. Grajower, R., Kaufman, E., and Rajstein, J.: Temperature in the pulp chamber during polishing of amalgam restorations, J. Dent. Res. **53**:1189, 1974.

31. Grajower, R., Kaufman, E., and Stern, N.: Temperature of the pulp during impression taking of full crown preparations with modelling compound, J. Dent. Res. **54**:212, 1975.

32. Greenhill, J.D., and Pashley, D.H.: The effects of desensitizing agents on the hydrodynamic conductance of human dentin in vitro, J. Dent. Res. **60**:686, 1981.

33. Heys, D.R., et al.: Histologic and bacterial evaluation of conventional and new copper amalgams, J. Oral Path. **8**:65, 1979.

34. Holden, G.P.: Some observations on the vibratory phenomena associated with high-speed air turbines and their transmission to living tissue, Br. Dent. J. **113**:265, 1962.

35. Hoppenbrouwer, P.M.M., Driessens, F.C.M., and Stadhouders, A.M.: Morphology, composition and wetting of dentinal cavity walls, J. Dent. Res. **53**:1255, 1964.

36. Jendresen, M., and Trowbridge, H.: Biologic and physical properties of a zinc polycarboxylate cement, J. Prosthet. Dent. **28**:264, 1972.

37. Jodaikin, A., and Austin, J.C.: The effects of cavity smear layer removal on experimental marginal leakage around amalgam restorations, J. Dent. Res. **60**:1861, 1981.

38. Johnson, N.W., Taylor, B.R., and Berman, D.S.: The response of deciduous dentine to caries studied by correlated light and electron microscopy, Caries Res. **3**:348, 1969.

39. Johnson, R.H., Daichi, S.F., and Haley, J.V.: Pulpal hyperemia—a correlation of clinical and histological data from 706 teeth, J. Am. Dent. Assoc., **81**:108, 1970.

40. Jones, J.C.G., Grieve, A.R., and Kidd, E.A.M: An in vitro comparison of marginal leakage associated with three resin based filling materials, Br. Dent. J. **145**:299, 1978.

41. Kakehashi, S., Stanley, H.R., and Fitzgerald, R.J.: The effects of surgical exposures of pulps in germ-free and conventional rats, Oral Surg. **20**:340, 1965.

42. Karjalainen, S.: Metabolic alterations in the odontoblast-predentine region during the propagation of caries, Finn. Dent. Soc. **75**(Suppl.):1, 1979.

43. Karjalainen, S., and Soderling, E.: The autoradiographic pattern of the in vitro uptake of proline by the coronal areas of intact and carious human teeth, Arch. Oral Biol. **24**:909, 1980.

44. Kawahara, H., Imanishi, Y., and Oshima, H.: Biological evaluation of glass ionomer cement, J. Dent. Res. **58**:1080, 1979.

45. Kelley, K.W., Bergenholtz, G., and Cox, C.F.: The extent of the odontoblast process in rheusus monkeys (Macaca mulatta) as observed by scanning electron microscopy, Arch. Oral Biol. **26**:893, 1981.

46. Kim, S.: Dynamic changes in the dental pulp circulation in response to dental procedures and materials. In Rowe, N.H., editor: Dental pulp reactions to restorative materials in the presence or absence of infection, Ann Arbor, Mich, 1982, University of Michigan.

47. Kim, S.: Ligamental injection: a physiological explanation of its efficacy, J. Endod. **12**:486, 1986.

48. Kim, S., et al.: Effects of local anesthetics on pulpal blood flow in dogs, J. Dent. Res. **63**:650, 1984.

49. Kuwabara, R.K., and Massler, M.: Pulpal reaction to active and arrested caries, J. Dent. Child. **33**:190, 1966.

50. Langeland, K., and Langeland, L.K.: Pulp reactions to crown preparation, impression, temporary crown fixation and permanent cementation, J. Prosthet. Dent. **15**:129, 1965.

51. Lin, L., et al.: Periodontal ligamental injection: effects on pulp tissue, J. Endod. **11**:529, 1985.

52. Lindholm, K.: The effect of crown preparation and compound impressions on the diameter of the pulp arteriole, Proc. Finn. Dent. Soc. **71**:10, 1975.

53. Magloire, H., et al.: Ultrastructural alterations of human odontoblasts and collagen fibers in the pulpal border zone beneath early caries lesions, Cell. Molec. Biol. **27**:437, 1981.

54. Massler, M.: Pulpal reaction to dentinal caries, J. Dent. Res. **17**:441, 1967.

55. Michelich, V.J., Schuster, G.S., and Pashley, D.H.: Bacterial penetration of human dentin in vitro, J. Dent. Res. **59**:1398, 1980.

56. Miller, W.A., and Massler, M.: Permeability and staining of active and arrested lesions in dentine, Br. Dent. J. **112**:187, 1962.

57. Möller, B.: Reaction of the human dental pulp to silver amalgam restorations: the modifying effect of treatment with calcium hydroxide, Acta Odont. Scand. **33**:233, 1975.

58. Mullaney, T.P., and Laswell, H.R.: Iatrogenic blushing of dentin following full crown preparation, J. Prosthet. Dent. **22**:354, 1969.

59. Nelson, R.J., Wolcott, R.B., and Paffenbarger, G.C.: Fluid exchange at the margins of dental restorations, J. Am. Dent. Assoc., **44**:288, 1952.

60. Newman, S.M.: Microleakage of a copal rosin cavity varnish, J. Prosthet. Dent. **51**:499, 1984.

61. Nordenvall, K-J., Brännström, M., and Torstensson, B.: Pulp reactions and microorganisms under ASPA and Concise composite fillings, J. Dent. Child. **46**:449, 1979.

62. Nyborg, H., and Brännström, M.: Pulp reaction to heat, J. Prosthet. Dent. **19**:605, 1968.

63. Okamura, K., et al.: Plasma components in deep lesions of human carious dentin, J. Dent. Res. **58**:2010, 1979.

64. Okamura, K., et al.: Dentinal response against carious invasion: localization of antibodies in odontoblastic body and process, J. Dent. Res. **59:**1368, 1980.

65. Okamura, K., et al.: Serum proteins and secretory component in human carious dentin, J. Dent. Res. **58:**1127, 1979.

66. Olgart, I., and Gazalius, B.: Effects of adrenaline and felypressin (Octapressin) on blood flow and sensory nerve activity on the tooth, Acta Odontol. Scand. **35:**69, 1977.

67. Olgart, L., et al.: Localization of substance p-like immunoreactivity in nerves in the tooth pulp, Pain **4:**153, 1977.

68. Parfitt, G.J.: The speed of development of the carious cavity, Br. Dent. J. **100:**204,1956.

69. Pashley, D.H.: The influence of dentin permeability and pulpal blood flow on pulpal solute concentrations, J. Endod. **5:**355, 1979.

70. Pashley, D.H.: Smear layer: physiological consideration, Operative Dent. **3:**13, 1984.

71. Pashley, D.H., and Livingston, M. J.: Effect of molecular size on permeability coefficients in human dentine, Arch. Oral. Biol. **23:**391, 1978.

72. Pashley, D.H., Michelich, V., and Kehl, T.: Dentin permeability: effects of smear layer removal, J. Prosthet. Dent. **46:**531, 1981.

73. Plant, C.G., and Jones, D.W.: The damaging effects of restorative materials. Part 1, Physical and chemical properties, Br. Dent. J. **140:**373, 1976.

74. Pohto, M., and Scheinin, A.: Microscopic observations on living dental pulp. IV. The effects of oil of clove and eugenol on the circulation of the pulp in the rats's lower incisor, Dent. Abst.**5:**405, 1960.

75. Qvist, V.: The effect of mastication on marginal adaptation of composite restorations in vivo, J. Dent. Res. **62:**904, 1983.

76. Reeves, R., and Stanley, H.R.: The relationship of bacterial penetration and pulpal pathosis in carious teeth, Oral Surg. **22.:**59, 1966.

77. Scott, J.N., and Weber, D.F.: Microscopy of the junctional region between human coronal primary and secondary dentin, J. Morphol. **154:**133, 1977.

78. Searls, J.C.: Light and electron microscope evaluation of changes induced in odontoblasts of the rat incisor by high-speed drill, J. Dent. Res. **46:**1344, 1967.

79. Seltzer, S., and Bender, I.B.: The dental pulp, ed. 3, Philadelphia, 1984, J.B. Lippincott Co.

80. Silverstone, L.M., et al.: Dental caries: aetiology, pathology and prevention, London, 1981, Macmillan Press, Ltd.

81. Silvestri, A.R., Cohen, S.N., and Wetz, J.H.: Character and frequency of discomfort immediately following restorative procedures, J. Am. Dent. Assoc. **95:**85, 1977.

82. Skogedal, O., and Ericksen, H.M.: Pulpal reactions to surface-sealed silicate cement and composite resin restorations, Can. J. Dent. Res. **84:**381, 1976.

83. Sneed, W.D., Hembree, J.H., and Welsh, E.L.: Effectiveness of three varnishes in reducing leakage of a high-copper amalgam, Operative Dent. **9:**32-34, 1984.

84. Son, H.G., Kim, S., and Kim, S.B.: Pulpal blood flow and bonding, IADR Abstract for The Hague Meeting, 1986.

85. Stanley, H.R.: Pulpal response to dental techniques and materials, Dent. Clin. North Am. **15:**115, 1971.

86. Stanley, H.R.: Pulpal response. In Cohen, S., and Burns, R., editors: Pathways of the pulp, ed. 3, St. Louis, 1984, The C.V. Mosby Co.

87. Stanley, H.R., Going, R.E., and Chauncey, H.H.: Human pulp response to acid pretreatment of dentin and to composite restoration, J. Am. Dent. Assoc. **91:**817, 1975.

88. Stanley, H.R., et al.: The detection and prevalence of reactive and physiologic sclerotic dentin, reparative dentin and dead tracts beneath various types of dental lesions according to tooth surface and age, J. Pathol. **12:**257, 1983.

89. Swerdlow, H., and Stanley, H.R.: Reaction of human dental pulp to cavity preparation. 1. Effect of water spray at 20,000 rpm, J. Am. Dent. Assoc. **56:**317, 1958.

90. Swerdlow, H. and Stanley, H.R.: Reaction of human dental pulp to cavity preparation, J. Prosthet. Dent. **9:**121, 1959.

91. Tönder, K., and Kvinnsland, I.: Micropuncture measurement of interstitial tissue pressure in normal and inflamed dental pulp in cats, J. Endod. **9:**105, 1983.

92. Torneck, C.D.: Changes in the fine structure of the dental pulp in human caries pulpitis. 2. Inflammatory infiltration, J. Oral Pathol. **3:**83, 1974.

93. Trowbridge, H.O.: Pathogenesis of pulpitis resulting from dental caries, J. Endod. **7:**52, 1981.

94. Trowbridge, H.O., Edwall, L., and Panopoulos, P.: Effect of zinc oxide–eugenol and calcium hydroxide on intradental nerve activity, J. Endod. **8:**403, 1982.

95. Trowbridge, H.O., et al.: Sensory response to thermal stimulation in human teeth, J. Endod. **6:**405, 1980.

96. Trowbridge, H., Scott, D., and Singer, J.: Effects of eugenol on nerve excitability, IADR Progr. Abst. **56:**115, 1977.

97. Van Hassel, H.J.: Physiology of the human dental pulp. In Siskin, editor: The biology of the human dental pulp, St. Louis, 1973, The C.V. Mosby Co.

98. Vojinovic, O., Nyborg, H., and Brännström, M.: Acid treatment of cavities under resin fillings: bacterial growth in dentinal tubules and pulpal reactions, J. Dent. Res. **52:**1189, 1973.

99. Watts, A.: Bacterial contamination and toxicity of silicate and zinc phosphate cements, Br. Dent. J. **146:**7, 1979.

100. Yamada, T., et al.: The extent of the odontoblast process in normal and carious human dentin, J. Dent. Res. **62:**798, 1983.

101. Yates, J.L., Murray, G.A., and Hembree, J.H.: The effect of cavity varnishes on certain insulating bases: a microleakage study, Operative Dent. **5:**43, 1980.

102. Zach, L.: Pulp liability and repair: effect of restorative procedures, Oral Surg. **33:**111, 1972.

103. Zach, L., and Cohen, G.: Pulp responses to externally applied heat, Oral Surg. **19:**515, 1965.

Self-assessment questions

1. Although each carious lesion is individual and influenced by multiple factors, the carious process is generally
   a. Continuous
   b. Rapid
   c. Intermittent
   d. Slow

2. A characteristic of the inflammatory reaction in the confined pulp tissue is
   a. Vasoconstriction of the vessels
   b. Increased vascular permeability
   c. Minimal cellular activity
   d. Stagnation of pulp circulation

3. Relatively few bacteria are found in a pulp abscess due to the
   a. Immune response of periapical tissue
   b. High tissue pH of the pulp
   c. Mechanical blockage of sclerotic dentin
   d. Antibacterial products of neutrophils

4. A ligamental injection of 2% lidocaine with 1:100,000 epinephrine will cause the pulp circulation to
   a. Cease for about 30 minutes
   b. Remain the same
   c. Increase markedly
   d. Decrease slightly

5. It is recommended to avoid a ligamental injection when the planned dental treatment is
   a. Pulp extirpation
   b. Class II amalgam preparation
   c. Pulpotomy
   d. Full crown preparation

6. The most severe stress that restorative procedures impart to the pulp is the
   a. Speed of the rotating bur
   b. Production of frictional heat
   c. Pressure exerted by the handpiece
   d. Transfer of bacteria through dentinal tubules

7. According to the hydrodynamic theory of dentin sensitivity, the movement of fluid through dentinal tubules will
   a. Stimulate the sensory nerve fibers of the underlying pulp
   b. Displace odontoblasts into the pulp tissue
   c. Have minimal effect on the odontoblasts
   d. Result in the death of many odontoblasts

8. The optimal amount of remaining dentin thickness (RDT) to protect the pulp from restorative procedures is
   a. 0.5 mm.
   b. 1.0 mm
   c. 1.5 mm.
   d. 2.0 mm

9. Recent studies have shown that acid-etching of dentin before insertion of the restorative material will
   a. Protect the pulp from bacterial invasion
   b. Enhance bacterial penetration of the dentin
   c. Destroy odontoblastic processes in the tubules
   d. Decrease pulpal blood flow

10. The major cause of pulpal injury resulting from the insertion of restorations is the
    a. Products of bacterial metabolism
    b. Desiccation of the pulp by restorative material
    c. Heat evolved during setting
    d. Acidity of the restorative materials

11. It is indicated to seal the dental tubules before placement of restorations in order to
    a. Allow a calcium bridge to form in the pulp
    b. Reduce the pathogenicity of the microorganisms
    c. Decrease the number of dentinal tubules
    d. Decrease the permeability of underlying dentin

12. Which of the following material has no inhibitory effect on bacterial growth?
    a. Amalgam
    b. Zinc oxide–eugenol
    c. Calcium hydroxide
    d. Zinc polycarboxylate cement

13. The smear layer on dentin walls acts to prevent pulpal injury by
    a. Reducing diffusion of toxic substance through the tubules
    b. Resisting the effects of acid-etching of the dentin
    c. Eliminating the need for a cavity liner or base
    d. Its bactericidal activity against oral microorganisms

14. Although the pulp is a very resilient tissue, the pulp
    a. Has little potential for healing following irritation
    b. Has a limit to its compensatory mechanism for healing
    c. Is not subject to increased tissue or vascular pressure
    d. Cannot recover from the effects of localized inflammation

PART THREE

RELATED CLINICAL TOPICS

15

TRAUMATIC INJURIES

STUART B. FOUNTAIN
JOE H. CAMP

Hindsight explains the injury that foresight would have prevented.

AUTHOR UNKNOWN

In considering dental traumatic injuries, it becomes quickly apparent that the majority of them are minor, consisting of cracked and chipped teeth. As such they could have been prevented by a little foresight on the part of each patient. However, dentists must be prepared to treat not only the minor cracked and chipped tooth injuries but also the more traumatic broken crowns, roots, bones, and missing teeth.

This chapter will discuss the epidemiology of traumatic injuries, the multiplicity of therapies available for the injuries, and a few preventive measures to lessen the incidence and severity of the injuries.

INCIDENCE

Although dental injuries occur at any age, one of the more likely times is ages 2 to 5 years. During this developmental period children are learning to walk and then to run. Because their coordination and judgment are not keenly developed, falling injuries are common. Approximately 30% of these young children suffer injuries to their primary teeth, generally fractured or displaced maxillary incisors.[2,18,26,70,175]

As children gain confidence and coordination, the incidence of dental injuries decreases; it then rises again during the very active 8- to 12-year age range, as a result of bicycle, skateboard, playground, or sports accidents.[26,206,130,134]

By the time students complete high school it is estimated that as many as one out of three boys or one out of four girls will have suffered a dental injury.[134] This seemingly high incidence of injuries to the permanent teeth is the result of the collective activities of young people throughout their school years. During high school the increased participation of boys and girls in sports creates a high risk of injury.

Prior to the 1960s, boys had three times as many injuries as did girls. The rapid increase in women's athletics during the 1970s has reduced this ratio, however, to one and one half injuries to boys for each injury to girls.[106,176]

In the teen and young adult years dental injuries result from motor vehicle accidents, sports, and accidental falls. A study of military personnel[114] showed the largest number of dental injuries to young male enlisted men occuring after hours as a result of fistfights. A fourth of the dental injuries in the public schools have been observed to be due to fighting and pushing.[51]

The most dangerous place in which tooth injuries are likely to occur is the home. Injuries at home or indoors account for 49% to 60% of tooth injuries.[62,74,122]

The dental injuries are predominantly enamel-only or enamel-and-dentin fractures of the maxillary incisors. Approximately 90% of dental injuries are chipped teeth,[106,173,176] with the remainder being severe crown fractures involving the pulp, tooth displacement, or avulsion.

The most vulnerable tooth is the maxillary central incisor, which sustains approximately 80% of the dental injuries, followed by the maxillary lateral and the mandibular central and lateral incisors.[70,106,134,173,176]

A major predisposing factor in dental injuries is incisal overjet of the maxillary incisors. As the dimension of incisal overjet increases from a normal 0 to 3 mm to a distinct 3 to 6 mm range, the incidence of injury to the maxillary incisors doubles. The severity of injury also increases with the overjet dimension. Children with an extreme overjet (6 mm) are twice as likely to injure two or more incisors.[104] A possible reason for this increase in severity of injury is the lack of lip closure over the overjet incisors, thereby reducing the impact absorbing protection of the lips.

Unfortunately dental injuries are a common finding among battered children. The abused child is generally very young (prekindergarten) and is injured by an enraged

462

parent who resorts to force to silence a crying or screaming child. The symptoms include multiple bruises all over the body as well as oral lacerations and fractured teeth.[160] For the protection of the child it is the responsibility of clinicians to report these suspicious symptoms to the proper authorities.

HISTORY AND CLINICAL EXAMINATION

Dental injuries are never convenient for either the patient or the clinician. Consequently, the emergency visit often consists of a distraught patient and/or parent meeting a hurried clinician. It is one of the challenges that face clinicans to control the scene, calm the patient and parents, and take the necessary time to conduct a qualitative evaluation of the patient's injuries. Without such control by the clinician, significant injuries can be easily missed in the haste of the moment.

The medical history (Fig. 9-2) is fundamental to all other evaluation and treatment of the patient. Local anesthesia cannot be administered safely without the completion of a standard medical questionnaire.

History of the accident

The *how, when,* and *where* of the accident are significant.[18]

Understanding *how* it occurred will assist the clinician in locating specific injuries. A blow to the lips and anterior teeth could possibly cause crown, root, or bone fractures to the anterior region and is less likely to injure the posterior regions. A blow under the chin or jaw could cause fractures to any tooth in the mouth. A padded blow (fall against a covered chair arm) could cause a root fracture or tooth displacement whereas a hard blow (concrete walk) would tend to cause coronal fractures.

When the accident occurred is most important. With the passage of time blood clots and collagen fibers begin to form, periodontal ligaments and teeth dry out, saliva contaminates the wound, and all these become factors in making decisions about the sequence of treatment.

Where the trauma occurred becomes significant for prognosis. A tooth avulsed on the bottom of a swimming pool has a much better chance for successful replantation than one found lying in a pool of gasoline and oil following an automobile accident. The necessity for prophylactic tetanus toxoid immunization is influenced by the location of the accident. Where the trauma occurred may also be significant because of insurance and possible litigation.

Another important question to ask is whether any treatment, of any kind, has been done for this injury by the parent, coach, physician, school nurse, teacher, or ambulance attendant. A normal-appearing tooth may have been replanted or repositioned 2 days previously by any of these or by the patient himself, and this will influence the prognosis for treatment and the sequence of treatment.

Clinical examination
Chief complaint

Aside from pain and bleeding, there may be a specific uncomfortable sensation. If the complaint is that the teeth "don't fit together now," the clinician must consider possible displacements or a bone fracture. Pain that occurs *only* when the patient closes the teeth together could indicate crown, root, or bone fractures or displacement.

Neurologic examination

While the clinician is obtaining the history of the accident and chief complaint, the patient should be observed for neurologic or other medical complications. Dental injuries may occur simultaneously with other head and neck injuries. Note should be made of whether the patient is communicating coherently. Does the patient have difficulty focusing or rotating his eyes, or in getting his breath? Airway obstruction by dental appliances must be considered.

Can the patient turn his head from side to side? Is there any paresthesia of the lips or tongue? Does the patient complain of ringing in the ears? Have there been persistent headaches, dizziness, drowsiness, or vomiting since the accident?

Before analgesics are prescribed or sedation by inhalation of nitrous oxide/oxygen is used, the clinician must be satisfied that there are no neurologic injuries.[55] If there is any question about this, the patient should be referred to appropriate medical treatment.

External examination

Before having the patient open his mouth for an intraoral examination, the clinician should first look for external signs of injury. Lacerations of the head and neck are easily detected. However, deviations of normal bone contours must be closely observed. The temporomandibular joint should be palpated externally while the patient opens and closes. Does the patient's opening and closing pattern deviate to either side? If so, this could indicate a unilateral mandibular fracture. Similarly the zygomatic arch, angle, and lower border of the mandible should be bilaterally palpated and note made of any areas of tenderness, swelling, or bruising of the face, cheek, neck, or lips. They could be clues to possible bone fractures.

Intraoral soft tissue examination

One next looks for lacerations of the lips, tongue, cheek, palate, and floor of the mouth. The facial and lingual gingivae and oral mucosa are palpated, with note made of areas of tenderness, swelling, or bruising. The anterior border of the ramus of the mandible is palpated. Any abnormal findings suggest possible tooth or bone injuries or fractures, and further radiographic examination of the area is indicated. Lacerations of the lips and tongue must be felt for embedded foreign objects.[43,93]

Hard tissue examination

One of the best examinations for evidence of traumatic injuries is simply to look carefully. Each tooth and its supporting structures must be examined with an explorer and periodontal probe. Basic questions such as "Is the occlusal plane disturbed?" and "Are there any missing teeth?" must be answered before any thermal or electric tests are begun.

The examiner looks for gross evidence of injury intially.

OUTLINE OF INITIAL NEUROLOGIC ASSESSMENT FOR THE PATIENT WITH TRAUMATIC DENTAL INJURIES

Notice unusual communication or motor functions.

Look for normal respiration without obstruction of the airway or danger of aspiration.

Replant avulsed teeth as indicated.

Obtain a medical history and information on the accident.

Determine blood pressure and pulse.

Examine for rhinorrhea or otorrhea.

Evaluate function of the eyes—is diplopia or nystagmus apparent, are pupillary activity and movement of the eyes normal?

Evaluate movement of the neck—is there pain or limitation?

Examine the sensitivity of the surface of the facial skin—is paresthesia or anesthesia apparent?

Confirm that there is normal vocal function.

Confirm ability to protrude the tongue.

Confirm hearing—is tinnitis or vertigo apparent?

Evaluate the sense of smell.

Assure follow-up evaluation.

From Croll, T.P., et al.: J. Am. Dent. Assoc. **100:**530, 1980.

If several teeth are out of alignment, a bone fracture is the most reasonable explanation. The mandible should be examined for fractures by placing the forefinger on the occlusal plane of the posterior teeth with the thumbs under the mandible and then rocking the mandible from side to side and from anterior to posterior. A mandibular fracture will cause discomfort with these motions and the grating sound of broken fragments might be heard.[43] Gentle but firm pressure should be used to prevent possible additional trauma to the inferior alveolar nerve and blood vessels.

Also one can try to move the individual teeth with finger pressure in the maxilla and mandible. Any looseness is indicative of displacement from the alveolar socket. Movement of several teeth together is evidence of an alveolar fracture. Mobility of the crown must be differentiated from the mobility of the tooth. In instances of crown fractures the crown will be mobile but the tooth will remain in position. Occasionally root fractures can be felt by placing a finger on the mucosa over the tooth and moving the crown.

Any freshly fractured cusps or incisal edge fractures should be recorded. Incomplete cusp fractures can be noted by using the tip of a dental explorer as a wedge in the occlusal grooves of the posterior teeth to elicit movement of any cusps. The patient may be asked to bite on a rubber polishing wheel with each tooth in succession to help locate tenderness that could mean an incomplete cusp fracture or displaced tooth.

Each incisal edge and cusp can be gently percussed with the mirror handle to locate imcomplete fractures or teeth that have been slightly displaced from the alveolar socket. Accumulation of extravasated fluid and tearing of periodontal fibers around a minimally displaced tooth will make the tooth tender to percussion.

Hemorrhage in the gingival sulcus may indicate a dis-placed tooth. Any discoloration of the teeth should be noted; viewing from the lingual surface of anterior teeth with a reflected light will help.

Obvious pulp exposures should be noted. Crown fractures with minute pulp exposures can be detected with a cotton pellet soaked in saline and pressed against the area of the suspected exposure.[18] The mechanical pressure of the cotton against an exposure will elicit a response. A dry cotton pellet can confuse the diagnosis by dehydrating dentinal tubules in a near exposure, causing a pain sensation, and should not be used.

When the visual examination is complete and all abnormal findings are noted, radiographs of the injured area should be exposed. These can be processed while additional tests are being conducted.

Thermal and electric tests

For decades controversy has surrounded the validity of thermal and electric tests on traumatized teeth. Only generalized impressions may be gained from these tests subsequent to a traumatic injury. They are, in reality, sensitivity tests for nerve function and do *not* indicate the presence or absence of blood circulation within the pulp. It is assumed that subsequent to traumatic injury the conduction capability of the nerve endings and/or sensory receptors is sufficiently deranged to inhibit the nerve impulse from an electric or thermal stimulus. This makes the traumatized tooth vulnerable to false-negative readings from these tests.

The reader is referred to Chapter 1 for specific descriptions of pulp tests, but a few general statements in regard to pulp tests on traumatized teeth may be helpful in trying to interpret the results.

Thermal and electric pulp tests of teeth in the traumatized area should be done at the time of the initial exami-

---

SAMPLE OF A PREPRINTED FORM TO BE GIVEN TO THE PATIENT WITH INJURY OF THE HEAD OR NECK OR TO THE PERSON ACCOMPANYING THE PATIENT

Attention!

When oral structures are injured, there can be additional injury that may not be evident immediately.

If any of these symptoms occur within 48 hours, please call your physician immediately for further examination:

Difficulty with breathing
Difficulty with vision
Dizziness
Pain in the region of the neck or inability to turn the head normally
Numbness of any area of the body
Ringing in the ears
Lethargy (unusual sleepiness)
Nausea or vomiting
Change in ability to function normally

If you do not have a physician whom you regularly see, please contact our office, and we will refer you for medical consultation.

Dentist's name

Address

Telephone

From Croll, T.P., et al.: J. Am. Dent. Assoc. **100:**530, 1980.

nation and carefully recorded to establish a basé line for comparison with subsequent repeated tests in later months. These tests should be repeated at 30-, 90-, and 180-day intervals and 1 year following the accident. The purpose of the tests is to establish a trend as to the physiologic status of the pulps of these teeth.

Teeth that give a positive response at the initial examination cannot be assumed to be healthy and continue to give a positive response. Teeth that yield a negative response or no response cannot be assumed to have necrotic pulps, because they may give a positive response later.

The transition from a negative to a positive response at a subsequent test may be considered a sign of a healthy pulp. The repetitious finding of positive responses may be taken as a sign of a healthy pulp. The transition from a positive to a negative response may be taken as an indication that the pulp is probably undergoing degeneration. The persistence of a negative response would suggest that the pulp has been irreparably damaged, but even this is not absolute.[35]

In testing teeth for response to cold, the dry ice pencil (CO_2 stick described in Chapter 1) gives more positive responses than does a water ice pencil. The intense cold ($-78°$ C) seems to penetrate the tooth and covering splints or restorations and reach the deeper areas of the tooth. In addition, dry ice does not form ice water, which could disperse over adjacent teeth or gingiva to give a false-positive response.

Radiographic examinations

Radiographs are essential to the thorough examination of traumatized hard tissue. They may reveal root fractures, subgingival crown fractures, tooth displacements, bone fractures, or foreign objects.

However, the fracture line may run in a mesial-distal direction in the tooth and not be evident on the radiograph. Also the fracture line may be diagonal in a faciallingual direction and not obvious on the film. Similarly, a hairline fracture may not be evident on the radiograph at the initial examination but later become obvious as tissue fluids and mobility spread the broken parts.

In instances of soft tissue laceration it is advisable to radiograph the injured area prior to suturing to be sure that no foreign objects have become enbedded. A soft tissue radiograph with a normal-size film briefly exposed at a reduced kilovoltage should reveal the presence of many foreign substances, including tooth fragments.

In reviewing the films of traumatized teeth, special attention should be directed to the dimension of the root canal space, the degree of apical closure of the root, the proximity of fractures to the pulp, and the relationship of root fractures to the alveolar crest. Whereas conventional periapical films are generally useful, an occlusal or Panorex film can supplement them when the examiner is looking for bone fractures or the presence of foreign objects.

In summary, the examination of traumatic injuries must be thorough and meticulously recorded. Most injuries are covered by some type of insurance, and many will eventually be involved in litigation. When asked to describe the condition of the patient at the time of the initial examination, months or years after the accident, the dentist will find a completely documented patient record, including quality radiographs, to be of immense assistance. These records form the basis for the justification of subsequent

A   B   C

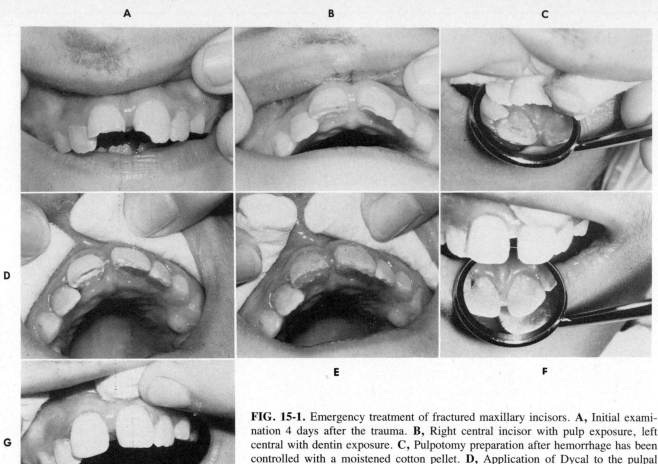

D

E   F

G

FIG. 15-1. Emergency treatment of fractured maxillary incisors. **A,** Initial examination 4 days after the trauma. **B,** Right central incisor with pulp exposure, left central with dentin exposure. **C,** Pulpotomy preparation after hemorrhage has been controlled with a moistened cotton pellet. **D,** Application of Dycal to the pulpal stump and exposed dentin. **E,** Acid-etching of enamel. **F** and **G,** Completed acid-etch resin restoration.

treatment and the associated professional fees. In addition, the rapid increase in professional liability claims against dentists further emphasizes the need for complete and accurate patient records (described in greater detail in Chapter 9).

CLASSIFICATIONS AND TREATMENT

Over the years various authors* have used a formal classification of traumatic injuries. While attempting to simplify discussion of traumatic injuries these authors were well intended; however, the result has been a confusing system of classes and subdivisions of classes that do not correspond from author to author. Therefore, to get back to basics, we have studiously avoided references to classes of traumatic injuries.

Crown fractures

The reported incidence of crown fractures varies from 26% to 92% of all traumatic injuries to the permanent den-

tition,* and from 4% to 38% of injuries to the primary dentition.[2,26] The wide variation in reported incidence is due to the diversity of sampling techniques and classifications of injuries.

Emergency treatment

All fractures of tooth structure must be treated as dental emergencies; thus the patient should be seen as soon as possible after injury. With crown fractures the immediate concern is pulpal protection. Rarely does a crown fracture occur without accompanying concussive or displacement injury. Therefore restoration of the tooth for esthetic purposes is not desirable or necessary at this time. Procedures involving mechanical preparation of the tooth, the application of forces such as wedge placement, and the seating of a stainless steel crown are contraindicated at this time unless necessary for pulpal protection because of the possibility of inflicting further damage to the pulpal or periodontal tissues.

*References 18,30,69,82,126,166,172.

*References 2,26,70,79,83,105,177.

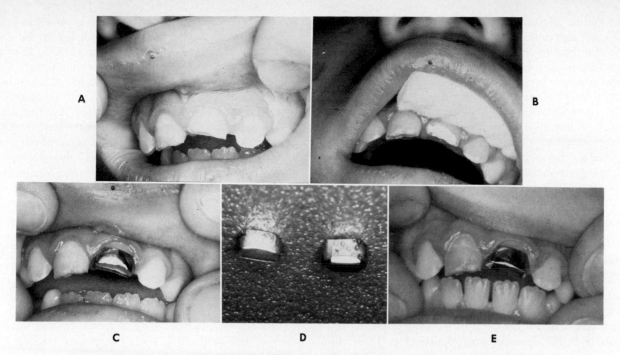

FIG. 15-2. Placement of a temporary stainless steel band to maintain a protective dressing over exposed dentin. **A,** Crown fracture of the left central incisor. Note the previous fracture of the right central. **B,** Application of Dycal to all exposed dentin. **C,** Selection of a loose-fitting band. **D,** Strip of stainless steel matrix material welded across the incisal edge to prevent loss of the protective dressing. **E,** Cemented band.

The acid-etch composite restoration is recommended whenever possible to maintain a protective pulpal dressing since it can be utilized without tooth preparation or the application of any forces, which might further damage the traumatized tooth (Fig. 15-1).

Since the introduction by Buonocore[45] of acid etching to increase the adhesion of resin to enamel, this technique has become widely accepted as the treatment of choice for restoring fractured teeth in children.[46,108,139] It does not adversely affect the pulp if proper protective measures are taken.[18,90] To protect the pulp adequately, a calcium hydroxide liner (e.g., Dycal or Life) must be placed on the exposed dentin before application of the phosphoric acid (Fig. 15-1). Eugenol-containing compounds (like ZOE) must be avoided when resin or composite restorations are being utilized since these interfere with the setting reaction of the restorations.

Because preparation of the tooth is usually necessary when a temporary crown is to be the emergency restoration, this technique should not be considered unless the fracture is so extensive that the acid-etch composite cannot be utilized. Preparation of the tooth will further damage the already traumatized tooth. Likewise, stainless steel crowns at this stage of treatment are contraindicated because of the forces necessary to fit them properly except as outlined below.

One of the prerequisites for using the acid-etch composite restoration is maintenance of a dry field during the application and curing of the composite. Although the application of a rubber dam is usually not advisable at the emergency appointment, it may be helpful if it can be done without further trauma to the teeth. Rubber dam clamps must not be applied to the traumatized teeth. Most injuries occur in the mixed dentition phase, when the teeth are not fully erupted and application of the rubber dam is difficult under ideal conditions. Therefore use of the rubber dam at the emergency appointment is usually not possible. Isolation is achieved by cotton rolls or sponges.

When gingival tissue seepage or hemorrhage prevents a dry working field, the use of a welded stainless steel or preformed orthodontic band is advocated. The tooth is momentarily dried, and a protective base of calcium hydroxide or ZOE is placed over the exposed dentin. A loose-fitting band is fabricated or selected from an assortment of preformed bands. A strip of stainless steel is welded across the incisal to close the opening and prevent the loss of the protective base. The band is checked to ensure that it does not interfere with the occlusion. It is then cemented to the tooth with zinc phosphate or polycarboxylate cement. A permanent-type cement is used because retention of the band is derived exclusively from the cementation. The enamel may be acid-etched before cementation to improve retention where necessary (Fig. 15-2).

An alternative to the band is the use of the incisal end of a stainless steel crown. The crown is trimmed to remove all undercuts and the incisal portion is fitted over the end of the tooth like a thimble. The crown should be large enough that it can be seated without any pressure. Otherwise, the technique is the same as for the band. When materials of this type are to be used, the patient and parents should be advised of the temporary nature of the restoration and that esthetics will be a more important consideration after healing has occurred.

Difficulty is encountered when proximal contacts with adjacent teeth are present and the acid-etch composite restoration cannot be utilized because of inadequate moisture control. In these cases it may be necessary to relieve the proximal contact slightly with a thin diamond bur. However, this rarely happens since most injuries occur during the mixed dentition phase and in individuals with prognathic maxillary incisors.

It is crucial that the occlusion be checked after placement of any form of temporary restoration. If the injured tooth is left high in occlusion, it will receive additional trauma and be prevented from healing properly.

Crown infraction

Crown infraction is an incomplete fracture or crack of enamel without loss of tooth structure. It results from traumatic impact to the enamel and appears as craze lines running parallel with the direction of the enamel prisms and terminating at the dentin-enamel juction (Fig. 15-3). Infraction lines are often associated with luxation injuries.[18]

The severest pulpal reaction is often seen in teeth with

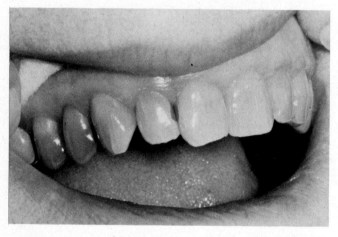

FIG. 15-3. Crown infraction lines resulting from trauma to the maxillary canine and lateral incisor.

the least apparent injury. Andreasen has shown that blows of low velocity, such a striking a tooth against the ground or with an elbow, are less apt to fracture the crown but cause the greatest damage to the supporting tissues. Crown fractures arc more apt to occur as a result of a high-velocity impact against the tooth. The force of the blow is dissipated in creating the fracture, with less resulting damage to the supporting tissues.[2,18] Frequently teeth sustaining fracture retain their vitality while the adjacent traumatized teeth, which remained intact, undergo pulpal necrosis.

Crown infraction injuries do not require treatment, but vitality tests are necessary to determine the extent of pulpal damage. These tests should be conducted at the emergency appointment and recorded for future reference. The patient must be periodically recalled to check for vitality of the involved teeth. Pulpal problems arising from these types of injury will be discussed in the section on concussion injuries.

Crown fracture involving enamel only

Emergency treatment after a crown fracture involving only enamel (Fig. 15-4, *A*) is confined to removal of the sharp edges to prevent injury to the lips and tongue and the performance of vitality tests. Shaping of the tooth and adjacent teeth for esthetic purposes should be postponed several weeks until the pulp and periodontal tissues have had adequate time to recover. Whereas most of these fractures can be corrected by selective grinding and recontouring of the adjacent teeth, if this is not possible the treatment of choice is an acid-etch composite restoration. The patient must be periodically recalled for vitality testing.

Crown fracture involving dentin

Crown fractures involving dentin expose large numbers of dentinal tubules through which bacteria and other harmful substances have a direct pathway to the pulp (Fig. 15-4, *B*). Emergency treatment consists of the application of a protective material over the exposed dentin to allow the pulp to form a protective barrier of reparative dentin. The restoration of choice to hold the protective dressing is the acid-etch composite. The exposed dentin should be covered with a layer of calcium hydroxide product (e.g., Dy-

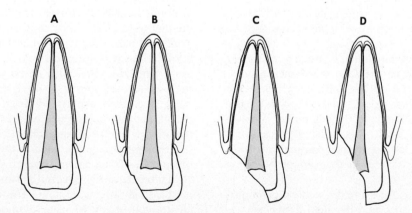

FIG. 15-4. Variations of crown fractures. **A,** Enamel only. **B,** Enamel and dentin. **C,** Enamel and dentin with pulpal exposure. **D,** Enamel, dentin, pulp, and root surface.

cal or Life) before application of the phosphoric acid (Fig. 15-1, *D*).

Although esthetics is an ultimate concern, it is of little importance at the emergency appointment. The tooth should not be prepared at this time to receive the final acid-etch composite. The use of rotary instruments will only further aggravate the injured tooth. Care should also be taken in placing the composite so that finishing of the restoration is not necessary. As little manipulation of the tooth as possible is desirable at this time. The tooth should not be restored to occlusion but left just out of occlusion.

Permanent restoration of the tooth may begin 6 to 8 weeks after the injury. This will allow sufficient time for pulpal healing, since it has been demonstrated that reparative dentin formation occcurs primarily during the first month after injury to the dentin and then decreased markedly after 48 days.[157] Also during this period any injury to the periodontal tissues will have completely healed.[11,31]

The acid-etch composite has been widely accepted as the restoration of choice for fractured crowns. In some cases, because of the extent of the fracture or for esthetic reasons, it may be necessary to restore the tooth with a crown.

The patient should be recalled at periodic intervals for vitality checks. These should be at 1, 3, and 6 months after the injury and every 6 months thereafter for several years. At each visit the tooth is examined, pulp tests are carried out, and a radiograph is made and compared with previous radiographs. Caution must be exercised in interpreting pulp tests since it is not uncommon for injured teeth to give abnormal responses for several months following injury.[140,148] If pulpal necrosis is determined, appropriate endodontic therapy should be provided.

Crown fracture exposing the pulp

In fractures involving exposure of the pulp when maintenance of vitality is desirable, the *best* prognosis is achieved if treatment is rendered as soon as possible after the injury (Fig. 15-4, *C*). Exposure of the pulp left untreated ultimately leads to pulpal necrosis from baterial infection. Experiments in germ-free (gnotobiotic) animals have shown the importance of bacterial contamination in the healing of exposed pulps; healing occurred in germ-free animals, regardless of the severity of the exposure, but failed in the presence of microorganisms.[112]

According to Cvek,[58,59] after traumatic exposure of the pulp there is immediate hemorrhage into the underlying tissue followed by a superficial inflammatory response to breakdown products and bacteria. Clotting subsequently occurs. In the ensuing days tissue changes can be either destructive (e.g., abscess formation or necrosis) or proliferative (hyperplasia). Up to 2 weeks, pulp exposure by mechanical means in teeth free of inflammation usually results in only proliferative response, with inflammation extending nor more than 2 mm from the exposure site. When superficial necrosis does occur, healthy pulp tissue is usually found several millimeters deeper within the pulp.[58,84,151] Therefore, if superficial layers of the pulp are removed, healthy pulp tissue is usually encountered that

will respond to vital conservative pulp procedures (Fig. 15-1).

Maintenance of pulpal vitality is especially important in the tooth with an incompletely developed root. In these teeth the treatment of choice should always be the procedure with the most favorable prognosis for retention of pulpal vitality so that completion of root development can be achieved.

After pulp exposure, when the objective of treatment is maintenance of vitality, this may be achieved by pulp capping or pulpotomy. When maintenance of vitality is not possible or practical, endodontic treatment should be performed.

Factors other than time affecting the outcome of pulp capping and pulpotomy procedures are (1) the accompanying injuries, (2) degenerative changes in the pulp, (3) the method of amputation of the coronal pulp, and (4) the type of dressing used for pulpal coverage.

Mature teeth with displacement injuries are poor candidates for pulp capping and pulpotomy procedures because of the impaired blood supply and the inflammation caused by the injury. However, this is not true for displaced teeth with immature roots.

Teeth with partial calcific pulpal obliteration indicative of degenerative and inflammatory changes within the pulp tissues resulting from caries or previous injuries are not candidates for pulp capping or pulpotomy.

The effects of tissue amputation and the type of capping agents used will be discussed later.

In practice, most clinicians reserve the pulpotomy procedure for treatment of teeth with incompletely formed roots. In mature teeth, if pulp capping is not feasible, a pulpectomy and root canal filling is usually the treatment of choice.

If fracture is so extensive that a post will be required for restoration of the tooth, a pulpectomy is the treatment of choice as long as the root is fully developed. If root formation is incomplete, a pulpotomy should be utilized, with a temporary post and crown until the root completes its development; then a pulpectomy and permanent post placement can be provided.

Pulp capping

Pulp capping is recommended for small traumatic exposures of the pulp that are treated within a few hours after the injury. Although pulp capping has been shown to be successful many days after exposure,[58] the maximum time at which this procedure will succeed has not been established. With longer times it has been shown[59] that more extensive tissue damage minimizes the chance for success especially when inflammation has resulted from contamination or debris at the exposure site.

Prior to placement of the dressing on the exposure site, the fractured tooth surface is cleaned with a moist cotton pellet and dried. Blowing of air directly on the exposure site should be avoided. The exposed dentin and pulp exposure are covered with a hard-setting calcium hydroxide material (e.g., Dycal or Life). The tooth is then acid-etched and a covering of composite resin placed following the criteria outlined in the previous section on fractures involving dentin.

For a complete discussion of pulp capping procedures and agents, please refer to Chapter 22.

Pulpotomy

In the pulpotomy procedure a portion of the pulp is removed to allow the application of a dressing in an area of healthy tissue. It may be desirable to remove the superficial pulp tissue to reach tissue free of inflammation, or as has been shown,[58] the removal of a small amount of tissue will form a preparation to receive the pulpal dressing and thereby simplify the retention of the dressing during subsequent restorative procedures (Fig. 15-1, C). Cvek has achieved 96% success with utilization of this procedure.

It is usually necessary to remove only a few millimeters of pulp tissue. However, the depth to which tissue is removed is determined by the dentist's clinical judgment. Traditionally the term *pulpotomy* has implied removal of tissue to the cervical line. This is not mandatory. All tissue judged to be inflamed should be removed so the pulpal dressing can be placed against healthy uninflamed pulp tissue.

Cvek[58] has shown that *the time between the accident and treatment is not critical so long as the superficially inflamed tissue is removed prior to treatment*. In exposures of long duration, where surface abscess formation or surface necrosis has occurred, it may be necessary to go quite deep. Obviously the deep pulpotomy would be attempted only in teeth with incompletely developed roots where further root development was desirable.

The instrument of choice for tissue removal in the pulpotomy procedure is an abrasive diamond bur utilizing high speed and adequate water cooling. This technique has been shown to create the least damage to the underlying tissue.[76]

All tissue coronal to the application of the dressing must be removed since this tissue would be deprived of blood supply and undergo necrosis, resulting in failure of the pulpotomy.[155] The amputation site must be clean with no shreads of tissue or dentin debris remaining. Copious amounts of water or physiologic saline lavage are necessary to clean the amputation site.

Hemorrhage is controlled by the application of wetted cotton pellets thoroughly blotted to remove most of the moisture. The use of dry cotton pellets is contraindicated since clotting will occur on the dry fibers and when removed stimulate further hemorrhage.

When hemorrhage is controlled, a dressing of calcium hydroxide is placed over the amputation site (Fig. 15-1, D). If the pulpal amputation extends into the tooth only a few millimeters, the use of a hard-setting material (e.g., Dycal or Life) is usually easiest. However, for deeper amputations, we have found calcium hydroxide powder carried to the tooth in an amalgam carrier to be easiest method of application. *Care must be exercised to avoid packing the calcium hydroxide into the pulp tissue.* A round-end plastic instrument is used to tease the calcium hydroxide powder gently against the pulp stump. If cal-

cium hydroxide powder is utilized for the dressing, one of the hard-setting bases must be applied over the dressing and the remaining dentin. The tooth is then acid-etched and restored with a composite resin according to the steps outlined in the section on fractures involving dentin.

For a complete discussion of the pulpotomy technique and other materials used as pulp dressings, please refer to Chapter 22.

Follow-up after pulp capping and pulpotomy

After pulp capping and pulpotomy the patient should be recalled periodically for 2 to 4 years to determine success. Although the normal vitality tests such as electric and thermal sensitivity are reliable after pulp capping and shallow pulpotomy, they are usually not helpful in the deeper pulpotomized tooth. Although histologic success cannot be determined, clinical success is judged by the absence of any clinical or radiographic signs of pathosis, the verification of a dentin bridge both radiographically and clinically, and the presence of continued root development in teeth with incompletely formed roots.

Controversy exists as to whether the pulp should be reentered after the completion of root development in the pulpotomized tooth. Many authors believe that pulp capping and pulpotomy procedures invariably lead to progressive calcification of the root canal; however, it has been our experience and the experience of others[58,115] that when careful techniques and good case selection are used this seldom happens. When pulps of clinically successful pulpotomies were removed 1 to 5 years following treatment, researchers reported histologically normal findings. They concluded on the basis of the histologic evidence that routine pulpectomy following pulpotomy of accidental pulp exposure is not warranted.[61] Thus the routine reentry to remove the pulp and place a root canal filling after completion of root development is contraindicated unless dictated by restorative considerations such as the necessity for retentive post placement. Nevertheless, canal calcification, internal resorption, and/or pulp necrosis are potential sequelae of pulp capping and pulpotomy procedures. Although unlikely, they are possible and the patient should be clearly informed.

Treatment of primary crown fractures

Fractures of primary crowns not involving the pulp are treated in the same manner as those in permanent teeth. For a complete description of pulpal treatment in the primary dentition, please refer to Chapter 22.

Root fractures

In the overall scope of traumatic injuries to teeth, root fractures are relatively uncommon, occurring in 7% or less of injuries to permanent teeth.[2,18] In primary and developing permanent teeth, root fractures are rare. These teeth, with very short roots, are more likely to be displaced or avulsed than to have fractured roots.

The diagnosis of a fractured root is based on the clinical mobility of the tooth, the displacement of the coronal segment, palpation tenderness over the root, and the radio-

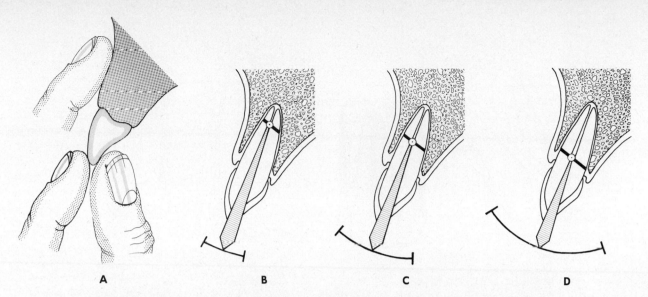

FIG. 15-5. Diagnosis of the location of a root fracture. **A,** Palpating the facial mucosa. By placing the forefinger of one hand on the mucosa and gently moving the crown of the injured tooth with the thumb and forefinger of the other hand, the dentist can often feel movement of the incisal segment of the root. **B** and **D,** Arc of mobility of the incisal segment of a tooth with a fractured root. As the location of the fracture moves incisally, the arc of facial-lingual mobility of the incisal segment increases. (**B,** apical third fracture; **C,** middle third; **D,** incisal third.)

graphic appearance. Careful examination is frequently necesssary to differentiate a root fracture from a subgingival crown fracture or a displaced tooth.

By placing the forefinger of one hand on the gingiva over the facial surface of the root of the affected tooth and gently moving the crown with the other hand, the clinician can often feel the location of the fracture. Also the arc of movement of the crown will aid in differentiating the injury. The closer the fracture is to the gingival crest, the longer will be the arc of movement of the crown; and the further the fracture is toward the apex, the shorter the arc of movement (Fig. 15-5).

The radiographic diagnosis of a root fracture requires careful review of radiographs of the site of injury, preferably with the aid of a magnifying glass. If the injury has caused a separation of the broken parts, the diagnosis is easy. If the central radiographic beam does not follow the direction of the fracture (Fig. 15-6), if the fracture runs in an oblique direction (Fig. 15-6), or if there has not been any separation of the broken segments of the root, then diagnosis becomes difficult at best or the fracture may be missed entirely. Fractures radiographed at an angle greater than ± 15 or 20 degress vertical to the fracture line have been shown to be of poor diagnostic quality.[18,63]

As the clinician runs through the sequence of tests, the tooth with a fractured root generally will be noted to be tender to percussion; there may be bleeding from the gingival sulcus, and frequently the tooth will not respond to thermal or electric pulp testing procedures.

The variable response of the traumatized tooth to pulp tests brings the clinician into the realm of the art of dentistry rather than the science.

There is a tendency for root-fractured teeth to remain vital. It is believed that the fractured area provides an avenue of escape for fluid pressure from edema and allows for possible collateral circulation from the periodontal ligament to assist in maintaining vitality of the traumatized pulp.[18,131,166,174] It has been shown that *only* 20% to 40% of teeth with fractured roots eventually undergo pulpal necrosis.[18,22,174]

If the fractured root is not apparent initially, it may become apparent days or weeks later as the patient continues to complain of sensitivity to biting pressure. This can be confirmed by percussion sensitivity. A follow-up radiograph may reveal a distinct fracture line at this later date due to separation of the broken root segments by edema and masticatory forces.[18]

Healing of fractured roots

Before beginning discussion of treatment of root fractures, it is essential that a basic understanding of the healing potentials of the fractured root be established. Given the background of these biologically normal healing patterns, the clinical decisions in regard to treatment become logical efforts to enhance the healing capacity of the tooth root. It is not our intent to describe the day-by-day histopathologic changes that occur at the fracture site but rather to present a general overview as a broad frame of reference. For a more detailed histopathologic description and references, the reader is referred to Andreasen[18] and Vanek.[166]

In the mechanism of root repair and separation of the broken segments in the alveolar socket, hemorrhage from broken capillaries in the pulp and periodontal ligament flows into the fracture site and clots. This clot gradually is organized by fibroblasts into fibrous connective tissue. The

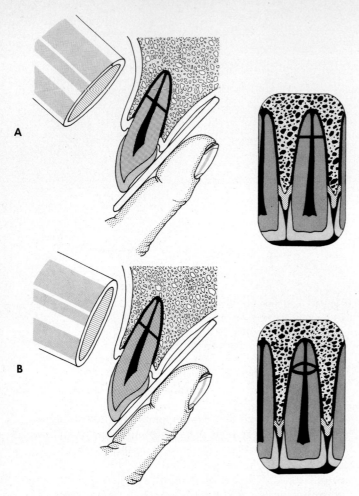

FIG. 15-6. Varying radiographic views of a root fracture depending on angulation of the central radiographic beam. **A,** Beam parallel with the fracture. **B,** Beam oblique to the fracture. This view gives an incorrect impression of an elliptical double fracture of the root.

fractured surfaces of dentin and cementum are gradually remodeled by surface resorption and apposition of calcific tissue.

Depending upon the amount of separation of the fragments, four alternative forms of repair have been classically described[18,22].

Calcific healing. If the fragments are in close apposition with little mobility of the parts, it is possible to get a calcific callus formation at the fracture site both externally on the root surface and internally on the root canal wall (Figs. 15-7, *A* 15-8, *D*, and 15-9). There may be a thin layer of fibrous connective tissue remaining in the fracture line and seen on the radiograph as a delicate fracture line across the root. The pulp will likely be vital but at a reduced level of responsiveness. Mobility will be within physiologic limits.

Connective tissue healing. If the broken parts are separated further or some mobility of the parts is present, the formation of a calcified callus is impeded and a fibrous attachment similar to a periodontal ligament may develop between the fractured segments (Fig. 15-10, *D* and *E*). The fractured dentin surfaces may be lined by cementum

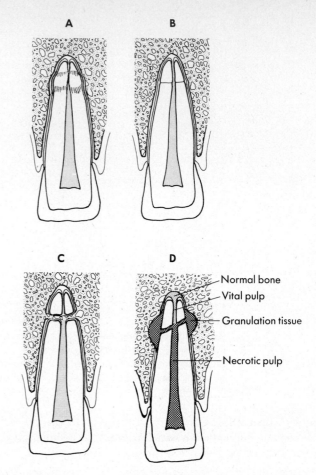

FIG. 15-7. Varying patterns of healing of a root fracture. **A,** Calcific callus union. **B,** Connective tissue union. **C,** Combination bone and connective tissue healing. **D,** Nonunion and granulation tissue formation. The apical pulp segment frequently remains vital.

and the sharp edges of the fracture may be rounded by surface resorption. The tooth will have little mobility after healing and pulp tests will be essentially normal. The connective tissue will be seen on the radiograph as a definite fracture line.

Combination bone and connective tissue healing. With further separation of the fragments and possible mobility of the broken parts, there may be growth of new bone between the fracture segments (Fig. 15-7, *C*). The fractured surfaces will be lined by cementum with a periodontal ligament between the tooth and the new bone. The tooth will be quite firm and the pulp will be vital to test procedures.

Healing with nonunion and granulation tissue formation. When there is severe dislocation of the fractured root and possible contamination of the pulpal tissues by oral fluids, the pulp may be sufficiently injured or infected to undergo necrosis. Generally the incisal portion of the pulp will undergo necrosis and the apical segment will remain vital.[22,174] The necrotic pulp will stimulate inflammation and granulation tissue formation in the fracture lines. The inflammation will spread to the alveolar bone adjacent to the fracture line, causing resorption of bone in

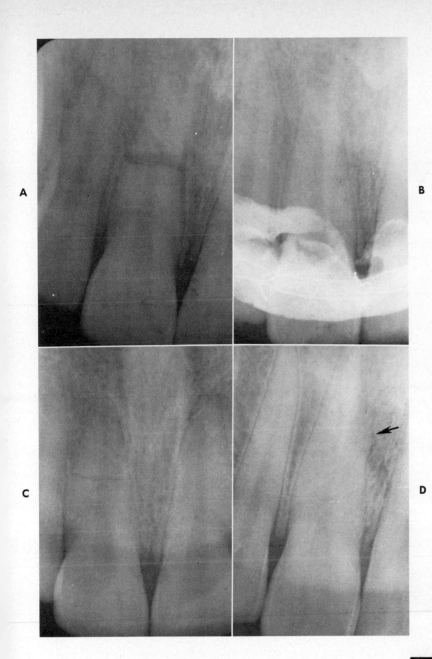

A

B

C

D

FIG. 15-8. Fracture in the middle third of a root treated by splinting only. **A,** Initial examination of the central incisor an hour after the trauma. Note the separation of segments. **B,** Wire and acrylic splint. **C,** Six-month follow-up. The tooth is vital to pulp testing. **D,** Nine-year follow-up. Both central incisors are equally responsive to pulp testing. Note the callus formation *(arrow)* and reduced pulpal lumen.

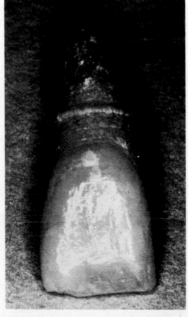

FIG. 15-9. Extracted tooth exhibiting callus formation of the root.

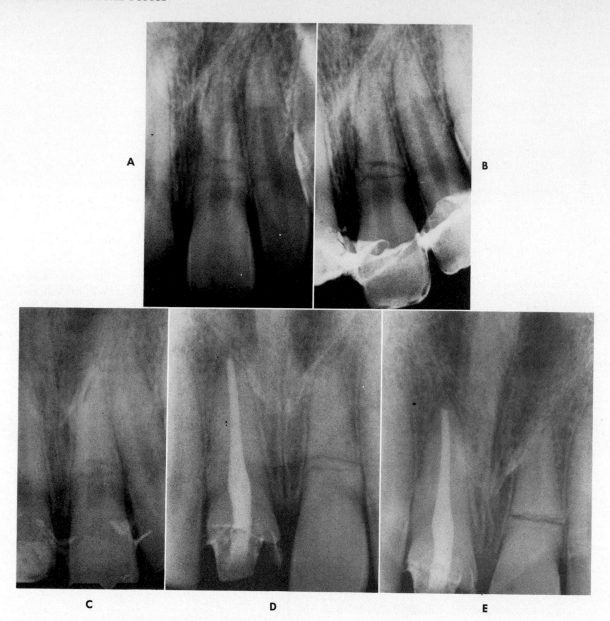

FIG. 15-10. Fractured incisal third of a root. **A,** Left central incisor with a fracture of both crown and root. **B,** Splinted with acrylic and cemented with zinc oxyphosphate. **C,** Three months after injury. **D,** Nine years after injury. Endodontic treatment was necessary on the right central incisor as well. Note the pulpal obliteration of the left central. **E,** Same as **D** but with a 10-degree variation in radiographic vertical angulation. Note the difference in appearance of the fracture. (Compare with Fig. 15-6).

this area. Radiographically the widening of the fracture line and the loss of alveolar bone adjacent to the fracture will be evident. The tooth will be loose, sensitive to percussion, perhaps turning dark, and slightly extruded (Fig. 15-7, *D*).

Treatment philosophy of teeth with fractured roots

Studies[18,131,166,174] have shown that the *majority of teeth with root fractures will maintain vitality of the pulpal tissues*. This has had a direct effect on the philosophy of treating root fractures. Given the tendency for the pulpal tissues to remain vital, the primary purpose of treatment is to enhance this natural tendency for healing.

It is obvious that a tooth root with a calcific callus formation reuniting the broken fragments is stronger than one without union of broken parts. The ultimate goal of the clinician faced with a broken tooth root problem should be to attempt to gain reunion of the broken root by calcified callus formation. Preservation of the vitality of the pulp will certainly enhance the prognosis for achieving that ultimate goal as opposed to immediately proceeding with root canal treatment, with the strong possiblity of extruding cement or sealer into the fracture site. Although the pulpal tissues are not essential to healing of the root fracture,[123] they are preferable to a foreign material in the fracture site. Therefore *the fracture should be reduced as soon as possible and the broken tooth firmly immobilized.* To avoid possible tearing of the pulpal tissues, excessive lateral pressure on the incisal portion of the fractured root should be avoided during repositioning of the broken parts. Contamination of the pulp through the fracture line with saliva or other contaminants should be carefully avoided. If necrosis of the incisal portion of the pulp occurs, reunion of the calcified tissues is not likely to occur. Every effort must be made to enhance healing of the delicate pulpal tissues.

With this philosophy of treatment as a basis, it becomes logical to divide root fractures into two types: those not communicating and those communicating with the oral cavity.

TREATMENT OF THE FRACTURED ROOT NOT COMMUNICATING WITH THE ORAL CAVITY

The noncommunicating fracture is generally in the apical or the middle third of the root. Diagnosis is dependent on possible mobility or displacement of the tooth, percussion sensitivity, and a correct angulation of the radiographic exposure.

The customary electric and thermal pulp tests should be done and carefully recorded. The degree of mobility and displacement as well as any tooth discoloration should also be noted on the chart. If the pulp is determined to be vital to clinical tests, the only treatment necessary is repositioning of the tooth to proper alignment and immobilizing by splinting to the adjacent teeth. The sooner the fracture is reduced prior to organization of a fibrin clot, the easier the fragments can be repositioned. If bone fragments interfere, they will have to be molded into position permitting realignment of the tooth. A radiograph should be taken after repositioning the fractured parts to confirm realignment.

The time for leaving the splint in position varies from 1 week to 3 months or more depending on the location of the fracture and the degree of mobility of the tooth. If the fracture is in the apical third of the root and there is minimal displacement or mobility, a splint may not be necessary. At the other end of the spectrum, if the fracture is at the crest of the alveolar bone with moderate displacement and mobility of the crown the splint may have to remain in position for 3 months. The clinician must exercise judgment in each instance. No good clinical studies of a sizable number of cases have been documented to determine the relationship between the time of splinting and the healing of fractured roots. A suggested rule of thumb for midroot fractures is 2 to 3 months. The tooth with the fractured root will need to be reevaluated as to the stability of the splint at 30 to 60 days following the accident.

When the splint is removed, the clinical status of the traumatized area must be determined. The degree of mobility, color of the crown, and percussion and palpation sensitivity need to be recorded as well as the responsiveness to electric and thermal tests. The depth of the gingival sulcus must be determined and recorded. Root fractures that retain vitality of the pulp have been shown to heal 77% of the time.[174] Closure of the root canal is an indicator of a vital pulp.

If the periodontal attachment has failed to heal and the probe penetrates the periodontal ligament space to the depth of the fracture site, the prognosis for healing of the fracture and retaining vitality of the pulp diminishes drastically.

If there is minimal mobility, the tooth responds positively to pulp tests and has not darkened in color, the patient is comfortable, and the radiograph indicates that healing is progressing, then no further treatment is necessary except to repeat the evaluation at 6-month and 1-year intervals. Any variations from this list of indicators of healing will indicate complications are occurring.

If mobility is present, the splint must be reapplied and the occlusion adjusted to eliminate stress on the tooth. If after 4 to 6 months the tooth continues to be mobile and the fracture site cannot be probed through the gingival sulcus, the tooth should be permanently splinted to the adjacent teeth.

All root fractures that do not communicate with the oral cavity after repositioning of the broken fragments should be treated as if the pulp is vital regardless of the results of the pulp tests at the initial emergency visit. If complications occur subsequently indicating pulp necrosis, endodontic treatment should be instituted at that time.[101,103]

Root fractures with evidence of pulpal necrosis

The radiographic appearance of bone destruction in or adjacent to the fracture site is the best indicator of pulpal necrosis.[101] and may take several months to develop. Lack of response to electric and thermal pulp tests without radiographic evidence of bone destruction adjacent to the fracture site does not warrant instituting endodontic therapy.[174] Darkening of the tooth and sensitivity to percussion and palpation are more reliable than electric and thermal pulp tests as indicators of pulpal necrosis.

Pulpal necrosis subsequent to root fractures has been shown to occur from 20% to 44% of the time. The occurrence of necrosis of the pulp seems to be related not to the location of the root fracture in the apical, middle, or incisal third but rather to communication with the oral cavity and the severity of displacement of the incisal segment.[18,174] If there is evidence of pulpal necrosis of the coronal portion of the pulp, it is generally believed that the apical segment will remain vital.[18,22,57,101] Endodontic treatment is therefore usually confined to the coronal segment of the root canal (Fig. 15-11).

Cvek[57,59] made the interesting observation that the displaced coronal segment of the root-fractured tooth should be treated similarly to a displaced intact tooth.

The coronal portion of the tooth with a fractured root and a necrosed pulp can be filled with gutta-percha after routine endodontic instrumentation of the coronal segment (Fig. 15-11) if it meets the following criteria:

1. There is no evidence of a periapical radiolucency at the end of the apical segment.
2. The space between the two fragments at the fracture site is minimal.
3. The root canal space is sufficiently constricted at the apical end of the coronal segment to permit creation

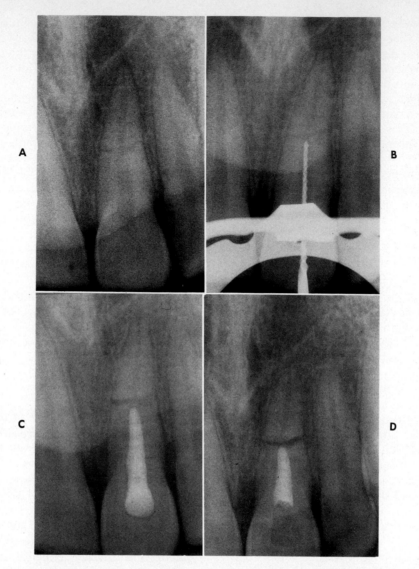

FIG. 15-11. Necrosis of the incisal segment of a pulp, with subsequent endodontics on the coronal segment only. **A,** Initial injury. **B,** Three months later the coronal pulp necrosed, and endodontic treatment was initiated. Vital tissue was noted in the apical segment. **C,** Treatment completed. **D,** Two years after treatment of the coronal segment.

of a mechanical stop for condensation of gutta-percha.

4. The apical segment of the pulp bleeds when touched with a paper point, indicating that vascularity is intact and permitting healing of the apical segment.

Filling the coronal portion of the pulpal space with calcium hydroxide seems to be indicated with the following criteria:[57,59,101]

1. There is no evidence of a periapical radiolucency at the end of the apical section.
2. The apical segment of the pulp seems vital as evidenced by bleeding on a paper point.
3. A radiolucent space is evident between or adjacent to the fractured segments.
4. A widened space can be detected between the broken fragments.
5. There is evidence of internal or external resorption of the coronal segment.

6. A wide root canal space makes a filling of the root canal with gutta-percha difficult, with a strong possibility of extrusion of the gutta-percha or cement into the fracture site.

Because pulp tests are not reliable in determining the vitality of the coronal pulp, endodontic treatment is generally not insituted until a radiolucency is visible at the fracture site. Therefore most teeth with fractured roots requiring endodontics in the coronal segment are treated with calcium hydroxide. When healing of the fracture site is evident after 6 months to a year, the calcium hydroxide can be replaced with gutta-percha.

As long as the periodontal attachment is intact, preventing leeching of the calcium hydroxide from the fracture site, and mobility is minimized, the prognosis for healing is excellent.[57,59,101,174]

If a radiolucency is present at the apex of the apical segment, this indicates pulpal necrosis in that segment as

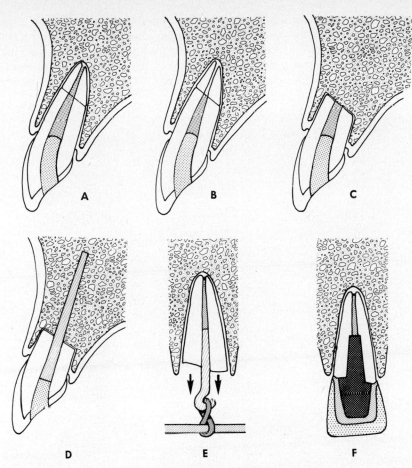

FIG. 15-12. Configurations of endodontic treatment of a fractured root. **A,** Coronal and apical segments. **B,** Coronal segment only. The apical segment pulp remains vital. **C,** Coronal segment with surgical removal of the abscessed apical segment. **D,** Endosseous implant for stabilization of the tooth with an excessively short root. **E,** Orthodontic extrusion of the apical segment after a fracture of the incisal third. **F,** Restoration of the orthodontically extruded apical segment.

well. Root canal treatment of both the coronal and the apical fragments is indicated (Fig. 15-12, *A*). This is feasible if both fragments are well approximated and access to the root canal of the apical fragment can be obtained through the coronal segment.

Various authors[77,126,170] have advocated the use of rigid filling materials to tie the two fragments together. The rigid filling materials may be necessary in instances of persistent mobility, generally in fractures involving the coronal third of the root. However, these concepts have slowly begun to change with the advent of the more esthetic acid-etch resin splint and greater documentation of healing capacity of root fractures that do not communicate with the oral cavity.* The prognosis is markedly reduced, with persistent mobility, and healing that utilizes the rigid internal splint is questionable (Fig. 15-13).

It has also been suggested[73] that the greater sealing capacity of gutta-percha makes it more appropriate as the filling material of choice. Furthermore, healing without a rigid internal splint has been documented.[123]

Adequate studies have not been done comparing the healing of teeth with fractured roots and pulpal necrosis of the coronal and apical segments utilizing gutta-percha, calcium hydroxide, or a rigid filling material as an internal splint. Less than 1% of dental injuries are of this type, making clinical studies difficult.

If pathosis exists in the apical segment and endodontic treatment is not possible, the apical segment must be removed surgically (Figs. 15-12, *C*, and 15-14). Frequently loss of the apical fragment does not create mobility problems.

The loss of the apical segment occasionally creates problems of an unfavorable crown root ratio. With improvements in the acid-etch composite resin techniques, it is possible to achieve permanent splinting for a tooth with minimal root structure. Placement of a "Maryland bridge" type of framework or direct interproximal bonding may be utilized for permanent splinting to the adjacent teeth.

The placement of an endodontic endosseous implant has been advocated to improve the stability of the coronal segment[18,72,73,146] (Fig. 15-12, *D*). However, in addition to the experimental status designation by the A.D.A., recent studies[18,143] have shown corrosion of the implants and

---

*References 18,22,57,100,101,103,174.

persistent inflammation around them. The Council of Dental Materials, Instruments, and Equipment of the American Dental Association[54] has recently stated that it does *not* currently recommend endosseous implants for routine clinical practice. Unfortunately the endodontic endosseous im-

plant, which has the advantage of utilizing a natural tooth with its periodontal attachment, has been grouped with implants for replacement of missing teeth that do not develop a periodontal attachment. However, in view of this official position of the A.D.A., it is advisable that the clinician

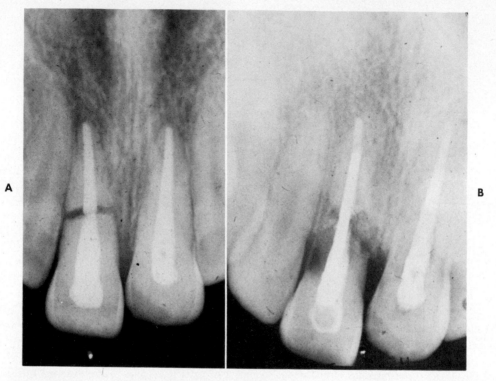

FIG. 15-13. Resorption subsequent to rigid internal splinting of root segments. **A,** Gutta-percha filling prior to placement of a rigid internal splint. **B,** One year later after placement of the splint. Note the root resorption at the fracture site.

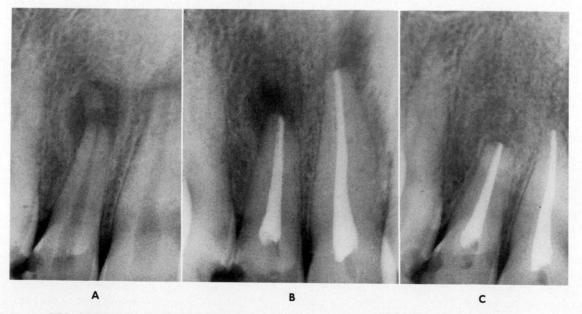

FIG. 15-14. Root fracture with pulpal necrosis and periapical pathosis. **A,** Initial examination. The patient reported a history of trauma approximately 1 year earlier. **B,** Endodontic treatment and surgical removal of the apical segment. **C,** Nine months subsequent to treatment. The periapical lesion is healing.

obtain written informed consent from the patient before utilizing the endodontic endosseous implant for tooth stabilization.

Root fractures with pulpal obliteration

After reduction of the fracture site and splinting and adjustment of the occlusion, the fracture will generally heal. One of the manifestations of healing is heavy calcification of the pulpal space, which has been reported in 69% to 86% of cases.[18,103] The obliteration seems to take two different patterns: partial obliteration occurs in the apical root canal space and the fracture site extending 1 or 2 mm into the coronal fragment, or the entire pulpal space becomes progressively obliterated.

The type of repair seems to be influenced by the severity of the fragment dislocation. As the severity increases, the likelihood of total pulpal obliteration increases.[103] Studies[101] have shown that 21% of root-fractured teeth undergoing total pulpal obliteration will also have pulpal necrosis. Since there are four out of five chances that the pulp will not necrose in the presence of heavy pulpal calcification, intervention with endodontic treatment to prevent calcific pulpal obliteration does not appear to be justified.[100,120]

Tooth color

After traumatic injuries a tooth may undergo a variety of color changes. These are frequently subtle and difficult to compare from one evaluation appointment to another. Lighting, adjacent restorations, dryness of the tooth, stains, and normal variations in tooth color all create errors in using color as a diagnostic criterion. Subjective judgment, varying from clinician to clinician, and different descriptive phrases also create inaccuracies.

In the face of these realistic variables, it may be stated that a dramatic change from normal tooth color to a distinct strong pink, purple, or dark gray can be taken as indicative of pulp necrosis when combined with tenderness to percussion and radiographic changes. A change to yellow or yellow-brown may indicate calcification of the pulp chamber as confirmed on the radiograph. Caution must be used in determining pulpal status by color. We have seen teeth with discoloration and no response to vitality tests in which the pulps were found to be vital.

Root fractures in permanent anterior teeth with incompletely developed roots are relatively unusual because of the tendency of these short-rooted teeth to be displaced rather than fractured. In these rare instances the large apical foramen seems to enhance healing. If the periodontal attachment is intact and adequate immobilization is attained, the tooth root will probably continue to develop normally.[99] However, obliteration of the pulp is more likely to occur in these teeth.

ROOT FRACTURES COMMUNICATING WITH THE ORAL CAVITY

Fractures of any part of the root coronal to the periodontal attachment have a poor prognosis for healing. There is periodontal breakdown along the fracture line with subsequent pulpal necrosis from the microbial contamination of the pulp through the fracture (Fig. 15-15).

The typical situation is the fractured maxillary incisor with the fracture on the labial surface 2 to 3 mm supragingival but tapering obliquely to 2 to 5 mm subgingivally on

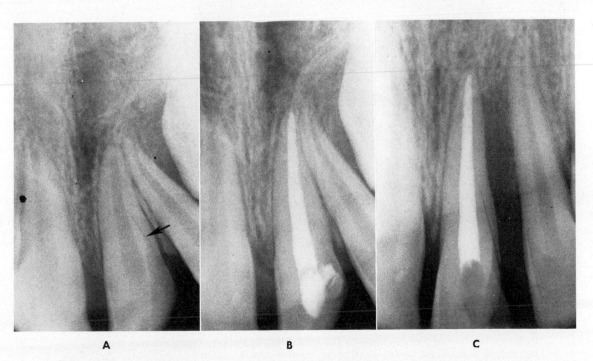

| A | B | C |

FIG. 15-15. Vertical root fracture communicating with the oral cavity. **A,** Immediately after the trauma. Note the vertical root fracture *(arrow).* **B,** Root canal filled with gutta-percha. **C,** Two years later a severe periodontal defect developed adjacent to the vertical root fracture.

the lingual. A similar fracture can occur with premolar and molar cusps. The emergency visit will require anesthetizing the patient facially and lingually and teasing off the broken crown from the residual periodontal attachment on the lingual. Endodontic treatment should be completed in one visit. Frequently the natural crown can be recemented on the tooth root with the aid of a temporary post or splinted to the adjacent teeth with acid-etch resin. It makes an excellent temporary covering and tends to prevent invagination of the lingual gingiva into the fracture site.

When the emergency has been resolved, plans must be made for restoring the tooth. In this instance clinical judgment becomes very important. The choices are (1) periodontal gingival and osseous surgery to expose an ade-

quate amount of tooth structure for a crown margin, (2) extrusion of the root until all the fracture site is supragingival sufficient for restoring the tooth (Figs. 15-12, *E* and *F*), (3) combined orthodontic extrusion and periodontal gingival and osseous recontouring for adequate margination, and (4) removing the clinical crown segment and retaining the submerged root with its vital pulp followed by placement of a fixed bridge across the space (Fig. 15-16). If the root pulp is necrotic, endodontic treatment must be accomplished. At the emergency appointment, removing the crown permits evaluation of the depth of the fracture. If the deepest aspect of the fracture is greater than approximately 2 mm below the bone level, extrusion of the tooth seems preferable to periodontal surgery. If less than 2 mm

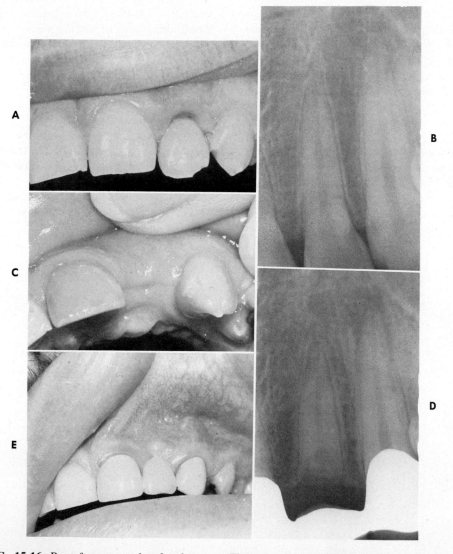

FIG. 15-16. Root fracture at the alveolar crest. The root was retained to preserve the alveolar ridge. **A,** Clinical view of a fractured lateral incisor with slight displacement of the crown. **B,** Radiographic view of the root fracture. The patient refused the opportunity for root extrusion but was willing to retain the root to preserve the alveolar ridge. **C,** Healed alveolar ridge after crown removal. **D,** Eighteen-month follow-up radiograph of the retained root after placement of a fixed bridge. Note the developing periapical lesion on the canine abutment. **E,** Clinical view of the bridge.

below bone on the lingual, periodontal gingival and osseous surgery seems indicated. The reason for this arbitrary distinction is that a minimal periodontal surgical procedure on the lingual will not compromise the support of the tooth, will not involve adjacent teeth, can be maintained hygienically, and will not alter the appearance of the tooth.

Periodontal procedures on the facial create an esthetic problem, and extrusion is preferable. When periodontal healing has occurred the tooth is restored with a post and crown. The reader is referred to Chapter 21 for these procedures.

Extrusion of the root is preferable if excessive periodontal surgery will be required to expose the fracture site. Heithersay[88,89] added the concept of combined endodontic-orthodontic treatment of fractured teeth to the treatment options (Fig. 15-12, E and F). Since then the technique has become a standard in the treatment of subcrestal defects.[64,147,171] A recent variation[56] suggests cementing the permanent post and core prior to beginning orthodontic treatment, thus eliminating the need for repeated post preparations.

Ingber[97] introduced an interesting concept into the treatment of cervical third root fractures. By utilizing small tatoo marks he showed that the marginal gingiva will follow the root as it is extruded orthodontically. The fractured root is extruded until the marginal gingiva and underlying bone have moved coronally beyond the level of the gingival crest of the adjacent teeth. Then the tooth is stabilized in the new position for 4 to 6 weeks to permit reorientation of the gingival fibers. During this stabilization period, the gingiva may migrate apically[36] and minimize the gingival and osseous surgical contouring required to align the height of the bone and gingiva with that of the adjacent teeth. However, periodontal surgery is almost invariably required before crown construction. This combined endodontic-orthodontic-periodontal technique has several advantages. By the surgical exposure of the root a better margin is obtained for restoring the tooth with less orthodontic movement. In contrast to a strictly periodontal surgical approach, the Ingber technique does not leave a residual periodontal defect on the broken tooth and does not affect adjacent teeth. When the periodontal and the orthodontic approaches are combined, the crown/root ratio of the result is stronger than with either technique alone. The coronal movement of bone requires less extrusion and less periodontal recontouring.

If for some reason the patient objects to wearing an orthodontic appliance an ''immediate'' surgical extrusion of the tooth may be utilized. This requires surgical access to the apex of the fractured tooth. The root is subluxated incisally with pressure on the apex, and the tooth is stabilized in its new position by bone chips packed at the apex to prevent retrusion and by sutures over the fractured surface of the root.[161].

Recent studies have suggested that the periapical surgery and bone chips packed at the apex are not necessary and may actually contribute to incipient root resorption.[110,111] After 6 weeks the tooth can be restored with a post crown.

Primary teeth with fractured roots

Primary teeth with root fractures are unusual, since they are short rooted and therefore are generally displaced.[3]

When root fractures occur, the primary root will heal if there is little dislocation of the coronal fragment and normal physiologic resorption will occur.[18]

If the coronal fragment is severely dislocated, the primary tooth should be extracted. Similarly a fracture that communicates with the oral cavity is an indication for extraction. Any small root fragments remaining in the socket should be left there, for they will be resorbed.[22]

Displaced teeth

Some authors[18,77,166] have referred to traumatized teeth as having concussions, subluxations, and partial or total luxations. There is confusion as to the differences among these terms. Different authors have used varying definitions. In the discussions to follow, concussion, displacement, and avulsion will be used since they seem to be adequate for clinical differentiation and treatment of traumatic conditions.

Concussion is an injury to a tooth and its attachment apparatus without displacement from its position in the alveolus. The most noticeable clinical finding is a markedly increased sensitivity to percussion. While there is no visible displacement, mobility may be present.

Displacement refers to an injury in which the tooth is moved from its position in the socket. If there is any movement of the tooth from its customary position, it has been displaced. The displacement may be lateral (facial, lingual, mesial, distal), extrusive (out of the socket), or intrusive (deeper into the alveolar bone) (Fig. 15-17).

Avulsion is the complete dislocation of the tooth from its socket.

Traumatic injuries to the tooth apparently cause obstruction of the major pulpal vessels at the apex. Subsequently there is diffusion of blood with dilation of the pulpal capillaries. The congestion of the capillaries is followed by capillary degeneration with release of erythrocytes and edema of the pulp. Because of the lack of collateral circulation in the pulp, there is little inflammatory response to the injury and the pulp may undergo partial or complete ischmemic infarction. With little or no circulation the pulp persists in this fashion for months or years. A transient bacteremia may penetrate small vessels at the apex and eventually become established in the infarcted pulpal tissues.

The infection that follows may be the first clinical indication of pulpal necrosis. Stanley et al.[156] noted that in some cases the infarction process is not total. A few vessels may remain functioning and transport fresh blood to parts of the pulp. These parts will remain vital. If pulp tests indicate negative responses but the pulp chamber has sensitive tissue and bleeding in the deeper parts, a persistent blood supply is supporting some nerve fibers. Apparently the thermal-mechanical receptors in the pulp are obstructed by the infarcted tissue, preventing transmission of a stimulus received through the enamel and dentin.[156]

It is inferred that if the trauma to the tooth and enclosed

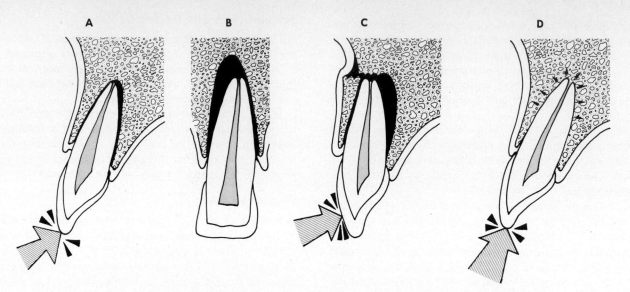

FIG. 15-17. Configurations of displaced teeth. **A,** Lateral displacement. In this instance the crown is forced lingually and the root facially. The same relationship would apply to mesial-distal lateral displacements. **B,** Extrusive displacement. **C,** Major lateral displacement with fracture of the alveolar bone. **D,** Intrusive displacement.

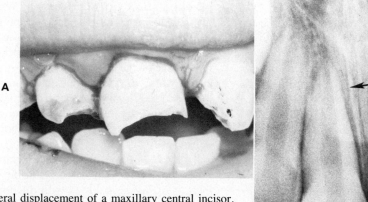

FIG. 15-18. Lateral displacement of a maxillary central incisor. **A,** Clinical view of the injury. Note the gingival sulcular hemorrhage and the crown fractures. **B,** Radiographic view of the injury. The periodontal ligament space is widened on the mesial of the right central incisor *(arrow).*

pulp is minimal the brief pulpal ischemia may cause reversible superficial infarcts. This might account for the return of positive pulpal responses weeks later.[140]

Concussion

In concussion injuries the blow to the tooth may be sufficient to cause bleeding in the periodontal ligament and pulpal edema.[18] The increased fluid in the periodontal ligament apparently increases the pressure of masticatory forces on the tooth and is uncomfortable to the patient because of the preexisting intraligamentary pressure.

The pulp may not respond to tests initially, but positive responses can return weeks or months later. Teeth that test vital immediately after the trauma tend to remain vital. At 3 months there is a high correlation between teeth testing vital and those remaining vital indefinitely.[33,140]

In concussion injuries the only treatment required is ad-

justing the tooth slightly out of occlusion. Pulp tests for vitality should be repeated and compared with the initial appointment base line at 1-, 3-, 6-, and 12-month intervals. If the tooth initially responds positively and subsequently responds negatively, this is a strong indicator of pulpal necrosis.

Displacement

If a tooth is displaced from its socket minimally, it will be slightly mobile and sensitive to percussion and biting pressure. There may be some bleeding from the gingival sulcus because of injury to the periodontal ligament. A slight thickening of the periodontal ligament may be noted radiographically. This tooth probably will not require splinting. If there is *any* doubt as to the necessity for a splint, one should be placed on the tooth.

It has been shown that tooth mobility in conjunction

with other injuries significantly increases the incidence of pulpal necrosis. Coronal fractures without concussion or mobility produced a 3% incidence of pupal necrosis. However, coronal fracture with concussion and mobility increased the incidence of pulpal necrosis to over 30%.[135,136,137]

Teeth with obvious clinical or radiographic displacement must be repositioned and splinted. Teeth with minor displacement are not routinely endodontically treated; however, approximately half of these will ultimately undergo pulpal necrosis and require root canal therapy.[141] Therefore these teeth must be followed clinically to determine pulpal status.

Major displacements

Teeth with major displacements (over 5 mm) from their position in the socket have sustained severe injuries. These injuries may be accompanied by alveolar bone fractures (Fig. 15-17, D). Diagnosis is obvious by extrusion of the tooth or facial-lingual displacement.

If multiple teeth are involved, as in an automobile accident, several teeth may be displaced and their normal positions may be confused. These teeth will have to be repositioned to occlude with the opposing arch.

Radiographically an extruded tooth will exhibit a markedly increased periodontal ligament space apically. If the root has been displaced in a mesial or distal direction, the widened space will be evident on the mesial or distal surface of the root (Fig. 15-18). If the root has been forced in a facial or lingual direction, the widened space may be masked by the tooth root in its new position.

Thermal and electric pulp tests are unpredictable in displaced teeth. The problem of reliable pulp tests with traumatized teeth has been discussed. Generally, the more severe the displacement and the greater the mobility the less likely the pulp will survive.[140]

Lateral and extrusive displacements. In detecting severe lateral displacements when the root is forced facially and the crown lingually, it is helpful to palpate the facial mucosa at the level of the root apex. With marked displacement the root end can be forced through the cortical plate of bone and can be felt with digital pressure. The tooth may be locked into the bone in the displaced position and will not be mobile. In repositioning the tooth it may be necessary to apply finger pressure on the root apex in a coronal direction to move it back through the fenestration into the socket. The fractured cortical bone can be molded back into place with fingers[18] (Fig. 15-19). The teeth should be radiographed immediately prior to splinting to confirm their correct repositioning.

Teeth with major lateral displacements or those extruded from the socket are repositioned in the socket and splinted for 7 to 14 days. They must be adjusted out of hyperocclusion. The time interval in repositioning displaced teeth is important because of the possibility of root resorption. Teeth repositioned in 90 minutes from the time of injury have less root resorption. There is also a greater possibility of loss of periodontal support with delayed repositioning.[3]

Teeth that have been displaced long enough for blood to be thoroughly clotted around them should not be repositioned forcefully, because of possible induction of root resorption. It is preferable to move them into their normal position orthodontically after healing has occurred. If a tooth is severely displaced and interfering with closure of the mouth, it should be adjusted to allow normal occlusion. When closure cannot be achieved by occlusal adjustment, it will be necessary to extract and replant the tooth. The socket should be irrigated with saline or water and aspirated to remove the blood clot. If curettage is necessary to remove the clot, care must be taken to prevent damage to the periodontal ligament. In this instance the tooth must be treated as one that has been avulsed.

Intrusive displacements. The intruded tooth is severely traumatized and requires special attention. This injury is second only to avulsion in severity. Depending upon the strength of the blow the intruded tooth may look short and be confused with a fractured crown. Sometimes it will be completely intruded into the bone and mistakenly assumed to be lost. The tooth is so firmly wedged in the bone that it is not mobile. Percussion will sound hard and harsh as compared to that of a normal tooth. If a permanent central incisor is completely intruded, it may have penetrated the floor of the nose and may even be seen in the nostril[18] (Fig. 15-20). The radiograph may show a loss of the periodontal space around a minimally intruded tooth. With a severe intrusive displacement the radiograph will show the location of the tooth and the severity of the intrusion.

Treatment of the intruded tooth is variable. A minimally intruded tooth will frequently reerupt spontaneously, particularly one with incomplete root formation. If the intrusion injury is severe, it will be necessary to retrieve the tooth with forceps and to splint it (Fig. 15-20) or move it into a position orthodontically. The least complications of root resorption and loss of crestal bone support occur when the intruded tooth is moved into position orthodontically over 3 to 4 weeks.

Ankylosis may occur as a sequel to root resorption. Recent evidence has shown that ankylosis occurs in as few as 5 to 6 days in experimental animals subjected to intrusive forces.[164] Orthodontic extrusion should be initiated promptly following injury in order to move the tooth into proper position prior to the onset of possible ankylosis.[153]

Another consideration is that pulpal necrosis will occur (seen in 96% of intruded teeth).[3] Also, external root resorption increases in the presence of necrotic pulps.[18] To *prevent the onset of inflammatory resorption, the fully formed intruded tooth must receive endodontic treatment within 2 to 3 weeks of the time of injury.* Therefore it must be in position to allow access to the root canal, which is another justification for proceeding with orthodontic treatment promptly rather than waiting for spontaneous eruption that might take several months. If the intrusion has not inhibited access to the pulp chamber, waiting for spontaneous eruption is a possiblity; however, ankylosis may occur preventing movement of the tooth into its proper position.

Complications of displacement injuries. The major complications of displacement injuries have been described by Andreasen.[3] They are pulpal necrosis, pulpal obliteration, root resorption, and loss of marginal bone support.

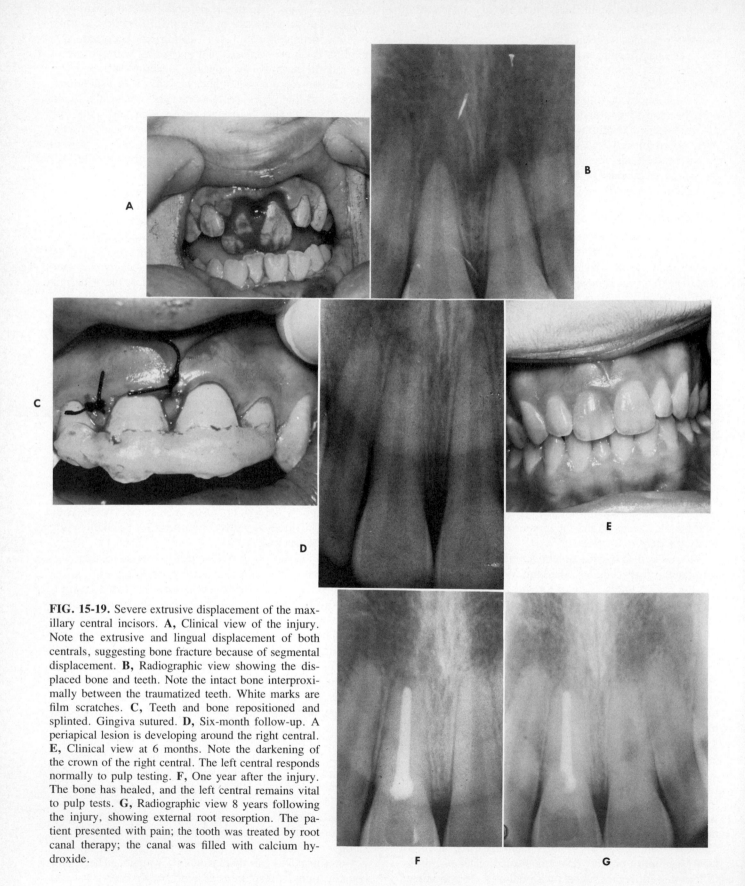

FIG. 15-19. Severe extrusive displacement of the maxillary central incisors. **A,** Clinical view of the injury. Note the extrusive and lingual displacement of both centrals, suggesting bone fracture because of segmental displacement. **B,** Radiographic view showing the displaced bone and teeth. Note the intact bone interproximally between the traumatized teeth. White marks are film scratches. **C,** Teeth and bone repositioned and splinted. Gingiva sutured. **D,** Six-month follow-up. A periapical lesion is developing around the right central. **E,** Clinical view at 6 months. Note the darkening of the crown of the right central. The left central responds normally to pulp testing. **F,** One year after the injury. The bone has healed, and the left central remains vital to pulp tests. **G,** Radiographic view 8 years following the injury, showing external root resorption. The patient presented with pain; the tooth was treated by root canal therapy; the canal was filled with calcium hydroxide.

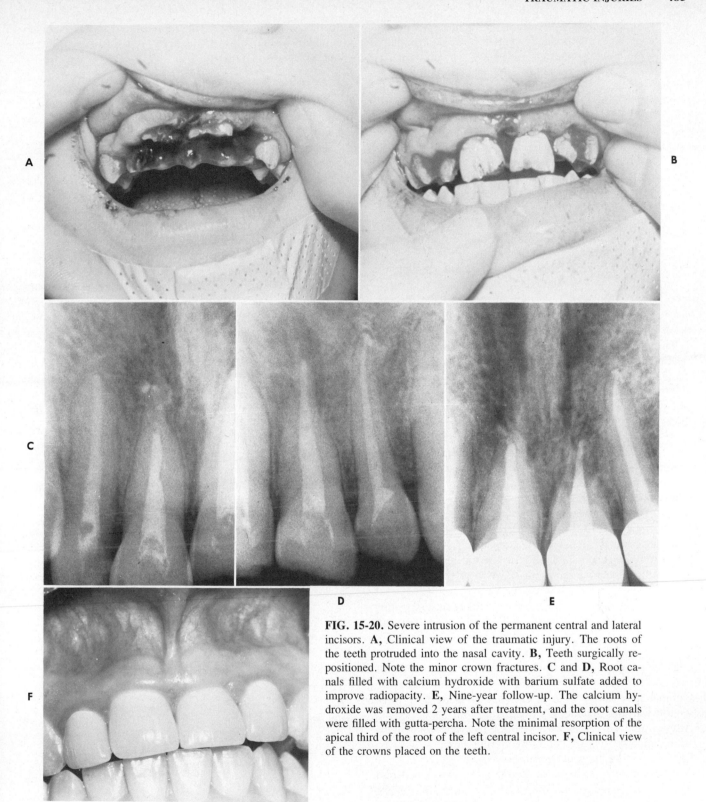

FIG. 15-20. Severe intrusion of the permanent central and lateral incisors. **A,** Clinical view of the traumatic injury. The roots of the teeth protruded into the nasal cavity. **B,** Teeth surgically repositioned. Note the minor crown fractures. **C** and **D,** Root canals filled with calcium hydroxide with barium sulfate added to improve radiopacity. **E,** Nine-year follow-up. The calcium hydroxide was removed 2 years after treatment, and the root canals were filled with gutta-percha. Note the minimal resorption of the apical third of the root of the left central incisor. **F,** Clinical view of the crowns placed on the teeth.

1. Pulpal necrosis, noted in 52% of displacement injuries, occurs in 96% of intrusive injuries. Reports vary in the incidence of pulpal necrosis following extrusive injury from 64% to 98%. It is also more likely to occur in teeth with fully developed roots than in those whose roots are incompletely developed.[3,67,68]

2. Pulpal obliteration with calcified tissue occurs approximately 20% to 25% of the time.[3] It is a response to a moderate injury such as minimal displacement. Severe displacement will probably lead to pulpal necrosis. The pulp is more likely to survive after trauma in teeth with incompletely formed roots, but these teeth are also more

likely to have pulpal obliteration. With intrusive injuries there is a high incidence of pulpal necrosis, so pulpal obliteration is uncommon.[3]

Pulpal necrosis subsequent to pulpal obliteration occurs in approximately 10% of traumatized teeth.[3,100] Therefore prophylactic pulp extirpation performed after evidence of pulpal obliteration with calcifications is not justified.[3,18,100,120] A successful rate of 80% in endodontically treated teeth with pulpal obliteration has been noted.[59]

3. Root resorption is usually seen after intrusive injuries; the next highest incidence follows extrusive injuries. Intrusions are also the injuries that have the higher incidence of pulpal necrosis. It is thought that the presence of the necrotic pulp contributes to root resorption.[18] Root resorption can be detected as early as 2 months after an injury, but it may also be delayed for several months.[3]

4. Loss of marginal bone support increases with the severity of the injury, particularly in intrusive and extrusive injuries. Delayed repositioning of the teeth also increases the risk of damage to the supporting periodontal tissues.[3]

Endodontic treatment of displaced teeth. Endodontic treatment of displaced teeth must be a clinical decision made on a case-by-case basis. Several factors may be helpful in deciding whether or not to enter the root canal. The primary determining factor for endodontic treatment is the diagnosis of pulpal necrosis. This is based on percussion sensitivity, marked discoloration, lack of pulpal responses to thermal and electric tests, and radiographic appearance (Fig. 15-19). Traumatized teeth are notoriously unreliable in responding to pulp tests.

In mature permanent teeth having severe displacement (over 5 mm) or intrusive injuries, pulpal necrosis is quite likely. Root canal treatment is therefore indicated in these teeth since the incidence of root resorption is particularly high. Applying calcium hydroxide as the temporary root canal filling material seems justified to prevent the onset of root resorption (Fig. 15-20).

Teeth with minimal displacement will require splinting and close monitoring of pulpal status and radiographic appearance at 1, 3, 6, and 12 months. If a periapical radiolucency appears or inflammatory resorption becomes evident, endodontic treatment should be started promptly. A periapical radiolucency occurring without simultaneous inflammatory resorption in a completely developed tooth would warrant endodontic treatment with gutta-percha. Any evidence of inflammatory root resorption would be justification for using calcium hydroxide temporarily to assist in arresting the root resorption.[59]

A displaced tooth with an incompletely developed root has a better prognosis for pulp survival.[3] Retention of the vital pulp is desirable to enhance normal development of the root. On the other hand, inflammatory root resorption in immature teeth progresses more rapidly.[18] Close monitoring of these teeth radiographically is therefore essential. When the decision is made that pulp necrosis has occurred or there is evidence of a periapical radiolucency or root resorption, endodontic treatment should begin promptly. Calcium hydroxide is used to fill the canal un-

til the apex has closed and root resorption has been arrested. This is followed later by a permanent filling of gutta-percha.

Displaced primary teeth

In young patients displacement occurs more frequently than crown or root fracture because of the resiliency of the alveolar bone and the shorter tooth roots.[2]

Determining the angle of displacement is critical in diagnosing displaced primary teeth since the primary roots are so close to the developing permanent teeth. The most typical displacement injury results in the crown's being tilted lingually while the root is forced facially but the tooth remains intact. If the root of the primary tooth has been forced facially, there is less likelihood of damage to the underlying permanent tooth (Fig. 15-21) than if the primary tooth has been forced lingually or intruded. Then the possibility of damage to the permanent tooth is greatly increased.

It has been noted that about 10% of the enamel hypoplasias in permanent anterior teeth are the result of trauma to the primary tooth. The enamel hypoplasias were primarily white and yellow-brown.[27] More serious injuries such as permanent crown or root malformations and sequestration of the permanent tooth germ are possible but not likely.[27]

Treatment of the concussed or minimally displaced primary tooth is confined to clinical and radiographic checkups.

Severe lateral or intrusive displacements will require radiographic ascertainment of the root position. An occlusal film held by the parent on the face of the child so that a lateral view of the traumatized tooth is obtained can be helpful in diagnosing the position of the root.[18,168]

If the root of the primary tooth has been displaced facially, the prevailing opinion[18,25,168] is that the tooth should be allowed to reerupt spontaneously. There seems to be no difference in complications for the permanent

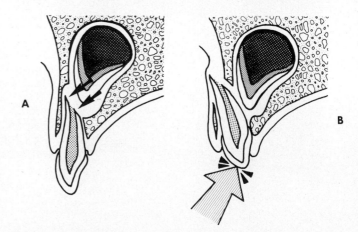

FIG. 15-21. Primary tooth displacement. **A,** Normal resorption of the primary root occurs on the lingual due to eruption of the permanent tooth. The apical portion of the primary root curves facially. **B,** Lateral displacement injuries to the primary tooth generally force the primary root facially with little injury to the erupting permanent tooth.

tooth if this is allowed to occur.[25] Furthermore, there is the possibility of increased damage to the permanent tooth by attempts to extract the traumatized primary tooth.[162] Reeruption will generally occur in 1 to 6 months.[18,133] If the intruded primary tooth does not reerupt in 2 to 3 months, it may be ankylosed and have to be extracted. Also, if cellulitis develops, the intruded primary tooth should be extracted.

If the primary root is displaced lingually into the developing permanent tooth, the primary tooth should be extracted.[18] The primary anterior tooth root is resorbed initially from the lingual. There is also a facial curvature to the remaining root. Since most traumatic accidents are from a frontal direction, we believe that primary anterior tooth displacements force the crown lingually and the root facially (Fig. 15-21). Consequently, the incidence of primary anterior teeth being driven into the developing permanent tooth is quite low.

The parent and child should be warned of the likelihood that serious damage to the developing tooth will occur when the primary tooth is driven into the developing permanent tooth. Insurance and litigation possibilities require careful records of the accident until the permanent teeth have erupted and have been carefully examined for developmental disturbances.

There is a distinct conflict of opinion concerning treatment of displaced primary teeth. One opinion is that these teeth should be extracted.[18,59] An opposing view, which we hold, is that displaced primary teeth should be retained (Fig. 15-22).

The reasoning behind our view is that for primary teeth endodontic therapy is a successful procedure. If the primary tooth is displaced rather than avulsed, it generally has a sufficient root to reattach in the socket. Therefore, if it can be repositioned and stabilized, it should be retained just as a permanent tooth is retained. In our experience the facial curvature of the primary tooth enables it to be snapped back into position, often not even requiring a splint. If the tooth is mobile, an acid-etch splint for 7 to 10 days is desirable.

The open apex of the primary tooth lends itself to revascularization.[102] Sometimes root canal treatment is not necessary. If signs of pulpal necrosis such as persistent percussion sensitivity, radiographic evidence of periapical radiolucency, or continuing darkening of the tooth occurs, endodontic treatment should be instituted.

Intruded primary teeth that have been permitted to reerupt will have pulpal necrosis in approximately one third of the cases.[133] The diagnosis of pulpal necrosis is based upon tenderness, periapical radiolucencies, and discoloration. One study[102] showed that 50% of graying discolorations were reversible in primary teeth. The gray discoloration subsequently turned yellow from pulpal obliteration. Caution in diagnosing pulpal necrosis should be exercised. Pulpal necrosis of 6 weeks' duration with associated periapical inflammation did not cause damage to the developing permanent tooth in monkeys.[28] When pulpal necrosis of the primary tooth has been diagnosed, endodontic treatment of the primary teeth should be initi-

ated promptly to eliminate the periapical inflammation.

It is thought that the initial impact of injury to the primary tooth causes the greatest damage to the developing permanent tooth.[25,162,168] Consequently, if the decision has been made to retain a primary tooth with facial displacement of the root, routine pedodontic-endodontic therapy is justified to eliminate periapical inflammation of extended duration.

Minor fractures of the alveolar process

If comminuted minor bone fractures occur simultaneously with trauma to the teeth, they should be molded

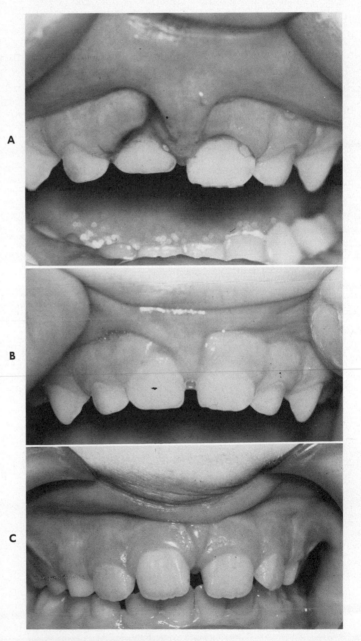

FIG. 15-22. Intruded primary tooth. **A,** Clinical view of the primary right maxillary central incisor. **B,** Six weeks later the tooth has reerupted spontaneously. **C,** Six-year clinical follow-up of the erupted permanent incisor. Note the very slight enamel hypoplasia defect at the gingival line.

back into place with the fingers (Fig. 15-19). No retained bone fragments should be discarded. The shorter the time interval between accident and repositioning of bone fragments, the greater will be the success rate.[3] This is due to the fact that the blood clot has not yet organized and exposure of bone to contamination has been minimized. If subsequent sequestration of bone occurs, the loss of periodontal support of involved teeth is permanent but the teeth may remain clinically functional.[3]

If the gingiva has been torn, it should be carefully sutured around the teeth at the cervical line. The teeth should be splinted for 7 to 10 days. However, if the fracture of bone is extensive, a longer splinting period may be required.

Complete avulsion and replantation

Complete avulsion or exarticulation occurs when a traumatic injury totally displaces a tooth from the socket. Variations in the reported incidence of complete avulsion range from 1% to 16% of all traumatic injuries to the permanent dentition and from 7% to 13% of traumatic injuries to the primary dentition.[2,66,75,138] Males experience complete avulsion three times as often as females; and the most frequently involved age groups are 7 to 11 years, as the permanent incisors are erupting.[20,21,78,118] According to Andreasen[18] the loosely structured periodontal ligaments surrounding erupting teeth favor complete avulsion.

The maxillary central incisors are the most frequently avulsed teeth in both the permanent and the primary dentition. Usually only one tooth is involved, and rarely are the mandibular teeth affected.

Factors affecting the success of replantation

Although there are reports of replanted teeth remaining in function over 40 years[20,34] replantation of avulsed teeth has generally been regarded as only a temporary measure. The average life span of the replanted tooth is reported to be 5 to 10 years; however, the period of retention may vary from a few weeks to a lifetime.[98] Despite the fact that reattachment usually occurs, most of the teeth are ultimately lost from progressive root resorption or problems associated with ankylosis in the growing child.

Many times the prognosis of the avulsed tooth is jeopardized by mismanagement of the situation. This is not surprising in light of the many conflicting techniques and philosophies contained in the replantation literature. Current techniques taught by various disciplines within dentistry differ greatly from those taught by other disciplines. Many of the previously accepted standards in treatment of avulsed teeth were based upon empiricism rather than scientific research, and numerous principles applied to the treatment of bony fractures had been erroneously adopted in the management of avulsed teeth. Although much remains to be discovered, the application of recent research has dramatically improved the prognosis for longer periods of retention of replanted teeth.

Extraoral time. Universal agreement exists that *the shorter the extraoral period the better the prognosis for retention of the replanted tooth.* Among the factors associated with root resorption, the length of extraoral time seems to be most critical.[2,7,20,60] The storage medium during extraoral time has also been shown to be critically related to the prognosis[12,40] (see below).

A well-documented clinical and radiographic study[20] with observation periods of 2 or more years showed that 90% of teeth replanted in less than 30 minutes exhibited no discernable resorption of the roots whereas 95% of teeth replanted after 2 hours demonstrated root resorption. These clinical findings have been substantiated by animal experiments.[1,12,18,71,113,119] The importance of extraoral time was summed up by Grossman and Ship,[78] who pointed out that success diminishes inversely with the length of time the tooth is out of the mouth; the longer the extraoral time, the less the success.

However, it should be noted that teeth may be replanted with success many hours or days after avulsion. Teeth replanted from 6 hours to 48 days after avulsion and treated endodontically were examined 1 to 7 years later and shown to be clinically functional. Although ankylosed and undergoing replacement resorption, there was no evidence of periapical infection.[86] Teeth replanted within a few minutes at the site where the injury occurred have the best prognosis for reattachment and prolonged retention. Consequently, when a parent or patient informs the dentist by telephone of an avulsed tooth, instructions should be given to replace the tooth in the socket. If the tooth is covered with debris, it can be cleaned by sucking on it or running cold tap water over it. The tooth should not be scrubbed or chemically cleansed in any manner. It is then teased into the socket and held in place until the patient reaches the dental office.

The education of allied professions as to the proper treatment to be rendered at the site of a dental injury is the responsibility of dentistry. Medical and allied personnel most likely to encounter injured persons after an accident should be able to render dental first aid and instruct patients as to the necessity of immediate dental care. Obviously medical injuries of a severe nature would take precedence over dental injuries. Individuals such as pediatricians, emergency room physicians and attendants, school nurses, athletic coaches and trainers, police officers, firemen, and other emergency personnel likely to be the first on the site of an injury or the first consulted following an injury should be instructed in proper first aid for dental injuries.[49]

Storage media and transportation of avulsed teeth.
Whenever possible, the avulsed tooth should be replanted at the site of the injury. If this is not possible, the tooth must be kept moist. A recent study by Andreasen[12] has shown that the storage medium may be more important than the extraoral time. Short periods of dry storage proved harmful, whereas prolonged storage in physiologic saline or saliva did not significantly impair periodontal healing. Surface resorption was found to be similar, regardless of the extraoral time or storage medium; however, inflammatory resorption was much more with dry storage. Replacement resorption was significantly increased with dry storage or storage in tap water. It was concluded that

physiologic saline or saliva offers good protection against root resorption during the extraoral period.[12]

Recent investigations[39-42] have shown that because of its physiologic osmolality and markedly fewer bacteria, milk may be superior to saliva for the storage of the avulsed tooth. While physiologic saline was satisfactory, it is not as readily available as milk. When teeth were stored in milk, much less root resorption, especially inflammatory resorption, was observed than when they were stored in saliva. Storage of avulsed teeth in saliva for 2 to 3 hours

causes swelling and membrane damage to periodontal ligament cells due to saliva's nonphysiologic osmolality.[39,42] Unfortunately, long-term studies are not available to confirm these short-term results.

Numerous investigations[12,14,23,38,154] have demonstrated the importance of keeping the avulsed tooth moist during the extraoral period. Allowing air drying of the periodontal ligament cells always increases resorption and ankylosis. While milk and physiologic saline are the best storage media, these may not readily be available when immediate

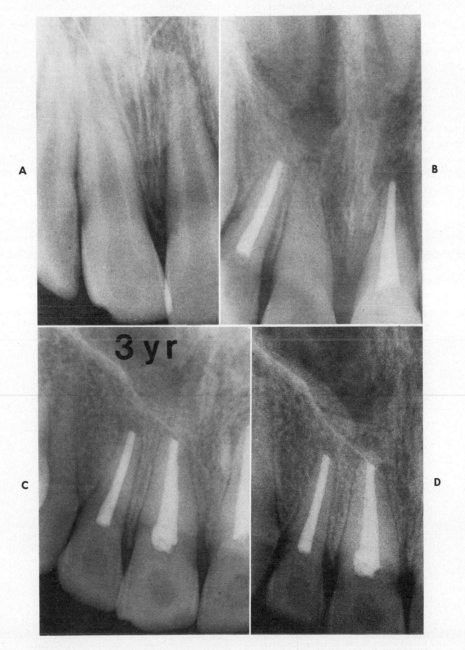

FIG. 15-23. Healing with a normal periodontal ligament after replantation. Extraoral time 30 minutes. **A,** Radiograph immediately after replantation of the left central incisor. **B,** Root canal of the replanted tooth filled with calcium hydroxide. Adjacent teeth required conventional root canal treatment due to pulpal necrosis. **C,** Three years after replantation. Calcium hydroxide was replaced with gutta-percha after 1 year. **D,** Seven years after replantation. Note the normal periodontal ligament space and the absence of root resorption.

replantation is impossible. In these cases, the tooth should be placed in the oral vestibule or under the tongue while the patient is transported to the dentist. If danger of aspiration exists because of the age of the patient or the extent of injury, the tooth may be placed in the mouth of the parent for transportation. At the very least, storage in a cup of tap water or a moist towel or sealing in plastic or foil to preserve the humidity is preferable to allowing the tooth to dry.

Using tissue culturing techniques, Söder et al.[152] demonstrated that after 2 hours of dry extraoral time, periodontal ligament cells will not demonstrate cell viability. As time increases, the number of viable cells declines very rapidly.

Preservation of the periodontal ligament and resorption. Preservation of a viable periodontal ligament around the replanted tooth is desirable. Extensive replacement resorption occurs when the periodontal tissues are removed before replantation.[15,18,23,119,167] It has been demonstrated that even after all the periodontal fibers are devitalized a tooth replanted with the periodontal tissues still attached resorbs more slowly than one replanted with denuded roots.[119] Therefore, regardless of the extraoral time, the periodontal ligament should not be removed or treated with any caustic chemicals prior to replantation of an avulsed tooth.

Andreasen[15] has concluded that the presence of an intact and viable periodontal ligament on the root surface is the *most* important factor in assuring healing without root resorption. He has also shown that resorption is more likely to occur on certain areas of the root surface of an avulsed

tooth than on others. These are the surfaces of the root receiving the most trauma during the removal of the tooth because the periodontal ligament is forced against the alveolar process, damaging cementoblasts. Resorption takes place on the root surfaces directly beneath the areas of cementoblastic damage.[16]

Following replantation a clot is formed in the torn periodontal ligament. Soon afterward, healing of the periodontal ligament begins with the proliferation of the connective tissue cells. The continuity of the periodontal ligament and supracrestal connective tissue is reestablished at 1 week. At 2 weeks new collagen fibers extend from the cementum to the alveolar bone. Periodontal healing is complete in 2 to 4 weeks when assessed histologically and by mobility tests. Surface resorption of the root was first recognized at 1 week and became prominent at 2 weeks.[11,21,125]

On the basis of histologic examination of replanted human and animal teeth, Andreasen[18] and Andreasen and Hjorting-Hansen[21] have divided periodontal healing into three types:

Healing with a normal periodontal ligament. Complete repair of the periodontal ligament occurs with this type of healing. Small areas of resorption representing localized areas of damage to the periodontal ligament, termed surface resorption, are present on the root. These usually involve only cementum but occasionally involve dentin. When dentin is resorbed, healing occurs with an altered root outline.[9,12,16] A normal-appearing periodontal space is seen radiographically. The tooth is not ankylosed (Fig. 15-23).

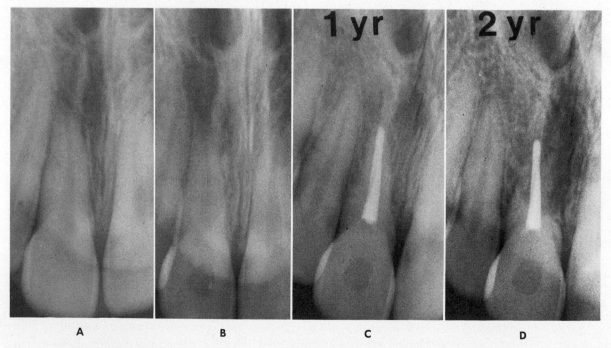

FIG. 15-24. Healing with replacement resorption and ankylosis. Extraoral time 90 minutes. **A,** Radiograph immediately after replantation of the right maxillary central incisor. **B,** Calcium hydroxide placement 1 month after replantation. **C,** Gutta-percha placed after removal of the calcium hydroxide 1 year after replantation. **D,** Two years after replantation. The tooth is resorbing and ankylosed. Note the lack of periodontal ligament space.

Healing with ankylosis or replacement resorption. Ankylosis occurs when areas of root resorption are repaired by the deposition of bone, resulting in a fusion of the root surface and the alveolar bone (Fig. 15-24). Andreasen[8,16] showed that ankylosis develops as a response in the periodontium to areas of damage to the periodontal ligament or root surface occurring as the tooth is avulsed or because of storage conditions before replantation. It may be temporary in areas of minor damage and later cease. Andreasen has termed this type transient replacement resorption.[18]

In more extensive injuries (i.e., denuded periodontal ligaments or teeth subjected to drying) the entire root is gradually resorbed and replaced by bone. Andreasen has termed this progressive replacement resorption[18] (Fig. 15-24).

Replacement resorption can be observed histologically in 2 weeks[11] and radiographically in 2 months.[20] Radiographically the normal periodontal space is absent and radiolucencies are not present. Clinically the tooth is immobile (Figs. 15-24 and 15-25).

Ankylosis usually does not present a problem in the fully formed jaw of an adult. Ankylosed teeth can be maintained until replacement resorption leads to loosening and exfoliation of the tooth. In younger patients, in whom maturation of the alveolar processes has not occurred, ankylosis may interfere with normal growth and development. When infraocclusion occurs in these patients, the tooth must be extracted and replaced prosthetically to prevent malocclusion.

Inflammatory resorption. Granulation tissue in the periodontal ligament adjacent to large areas of root resorption characterizes this type[21] (Fig. 15-26). Andreasen[9] has shown that these resorption defects occur on the root surface adjacent to areas of damage to the periodontal ligament during avulsion or extended drying before replanta-

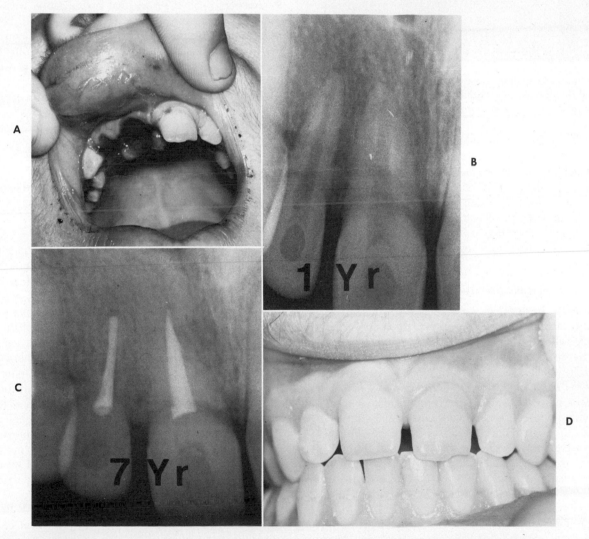

FIG. 15-25. Ankylosis subsequent to replantation 3½ hours after avulsion. **A,** Clinical view. **B,** Radiograph at 1 year. Canals have been repacked several times with calcium hydroxide. Note the loss of periodontal ligament space and the minor root resorption. **C,** Seven-year follow-up showing progressive replacement, resorption, and ankylosis. **D,** Clinical view 7 years after replantation. Despite ankylosis, the teeth are functioning normally.

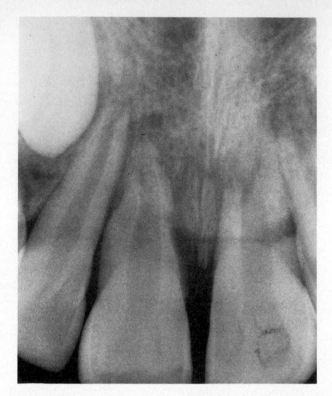

FIG. 15-26. Inflammatory root resorption after replantation. Root canal therapy was not instituted. Extensive root resorption has occurred within 3 months.

tion. The etiology is communication between the surface resorption and the pulp via the dentinal tubules. The mechanism of action is toxic products and bacteria penetrating from the root canal, which contains necrotic tissue, into the periodontal tissues, causing the inflammatory process.[5] Resorption, in turn, is accelerated. Root resorption may progress rapidly, resulting in loosening and early loss of the tooth. Endodontics may lead to evidence of repair in some cases.

Endodontic treatment of replanted teeth

Teeth with incomplete root formation. In avulsed teeth with incomplete root formation, revascularization may occur following replantation. Chances for revitalization are improved if replantation is achieved immediately or within 30 minutes. Studies[20,118,129] have shown that *the pulp will not survive after an extraoral time of 2 hours.*

Therefore in avulsed teeth with incomplete root formation replanted within 2 hours, pulp removal should be delayed until signs of pulpal necrosis are evident (Fig. 15-27). These teeth must be followed closely and, if signs of pulpal necrosis occur, endodontic treatment should immediately be instituted (Fig. 15-28). It is recommended that these patients be seen monthly until continued root development is evident or pulpal necrosis confirmed.

It is possible to achieve further root development in the replanted tooth with an incomplete root following revascularization; however, in most cases root formation ceases and obliteration of the pulp canal with dentin or bone occurs.[18,150] (Fig. 15-27).

The usual vitality tests are not very reliable following replantation. The radiograph should be checked carefully for any signs of developing pathosis. Vitality may be checked by oral examination for color changes by transillumination or tissue changes (e.g., inflammation or sinus tract formation) or by percussion sensitivity or mobility. Although functional repair of pulp nerve fibers has been shown to be reestablished in approximately 35 days following replantation,[129] the electric pulp tester is unreliable in teeth with incompletely formed roots.

If more than 2 hours has elapsed before replantation is achieved in the tooth with incomplete root development, the pulp should be removed following replantation and splinting. The treatment is with calcium hydroxide, the same as that outlined later for the avulsed tooth with a fully formed root. In our experience the prognosis for such teeth is poor.

Teeth with complete root formation. Although reported,[20,129] revascularization of the pulp following replantation of avulsed teeth with fully formed roots is rare. Researchers[117] have shown that revitalization was significantly related to the stage of root development, being almost complete in immature teeth while almost totally lacking in young mature or mature teeth. With fully formed roots, the usual sequelae are pulpal necrosis and accompanying inflammatory resorption. Therefore *all replanted teeth with complete root formation must be treated endodontically.*

Numerous investigations comparing fully developed replanted teeth with and without endodontic treatment have shown more favorable results in the former.* Periapical abscess formation invariably formed when the pulp tissue was not removed (Fig. 15-26), whereas teeth with root canal fillings did not show such abscesses (Figs. 15-23 and 15-25).

Andreasen[13,17] has shown the mechanism of action to be communication with infected dentinal tubules under areas of surface resorption on the root adjacent to injury to the periodontal ligament. When the resorptive defect is deep enough to communicate with dentinal tubules, toxic elements enter the periodontal ligament through the exposed tubules and create an inflammatory response. Inflammatory root resorption was always related to either a leukocytic zone or necrotic pulp tissue adjacent to the dentinal tubules communicating with the resorption site. Vital pulp tissue was never found in relation to active inflammatory root resorption. When bacteria were present, inflammatory resorption was worse. If the resorptive defect is shallow and does not penetrate the cemental surface, inflammatory resorption does not occur since the toxic elements do not reach the periodontal ligament but are arrested by the cementum. If the pulp contains vital tissue or if root canal filling has been done, only surface resorption occurs irrespective of the depth of the resorptive cavities.[13,17] Therefore early removal of pulp tissue and placement of a root canal filling should be part of the replantation procedure.

---

*References 5,13,17,20,21,31,60.

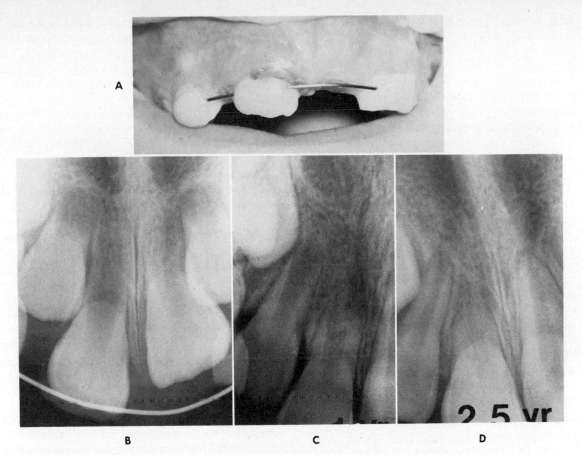

FIG. 15-27. Replantation of a tooth with incomplete root formation. Extraoral time 15 minutes. **A,** Clinical view with acid-etch resin and wire splint immediately after replantation and splinting. **B,** Radiograph same day. **C,** Continued root development and pulpal obliteration 1 year later. **D,** Complete pulpal obliteration and blunting of root development 2 years after replantation.

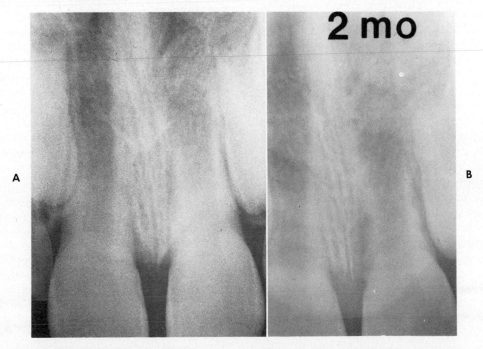

FIG. 15-28. Replantation of a tooth with incomplete root formation. Extraoral time 30 minutes. **A,** Immediately after replantation. **B,** Two months later root resorption is apparent. If root resorption is to be arrested, endodontic treatment with calcium hydroxide must be started immediately. However, the prognosis is poor due to advanced root resorption in an immature root.

When inflammatory resorption has begun, it can sometimes be arrested by removal of the necrotic pulp tissue and placement of a calcium hydroxide filling within the root canal.[4] (See below.)

In the past, controversy has existed over whether to perform endodontic treatment before or after replantation. It is now known that since root canal treatment would prolong the extraoral period it should be accomplished *after* replantation. Further damage to the periodontal ligament from handling the tooth or exposure to chemicals during the endodontic procedure can be avoided. Also, a source of bacterial contamination, which Andreasen believes may be significantly related to resorption, may be eliminated by decreased manipulation of the avulsed tooth.[19]

Although some workers[37,53,145] have found that immersion of the roots of replanted teeth of experimental animals in 1% to 2% solutions of sodium fluoride or acidulated sodium fluoride before replantation decreased the amount and severity of root resorption, others[32] have found no significant reduction in resorption. Adequate research does not exist to warrant recommending this procedure. Coating of the roots of avulsed teeth with a biodegradable compound, polylactic acid, in an attempt to inhibit resorption and ankylosis has also been shown to be ineffective.[81]

Replantation technique

The avulsed tooth must be replanted as soon as possible, preferably at the site where the injury occurred. Care must be taken to avoid further damage to the periodontal tissues. Obvious contamination with soil or foreign matter should be cleaned with physiologic saline or water. The periodontal ligament should not be removed or the root altered in any manner, and *no* attempt should be made to sterilize the tooth.

The pulp should not be removed, and alternative treatments such as apical seal of the root with alloy or other materials are contraindicated. Removal of the apex and creation of openings in the root surface to encourage revascularization have proved fruitless.[149]

Venting or raising a tissue flap for purposes of creating a vent through the cortical bone is unnecessary and only causes more tissue damage and inflammation.

The alveolar socket should be examined; and if fracture has occurred, it may be necessary to reposition the fractured bone prior to replantation. Fracture of the alveolar bone has been shown to lead to earlier and more rapid progression of root resorption in replanted teeth.[20] However, Andreasen has shown that vital periodontal ligament is able to induce the formation of new alveolar bone.[14] Therefore it is possible to obtain reattachment of replanted teeth if part of the alveolar socket is destroyed during the accident.

Maintenance of the periodontal tissues within the socket is important and has been shown to play a role in resorption and ankylosis.[124] Therefore, one must not curette the socket. If a blood clot is present, it should be removed by irrigation rather than curettage. Andreasen[10] found similar results in animals whether the coagulum was removed before replantation or the tooth was replanted with the coagulum in situ.

The use of local anesthetic is usually not necessary. Often the pain associated with the injection is more severe than the pain from replantation. Even when soft tissue lacerations necessitate the use of anesthetic, the tooth should be replanted immediately to minimize the extraoral time.

The tooth is replanted and repositioned with light finger pressure. A radiograph should be exposed to verify the adequacy of the repositioning. Any soft tissue lacerations are sutured to arrest seepage of hemorrhage prior to splinting of the tooth.

Antibiotics and tetanus prophylaxis. Although Andreasen[19] has presented some preliminary evidence to warrant their use, the administration of antibiotics has not been shown to promote healing of replanted teeth in experimental animals.[121] Since acute infections rarely occur with replantation of avulsed teeth, the routine administration of antibiotics is not justified when the pulp tissue is to be removed within the first 2 weeks. Patients with obviously contaminated teeth or medical indications for prophylactic antibiotics are exceptions.

If the avulsed tooth or wound has been contaminated with soil, the patient must receive a tetanus injection. In other situations clinical judgment may be used in making this determination.

Pulp extirpation and calcium hydroxide root canal filling. The use of calcium hydroxide in the treatment of inflammatory root resorption was first reported by Andreasen.[4] The material was used in replanted teeth with incomplete root formation in which inflammatory root resorption had begun following pulp necrosis. This technique evolved from the use of calcium hydroxide to promote apexification in pulpless teeth with undeveloped apices. Calcium hydroxide was later reported to inhibit root resorption when endodontic treatment was performed and the canals temporarily filled with calcium hydroxide paste.[60] Since that time the use of these pastes to inhibit root resorption has become the accepted treatment.[50] The exact mode of action of calcium hydroxide in inhibiting resorption is unknown. A number of theories have been proposed. Webber's report[169] on the expanded endodontic role of calcium hydroxide provides a thorough review of these theories.

Endodontics should be instituted within 1 or 2 weeks after replantation to prevent the development of inflammatory root resorption. As stated earlier, root canal treatment is achieved after replantation of the avulsed tooth to avoid further damage to the periodontal ligament and to minimize extraoral time.

Andreasen[13] has shown that there is increased replacement and surface root resorption when gutta-percha fillings are placed in avulsed teeth prior to replantation compared to those left untreated or with extirpated pulps. This is due to increased extraoral time and further damage to the periodontal ligament from handling and/or chemical contact. Pulp extirpation did not increase resorption in these teeth as compared to those with nonextirpated pulps.

To prevent inflammatory root resorption, the pulp must be extirpated within 1 or 2 weeks following replantation. This may be achieved through the splint placed during the emergency appointment. Since the tooth will not be firmly attached, extirpation should be done before the splint is removed. The presence of the splint may make use of the rubber dam difficult. As in all endodontic procedures, however, isolation of the tooth is essential; therefore, if placing the rubber dam is difficult, an alternative is to use sponges and cotton rolls with the patient seated upright.

When endodontic treatment is rendered without the rubber dam, strong precautionary measures must be taken to avoid the accidental swallowing or aspiration of endodontic instruments or irrigants. This is achieved by tying dental floss on the handles of the instruments. In cases of accidental dropping, the floss serves as a means of retrieval. A more desirable alternative is to prepare a large opening in the rubber dam that allows several teeth to fit through. A rubber dam clamp is placed on the teeth mesial and distal to the tooth undergoing endodontic treatment.

The usual access cavity is made, the pulp extirpated, and the access cavity sealed with a sterile cotton pellet and a temporary restoration placed. The tooth should *never* be left open to drain, as this will allow the ingress of bacteria and debris, leading to inflammatory root resorption.

Placement of calcium hydroxide in the root canal should be delayed 1 to 2 weeks following replantation. Andreasen[11] has shown that immediate insertion of the calcium hydroxide in replanted teeth causes noticeably more replacement resorption than is seen in teeth with extirpated pulps or gutta-percha fillings. He postulates that calcium hydroxide diffuses through the apical foramen, further injuring the periodontal ligament. He has also pointed out[11] that inflammatory resorption is initiated at around 2 weeks, about the time that periodontal healing is occurring[7]; therefore, this seems to be the ideal time for placement of the calcium hydroxide (Figs. 15-23 to 15-25).

Before the calcium hydroxide is placed, the root canal is thoroughly cleaned by routine endodontic treatment. As with any endodontic procedure, the use of the rubber dam is advisable. The working length is established radiographically or with the Neo-Sono, care being taken to avoid overextension of instruments through the apex of the tooth into the periapical tissues. The canal is cleaned with endodontic instruments and frequently irrigated with sodium hypochlorite.

After mechanical debridement of the canal, it is thoroughly dried and filled with a thick paste of calcium hydroxide and water. The paste is carried into the canal with an amalgam carrier and packed with blunt-ended pluggers until it reaches the apex. The addition of some dry calcium hydroxide powder within the canal will aid in condensing the material to the apex. The use of a Lentulo spiral, the McSpadden compactor, or syringes to carry the material into the canal is also an acceptable method of filling.

Vehicles other than water that have been used to form the paste with calcium hydroxide include camphorated parachlorophenol (CMCP), Cresanol, physiologic saline, and anesthetic solution. Although clinically the results with these agents seem to be the same, Cvek[59] has warned against combining calcium hydroxide with intracanal medicaments because of their proved damage to periapical tissues.

Commercial preparations of calcium hydroxide (e.g.,

Pulpdent, Hypo-Cal, Calxyl) are acceptable as the filling paste, but their consistency makes them more difficult to use. Calcium hydroxide preparations that set into a hard mass and have a short working time (e.g., Dycal) are *unacceptable* since the filling procedure cannot be completed before the material sets and they are more difficult to remove from the canal prior to final placement of gutta-percha. Small amounts of barium sulfate may be added to aid in radiographic interpretation without altering the reaction of the calcium hydroxide. (Fig. 15-20, *C* and *D*).

The canal is generally filled without the use of local anesthetic. The patient's feeling is used as a guide in determining the depth of the filling paste. An attempt is made to fill the canal completely but to avoid overfilling. If overfilling occurs, no attempt is made to remove the excess since the material is absorbable.[94] Radiographic checks are made to verify the depth of the filling.

If conditions are not ideal for placement of the root canal filling after instrumentation (i.e., the canal cannot be dried thoroughly), the tooth may be temporarily closed again. Usually when these circumstances occur, the canal is medicated with calcium hydroxide paste and closed for a few weeks, after which the canal is recleaned and repacked.

When the canal is satisfactorily filled, the outer 3 to 4 mm of the access opening is sealed with a permanent filling material. Silicate cement or composite resin is the material of choice in anterior teeth, and amalgam for posterior teeth. It is necessary to place a permanent-type restoration in the access cavity since loss of the outer seal will quickly lead to loss of the root canal filling paste and the initiation of an infection with inflammatory root resorption.

Since calcium hydroxide is an absorbable material, it will eventually begin to dissipate out of the canal in some teeth. If this happens, the canal may become infected and an inflammatory resorption may be initiated. Therefore it is necessary to reclean and repack the canal periodically. The optimum time for this has not been established, and probably varies among individuals, but it is generally agreed that it should be done every 3 to 6 months until the decision is made to fill the canal with a permanent filling of gutta-percha.

We have noted that radiographically visible resorption terminates after the canals are filled with calcium hydroxide. In teeth treated endodontically within 2 weeks after replantation and filled with calcium hydroxide, there is usually no radiographic evidence of resorption as long as the calcium hydroxide filling remains intact. The mode of action of calcium hydroxide in inhibiting resorption is unknown. Investigators[163] have shown an increase in the pH of dentin in teeth in which the canals have been filled with calcium hydroxide. They have speculated that the rise in pH stimulates the repair processes of the tissues while reducing the resorptive process, since an acidic environment is necessary for osteoclastic activity.

While calcium hydroxide is present in the canal, the patient is recalled every 3 months and instructed to return immediately if any adverse symptoms occur before that time. If evidence of periapical involvement due to breakdown of the filling material exists, the canal is immedi

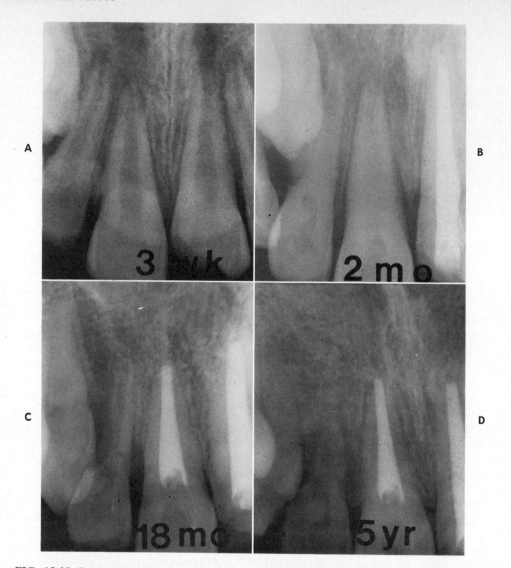

FIG. 15-29. Replantation of a permanent tooth adjacent to an erupting permanent tooth. **A,** Three weeks after replantation of the right maxillary central and lateral incisors adjacent to the erupting canine. **B,** Placement of calcium hydroxide in the replanted teeth. Routine endodontics has been completed on the left central incisor. **C,** Canine erupted. Note the advanced resorption of the lateral incisor. Calcium hydroxide was repacked every 3 months in the right lateral incisor. Gutta-percha has been placed in the right central. **D,** Massive root resorption of the right lateral incisor 5 years after replantation.

ately recleaned and refilled. Otherwise, it is recleaned and refilled every 3 to 6 months. The optimum time for retention of the calcium hydroxide prior to placement of a permanent gutta-percha filling is unknown. Empirically the minimum time for retention has been established as 1 year.

When a replanted tooth is adjacent to an erupting tooth, as in the case of a lateral incisor before eruption of the canine, there is acceleration of the resorptive process. In these cases it is advised that calcium hydroxide be left in the canal until the adjacent tooth has erupted (Fig. 15-29).

Permanent root canal filling with gutta-percha. Since calcium hydroxide is not a permanent root canal filling, the replanted tooth must ultimately be filled with gutta-percha (Figs. 15-23 and 15-25). As stated, the optimum time for retention of the calcium hydroxide filling has not

been determined but empirically a minimum of 1 year seems to be adequate in most cases.[169]

After calcium hydroxide is removed from the root canal and gutta-percha placed, replacement resorption begins in many replanted teeth. This may be followed by ankylosis and possible loss of the tooth. However, many teeth show little evidence of resorption, or very slow resorption, and the prognosis for long retention of these is excellent (Fig. 15-25).

Although much has been learned about the replanted tooth, many unanswered questions remain. Numerous areas of replantation have had little or no scientific investigation, among them the role of immunology. It is hoped that continued research will develop treatments that enable practitioners to retain these replanted teeth permanently.

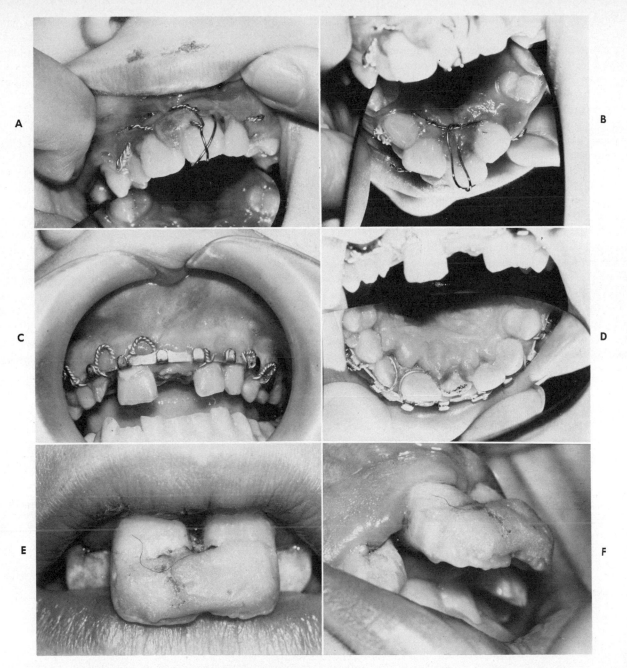

FIG. 15-30. Improper splinting. **A** and **B,** Maxillary left central incisor replanted. Note the inflammation of gingival tissues around the improperly placed wires. **C** and **D,** Improper use of an arch bar. The wires caused gingival inflammation and pressures on the teeth, resulting in facial displacement. **E** and **F,** Splinting. Maxillary central incisors replanted and splinted with fixation to an adjacent sound tooth. Note the incorporation of hair in the resin.

Splinting

The development of the acid-etch technique and the application of scientific research in the area of tooth-related injuries have revolutionized splinting. For years the principles and practice of treating bone fractures were erroneously applied to traumatized teeth. Many of the splinting techniques previously advocated were time consuming. Not only were the splints difficult to fabricate and difficult to remove, they also contributed to injury of the soft and hard supporting tissues.

Splinting techniques that cause gingival inflammation prevent the inflammatory response from resolving in the marginal gingiva and possibly around the replant. Splints that subject the teeth and alveolar bone to pressures and tensions in the same manner as active orthodontic appliances cause inflammation and resorption. Interdental wiring and arch bars ligated to the teeth cannot be passively placed and therefore have no place in treating tooth trauma unless as techniques of last resort. Wire ligatures activate the resorptive mechanism, create gingival irritation, and are difficult to apply as well as to remove and clean (Fig. 15-30).

The exact value and influence of splinting on pulpal and periodontal healing have not been determined.[18] It has been shown that splinting failed to improve healing and exerted a harmful effect upon periodontal healing by increasing the extent of pulpal necrosis and inflammatory root resorption when compared to nonsplinting.[116]

Studies[6] have shown that rigid splinting of replanted teeth increases the amount of root resorption. Rigid splinting after replantation is a detriment rather than an asset.[96] Poor formation of collagen fibers has been found with prolonged and rigid splinting and the postulation advanced that since little tension can be transmitted during rigid fixation this may cause atrophy and increased susceptibility to ankylosis.[96] However, some degree of mobility is desirable for proper regeneration, functional orientation, and development after the initial attachment occurs.[96] Consequently Andreasen[18] has advised that replanted teeth be splinted for a minimum of 1 week since this time is sufficient to secure adequate periodontal healing.

The requirements for an acceptable splint are as follows[49]:

1. Easy to fabricate directly in the mouth without lengthy laboratory procedures
2. Can be placed passively without causing forces on the teeth
3. Does not contact the gingival tissues, causing gingival irritation
4. Does not interfere with normal occlusion
5. Is easily cleaned and allows for proper oral hygiene
6. Should not traumatize the teeth or gingiva during application
7. Allows approach for endodontic therapy
8. Is easily removed

The acid-etch resin and arch wire splint, as advocated by Heiman et al.,[85] usually satisfies all the above requirements (Fig. 15-31). The use of a 20 or 30 pound test monofilament nylon line as a substitute for the arch wire has been advocated since this would allow a degree of physiologic movement and possibly result in less resorption[29] (Fig. 15-31).

In this technique an orthodontic wire is bent to passively conform to the facial surfaces of the teeth, encompassing at least one sound tooth on each side of the injured tooth or teeth. Any size or shape of the wire is acceptable as

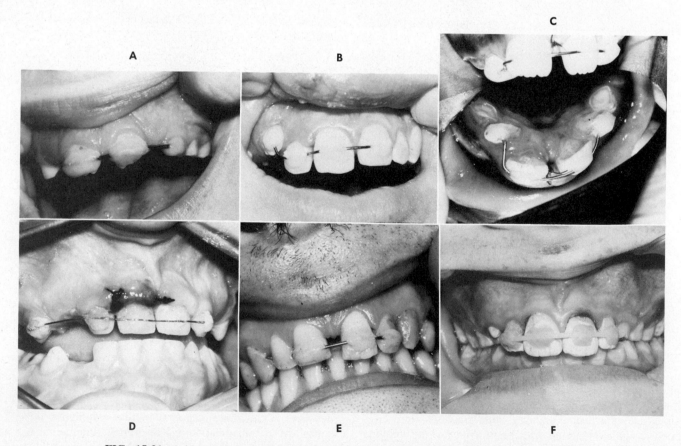

FIG. 15-31. Acid-etch-resin-and-arch-wire splint. **A,** Splinting in the mixed dentition utilizing primary and permanent tooth abutments. **B** and **C,** Splints attached to erupting teeth. **D,** Splinting across an edentulous space. **E,** Use of a paper clip for the arch wire. **F,** A Monofilament nylon line used as a substitute for the arch wire allows a degree of physiologic movement.

long as it is at least 0.015 or larger. The middle third of the facial surfaces of the crowns is etched with phosphoric acid for 1 to 2 minutes. The etching gels work better than liquids, since tissue seepage is generally a problem. After the teeth are thoroughly washed and dried, the arch wire is attached to the facial surfaces with resin. Any form of resin or composite is acceptable for attaching the wire to the teeth.

The wire is attached to the uninjured teeth first and the resin allowed to cure. Only a small amount of resin in the middle third of the exposed crown is necessary to hold the splint. The injured teeth are then attached to the wire with resin, care being taken to ensure that they are in the proper position. A radiograph is taken for verification.

An alternative to this technique is the use of direct-bonded orthodontic brackets and the application of an arch wire.[95] However, this is more time consuming and requires measures to ensure that the arch wire is totally passive.

Although it is possible that some injuries are so extensive that this type of splint cannot be utilized to treat traumatized teeth, we have not encountered such a situation. Extensive injuries in which tissue seepage prevents drying of the teeth may require fabrication of acrylic or cast metal splints that are cemented or held by interdental wiring. However, these types of splints are reserved for situations in which direct-bonding techniques are impossible or impractical.

When one is splinting in the primary dentition with acid-etch techniques, the bonding must be enhanced by roughening the facial surface of the teeth to be etched with a rough diamond stone prior to placing the etching gel. After splint removal the roughened teeth should be polished.

The use of the acid-etch-resin-and-arch-wire splint does not interfere with the occlusion; therefore mastication on the posterior teeth is possible. On mandibular anterior splints, where the wire on the facial would interfere with occlusion, the arch wire is placed on the lingual surface. The patient is instructed not to bite on the injured tooth for several weeks. Food should be cut into bite-sized pieces and placed in the mouth rather than incised.

The patient is instructed in proper oral hygiene and the importance of keeping the area clean. It is usually possible to continue brushing and flossing immediately after the splint is placed.

Removal of the acid-etch-resin-and-arch-wire splint is simple (Fig. 15-32). A high-speed diamond with copious water supply is used to grind through the resin to expose and free the wire. It is not necessary or advisable to remove all fragments of the resin at the time of splint removal. Since complete healing of the periodontal tissues has not occurred at 1 week, excessive manipulation may cause displacement of the teeth. When the wire is removed, the remaining resin is smoothed and left in place for several weeks. After healing is complete, the resin can be removed with a sharp scaler or carver.

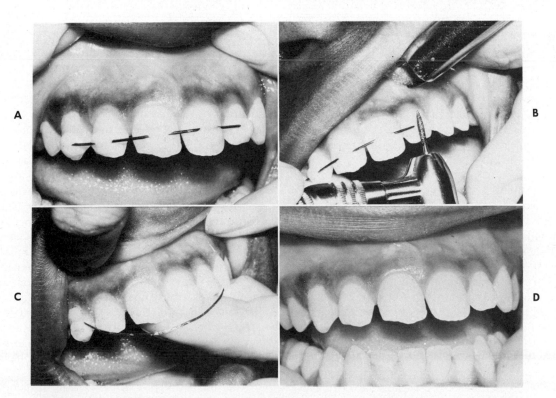

FIG. 15-32. Removal of acid-etch-resin-and-arch-wire splint. **A,** Splint ready for removal. **B,** High-speed diamond with copious water spray used to grind through the resin and free the arch wire. **C,** Wire removed. **D,** Resin smoothed. Remnants will be removed after healing is completed.

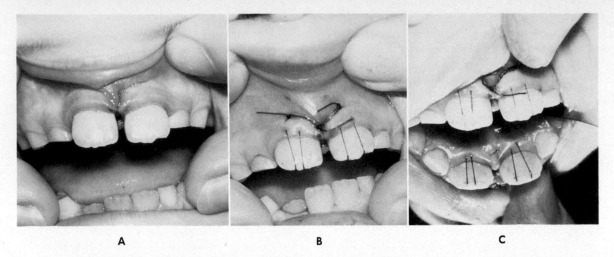

FIG. 15-33. Suture splint. **A,** The maxillary central incisors have been replanted. The short clinical crowns of the primary teeth make it difficult to place the acid-etch-resin-and-arch-wire splint. The facial surfaces of the central incisors are acid-etched. **B** and **C,** A suture is placed in the facial tissue 5 to 6 mm above the gingival margin and is passed over the incisal of the tooth and into the lingual tissue. It then recrosses the incisal edge into the facial tissue and is tied. Resin is placed on the facial surface to maintain the suture in position.

Problems may be encountered in very young or retarded patients who will not tolerate a foreign material such as a splint in their mouth. Occasionally in the primary or early mixed dentition there are no adjacent teeth or not enough exposed tooth structure on which to attach acid-etch resin. In these cases a suture splint (as advocated by Rand[132] and modified by Camp[49]) is easily applied and provides good stabilization. After the injured tooth is repositioned, its facial surface is acid-etched. Next a suture is passed through the gingiva above the facial surface, carried over the incisal edge of the tooth and into the lingual gingival tissue, and brought out again. The suture is then passed over the incisal edge and again into the facial gingival tissue, where it is drawn tight and tied. A small amount of resin is cured over the facial surface and the suture to assure retention of the suture on the incisal edge (Fig. 15-33).

Duration of splinting

Confusion exists as to the optimum time that a splint should be left in place. This confusion is related to the diversity of situations requiring splinting.

Recent studies[6,96] have shown that rigid splinting of replanted teeth *increases* resorption and ankylosis. Therefore replanted teeth should be splinted for a minimum length of time. Andreasen[18] has pointed out that 1 week is sufficient to secure adequate periodontal support, since gingival fibers are healed during this time. The recommended splinting time for displaced and avulsed teeth is 7 to 10 days.

The optimum time for leaving a splint in place for displaced or avulsed teeth in combination with alveolar fracture has not been determined. We suggest 14 to 21 days. More extensive bone fractures may require longer splinting times. Root fractures require the longest splinting period (10 to 12 weeks) because of the time required for callus formation on the root.

PREVENTION OF TRAUMATIC INJURIES TO THE TOOTH

At the beginning of this chapter is the oft quoted statement: "Hindsight explains the injury that foresight would have prevented." In all previous sections of the chapter we have looked at injuries that have already occurred (i.e., hindsight) and discussed methods of treating them. We must now use foresight and discuss ways to prevent some of these injuries. Because of the variety of ways they occur, however, it is unlikely that most of them can be prevented.

The remarkable story of prevention of dental injuries in football should encourage the profession to continue to look for ways to prevent traumatic oral injuries. In the 1940s and 1950s it was a source of pride among tough football players while talking to younger boys and girls to slip their "flipper" or "clicker" out of position with their tongue. The remaining gap-toothed grin was sufficiently startling that it invariably stimulated gasps of amazement among the boys and squeals of shock among the girls.

In those days of unprotected hard-nose football, oral or facial injuries constituted 50% of football mishaps. There was a 10% chance each year that a player would have such an injury. However, with the introduction of the face guard and padded helmets, approximately half of these injuries have been eliminated.[87] In 1962 the National High School Alliance Football Rules Committee adopted a ruling requiring high school football players to wear mouth guards. Within 5 years the incidence of dental injuries dropped to less than 0.3%.[159]

After documentation of the benefits of mouth guards in reducing head and neck injuries[92,158] as well as dental injuries, the National Collegiate Athletic Association Football Rules Committee adopted a mouth protector requirement in 1973. The mandatory use of mouth guards has

EMERGENCY PROCEDURES FOR INJURED TEETH

Fractured anterior tooth

1. Pulp *not* exposed
   a. Cover exposed dentin with $Ca(OH)_2$ or ZOE.
   b. Place acid-etch resin (resin will not set in contact with ZOE) or band over dressing to maintain seal.
   c. Restore tooth permanently in 6 to 8 weeks.
2. Pulp exposed in tooth with *open apex*
   a. Pulp cap with $Ca(OH)_2$ if treatment performed within 3 to 4 hours after injury.
   b. If massive pulp exposure or exposure over 3 to 4 hours, perform pulpotomy to maintain vitality and allow root completion. After root completion, perform root canal filling as necessary.
   c. If pulp necrotic, perform apexification procedure ($Ca(OH)_2$ powder) to induce apical closure. After root completion, fill canal with gutta-percha as permanent filling.
3. Pulp exposed tooth with fully formed root
   a. Perform root canal therapy, if you do not wish to try to preserve pulpal vitality with pulp capping.

Root fracture

1. Time critical
   a. Reposition segment as soon as possible and maintain vitality of pulp.
   b. Must achieve repositioning before blood clots.
2. Acid-etch resin arch wire splint for 10 to 12 weeks
3. No root canal therapy *unless* evidence of pulpal pathosis
4. If root fracture communicates with oral cavity, prognosis is poor for reuniting segments

Displaced tooth

1. Time critical—reposition immediately (within 1 to 2 hours)
   a. Reposition the tooth correctly.
   b. Splint with acid-etch resin arch wire for 7 to 10 days.
   c. Perform endodontic therapy if pulpal pathosis is confirmed during recalls.
      (1) Severe displacements (more than 5 mm) will usually require root canal therapy and $Ca(OH)_2$ powder filling. (See "$Ca(OH)_2$ root canal filling technique.")
      (2) Minor displacements should be followed closely to determine vitality. These teeth may not respond normally to electric pulp testing for several months.
   d. If bony involvement, see section on alveolar fractures.

Intruded tooth

1. Open apex, divergent canals
   a. If minor, leave alone.
   b. If severe, can surgically or orthodontically reposition.
      (1) May need to perform endodontic treatment.
      (2) Prognosis guarded.
2. Fully formed root
   a. Reposition surgically or orthodontically promptly.
   b. If surgically repositioned, splint with acid-etch resin arch wire for 7 to 10 days.
   c. Pulp must be removed during first 2 weeks.
   d. Clean canal and fill with $Ca(OH)_2$ powder.
   e. After 6 to 12 months, fill canal permanently with gutta-percha.

Minor fractures of the alveolar process associated with traumatized teeth

1. Bony fragments repositioned
2. Soft tissues sutured as necessary
3. Teeth splinted with acid-etch resin arch wire, left in place 7 to 14 days
4. *More extensive fractures* of bone require longer splinting period

Continued.

EMERGENCY PROCEDURES FOR INJURED TEETH—cont'd

Avulsed, tooth out of mouth

1. Replantation immediately at time of injury, if possible
   a. Time critical. Prognosis deteriorates rapidly as extraoral time increases.
   b. Instruct patient or parent by telephone to replant tooth immediately at site of injury.
      (1) If tooth dirty, rinse under tap water. Do not scrub, Plug sink.
      (2) Gently tease tooth back into socket.
      (3) Patient to hold tooth in socket while being transported to dental office.
   c. If replantation at site not possible.
      (1) Place tooth in glass of milk or physiologic saline, if available.
      (2) If milk or physiologic saline is not available, hold tooth in bucal vestibule while coming to office. If danger of swallowing or if patient medically impaired from injury, do not allow tooth to air dry. Place tooth in glass of water, wet towel, or plastic wrap.
      (3) As soon as patient arrives, replant tooth immediately.
   d. For alveolar fracture, refer to section above.
   e. Place acid-etch-resin-and-arch-wire splint for 7 to 10 days.
2. Replantation of tooth with open apex (blunderbuss apex)
   a. If *less* than 2 hours, replant and do not perform endodontics.
      (1) Revitalization is desired.
      (2) During recalls, if pulp becomes necrotic clean root canal and fill with $Ca(OH)_2$ powder. (See "$Ca(OH)_2$ root canal filling technique.")
   b. If *longer* than 2 hours, during first 2 weeks following replantation clean root canal and fill with $Ca(OH)_2$ powder.
3. Replantation with completed root development
   a. Remove pulp during first 2 weeks.
   b. Fill canal with $Ca(OH)_2$ powder. (See "$Ca(OH)_2$ root canal filling technique.")
   c. Endodontic therapy must *always* be performed in tooth with completed root development.

---

now extended to professional football.[44] It is estimated that over 200,000 injuries are being prevented annually.[48]

A particularly satisfying major side benefit of the mouth guard has been the reduction of head concussions and neck injuries requiring cervical traction.[158] One collegiate team reported elimination of head concussion injuries while players were wearing mouth guards during the season.[127]

The dental profession can take considerable pride in this outstanding accomplishment over the last 20 years. Football mouth guards for high school players have been fabricated as a voluntary public service by practicing dentists across the United States under the sponsorship of local dental societies at no cost, or perhaps minimal expense for materials, to the schools. A mouth guard program for the local high schools is an excellent project for a local dental society and enhances the stature of the profession of dentistry immeasurably.

The success of the football mouth guard program has not been duplicated in other sports. Although most boxers use mouth guards, not all ice hockey leagues require them. The rate of injury in ice hockey may be three to six times as great as that in football[52,109] The use of mouth guards must be encouraged in basketball, wrestling, soccer, rugby, lacrosse, auto racing, karate, judo, field hockey, and baseball.[47]

With the enormous growth in female athletics, attention must be given to prevention of dental injuries in female athletes. Currently, mouth protectors are not mandatory for any organized female sports.[48] Similarly, more emphasis needs to be placed on wearing mouth guards in unorganized sports.[107]

There is the oft repeated quote from the late football coach Vince Lombardi that "kissing is a contact sport, football is a collision sport.[159] If in a collision sport like football dental injuries can be reduced so dramatically, these other contact sports should also be able to enjoy a similar reduction in traumatic dental injuries. Individual sports like skiing, parachuting, gymnastics, hurdling, and diving should also require mouth guards.

It has been noted that currently more injuries occur from noncontact sports than from contact sports, because many contact sports participants are wearing mouth guards.[62] Stevens[159] has described the functions of mouth guards as follows:

1. They hold the soft tissues of the lips and cheeks away from the teeth and prevent laceration and bruising of the lips and cheeks against the hard and irregular teeth during impact.
2. They cushion and distribute the forces from direct frontal blows that would otherwise cause fracture or dislocation of anterior teeth.
3. They prevent the teeth in opposing arches from violent contact, which might chip or fracture teeth or damage supporting structures.
4. They provide the mandible with resilient but braced support, which absorbs impacts that might fracture

---

EMERGENCY PROCEDURES FOR INJURED TEETH—cont'd

Ca(OH)₂ root canal filling technique

1. Pulp extirpated, root canal thoroughly instrumented
2. Ca(OH)₂ powder to fill canal
   a. May use dry powder.
   b. Some prefer to make paste of Ca(OH)₂ with water.
   c. Others prefer a paste of Ca(OH)₂ with CMCP.
3. Canals recleaned and repacked with Ca(OH)₂ at 3-month intervals for *minimum* of 1 year
4. After completion of step 3, if resorption is arrested or nonexistent, canal filled with gutta-percha

The acid-etch resin arch wire splint

1. Orthodontic wire bent to conform to facial surfaces of teeth to be splinted
   a. At least one sound tooth on each side of displaced tooth or teeth must be included.
   b. Size or shape of wire is unimportant.
2. Arch wire attached to teeth with acid-etch resin
   a. Middle half of facial surfaces of teeth is etched with phosphoric acid gel or solution for 1 to 2 minutes.
   b. Teeth are thoroughly washed and dried.
   c. Arch wire is attached to facial surfaces of teeth with resin.
      (1) Any form of resin, composite, or light-cured resin is acceptable.
      (2) Only a small amount of resin in facial half of crown is necessary to hold arch wire.
      (3) Take care to avoid contact of resin with gingiva.
   d. During attachment of arch wire, one must ensure that injured tooth is in correct position.
      (1) Take radiograph following placement to verify correct position of injured tooth.
3. Instructions to patient
   a. Avoid biting on splinted teeth. Cut food into bite size and chew on posterior teeth.
   b. Remember to keep the area clean.
4. Removal of splint
   a. Resin and wire are drilled through and wire is freed.
   b. It is not advisable to remove all resin from injured teeth at time of splint removal.
      (1) Excessive manipulation of injured teeth may cause displacement.
      (2) Smooth resin and leave remnants for several months.
      (3) After teeth are firmly attached (2 to 3 months), fragments of remaining resin can be removed with sharp carver or scaler.

---

the unsupported angle or condyle of the mandible.

5. They help prevent concussions, cerebral hemorrhage, and possible death by holding jaws apart and acting as shock absorbers to prevent upward and backward displacement of the mandibular condyles against the base of the skull.
6. They give protection against neck injuries.
7. They are psychologic assets to contact sport athletes by increasing confidence and aggressiveness.
8. They fill the space and support adjacent teeth so that removable partial dentures can be removed during contact sports, preventing possible swallowing or aspiration of loose appliances.

Acceptance of mouth guards by athletes is very important. Adolescents accept mouth guards more readily than adults.[65] The qualities of a good mouth guard are adequate retention, comfort, ease of speech, resistance to wear and tear, ease of breathing, and protection for the teeth, gingiva, and lips.

The three most common types of mouth protectors are stock, mouth-formed, and custom-made.

The *stock* mouth guards come in one size and supposedly fit everyone. Therefore they are likely to be loose and ill-fitting. The protection afforded by them is questionable and it has been recommended that they be withdrawn from use.[165]

The *mouth-formed* protectors come in a manufacturer's kit and consist of an outer shell of plastic and an inner liner that can be adapted to the teeth by biting into the material after warming in hot water. These are the most popular of the three types because of their minimal expense and the fact that they can be produced for an entire team in a short time.

The *custom-fitted* mouth guards require an initial impression to make a stone model of the arches. The mouth guard is then individually custom made on the model. These offer the most protection but take more time and expense in preparation (Fig. 15-34).

• • •

Mouth guards have also been advocated for use in the operating room during general anesthesia.[91,128,142] Anterior

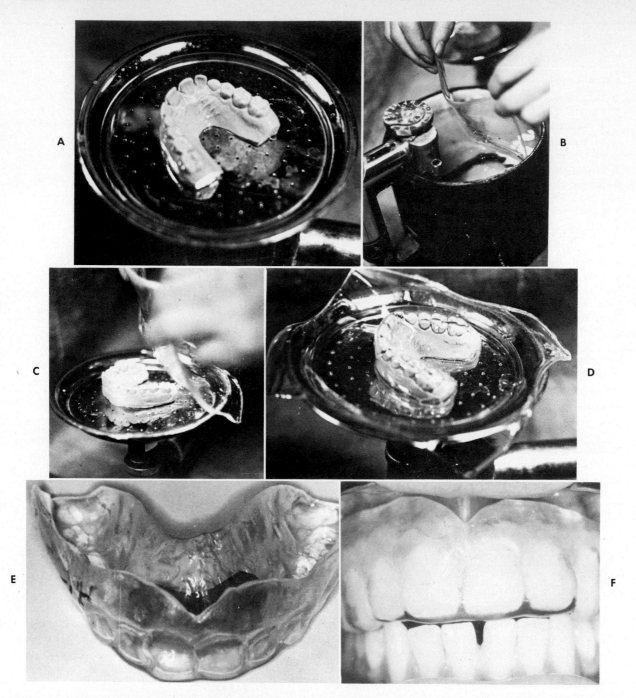

FIG. 15-34. Fabrication of a mouth protector. **A,** Stone model trimmed to obtain the best vacuum results. **B,** Sta-Guard material softened in a boiling water bath. **C,** Softened material placed over the cast with the vacuum activated. **D,** Vacuum-formed mouth protector. **E,** Finished implement. **F,** In place. (Courtesy Dr. Paul Vanek.)

teeth are vulnerable to chipping or displacement during orotracheal or nasotracheal intubation procedures. With the increase in microlaryngoscopic and esophagoscopic procedures anterior teeth and fixed prostheses are more frequently at risk. Simple acrylic mouth guards can be prepared preoperatively if the operating room procedure is of a nonemergency nature.

Custom-made mouth guards should be fabricated for handicapped children subject to frequent falls. Excellent retention is mandatory for these appliances.

Another preventive measure that can reduce traumatic injuries is prophylactic orthodontics. People with extreme overjet are two to five times as likely as other persons to suffer injury to their maxillary incisors.[104,159]

The use of seat belts and shoulder harnesses in automobiles is another common-sense precaution.

Education of the public is very important. The North Carolina Dental Society has developed a public-awareness campaign to educate coaches, teachers, industrial and school nurses, emergency medical personnel, and parents as to the proper procedures for handling dental emergencies, particularly the avulsed tooth. The outline on pp. 501 to 503 was distributed to all North Carolina dentists as a quick reminder of appropriate treatment.

REFERENCES

1. Anderson, A.W., Sharav, Y., and Massler, M.: Periodontal reattachment after tooth replantation, Periodontics **6**:161, 1968.
2. Andreasen, J.O.: Etiology and pathogenesis of traumatic dental injuries: a clinical study of 1,298 cases, Scand. J. Dent. Res. **78**:329, 1970.
3. Andreasen, J.O.: Luxation of permanent teeth due to trauma: a clinical and radiographic follow-up study of 184 injured teeth, Scand. J. Dent. Res. **78**:273, 1970.
4. Andreasen, J.O.: Treatment of fractured and avulsed teeth, J. Dent. Child. **38**:29, 1971.
5. Andreasen, J.O.: Effect of pulpal necrosis upon peridontal healing after surgical injury in rats, Int. J. Oral Surg. **2**:62, 1973.
6. Andreasen, J.O.: The effect of splinting upon periodontal healing after replantation of permanent incisors in monkeys, Acta Odontol. Scand. **33**:313, 1975.
7. Andreasen, J.O.: Periodontal healing after replantation of traumatically avulsed human teeth: assessment by mobility testing and radiography, Acta Odontol. Scand. **33**:325, 1975.
8. Andreasen, J.O.: Analysis of pathogenesis and topography of replacement root resorption (ankylosis) after replantation of mature permanent incisors in monkeys, Swed. Dent. J. **4**:231, 1980.
9. Andreasen, J.O.: Analysis of topography of surface and inflammatory root resorption after replantation of mature permanent incisors in monkeys, Swed. Dent. J. **4**:135, 1980.
10. Andreasen, J.O.: The effect of removal of the coagulum in the alveolus before replantation upon periodontal and pulpal healing of mature permanent incisors in monkeys, Int. J. Oral Surg. **9**:458, 1980.
11. Andreasen, J.O.: A time-related study of periodontal healing and root resorption activity after replantation of mature permanent incisors in monkeys, Swed. Dent. J. **4**:101, 1980.
12. Andreasen, J.O.: Effect of extra-alveolar period and storage media upon periodontal and pulpal healing after replantation of mature permanent incisors in monkeys,, Int. J. Oral Surg. **10**:43, 1981.
13. Andreasen, J.O.: The effect of pulp extirpation or root canal treatment on periodontal healing after replantation of permanent incisors in monkeys, J. Endod. **7**:245, 1981.
14. Andreasen, J.O.: Interrelation between alveolar bone and periodontal ligament repair after replantation of mature permanent incisors in monkeys, J. Periodont. Res. **16**:228, 1981.
15. Andreasen, J.O.: Periodontal healing after replantation and autotransplantation of incisors in monkeys, Int. J. Oral Surg. **10**:54, 1981.
16. Andreasen, J.O.: Relationship between cell damage in the periodontal ligament after replantation and subsequent development of root resorption: a time related study in monkeys, Acta Odontol. Scand. **39**:15, 1981.
17. Andreasen, J.O.: Relationship between surface and inflammatory resorption and changes in the pulp after replantation of permanent incisors in monkeys, J. Endod. **7**:294, 1981.
18. Andreasen, J.O.: Traumatic injuries of the teeth, ed. 2, Philadelphia, 1981, W.B. Saunders Co.
19. Andreasen, J.O.: Root fractures, luxation and avulsion injuries—diagnosis and management, Presented at the International Conference on Oral Trauma, Dallas, Texas, November 9, 1984.
20. Andreasen, J.O., and Hjorting-Hansen, E.: Replantation of teeth. I. Radiographic and clinical study of 110 human teeth replanted after accidental loss, Acta Odontol. Scand. **24**:263, 1966.
21. Andreasen, J.O., and Hjorting-Hansen, E.: Replantation of teeth. II. Histological study of 22 replanted anterior teeth in humans, Acta Odontol. Scand. **24**:287, 1966.
22. Andreasen, J.O., and Hjorting-Hansen, E.: Intraalveolar root fractures; radiographic and histological study of 50 cases, Oral Surg. **25**:414, 1967.
23. Andreasen, J.O., and Kristensson, L.: The effect of limited drying or removal of the periodontal ligament: periodontal healing after replantation of mature permanent incisors in monkeys, Acta Odontol. Scand. **39**:1, 1981.
24. Andreasen, J.O., and Kristerson, L.: The effect of extra-alveolar root filling with calcium hydroxide on periodontal healing after replantation of permanent incisors in monkeys, J. Endod. **7**:349, 1981.
25. Andreasen, J.O., and Ravn, J.J.: The effect of traumatic injuries to the primary teeth on their permanent successors, Scand. J. Dent. Res. **79**:284, 1971.
26. Andreasen, J.O., and Ravn, J.J.: Epidemiology of traumatic dental injuries to primary and permanent teeth in a Danish population sample, Int. J. Oral Surg. **1**:235, 1972.
27. Andreasen, J.O., and Ravn, J.J.: Enamel changes in permanent teeth after trauma to their primary predecessors, Scand. J. Dent. Res. **81**:203, 1973.
28. Andreasen, J.O., and Riis, I.: Influence of pulp necrosis and periapical inflammation of primary teeth on their permanent successors, Int. J. Oral Surg. **7**:178, 1978.
29. Antrim, D.D., and Ostrowski, J.S.: A functional splint for traumatized teeth, J. Endod. **8**:328, 1982.
30. Bakland, L.K.: Traumatic injuries. In Ingle, J.I., and Taintor, J.F., editors: Endodontics, ed. 3, Philadelphia, 1985, Lea & Febiger.
31. Barbakow, F.H., Austin, J.C., and Cleaton-Jones, P.E.: Experimental replantation of root-canal-filled and untreated teeth in the vervet monkey, J. Endod. **3**:89, 1977.
32. Barbakow, F.H., Cleaton-Jones, P.E., and Austin, J.C.: Healing of replanted teeth following topical treatment with fluoride solution and systemic admmission of thyrocalcitonin: a histometric analysis, J. Endod. **7**:302, 1981.
33. Barkin, P.R.: Time as a factor in predicting the vitality of traumatized teeth, J. Dent. Child. **40**:188, 1973.
34. Barry, G.N.: Replanted teeth still functioning after 42 years: report of a case, J. Am. Dent. Assoc. **92**:412, 1976.
35. Bhaskar, S.N., and Rappaport, H.M.: Dental vitality tests and pulp status, J. Am. Dent. Assoc. **86**:409, 1973.
36. Bielak, S., Bimstein, E., and Eidelman, E.: Forced eruption: the treatment of choice for subgingivally fractured permanent incisors, J. Dent. Child. **49**:186, 1982.
37. Bjorvatn, K., and Massler, M.: Effect of fluoride on root resorption in replanted rat molars, Acta Odontol. Scand. **29**:17, 1971.
38. Blomlöf, L., et al: Periodontal healing of replanted monkey teeth prevented from drying, Acta Odontol. Scand. **41**:117, 1983.
39. Blomlöf, L., et al.: Storage of experimentally avulsed teeth in milk prior to replantation, J. Dent. Res. **6**:912, 1983.
40. Blomlöf, L., Lindskog, S., and Hammarström, L.: Periodontal healing of exarticulated monkey teeth stored in milk or saliva, Scand. J. Dent. Res. **89**:251, 1981.
41. Blomlöf, L., and Otteskog, P.: Viability of human periodontal ligament cells after storage in milk or saliva, Scand. J. Dent. Res. **88**:436, 1980.
42. Blomlöf, L., Otteskog, P., and Hammarström, L.: Effect of storage in media with different ion strengths and osmolalities on human periodontal ligament cells, Scand. J. Dent. Res. **89**:180, 1981.
43. Braham, R.L., Roberts, M.W., and Morris, M.E.: Management of dental trauma in children and adolescents, J. Trauma **17**:857, 1977.
44. Brotman, I.N., and Rothschild, H.L.: Report of a breakthrough in preventive dental care for a National Football League team, J. Am. Dent. Assoc. **88**:553, 1974.
45. Buonocore, M.G.: A simple method of increasing the adhesion of acrylic filling material to enamel surfaces, J. Dent. Res. **34**:849, 1955.

46. Buonocore, M.G., and Davila, J.: Restoration of fractured anterior teeth with ultraviolet-light polymerized bonding materials: a new technique, J. Am. Dent. Assoc. **86**:1349, 1973.

47. Bureau of Dental Health Education, Council on Dental Materials and Devices: Mouth protectors: 11 years later, J. Am. Dent. Assoc. **86**:1365, 1973.

48. Bureau of Health Education and Audiovisual Services, Council on Dental Materials, Instruments and Equipment: Mouth protectors and sports team dentists, J. Am. Dent. Assoc. **109**:84, 1984.

49. Camp, J.H.: Replantation of teeth following trauma. In McDonald, R.E., et al., editors: Current therapy in dentistry, vol. 7, St. Louis, 1980, The C.V. Mosby Co.

50. Camp, J.H., et al.: Recommended guidelines for treatment of the avulsed tooth, J. Endod. **9**:571, 1983.

51. Carter, A.P., et al.: Dental injuries in Seattle's public school children: school year 1969-70, J. Public Health Dent. **32**:251, 1972.

52. Castaldi, C.: Injuries to the teeth. In Vinger, P.F., and Hoerner, E.F., editors: Sports injuries: the unthwarted epidemic, Littleton, MA, 1981, PSG Publishing Co., Inc.

53. Coccia, C.T.: A clinical investigation of root resorption rates in reimplanted young permanent incisors: a five-year study, J. Endod. **6**:413, 1980.

54. Council on Dental Materials, Instruments, and Equipment: Council reevaluates position on dental endosseous implants, J. Am. Dent. Assoc. **100**:247, 1980.

55. Croll, T.P., et al.: Rapid neurologic assessment and initial management for the patient with traumatic dental injuries, J. Am. Dent. Assoc. **100**:530, 1980.

56. Cronin, R.J.: Prosthodontic management of vertical root extrusion, J. Prosthet. Dent. **46**:498, 1981.

57. Cvek, M.: Treatment of nonvital permanent incisors with calcium hydroxide, Odontol. Rev. **25**:239, 1974.

58. Cvek, M.: A clinical report on partial pulpotomy and capping with calcium hydroxide in permanent incisors with complicated crown fractures, J. Endod. **4**:232, 1978.

59. Cvek, M.: Endodontic treatment of traumatized teeth. In Andreasen, J.O.: Traumatic injuries of the teeth, ed. 2, Philadelphia, 1981, W.B. Saunders Co.

60. Cvek, M., Granath, L.E., and Hollender, L.: Treatment of nonvital permanent incisors with calcium hydroxide. 2. Variation of occurrence of ankylosis of reimplanted teeth with duration of extra-alveolar period and storage environment, Odontol. Rev. **25**:43, 1974.

61. Cvek, M., and Lundberg, M.: Histological appearance of pulps after exposure by a crown fracture, partial pulpotomy, and clinical diagnosis of healing, J. Endod. **9**:8, 1983.

62. Davis, G.T., and Knott, S.C.: Dental trauma in Australia, Aust. Dent. J. **29**:217, 1984.

63. Degering, C.I.: Radiography of dental fractures, Oral Surg. **30**:213, 1970.

64. Delivanis, P., Delivanis, H., and Kuftinec, M.M.: Endodontic-orthodontic management of fractured anterior teeth, J. Am. Dent. Assoc. **97**:483, 1978.

65. deWet, F.A.: The prevention of orofacial sports injuries in the adolescent, Int. Dent. J. **31**:313, 1981.

66. Down, C.H.: The treatment of permanent incisor teeth of children following traumatic injury, Aust. Dent. J. **2**:9, 1957.

67. Dumsha, T. and Hovland, E.J.: Pulpal prognosis following extrusive luxation injuries in permanent teeth with closed apexes, J. Endod. **8**:410, 1982.

68. Eklund, G., Stalhane, I., and Hedegard, B.: A study of traumatized permanent teeth in children aged 7-15 years, Swed. Dent. J. **69**:179, 1976.

69. Ellis, R.G., and Davey, K.W.: The classification and treatment of injuries to the teeth of children, ed. 5, Chicago, 1970, Year Book Medical Publishers, Inc.

70. Ferguson, F.S., and Ripa, L.W.: Prevalence and type of traumatic injuries to the anterior teeth of preschool children, J. Pedod. **4**:3, 1979.

71. Flanagan, V.O., and Myers, H.I.: Delayed reimplantation of second molars in the Syrian hamster, Oral Surg. **11**:1179, 1958.

72. Frank, A.L.: Improvement of the crown-root ratio by endodontic endosseous implants, J. Am. Dent. Assoc. **74**:451, 1967.

73. Frank, A.L.: Resorption, perforations, and fractures, Dent. Clin. North Am. **18**:465, 1974.

74. Galea, H.: An investigation of dental injuries treated in an acute care general hospital, J. Am. Dent. Assoc. **109**:434, 1984.

75. Gelbier, S.: Injured anterior teeth in children: a preliminary discussion, Br. Dent. J. **123**:331, 1967.

76. Granath, L.E., and Hagman, G.: Experimental pulpotomy in human bicuspids with reference to cutting technique, Acta Odontol. Scand. **29**:155, 1971.

77. Grossman, L.I.: Endodontic practice, ed. 10, Philadelphia, 1981, Lea & Febiger.

78. Grossman, L.I., and Ship, I.I.: Survival rate of replanted teeth, Oral Surg. **29**:899, 1970.

79. Haavikko, K., and Rantanen, L.: A follow-up study of injuries to permanent and primary teeth in children, Proc. Finn. Dent. Soc. **72**:152, 1976.

80. Hallet, G.E.M.: Problems of common interest to the pedodontist and orthodontist with special reference to traumatized incisor cases, Trans. Eur. Orthod. Soc., p. 266, 1953.

81. Hardy, L.B., O'Neal, R.B., and del Rio, C.E.: Effect of polylactic acid on replanted teeth in dogs, Oral Surg. **51**:86, 1981.

82. Hargreaves, J.A., and Craig, J.W.: The management of traumatized anterior teeth of children, Edinburgh, 1970, E. & S. Livingstone, Ltd.

83. Hedegard, B., and Stalhane, I.: A study of traumatized permanent teeth in children aged 7-15 years, Swed. Dent. J. **66**:431, 1973.

84. Heide, S.: Pulp reactions to exposure for 4, 48, or 168 hours, J. Dent. Res. **59**:1910, 1980.

85. Heiman, G.R., et al.: Temporary splinting using an adhesive system, Oral Surg. **31**:819, 1971.

86. Heimdahl, A., von Konow, L., and Lundquist, G.: Replantation of avulsed teeth after long extraalveolar periods, Int. J. Oral Surg. **12**:413, 1983.

87. Heintz, W.D.: Mouth protectors: a progress report, J. Am. Dent. Assoc. **77**:632, 1968.

88. Heithersay, G.S.: Combined endodontic-orthodontic treatment of transverse root fractures in the region on the alveolar crest, Oral Surg. **36**:404, 1973.

89. Heithersay, G.S., and Moule, A.J.: Anterior subgingival fractures: a review of treatment alternatives, Aust. Dent. J. **27**:368, 1982.

90. Helle, A., Sirkkanen, R., and Evalahti, M.: Repair of fractured incisal edges with UV-light polymerized and self-polymerized fissure sealants and composite resins: two-year report of 93 cases, Proc. Finn. Dent. Soc. **71**:87, 1975.

91. Henry, P.J., and Barb, R.E.: Mouth protectors for use in general anesthesia, J. Am. Dent. Assoc. **68**:569, 1964.

92. Hickey, J.C., et al.: The relation of mouth protectors to cranial pressure and deformation, J. Am. Dent. Assoc. **74**:735, 1967.

93. Hill, F.J., and Picton, J.F.: Fractured incisor fragment in the tongue: a case report, Pediatr. Dent. **3**:337, 1981.

94. Holland, R., et al.: Root canal treatment with calcium hydroxide. 1. Effect of overfilling and refilling, Oral Surg. **47**:87, 1979.

95. Hovland, E.J., and Gutmann, J.L.: Atraumatic stabilization for traumatized teeth, J. Endod. **2**:390, 1976.

96. Hurst, R.B.: Regeneration of periodontal and transseptal fibers after autografts in Rhesus monkeys; a qualitative approach, J. Dent. Res. **51**:1183, 1972.

97. Ingber, J.S.: Forced eruption. 2. A method of treating nonrestorable teeth—periodontal and restorative considerations, J. Periodontal. **47**:203, 1976.

98. Ingle, J.I., et al.: Diagnosis and treatment of traumatic injuries and their sequelae. In Ingle, J.I., and Beveridge, E.E., editors: Endodontics, ed. 2, Philadelphia, 1976, Lea & Febiger.

99. Jacobsen, I.: Root fractures in permanent anterior teeth with incomplete root formation, Scand. J. Dent. Res. **84**:210, 1976.

100. Jacobsen, I., and Kerekes, K.: Long-term prognosis of traumatized permanent anterior teeth showing calcifying processes in the pulp cavity, Scand. J. Dent. Res. **85**:588, 1977.

101. Jacobsen, I., and Kerekes, K.: Diagnosis and treatment of pulp necrosis in permanent anterior teeth with root fracture, Scand. J. Dent. Res. **88**:370, 1980.

102. Jacobsen, I., and Sangnes, G.: Traumatized primary anterior teeth, Acta Odontol. Scand. **36**:199, 1978.

103. Jacobsen, I., and Zachrisson, B.V.: Repair characteristics of root fractures in permanent anterior teeth, Scand. J. Dent. Res. **83**:355, 1975.

104. Jarvinen, S.: Incisal overjet and traumatic injuries to upper permanent incisors: a retrospective study, Acta Odontol. Scand. **36**:359, 1978.

105. Jarvinen, S.: Extent to which treatment is sought for children with traumatized permanent anterior teeth: an epidemiologic study, Proc. Finn. Dent. Soc. **75**:103, 1979.

106. Jarvinen, S.: Fractured and avulsed permanent incisors in Finnish children: a retrospective study, Acta Odontol. Scand. **37**:47, 1979.

107. Jarvinen, S.: On the causes of traumatic dental injuries with special reference to sports accidents in a sample of Finnish children: a study of a clinical patient material, Acta Odontol. Scand. **38**:151, 1980.

108. Jordan, R.E., et al.: Restoration of fractured and hypoplastic incisors by the acid-etch resin technique: a three-year report, J. Am. Dent. Assoc. **95**:795, 1977.

109. Josell, S.D., and Abrams, R.G.: Traumatic injuries to the dentition and its supporting structures, Pediatr. Clin. North Am. **29**:717, 1982.

110. Kahnberg, K.-E.: Intraalveolar transplantation of teeth with crown-root fractures, J. Oral Maxillofac. Surg. **43**:38, 1985.

111. Kahnberg, K., Warfvinge, J. and Birgersson, B.: Intraalveolar transplantation, Int. J. Oral Surg. **11**:372, 1982.

112. Kakehasi, S., Stanley, H.R., and Fitzgerald, R.T.: The effects of surgical exposures of dental pulps in germ free and conventional laboratory rats, Oral Surg. **20**:340, 1965.

113. Kaqueler, J.C., and Massler, M.: Healing following tooth replantation, J. Dent. Child. **36**:303, 1969.

114. Katz, R.V., et al.: Epidemiologic survey of accidental dentofacial injuries among U.S. Army personnel, Community Dent. Oral Epidemiol. **7**:30, 1979.

115. Krakow, A.A., Berk, H., and Grøn, P.: Therapeutic induction of root formation in the exposed incompletely formed tooth with a vital pulp, Oral Surg. **43**:755, 1977.

116. Kristerson, L., and Andreasen, J.O.: The effect of splinting upon periodontal and pulpal healing after autotransplantation of mature and immature permanent incisors in monkeys, Int. J. Oral Surg. **12**:239, 1983.

117. Kristerson, L., and Andreasen, J.O.: Influence of root development on periodontal and pulpal healing after replantation of incisors in monkeys, Int. J. Oral Surg. **13**:313, 1984.

118. Lenstrup, K., and Skieller, V.: A follow-up study of teeth replanted after accidental loss, Acta Odontol. Scand. **17**:503, 1959.

119. Löe, H., and Waerhaug, J.: Experimental replantation of teeth in dogs and monkeys, Arch. Oral Biol. **3**:176, 1961.

120. Lundberg, M., and Cvek, M.: A light microscopy study of pulps from traumatized permanent incisors with reduced pulpal lumen, Acta Odontol. Scand. **38**:89, 1980.

121. Massler, M.: Tooth replantation, Dent. Clin. North Am. **18**:445, 1974.

122. Meadow, D., Needleman, H., and Lindner, G.: Oral trauma in children, Pediatr. Dent. **6**:248, 1984.

123. Michanowicz, A.E., Michanowicz, J.P., and Abou-Rass, M.: Cementogenic repair of root fractures, J. Am. Dent. Assoc. **82**:569, 1971.

124. Morris, M.L., et al.: Factors affecting healing after experimentally delayed tooth transplantation, J. Endod. **7**:80, 1981.

125. Nasjleti, C.E., et al.: Healing after tooth reimplantation in monkeys, Oral Surg. **39**:361, 1975.

126. Natkin, E.: Diagnosis and treatment of traumatic injuries and their sequelae. In Ingle, J.I., editor: Endodontics, Philadelphia, 1965, Lea & Febiger.

127. News of dentistry: Fitted mouthguards afford key protection, J. Am. Dent. Assoc. **84**:531, 1972.

128. Noyek, A.M., and Winnick, A.N.: An acrylic dental protector in peroral endoscopy, J. Otolaryngol. **5**:1, 1976.

129. Ohman, A.: Healing and sensitivity to pain in young replanted human teeth: an experimental, clinical, and histological study, Odontol. Tidskr. **73**:165, 1965.

130. O'Mullane, D.M.: Injured permanent incisor teeth: an epidemiological study, J. Irish Dent. Assoc. **18**:160, 1972.

131. Pindborg, J.J.: Clinical, radiographic, and histological aspects of intra-alveolar fractures of upper central incisors, Acta Odontol. Scand. **13**:41, 1955.

132. Rand, A.: Suture splint for displaced teeth, J. N.J. Dent. Assoc. **46**:30, 1975.

133. Ravn, J.J.: Sequelae of acute mechanical traumata in the primary dentition, J. Dent. Child. **35**:281, 1968.

134. Ravn, J.J.: Dental injuries in Copenhagen school children, school years 1967-1972, Community Dent. Oral Epidemiol. **2**:231, 1974.

135. Ravn, J.J.: Follow-up study of permanent incisors with enamel cracks as a result of an acute trauma, Scand. J. Dent. Res. **89**:117, 1981.

136. Ravn, J.J.: Follow-up study of permanent incisors with enamel-dentin fractures after acute trauma, Scand. J. Dent. Res. **89**:355, 1981.

137. Ravn, J.J.: Follow-up study of permanent incisors with enamel fractures as a result of an acute trauma, Scand. J. Dent. Res. **89**:213, 1981.

138. Ravn, J.J., and Rossen, I.: Prevalence and distribution of traumatic tooth injuries among Copenhagen school children, 1967–68, Tandlaegebladet **73**:1, 1969.

139. Roberts, M.W., and Moffa, J.P.: Repair of fractured incisal angles with an ultraviolet-light-activated fissure sealant and a composite resin: two year report of 60 cases, J. Am. Dent. Assoc. **87**:888, 1973.

140. Rock, W.P., et al.: The relationship between trauma and pulp death in incisor teeth, Br. Dent. J. **136**:236, 1974.

141. Rock, W.P., and Grundy, M.C.: The effect of luxation and subluxation upon the prognosis of traumatized incisor teeth, J. Dent. **9**:224, 1981.

142. Salisbury, P.L., Curtis, J.W., and Kohut, R.I.: Appliance to protect maxillary teeth and palate during endoscopy, Arch. Otolaryngol. **110**:106, 1984.

143. Seltzer, S., et al.: Titanium endodontic implants: a scanning electron microscope, electron microprobe, and histologic investigation, J. Endod. **2**:267, 1976.

144. Shulman, L.B., Gedalia, I., and Feingold, R.M.: Fluoride concentration in root surfaces and alveolar bone of fluoride-immersed monkey incisors three weeks after replantation, J. Dent. Res. **52**:1314, 1973.

145. Shulman, L.B., Kalis, P.J., and Goldhaber, P.: Fluoride inhibition of tooth-replant root resorption in Cebus monkeys, J. Dent. Res. (abstr. 440), 1968.

146. Silverband, H., Rabkin, M., and Cranin, A.N.: The uses of endodontic implant stabilizers in posttraumatic and periodontal disease, Oral Surg. **45**:920, 1978.

147. Simon, J.H.S., et al.: Extrusion of endodontically treated teeth, J. Am. Dent. Assoc. **97**:17, 1978.

148. Skieller, V.: The prognosis for young teeth loosened after mechanical injuries, Acta Odontol. Scand. **18**:171, 1980.

149. Skoglund, A.: Pulpal survival in replanted and autotransplanted apicoectomized mature teeth of dogs with prepared nutritional canals, Int. J. Oral Surg. **12**:31, 1983.

150. Skoglund, A., and Tronstad, L.: Pulpal changes in replanted and autotransplanted immature teeth of dogs, J. Endod. **7**:309, 1981.

151. Smukler, H., and Tagger, N.: Vital root amputation: a clinical and histological study, J. Periodontol. **47**:324, 1976.

152. Söder, P.O., et al.: Effect of drying on viability of periodontal membrane, Scand. J. Dent. Res. **85**:164, 1977.

153. Spalding, P.M., et al.: The changing role of endodontics and orthodontics in the management of traumatically intruded permanent incisors, Pediatr. Dent. **7**:104, 1985.

154. Stanley, H.R., Laskin, J., and Broom, C.A.: Moistness, more than temperature variations, prevents autolysis of pulp tissue in avulsed teeth, J. Endod. **9**:360, 1983.

155. Stanley, H.R., and Lundy, T.: Dycal therapy for pulp exposures, Oral Surg. **34**:818, 1972.

156. Stanley, H.R., et al.: Ischemic infarction of the pulp: sequential degenerative changes of the pulp after traumatic injury, J. Endod. **4**:325, 1978.

157. Stanley, H.R., White, C.L., and McCray, L.: The rate of tertiary (reparative) dentin formation in the human tooth, Oral Surg. **21**:180, 1966.

158. Stenger, J.M., et al.: Mouthguards: protection against shock to head, neck, and teeth, J. Am. Dent. Assoc. **69**:273, 1964.

159. Stevens, O.O.: Prevention of traumatic dental and oral injuries. In Andreasen, J.O.: Traumatic injuries of the teeth, ed. 2, Philadelphia, 1981, W.B. Saunders Co.

160. Tate, R.J.: Facial injuries associated with the battered child syndrome, Br. J. Oral Surg. **9**:41, 1971.

161. Tegsjö, U., Valerius-Olsson, H., and Olgart, K.: Intra-alveolar transplantation of teeth with cervical root fractures, Swed. Dent. J. **2**:73, 1978.

162. Thylstrup, A., and Andreasen, J.O.: The influence of traumatic intrusion of primary teeth on their permanent successors in monkeys, J. Oral Pathol. **6**:296, 1977.

163. Tronstad, L., et al.: pH changes in dental tissues after root canal filling with calcium hydroxide, J. Endod. **7**:17, 1981.

164. Turley, P.K., Joiner, M.W., and Hellstrom, S.: The effect of orthodontic extrusion on traumatically intruded teeth, Am. J. Orthod. **85**:47, 1984.

165. Turner, C.H.: Mouth protectors, Br. Dent. J. **143**:82, 1977.

166. Vanek, P.M.: Traumatic injuries, In Cohen, S., and Burns, R.C., editors: Pathways of the pulp, ed. 2, St. Louis, 1980, The C.V. Mosby Co.

167. Van Hassel, H.J., Oswald, R.J., and Harrington, G.W.: Replantation. 2. The role of the periodontal ligament, J. Endod. **6**:506, 1980.

168. Wald, C.: Consequences of intrusive injuries to primary teeth, J. Pedod. **3**:67, 1978.

169. Webber, R.T.: Traumatic injuries and the expanded endodontic role of calcium hydroxide. In Gerstein, H., editor: Techniques in clinical endodontics, Philadelphia, 1983, W.B. Saunders Co.

170. Weine, F.S. Endodontic therapy, ed. 3, St. Louis, 1982, The C.V. Mosby Co.

171. Worfson, E.M., and Seiden, L.: Combined endodontic-orthodontic treatment of subgingivally fractured teeth, J. Can. Dent. Assoc. **11**:621, 1975.

172. World Health Organization: International classification of diseases: application to dentistry and stomatology, ICD-DA, Copenhagen, 1969, W.H.O.

173. York, A.H., et al.: Dental injuries to 11-13 year old children, N.Z. Dent. J. **74**:218, 1978.

174. Zachrisson, B.V., and Jacobsen, I.: Long-term prognosis of 66 permanent anterior teeth with root fracture, Scand. J.. Dent. Res. **83**:345, 1975.

175. Zadik, D.: A survey of traumatized primary anterior teeth in Jerusalem preschool children, Community Dent. Oral Epidemiol. **4**:149, 1976.

176. Zadik, D., Chosack, A., and Eidelman, E.: A survey of traumatized incisors in Jerusalem school children, J. Dent. Child. **39**:185, 1972.

177. Zadik, D., et al.: Traumatized teeth: two-year results, J. Pedod. **4**:116, 1980.

Self-assessment questions

1. Which of the following symptoms may be a neurologic complication of head and neck injuries?
   a. Inability to turn head normally
   b. Nausea or vomiting
   c. Dizziness
   d. All of the above

2. Initial thermal and electric testing of traumatized teeth
   a. Establishes a base line as to the physiologic status of the pulp
   b. If positive, can be assumed to indicate a healthy pulpal state
   c. If negative, signifies that root canal treatment should be initiated
   d. Should be repeated one additional time in 30 days to finalize the pulp status

3. Initial radiographic examination of dental injuries
   a. Will reveal hairline root fractures
   b. Will show fracture lines that are diagonal in a facial-lingual direction
   c. Should include a soft tissue radiograph in areas of lip lacerations
   d. Does not indicate the supplemental need of occlusal or panoramic films

4. The most desirable emergency restorative procedure for a crown fracture is
   a. Full veneer crown preparation with a stainless steel crown
   b. A stainless steel or preformed orthodontic band
   c. An acid-etch composite restoration
   d. A pin-retained composite restoration

5. For a crown fracture involving dentin
   a. Emergency treatment consists of protecting the pulp
   b. A pin-retained composite buildup is the restoration of choice
   c. Permanent restoration may be accomplished immediately or within 4 weeks
   d. Periodic recalls to check pulp vitality are usually not required

6. Maintenance of pulpal vitality in exposed pulp-crown fractures
   a. Improves the prognosis with elapsing time before treatment
   b. Is the treatment of choice for teeth with incompletely formed roots
   c. Is generally reserved for mature teeth
   d. Is recommended for teeth with partial calcific pulpal obliteration

7. The pulpotomy procedure
   a. Is limited to teeth with necrotic pulps
   b. Requires the removal of all pulp tissue judged to be inflamed
   c. Utilizes a low-speed round bur to minimize damage to the underlying tissue
   d. Should not be carried any deeper than the cervical line

8. The initial priority in treatment of a root fracture is
   a. Preservation of the pulp
   b. Reduction and immobilization
   c. Root canal therapy
   d. Calcium hydroxide pulp therapy

9. A stabilized, healed root fracture with evidence of hypercalcification of the pulpal space generally requires
   a. No further treatment
   b. Endodontic therapy with gutta-percha
   c. Endodontic therapy with calcium hydroxide
   d. Surgical removal of the apical segment

10. Root fractures communicating with the oral cavity
    a. Have an excellent prognosis of healing with a vital pulp if well stabalized
    b. Require periodontal surgery as the treatment of choice if more than 2 mm below the bone
    c. Require root canal therapy of the vital pulp if root submergence is considered
    d. Will necessitate root extrusion if excessive periodontal surgery is required for restoration

11. Endodontic treatment of displaced mature teeth
    a. Is dependent on response to pulp testing
    b. Justifies the preventive application of calcium hydroxide for severe displacements
    c. Requires filling with gutta-percha in the presence of inflammatory root resorption
    d. Is required following evidence of calcific pulpal obliteration

12. A displaced primary tooth
    a. With the root forced lingually faces the increased possibility of injury to the permanent tooth
    b. Is less frequent than root fracture of a primary tooth
    c. If minimal, is treated by endodontic therapy and splinted
    d. Will exfoliate in a normal fashion if ankylosed in an intruded position

13. Replantation of mature avulsed teeth
    a. Is generally regarded as a permanent successful procedure
    b. Has been reported to last an average 1 to 5 years
    c. Is most successful with a longer extraoral period
    d. Is affected by the storage medium during the extraoral period

14. Replantation technique of avulsed mature teeth requires
    a. Removal of any soil contamination or foreign matter by rinsing with water followed by sterilization
    b. Leaving the pulp tissue intact and sealing the apex with an alloy prior to replantation
    c. Removal of any blood clot present in the socket by curettage
    d. Repositioning with light finger pressure, verifying by radiograph, and splinting

16

ROOT RESORPTION

NOAH CHIVIAN

This chapter is directed toward the diagnosis and treatment of problems presented by root resorption.

The following definitions will provide a common ground of understanding:[5]

resorption A condition associated with either a physiologic or a pathologic process which results in a loss of substance from a tissue, such as dentin, cementum, and alveolar bone.

root resorption Resorption affecting the cementum and/or dentin of the root of a tooth. On the basis of the site of origin of the resorption, it may be referred to as internal, external, or root-end resorption.

idiopathic resorption Resorption occurring without apparent cause.

internal resorption A type of tooth resorption initiated within the pulp cavity. When the resorption process occurs within the crown of the tooth and reaches the enamel, a pink spot may be seen.

external resorption Resorption initiated in the periodontium and affecting the external or lateral surfaces of a tooth.

Diagnosis

An examination of the definition of root resorption can provide a clue to establishing the diagnosis of internal or external resorption. "On the basis of site of origin . . . it may be referred to as internal or external. . . ."[5]

Kronfeld[80] said:

As a rule the clinical diagnosis of internal resorption is not difficult. Any radiographically visible defect in a tooth that is not caused by caries must be the result of a resorptive process of some kind. More difficult is the pathological interpretation. Two possibilities exist: Either the resorption originated from the pulp, began inside of the tooth, and progressed from the pulp cavity outward, or it originated in the periodontal membrane and invaded the pulp chamber from without.

Histologic examination of the tooth would provide a definitive diagnosis,[140] but this is not a practical approach.

Therefore the radiograph has proved to be an essential clinical tool in establishing the differential diagnosis between internal and external resorption.

Supplemental radiographs from different horizontal angles (i.e., from mesial or distal projections) will aid in the diagnosis (Fig. 16-1). If the resorption defect does not change position in a comparison of multiple radiographs, it is within the confines of the root and therefore is *internal* resorption. Labial or lingual external resorption superimposed over the canal can mimic internal resorption but it will change position on the multiple radiographs[11] (Figs. 16-2 and 16-46). (See discussion of the buccal object rule, Chapter 4.) Tamse et al. have described the roentgenographic features of external root resorption.[133]

Gartner et al.[49] simplified the diagnostic process by summarizing the radiographic appearance of the lesions. The key to their criteria is as follows:

external resorption The lesion may be superimposed over the canal and the *unaltered canal* can be followed all the way to the apex (Fig. 16-2).

internal resorption The canal or chamber shows an enlarged area and is not present in the area of the lesion (Fig. 16-3).

Previous editions of this text utilized a 1958 classification[23] of internal resorption to clarify treatment modalities for the condition. However, a study of the radiographs of cases used to illustrate symmetric and asymmetric internal resorption showed these entities to be different. Cases that were designated as symmetric internal resorption were, in fact, internal resorption. And cases that were called asymmetric internal resorption were actually external resorption. By definition, they started in the periodontal ligament and an unaltered canal could be followed all the way to the apex. In this edition some cases that were previously classified as internal resorption are now in the external resorption section. Although the designations may have changed, the treatment procedures have stood the test of time and are still viable methods.

510

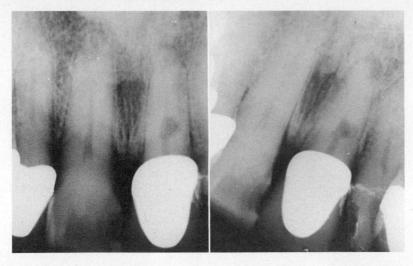

FIG. 16-1. Internal resorption. Radiographs from two different horizontal projections depict the lesion within the confines of the root.

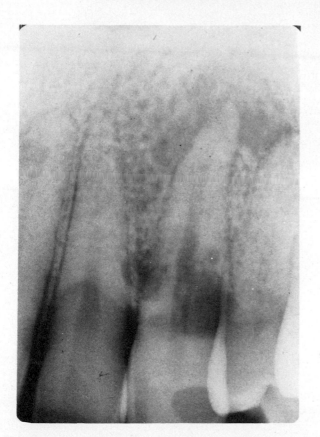

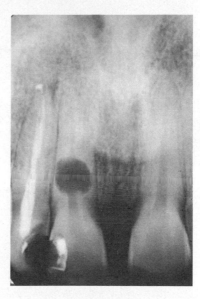

FIG. 16-3. Internal resorption. No outline of the canal present in the affected area.

FIG. 16-2. External resorption. Canal superimposed over the lesion.

Frank[46] has described a category of resorption, "external-internal progressive resorption," that he feels is distinct from previously reported designations. Pomeranz reported a case of active external-internal root resorption.[109] Andreasen[11] uses the terms internal replacement and internal inflammatory root resorption. These may be different stages of the same process. By definition, both entities are internal resorption and the treatment procedures are similar.

This refinement of the differential diagnostic procedure has resulted from a distillation of the literature coupled with a critical evaluation of 25 years of clinical experience. The intent of the rigid definitions of the clinical entities in the previous editions was an attempt to simplify the treatment procedures. In fact, they probably confused the issue. A philosopher once said, "Maturity can be measured by the amount of pain experienced when accepting a new idea." The ability to accept change is part of the educational process, to which we as practitioners in the healing arts must be committed.

INTERNAL RESORPTION

"Internal resorption has been one of dentistry's major mysteries. Why should one tooth suddenly start to resorb when thousands of other teeth do not? What triggers the

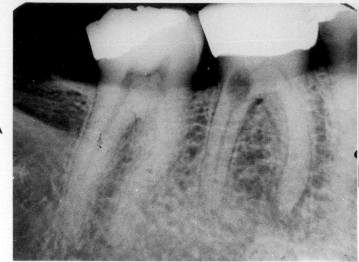

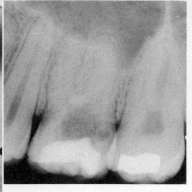

FIG. 16-4. A, Internal resorption of a mandibular first molar. No outline of the canal is present in the affected area. **B,** Internal resorption of a maxillary first molar 15 years after a pulp cap.

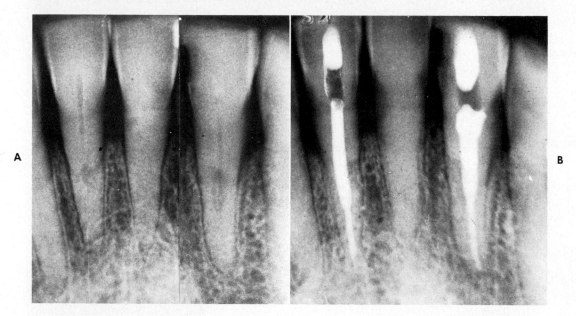

FIG. 16-5. Multiple internal resorption 22 years after an auto accident. **A,** Preoperative. **B,** Postoperative.

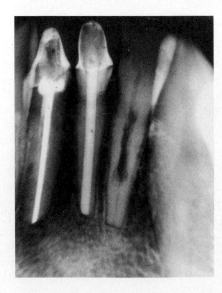

FIG. 16-6. Internal resorption due to trauma. The left central incisor had undergone endodontic therapy 18 years previously, the right central 10 years previously. Both teeth fractured. The right lateral incisor, which had been displaced in the same injury (20 years earlier), suffered internal as well as apical external resorption.

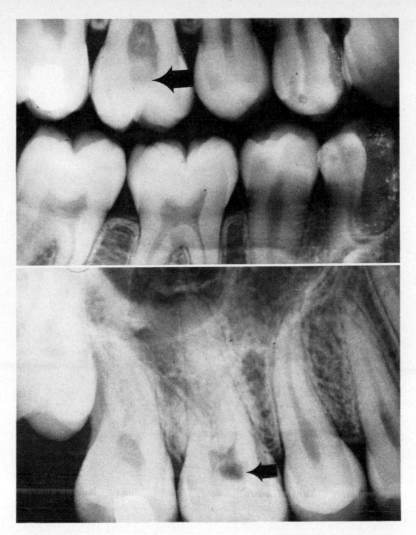

FIG. 16-7. Internal resorption due to orthodontics. There is perforating internal resorption on the palatal surface of the crown at the gingival margin *(arrow)*. Orthodontia was the only dental treatment. No history of trauma.

mechanism?'' Sweet[132] researched these questions and presented a few hypotheses but came up with no definite conclusions; other authors have had similar experience.

Internal resorption has been found to exist more often than was previously suspected. It can affect one tooth (Fig. 16-4) or many teeth (Fig. 16-5). Incisors show the highest incidence, however, it is also seen in posterior teeth. Although there is no known etiology for it, trauma (Fig. 16-6) has been frequently suggested as a cause.[35,55,58,116] A 2% incidence following luxation injuries has been reported,[6] and it can follow vital root resection[4] as well as calcium hydroxide pulpotomy.[34,67] It has been produced experimentally by the application of diathermy,[56] and even anachoresis[107] has been mentioned as a cause of it. Weine[143] suggests that orthodontics may be an etiologic factor (Fig. 16-7).

Internal with external root resorption has also been observed.[40] Internal resorption is not usually associated with any systemic disease.[126] As early as 1830,[21] inflammation within the pulp was cited as a cause of internal resorption,

and 90 years later[97] it was concluded that internal resorption was a result of a ''chronic productive pulpitis.'' Today it is believed that internal resorption is indeed probably caused by a chronic irreversible pulpitis[26,35,113,117,143] (Fig. 16-8).

Numerous diverse aspects of internal resorption have been studied; however, the actual mechanism is still a matter of speculation. A root canal provides an atmosphere well suited for the development of hard tissue-resorbing cells. This can occur after a traumatic episode, whether it be a crown preparation or an impact injury. Circulation changes influence cell metabolism to a large degree. Root resorptions appear to be more frequent close to blood vessels.[111] It has also been observed that active hyperemia with high oxygen pressure supports and induces odontoclastic activity. Electrical activity such as piezoelectricity and streaming potentials (charges arising from blood flow through the vessels) may add to the resorptive process.

Cytologic alterations occur within the pulp when odontoclasts form from undifferentiated reserve connective tis-

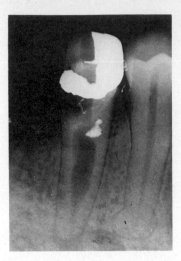

FIG. 16-8. Internal resorption due to chronic irreversible pulpitis.

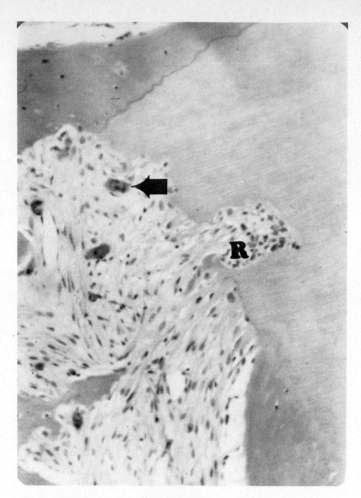

FIG. 16-9. Internal resorption. Histologic section. Arrow shows a multinucleated giant cell. *R,* Resorptive lacunae in dentin. (x 100.) (Courtesy Dr. Harold Stanley.)

sue cells.[137] (This agrees with the earlier findings of Thoma.[55]) Histochemical changes have been documented in teeth undergoing internal resorption.[61] Multinucleated cells lying in resorptive lacunae (Fig. 16-9) in dentin were of similar morphology to bone resorbing cells and had similar enzymes (acid phosphatase and β-glucuronidase).[65]

The scanning electron microscope has revealed yet another possible cause of internal resorption. Evidence has been uncovered[79] that there are organic materials and microorganism-like structures in a resorbed root. According to Stanley,[127] concomitant with resorption of the dental structure is the frequent deposition of a hard tissue resembling bone or cementum. The resultant structure bears no relationship to the normal form of the tooth and consequently has been termed ''metaplastic'' tissue. It has also been postulated that all resorption develops in the following sequence of events[24]: Sudden trauma to the tooth produces intrapulpal hemorrhage. Internal resorption is preceded by the disappearance of odontoblasts and a pulpal invasion of macrophage-like cells.[61] The hemorrhage organizes (i.e., is replaced by granulation tissue). The proliferating granulation tissue compresses the dentin walls, predentin formation ceases, odontoclasts differentiate from the connective tissue, and resorption begins. Necrosis of the pulp may occur as the destruction becomes extensive and the pulp communicates with the oral fluids after perforation of the root or crown surface.

Heithersay[67] postulates a possible reason for internal resorption may be the effect of a collateral blood supply via an interconnecting and large lateral accessory canal. This would provide a sufficient vascular bed for the resorptive process to occur. He points out that a large accessory canal can usually be demonstrated in cases treated endodontically (Figs. 16-14 and 16-16).

Internal resorption is usually asymptomatic, first recognized clinically through routine full-mouth radiographs. Several radiographs taken from different horizontal angles are necessary to examine the extent of the tooth loss and to determine a treatment plan. Pain may become a factor

when perforation of the crown occurs and the metaplastic tissue is exposed to the oral fluids. Perforation of the root, resulting in the formation of a periodontal lesion, usually produces immediate symptoms. When resorption in the crown is extensive, the patient may become aware of a pink spot.[41]

Internal resorption may be rapid, destroying the tooth in months (Fig. 16-10); or it may take years (Fig. 16-11). Since there is no way of predicting the rate of devastation, it is imperative that the altered pulp tissue be removed when the pathosis is first discovered. With internal resorption of the plan of ''careful watching'' may quickly become one of ''supervised neglect'' unless the pulp is extirpated. Spontaneous repair is extremely rare.[63,144] *Therefore prompt endodontic treatment is imperative in all diagnosed cases of internal resorption.*

Treatment

To establish treatment guidelines for internal resorption, this discussion is divided into three sections: non-surgical, recalcification with calcium hydroxide, and surgical. The choice of approach will be determined by the ability of the dentist to fulfill the endodontic triad requirements (saniti-

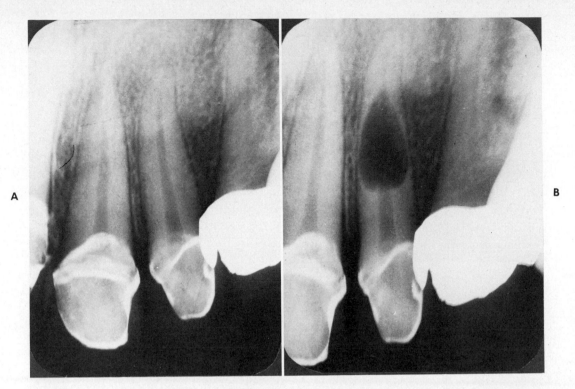

FIG. 16-10. Rapid tooth destruction due to internal resorption. **A,** Immediately after crown preparation. **B,** Four months later.

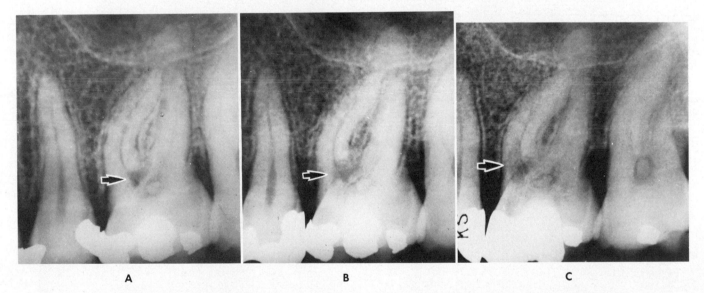

FIG. 16-11. Slow tooth destruction due to internal resorption *(arrows)*. **A,** Lesion first observed. **B,** Four years later. **C,** Fifteen years later.

zation, debridement, and obturation) and by the extent and position of the pathologic defect.

If the requirements can be met and the resorptive defect does not perforate the canal wall, a nonsurgical approach is the treatment of choice.

If the three basic endodontic tenets can be met but there is perforation of the canal wall apical to the epithelial attachment, the calcium hydroxide technique should be used.

When there is extensive root destruction or uncontrolla-

ble bleeding or the perforation is coronal to the epithelial attachment, a surgical approach is demanded; extraction may be necessary in some cases (Fig. 16-12).

Nonsurgical treatment

After initial penetration into the chamber and establishing working length (Fig. 16-13, *A*), the access cavity modified to treat resorption should be widened into the coronal part of the root with round burs, Gates-Glidden burs (Fig. 16-13, *B*), or Peeso drills. Considerable bleeding is usually

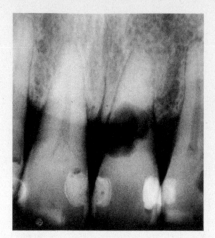

FIG. 16-12. Internal resorption with extensive root destruction. Extraction is indicated. (Courtesy Dr. Robert Uchin.)

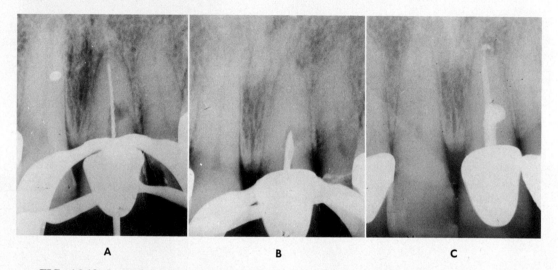

A   B   C

FIG. 16-13. Internal resorption. **A,** Working length measurement. **B,** Canal coronal to defect enlarged with Gates-Glidden bur. **C,** Canal and defect filled with thermoplastic injection molded gutta-percha and sealer.

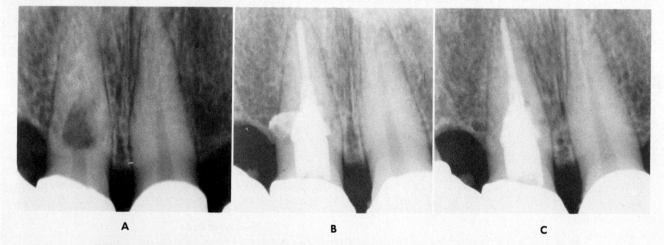

A   B   C

FIG. 16-14. Internal resorption. Nonsurgical treatment of a central incisor. **A,** Pretreatment. **B,** Immediate posttreatment. Defect sealed with vertical condensation, sealer expressed through an undetected perforation. **C,** Two years postoperative. Excess cement has been absorbed.

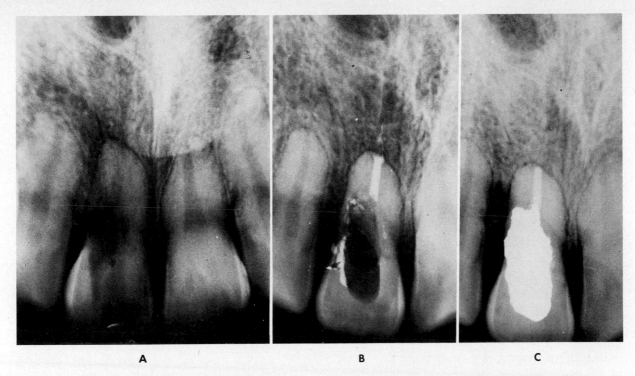

FIG. 16-15. Nonperforating internal resorption. **A,** Pretreatment. **B,** Apical section of the canal sealed with warmed gutta-percha. Osteoid tissue has been removed from the remainder of the canal. **C,** One year later. The resorption defect was filled with silver amalgam via the access cavity.

encountered when the highly vascularized mass of granulomatous tissue is uncovered. Irrigation with copious amounts of undiluted 5.25% sodium hypochlorite solution will assist in controlling the hemorrhage and dissolving the pulp tissue in the inaccessible recesses. The use of endodontic ultrasonics also will be of great value. Vasoconstrictors (Orastat), astringents (Hemodent), or very cautiously applied oxygenating agents (Superoxol) effectively control excess bleeding. It may be necessary to remove the pulp and granulomatous tissue to achieve a clear field of operation. This can be accomplished with long shank no. 4 or 6 round burs in a low-speed handpiece or a 33L endodontic explorer. If the bleeding cannot be stopped, a change to the surgical approach will be necessary.

Once a dry field can be established, the apical portion of the canal should be instrumented. As mentioned previously, both resorption and deposition of tooth structure may appear concurrently in the defect. In many cases this results in calcification of the canal apical to the defect, preventing easy access. Probing with a DG 16 explorer or a file will aid in locating the canal. Further judicious drilling with the no. 2 or 4 long round bur may uncover the opening. If stymied at this juncture expose another radiograph and reassess the canal position. When penetration to the apical part of the canal is achieved, cleaning and shaping can proceed in the usual manner. The canal is dried with paper points and the defect dried with cotton pellets or a swab made by wrapping loose cotton around a barbed broach.

The canal apical to the resorbed area may be sealed with

gutta-percha by lateral or vertical condensation. Remove excess gutta-percha from the defect and examine once again for perforations. If there is no bleeding, the pathologic void is ready for sealing with warm gutta-percha by thermoplastic injection molding (Figs. 16-13, *C*, and 16-14) or thermatic condensation. Silver amalgam to serve as a core (Fig. 16-15), fast-setting zinc oxide–eugenol cement[22] (I.R.M.), eucapercha,[29] and a hydrophilic plastic material (Hydron)[87] have also been used at this stage.

It is important to remember that the success of the case depends not only on sealing the canal but on filling the entire void as well. This is necessary because the full extent of the resorptive defect is not always visible clinically or radiographically (Fig. 16-16).

In all cases of root resorption, consideration should be given to reinforcing the tooth with a preformed stainless steel post. Such reinforcement may double the resistance to fracture[78] (Figs. 16-17 and 16-18).

Recalcification with calcium hydroxide. When perforating internal resorption occurred in an inoperable site, extraction, root resection, or intentional replantation[27] may have been the only available options until recently. When filling the void via the pulp chamber, one was faced with the liability of extruding the filling material into the periodontal attachment apparatus. Healing sometimes occurred in spite of treatment (Fig. 16-19).

It is now known that a thick paste of $Ca(OH)_2$ and a biologically compatible vehicle may be used to promote physiologic repair of small perforations.

Since $Ca(OH)_2$ was introduced in 1930 as a pulpotomy

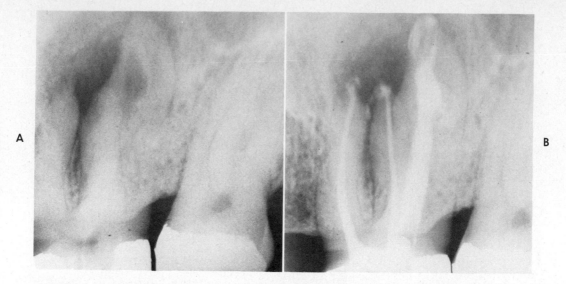

FIG. 16-16. Internal resorption. Nonsurgical treatment of a maxillary first molar. **A,** Pretreatment. **B,** Posttreatment. The defect has been sealed with vertical condensation. Note the accessory canals and the extent of the defect.

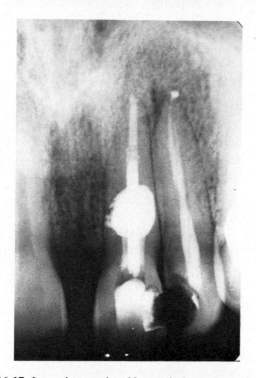

FIG. 16-17. Internal resorption. Nonsurgical treatment of a maxillary central incisor. Apical section of the canal and the defect sealed with gutta-percha, thermatic condensation. Post room was prepared through the gutta-percha. A stainless steel post has been cemented with zinc phosphate cement. The lateral incisor was previously treated elsewhere.

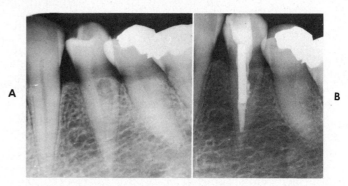

FIG. 16-18. External cervical resorption. Tooth is in buccal version with a wear facet on buccal aspect of buccal cusp. **A,** Pretreatment radiograph. An 11 mm periodontal pocket is present. Resorptive defect is superimposed over root canal. **B,** Posttreatment. Root canal therapy was completed with gutta-percha and cementation of a stainless steel parapost. The defect was sealed during surgery with a composite resin.

agent by Hermann,[69] the dental profession has continued to find new uses for this material, alone or in combination with other substances. Besides its use in pulp capping and pulpotomy procedures, some clinicians [30,42] have advocated that it be used in combination with a vehicle for stimulating further root development in pulpless teeth with immature apices. The clinical findings of these authors are corroborated by histologic studies.[38,136] This $Ca(OH)_2$-vehicle mixture has been used to arrest resorption in replanted teeth exhibiting inflammatory resorption, and it has been used as well in the deposition of new root structure and in halting external resorption in traumatized teeth.[129] The successful regeneration of tooth structure and the reestablishment of an intact canal with $Ca(OH)_2$ and camphorated parachlorophenol (CMCP) in teeth that had developed a vertical fracture as a result of the torquing action of posts have also been demonstrated.[129]

The $Ca(OH)_2$-vehicle can serve as an intracanal dressing between appointments,[138] in the repair of mechanical perforations[45] and furcation problems,[143] and in the treatment of horizontal root fractures[33,83] and persistent periapical inflammations.[125] Thus its expanded role to aid in hard tissue repair has added a new dimension to dental care.

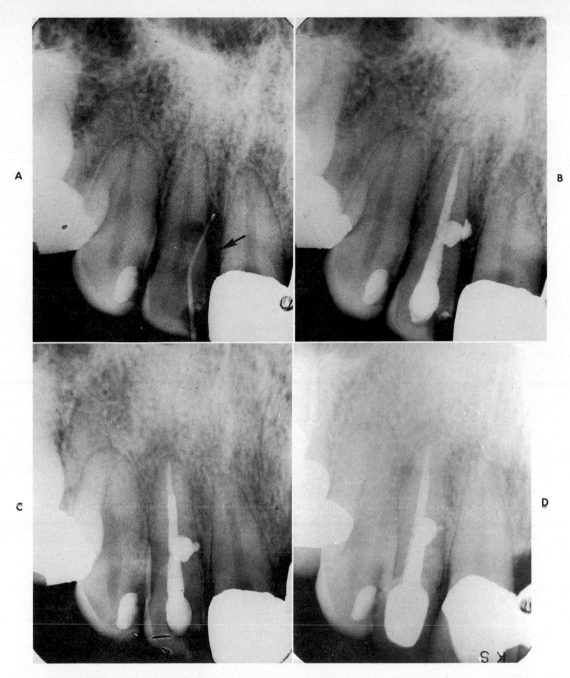

FIG. 16-19. Perforating internal resorption at an inoperable site. **A,** Gutta-percha point in a sinus tract. (Surgery would require removal of crestal bone, setting up a potential periodontal defect.) **B,** Canal and defect sealed with warmed gutta-percha. **C,** Two years later the excess gutta-percha is absorbing, and there is bone regeneration at the lateral defect. The crestal bone is intact. **D,** Four years later. The tooth is asymptomatic with no gingival defects. (Courtesy Dr. Stanley M. Baer.)

There have also been positive predictable results with the use of $Ca(OH)_2$ in a biologically compatible vehicle—e.g., anesthetic solution,[142] saline, methyl cellulose, distilled water, or even CMCP (although the biologic acceptability of CMCP is doubtful)—to promote physiologic repair of small perforations. Possibly other medicaments produce similar results.

Mode of action. The rationale for the use of $Ca(OH)_2$ appears to be well grounded after 50 years. However, the exact mode of action of $Ca(OH)_2$ is unknown. We use it because clinically it works and apparently does no harm.

As a pulp capping and vital pulpotomy agent $Ca(OH)_2$ has been shown to stimulate vital pulp tissue cells to produce reparative dentin.[128] When it is used experimentally to fill root canals after vital pulp extirpation, periapical histologic sections show the healing process to be similar to pulpal healing when the same material is used.[71] Teeth with incompletely formed roots and necrotic pulps produced an apical barrier of hard tissue after canal debridement and placement of a $Ca(OH)_2$ paste for varying lengths of time.[33,136] In this instance no vital pulp tissue is present. Healing results from the stimulation of undifferentiated mesenchymal cells in the apical periodontal ligament.

In the repair of perforating internal resorption and iatrogenic perforations the same connective tissue (the periodontal ligament) is brought into the picture. In these cases the affected PDL is on the lateral aspect of the root rather than at the apex. It still provides the same rich source of healing potential—the undifferentiated mesenchymal cells generally present in all connective tissue. As long as the perforation is part of a closed system (i.e., apical to the epithelial attachment) and covered by bone, and as long as no communication exists with the oral fluids, $Ca(OH)_2$ will reduce the inflammatory response and promote healing with a hard tissue barrier.

$Ca(OH)_2$ has an antibacterial effect.[34] Microorganisms coming in contact with the paste are probably destroyed by its high pH.[75] It has an active influence on the local environment of resorption area by making osteoclastic activity impossible and stimulating repair.[139] This is directly related to the alkaline pH of the $Ca(OH)_2$, which spreads through the dentin after placement in the pulp chamber. Hard tissue resorption, with its enzymatic activity, takes place in an acid pH. $Ca(OH)_2$ creates an alkaline environment in which this reaction is reversed and hard tissue deposition can take place. The phenomenon of pH change to the periphery is increased, especially where resorption has exposed the dentin.[139] This research finding provides an understanding for the use of $Ca(OH)_2$ in the treatment of external resorption.

Although the exact mode of action of $Ca(OH)_2$ is not understood, recent research shows that we are on the right track in using it.

Standard technique. In the previous editions of this text the use of $Ca(OH)_2$ with CMCP was recommended, even though its biologic acceptability was doubtful. Currently use of the more biologically acceptable anesthetic solutions[142] as the vehicle for mixing with $Ca(OH)_2$ is recommended.

The $Ca(OH)_2$ is mixed with a few drops of anesthetic solution in a Dappen dish or on a mixing slab to the consistency of a resin filling. It may be introduced into the chamber with a plastic instrument, a specifically designed Teflon-coated amalgam carrier, or a rubber-base impression syringe. Because it must be present at the site of resorption, the material is delivered to the desired level with a long-handled endodontic plugger. The Schilder plugger* in various diameters with 5 mm incremental markings (Chapter 5) is most helpful in compressing the paste to the working length. Controlled pressure is needed to fill the canal completely with the $Ca(OH)_2$–anesthetic paste. The mixture has a radiographic density similar to that of dentin and can easily be differentiated from the unfilled canal space; radiographs are used to determine when the canal is

filled completely. To provide increased opacity to the paste,[142] $BaSO_4$ may be added in a ratio of one part to eight parts of $Ca(OH)_2$. Because the reaction of the periodontium adjacent to the defect is one of repair, the material should be placed in direct contact with these tissues. Although not yet confirmed histologically, the mechanism of repair appears to be similar to apexification (Chapter 15).

A radiograph is essential at the completion of this phase. The patient should be recalled in 6 weeks for another film and dressing change. If the radiograph shows the material to be washed out or the material appears to be soft and moist, this is indicative of an active interchange with the reparative cells. Then another mixture of the $Ca(OH)_2$-anesthetic paste is placed in the defect area and checked again at 6-week intervals until it is dry upon direct examination. If at the first recall there is no radiographic change in the density of the paste and the material is firm and dry on clinical examination, the paste is replaced and checked at 3-month intervals.

The anesthetic solution acts as a vehicle and does not change the chemical formulation of the $Ca(OH)_2$. There is no reaction between the two ingredients. The paste does not set up like a dental cement and therefore is easily removed with endodontic excavators, irrigation, and finally a swab made of loose cotton fibers wrapped around a barbed broach.

The defect should be sealed when there is both clinical and radiographic evidence of healing (i.e., apposition of a barrier at the site of the perforation). Repair may be observed as early as 6 months postoperative and as late as 20 months.

Use with perforating resorption. Frank and Weine[47] reported on a technique using the $Ca(OH)_2$-CMCP mixture for the nonsurgical treatment of perforating internal resorption. In such situations other similar techniques have been used in which the deposition of a cementum-like or osteoid tissue at the site of the defect is the end result. The intention of these techniques is to effect periodontal repair at the site of the defect. The biologic repair should serve as a limiting barrier for the gutta-percha and sealer.

The key to success in these situations is control of bleeding. If this can be accomplished with the aid of an aluminum chloride solution (Hemodent) or with Orastat, the usual treatment can be followed: canal debridement and obturation with gutta-percha apical to the level of the perforation (Fig. 16-20, *A* and *B*). The rest of the canal and void are then filled with the $Ca(OH)_2$-anesthetic solution paste. The access cavity is then sealed with zinc oxide-eugenol or Cavit and covered with a layer of zinc phosphate cement or a composite restoration. The procedure should be checked at 3-month intervals (Fig. 16-20, *C*) with a radiograph and clinical examination. If bleeding occurs when the tooth is probed through the access cavity with an endodontic explorer, the paste should be replaced and the coronal opening resealed for another 3 months. When sufficient ''new tooth structure'' has been deposited in the defect area and the perforation cannot be probed, the rest of the canal may be obturated with gutta-percha (Fig. 16-20, *D* to *G*).

If the perforation is at a level apical to the epithelial

L.D. Caulk Co., Milford, Del.

A B C

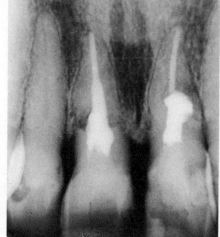

D

G

E F

FIG. 16-20. Perforating internal resorption. Recalcification treatment of the maxillary central incisors. **A,** Pretreatment. Intact epithelial attachments on both teeth. **B,** Left central incisor repaired after 6 months of calcium hydroxide treatment. Recalcification complete. Sealer was not expressed through the repaired defect. Clinical examination of the right central incisor 6 months after $Ca(OH)_2$ paste placement showed an opening into the periodontal ligament. **C,** Right central incisor 9 months after initial treatment. $Ca(OH)_2$-anesthetic solution paste placed in the defect. **D,** Right central incisor 15 months after treatment with $Ca(OH)_2$ paste. The perforation repair is complete. **E and F,** Right central incisor (two views). Defect sealed with gutta-percha, vertical condensation. Cement was expressed through the cementoid barrier even though no clinical opening was evident. **G,** One year later the left central incisor showed further calcification of bone and tooth structure. (Compare with **B.**) In the right central incisor the excess cement was absorbed. Lamina dura is intact.

attachment, where it is protected by the alveolar bone, the chances of success with this technique are considered favorable. The converse is also true. Failure will occur if the perforation is coronal to the attachment apparatus. The $Ca(OH)_2$ most likely will be washed out by the oral fluids, rendering the treatment ineffective. In such cases a surgical approach to the repair of the defect will probably be necessary.

The $Ca(OH)_2$–anesthetic solution mixture may be used with internal resorption and an immature apex (Fig. 16-21, A and B). The technique will encourage physiologic repair of the defect and further apical maturation. When this is done, the canal and defect are sealed with gutta-percha (Fig. 16-21, C and D).

Treatments utilizing the $Ca(OH)_2$–anesthetic solution paste may aid in salvaging previously "hopeless" cases.

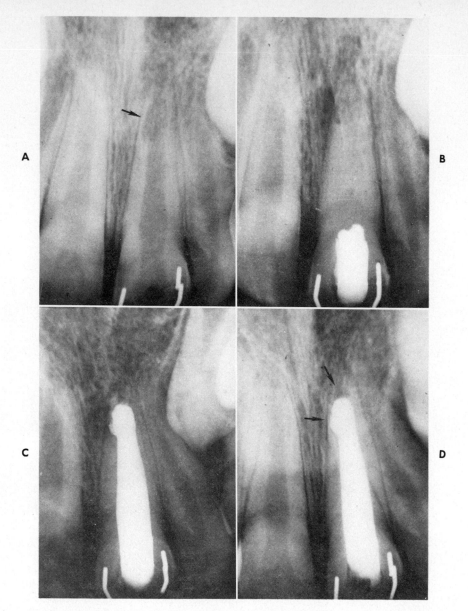

FIG. 16-21. Incompletely formed apex and internal resorption. **A,** Pretreatment. Arrow denotes the resorbing apical third. **B,** Entire canal filled with a Ca(OH)$_2$-vehicle mixture. **C,** Six months later, further apical development. The canal was sealed with warmed gutta-percha. **D,** Two years later, further apical development and bone regeneration *(arrows)* at the site of resorption.

Surgical treatment

When the nonsurgical and recalcification requirements cannot be met or have been unsuccessful, a surgical approach is required to correct internal resorption problems (Fig. 16-22). Debridement and sealing of the canal and defect are also essential in this course of action. Surgery may provide a means to accomplish these goals.

Most surgical cases fall into the following categories:

1. Altered anatomy of the root apex by the resorption process[17] (Fig. 16-23)
2. Uncontrollable bleeding from the perforation defect
3. Perforation near or at the epithelial attachment (Fig. 16-24)

Direct examination of the defect via the surgical flap may reveal the tooth loss to be more extensive than originally anticipated. If it cannot be corrected or there is insufficient tooth structure remaining, extraction may be required. In multirooted teeth a hemisection may be in order (Fig. 16-25).

Careful treatment planning, including the allocation of sufficient chair time, is essential prior to the actual procedure. The anticipation of problems and the preparations for solving them are necessary before using the scalpel. Whenever possible, the canal and defect should be instrumental prior to the surgical appointment. This will give the dentist a preview of what is in store at the time of surgery.

Examination of the gingival tissues with a periodontal probe provides a wealth of information needed to deter-

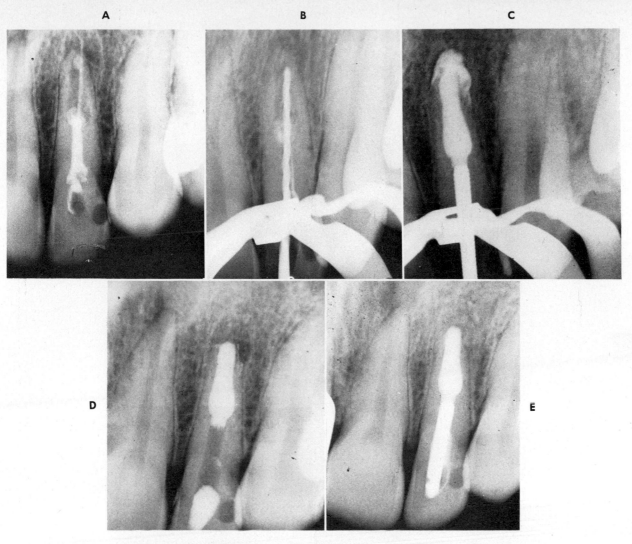

FIG. 16-22. Internal resorption. Surgical treatment of a nonsurgical failure. **A,** Pretreatment. Canal and defect not filled properly. Gutta-percha extends beyond the root. **B,** Gutta-percha removed. Measurement radiograph. **C,** Canal and defect sealed with gutta-percha, vertical condensation. Tryin of a Para Post. **D,** Postsurgical. Apical curettage, excess sealer removed. The apical gutta-percha seal was intact. **E,** Two years posttreatment. Bone remineralized.

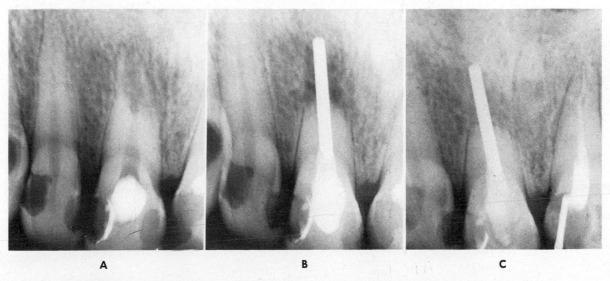

FIG. 16-23. Internal resorption. Surgical treatment of a maxillary central incisor. **A,** Pretreatment. **B,** Apicoectomy and a Vitallium pin placed with zinc phosphate cement. **C,** Five years posttreatment. The right central incisor was previously treated elsewhere.

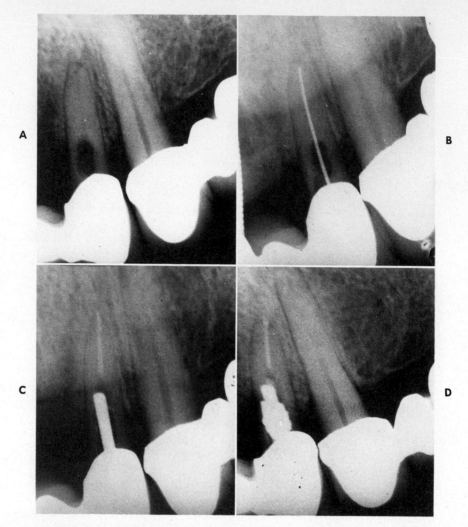

FIG. 16-24. Perforating internal resorption. Surgical treatment of a perforation at the labial surface of a root. **A,** Pretreatment. **B,** Canal length established with a test file, followed by thorough cleaning and shaping. **C,** Apical half of the canal sealed with gutta-percha, lateral condensation. Post tryin. Note that the palatal wall of the defect is intact. **D,** Postsurgical. The post has been cemented and the defect filled with silver amalgam.

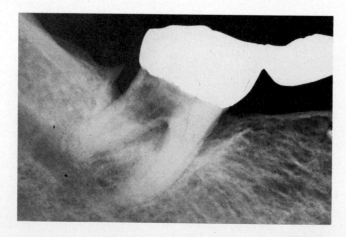

FIG. 16-25. Extensive internal resorption of a mandibular molar, requiring hemisection.

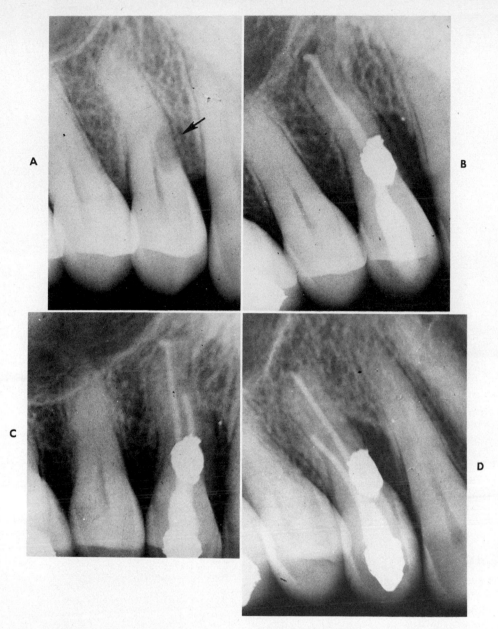

FIG. 16-26. External resorption *(arrow),* requiring surgical endodontic therapy. (Similar to the concept for internal resorption.) **A,** Pretreatment. **B,** Immediately after the procedure. **C,** Two years later. **D,** Twelve years after the procedure. The periodontal defect was manageable, with minimal apical migration.

mine the proper treatment sequence and choice of flap design. With the probe the dentist locates the perforation on the labial aspect of the root coronal to the epithelial attachment (Fig. 16-24). Therefore the exposure, curettage, and cleaning of the defect are performed before access to the crown is gained. A triangular flap is used because the area of operation is in the coronal third of the root. Since a dry field has been established, the instrumentation and sealing of the apical section of the root are completed routinely. A stainless steel post is cemented in place, and the defect is repaired with silver amalgam.

A periodontal defect may result from any endodontic repair surgery near the epithelial attachment. This will occur if the crestal bone is lost because of the pathologic process or is necessarily removed to expose the defect. The bone loss usually extends to the apical level of the repair material (i.e., amalgam) (Fig. 16-26). This is an important consideration in determining a course of action, and the patient should be informed of the possibility. When the resorption is in the apical third of the root, a root resection coronal to the defect should be employed (Fig. 16-27). An endodontic implant has been suggested when extensive root destruction has occurred in the middle or apical third of the root[43] (Fig. 16-23).

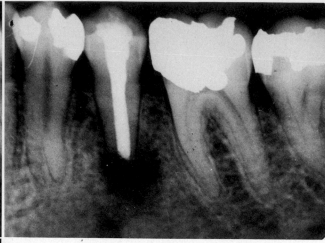

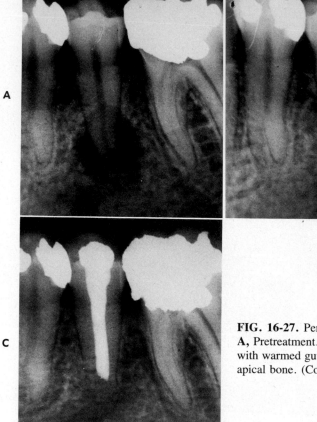

FIG. 16-27. Perforating internal resorption in the apical third of the root. **A,** Pretreatment. **B,** Posttreatment. Apicoectomy after the canal was sealed with warmed gutta-percha. **C,** Eighteen months later. Regeneration of periapical bone. (Courtesy Dr. Michael Anker.)

EXTERNAL RESORPTION

The loss of cementum and/or dentin from the roots of the teeth originating in the periodontal ligament is defined as external resorption. Although the etiology of internal resorption is unknown, many situations are cited as causes of external resorption. Shafer et al.[119] designated the following etiologic factors:

Periapical inflammation
Excessive mechanical or occlusal forces
Replantation of teeth
Impaction of teeth
Tumors and cysts
Idiopathic

Radiation therapy, luxation injuries (Fig. 16-28), and periodontal disease are frequent causes of this pathologic process. Recently, the bleaching of endodontically treated teeth (Fig. 16-29) has been mentioned on numerous occasions.* Galvanic corrosion of nonprecious posts[92] and bacterial invasion have also been mentioned.[109]

External resorption may be found in hypoparathyroid-

*References 16, 54, 62, 74, 76, 81, 82a, 93.

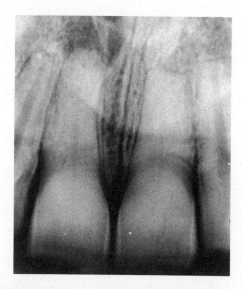

FIG. 16-28. External resorption as a result of a concussion injury 10 years earlier. Left central incisor—pulp necrosis and periapical pathosis. Right central incisor—apical root resorption and calcification of canal space; no response to vitality testing. Right lateral incisor—apical root resorption; positive response to vitality testing.

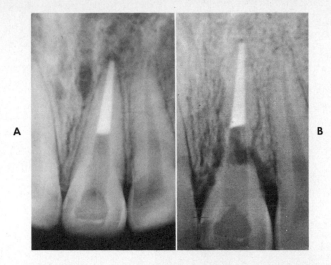

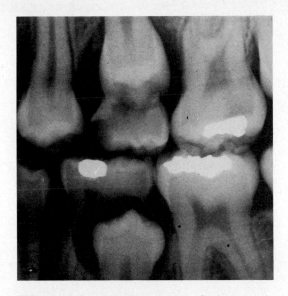

FIG. 16-29. External resorption following bleaching. **A,** Completion of root canal therapy immediately followed by walking bleach procedure. **B,** External resorption 16 months following bleaching procedure. The tooth was extracted 6 months later. (Courtesy Drs. William Goon and Stephen Cohen.)

FIG. 16-30. Physiologic resorption of primary teeth.

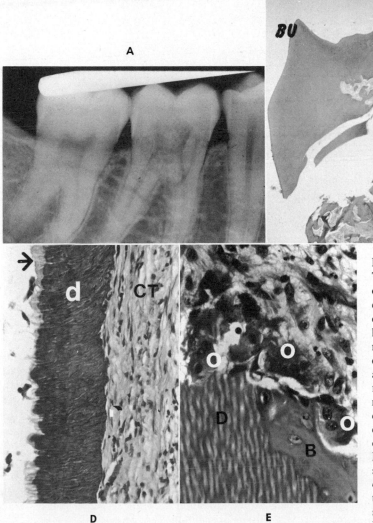

FIG. 16-31. Idiopathic external resorption. There was no recalled history of trauma, pernicious habits, orthodontia, periodontal disease or carics. **A,** Radiograph of mandibular first molar; defect on lingual surface of tooth. **B,** Low-power histologic section of tooth. *BU,* Buccal; *Arrow,* rim of dentin adjacent to pulp chamber apparently resistant to resorption; *1 to 3,* sections examined in subsequent figures. **C,** Higher magnification of curea 1. *Arrow,* Ingrowth of replacement bone. **D,** Higher magnification of curea 2. *Arrow,* predentin free of resorption; *d,* dentin not affected by resorptive process; *ct,* connective tissue showing slight inflammation. **E,** Higher magnification of area 3. Active resorption and deposition are taking place. *O,* odontoclasts in lacunae resorbing dentin; *D,* dentin; *B,* bone deposited in area of previously resorbed dentin. (Courtesy Drs. John Creech and Richard E. Walton.)

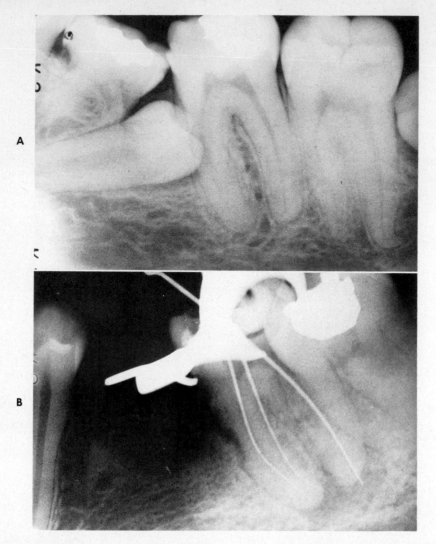

FIG. 16-32. External resorption due to an impacted tooth. **A,** Crown of the premolar contacting the distal root of the molar. **B,** Six months postsurgical. Deciduous molar and impacted premolar extracted. Note the regeneration of alveolar bone in the site of external resorption. The periapical pathosis resulted from caries not related to the resorption. (Courtesy Drs. Michael Chusid and Robert Strausberg.)

ism, calcinosis, Gaucher's disease, hyperparathyroidism, Turner's syndrome, and Paget's disease.[121]

Morse[95] states, "The resorption . . . in systemic disturbances usually occurs at the apex of several teeth and is bilateral." The treatment of the underlying systemic disease may cause the resorption to cease.

External resorption of primary teeth during the eruption of their permanent successors is considered physiologic (Fig. 16-30). Three separate phases have been described: active, partial, and reparative.[2,3] Fibroblastic activity within the periodontal ligament is responsible for the production of a mucopolysaccharidase-like enzyme during primary tooth resorption. There is a definite increase of hydroxyproline in resorbing teeth, and there is no inflammatory infiltrate.

External resorption without an apparent cause (Fig. 16-31) (idiopathic) continues to be mentioned as an etiologic factor.[31,72,96,112] For example, one article[31] presented a pa-

tient in whom nine premolar and molar teeth had undergone apical root resorption without apparent cause. There was no history of trauma or orthodontic treatment and the blood chemistry was normal.

Pressure from an impacted tooth[18,57,59,101,134] (Fig. 16-32) may cause root resorption. A comprehensive study[101] of impacted teeth reported a 7.5% incidence of external root resorption at the contact area of the roots of the adjacent teeth. The incidence was highest in the younger age group (21 to 30 years), and males were twice as susceptible as females. The authors concluded that inflammation in addition to pressure may play a role in the resorption (Fig. 16-33).

Clinically the resorption ceases when the impacted tooth is removed. If the resorption is not severe and the site is apical to the epithelial attachment, repair can be expected with cellular cementum (Fig. 16-34).

External resorption is almost universal. In a study using

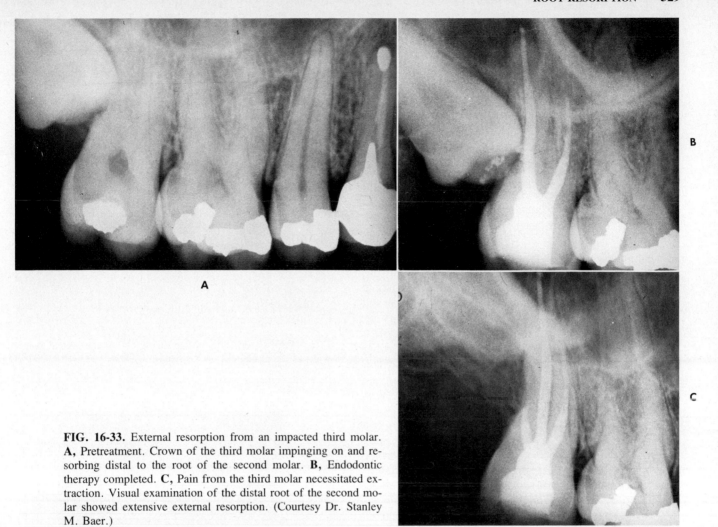

FIG. 16-33. External resorption from an impacted third molar. A, Pretreatment. Crown of the third molar impinging on and resorbing distal to the root of the second molar. B, Endodontic therapy completed. C, Pain from the third molar necessitated extraction. Visual examination of the distal root of the second molar showed extensive external resorption. (Courtesy Dr. Stanley M. Baer.)

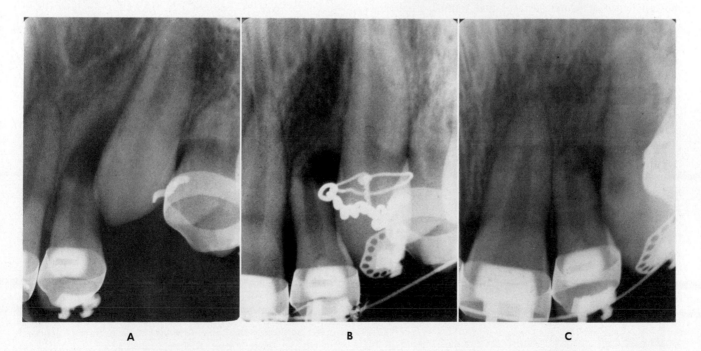

FIG. 16-34. External resorption due to an impacted canine. A, Resorption of the apex of the lateral incisor. The canine was surgically exposed to facilitate orthodontic treatment. B, Extrusive force was applied to the canine, moving it away from the apex of the lateral incisor. C, Repair of the apex. (Courtesy Dr. Issac Post.)

radiographs of 5800 teeth in 301 young adults[88] all the patients examined showed evidence of resorption in four or more permanent teeth. These ranged from mild cases, with the apex blunted at least 1 or 2 mm, to situations in which more than half the root length was lost. Another study[68] found that 90% of 261 teeth from 15 adult cadavers exhibited root resorption. External resorption was found in 49.6% of the permanent pulpless teeth studied. The degree of resorption was significantly related to the presence and size of the periapical lesion. Much more resorption was reported[77] in the roots without root canal filling than in those that were filled.

Microscopic areas of lateral resorption are common in the elderly. In some instances these foci show repair by cementum.[24]

When a light microscope was used, one study[64] found that 80% of healthy teeth and 90% of periodontally involved teeth showed root resorption. In another study[118] resorption of dentin was seen within the root canal and periapical portion of the root in 62% of the cases examined. Another phase of the same investigation reported root resorption in 100% of the cases involving extractions for periodontal reasons. In both groups repair by cementum had occurred in most cases.

It has also been proposed[122] that root resorption may be an intermediate step in the progression of periodontal disease, not necessarily a cause or effect. When teeth are lost because of periodontal disease, shifting of the remaining dentition occurs. The resultant occlusal forces become more lateral than vertical, and saucer-shaped resorptions are usually observed on the pressure side of these roots. As the disease process migrates apically, salivary calculus may invade the lateral resorbed areas before cemental repair can take place. The calculus adheres tenaciously to the roughened cemental surfaces and routine prophylaxis is usually insufficient to remove these deposits. Thus the disease progresses further as the bone loss and root resorption are combined with occlusal forces and local irritants.

Periapical inflammation
Apical resorption

Because apical external resorption is widespread in the population, its effect on the prognosis of endodontic therapy should be examined. Two authors[48,130] reported a poorer prognosis when apical resorption was observed. For years investigators[58,66,70] have believed that apical resorption is a contraindication to nonsurgical treatment. These investigators concluded that the apex was denuded of its periodontal ligament, resulting in such consequences as necrotic cementum, the likelihood of a persistent bacterial nidus in the necrotic dentin, and an inability to seal the enlarged apex. Others,[44,91,106] however, have stated that teeth with eroded apices are candidates for nonsurgical root canal therapy. One author[100] suggested that root resorption before treatment was *not* associated with a particularly poor prognosis.

A histologic analysis[117] showed cemental repairs of resorptive areas in both cementum and dentin. It also demonstrated that the presence of extensive apical resorption is

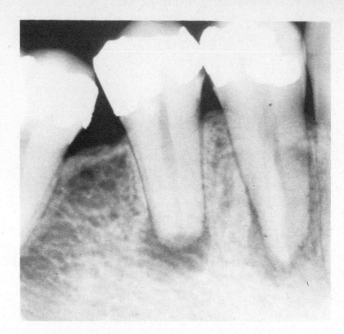

FIG. 16-35. External resorption due to chronic periapical lesions with necrotic pulps.

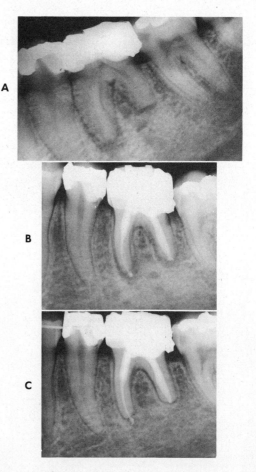

FIG. 16-36. External apical resorption. Nonsurgical endodontic therapy. **A,** Pretreatment. **B,** Immediately posttreatment. **C,** One year later, good bone remineralization. Note the physiologic rounding of the distal root.

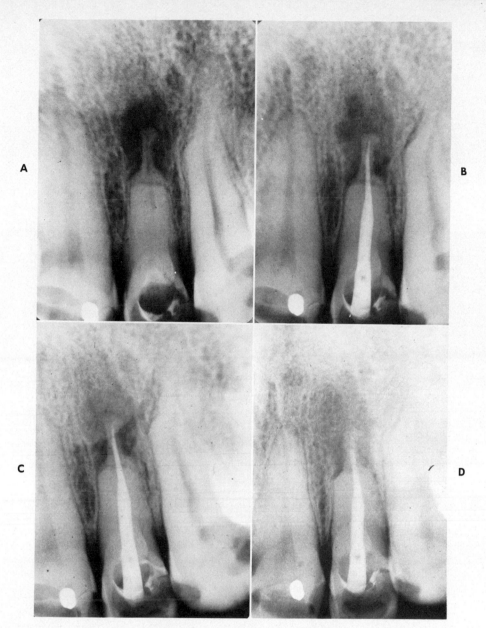

FIG. 16-37. Severe external apical resorption. Nonsurgical therapy. **A,** Pretreatment. Extensive resorption in the apical third, but the canal appears intact. **B,** Posttreatment. Lateral condensation with finger spreaders. No lateral defects were seen in the apical region. **C,** Six months after treatment there is evidence of some bone remineralization. **D,** Five years after treatment, clinically asymptomatic with continuing bone remineralization.

usually indicative of severe pulpal involvement wherein the pulp is either chronically inflamed or necrotic (Fig. 16-35). Because extirpation of the pulp and complete canal debridement are necessary in these situations, attempts to preserve the pulp are contraindicated. Apical resorption is associated with chronic apical periodontitis.[73]

Root resorption, among other reactions, will result if the root end is perforated during routine cleaning and shaping. The intensity of the periapical response is markedly increased if bacterial endotoxins infiltrate the apex.[108] Conversely, mild periapical reactions will be present without root resorption, even in the presence of bacterial endotox-

ins, if the root end is not perforated. Therefore it would be prudent for the dentist to confine instrumentation to the canal. Instrumentation rather than canal disinfectants is the most important factor for hard tissue resorption at the root canal wall.[120]

In the opinion of Strindberg,[130] "since the canal is generally open at the apex there is a fairly pronounced overfilling, a circumstance that may itself imply a poorer prognosis." With current treatment methods, however, this old stumbling block to nonsurgical treatment in the presence of external root resorption is no longer present. With newer gutta-percha techniques emphasizing coronal shap-

A   B   C

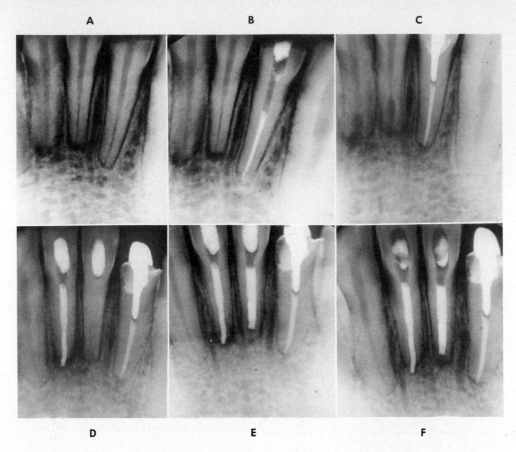

D   E   F

FIG. 16-38. External apical resorption. Apexification technique. **A,** Pretreatment. Same day as a baseball injury. The right lateral incisor has a crown fracture and pulp exposure. The central incisors have vital pulps. **B,** Posttreatment. Right lateral incisor, same day. **C,** Six-month recall. The right lateral incisor is asymptomatic. A cast post has been cemented. Both central incisors have external apical and internal resorption. **D,** One month later. The attempt to confine gutta-percha to the canal of the left central incisor was unsuccessful. In the right central incisor apexification was accomplished with Ca(OH)$_2$ paste. **E,** Six months later bone is regenerating in the left central incisor. In the right central incisor an apical barrier has been established and the canal sealed by vertical condensation of gutta-percha. **F,** One year later (25 months after injury) there is almost complete bone repair around all teeth.

ing with an apical constriction, most canals can be adequately shaped to confine the filling material within the canal. After proper canal preparation the canal (Fig. 16-36) is sealed with gutta-percha by lateral, vertical, or thermatic condensation, even in cases of severe apical resorption (Fig. 16-37).

When resorption has enlarged the apical portion of the canal, precluding proper instrumentation and sealing, apical closure techniques should be used to ensure a better prognosis for nonsurgical endodontic therapy (Fig. 16-38)

When recall radiographs 6 months or 1 year later show continued resorption or persistent periapical pathosis, apical surgery should be performed. If from the outset the surgical approach would allow for sealing of lateral defects in a case of external resorption (Fig. 16-24), the clinician would be justified in using it. Usually. however, nonsurgical treatment is the initial approach for external resorption.

Cervical resorption

External resorption in the coronal third of the root near the cementum-enamel junction is usually the result of an inflammatory reaction in the surrounding tissues, the periodontal ligament. It may occur years after a traumatic incident that the patient no longer remembers. It is primarily seen in replanted and ankylosed teeth in infraposition but can occur in luxated teeth.[33] It may be a consequence of orthodontic movement (Fig. 16-39) and it can occur in teeth with vital pulps as well as those that have undergone endodontic therapy.

Cervical resorption can undermine the crown. It has been shown that extensive external resorption may surround the pulp chamber and canal and not penetrate it. The odontoblastic layer and underlying predentin seem to act in concert as a barrier against resorption[61] (Fig. 16-31). In advanced stages it creates the classic "pink spot" (Fig. 16-40). It is often mistaken for internal resorption and was

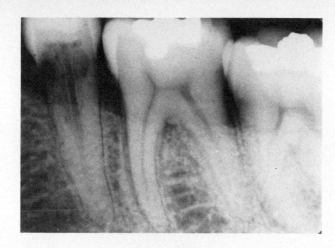

A

FIG. 16-39. Cervical external resorption 6 years after the completion of orthodontic treatment.

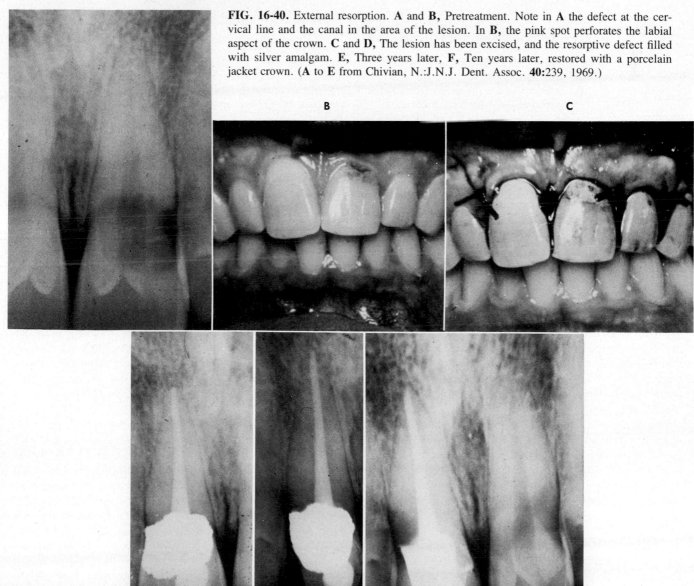

FIG. 16-40. External resorption. **A** and **B,** Pretreatment. Note in **A** the defect at the cervical line and the canal in the area of the lesion. In **B,** the pink spot perforates the labial aspect of the crown. **C** and **D,** The lesion has been excised, and the resorptive defect filled with silver amalgam. **E,** Three years later, **F,** Ten years later, restored with a porcelain jacket crown. (**A** to **E** from Chivian, N.:J.N.J. Dent. Assoc. 40:239, 1969.)

B   **C**

D   **E**   **F**

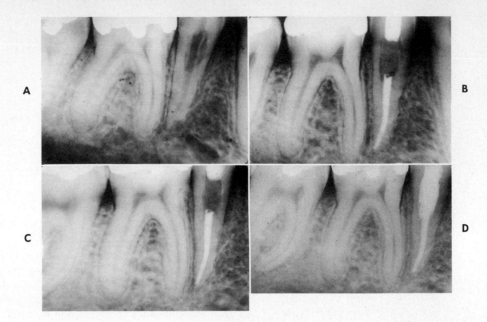

FIG. 16-41. External cervical resorption 5 years after completion of orthodontics. **A,** Pretreatment. **B,** Apex sealed with lateral condensation of gutta-percha. Perforation apical to the epithelial attachment located a lingual surface through the enlarged access cavity. Calcium hydroxide past was placed in the defect. **C,** Nine months after treatment. No perforation evident clinically. **D,** Coronal defect sealed with vertical condensation.

recently classified as a new entity.[46] However, because an intact canal follows the entire length of the tooth and the resorption starts in the periodontium, it is correctly classified as external resorption.

The treatment approaches are similar to those described for internal resorption. Once again, the position of the resorption in relation to the epithelial attachment dictates the choice:

1. If the defect extends from above the attachment to below it, a nonsurgical approach may be attempted.[50] Pulp extirpation, cleaning, shaping, and sealing the canal follow the standard course of treatment. Access to the lesion, which is outside the canal and chamber, is obtained with a large round bur from within the tooth. Amalgam or composite is the defect-filling material of choice. The tooth should be reinforced with a post.[15]

The nonsurgical approach for cervical resorption, however, has its limitations. It can be used only if the perforation to the periodontal ligament is small and the filling material can be confined to the defect. It may serve as an intermediate step to surgery if there is extrusion of the repair material outside the tooth. It is a convenient way to fill the defect; the surgery is then directed toward removing the excess.

2. If the perforation is apical to the attachment, a recalcification procedure is used (Fig. 16-41). If it is coronal, then surgery is indicated to seal the defect Figs. 16-18, 16-40, and 16-42).

Pulp extirpation is required in these cases. The extent of the resorption and subsequent repair procedure, in the surgical method, will have an irreversible effect on the pulp tissue.

Bleaching. There are numerous reports recently* that external resorption in the cervical region of the tooth is a possible consequence of bleaching (Fig. 16-43). Harrington and Natkin[62] hypothesized that seepage of the Superoxol through the dentinal tubules created the inflammatory process in the adjacent gingival tissues. Others[81] pointed out that cementum and enamel do not join at the cementoenamel junction in approximately 10% of all teeth. They also noted that the bleaching procedure denatures the dentin exposed at the cervical line and renders it an immunologically different tissue. This creates a foreign body reaction. Patent dentinal tubules, prior history of trauma, and etching the dentin prior to bleaching may also contribute to the problem. Probably the number of cases reported would increase many times if all dentists who bleach teeth were questioned.

Until recently the dental profession was not aware of the problem. Either the resorption was not associated with bleaching, or it was attributed to other causes, or it was called idiopathic. The problem is with us; our bleaching technique must be directed toward reducing its probability.

1. Protection of the dentinal tubules. Remove the gutta-percha apical to the cervical line to remove discolored dentin. However, do not extend the preparation into the root. Use the crestal bone as a guide. Place a layer of cement, (IRM, CAVIT, or glass ionomer) over the gutta-percha to prevent the ingress of the bleaching materials alongside the gutta-percha.

2. Eliminate the use of heat. Walking bleaches[102,123]

---

*References 16, 54, 62, 74, 76, 81, 82a, 93.

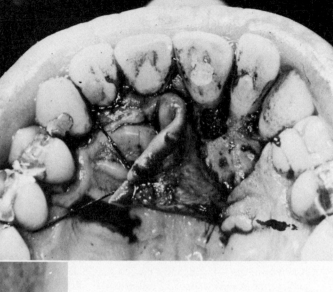

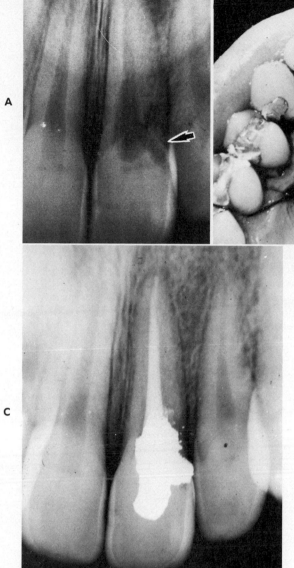

FIG. 16-42. Cervical external resorption *(arrow).* **A,** Pretreatment. **B,** Palatal surgical approach. A triangular flap tied to the premolar teeth gives clear vision. **C,** Posttreatment. (Courtesy Dr. Hyman R. Baer.)

have been effective for over a quarter of a century. Repeated treatments will produce results equal to a one-sitting thermocatalytic procedure.

3. *Avoid etching of the dentin.* Some techniques suggest etching the dentin prior to bleaching.[25] Phosphoric or citric acid will open the dentinal tubules, and may lead to a direct path to the gingival tissues. Avoid this potential liability.

4. *Beware of the caustic nature of Superoxol.*[114] Many of the cases reported a previous history of trauma in youngsters with varying degrees of tooth development. The dentin walls may not have been fully developed and the Superoxol would have greater ease of penetrating on. Spasser advocates sodium perborate (USP) and water for the walking bleach. His considerable experience produces excellent results with no history of external resorption.[123,124] Because the desired end result can be achieved

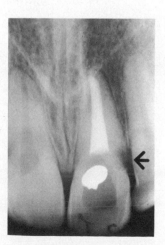

FIG. 16-43. External cervical resorption following bleaching *(arrow)* at defect on distal surface of the cementoenamel junction. (From Montgomery, S.: Oral Surg. **57:**203, 1984.)

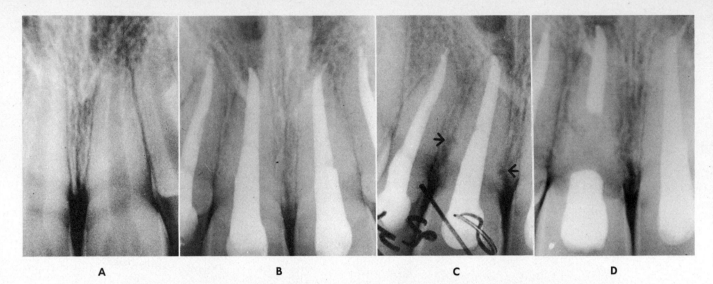

FIG. 16-44. External cervical resorption following intentional endodontics and walking bleach. **A,** Pretreatment—4 years after unsuccessful external (vital) bleaching to improve the esthetics of tetracycline-stained teeth. **B,** Posttreatment. Intentional endodontics was completed on maxillary anterior teeth. The gutta-percha was removed coronal to the cementoenamel junction and the tooth structure was washed with 50% citric acid. Walking bleaches were performed on three separate occasions. **C,** Two years posttreatment. Note external resorption on central incisor *(arrows).* **D,** One year later following calcium hydroxide therapy. Periodontal healing appears on mesial surface: but there is further extension of lingual cervical resorption. (Courtesy Drs. Bryce W. Bonness and William T. Johnson.)

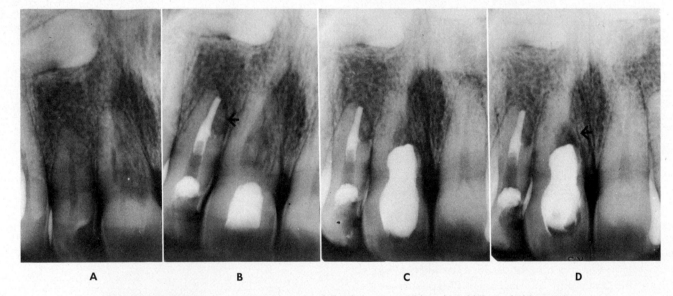

FIG. 16-45. External resorption 11 years following auto accident in which teeth hit steering wheel. **A,** *Lateral incisor*—small area of resorption on mesial surface in apical third of root. *Central incisor*—extensive resorption on incisor two thirds of root. **B,** One month later. *Lateral incisor*—nonsurgical root canal therapy. Canal is filled with gutta-percha and sealer extruded through small perforation *(arrow)*. *Central incisor*—access through chamber to resorption location revealed extensive perforation on mesiolabial surface of the root. Calcium hydroxide therapy was instituted. It was changed at 3-month intervals for 1½ years. The canal coronal to the defect was not penetrated. **C,** Thirty months later. *Lateral incisor*—absorption of excess sealed. There is evidence of bone regeneration at apex. *Central incisor*—since there was no evidence of repair a surgical approach was used. The canal coronal to the defect was filled with IRM. The defect was sealed with composite resin. **D,** Twenty-six months following surgery. *Lateral incisor*—complete regeneration of apical lamina dura. *Central incisor*—evidence of regeneration of lamina dura at surgical site *(arrow)*.

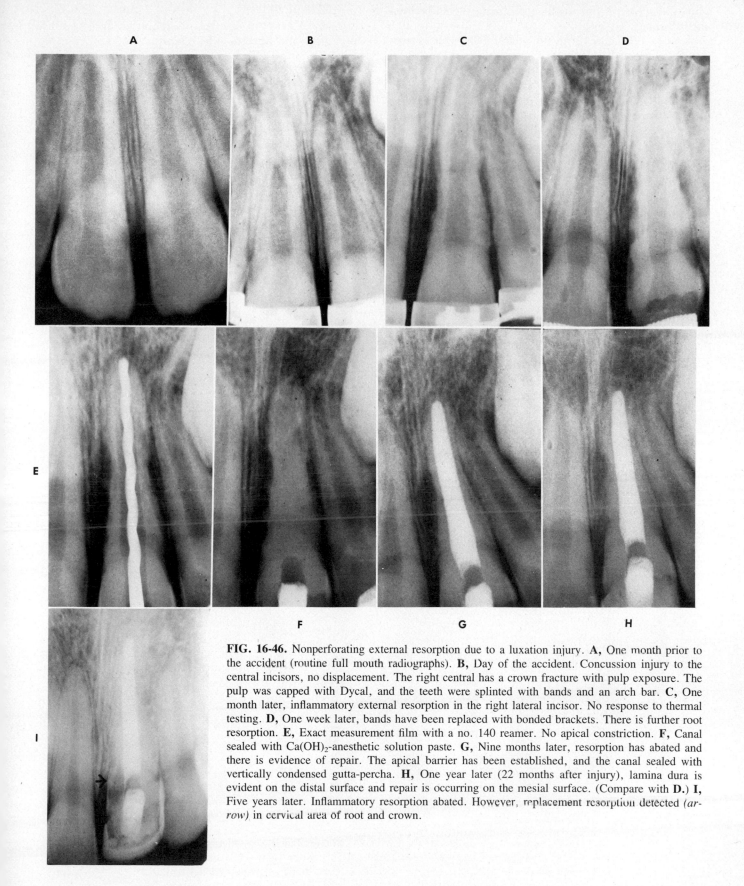

FIG. 16-46. Nonperforating external resorption due to a luxation injury. **A,** One month prior to the accident (routine full mouth radiographs). **B,** Day of the accident. Concussion injury to the central incisors, no displacement. The right central has a crown fracture with pulp exposure. The pulp was capped with Dycal, and the teeth were splinted with bands and an arch bar. **C,** One month later, inflammatory external resorption in the right lateral incisor. No response to thermal testing. **D,** One week later, bands have been replaced with bonded brackets. There is further root resorption. **E,** Exact measurement film with a no. 140 reamer. No apical constriction. **F,** Canal sealed with Ca(OH)$_2$-anesthetic solution paste. **G,** Nine months later, resorption has abated and there is evidence of repair. The apical barrier has been established, and the canal sealed with vertically condensed gutta-percha. **H,** One year later (22 months after injury), lamina dura is evident on the distal surface and repair is occurring on the mesial surface. (Compare with **D.**) **I,** Five years later. Inflammatory resorption abated. However, replacement resorption detected (*arrow*) in cervical area of root and crown.

without Superoxol, only sodium perborate should be used for bleaching.

A recent procedure for treating tetracycline-stained teeth has been reported.[1] It involves intentional root canal therapy and bleaching from within the crown. The bleaching results were successful. However, a recent report[76] (Fig. 16-44) following this technique resulted in external resorption in the cervical region in one of the six teeth treated. It has not responded to calcium hydroxide therapy and will probably be lost in the near future. The concept of treating tetracycline-stained teeth with root canal therapy and bleaching should be reevaluated.

Lateral resorption

A major cause of external resorption on the lateral aspect of the root appears to be a luxation injury wherein the tooth has been displaced but not avulsed. Intrusion trauma produces a higher frequency of external root resorption than do other types of luxation injury because of the crushing of the periodontal ligament.[11] Pulp death usually occurs, requiring endodontic intervention.

Nonperforating resorption. When lateral external resorption does not perforate the root canal, nonsurgical treatment with a gutta-percha filling can be used successfully to stop the destruction. Cvek[32] stated that "the arrest

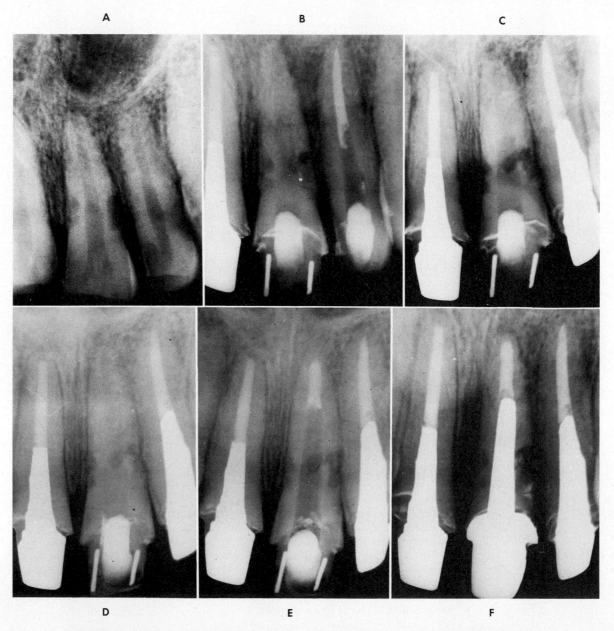

FIG. 16-47. External root resorption of a maxillary right central incisor. **A,** Pretreatment. **B,** One month later. Endodontic therapy has been completed on adjacent teeth. The canal has been debrided and filled with a Ca(OH)$_2$-vehicle mixture. **C,** Two months later, further resorption. **D,** Six months later, resorption abating. **E,** Apical section of the canal sealed with warmed gutta-percha. Note the regeneration of alveolar bone and the growth of new tooth structure. **F,** Post and core cemented. Cement was extruded through a pinpoint defect distally.

of external root resorption related to pulpal necrosis can be ascribed exclusively to removal of necrotic pulp and anti-bacterial treatment of the root canal'' (Fig. 16-45). The extrusion of a radiopaque paste (root canal cement) into the periodontal ligament through the root canal, under pressure, will aid in the confirmation of perforating root resorption.[39]

I pretreat all luxation injury cases with $Ca(OH)_2$ and anesthetic solution for 6 to 12 months.[142] If no resorption is seen radiographically by that time, the root canal is sealed with gutta-percha. When lateral resorption is noticed from the outset, pulp extirpation, debridement, and $Ca(OH)_2$ therapy are obligatory (Fig. 16-46). The effect of the

$Ca(OH)_2$ on areas of inflammation in the periodontal ligament is increased when the cementum is resorbed from the root.[139]

Perforating resorption. When the lateral resorption process reaches the dentin or perforates the root canal, the $Ca(OH)_2$ procedure should be attempted after canal debridement. In addition to halting the destruction, it will promote the deposition of new tooth structure to repair the defect physiologically (Fig. 16-45).[129]

Calcium hydroxide should be placed into the resorption defect at 3-month intervals until there is evidence of hard tissue repair. This is confirmed by both radiographs and direct examination through the access cavity. When a

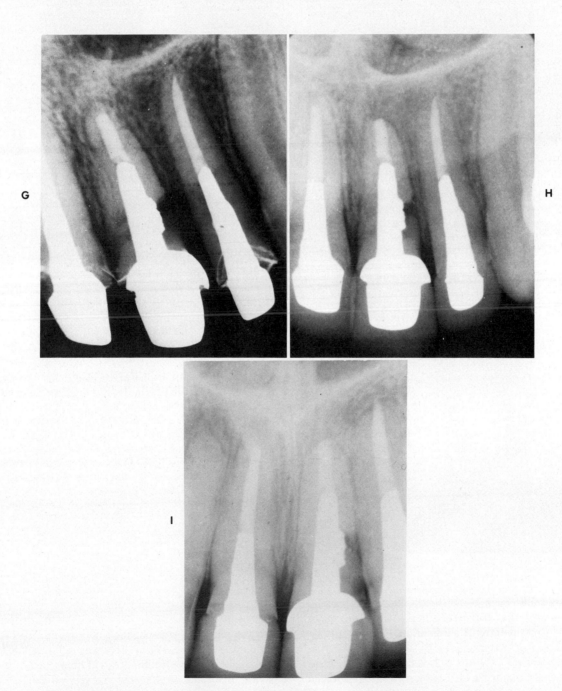

FIG. 16-47, cont'd. G, Amalgam sealed in the defect via a surgical approach. **H,** Twenty-four months later, bone regeneration. **I,** Forty-eight months later.

A   B   C

D

E   F

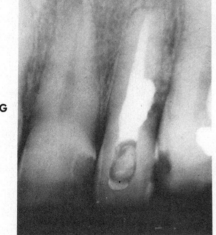

G

FIG. 16-48. Perforating external resorption treatment, recalcification technique. **A** and **B** Pretreatment (two views). The lesion moved when the horizontal angle of the x-ray cone was changed. The perforation is apical to the epithelial attachment, covered by bone, and too apical for root extension. Therefore a recalcification procedure was used. **C,** Apical section filled with gutta-percha. **D,** Access cavity enlarged. The defect was filled with $Ca(OH)_2$-anesthetic solution paste. **E,** One year later a lateral calcific barrier has been established. No perforation was noted clinically. **F,** Defect sealed with vertically condensed gutta-percha. Excess cement was expressed through the barrier. **G,** One year later there is evidence of bone repair at the site of the lateral defect.

physical barrier has been established, the defect can be filled with gutta-percha. If hard tissue repair has not taken place after 24 to 30 months, a surgical approach should be used. The choice of material used to seal the perforation (i.e., amalgam, IRM, Cavit, composite resin, or glass isonomer cement) should be determined by its location in relation to the marginal gingiva (Fig. 16-45).

Fig. 16-47 illustrates the treatment of a tooth that was

luxated but not displaced from its socket. After canal debridement a paste of $Ca(OH)_2$ and CMCP was introduced into the canal. It was changed at 3-month intervals for a period of 9 months. When there was radiographic evidence of repair and no perforations could be probed in the access cavity, the canal was sealed by vertical condensation of warmed gutta-percha. No gutta-percha or sealer penetrated through any defects. To prepare for a post and core, the

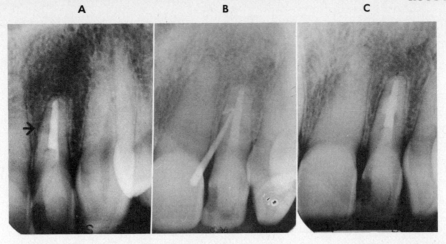

FIG. 16-49. Perforating external resorption: surgical approach. **A,** Pretreatment 3 years after luxation injury and nonsurgical root canal therapy *(arrow)* defect on mesial surface of root. **B,** Pretreatment. Gutta-percha cone was inserted through sinus tract to defect. **C,** Posttreatment. A surgical approach was used to uncover the defect, which extended to the canal space. It was sealed with light-cured composite resin.

coronal two thirds of the gutta-percha was removed. (Where feasible, preparation for the post should extend *apical* to the area of repaired resorption to reduce the chances of fracture of the root.) Cement was expressed through a previously healed defect when the post was inserted. (To reduce cementation pressure, the post should be vented adjacent to the area of repair.) Surgery was used to remove the cement and to repair the pinhole opening. An enlarged undercut preparation was used for amalgam retention. No effort was made to rebuild the contour of the root once the defect was sealed. Twenty-four months later, bone repair was seen.

If the cause of external resorption is pulpal or periapical inflammation that can be eliminated by endodontic therapy using new treatment modalities, the prognosis is favorable.

Sports-related injuries may be the cause of latent areas of root resorption (Fig. 16-48). The patient recalls being struck in the mouth with a hockey puck 12 years before the initial examination. The luxation injury was one of concussion without displacement. The teeth were sensitive to temperature change for several weeks; no dental treatment was required. A shallow silicate cement restoration on the distal surface of the tooth did not appear to contribute to the external resorption. A recalcification procedure was used. There are situations when a surgical approach is required because of location of the defect or its time of discovery (Fig. 16-49).

Excessive mechanical forces: orthodontic movement

Root resorption following orthodontic treatment has long been recognized. (See Chapter 20.) Some root resorption will occur in all malocclusion cases managed orthodontically.* Caution has been suggested in both time of treatment and movement attempted on teeth exhibiting pretreatment root shortening. This resorption potential, a pre-

*References 20, 37, 60, 82, 84, 86, 127, 131, 141, 147.

disposition for frequent and severe postorthodontic root resorption, has been linked to genetic factors.[99] These teeth develop more than average resorption during orthodontic treatment.[52] Orthodontic literature usually states that the amount of tooth loss is clinically insignificant and that neither the stability nor the function of the teeth is affected by resorption. However, a resorptive index has been reported that permits a quantitative assessment of the occurrence and the degree of root resorption during orthodontic treatment. Six months after treatment the highest incidence of root resorption was found in the mandibular central incisors (95%), maxillary central incisors (90%), and maxillary lateral incisors (87%). The lowest incidence was in the mandibular premolars (53%).[52]

A statistical analysis of postorthodontic patients has indicated that apical root resorption is a greater risk when orthodontic treatment is started after 11 years of age than with patients starting earlier. In the same study it was noted that fixed appliances caused significantly more apical root resorption than removable appliances.[84] It has been hypothesized that traumatized teeth have a greater tendency toward root resorption during orthodontic treatment than uninjured teeth. This assumption was not supported by this study. It was noted that traumatized teeth with signs of root resorption before orthodontic treatment may be more prone to root resorption during treatment.[86]

The logical question to ask at this juncture is, Do endodontically treated teeth become more susceptible than vital teeth to root resorption during orthodontic treatment? In one study[53] it was stated that an endodontically treated tooth was less likely to resorb than a vital tooth in the same patient. However, in another study[146] a greater frequency of root resorption was found in endodontically treated teeth than in nontreated teeth. Yet another study[145] found no significant difference in the amount of root resorption between endodontically treated and vital teeth when both were subjected to orthodontic movement (Fig. 16-50). A recent in vivo study[89] showed no significant difference between external root resorption of endodontically

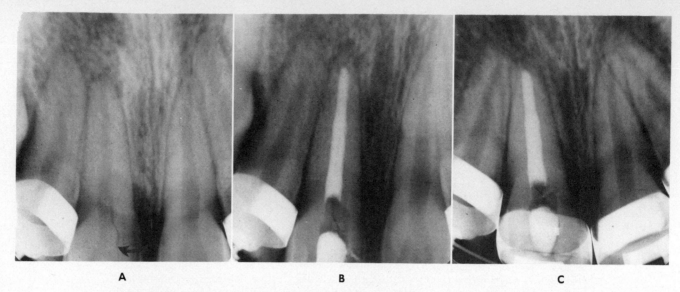

A   **B**   **C**

FIG. 16-50. Root resorption due to orthodontics. **A,** Pretreatment. Left central incisor with a vertical fracture in the crown *(arrow)* and a necrotic pulp. Other incisors responded to thermal testing. **B,** Posttreatment. **C,** One-year recall. Periapical bone remineralization, apical root resorption in the left central and lateral incisors. Active movement was initiated 6 weeks after endodontic therapy was completed.

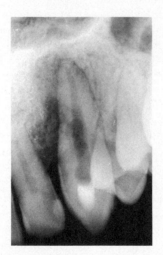

FIG. 16-51. External resorption 10 years after surgical exposure of impacted canine and orthodontic treatment.

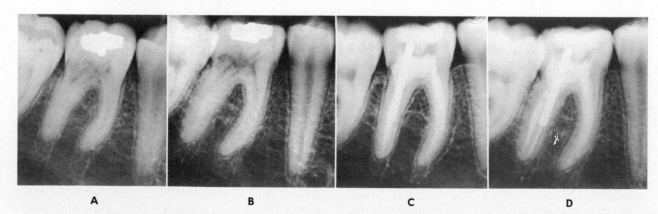

A   **B**   **C**   **D**

FIG. 16-52. External resorption 2 years after completion of orthodontic treatment. **A** and **B,** Pretreatment—two different horizontal angles. Outline of pulp chamber is evident. Occlusal amalgam is of 7 years duration. **C** and **D,** Posttreatment. Access to *the* defect was obtained through occlusal surface. There was a supracrestal perforation at the distolingual gingival point angle *(arrow).* Canals were filled with gutta-percha and sealer and a Parapost was cemented into distolingual canal. The defect was sealed with a composite resin.

treated teeth and vital teeth when both were subjected to orthodontic forces. Although there is mixed opinion on the subject, the conclusion to be drawn from the literature is that virtually all teeth show some resorption during orthodontic treatment.

Root resorption associated with orthodontic treatment usually ceases at the completion of the active and retentive phases. However, in some situations the process continues. Intentional extirpation and calcium hydroxide therapy have been successful in abating apical inflammatory resorption that continued after the completion of orthodontic therapy.[51,90]

Because apical resorption frequently occurs during orthodontic treatment, it behooves the clinician to fill root canals in three dimensions[23] with gutta-percha rather than with silver points, especially in patients who may need orthodontics. Only with well-condensed gutta-percha will the canal remain sealed, even if a few millimeters of the root resorb.

Surgical exposure and subsequent orthodontic movement increase the risk of cervical and lateral external resorption (Fig. 16-51). Extensive external resorption of the crown and root may occur from bodily movement or tipping forces (Fig. 16-52). Extraction may be necessary in some extreme cases (Fig. 16-53).

Orthodontic treatment has been suggested as a cause of internal resorption; however, this has not been confirmed[143] (Fig. 16-7).

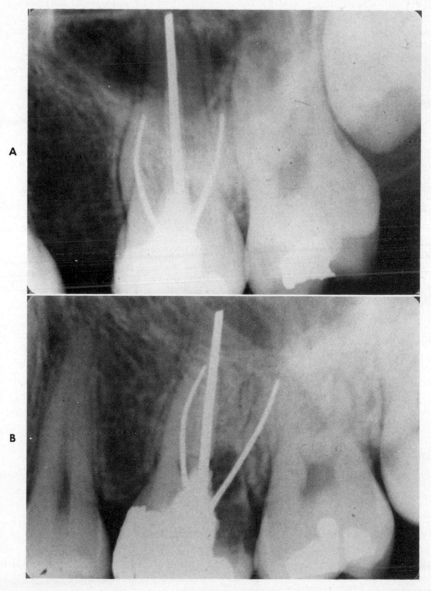

FIG. 16-53. External root resorption after completion of orthodontics. **A,** Endodontic therapy accomplished 6 months prior to tooth movement. Note the distance between the distal surface of the molar and the mesial surface of the premolar. **B,** Eight years later (6 years after completion of orthodontics) there is extensive cervical resorption at the distal gingival surface of the tooth. No evidence of decay.

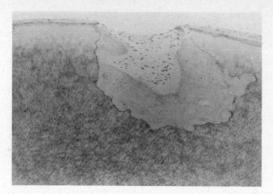

FIG. 16-54. Surface resorption of root as result of traumatic injury. Resorption has stopped and repair is evident (Cellular cementum has formed on the walls of the resorption lacuna). (Courtesy of Dr. Leif Tronstad.)

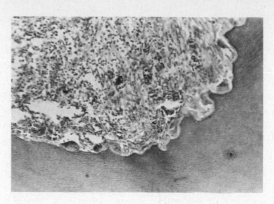

FIG. 16-56. Dentoalveolar ankylosis with replacement resorption of traumatically injured tooth. Ankylosis occurs in areas of necrosis of periodontal ligament. This type of resorption leads to replacement of root by bone, and crown of tooth will finally fall out. (Courtesy Dr. Leif Tronstad.)

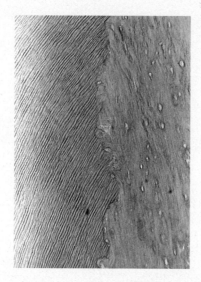

FIG. 16-55. External inflammatory root resorption of traumatically injured tooth. The resorptive process has started because of injury to root surface. The resorption is sustained by infection of necrotic pulp tissue and penetration of certain bacterial metabolites (toxins) from the root canal to the root surface. (Courtesy Dr. Leif Tronstad.)

Replantation of teeth

Root resorption following replantation of avulsed teeth is a postoperative response that must be anticipated. One author[11] reviewed the frequency of progressive root resorption after replantation of avulsed permanent teeth and reported that it ranged from 80% to 96%.

It should be understood by the dentist and patient that replantation is a temporary, stopgap procedure. On rare occasion, replanted teeth have had extended ''second lives.'' However, tooth retention that lasts 5 to 7 years can with justification be considered successful.

Resorption in replanted teeth is usually external. The degree of tooth loss is directly related to the severity of injury to the periodontal ligament at the time of luxation. The insult to the tooth may be compounded by replantation

procedures that are injurious to the teeth and attachment apparatus.

In an intentional replantation study of over 1000 teeth,[36] the greatest degree of root resorption was found to be caused by

The use of peroxide and sodium hypochlorite for canal irrigation

The trauma of excessive manipulation

Curettement of the periodontal ligament

All these procedures are detrimental to periodontal structures and should be avoided. The immersion of teeth in a 2% sodium fluoride solution does not retard the rate of root resorption[110] and may, in fact, increase the incidence of replacement resorption.[8] A short-term study[98] showed promise in reducing post-replantation resorption by altering the cementum with enzymes.

Recent research on avulsed teeth has focused on the role of the socket,[104] extraoral time,[10] the effect of the storage medium,[10,103] calcium hydroxide,[14,28] and the treatment of the periodontal ligament.[11,105] Specific clinical methods to prevent and treat resorption on avulsed teeth are outlined in Chapter 15.

Andreasen[7,12] classified the three types of periodontal reaction that occur following replantation of avulsed teeth as

1. Healing with a normal periodontal ligament (Fig. 16-54)
2. Replacement resorption (Fig. 16-55)
3. Inflammatory resorption (Fig. 16-56)

More than one type may be seen radiographically in the same tooth.

Healing with a normal periodontal ligament. When there is healing with a normal periodontal ligament (Fig. 16-57), the replantation has been successful. Clinically the tooth is stable and asymptomatic, and the gingiva is free of inflammation. According to Andreasen,[7] ''Small areas of the root surface may show superficial resorption lacunae repaired by cementum. This condition, which has been

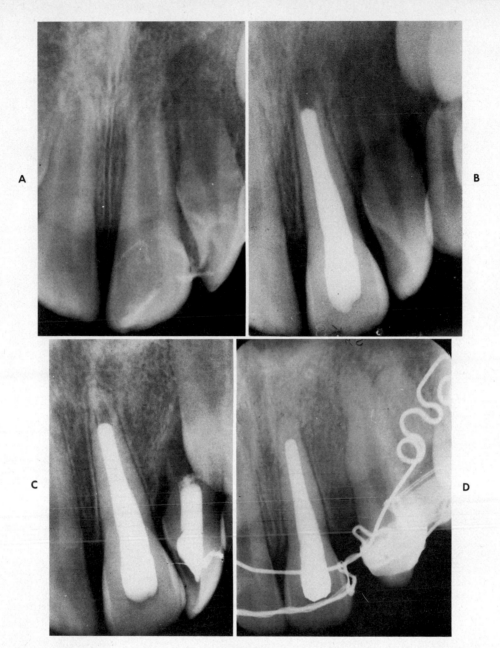

FIG. 16-57. Replantation followed by healing with a normal periodontal ligament. **A,** Day of replantation. **B,** Three months later, canal filled. **C,** Twenty-four months later, further apical development. *Note:* The lateral incisor was traumatized but not avulsed in a previous accident. **D,** Nine years later, apical development complete, tooth undergoing orthodontic movement.

termed surface resorption, is self-limiting and shows spontaneous repair.'' Radiographically no resorption is visible.

Replacement resorption. Ankylosis occurs in cases of replacement resorption. The root is resorbed, and alveolar bone is deposited in its place. This progressive phenomenon is most frequently encountered following replantation (Fig. 16-58). Resorption, when present, usually starts within 1 year of replantation.[8,13] At present there is no known treatment that will stop the process, which fortunately occurs at a slow rate. The tooth remains stable in the arch until there is very little root remaining; when the epithelial attachment alone is left to retain the crown, extraction is indicated.

Attempts at orthodontic movement are unsuccessful in ankylosed teeth. The lock-and-key adaptation of the bone to the resorbed tooth will resist efforts toward realignment.

Inflammatory resorption. A two-edged sword is an apt description of inflammatory resorption. On one edge there can be rapid dissolution of root structure. On the other edge this progressive reaction is often amenable to treatment. Radiographically there may be root resorption and bone radiolucency (Fig. 16-59). Histologically the lesion

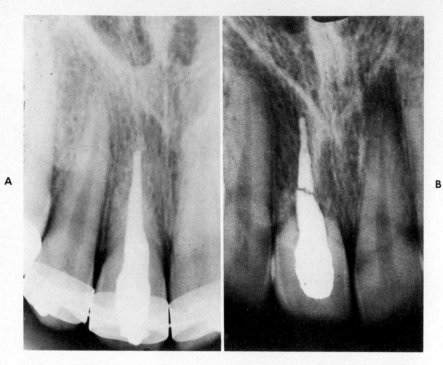

A

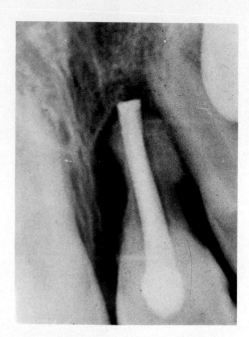

B

FIG. 16-58. Replacement resorption. **A,** 1 year and, **B,** 6 years after replantation.

FIG. 16-59. Inflammatory resorption 6 months after replantation. Inadequate root canal filling is a contributing factor.

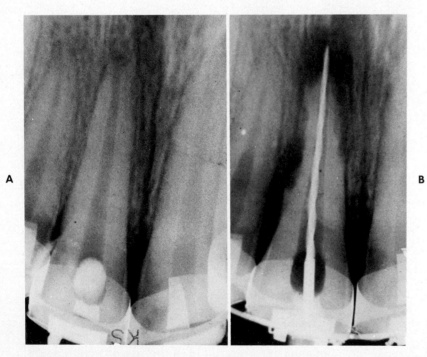

A

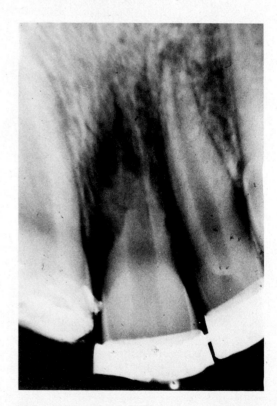

B

FIG. 16-60. Inflammatory resorption. **A,** Immediately and, **B,** 3 weeks after replantation. The resorption is advanced and extensive after only 3 weeks.

FIG. 16-61. Three months after replantation. Pathognomonic picture of inflammatory resorption when a tooth is replanted without pulpectomy shortly thereafter.

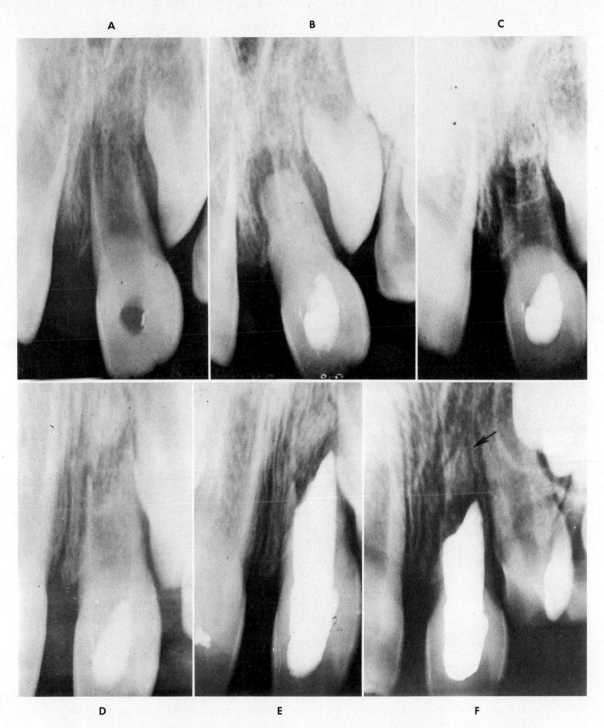

FIG. 16-62. Open apex replantation, Ca(OH)$_2$ treatment. **A,** One week after replantation. **B,** Six weeks after replantation, apical radiolucency. The canal has been filled with Ca(OH)$_2$-vehicle. **C,** Five months after replantation. The dressing appears washed out; Ca(OH)$_2$-vehicle replaced. **D,** Nine months after replantation, no apical radiolucency. The clinician was able to probe a definite apical shelf. **E,** Nine months after replantation. The canal has been filled with warmed gutta-percha to the oblique shelf. **F,** Twenty-one months after replantation, preliminary maturation of the apical segment *(arrow)*.

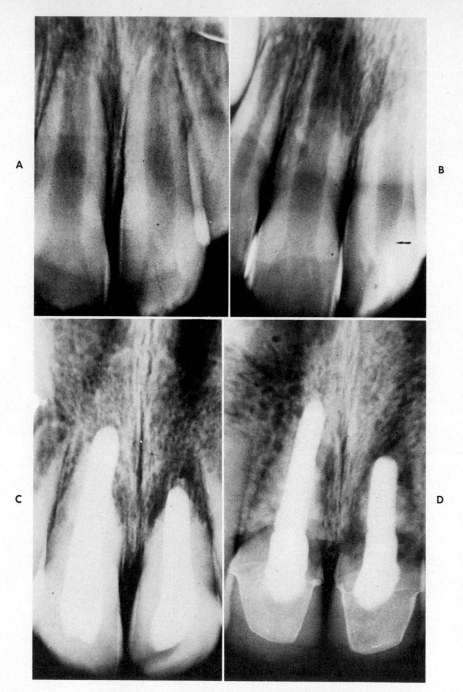

FIG. 16-63. Inflammatory resorption, nonsurgical treatment. **A,** Immediately after replantation. **B,** Three months after replantation. Note the inflammatory resorption. **C,** Five months after replantation. Endodontic therapy has been completed. **D,** Ten years after replantation. Rapid inflammatory resorption has been followed by the slower process of replacement resorption. (**B** and **C** courtesy Dr. Calvin Reeman.)

demonstrates "bowl-shaped areas of resorption involving cementum and dentin. Intensive inflammatory reaction [is] found in the periodontal ligament with the presence of lymphocytes, plasma cells, and polymorphonuclear leukocytes in granulation tissue.''[7,9] As the condition progresses, the teeth become mobile unless definite therapy is instituted. The resorption may take place with mercurial speed (Fig. 16-60).

Pulp necrosis. An unusual inflammatory pattern is seen in teeth replanted without pulpectomy when pulp necrosis has occurred. The radiographic picture of diffuse radiolucency and extensive root resorption is pathognomonic for this situation (Fig. 16-61). Pulp extirpation and canal debridement are essential to arrest the process.[19] If the clinical situation can be kept under control, the $Ca(OH)_2$–biologically compatible vehicle technique can be used to fill the canal for as long as 1 year. Andreasen[7] was able to arrest inflammatory resorption in nine out of ten cases of apical involvement by using this technique, and Burke[26] produced calcific healing of external root resorption with the Ca(OH)$_2$ paste. (See p. 534 for further information.)

Reexamination at 3-month intervals allows for inspection of apical closure in immature apices for evaluation of the progress of resorption and of root structure regeneration when lateral perforations have occurred. Sealing the canals with conventional gutta-percha techniques is facilitated by this biologic healing process (Fig. 16-62).

Before the development of the Ca(OH)$_2$ technique in the treatment of avulsed teeth with inflammatory resorption, when pulp extirpation and canal debridement were performed before the canals were sealed with gutta-percha the postoperative picture changed from rapid destruction by inflammatory resorption to slow replacement resorption (Fig. 16-63). When inflammatory resorption is noted after the filling of the canal, surgery may be indicated to arrest the process.

With the accumulation of further data on the replantation of avulsed teeth, newer treatment concepts and procedures may become available.

REFERENCES

1. Abou-Rass, M.: The elimination of tetracycline discoloration by intentional endodontics and internal bleaching, J. Endod. **8**:101, 1982.
2. Alexander, S.A., and Swerdloff, M.: Mucopolysaccharidase activity during human deciduous root resorption, Arch. Oral Biol. **24**:735, 1979.
3. Alexander, S.A., and Swerdloff, M.: Collagen activity of the periodontal ligament and hydroxyproline content during human deciduous root resorption, J. Periodont. Res. **15**:434, 1980.
4. Allen, A.L., and Gutman, J.L.: Internal root resorption after vital root resection, J. Endod. **3**:438, 1977.
5. American Association of Endodontists: Annotated glossary of terms used in endodontics, ed. 4, Chicago, 1984, The Association.
6. Andreasen, J.O.: Luxation of permanent teeth due to trauma: a clinical and radiographic follow-up study of 189 injured teeth, Scand. J. Dent. Res. **78**:273, 1970.
7. Andreasen, J.O.: Treatment of fractured and avulsed teeth, J. Dent. Child. **38**:29, 1971.
8. Andreasen, J.O.: Personal communication, April, 1976.
9. Andreasen, J.O.: Analysis of topography of surface and inflammatory root resorption after replantation of mature permanent incisors in monkeys, Swed. Dent. J. **4**:135, 1980.
10. Andreasen, J.O.: A time-related study of periodontal healing and root resorption activities after replantation of mature permanent incisors in monkeys, Swed. Dent. J. **4**:101, 1980.
11. Andreasen, J.O.: Traumatic injuries of the teeth, ed. 2, Philadelphia, 1981, W.B. Saunders Co.
12. Andreasen, J.O.: External root resorption: its implications in dental traumatology, Paed. Periododon. Orthododon. Endod. **18**(2):109, 1985.
13. Andreasen, J.O., and Hjorting-Hansen, E.: Replantation of teeth. I. Radiographic and clinical study of 110 human teeth replanted after accidental loss, Acta Odontol. Scand. **24**:263, 1966.
14. Andreasen, J.O., and Kristerson, L.: The effect of extra-alveolar root filling with calcium hydroxide on periodontal healing after replantation of permanent incisors in monkeys, J. Endod. **7**:349, 1981.
15. Antrim, D.D., Hicks, M.L., and Altaras, D.E.: Treatment of subosseous resorption: a case report, J. Endod. **8**(12):567, 1982.
16. Arens, D.E.: Bleaching—an asset or a liability? American Academy of Esthetic Dentistry Annual Meeting, August, 1985.
17. Arens, D.E., Adams, W.R., and DeCastro, R.A.: Endodontic surgery, New York, 1981, Harper & Row, Publishers, Inc.
18. Azaz, B., and Shtayer, A.: Resorption of the crown in the impacted maxillary canines, Int. J. Oral Surg. **7**:167, 1978.
19. Barbakow, F.H., Austin, J.C., and Cleaton-Jones, P.E.: Experimental replantation of root canal filled and untreated teeth in the vervet monkey, J. Endod. **3**:89, 1977.
20. Barber, A.F., and Sims, M.R.: Rapid maxillary expansion and external root resorption in man: a scanning electron microscope study, Am. J. Orthod. **79**(6):630, 1981.
21. Bell, T.: The anatomy, physiology, and diseases of the teeth, Philadelphia, 1830, Carey & Lea.
22. Bellizzi, R., and Cias, W.L.: Endodontic management of extensive root resorption, Oral Surg. **49**:165, 1980.
23. Berning, H.P., and Lepp, F.L.: Progressive internal resorption in permanent teeth, Dent. Abstr. **3**:607, 1958.
24. Bhaskar, S.N.: Synopsis of oral pathology, ed. 7, St. Louis, 1986, The C.V. Mosby Co.
25. Boksman, R., Jordan, R.E., and Skinner, D.H.: A conservative bleaching treatment for the nonvital discolored tooth, Compend. Contin. Ed. **5**(6):471, 1984.
26. Burke, J.H.: Reversal of external root resorption. J. Endod. **2**:87, 1976.
27. Chivian, N.: Intentional replantation, J. N.J. Dent. Soc. **38**:247, 1967.
28. Coccia, C.T.: A clinical investigation of root resorption in replanted young permanent incisors: a five year study. J. Endod. **6**:413, 1980.
29. Collins, N.A., and Murrin, J.R.: Endodontic treatment of internal resorption using a gutta percha-euchapercha technic: report of a case, J. Ky. Dent. Assoc. **31**:19, 1979.
30. Cooke, C., and Rowbotham, T.C.: Root canal therapy in non-vital teeth with open apices, Br. Dent. J. **108**:147, 1960.
31. Cowie, P., and Wright, B.A.: Multiple idiopathic root resorption, Can. Dent. Assoc. J. **47**:111, 1981.
32. Cvek, M.: Clinical procedures promoting apical closure and arrest of external root resorption in non-vital permanent incisors. In Transactions, Fifth International Conference on Endodontics, Philadelphia, 1973, University of Pennsylvania.
33. Cvek, M.: Endodontic treatment of traumatized teeth. In Andreason, J.O.: Traumatic injuries of the teeth, ed. 2, Philadelphia, 1981, W.B. Saunders Co.
34. Cvek, M., Hollander, L., and Nord, C.E.: Treatment of non-vital permanent incisors with calcium hydroxide. VI. A clinical, microbiological, radiological evaluation of treatment in one sitting of teeth with mature and immature roots, Odontol. Rev. **27**:93, 1976.
35. Dargent, P.: A study of root resorption, Actual. Odontostomatol. **117**:47, 1977.
36. Deeb, G., Prietto, P.P., and McKenna, R.C.: Reimplantation of luxated teeth in humans, J.S. Calif. Dent. Assoc. **33**:194, 1965.
37. Dougherty, H.L.: The effect of mechanical forces upon the mandibular buccal segments during orthodontic treatment, Am. J. Orthod. **54**:83, 1968.
38. Dylewski, J.J.: Apical closure of nonvital teeth, Oral Surg. **32**:82, 1971.
39. England, M.C.: Diagnostic procedure for confirmation of a suspected resorptive defect of the root, J. Endod. **3**:157, 1977.
40. Fischer, W.G., and Guggenheimer, J.: Concurrent external and internal resorption, Oral Surg. **43**:161, 1977.
41. Fothergill, J.A.: In Hutchinson, S.J., et al.: Casual communications, Trans. Odontol. Soc. G.B. **32**:213, 1900.
42. Frank, A.L.: Therapy for the divergent pulpless tooth by continued apical formation, J. Am. Dent. Assoc. **72**:87, 1966.
43. Frank, A.L.: Improvement of the crown-root ratio by endodontic endosseous implants, J. Am. Dent. Assoc. **74**:451, 1967.

44. Frank, A.L.: Resorptions, perforations, and fractures, Dent. Clin, North Am. **18**:465, 1974.

45. Frank, A.L.: Calcium hydroxide: the ultimate medicament? Dent. Clin, North Am. **23**:691, 1979.

46. Frank, A.L.: External-internal progressive resorption and its non-surgical correction, J. Endod. **7**(10):473, 1981.

47. Frank, A.L., and Weine, F.S.: Non-surgical therapy for the perforating defect of internal resorption, J. Am. Dent. Assoc. **87**:863, 1973.

48. Frostell, G.: Factors influencing the prognosis of endodontic therapy. In Grossman, L.I., editor: Transactions, Third International Conference on Endodontics, Philadelphia, 1963, University of Pennsylvania.

49. Gartner, A.H., et al.: Differential diagnosis of internal and external resorption, J. Endod. **2**:329, 1976.

50. Gelman, R.A.: External (cervical) root resorption; a case report, J. N.J. Dent. Assoc. **55**(1):57, 1984.

51. Gholston, L.R., and Mattison, G.D.: An endodontic-orthodontic technique for esthetic stabilization of externally resorbed teeth, Am. J. Orthod. **83**(5):435, 1983.

52. Goldson, L., and Henrikson, C.O.: Root resorption during Begg treatment: longitudinal roentgenologic study, Am. J. Orthod. **68**:55, 1975.

53. Goldson, L., and Malmgren, O.: Orthodontic treatment of traumatized teeth. In Andreasen, J.O.: Traumatic injuries of the teeth, ed. 2, Philadelphia, 1981, W.B. Saunders Co.

54. Goon, W., Cohen, S., and Boner, R.F.: External cervical root resorption following bleaching, J. Endod. **12**:414, 1986.

55. Gorlin, R.J., and Goldman, H.M., editors: Thoma's oral pathology, ed. 6, St. Louis, 1970, The C.V. Mosby Co.

56. Gottlieb, B., and Orban, B.: Veränderungen im Periodontium nach chirurgischer Diathermie, Z. J. Stomatol. **28**:1208, 1930.

57. Goultschin, J., Nitgan, D., and Azaz, B.: Root resorption—review and discussion, Oral Surg. **54**(5):586, 1982.

58. Grossman, L.I.: Endodontic practice, ed. 10, Philadelphia, 1981, Lea & Febiger.

59. Halcomb, J.B., Dodds, R.N., and England, M.C.: Endodontic treatment modalities for external root resorption associated with impacted mandibular third molars, J. Endod. **9**(8):335, 1983.

60. Hall, A.M.: Upper incisor root resorption during stage II of the Begg technique: two case reports, Br. J. Orthod. **5**:47, 1978.

61. Hammarström, L., and Lindskog, S.: General morphologic aspects of resorption of teeth and alveolar bone, Int. Endod. J. **18**:293, 1985.

62. Harrington, G.W., and Natkin, E.: External resorption associated with bleaching of pulpless teeth, J. Endod. **5**:344, 1979.

63. Hartness, J.D.: Fractured root with internal resorption, repair and formation of callus, J. Endod. **1**:73, 1975.

64. Harvey, B.L., and Zander, H.A.: Root surface resorption of periodontally diseased teeth, Oral Surg. **12**:1439, 1959.

65. Hasselgren, G., and Stomberg, T.: Histochemical demonstration of acid hydrolase activity in internal dentinal resorption, Oral Surg. **42**:381, 1976.

66. Healy, H.J.: Endodontics: selection of case treatment procedures, J. Am. Dent. Assoc. **53**:434, 1956.

67. Heithersay, G.S.: Clinical endodontic and surgical management of tooth and associated bone resorption, Int. Endod. J. **18**(2):93-108, 1985.

68. Henry, J.L., and Weinmann, J.P.: Pattern of root resorption and repair of human cementum, J. Am. Dent. Assoc. **42**:270, 1951.

69. Hermann, B.W.: Dentinobliteration der Wurzelkanale nach der Behandlung mit Kalzium, Zahnaerztl. Rund. **39**:888, 1930.

70. Hinman, T.P.: The interpretation of x-ray pictures of apical granulations, giving differential diagnosis of cases favorable and cases unfavorable for treatment and root canal filling. J. Natl. Dent. Assoc. **8**:83, 1921.

71. Holland, R., et al.: Reaction of human periapical tissue to pulp extirpation and immediate root filling with calcium hydroxide, J. Endod. **3**:63, 1977.

72. Hopkins, R., and Adams, D.: Multiple idiopathic resorption of teeth, Br. Dent. J. **146**:305, 1979.

73. Hoyer, I.: Pathologische Zahnwurzelresorption und ihr klinische Bedeutung, Stomatol. D.D.R. **27**:46, 1977.

74. James, G.: Personal communication, 1985.

75. Jansen, H.: Ueber die bakterizide Wirkung des Hermann schen Calxyl-Präparates, Vergleichen mit dem Schweizer Präparat Endoxyl. Unpublished dissertation, University of Bonn, 1949.

76. Johnson, W.T.: External cervical resorption: a case report, Iowa City, 1985, Iowa Association of Endodontics.

77. Kaffe, I., et al.: A radiographic survey of apical root resorption in pulpless permanent teeth, Oral Surg. **58**(1):109, 1984.

78. Kantor, M.E., and Pines, M.S.: A comparative study of restorative techniques for pulpless teeth, J. Prosthet. Dent. **38**:405, 1977.

79. Kaufman, A.Y., Tal, M., and Binderman, K.: Internal root resorption: a report of a case with scanning electron microscopic study, J. Endod. **3**:236, 1977.

80. Kronfeld, R.: Histopathology of the teeth, Philadelphia, 1939, Lea & Febiger.

81. Lado, E.A., Stanley, H.R., and Weissman, M.I.: Cervical resorption in bleached teeth, Oral Surg. **55**:78, 1983.

82. Langford, S.M., and Sims, M.R.: Root surface resorption and periodontal attachment following rapid maxillary expansion in man, Am. J. Orthod. **81**:108, 1982.

82a. Latcham, N.L. Postbleaching cervical resorption, J. Endod. **12**:262, 1986.

83. Leubke, R.: Personal communication.

84. Linge, B.O., and Linge, L.: Apical root resorption in upper anterior teeth, Euro. J. Orthod. **5**:173, 1983.

85. Lustman, J., and Ehrlich, J.: Deep external root resorption treatment by combined endodontic and surgical approach, Int. Dent. J. **2**:203, 1974.

86. Malomgren, O., et al.: Root resorption after orthodontic treatment of traumatized teeth, Am. J. Orthod. **82**(6):487, 1982.

87. Mandor, R.B.: A tooth with internal resorption treated with a hydrophilic paste material: a case report, J. Endod. **7**:430, 1981.

88. Massler, M., and Perreault, J.G.: Root resorption of the permanent teeth of young adults, J. Dent. Child. **21**:158, 1954.

89. Mattison, G.D., et al.: Orthodontic root resorption of vital and endodontically treated teeth, J. Endod. **10**(8):354, 1984.

90. Mattison, G.D., Gholston, L.R., and Boyd, P.: Orthodontic external resorption root resorption—endodontic considerations, J. Endod. **9**(6):253, 1983.

91. Maurice, C.G.: Selection of teeth for root canal treatment, Dent. Clin. North. Am., p. 761, November 1957.

92. Metzger, P.R.: Externe wortelresorptie bij endodontisch behandelde elementen, Ned. Tijdschr. Tandhldkd. **88**:256, 1981. (P.R. Wesselink, translator.)

93. Montgomery, S.: External cervical resorption after bleaching a pulpless tooth, Oral Surg. **57**:203, 1984.

94. Morris, M.L., et al.: Factors affecting healing after experimentally delayed tooth transplantation, J. Endod. **7**:80, 1981.

95. Morse, D.R.: Clinical endodontology, Springfield, IL, 1974, Charles C Thomas, Publisher.

96. Mount, G.J.: Idiopathic internal resorption, Oral Surg. **33**:80, 1972.

97. Mummery, F.J.H.: The pathology of "pink spots" on teeth, Br. Dent. J. **41**:7, 1920.

98. Nevins, A.J., et al.: Replantation of enzymatically treated teeth in monkeys. 1, Oral Surg. **50**:277, 1980.

99. Newman, G.W.: Possible etiologic factors in external root resorption, Am. J. Orthod. **67**:522, 1975.

100. Nichols, E.: An investigation into the factors which may influence the prognosis of root canal therapy. Master's thesis, London, 1960, Faculty of Medicine, University of London.

101. Nitzen, D., Kernan, T., and Marmany, Y.: Does an impacted tooth cause root resorption of the adjacent one? Oral Surg. **51:**221, 1981.
102. Nutting, E.B., and Poe, G.S.: A new combination for bleaching teeth, J. South Calif. Dent. Assoc. **31:**289, 1963.
103. Oswald, R.J., Harrington, G.W., and Van Hassel, H.J.: A post-replantation evaluation of air-dried and saliva-stored avulsed teeth, J. Endod. **6:**546, 1980.
104. Oswald, R.J., Harrington, G.W., and Van Hassel, H.J.: Replantation. 1. The role of the socket, J. Endod. **6:**479, 1980.
105. Oswald, R.J., Harrington, G.W., and Van Hassel, H.J.: Replantation. 2. The role of the periodontal ligament, J. Endod. **6:**506, 1980.
106. Penick, E.C.: The endodontic management of root resorption, Oral Surg. **16:**344, 1963.
107. Penido, R.S., Carrel, R., and Chialastri, A.J.: The anachoretic effect in root resorption: report of a case, J. Pedod. **5:**85, 1980.
108. Pitts, D.L., Williams, L., and Morton, T.H.: Investigation of the role of endotoxin in periapical inflammations, J. Endod. **8:**10, 1982.
109. Pomeranz, H.: A very active case of idiopathic external root resorption, Oral Surg. **55**(5):521, 1983.
110. Robinson, P.J., and Shapiro, I.M.: Effect of diphosphonates on root resorption, J. Dent. Res. **55:**166, 1976.
111. Rygh, P.: Orthodontic root resorption studied by electron microscopy, Angle Orthod. **47:**1, 1977.
112. Sadler, A., and Ritchie, G.M.: Odontoclastoma or idiopathic external resorption, Oral Surg. **52:**304, 1981.
113. Schroeder, A.: Endodontics—science and practice, Chicago, 1981, Quintessence Publishing Co., Inc.
114. Seale, N.S., McClintoch, J.E., and Taylor, A.N.: Pulpal reactions to bleaching of teeth in dogs, J. Dent. Res. **60:**948, 1981.
115. Deleted in proofs.
116. Seltzer, S.: Endodontology, New York, 1971, McGraw-Hill Book Co.
117. Seltzer, S., and Bender, I.B.: The dental pulp, ed. 2, Philadelphia, 1975, J.B. Lippincott Co.
118. Seltzer, S., et al.: Biologic aspects of endodontics. I. Histologic observations of the anatomy and morphology of root apices and surrounding structures, Oral Surg. **22:**375, 1966.
119. Shafer, W.G., Hine, M.K., and Levy, B.M.: A textbook of oral pathology, ed. 3, Philadelphia, 1974, W.B. Saunders Co.
120. Simon, M., et al.: Hard tissue resorption and deposition after preparation and disinfection of the root canal, Oral Surg. **56**(4):421, 1983.
121. Smith, N.H.H.: Monostotic Paget's disease of the mandible presenting with progressive resorption of the teeth, Oral Surg. **46:**246, 1978.
122. Sottosanti, J.S.: A possible relationship between occlusion, root resorption, and the progression of periodontal disease, Periodont. Abstr. **25:**69, 1977.
123. Spasser, H.F.: A simple bleaching technique using sodium perborate, N.Y. State Dent. J. **27:**332, 1961.
124. Spasser, H.F.: Personal communication, 1986.
125. Spolnick, K.: Personal communication.
126. Stafne, E.C., and Slocumb, C.H.: Idiopathic resorption of teeth, Am. J. Orthod. **30:**41, 1944.
127. Stanley, H.R.: Diseases of the dental pulp. In Tiecke, R.W., editor: Oral pathology, New York, 1965, McGraw-Hill Book Co.
128. Stanley, H.R., and Lundy, T.: Dycal therapy for pulp exposures, Oral Surg. **34:**818, 1972.
129. Stewart, G.G.: Calcium hydroxide–induced root healing, J. Am. Dent. Assoc. **90:**793, 1975.
130. Strindberg, L.Z.: Dependence of the results of pulp canal therapy on certain factors; an analytic study based on radiographic and clinical follow-up examination, Dent. Abstr. **2:**176, 1956.
131. Stuteville, O.H.: Injuries caused by orthodontic forces and the ultimate result of these injuries, Am. J. Orthod. Oral Surg. **24:**105, 1938.
132. Sweet, A.F.S.P.: Internal resorption, Dent. Radiogr. Photogr. **38:**4, 1969.
133. Tamse, A., Littner, M.M., and Kaffe, I.: Roentgenographic features of external root resorption, Quint. Int. **13**(1):51, 1982.
134. Tasch, E.G., and Kennon, S.: Implications of related impacted third molars, J. Ky. Dent. Assoc. **30:**13, 1978.
135. Torabinejad, M.: Personal communication, 1985.
136. Torneck, C.D., Smith, J.S., and Grindall, P.: Biologic effect of endodontic procedures on developing incisor teeth. IV. Effect of debridement procedures and calcium hydroxide–camphorated parachlorophenol paste in the treatment of experimentally induced pulp and periapical disease, Oral Surg. **35:**541, 1973.
137. Toto, P.D., and Restarski, J.S.: The histogenesis of pulpal odontoclasts, Oral Surg. **16:**172, 1963.
138. Tronstadt, L.: Personal communication.
139. Tronstadt, L., et al.: pH changes in dental tissues after root canal filling with calcium hydroxide, J. Endod. **7:**17, 1981.
140. Warner, G.R., et al.: Internal resorption of teeth: interpretation of histologic findings, J. Am. Dent. Assoc. **34:**468, 1947.
141. Watson, W.B.: Expansion and fenestration or dehiscence, editorial, Am. J. Orthod. **77:**330, 1980.
142. Webber, R.T.: Traumatic injuries and the expanded endodontic roll of calcium hydroxide. In Gerstein, H., editor: Techniques in clinical endodontics, Philadelphia, 1983, W.B. Saunders Co.
143. Weine, F.S.: Endodontic therapy, ed. 3, St. Louis, 1982, The C.V. Mosby Co.
144. Weisman, M.I., and Rackley, R.H.: Recalcification of internal resorption: a rare case, J. Ga. Dent. Assoc. **41:**15, 1978.
145. Weiss, S.D.: Root resorption during orthodontic treatment in endodontically treated and vital teeth. Master's thesis, Memphis, 1969, University of Tennessee, College of Dentistry, Department of Orthodontics.
146. Wickwire, N.A., et al.: The effects of tooth movement upon endodontically treated teeth, Angle Orthod. **44:**235, 1974.
147. Williams, S.: A histomorphometric study of orthodontically induced root resorption, Eur. J. Orthod. **6**(1):35, 1984.

Self-assessment questions

1. Internal resorption
   a. Will appear as a lesion superimposed over an unaltered canal in a radiograph
   b. Is associated with a systemic disease
   c. Is frequently associated with trauma
   d. Requires deferment of treatment with "careful watching"

2. According to Chivian internal resorption is probably the result of
   a. A necrotic pulp
   b. An acute pulpitis
   c. A reversible pulpitis
   d. An irreversible chronic pulpitis

3. Which of the following may be used to fill the pathologic void of a nonperforating internal resorption?
   a. Silver amalgam
   b. Gutta-percha
   c. Zinc oxide–eugenol
   d. All of the above

4. Surgical treatment of internal resorption is indicated when
   a. The resorption process alters the anatomy of the apical third
   b. There is uncontrolled bleeding from the perforation defect
   c. The perforation is near or at the epithelial attachment
   d. All of the above

5. When a small perforating internal resorption area occurs in a surgically inoperable site, what is the suggested treatment?
   a. "Wait-and-see" observation
   b. Conventional endodontics
   c. Calcium hydroxide therapy
   d. Extraction

6. The rationale for using calcium hydroxide to repair perforating internal resorption is that
   a. It reduces the inflammatory response and promotes healing with a hard tissue barrier
   b. It promotes osteoclastic activity
   c. An acid pH environment is created, allowing hard tissue deposition
   d. Its success is directly attributable to its antibacterial effect

7. The causes of external resorption include
   a. Periapical inflammation
   b. Excessive mechanical or occlusal forces
   c. Impaction of teeth
   d. All of the above

8. External resorption may be found in one of the following systemic diseases:
   a. Hypoparathyroidism
   b. Diabetes
   c. Leukemia
   d. Parkinson's disease

9. Apical external resorption
   a. Requires surgical intervention for healing
   b. Is usually associated with a vital pulp
   c. Is initially treated nonsurgically
   d. Has a poor prognosis requiring extraction

10. Cervical resorption
    a. Is usually the result of a pulpal inflammatory reaction
    b. In advanced stages may create the classic "pink spot"
    c. Is a form of internal resorption
    d. Requires a recalcification procedure when the perforation is coronal to the gingival attachment

11. Lateral root resorption
    a. Is usually a result of concussive type tooth injuries
    b. Will usually require calcium hydroxide therapy prior to obturation of canal
    c. Is most often associated with a vital pulp
    d. When observed, requires extraction

12. Which of the following statements regarding replanted teeth is true?
    a. Curettement of the periodontal ligament increases the degree of root resorption
    b. Of avulsed permanent teeth, 20% undergo root resorption
    c. Resorption is usually of the internal type
    d. Immersion in 2% sodium fluoride prior to replantation retards the rate of resorption

17

ENDODONTIC-PERIODONTAL RELATIONS

JAMES H.S. SIMON
QUINTILIANO DINIZ De DEUS

The function of a tooth depends on the health of the periodontium: the gingival unit, cementum, periodontal ligament, and alveolar bone. Disease in this area usually results from the direct extension of pulpal disease or from the apical progression of gingival inflammation that can affect the cementum, periodontal ligament, and alveolar bone in its course.

EFFECT OF PULPAL INFLAMMATION ON THE ATTACHMENT APPARATUS

As described in Chapter 11, pulpal disease can progress beyond the apical foramen and involve the periodontal ligament. The inflammatory process results in replacement of the periodontal ligament by inflammatory tissue, usually with accompanying resorption of alveolar bone, cementum, or dentin. The apical foramen, however, may not be the only opening of the tooth that communicates with the periodontal ligament.

Lateral canals

It is well established that lateral (accessory) canals are a normal anatomic component of many teeth, especially in the apical third of the root and in the furcation area of molars. Thus the same inflammatory response occurring at the apex may occur in the periodontal ligament at the openings of lateral canals. The results of this process may appear as a lateral radiolucency on the root (Figs. 17-1 to 17-3). The apical area may or may not be similarly in-

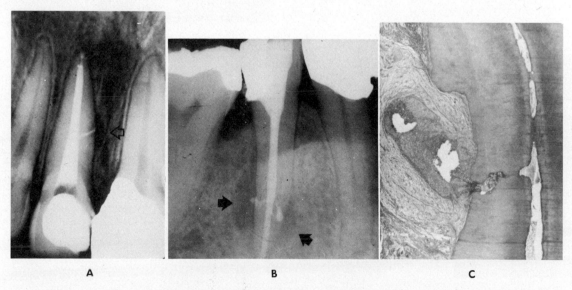

A B C

FIG. 17-1. A and **B,** Lateral canals filled with sealer and/or gutta-percha with adjacent radiolucencies. **C,** Histologic section showing inflammatory response in periodontal ligament opposite necrotic contents of lateral canal.

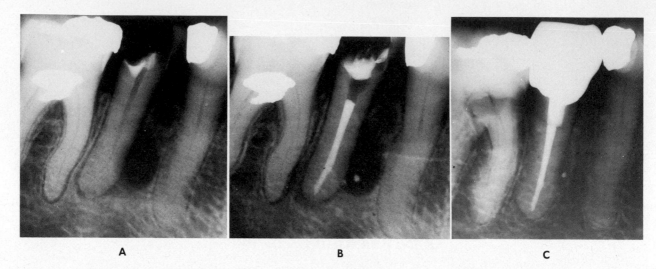

FIG. 17-2. Mandibular second premolar with a lesion that appears to be a lateral periodontal cyst. **A,** Pretreatment. **B,** Posttreatment. Root canal sealer is present in the radiolucency. **C,** One year later, evidence of healing. This lesion as apparently of endodontic origin.

FIG. 17-3. Two upper first molars that have been endodontically treated and then cleared. Lateral canals in mesiobuccal roots are filled with gutta-percha but because of the angulation would not be visible on an x-ray.

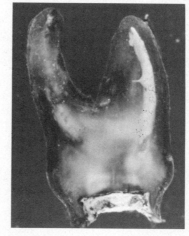
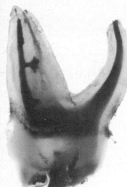

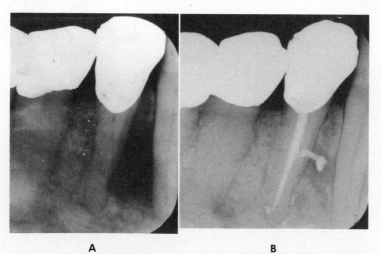

FIG. 17-4. A, Preoperative radiograph with a large lateral radiolucency almost up to the crestal bone. **B,** Eighteen-month recall showing a large lateral and smaller apical canal with almost complete healing of radiolucency. (Courtesy Dr. Anthony D. Goodman.)

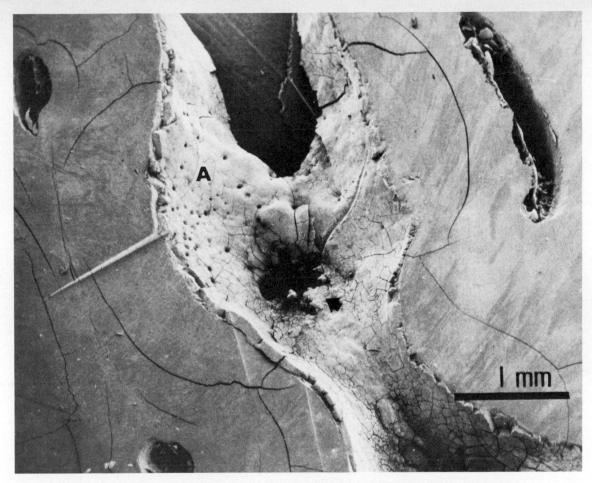

FIG. 17-5. Human molar bifurcation area (scanning electron micrograph). Large accessory foramen *(A)* visible in the bifurcation surrounded by numerous small accessory foramina. (×20.) Cracks in the specimen are due to dehydration during preparation. (Courtesy Dennis W. Foreman, Jr., Ph.D., College of Dentistry, Ohio State University.)

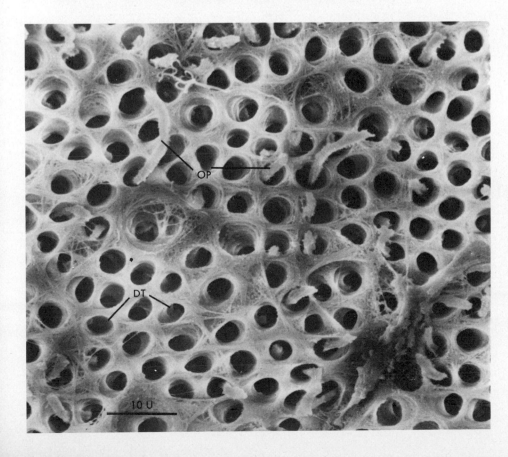

FIG. 17-6. Pulp-dentin border of a human incisor. (Scanning electron micrograph, ×2000.) Numerous dentinal tubules *(DT)* and odontoblastic processes *(OP)* are evident. (Courtesy Dennis W. Foreman, Jr., Ph.D., College of Dentistry, Ohio State University.)

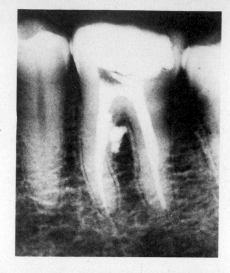

FIG. 17-7. Mandibular molar showing stripping of the mesial root during canal preparation. At times these perforations appear to be lateral canals opening into the bifurcation area.

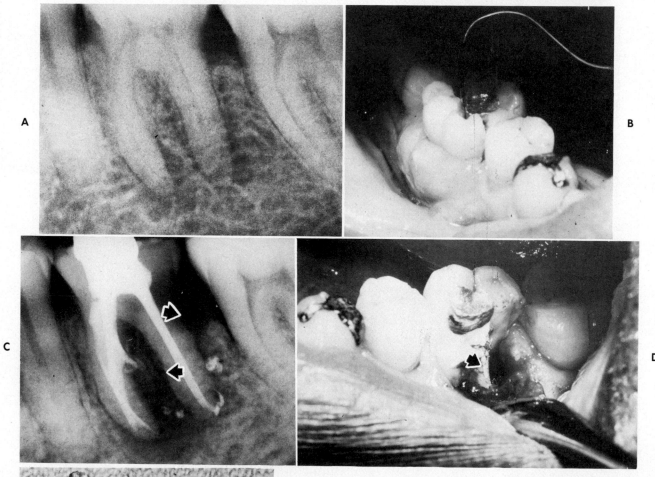

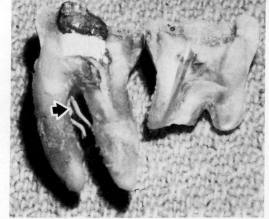

FIG. 17-8. Mandibular first molar. **A,** Pretreatment. **B,** and **C,** Five months after therapy. A buccal cusp fracture and large buccal swelling have occurred. Note in **C** the distal bone loss *(top arrow)* and the bifurcation involvement due to mesial root stripping *(bottom arrow).* **D,** Fracture segment removed. Note the exposure of gutta-percha in the distal canal *(arrow).* **E,** Extracted tooth. Note the extent of the fracture and the gross overfilling of the stripped area with gutta-percha *(arrow).*

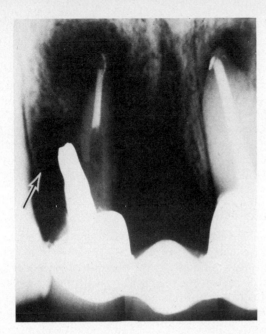

FIG. 17-9. Maxillary lateral incisor with a distal perforation. Note the radiolucency *(arrow)* developing around the exposed post.

volved. Inflammatory involvement of the apex and lateral canals may also extend crestally along the lateral aspects of the root and ultimately involve the furcation or crestal area of the attachment apparatus, or both (Figs. 17-4 and 17-5).

Dentinal tubules

Another avenue of the pulpal pathologic effect on the periodontium was demonstrated by Seltzer et al.[35] when they were able to induce interradicular periodontal changes in dogs and monkeys. By simulating pulpotomies, using various pulp-capping agents, and exposing the coronal pulps, they were able to show periodontitis (inflammation and resorption of dentin, cementum, and the alveolar crest of bone) in the furcation area of 21 out of 100 teeth examined. They concluded that interradicular lesions of the attachment apparatus could be created and maintained by inflamed and necrotic pulp tissue, not only through lateral canals but also through dentinal tubules (Fig. 17-6). Thus pulpal disease may have a direct inflammatory effect on the periodontal ligament by direct extension through the apical foramen, lateral canals, and dentinal tubules.[46] Iatrogenic involvement of the attachment apparatus can result from root perforations caused by overzealous endodontic access instrumentation (Figs. 17-7 and 17-8) or by lateral perforation during post preparation[12,37] (Fig. 17-9).

EFFECT OF PERIODONTAL INFLAMMATION ON THE PULP

The effect of periodontal disease on the pulp is not as clear-cut as the effect of pulpal disease on the periodontium. Periodontal inflammation may exert a direct effect on the pulp through the same lateral canal or dentinal tubule pathways. Seltzer et al.[36] extracted periodontally in-

volved teeth without caries or restorations and found that 37% had some degree of pulpal inflammation, or necrotic pulp tissue, or both. Others[19,32] have also demonstrated direct inflammatory extension of periodontal inflammation through lateral canals. However, they did not demonstrate that total pulpal necrosis would result from inflamed lateral canals. Some researchers[19] have stated that as long as the main canal is not seriously damaged the pulp might not succumb. Other researchers[5] created periodontal disease in six monkeys by placing ligatures around the necks of teeth. After 5 to 7 months of exposure to plaque, 30% to 40% of the root length was exposed and involved in periodontitis. When these teeth were sectioned and compared to normal, 57% of the teeth exposed to periodontitis had pathologic changes. Inflammatory cells and secondary dentin were found. However, only one tooth was necrotic and these changes were considered mild.

That periodontal therapy may increase this pulpal inflammatory effect has been shown.[22] By planing the roots of molars and then drawing a dye through the canals, these authors demonstrated the presence of patent canals in 59% of the molars. The incidence of patent canals in the coronal and middle third of maxillary molars was 55%; it was 63% in mandibular molars. The unplaned teeth had a significantly lower percentage of patent canals. However, in another study investigators[5] created periodontal disease in monkeys, scaled the teeth, and then let plaque accumulate for up to 30 days. In comparing the histologic status of the pulp to those teeth where only peridontitis was created, no difference was detected. Thus they concluded that scaling and/or root planing followed by plaque accumulation did not cause severe changes in the pulp tissue. However, the findings implied that the pulp may be susceptible to plaque substances only where external resorptions are present. Other investigators[13] found similar pulpal changes when they root planed the mesial surface of the maxillary first molar in rats. The rats were sacrificed at various intervals up to 1 year. In 32 of the 35 rats the prevalent finding was reparative or secondary dentin formation.

In a long-term clinical study (from 5 to 24 years follow-up) researchers[31] evaluated 387 maxillary molars that all had periodontal disease involving the furcation and were all treated with periodontal therapy. They found that 366 (94%) teeth did not have endodontic therapy at any time. Only 14 (4%) had endodontic treatment subsequent to periodontal therapy. They ascribed the etiology of these to caries or pulpal degeneration under restorations and therefore concluded that endodontic therapy was not a significant factor in the retention of the 341 teeth.

Degeneration

The direct extension of inflammation does not appear to be the initial effect of periodontal disease on the pulp. Two studies[44,45] of the effects of gingival wounds on the pulp in rats found irregular dentin formation in the pulp opposite the wound site; this might be transmitted through irritation of the odontoblastic process. This irregular dentin formation may be aided by cemental resorption in periodontal inflammation.

These findings have been confirmed by other

studies[19,34,42]: the initial effect of periodontal inflammation on the pulp may be degenerative. Irregular or reparative dentin formation was found with some resorption of dentin. It has been shown that if the nutritional supply to the pulp is hampered the effect is a reduction in the number of cells and an increase in dystrophic calcifications, fibrosis, collagen resorption, and inflammation.[34] Investigators[42] reported that the periodontal effect on the pulp occurs later and less frequently than does the pulpal effect on the periodontium. Thus there is mounting evidence that periodontal disease can have an effect not only on the pulp through lateral canals but also apparently across the untreated tooth surface.

On the other hand, other researchers[24] stated that pathologic pulpal changes occurred as often in teeth without periodontitis as with periodontitis. Even in the same patient there was no difference in the pulpal findings regardless of the severity of periodontal disease. In essence, the study concluded that periodontal disease had no effect on the pulp. Another study[43] also concluded that chronic inflammatory disease of the periodontium does not affect the pulp. In another study [8] on 38 human teeth (caries free and intact) and 12 teeth with caries or fillings it was found that in 34 teeth with periodontitis, six teeth had pathologic changes. The normal periodontal group had no changes, and of eight teeth in the gingivitis group one tooth was pathologic. The pathologic changes they attributed to caries or operative procedures. They could not identify periodontal disease as a causative factor in pulpal pathosis.

None of these teeth had been treated with periodontal therapy.

In support of these findings other investigators[49] sectioned 25 teeth from one patient who had varying amounts of periodontal disease on all the teeth. All teeth had pulps that were free of pathosis. Although most teeth had foci of calcification, the tissues were within normal limits. They also could not show a cause and effect relationship between periodontal disease and the pulp. Thus conflicting studies have been reported, showing that the effect of periodontal disease on the pulp is controversial.

THEORETICAL PATHWAYS OF OSSEOUS LESION FORMATION

Applying the previous discussion and findings* to clinical conditions, we may theorize the pathways of bony lesion formation. Perhaps, as a result, the reader will have a better understanding of the pathogenic interreactions between pulpal and periodontal disease and be able to evaluate more accurately the results of diagnosis and treatment.

Primary endodontic lesions

Sinus tract formation through the periodontal ligament has been shown to be a part of the natural history of pulpal disease.[48] A sinus tract originating from the apex or a lat-

---

*References 4, 6, 30, 33, 39, 41, 47.

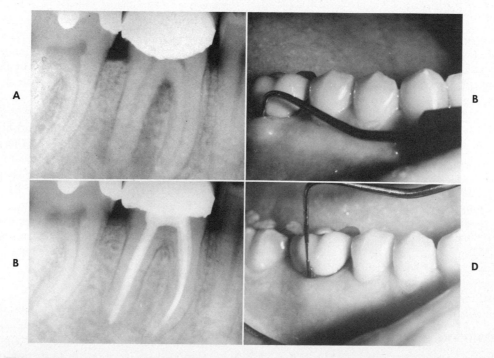

FIG. 17-10. Primary endodontic lesion. **A,** Preoperative radiograph with periapical and furcal radiolucency. **B,** Clinical photograph with periodontal probe in place. Note small gingival swelling that simulates a periodontal abscess. **C,** Radiograph 6 months after endodontic treatment only. The lesion has healed. **D,** Clinical photograph showing healing with periodontal probe in place. (Courtesy Dr. Frank J. Wilkinson.)

eral canal may form along the root surface and exit through the gingival sulcus (Fig. 17-10). This is not a true periodontal pocket but a fistula that, instead of opening on the buccal or lingual mucosa, drains along the periodontal ligament into the sulcus. This drainage through the sulcus often shows as a radiolucency along the mesial or distal root surface or in the bifurcation area (Figs. 17-11 to 17-13). The tract usually involves only one aspect of the tooth. For example, if the fistula goes through the bifurcation area, the mesial and distal crestal bone levels may be normal.

Clinically, drainage may be evident in the sulcus area and some swelling may be present, especially in the bifurcation area, simulating a periodontal abscess. However, this may be the only area of apparent periodontal involve-ment (Fig. 17-10). The tract can usually be probed with a gutta-percha cone, silver cone, or periodontal probe that will go toward the source of irritation, generally the root apex or a lateral canal. This tract is usually more tubular and thinner than an infrabony periodontal pocket. Pain is not often present, although the patient may have some minor discomfort. Endodontic testing procedures should reveal a necrotic pulp or, in multirooted teeth, at least an altered response, indicating that at least one canal is necrotic. Because this lesion is an endodontic problem that has merely fistulated through the periodontal ligament, complete resolution is usually anticipated after routine endodontic treatment.

Primary endodontic lesions with secondary periodontal involvement. If the primary lesion is untreated, it may

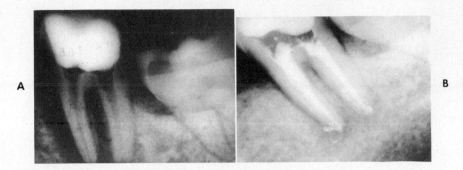

FIG. 17-11. Primary endodontic lesion. **A,** Preoperative radiograph with radiolucency along entire mesial root, giving the appearance of periodontal disease. **B,** Nine months after endodontic therapy the mesial bone appears to have almost completely remineralized.

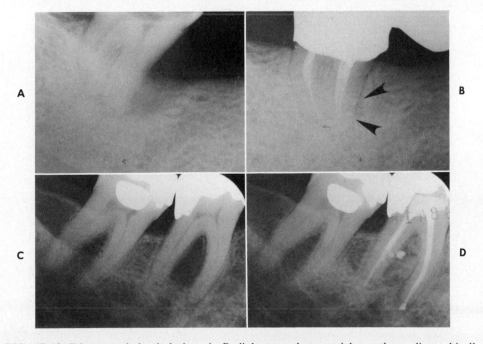

FIG. 17-12. Primary endodontic lesion. **A,** Radiolucency along mesial root that radiographically appears to be periodontal disease. **B,** Twenty-two months recall after only endodontic treatment, the lesion healed. Note two lateral canals in the mesial root *(arrows).* **C,** Preoperative radiograph with a furcal radiolucency. **D,** Six-month recall with furca healed in and lateral canal apparent in the distal root. (Courtesy Dr. Anthony D. Goodman.)

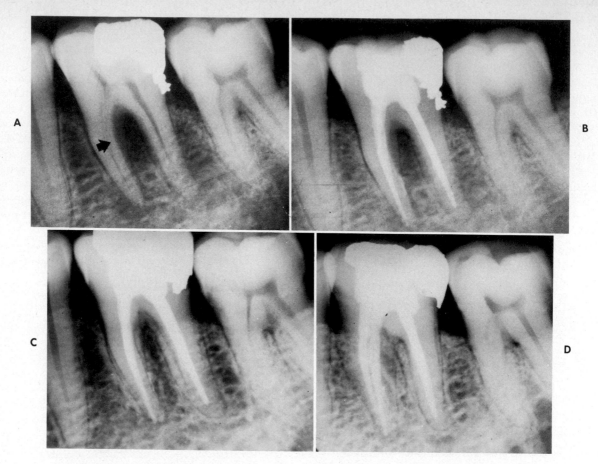

FIG. 17-13. Mandibular first molar. **A,** Note the radiolucency in the bifurcation area *(arrow).* The patient also had buccal gingival swelling and purulent drainage. Mesial and distal bone is high (except where there is for overhanging amalgam). **B,** Posttreatment. **C,** and **D,** One-year recall, evidence of bony healing. *Note:* **D** is at a different angulation to separate the two mesial roots.

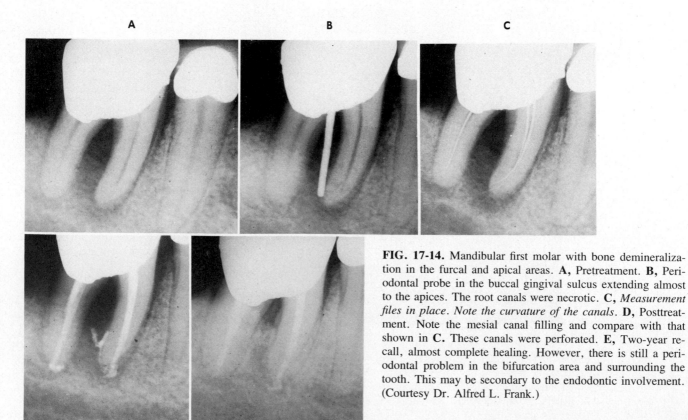

FIG. 17-14. Mandibular first molar with bone demineralization in the furcal and apical areas. **A,** Pretreatment. **B,** Periodontal probe in the buccal gingival sulcus extending almost to the apices. The root canals were necrotic. **C,** *Measurement files in place. Note the curvature of the canals.* **D,** Posttreatment. Note the mesial canal filling and compare with that shown in **C.** These canals were perforated. **E,** Two-year recall, almost complete healing. However, there is still a periodontal problem in the bifurcation area and surrounding the tooth. This may be secondary to the endodontic involvement. (Courtesy Dr. Alfred L. Frank.)

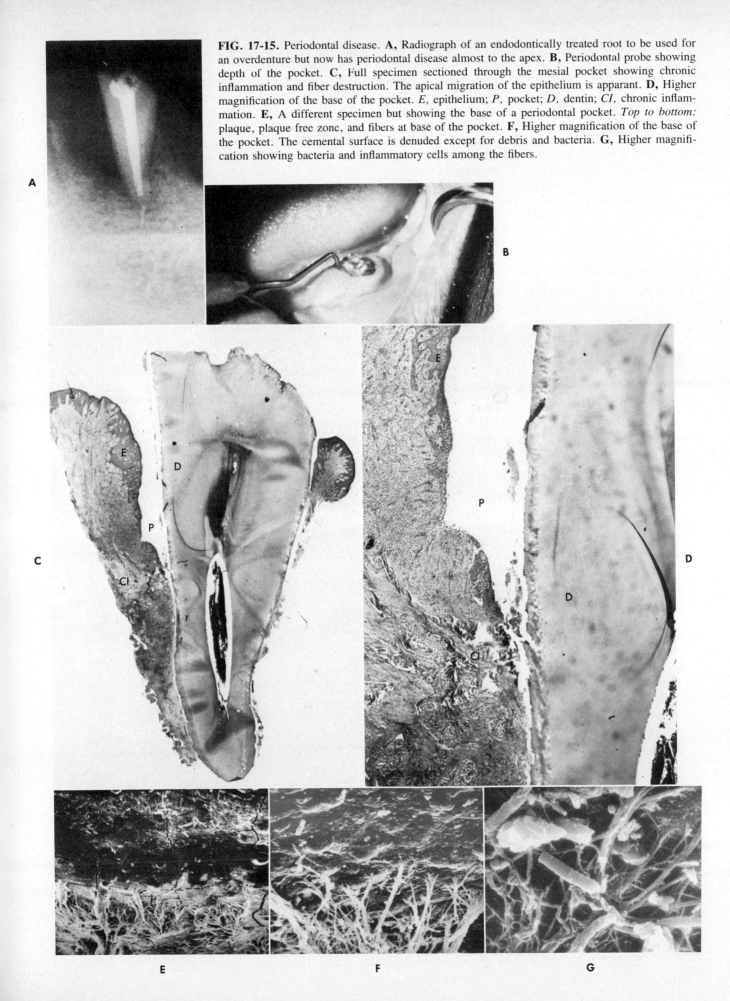

FIG. 17-15. Periodontal disease. **A,** Radiograph of an endodontically treated root to be used for an overdenture but now has periodontal disease almost to the apex. **B,** Periodontal probe showing depth of the pocket. **C,** Full specimen sectioned through the mesial pocket showing chronic inflammation and fiber destruction. The apical migration of the epithelium is apparant. **D,** Higher magnification of the base of the pocket. *E,* epithelium; *P,* pocket; *D,* dentin; *CI,* chronic inflammation. **E,** A different specimen but showing the base of a periodontal pocket. *Top to bottom:* plaque, plaque-free zone, and fibers at base of the pocket. **F,** Higher magnification of the base of the pocket. The cemental surface is denuded except for debris and bacteria. **G,** Higher magnification showing bacteria and inflammatory cells among the fibers.

become secondarily involved with periodontal disease. For example, plaque formation beginning at the tract opening may be followed by calculus formation and gingivitis leading to periodontitis. If this occurs, not only does the diagnosis become more difficult but the prognosis and treatment may also be altered.

Diagnostically these lesions have a necrotic root canal and plaque or calculus, or both, demonstrable by a probe or radiograph. At this point both endodontic therapy and periodontal therapy are necessary.[14,15] If the endodontic therapy is adequate, the prognosis depends on the severity of periodontal involvement and the efficacy of periodontal therapy. With endodontic therapy alone, only part of the lesion can be expected to heal (Fig. 17-14).

Primary periodontal lesions

The progression of periodontal disease to the formation of osseous lesions and their radiographic appearance along the lateral aspects of roots and in the furcation areas are well known. These may or may not be in conjunction with trauma from occlusion. In periodontally involved teeth, however, endodontic testing procedures usually reveal a clinically normal pulpal response. In addition, careful peri-

odontal examination will usually reveal probable pocket depths and an accumulation of plaque and calculus. The bony lesion is usually more widespread and generalized than are lesions of endodontic origin (Fig. 17-15). Because this is purely a periodontal problem, the prognosis rests exclusively with the periodontal therapy.

Primary periodontal lesions with secondary endodontic involvement. As stated earlier, periodontal disease may have an effect on the pulp through dentinal tubules or lateral canals, or both. Thus endodontic pulp testing procedures should be an integral part of periodontal diagnosis. If the tooth does not respond to periodontal treatment as anticipated, a necrotic pulp may be the reason. Once the pulp becomes secondarily inflamed, it can in turn (by the mechanism described earlier) affect the primary periodontal lesion. This lesion is now similar to the primary endodontic lesion that has been secondarily involved with periodontal disease. The difference lies only in the sequence of formation.

Periodontal therapy procedures themselves may lead to secondary endodontic involvement. Scaling, curettage, and flap procedures may open lateral canals or dentinal tubules, or both to the oral environment, resulting in pulpal

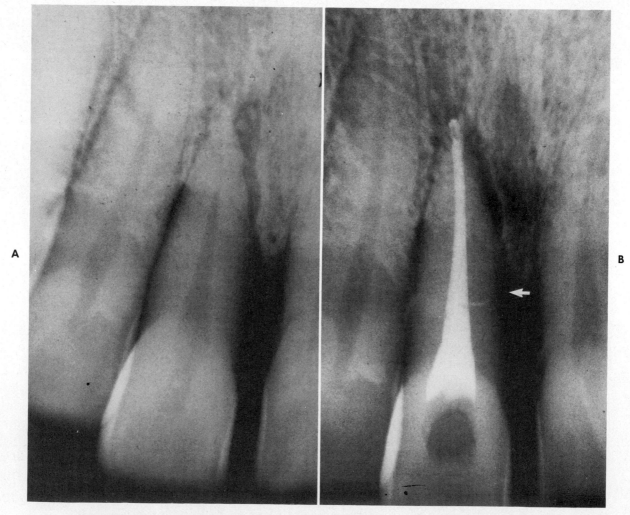

FIG. 17-16. A, Preoperative, periodontal involvement. **B,** Postoperative, lateral canal opening to the oral environment *(arrow)*.

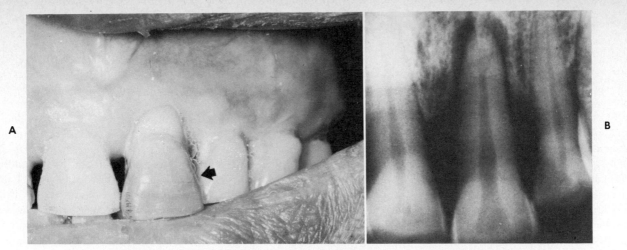

FIG. 17-17. A, Discolored incisor *(arrow)* with gingival recession. B, Periapical radiolucency and evidence of periodontal bone disease. The tooth had a necrotic root canal. This is thought to show the formation of "true" combined lesions wherein separate endodontic and periodontic lesions may join.

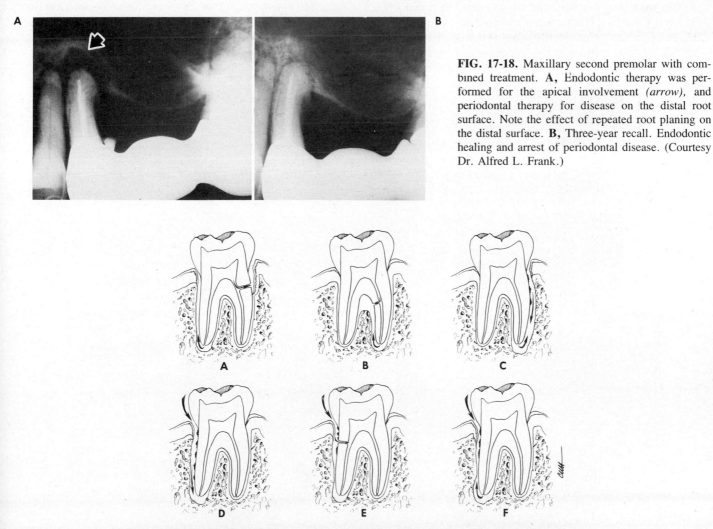

FIG. 17-18. Maxillary second premolar with combined treatment. A, Endodontic therapy was performed for the apical involvement *(arrow)*, and periodontal therapy for disease on the distal root surface. Note the effect of repeated root planing on the distal surface. B, Three-year recall. Endodontic healing and arrest of periodontal disease. (Courtesy Dr. Alfred L. Frank.)

FIG. 17-19. A to C, Endodontic lesions. A, The pathway of fistulation is evident through the periodontal ligament from the apex or a lateral canal. B, Fistulation through the apex or a lateral canal, causing bifurcation involvement. C, Secondary periodontal involvement. The existing pathway, as in A, is shown; with the passage of time, however, periodontitis, with plaque and calculus formation begins at the cervical area. D to F, Periodontal lesions. D, This is the progression of periodontitis to apical involvement. Note the vital pulp. E, Secondary endodontic involvement. The primary periodontal involvement at the cervical margin and the resultant pulpal necrosis once the lateral canal is exposed to the oral environment produce this picture. F, True combined lesions—coalescence.

disease.[22] However, this is a controversial point.[5,13-15,31] It is also possible for the blood vessel within a lateral canal to be severed by a currette during treatment. Postoperatively, these teeth may demonstrate necrotic pulps or symptoms of pulpitis. Severe pain is usually indicative of pulpal involvement.[4] The progression of periodontal disease alone may lead to a necrotic pulp. If the apical migration of the epithelial attachment uncovers or opens a lateral canal to the oral environment, necrosis of the pulp may ensue. Endodontic therapy in addition to periodontal procedures would then be indicated. Because no cause could be determined for the necrotic pulp in Fig. 17-16, the periodontal disease was suspected of having progressed apically to a point where the lateral canal was exposed to the oral environment with resulting pulpal necrosis. Upon completion of endodontic treatment the canal was sealed.

"True" combined lesions

In and around many teeth both pulpal and periodontal disease may be present independently. In these cases each disease may progress until the lesions unite to produce a radiographic and clinical picture similar to that of other lesions with secondary involvement (Figs. 17-17 and 17-18). A necrotic pulp, plaque, calculus, and periodontitis will be present in varying degrees. Once the endodontic and periodontal lesions join, they may be indistinguishable from endodontic and periodontal lesions that are secondarily involved.

Thus with the application of research findings and clinical experience, the pathways of osseous lesion formation may be theorized (Fig. 17-19). This theorization is intended as a guide for the evaluation and understanding of both our successes and failures in treating teeth with osseous lesions. By understanding their formation, we can better anticipate the potential for healing after treatment.

HEALING POTENTIAL

Many bony lesions are seen before they are able to complete their progression and are thus easier to treat both periodontally and endodontically. Clinically, primary endodontic lesions will usually heal completely. With lesions having an endodontic component, we anticipate that what is of endodontic origin may heal. Thus bony destruction of endodontic origin can usually be expected to heal. However, this is not usually the case with bony destruction of periodontal disease. Bone destruction from periodontal disease is reversible only in a three-walled infrabony pocket and only immediately following an acute periodon-

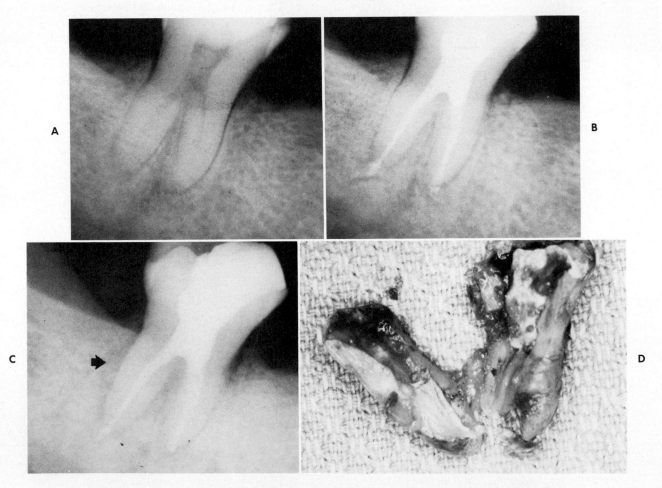

FIG. 17-20. A, Pretreatment. **B,** Posttreatment. **C,** Recall 9 months later. Note the distal radiolucency *(arrow).* Clinically the patient complained of discomfort when chewing; a mesiodistal fracture was apparent. **D,** After extraction and separation of the fracture segments. Note the extent of involvement.

tal (lateral) abscess.[27] Although much work is being done on periodontal healing, no studies have shown how endodontic lesions fistulating through the periodontal ligament heal. We may speculate on some of the possibilities.

With primary endodontic lesions there is apparently no resultant apical migration of the epithelial attachment,[40,46] possibly because apical migration is retarded in the presence of extensive local inflammation. In addition, if the cemental fibers are removed from the root surface, the epithelial attachment will migrate apically until new fiber support is found. If there is no long-term exposure to the oral environment (bacteria, toxins, and antigenic material), it is possible that when (or if) the endodontic lesion fistulates through the periodontal ligament space the cementum and its fibers may not be irreversibly disturbed.

Authors conducting periodontal studies[25,26,28,46] have proposed that the induction mechanism for healing may be in the fibers, cementum, or dentin. Thus if the fibers are disturbed, the cementum may induce new cementum and fiber formation to effect healing; or, if the fibers and cementum are affected, the dentin may induce new cementum and fiber formation. It has been suggested that the root does not contain a bone inductive principle but that, in fact, it may be a co-inducer with bone.[25] Although the mechanism of healing of endodontic lesions is not clear, clinically these lesions heal after endodontic treatment.

With lesions secondarily involved by periodontal disease, healing of the portion of the lesion not affected by periodontal disease can occur following endodontic treatment. Thus the prognosis of lesions with secondary periodontal involvement usually depends on the efficacy of the periodontal therapy. In general, it may be stated that the greater the periodontal involvement, the poorer the prognosis. Conversely, the more the lesion is the result of pulpal disease, the better the prognosis. The healing potential dictates the treatment.

DIFFERENTIAL DIAGNOSIS

In diagnosing these radiographic osseous lesions, one must resist the temptation to label everything a combined lesion. A variety of problems can mimic these lesions.

A tooth with a long-standing crack or vertical fracture

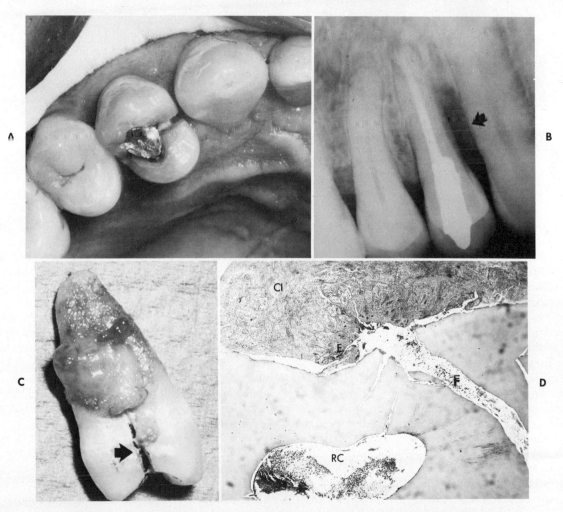

FIG. 17-21. A, Mesial-distal fracture of a maxillary first premolar. **B,** Mesial radiolucency *(arrow)* simulating periodontitis. **C,** Fracture *(arrow)* and attached soft tissue. **D,** Horizontal histologic section through the base of the soft tissue attached to the tooth. Note the epithelium directly opposite the fracture. *RC,* Root canal; *F,* fracture; *E,* epithelium; *CI,* chronic inflammation.

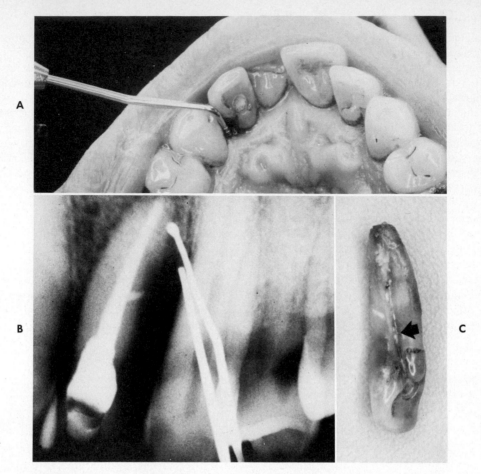

FIG. 17-22. A, Maxillary lateral incisor with a periodontal probe along the groove. **B,** Lateral radiolucency with silver cones in two labial sinus tracts. **C,** Note the apical extent of the lingual developmental groove *(arrow)*.

may have a radiographic picture of vertical bone loss along the root surface (Figs. 17-20 and 17-21). It may be barely discernible or a dark, teardrop radiolucency. Clinically these teeth can exhibit the spectrum of pulpal and periodontal disease, depending on the severity and length of time the tooth has been fractured. The diagnosis of fractured teeth is usually fairly straightforward; however, cracked teeth may demonstrate the most bizarre symptoms and pose a difficult diagnostic challenge as described in Chapter 1. In a sense, these lesions resulting from vertical fracture may be considered "true" combined lesions and have a poor prognosis.

Developmental grooves, principally in maxillary central and lateral incisors, are also capable of causing localized periodontitis and bone destruction along the root surface.[9,21,38] These grooves or morphologic invaginations usually run from the cingulum apically through the enamel, cementum, and dentin (Fig. 17-22). It is thought that they may be an attempt to form an accessory root. However, once plaque and calculus breach the epithelial attachment, the groove becomes a haven for bacteria and debris, leading to self-sustaining periodontal problem. The

bone destruction is usually tubular in effect and follows the path of the groove.

It is easy to diagnose these conditions if one is aware of their existence. Clinically, they may be asymptomatic or demonstrate acute or chronic periodontal symptoms. It is also conceivable that the pulp of these teeth may become secondarily involved and demonstrate symptoms of pulpal disease. These lesions are somewhat analogous to the enamel projections in the furcation area of mandibular molars.[23] Depending on the apical extent of these grooves, the periodontal prognosis may be good (tooth may be retainable) to poor. It must also be emphasized that systemic diseases and lesions of origin other than pulpal or periodontal can cause similar lesions.

TREATMENT

Osseous lesions are not the only periodontal consideration in endodontics. It has been suggested[33] that, because endodontists are in a sense apical periodontists, the periodontal evaluation of a tooth cannot be minimized. After all, if a tooth cannot be made periodontally sound, endodontic efforts may be for naught.

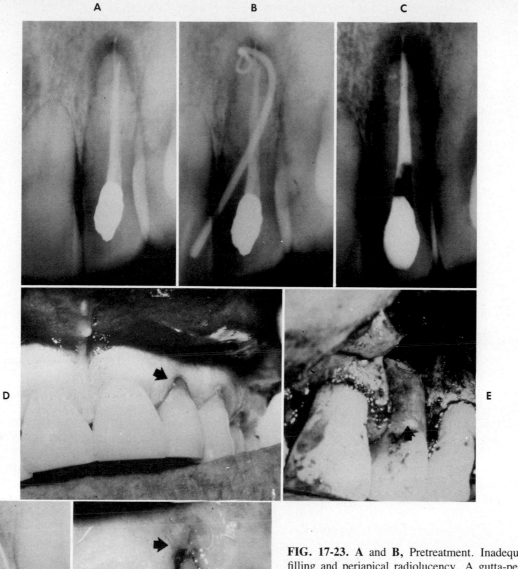

FIG. 17-23. A and **B,** Pretreatment. Inadequate root canal filling and periapical radiolucency. A gutta-percha probe inserted through the labial gingival sulcus extends to the apical region. **C,** Continued labial drainage, making an attempt to re-treat the root canal unsuccessful. **D,** Note the position of the gingival margin *(arrow)*. **E,** Full flap raised. Total lack of labial bone from crown to apex *(arrow)*. **F,** Postsurgical recall 3 months later. A silver cone probe extends through the gingival sulcus to the apex. **G,** Three months later, beginning gingival recession and pocket formation *(arrow)*. The prognosis for this tooth is poor.

Surgical considerations

Periodontal evaluation plays a very important role in surgical endodontics. Usually the flap design will be dictated by the health of the periodontal attachment and gingiva (Figs. 18-8 to 18-12). With envelope-type flaps, the horizontal incision is made in the attached gingiva. If little or no attached gingiva exists, a full flap should be raised and then possibly repositioned apically to create a new attached gingiva. Another consideration with this type of flap is the underlying bone. The flap edges should be sutured over sound bone to promote healing and to avoid the formation of postsurgical gingival recession or soft tissue defects (Fig. 17-23).

When a full flap is raised in the presence of periodontal

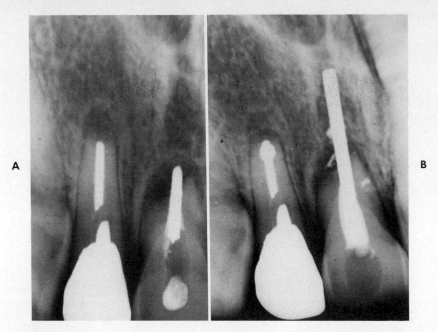

FIG. 17-24. A, Pretreatment. Poor crown/root ratio in the central incisor and inadequate root canal fillings in the central and lateral incisors. **B,** Posttreatment. An endodontic implant in the central incisor improves the crown/root ratio and stability.

disease, the clinician should perform the necessary scaling, curettage, or osseous-contouring procedures at the same time. Because a flap is being raised, it makes sense to perform local periodontal therapy rather than subject the patient to another procedure strictly for periodontal reasons. Any surgical endodontic procedure entails careful evaluation and possible treatment of periodontal structures as described in Chapter 18.

A further aid in periodontal treatment is the endodontic implant. This is usually indicated when increased crown root ratio is desired for stabilization in advanced periodontally involved teeth or to eliminate secondary occlusal trauma. However, the endodontic implant does not cure periodontal disease.[10-12] Furthermore, it can easily be abused. Currently, the American Dental Association classifies the endodontic implant as an experimental procedure[29] (Fig. 17-24).

Hemisection and root amputation

Recently there has been interest in maintaining roots and portions of teeth. This concept is not new, as shown by G.V. Black's attempt at root amputation in the 1880s. However, interest was not shown by the dental profession until the late 1950s. Teeth that formerly were considered hopeless now may be retained by alteration of form.

With both hemisection and root amputation, whenever possible the endodontic treatment should be completed before surgery; it is usually easier to isolate a tooth and prevent saliva leakage and contamination when this treatment sequence is followed.

Hemisections and root amputations are usually indicated when one or two roots become untreatable because of the following:

1. Endodontic reasons (separated instruments, root perforations [from resorption], obstructed canals)
2. Periodontal reasons (furcation involvement, severe involvement of one root)
3. Restorative reasons (caries destruction or erosion of a large portion of the crown and root, perforations during post preparation or fracture)
4. Combinations of these[1-3]

Hemisection. It may be desirable to retain half the tooth—in essence, convert a molar into a premolar. At this point the endodontic therapy can be accomplished by cleaning, shaping, and filling the root canal system to be retained and filling the entire pulp chamber with amalgam. The tooth may then be sectioned and restored (Figs. 17-25 and 17-26).

The sectioning can be done with a pencil diamond or long-shanked fissure bur. The initial cut, however, should not be directly in half but rather a little toward the root to be sacrificed. (Exposing a radiograph is usually helpful to ensure a proper angulation of the cut.) This procedure leaves enough tooth structure for the clinician to complete the crown preparation. A flap may or may not be necessary for hemisection, depending on the situation. (For example, periodontal involvement of the furca usually allows sufficient access for sectioning and root removal without requiring a flap.) After hemisection a radiograph should be exposed to ensure that there are no sharp edges of tooth structure or bone. The remaining root is restored with a post-crown preparation resembling a premolar (Chapter 21). It may or may not be part of a splint. In some instances the root can be used to support an overdenture. The occasion may also arise when both roots can be retained and the tooth sectioned to open the furcation area

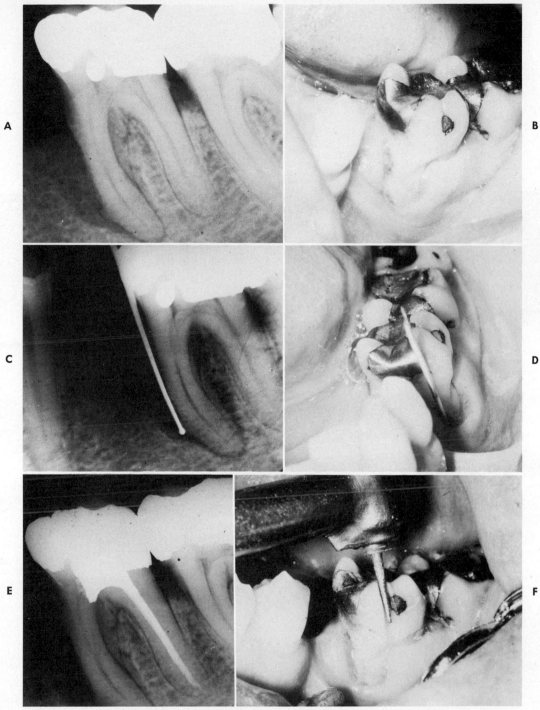

Continued.

FIG. 17-25. Mandibular first molar. **A** and **B**, Pretreatment. Severe periodontal disease with gingival recession on the mesial root. **C** and **D**, Silver cone probe through the mesial gingival sulcus almost to the apex. The tooth responded within normal limits to endodontic pulp-testing procedures. **E**, Completed root canal filling. **F**, Beginning hemisection cut with a high-speed diamond bur. **G**, Completed hemisection cut. **H**, Clinical appearance after the cut. **I**, Direct view and mirror reflection showing soft tissue healing of the extraction socket 1 week after hemisection. **J**, Abutments prepared for the bridge. **K**, Mirror reflection showing the bridge in place. **L**, Three-month recall. **M**, Five-month recall.

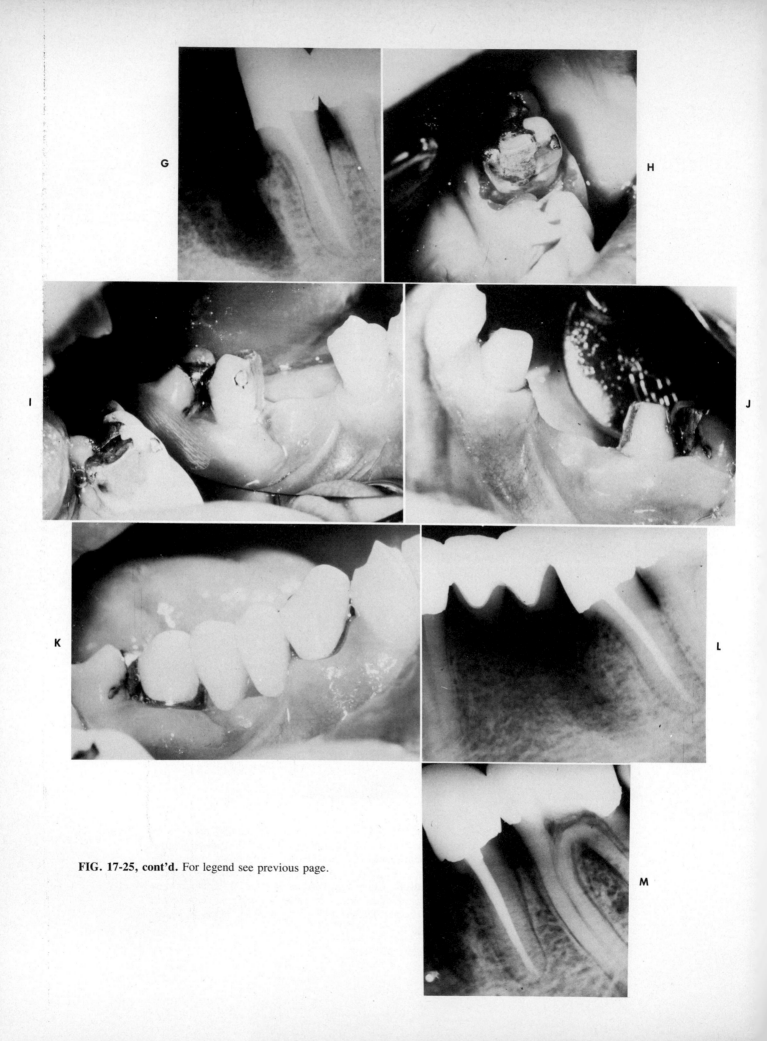

FIG. 17-25, cont'd. For legend see previous page.

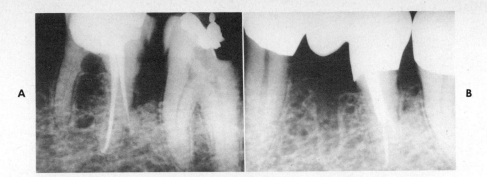

FIG. 17-26. A, Radiograph of mundibular molar with two distal roots. Extensive decay perforated into the furcal area. **B,** After hemisection a three-unit bridge was used for replacement. Note that mesial margin for the crown does not leave an overhang.

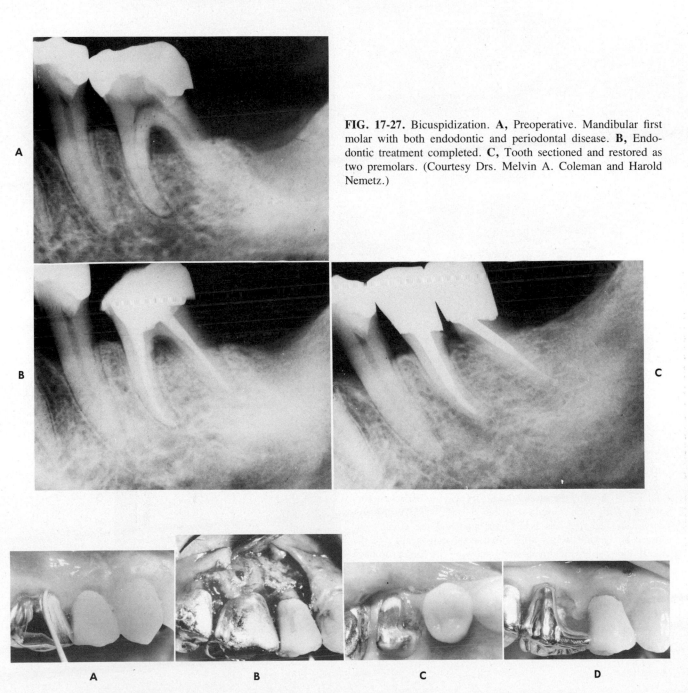

FIG. 17-27. Bicuspidization. **A,** Preoperative. Mandibular first molar with both endodontic and periodontal disease. **B,** Endodontic treatment completed. **C,** Tooth sectioned and restored as two premolars. (Courtesy Drs. Melvin A. Coleman and Harold Nemetz.)

FIG. 17-28. A, Clinical photograph with a gutta-percha probe in place alongside the mesiobuccal root. **B,** With the flap raised a vertical fracture in the mesiobuccal root is apparent. The decision to amputate the root was made. **C,** After root amputation, the entire crown was contoured to have root support for all remaining tooth structure. **D,** Final restoration in place.

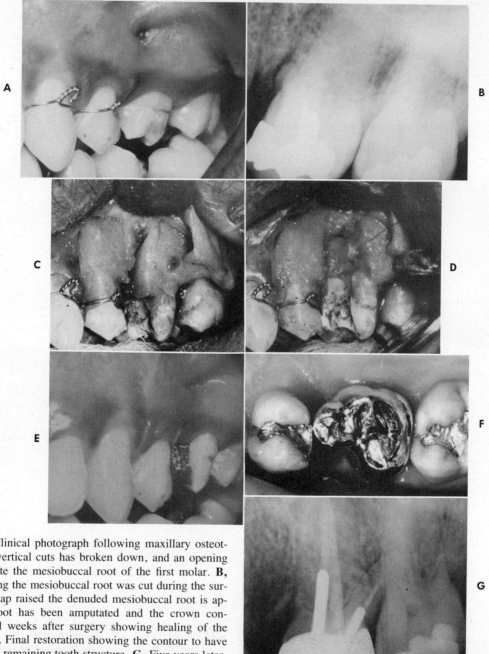

FIG. 17-29. A, Clinical photograph following maxillary osteotomy. One of the vertical cuts has broken down, and an opening is apparent opposite the mesiobuccal root of the first molar. **B,** Radiograph showing the mesiobuccal root was cut during the surgery. **C,** With a flap raised the denuded mesiobuccal root is apparent. **D,** The root has been amputated and the crown contoured. **E,** Several weeks after surgery showing healing of the buccal opening. **F,** Final restoration showing the contour to have root support for all remaining tooth structure. **G,** Five years later. Note the two palatal canals.

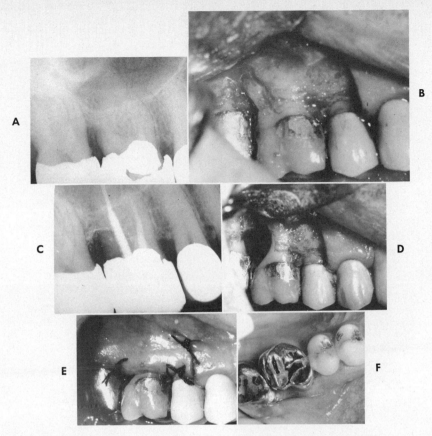

FIG. 17-30. A, Preoperative radiograph showing periodontal defect on distobuccal root of first molar. **B,** Flap raised to reveal the extent of periodontal disease. **C,** Endodontic therapy completed on remaining two roots. **D,** Amputation of the distobuccal root. **E,** Flap replaced. **F,** Final restoration.

for periodontal reasons. Both roots are then restored to form two premolars (bicuspidization) (Fig. 17-27).

Root amputation. The endodontic phase of treatment consists of cleaning and shaping the root (or roots) to be retained with files and Gates-Glidden burs. After the root canal system has been obturated with gutta-percha, a no. 4 to 6 slow-speed, long-shanked, round bur is used to drill 2 to 3 mm into the root (or roots) to be amputated. The root and the entire pulp chamber are then filled thoroughly with well-condensed amalgam to ensure a continued seal of the pulp chamber after the root is removed.

In some cases the extent of bone loss and the periodontal involvement are so severe that a flap does not have to be raised; other cases require a small triangular flap, as described on p. 588.

In maxillary molars one or even two roots may be amputated. The procedure is similar to hemisection except the contouring of the remaining crown is more complex. The root itself should not simply be cut away; the crown portion supported by the root must be recontoured to accept new occlusal demands[3,17,50] and to ensure good oral hygiene. The crown may be contoured first and the underlying root then removed, or the crown and root cut off together (Figs. 17-28 to 17-31).

Again, root sectioning may be accomplished with pencil diamond burs or with long-shanked fissured burs. The amputated root is most easily removed with an elevator. After the root has been amputated, the remaining crown and root(s) should be examined clinically and checked radiographically to confirm complete root removal and ensure a smooth furca with no sharp edges. A knowledge of root anatomy is necessary to ascertain that root removal is completed and to avoid gouging of the crown or furca. Fused roots usually preclude hemisection and root amputation. However, in both procedures the remaining tooth portion must be restorable so its function can be returned.

Both these procedures are excellent if used when indicated and if used properly. If abused, the techniques can lead to predictable failure both periodontally and restoratively.

However, in a 10-year study on 50 hemisected mandibular molars and 50 resected maxillary molars with root amputation, these teeth were treated for pocket elimination with furcation involvements.[20] After 10 years 38% of the teeth failed. However, in the first 5 years only 15.8% of the failures occurred, but in the next 2 years 55.3% of the failures happened. The mandibular teeth failed 2:1 over the maxillary molars. The most prevalent cause of failure

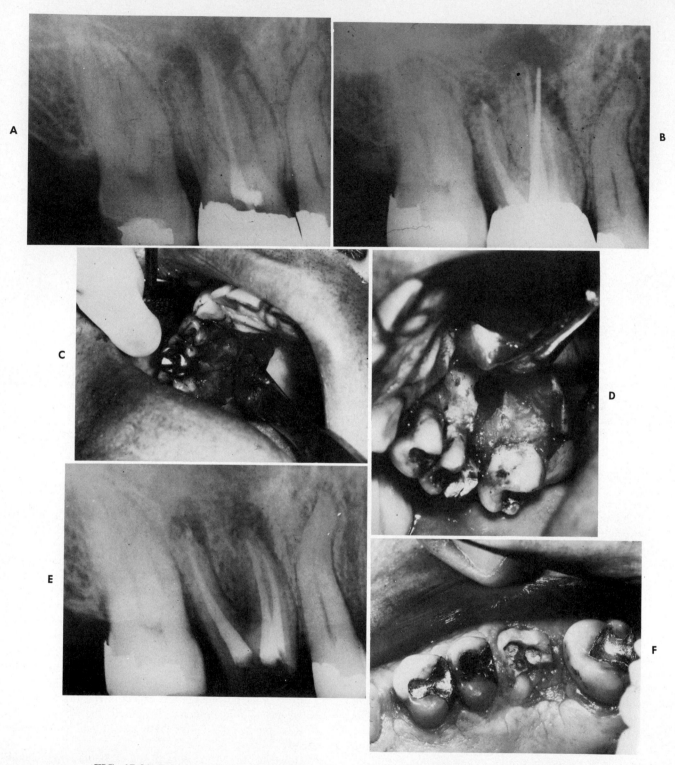

FIG. 17-31. Palatal root amputation. **A,** Preoperative. Endodontic treatment is incomplete. Note the periapical lesions. **B,** Immediately posttreatment. Periodontal probe inserted along the palatal root. **C,** A palatal flap has been reflected to expose the periodontal defect involving the palatal root. **D,** The palatal root has been amputated. **E,** Posttreatment. Palatal root amputated. Note the two canals in the mesial-buccal root. **F,** Approximately 10 days later, soft tissue healing.

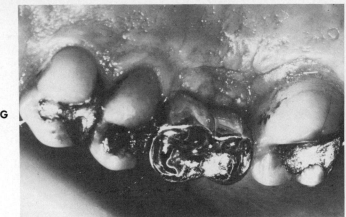
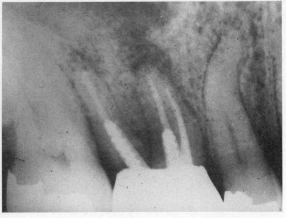

FIG. 17-31, cont'd. G, Final restoration of the remaining two buccal roots. **H,** Case completed.

was root fracture. They attributed this to parafunctional occlusal habits, small size of the root, and weakening the lateral walls with endodontics, post preparation, or poor post design. Most failures were attributed to endodontic or restorative problems, not periodontal disease.

With all phases of dentistry, it is mandatory to diagnose and understand the presenting clinical situation before starting treatment. The interaction of endodontics and periodontics is no exception. Although we are able to provide excellent benefits to patients in these areas, the potential for abuse exists. Only a thorough knowledge and understanding of the interrelationships of all phases of dentistry will enhance the benefits our patients derive.

REFERENCES

1. Abrams, L., and Trachtenberg, D.O.: Hemisection—technique and restoration, Dent. Clin. North Am. **18:**415, 1974.
2. Amsterdam, M., and Rossmann, S.: Technique of hemisection of multirooted teeth, Alpha Omegan **53:**4, 1960.
3. Basaraba, N.: Root amputation and tooth hemisection, Dent. Clin. North Am. **13:**121, 1969.
4. Bender, I.B., and Seltzer, S.: The effect of periodontal disease on the pulp, Oral Surg. **33:**458, 1972.
5. Bergenholtz, G., and Lindhe, J.: Effect of experimentally induced marginal periodontitis and periodontal scaling on the dental pulp, J. Clin. Periodontol. **5:**59, 1978.
6. Blair, H.A.: Relationships between endodontics and periodontics, J. Periodontol. **43:**209, 1972.
7. Cameron, C.E.: Cracked-tooth syndrome, J. Am. Dent. Assoc. **68:**405, 1964.
8. Czarnecki, R.T., and Schilder, H.: A histological evaluation of the human pulp in teeth with varying degrees of periodontal disease, J. Endod. **5:**242, 1979.
9. Everett, F.G., and Kramer, G.M.: The disto-lingual groove in the maxillary lateral incisor; a periodontal hazard, J. Periodontol. **43:**352, 1971.
10. Frank, A.L.: Endodontic endosseous implants and treatment of the wide open apex, Dent. Clin. North Am. **11:**675, 1967.
11. Frank, A.L.: Improvement of the crown-root ratio by endodontic endosseous implants, J. Am. Dent. Assoc. **74:**451, 1967.
12. Frank, A.L.: Resorption, perforations, and fractures, Dent. Clin. North Am. **18:**465, 1974.
13. Hattler, A.B., and Listgarten, M.A.: Pulpal response to root planing in a rat model, J. Endod. **10:**471, 1984.
14. Hiatt, W.H.: Regeneration of the periodontium after endodontic therapy and flap operation, Oral Surg. **12:**1471, 1959.
15. Hiatt, W.H.: Periodontal pocket elimination by combined therapy, Dent. Clin. North Am., p. 133, March 1964.
16. Kipioti, A., et al.: Microbiological findings of infected root canals and adjacent periodontal pockets in teeth with advanced periodontitis, J. Oral Surg. **58:**213, 1984.
17. Kirchoff, D.A., and Gerstein, H.: Presurgical crown contouring for root amputation procedures, Oral Surg. **27:**379, 1969.
18. Koenigs, J.F., Brillant, J.D., and Foreman, D.W., Jr.: Preliminary scanning electron microscope investigations of accessory foramina in furcation areas of human molar teeth, Oral Surg. **38:**773, 1974.
19. Langeland, K., Rodriques, H., and Dowden, W.: Periodontal disease, bacteria and pulpal histopathology, Oral Surg. **37:**257, 1974.
20. Langer, B., Stein, S.D., and Wagenberg, B.: An evaluation of root resections: a ten-year study, J. Periodontol. **52:**719, 1981.
21. Lee, K.W., Lee, E.C., and Poon, K.Y.: Palato-gingival grooves in maxillary incisors, Br. Dent. J. **124:**14, 1968.
22. Lowman, J.V., Burke, R.S., and Pelleu, G.B.: Patent accessory canals: incidence in molar furcation region, Oral Surg. **36:**580, 1973.
23. Masters, D.H., and Hoskins, S.W.: Projection of cervical enamel into molar furcations, J. Periodontol. **35:**49, 1964.
24. Mazur, B., and Massler, M.: The influence of periodontal disease on the dental pulp, Oral Surg. **17:**598, 1964.
25. Morris, M.L.: A study of the inductive properties of the organic matrix of dentin and cementum, J. Periodontol. **43:**10, 1972.
26. Morris, M.L.: The subcutaneous implantation of periodontally diseased roots, J. Periodontol. **43:**737, 1972.
27. Prichard, J.F.: Advanced periodontal disease, ed. 2, Philadelphia, 1972, W.B. Saunders Co.
28. Register, A.A., et al.: Human bone induction by allogeneic dentin matrix, J. Periodontol. **43:**459, 1972.
29. Reports of Councils and Bureaus, J. Am. Dent. Assoc. **88:**394, 1974.
30. Ross, I.F.: The relations between periodontal and pulpal disorders, J. Am. Dent. Assoc. **84:**134, 1972.
31. Ross, I.F., and Thompson, R.H.: A long term study of root retention in the treatment of maxillary molars with furcation involvement, J. Periodontol. **49:**238, 1978.
32. Rubach, W.C., and Mitchell, D.F.: Periodontal disease, accessory canals and pulp pathosis, J. Periodontol. **36:**34, 1965.
33. Schilder, H.: The relationship of periodontics to endodontics. In Grossman, L.I., editor: Transactions, Third International Conference on Endodontics, Philadelphia, 1963, University of Pennsylvania.
34. Seltzer, S.: Endodontology, New York, 1971, McGraw-Hill Book Co.
35. Seltzer, S., et al.: Pulpitis-induced interradicular periodontal changes in experimental animals, J. Periodontol. **38:**124, 1967.
36. Seltzer, S., Bender, I.B., and Ziontz, M.: The interrelationship of pulp and periodontal disease, Oral Surg. **16:**1474, 1963.
37. Seltzer, S., Sinai, I., and August, D.: Periodontal effects of root perforations before and during endodontic procedures, J. Dent. Res. **49:**332, 1970.
38. Simon, J.H., Glick, D.H., and Frank, A.L.: Predictable endodontic

and periodontic failures as a result of radicular anomalies, Oral Surg. **31**:823, 1971.

39. Simon, J.H., Glick, D.H., and Frank, A.L.: The relationship of endodontic-periodontic lesions, J. Periodontol. **43**:202, 1972.

40. Simon, P., and Jacobs, D.: The so-called combined periodontal-pulpal problem, Dent. Clin. North Am. **13**:45, 1969.

41. Simring, M., and Goldberg, M.: The pulpal pocket approach: retrograde periodontitis, J. Periodontol. **35**:22, 1964.

42. Sinai, I.H., and Soltanoff, W.: The transmission of pathologic changes between the pulp and the periodontal structures, Oral Surg. **36**:558, 1973.

43. Smukler, H., and Tagger, M.: Vital root amputation, a clinical and histologic study, J. Periodontol. **47**:324-330, 1976.

44. Stahl, S.S.: Pulpal response to gingival injury in adult rats, Oral Surg. **16**:1116, 1963.

45. Stahl, S.S.: Pathogenesis of inflammatory lesions in pulp and periodontal tissues, Periodontics **4**:190, 1966.

46. Stahl, S.S., et al.: Speculations about gingival repair, J. Periodontol. **43**:395, 1972.

47. Stallard, R.E.: Periodontal disease and its relationship to pulpal pathology, Annual Meeting, American Institute of Oral Biology, 1967.

48. Taggar, M., and Massler, M.: Periapical tissue reactions after pulp exposure in rat molars, Oral Surg. **39**:304, 1975.

49. Torabinejad, M., and Kiger, R.D.: A histologic evaluation of dental pulp tissue of a patient with periodontal disease, Oral Surg. **59**:198, 1985.

50. Weine, F.S.: Endodontic therapy, ed. 3, St. Louis, 1982, The C.V. Mosby Co.

Self-assessment questions

1. Pulpal inflammation may extend to which area of the attachment apparatus?
   a. Lateral aspect of the root
   b. Apical area of the root
   c. Furcation area
   d. All of the above

2. Which route of pulpal disease may not have a direct inflammatory effect on the periodontal ligament?
   a. Lateral canals
   b. Dentinal tubules
   c. Overinstrumentation
   d. Post perforation

3. Studies indicate that the periodontal inflammatory effect on the pulp causes
   a. Decreased reparative dentin formation
   b. Decrease in the cellular component of the pulp
   c. Decrease in dystrophic calcification
   d. Decrease in fibrosis

4. Which of the following characteristics is true of a sinus tract fistula of pulpal origin?
   a. It usually involves more than one aspect of the tooth
   b. Generally endodontic testing will reveal a vital pulp
   c. A poor prognosis is anticipated with endodontic therapy
   d. The tract can usually be probed to the source of the irritation

5. Primary endodontic lesions with secondary periodontal involvement
   a. Can be expected to heal completely with endodontic therapy alone
   b. Clinically reveal only a necrotic root
   c. Are usually treated with periodontal surgery before endodontic therapy
   d. Have a prognosis that depends on the periodontal involvement and the efficacy of periodontal treatment

6. The following is true of primary periodontal lesions:
   a. The prognosis is based on the success of periodontal therapy
   b. The bony lesion is usually more widespread than the lesion of pulpal origin
   c. A probeable pocket usually has evidence of plaque and calculus formation
   d. All of the above

7. Which statement is false regarding primary periodontal lesions with secondary pulpal involvement?
   a. Periodontal therapy alone is successful
   b. Postoperatively the tooth develops a necrotic pulp
   c. Postoperatively severe pain may develop
   d. The tooth does not respond to periodontal treatment as expected

8. With "true" combined lesions
   a. A vital pulp is usually present
   b. There is a distinction between periodontal lesions and pulpal lesions that are secondarily involved
   c. A necrotic pulp, calculus, and periodontitis will be present in varying degrees
   d. Pulpal and periodontal diseases generally do not progress to unite

9. Developmental grooves
   a. Usually create primary endodontic lesions with secondary periodontal involvement
   b. Are found generally throughout the mouth
   c. Have a prognosis dependent on the endodontic extent of involvement
   d. Can lead to a self-sustaining periodontal condition with secondary pulpal involvement

10. A tooth with a long-standing crack or vertical fracture
    a. May present a radiographic picture of vertical bone loss along the root surface
    b. Can present bizarre symptoms and cause difficulty in diagnosis
    c. May be considered a "true" combined lesion with a poor prognosis
    d. All of the above

11. Which of the following conditions may not be a candidate for a hemisection or root amputation procedure?
    a. A pathologic root perforation of a multirooted tooth
    b. A furcation involvement with severe bone loss of one root
    c. Caries destruction of a large portion of the crown and root of a lower molar
    d. Root perforation during post preparation of a maxillary canine

12. Before a root amputation procedure, the canal orifice of the root to be amputated is filled with
    a. Gutta-percha
    b. Polycarboxylate cement
    c. Amalgam
    d. A composite

18

SURGICAL ENDODONTICS

DONALD E. ARENS

Techniques for cleaning, shaping, and filling the root canal system have been described in Chapters 7 and 8. However, there are situations in which the root canal system cannot be thoroughly debrided or properly obturated. In these cases a surgical approach is the only reasonable alternative to extraction.* Surgical endodontics should be considered merely another treatment alternative and not a radical endodontic procedure.[21]

CONTRAINDICATIONS TO SURGICAL ENDODONTICS

The restorability and the periodontal prognosis of a tooth are important in deciding on treatment; however, the medical condition of the patient is paramount. Because a surgical entry obviously requires an incision of soft tissue and the removal of bone, the patient must be physically and mentally capable of enduring the procedure and physiologically healthy enough to permit uneventful healing. Hence a thorough medical history (as described in Chapter 1) should be recorded, reviewed, and discussed with the patient to determine if any potential health hazards exist.

When doubt arises from an evaluation of the history, medical consultation with the attending family physician is indicated. Because the patient's welfare becomes the clinician's responsibility once treatment begins, all questions should be answered *prior* to the surgery. Neglect of existing medical contraindications may constitute malpractice. Attention must also be given to the patient's daily pharmacologic regimen. To avert any drug antagonism or synergism, all medications must be appraised and the proper precautions instituted. It is inadvisable to change or discontinue a patient's medication without consulting with the prescribing physicians.

ANTIBIOTIC PROPHYLACTIC THERAPY

The following information is extracted from the December 1984 publications of the policies established by the Committee on Rheumatic Fever and Infective Endocarditis of the Council on Cardiovascular Disease.*

Any dental treatment, surgical procedure, or instrumentation that involves mucosal surfaces or contaminated tissue will most likely cause a transient bacteremia. Blood-borne bacteria may lodge on damaged, abnormal or prosthetic valves or on endocardium near congenital defects and result in bacterial endocarditis or endarteritis. Since it is impossible to predict which patients may develop these sequelae, prophylactic antibiotic therapy should be prescribed for any dental condition in which gingival bleeding may be induced and the increased bacteremia might stimulate a secondary infection remote from the surgical site. Specifically, but not all inclusive, the following recommendations have been established by the committee.

Cardiac conditions
Endocarditis prophylaxis recommended:
  Prosthetic cardiac valves (including biosynthetic valves)
  Most congenital cardiac malformations
  Surgically constructed systemic-pulmonary shunts
  Rheumatic and other acquired valvular dysfunction
  Idiopathic hypertrophic subaortic stenosis (IHSS)
  Previous history of bacterial endocarditis
  Mitral valve prolapse with insufficiency
Endocarditis prophylaxis not recommended:
  Isolated secundum atrial septal defect
  Secundum atrial septal defect repaired without a patch 6 or more months earlier
  Patent ductus arteriosus ligated and divided six or months earlier
  Postoperative coronary artery bypass graft (CABG) surgery

Procedures for which endocarditis prophylaxis is indicated
  All dental procedures likely to induce gingival bleeding (not simple adjustment of orthodontic appliances or shedding of deciduous teeth)
  Tonsillectomy and/or adenoidectomy

---

*References 29, 34, 37-39, 48, 62, 92.

*Prepared by the Committee on Prevention of Rheumatic Fever and Bacterial Endocarditis of the American Heart Association, Circulation **70:**1123A, 1984. By permission of the American Heart Association, Inc.

SUMMARY OF RECOMMENDED ANTIBIOTIC REGIMENS
FOR DENTAL/RESPIRATORY TRACT PROCEDURES

Standard Regimen

For dental procedures that cause gingival bleeding, and oral/respiratory tract surgery	Penicillin V 2.0 g orally 1 hour before, then 1.0 g 6 hours later. For patients unable to take oral medications. 2 million units of aqueous penicillin G IV or IM 30-60 minutes before a procedure and 1 million units 6 hours later may be substituted

Special Regimens

Parenteral regimen for use when maximal protection desired: e.g., for patients with prosthetic valves	Ampicillin 1.0-2.0 g IM or IV plus gentamicin 1.5 mg/kg IM or IV, ½ hour before procedure, followed by 1.0 g oral penicillin V 6 hours later. Alternatively, the parenteral regimen may be repeated once 8 hours later
Oral regimen for penicillin-alllergic patients	Erythromycin 1.0 g orally 1 hours before, then 500 mg 6 hours later
Parenteral regimen for penicillin-allergic patients	Vancomycin 1.0 g IV *slowly* over 1 hour, starting 1 hour before. No repeat dose is necessary

Note: *Pediatric doses:* Ampicillin 50 mg/kg per dose: erythromycin 20 mg/kg for first dose, then 10 mg/kg, gentamicin 2.0 mg/kg per dose; penicillin V full adult dose if greater than 60 lb (27 kg), one-half adult dose if less than 60 lb (27 kg); aqueous penicillin G 50,000 units/kg (25,000 units/kg for follow-up); vancomycin 20 mg/kg per dose. The intervals between doses are the same as for adults. Total doses should not exceed adult doses.

Surgical procedures or biopsy involving respiratory mucosa
Bronchoscopy, especially with a rigid bronchoscope
Incision and drainage of infected tissue
Genitourinary and gastrointestinal procedures as listed in text

The committee also recognized that antibiotic regimens used to prevent recurrences of acute rheumatic fever are inadequate for the prevention of bacterial endocarditis and that practioners must exercise clinical judgment in determining the duration and choice of antibiotics when special circumstances present. It also recommends special attention be given to unusual clinical events following dental or surgical procedures.

The specific recommendations relative to the antibiotic regimens for Dental/Respiratory Tract procedures are as follows.

1. Standard regimen

Oral penicillin. For adults and children over 60 lb (27 kg): Penicillin V 2.0 g 1 hour prior to the procedure and then 1.0 g 6 hours later. For children less than 60 lb: 1.0 g 1 hour prior to the procedure and then 500 mg 6 hours later.

For patients unable to take oral antibiotics prior to a procedure, 2 million units of aqueous penicillin G (50,000 units/kg for children) IV or IM 30-60 minutes prior to the procedure and 1 million units (25,000 units/kg for children) 6 hours later may be substituted.

2. For patients with prosthetic valves and others with highest risk of endocarditis

Parenteral ampicillin and gentamicin. Ampicillin 1.0 to 2.0 g (50 mg/kg for children) plus gentamicin 1.5 mg/kg (2.0 mg/kg for children) both IM or IV ½ hours prior to the procedure, followed by 1 g oral penicillin V 6 hours later. Alternatively, the parenteral regimen should be repeated once 8 hours later.

3. Standard regimen for patients allergic to penicillin

Oral erythromycin. Erythromycin 1.0 g (20 mg/kg for children) one hour prior to the procedure and then 500 mg (10 mg/kg for children) 6 hours later.

For patients unable to tolerate oral erythromycin, changing to a different erythromycin preparation may be beneficial. For those who cannot tolerate either penicillin or erythromycin, an oral cephalosporin (1.0 g 1 hour prior to the procedure plus 500 mg 6 hours later) may be useful, but data are lacking to allow specific recommendation of this regimen. Tetracyclines *cannot* be recommended for this purpose.

4. Regimen for high-risk patients allergic to penicillin

IV vancomycin. Vancomycin 1 g (20 mg/kg for children) IV *slowly* over 1 hour starting 1 hour prior to procedure. Because of the long half-life of vancomycin, a repeat dose should not be necessary.

Notes. In unusual circumstances or in the case of delayed healing, it may be necessary to provide additional doses of antibiotics even though bacteremia rarely persists longer than 15 minutes after the procedure. Penicillin V is the preferred form of oral penicillin because it is relatively resistant to gastric acid.

For those patients taking an oral penicillin for secondary prevention of rheumatic fever or for other purposes, viridans streptococci relatively resistant to penicillin may be present in the oral cavity. In such cases, the physician or dentist should select erythromycin or one of the parenteral regimens.

Some patients with a prosthetic heart valve in whom a high level of oral health is being maintained may be offered oral antibiotic prophylaxis for routine dental procedures. Parenteral antibiotics are recommended, however, for patients with prosthetic valves who require extensive dental procedures, especially extractions, or oral or gingival surgical procedures.

Other indications for antibiotic prophylaxis to prevent endocarditis

1. In susceptible patients, prophylaxis to prevent endocarditis is also indicated for surgical procedures on any infected or contaminated tissues, including incision and drainage of abscesses. In these circumstances, regimens should be individualized but in most instances should include antibiotics effective against *Staphylococcus aureus*.

2. Antibiotic prophylaxis for the surgical and dental procedures indicated above should also be given to patients with a documented previous episode of bacterial endocarditis, even in the absence of clinically detectable heart disease.

3. Patients with indwelling transvenous cardiac pacemakers appear to present a low risk of endocarditis; when such cases occur they are predominantly due to staphylococci. However, dentists and physicians may choose to employ prophylactic antibiotics when dental and surgical procedures are performed in these patients. The same recommendations apply to renal dialysis patients with arteriovenous shunt appliances.

4. Endocarditis prophylaxis also deserves consideration in patients with ventriculo atrial shunts for hydrocephalus, because there are documented cases of bacterial endocarditis in these patients.

ANATOMIC CONSIDERATIONS

Local conditions that may influence one's decision to perform apical surgery can be anatomic or neurovascular. Because of poor access and visibility the lingual aspect of the mandible often presents almost impossible treatment situations. The thickness of the buccal plate of bone in the posterior molar region of the mandible may require such extensive bone removal to gain access to the apex that entry is not judicious. Similarly, perforations of the lateral surfaces of a root caused by internal or external resorption or an iatrogenic incident require the removal of strategic periodontal bone. Thus the patient is left with an undesirable and unesthetic periodontal defect.

Normally the neurovascular supply in the anterior aspect of the palate does not present a major problem because the vessels and nerves are small and, when cut, readily unite and reinnervate. However, the vessels in the greater palatine region are more delicate; although the nerves will reinnervate, the severed blood vessels can present difficult-to-manage bleeding problems. Other bundles of concern are the vessels within the mandibular canal. Although they are usually inferior to the apices of the molars and premolars, it is possible for the inferior alveolar nerves and blood vessels to be found at or even above the root tips. When operating in the posterior mandibular region, it is advisable for the clinician to expose frequent radiographs to check orientation. Neurovascular branches exit from bone through the mental foramen, so the tissue in this region when incised and elevated requires careful attention and concentration. The foramen is usually found around the apex of the premolars; and before bone is drilled, these vessels should be identified, dissected, and carefully displaced. Only after the location of the neurovascular bundle is known can the involved tooth or teeth be confidently approached. Because paresthesia may result when these major vessels are involved with the surgery it is imperative the patient be forewarned. In exposing the root tips of maxillary teeth the sinus floor may be perforated. Care must be exercised to prevent debris, root tips, or filling materials from being pushed through the opening. Invading pathologic lesions will often drain through the nasal passage. When this happens excessive bleeding will be noticed during and after the surgery. Both situations should heal uneventfully if the proper flap design was chosen.

Again, the patient should be informed of these possibilities before surgery and special postoperative instructions should be given following surgery. The remaining consideration before surgery is the surgical skill of the clinician. A certain degree of knowledge, dexterity, and confidence is required for safe and successful surgery. If one feels uncomfortable about performing a particular surgical procedure, he or she should refer the case to a specialist. The general dentist and the patient both benefit when a referral is made under these circumstances.

Further consideration will be given to anatomical variances and precautions later in this chapter when surgery is discussed by area.

INDICATIONS FOR SURGERY

When nonsurgical treatment is impossible or ineffective in resolving a canal or periapical problem, the skillful application of sound surgical principles offers many distinct advantages.[6] Such surgical considerations can be grouped into the following categories.

Relief of pain

When toxic products from a necrotic tooth enter the periapical area, inflammation results. As the blood vessels expand and fluids accumulate, the periapical tissue pressure begins to increase. Because the cortical bone has not been sufficiently demineralized in an acute apical periodontitis, the situation may not be radiographically apparent (Fig. 18-1, A); the restraint of these fluids will often cause the pressure to become unbearable. If not relieved, severe pain may reach levels that even strong narcotic therapy cannot relieve. Merely extirpating the pulpal remnants may prove inadequate and a direct apical approach through bone becomes the only reasonable alternative. Such a procedure, commonly known as trephination, has been a reported dental practice as early as the year 1500 BC.[46] Anthropologists found substantial evidence of holes bored in ancient Egyptian mandibles that are believed to have been made to drain abscesses.[65,74] Although the purpose of trephination remains unchanged, the introduction of anesthetics and the sophistication of surgical techniques certainly have improved the procedure.[65,71]

Technique for trephination. Because the inflammatory exudate has not entered the soft tissues, routine local anesthetic administration is effective in cases of acute apical periodontitis.

Because these patients are in great pain and under great stress the diseased tooth should be identified, diagnosed, and anesthetized as quickly as possible.

In addition to the routine infiltration or block injection, the intraligamentory injections are recommended to assure the required depth of anesthesia. Intraligamentary injections should be administered just prior to the surgery. To further enhance patient comfort and cooperation, a systemic relaxant or sedative can be administered orally. For an adult 10 mg of diazepam (Valium) or 120 mg of secobarbital (Seconal) or sodium pentobarbital (Nembutal) will help reduce apprehension and fear. Such doses will not render the adult patient unconscious but will provide tran-

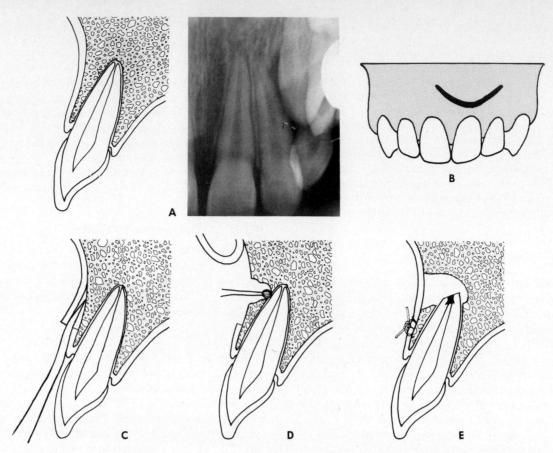

FIG. 18-1. Acute apical periodontitis. **A,** Graphic and radiographic demonstration of only a thickening of the periodontal ligament but no hard tissue resorption. **B,** A half-moon incision is made by a no. 15 Bard-Parker scalpel in the attached gingiva. **C,** A periosteal elevator is inserted into the incision and the flap is reflected. **D,** A large (no. 6 to 8) round bur is used to remove the cortical and cancellous bone covering the inflamed apex. **E,** When the correct apex is identified and curretted and amalgam is placed in the apex, the flap is respositioned and sutured closed.

quility, and ease fears, thereby enhancing the effects of the local anesthetic. Nitrous oxide analgesia is also very useful because its effect is short acting and it thus can be used when the patient is unaccompanied.

When the practitioner is assured the patient is anesthetized, the offending tooth is opened and the pulpal remnants are extirpated. A file positioned to the apical foramen is measured radiographically or electronically and the canal is cleaned and shaped as described in Chapter 7. A cotton pellet is placed over the chamber entry and the crown opening is sealed with zinc oxide–eugenol cement. Attention is now directed to the surgery. A small half-moon incision is made with a no. 15 scalpel (Fig. 18-1, *B*). The incision should begin 1 mm gingival to the mucobuccal fold one tooth lateral to the diseased tooth and proceed gingivally to a point 4 to 6 mm below or above the known length of the tooth. This point can be accurately determined because the canal has been previously measured. The incision is completed by directing the blade toward the mucobuccal fold over the adjacent tooth on the opposite side.

A full mucoperiosteal flap is firmly but carefully reflected by a no. 9 Molt periosteal elevator (Fig. 18-1, *C*).

It is imperative that the sharp edge of the elevator remain on bone throughout this maneuver so the periosteum will be an integral part of the flap. After the bone has been exposed, a no. 6 round bur will be used to bore through the cortex and cancellous bone 1 or 2 mm beneath the suspected apical tip (Fig. 18-1, *D*). Locating the apex when the canal has not been premeasured and instrumented is difficult. The root approach depends upon knowing root length averages, palpating the topography of the bone for the convexities created by the root mass, and maintaining an unrestricted view of the surgical field as the cortical bone is removed.[5]

Note: No surgical procedure should be attempted blindly, and for this reason artificial fistulators have no place in modern dentistry.[76,82] If the initial bone entry proves unsuccessful in locating the root, a piece of sterile x-ray lead foil can be temporarily inserted into the bone opening and radiographed. The opaque foil will reorient the clinician to the root and the necessary directional adjustment can then be made. When the root has been identified, the apex is uncovered and the inflamed periapical tissue is curetted. This incision need not remain open and can be closed by one or two sutures (Fig. 18-1, *E*).

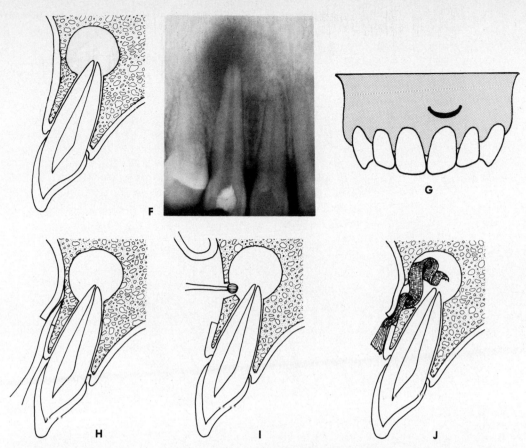

FIG. 18-1, cont'd. Acute apical abscess. **F,** Graphic and radiographic demonstration showing demineralization of the cancellous bone but no resorption of the cortical plate. **G** and **H,** Incision and elevation for exposure. **I,** The round bur prepares an opening through the cortical plate, but the apex is more easily identified because of the cancellous destruction. **J,** The incision edges are kept apart by a gauze drain inserted into the lesion and extending out the path of entry.

When sufficient time is available at this appointment to include the sterilization and filling of the canal, the surgery will actually conclude treatment. This is no more difficult for the patient or the doctor and obviously eliminates the need for future visits. However, these procedures are usually called for at unscheduled times, making complete treatment difficult and inconvenient. Consequently, in the majority of acutely symptomatic teeth the periapical area is trephinated and the canal is left semi-treated until the acute symptoms subside.

Prescribing antibiotics is a matter of clinical judgment (Chapter 12); however, it is prudent to prescribe an analgesic that will relieve moderate-to-severe pain. Postoperative instructions should be given, with emphasis on external cold packs, diet, supplemental vitamin intake, and thorough oral hygiene.

Establishing drainage

When acute periapical inflammation remains untreated, cancellous bone is destroyed[91] (Fig. 18-1, *F*) and a thick acidic purulent exudate begins to accumulate. The bone continues to demineralize and the patient's condition worsens,[9,13,54] eventually causing systemic symptoms to develop. The patient may become febrile, chilled, and nauseated and exhibit symptoms of malaise. An apical radiolucency may become apparent when the suppurative material erodes the cortical plate. The patient is probably experiencing unrelenting moderate to intense pain. It is conceivable that draining the abscess through the canal may eliminate the need for a surgical entry. Therefore the canal is opened and instrumented. The canal is irrigated until the pressure is reduced and the flow stops. The patient usually notices immediate improvement and quickly becomes more comfortable. However, to prevent the entry of food, debris, and additional strains of bacteria, most authorities[14,44] agree the canal should be closed even at the risk the acute symptoms might return. When to close the access cavity can be influenced by a number of circumstances. If apical surgery is anticipated, regardless of drainage, it may not be essential to close the access cavity. If the patient is in transit, has pressing business or social appointments, or lacks understanding of the reasons to close the access cavity, simply closing the canal and trephining the bone will assure relief of the symptoms. The trephination technique is the same as that used for acute periodontitis (Fig. 18-1, *B* to *D*). However, to minimize the risk of swelling, the incision is kept open by suturing in an iodoform gauze wick or rubber dam material cut to

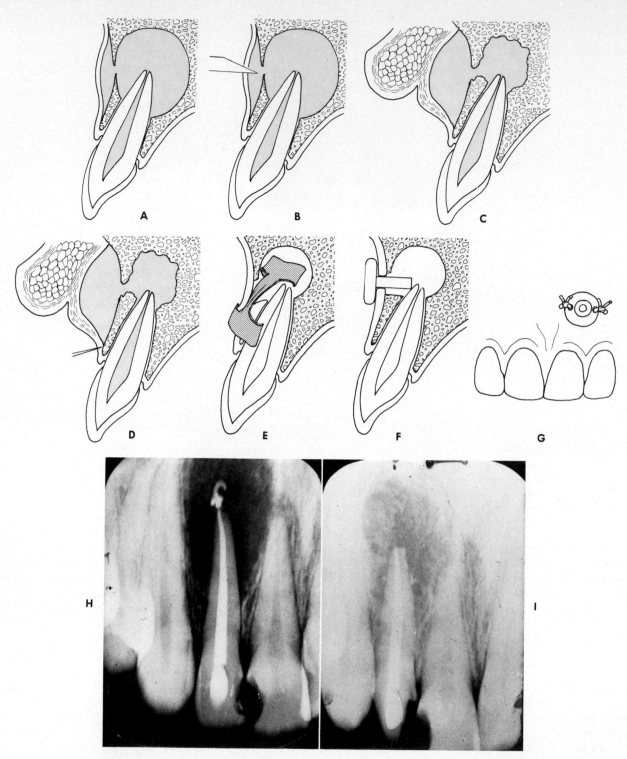

FIG. 18-2. *Phoenix abscess.* **A,** Graphic appearance of the cortical plate perforation and the fluid pressure forcing the periosteum to distend. **B,** A no. 11 Bard-Parker scalpel blade is inserted through the mucosa. *Cellulitis.* **C,** The liquefaction process continues to produce and force the purulent matter into the facial planes, causing severe swelling of the lip and face. **D,** A no. 15 Bard-Parker scalpel incises the attached gingiva coronal to the swelling, and the flap is elevated. **E,** The edges of the incision are kept apart by gauze or a rubber dam drain. **F** and **G,** For drainage over longer periods a plastic chuck is inserted and sutured in position. When the lesion size is reduced and symptoms subside, the drain can be removed. **H** and **I,** Preoperative and postoperative radiographs demonstrating lesion reduction by marsupialization.

the shape of the letter I between the edges of the incision (Fig. 18-1, *J*).

The patient is instructed in postoperative care, and the medication prescribed should include a 5-day regimen of antibiotics. The patient is reappointed in a week and the root canal is cleaned, shaped, and (if dry and not malodorous) filled with gutta-percha and sealer. The drain is left for an additional week; and if the area remains asymptomatic, the wick is removed. If a sinus tract appears in future postoperative examinations, the patient is scheduled for an apical curettage and apicoectomy and, when warranted, an apical reverse fill.

If an apical abscess is allowed to continue unattended, the resorptive process of inflammation will ultimately perforate the cortical plate. The periosteum becomes the next tissue barrier, and the pressure of the suppurative exudate causes the mucoperiosteal tissues to swell. If the roots are short or the mucobuccal fold is high in the maxilla or low in the mandible, the patient may observe a parulis or gumboil. At this point the pain will subside because nature has now performed the trephination. In these situations, opening, cleaning, and shaping the canal will often be all that is required to eliminate the irritants and allow the periapical area to repair. If the swelling is localized, piercing the central zone with a no. 11 scalpel (Fig. 18-2, *B*) will drain the lesion without exerting pressure on the abscess base. Both the instrumentation of the canal and the piercing can usually be accomplished without anesthesia. Infiltrating anesthetics into these swollen tissues usually intensifies the pain by increasing the fluid pressure; but whenever block anesthesia can be administered with minimal discomfort, it should be used.

Injecting anesthetic into localized areas of infection is often ineffective because (1) the anesthetic solution is rapidly diluted; (2) there is a tendency to minimize the amount given; (3) it is more quickly absorbed because of the inflammation; and (4), most important, the pH differential between the anesthetic solution and the purulent matter inhibits the hydrolysis of the salt and prevents the liberation of the free alkaloidal base. Therefore *attempting to anesthetize a localized swollen area by infiltrating anesthetic directly into the inflamed area is not recommended.*

Because suppurative and hemorrhagic drainage with acute abscesses can be quite heavy, high-volume aspiration should accompany the stab incision. Once the purulent flow has subsided, the puncture is enlarged by inserting the no. 11 tip into the opening and lifting the cutting edge. The point on this blade is designed perfectly for incising these swollen tissues.

If the purulent exudate does not localize, it can pass from the superficial to the deep spaces, distending the lip (Fig. 18-2, *C*), face, or neck. Such swellings are indurated, diffuse, and uncomfortable; but because the pressure is no longer trapped, they are usually less painful. The spread of infection can be by way of the lymphatic system, the venous or hematogenous route, or direct extension between the fascial planes. The severity of the cellulitis is dependent upon several factors, particularly location. The closer the accumulation of purulent fluid comes to the angular or pterygoid veins, the more dangerous the infection becomes. These emissary veins are not shunted and therefore may carry the infection to the brain, spinal cord, or cavernous sinus.

With mandibular infections, as the purulence spreads from one anatomic space to the next, the swelling may interfere with breathing and possibly close off the airway. These spreading purulent infections, if not properly and quickly treated, are potentially fatal. Accordingly, one cannot be complacent or uncertain about treatment. Large doses of antibiotics, even combinations of antibiotics, should be immediately instituted (see Chapter 12) and, even if the exudate is primarily hemorrhagic rather than purulent, when possible the swelling should be incised.

Fortunately the great majority can be drained intraorally, but on rare occasion it becomes necessary to make an extraoral puncture. This intentional incision is far better than the unesthetic, irregular opening and scar that nature would produce.

Cellulitis victims appear ill, irritable, lethargic, and possibly febrile; and they may present communication problems. They should be notified beforehand that a responsible adult who is capable of driving must accompany them on this emergency visit. When the patient has been examined, the diagnosis and treatment plan should be thoroughly discussed. Some patients may need to be premedicated, as previously mentioned, with 120 mg of secobarbital (Seconal) or sodium pentobarbital (Nembutal) and then allowed to relax for 20 to 30 minutes. Local anesthetics should be infiltrated into the tissues surrounding but not directly involved in the swelling. The attached gingiva is usually uninvolved and is an excellent tissue to anesthetize and incise. While waiting for the anesthetic to take effect, one can open, clean, and shape the diseased canal(s). If the tooth is somewhat mobile, it may need to be splinted or held firmly during the endodontic procedures. The decision to close the tooth is determined by the presence or absence of drainage. If there is no drainage, or drainage that quickly ceases the tooth can be closed. On occasion the drainage is continuous and unstopable requiring that the tooth be left open to drain for at least 24 hours.

The patient should be forewarned as to the possibility of some discomfort during the surgical entry. However, any discomfort can be reduced substantially by a compassionate, understanding, and communicative approach. A clinician who is gentle and caring will produce enough placebo effect to perform the incision and drainage of the distended tissues, even in the absence of profound anesthesia. A small semilunar incision is made incisal to the swelling (Fig. 18-2, *D*). The first exudate may be only hemorrhagic, but a small curette passed into the incision and slid on bone under the periosteum toward the central zone of infection will enable the purulent exudate to flow profusely.

If the incision is made too early in a developing cellulitis, this purulent flow may not happen; however, when the infection does localize sufficiently, the pathway has been provided. The edges of the incision are kept apart by

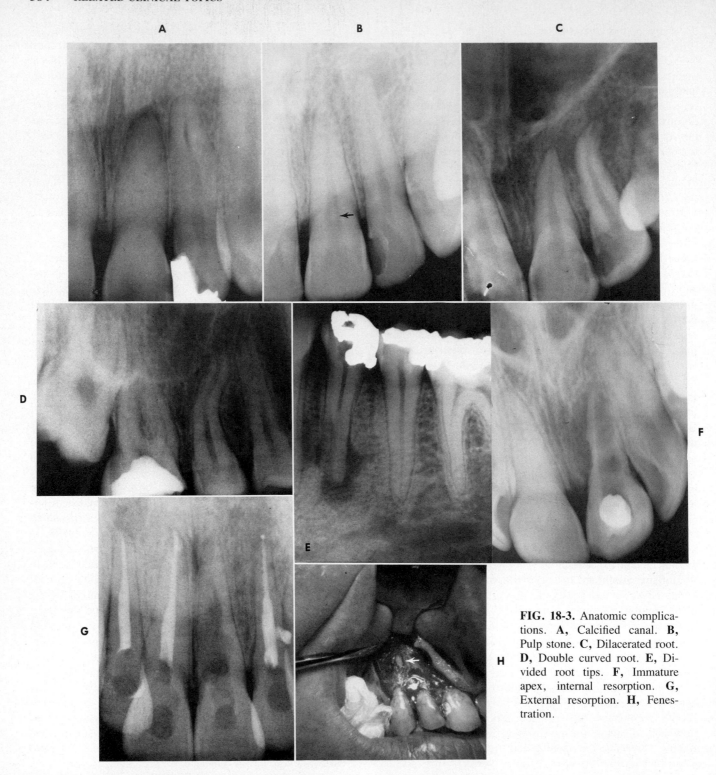

A   B   C

D   F

E

G   H

FIG. 18-3. Anatomic complications. **A,** Calcified canal. **B,** Pulp stone. **C,** Dilacerated root. **D,** Double curved root. **E,** Divided root tips. **F,** Immature apex, internal resorption. **G,** External resorption. **H,** Fenestration.

inserting gauze or rubber dam into the opening. Because gauze may inhibit the flow of viscous fluid, use of the rubber **I** is recommended (Fig. 18-2, *E*). If drainage from the incision has been clearly established, there is no benefit to leaving the tooth open.

Postoperative care includes good oral hygiene, increased protein and vitamin intake, antibiotic therapy (heavier than normal dosage), and an analgesic of moderate strength.

Contrary to most beliefs, incision and drainage cases do not necessarily require subsequent apical surgery.[33,93]

Continued conventional canal treatment that eliminates the source of the infection often ends the episode. If the signs and symptoms subside, the canal can be routinely filled and the area will probably heal uneventfully.

If during treatment the canal or the incision continues to exude or in subsequent examinations one notices an increase in the size of the radiolucency, or the reappearance of a sinus tract, then apical surgery should be performed.

When patients do not seek treatment during these inflammatory stages, the chronic destructive processes of the body often take a heavy toll on teeth and bone. Inflammatory resorption can produce massive lesions within the jawbone, and such cases in the past were thought to require surgery to succeed. This was an incorrect assumption. Removing all the necrotic debris from the infected canal and inserting and retaining a mucosal drain often reduces the size of these lesions and minimizes the surgical area needing curetting. It may even eliminate the need for surgery entirely. These long-duration draining techniques, often referred to as marsupialization, have been advocated by some authorities[18]; but because the drains must be inserted and maintained for extended periods, a rigid tube is recommended. Polyethylene tubing or plastic (Mid-West) handpiece chucks (Fig. 18-2, *F* and *G*) with or without stents have been successful in this endeavor. The patients are instructed in oral hygiene and soon learn to remove, clean, and replace the tubing with little or no difficulty.

Selecting cases for marsupialization requires careful diagnosis. The following conditions should be considered:

1. The radiolucency must be associated with one or more nonvital teeth.
2. Apical surgery without marsupialization may harm adjacent teeth or anatomic structures.
3. Drainage must have been established and the case be asymptomatic.
4. The lesion, when probed, must not be firm.
5. If any doubt exists, a small sample should be curetted and submitted for biopsy at the time the tube is inserted. If the histopathologic diagnosis demands total excision, the patient should be rescheduled for a total curettage.

When the case has been accepted for tubing and the drain has been inserted, endodontic therapy can be completed. The tooth and periapical area should remain asymptomatic during and after the endodontic therapy, and within 12 to 14 weeks some evidence of peripheral bone deposition should be seen radiographically (Fig. 18-2, *H* and *I*). If it does, the drain can be removed; if it remains asymptomatic, no further treatment will be required. If the sinus tract remains open, if symptoms reappear, or the lesion does not continue to remineralize, then apical surgery is scheduled.

Anatomic complications

Through various aberrations, the root canal system of teeth can be altered by calcification, growth, and development. Dystrophic calcifications; impassable denticles; bizarre root shapes, sizes, and directions; and root resorp-

tions can challenge the most skilled clinician[5,22,24,43] (Fig. 18-3, *A* to *G*). Although improved techniques and materials have removed the need for apical surgery in some cases, the majority of these teeth require an apicoectomy and frequently require a filling in the apical foramen or any other root opening that exists.

The buccal roots of maxillary molars, premolars, and canines often fenestrate the buccal plate (Fig. 18-3, *H*); and although conventional endodontic therapy appears radiographically to be successful, the patient's symptoms linger. Unless the root tips are reduced in length, the resorbed bone over the tip may never regenerate. When the root has been surgically reduced to lie entirely within bone, the cortical plate repairs and the symptoms subside.

Iatrogenic problems

At times we clinicians err. We may ignore the criteria suggested by manufacturers and others for instrument and material usage; we may obturate canals with sealers and fillers that are insoluble and impossible to remove from canals; we may break instruments; we occasionally cause ledges, root perforations, and periapical abuses by injudicious or thoughtless zeal (Fig. 18-4). Such cases are embarrassing and unfortunate; and to correct them, apical alteration and the placement of retrograde fillings often become the only solution.[1,2]

Trauma

When teeth are intruded, extruded, or otherwise displaced, finger pressure alone may not be sufficient for repositioning (Fig. 18-5, *A*). Arch bars, wires, or forceps may be more effective but potentially more damaging. Reflecting a flap and exposing the damaged alveolus sometimes solves the problem and allows for gentle atraumatic replacement and repositioning. When roots are fractured (Fig. 18-5, *B*) and the pulp becomes necrotic, the treatment options are relative to the level of the fracture (as described in Chapter 15).

Need for biopsy (Fig. 18-6)

Although the most common radiolucent lesions treated by dentists are periapical granulomas and apical cysts, other conditions can mimic their appearance and can only be diagnosed microscopically.[43,54] Such radiolucencies can be developmental, infectious, metabolic, traumatic, odontogenic, or neoplastic. Most lesions associated with vital teeth or in unusual locations raise doubts, and, because of their appearance or response, qualify for histologic evaluation.[84] This holds true for any tissue curetted from periapical areas. *If tissue warrants removal, it warrants microscopic diagnosis.*[5]

Failure of endodontically treated teeth (Fig. 18-7)

Whenever possible, the nonsurgical re-treatment of failing canals should be attempted before the case is subjected to surgery.[16,33,93]

Studies indicate that the incidence of failure is highest with poorly filed or filled canals.[41,43,77] If the canal cannot

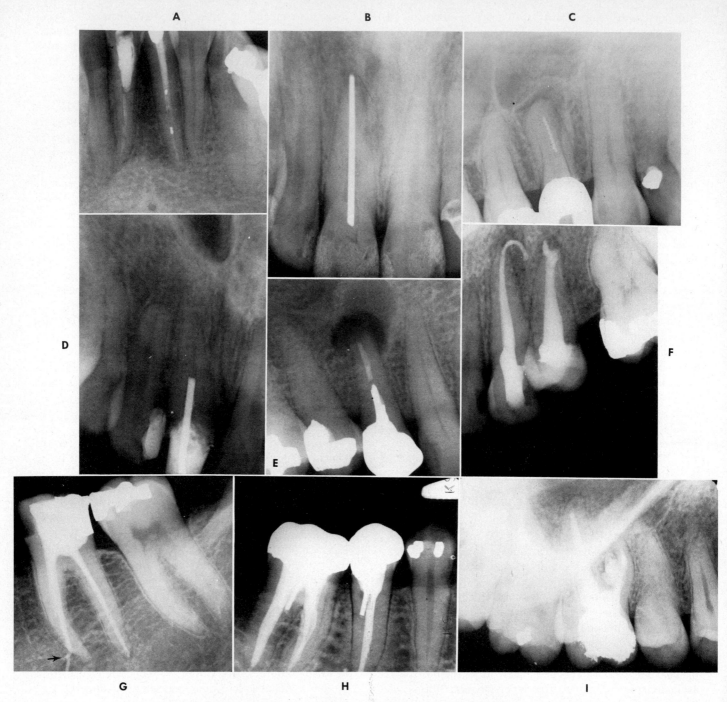

FIG. 18-4. Iatrogenic complications. **A,** Canals obstructed by nonsoluble nonremovable materials that cannot be bypassed. **B,** Nonremoveable silver point. **C,** Lodged fragmented instrument. **D,** Post without obturation of the root canal system. **E,** Post, core, and crown with the root canal incompletely filled. **F,** Overextended canal filling material. **G,** Ledging and perforation *(arrow).* **H,** Perforated restoration pin. **I,** Overenlargement with eventual stripping of root surface.

be re-treated, curettage alone may also prove inadequate. For this reason, when one assumes the responsibility of a tooth and the canal(s) cannot be ideally retreated a retrograde filling is indicated.

Expedience

One-appointment complete endodontic treatment has proved to be successful for several types of cases and has been very well accepted by the profession and the public. However, necrotic cases, particularly those with periapical radiolucencies and no visible sinus tract, usually require multiple appointments. When time, cost, travel distance, or patient management affect treatment planning, endodontics combined with apical surgery for nonvital cases becomes advantageous. The same holds true if repeated exacerbations jeopardize the doctor-patient relationship

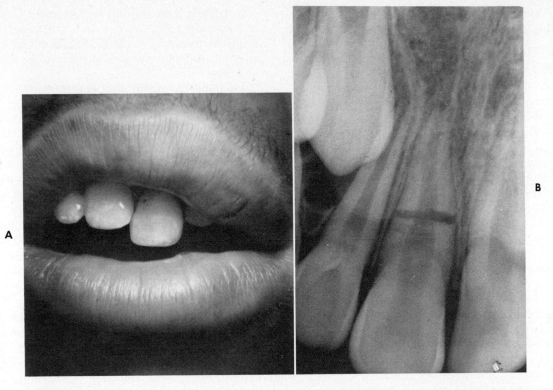

FIG. 18-5. Trauma. **A,** Displaced anterior teeth that require repositioning. **B,** Midroot fracture with separation.

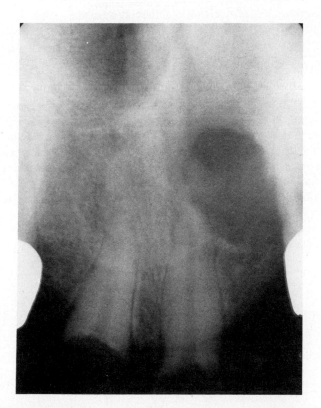

FIG. 18-6. Biopsy. Because of their location, appearance, or symptoms, some lesions should be diagnosed microscopically.

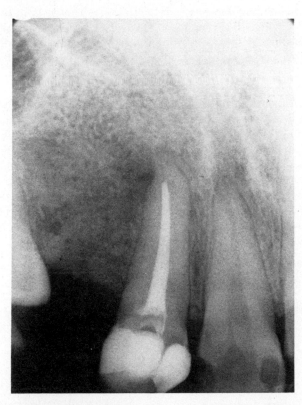

FIG. 18-7. Endodontic failure. Due to unusual aberrations in root canal development or underextension of the root canal filling material, certain cases will not heal without re-treatment or surgical repair.

and patient confidence and respect begin to dwindle because of recurring difficulties.

ENDODONTIC SURGERY
Flap design

After a case has been carefully selected for surgery, attention must be focused on flap design. The following conditions should be evaluated:

1. Number of teeth involved
2. Length and shape of the roots involved
3. Presence or absence of periapical pathosis
4. Extent of the periapical lesion
5. Depth of the sulcus
6. Location and size of the frenum and muscle attachments
7. Approximating anatomic structures
8. Thickness of bone at the surgery site
9. Height and depth of the vestibule
10. Access needed
11. Types of restorations in the surgical area

When these conditions have been assessed, the dental surgeon must design a flap that will fulfill these objectives. With minor modifications the following designs are most commonly used.[45]

1. Semilunar
2. Luebke-Ochsenbein
3. Triangular
4. Trapezoidal
5. Gingival

Semilunar flap (curved) (Fig. 18-8). This incision begins 1 mm above the mandibular or below the maxillary mucobuccal fold and follows a half-moon path with its convexity toward the gingiva. The major portion of the incision should be in the attached gingiva and at least 3 mm apical to the sulcus depth.

Although this design is the most popular and most often used flap, it may have the most disadvantages. The incision is difficult to reapproximate and suture. It offers the least amount of access and convenience to the operative site. It is not adaptable to enlargement or extension if greater dimension and visibility are required. It may cross the bony cavity extension, inviting delayed or incomplete healing. Greater force is required to maintain flap retraction. Finally, it almost always produces unesthetic, extensive scarring of the alveolar mucosa.

Its popularity stems from the fact that it is fast and easy to incise and reflect. It can only be recommended when surgically treating a single tooth with a long root, a large mucosal vestibule, excellent attached gingiva, and little or no lesion.

Luebke-Ochsenbein flap (submarginal) (Fig. 18-9). This is a modification of the semilunar design. A vertical incision is made on each side of the surgical site; the vertical incisions are joined by a scalloped horizontal incision in the gingiva, 3 mm apical to the depth of the sulcus. It is important that the vertical and horizontal incisions join at an obtuse angle. This will ensure that the base is wider than the free edge, thereby assuring an adequate blood supply to the flap.

This design not only offers the simplicity and speed of the semilunar but also releases tension to the flap. It magnifies visibility and increases access. It provides definitive landmarks that can be accurately repositioned and sutured. This will enhance primary healing and reduce the potential for scar. It is primarily indicated whenever the gingival tissues and attachments are not to be disturbed, particularly when the offending or adjacent teeth are restored with veneered crowns.

The design still presents problems when the periapical lesion is large, when extension is needed during the surgery, when the roots are short, or when the blood supply to the flap is endangered by the deficiency of the geometric design.

Triangular flap (intrasulcular) (Fig. 18-10). A single angling vertical incision is joined at an obtuse angle by a gingival horizontal incision. The gingival incision is made in the gingival sulcus and frees the radicular tissue as well as the entire papilla. The vertically angling incision is made in the trough between the root eminences and extends from the gingival crest to the mucobuccal fold.

Although this design is a little more difficult to incise, suture, and retract, it is the least confining; offers the convenience of extension during surgery; is excellent for any length of tooth; offers excellent landmarks for repositioning; and will allow for simultaneous periodontal curettage and alveoloplasty.[23] In addition, it assures an adequate blood supply to the flap and is therefore the least likely to scar. Although unpredictable, there is always the risk of marginal gingival recession with an intrasulcular incision. Because healing most likely will be by second intent, the

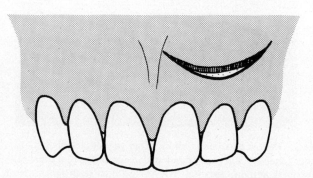

FIG. 18-8. The semilunar flap is a curved incision with its most convex point toward the gingival sulcus.

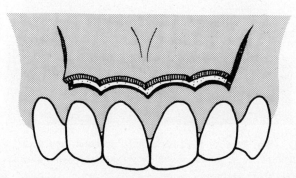

FIG. 18-9. The Luebke-Ochsenbein flap is modified scalloped semilunar incision.

submarginal flap should be chosen when veneered crowns will be directly involved. To promote healing oral hygiene must be emphasized.

Trapezoidal flap (Fig. 18-11). This design is a gingival horizontal incision connecting two vertical releasing incisions. Since the angles formed at the junction of the incision must be obtuse, the geometric appearance is that of a trapezoid.

This design resembles the Luebke-Ochsenbein flap except that the horizontal component is made at the gingival crest. It has all the advantages of the triangular design, but its main advantage is the reduction of tension on the flap, making it less fatiguing to the dentist and less traumatic to the tissue. Its success is predicated on maintaining an adequate blood supply to the flap and tissue slough can only be prevented when the base width exceeds the free edge width.

The palate is an excellent area to utilize a modified trapezoidal flap. For access to the apexes of the anterior teeth palatally, a bilateral vertical incision is placed from the distal lingual line angle of the cuspids to the junction of the horizontal and alveolar bone of the vault.

The length of the vertical incisions will depend on the demands of access. The blood supply to the palatal tissue is very delicate and every attempt to minimize the size of the flap should be considered. These vertical incisions are joined by a horizontal intrasulcular incision. The nasopalatine nerves are small and when severed readily unite and

heal. Minimal bleeding can be expected, as the vessels of this area are also minor.

To approach posterior palatal roots a horizontal intrasulcular incision releases the gingiva from the distal line angle of the cuspid to an area one or two teeth posterior to the offending tooth. An anterior vertical incision extending from the distal line angle of the cuspid to the junction of the horizontal and alveolar bone in the vault will be made from the horizontal incision.

To avoid the greater palatine vessels as they trace anteriorly in the junction, the posterior vertical incision is designed to be a relaxing incision cut from the horizontal incision to a point short of the junction and only as long as required for access. The vessels that extend from the greater palatine canal should be avoided for they are large and, when cut, bleed extensively. Fortunately as they traverse the bone anteriorly, they are continually branching and reducing in size, accounting for the greater security when extending the anterior vertical incision to the junction.

Gingival flap (Fig. 18-12). This design is the result of a continuous and extended release of the gingiva without any vertical relaxing incisions. Because it is so confining, it offers no advantage in endodontic surgery. It is used primarily for periodontal treatment where apical root exposure is not required.

Surgical principles. Until the twentieth century, dental surgery was fraught with problems.[75] Following the advent of local anesthesia, antibiotics, and reliable sterilization techniques and materials, surgery quickly became a predictable successful treatment. The following "tenets of Halsted" form the basis of modern surgery.

1. Tissue should be handled gently.
2. Sharp anatomical dissection should be used.
3. Aseptic techniques should prevail.
4. Careful hemostasis should be attained.
5. Suturing material should be fine and nonirritating, and only a minimal amount of suturing should be done.
6. All dead spaces should be obliterated.
7. Tension should be avoided.
8. A period of rest should follow surgery.

Regardless what surgical movement is performed, every effort should be made to adhere to these tenets.

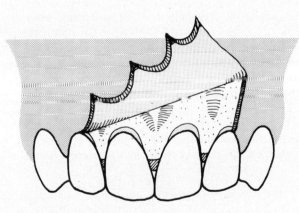

FIG. 18-10. The triangular flap is a single vertical incision from the mucobuccal fold to the gingival sulcus joining a horizontal gingival incision along the crest.

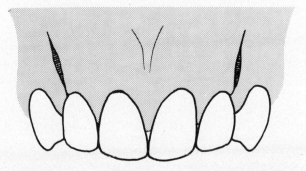

FIG. 18-11. The trapezoidal flap is a triangular flap modified at the most distal point of the horizontal sulcular incision by a second vertical releasing incision.

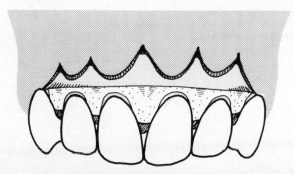

FIG. 18-12. The gingival flap is a horizontal sulcular incision that has no vertical releasing extensions.

Surgical movements

Incision

An incision is a cut made with a sharp instrument that separates tissue.[27,45] To gain access to cortical bone, an incision must be made. For cutting tissue against a bony base a no. 15 Bard-Parker scalpel blade offers the greatest efficiency. The last 2 mm of the blade is pressed firmly against the bone. The cut is made through the mucosa, connective tissue, and periosteum (Fig. 18-13). The blade edge should not be lifted or removed from the incision until the cut is complete. This avoids making a ragged incision, which is difficult to elevate, reapproximate, and suture. A precise cut would invite healing by primary intention rather than by granulation tissue and scar. The pen grasp gives the greatest control to the surgeon when incising.

Since bone must be completely exposed for apical surgery, full-thickness flaps have definite advantages over split-thickness flaps (Fig. 18-14, A and B). A full-thickness mucoperiosteal flap refers to the fact all layers of soft tissue are included in the flap. It has nothing to do with the location of the flap, which has often been confusing in the literature. Incisions for full-thickness flaps are easier to make because the bone provides a solid landmark to firmly press the scapel blade. Because the intact periosteum will remain a part of the flap, full flaps heal with fewer complications.

For simplicity incisions are classified by their direction in relation to the teeth. Vertical as well as horizontal incisions are made in the attached gingiva by holding the blade at a right angle to the cortical plate. The blunt edges of these incisions are more easily repositioned than beveled edges because they leave less chance for gaps or overlaps.

The apically directed incision is executed by placing the knife in the sulcus in the area of the gingival margin and advancing the edge of the blade apically until it contacts bone.[3,27,50] The incision will separate the labial and lingual tissue as it relieves the radicular and papillary tissue.[51] Also known as the sulcular incision, it is used when the triangular or trapezoidal flap design has been selected. When the apical incision is made within the gingival tissue and the sulcular tissue attachment is left undisturbed we create the split or partial-thickness flap. This is used primarily for periodontal surgery but recently interest has been directed toward combining the two techniques. Here the split-thickness cut is made at the crest and continues to the attached gingiva. From that point the flap will include the periosteum to gain access to the osseous defect. This dual incision is extremely difficult to execute since there are no tissue landmarks to follow when separating the periosteum from the gingival tissue. If one layer or the other is overly thinned, the circulation is endangered and necrosis is inevitable. In addition, separating these layers can be abusive and, if tissue tears, healing is impaired (see Fig. 18-14, A).

The vertical incisions should be made in the concavities between the root bodies, where the tissue is thickest and has the best blood supply. All incisions must be made on

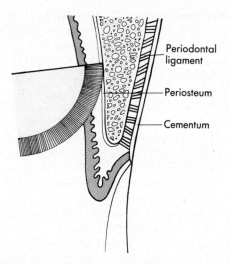

FIG. 18-13. The no. 15 Bard-Parker blade is most efficient when its last 2 mm are pressed firmly against bone. The incision for all endodontic surgery should be firm and continuous.

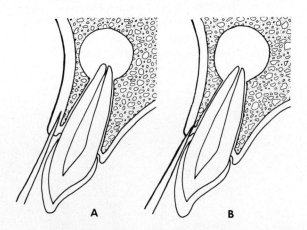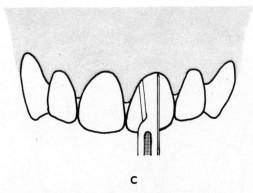

FIG. 18-14. The split-thickness incision, **A,** will separate periosteum from the outer mucosal layer whereas the full-thickness incision, **B,** will enable periosteum to become an integral part of the flap. The apically directed incision. **C,** will free the radicular tissue along with the papilla by insertion of the blade edge into the sulcus until it contacts the crest.

bone and must never cross an existing osseous defect or one that will be produced during the surgery. For this reason one should never underestimate the bone destruction caused by a periapical lesion. A radiolucency represents cortical destruction and does not reflect the true extent of cancellous demineralization.[9,54,83] Lesions can far exceed their radiographic dimensions, and the medullary extension may require that large amounts of surrounding cortical bone be removed to gain sufficient access. Accordingly, when doubt exists concerning the size of a periapical lesion, the vertical incision(s) should be made two or three teeth lateral to the involved tooth (Fig. 18-15). Because all incisions heal across the incision line, healing potential is not affected by incision length.[70,87] Therefore the span of the flap should be increased in preference to restricting the operative field. For conservatism, attention must also be focused on the gingival-apical osseous destruction. This aspect may be more difficult to determine radiographically because it is often masked by the root. These possibilities emphasize the disadvantages of selecting the semilunar or Luebke-Ochsenbein designs and support the advantages of the triangular or trapezoidal flaps.

Whichever flap is chosen, the incision should begin coronal to the mucobuccal fold and, whenever possible, should never extend into the muscle attachments of the lip and cheek. These tissues are highly vascular and, when cut, present a continuous hemorrhage problem throughout the surgery. Furthermore, the patient will experience increased soreness, swelling, and perhaps even ecchymosis postoperatively.

When the triangular or trapezoidal design is selected, one must carefully locate the gingival junction of the vertical and horizontal incisions. Terminating the vertical incision at the line angle of a tooth (Fig. 18-16) will preserve the integrity of both the radicular gingival tissue and the papilla. This provides firm tissue for suturing and minimizes the potential of clefting.

Elevation

A sharp and distinct incision simplifies elevation of the flap. A Molt no. 9 periosteal elevator with a sharp edge will easily separate tissue from bone. With the concave surface down, the sharp edge is inserted between the incision edges until it contacts bone. Using a firm apical force and moving along the incision line, one strips the flap (including periosteum) away from the cortical plate (Fig. 18-17, A and B). The elevation should continue apically until solid bone is exposed on all sides of the lesion (Fig. 18-17, C). If the lesion is not at first apparent, the tissue should be retracted a few millimeters apical to the suspected root length. Because the granulation tissue of the

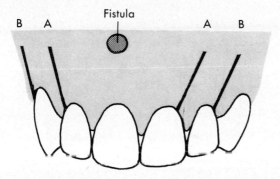

FIG. 18-15. The dimensions of a lesion cannot be fully identified radiographically, and for this reason vertical incisions should be extended more laterally to provide greater access. *A,* Narrow flap; *B,* wider flap for improved access.

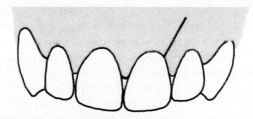

FIG. 18-16. The vertical incision terminates at the line angle of a tooth, thereby preserving the papilla for suturing.

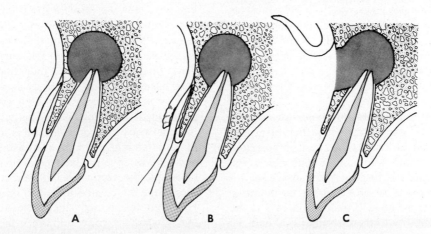

FIG. 18-17. A, If the incision is sharp and to bone, the periosteal elevator should contact the bone and strip periosteum from its attachment. **B,** If it is ragged or incomplete, the tissue will tear and healing will be impeded. **C,** Elevation should continue until the *entire* lesion is uncovered and solid bone can be identified on all sides.

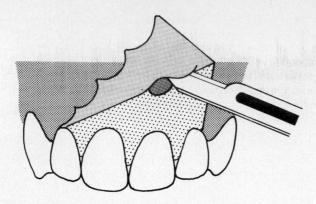

FIG. 18-18. Chronic lesions of long duration occasionally prevent elevation because the granulation tissue grows out of its bony crypt and becomes an integral part of the overlying mucoperiosteum. A scapel is required to release the lesion from the mucoperiosteum.

lesion quite often grows out of its bony crypt and becomes an integral part of the mucoperiosteum, elevation may be resisted. Rather than tear the flap or granulation tissue, a gentle dissection with a scalpel should be performed to free the flap and allow elevation to continue uninhibited (Fig. 18-18). This is preferable to creating a hole in the body of the flap, thereby inviting an ingress of food and bacteria to the bony cavern. The intact periosteum will begin its reattachment to bone immediately after its replacement. This permits uneventful healing and reduces postoperative pain and discomfort.

If bleeding becomes a problem during the retraction, infiltrating anesthetics that contain a vasoconstrictor along the incision will help reduce the flow. When bone ledges or exostoses are encountered one must be especially careful because the soft tissue covering these eminences is especially thin and delicate. When impediments are met, changing cleaving directions and instrument angulation and maintaining constant contact with bone will minimize the chances of slipping or tearing. This approach is also advantageous when peeling the tissue from the nasal spine. Stripping muscle attachments and frena from bone presents more psychologic than surgical problems. The same holds true when uncovering the mental vessels. When flap elevation is done cleanly and delicately, reattachment is inevitable and paresthesia a rarity.

Retraction

The purpose of a tissue retractor is to hold soft gingival tissue away. Retractors vary from blunt flat blades to sharp-toothed claws; and as long as they rest on bone and do not impinge tissue, it makes little difference which type is used. If the flap tissue has been elevated above the lesion, a solid bone base wil be provided for the retractor (Fig. 18-19). Proper retraction will maintain access to the lesion and improve visibility to the entire surgical area.

Osteotomy

The objective of apical surgery is to uncover the apex of a diseased tooth. Although the resorptive process of inflammation demineralizes bone and often provides this ac-

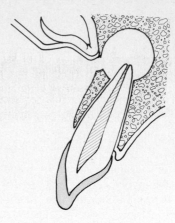

FIG. 18-19. The purpose of a retractor is to hold tissue back from the surgical site. It should rest on bone and not impinge on the tissue.

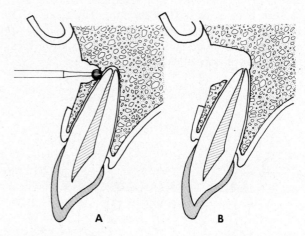

FIG. 18-20. A large round bur is used to remove cortical and cancellous bone. The initial approach is, **A,** to identify the correct root and then, **B,** enlarge the window to expose the lesion and the apex, facilitating curettage.

cess, most cases require a trephination through the cortical plate. This can be accomplished with large carbide round burs in a slow or variable-speed handpiece. All bone cutting should be accompanied by a continuous flow of water to clean the area of shavings, clean the bur of bone mud, and protect the bone from frictional burn. If the bone is dense or thick, high-speed reduction with the new sealed-head handpieces pressurized by compressed air or nitrogen is very acceptable as long as a copious water lavage is maintained. A major problem is where to make the entry in bone when the cortical plate is intact. Prior knowledge of the offending root length, measurements of radiographs, and a knowledge of the average lengths of teeth will help determine the vertical height; the convexities and concavities of the bone can often direct one to the lateral position. However, this is not dependable, for the topography flattens toward the apex, and when the line axis of the roots are not perpendicular to the ridge the lateral position can become confused.

The most reliable method involves placing a piece of sterile lead x-ray foil (or equivalent radiopaque material) in a small bur hole made where the apex is believed to lie.

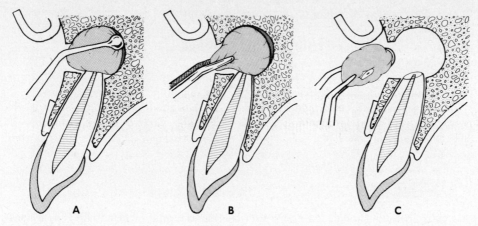

FIG. 18-21. A, When the lesion is completely exposed, the concave surface of a sharp curette will strip the tissue from bone; and once the tissue is free, it can be spooned from the bone cavity. The specimen should not be pulled from the crypt, **B,** so that when resistance is met (because of its attachment to the root), **C,** the apex can be included in the biopsy by cutting off the last few millimeters of the root with a fissure bur and removing it with the tissue.

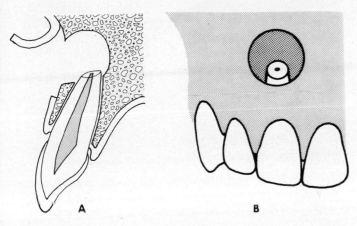

FIG. 18-22. A, Whenever the apex of a root is removed, it should be cut on a bevel facing the clinician. **B,** This will provide greater visibility and access to the canal.

Once radiographed, the foil will orient the clinician to the apex and entry adjustments can be made.

Preliminary bone removal should be done only to locate the offending root (Fig. 18-20, *A*). Because of the varied angulations and directions that roots take, apices should not be uncovered until positive root identification has been made. This is particularly important in the premolar-canine areas, where the arch curvature can disorient the entrance. When the offending root is accurately identified, apical bone is removed until the lesion and root tip are uncovered (Fig. 18-20, *B*).

Curettage

Once the lesion is exposed attention is directed to removing the pathosis for biopsy. An intact enucleation of the entire lesion will give the pathologist the greatest opportunity to make an accurate diagnosis. This is easily accomplished by increasing the dimensions of the bony window until a sharp curette can contact all sides of the bony crypt.

The curette, with its concave surface facing the bone, is inserted into the crypt and the diseased tissue is cleaved from the bone and spooned out of the hole (Fig. 18-21, *A*). Preservation of the tissue in a 10% formalin solution will prevent cellular breakdown until a pathologist can conduct a histologic examination.

Many times the tissue is so tenaciously attached to the root surface that it resists removal (Fig. 18-21, *B*). By using a tapered fissured bur and cutting the apical 2 to 3 mm free of the root, one can remove the tissue and root segment in its entirety (Fig. 18-21, *C*). Even though there is controversy concerning the need to remove all inflammatory tissue, it is certainly prudent to do so whenever possible. Although over 90% of the lesions will be periodontal granulomas or cysts, there are other more serious possibilities that exist.[84] Therefore *tissue that warrants removal warrants diagnosis*.[5]

Apicoectomy

The removal of root tips is indicated in the following circumstances: (1) when the anatomy of the canal system has not been conducive to nonsurgical treatment; (2) when iatrogenic perforation or ledges prevent apical sealing; (3) when the root tip is resorbed or fractured; or (4) when a retrograde filling must be placed in an apex because an irremovable obstruction exists in the canal, preventing treatment by conventional therapy.

After the root tip is reduced, it should be cut at a 45-degree lingual and labial bevel facing the clinician (Fig. 18-22). This will furnish the best view of the apex, uncover second canals, and provide a flat surface for a retrograde filling.

Closure

After apical treatment, attention is focused on closing the flap; final radiographs should be exposed *before* suturing. Often small particles of root and root canal filling materials will be left or scattered to other areas of the site and not evacuated. When searching for displaced particles the

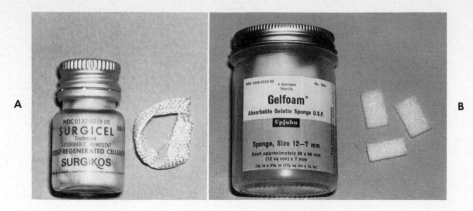

FIG. 18-23. Because bleeding is a natural sequela of surgery, artificial hemostasis is occasionally required. Two agents used for this purpose are, **A,** Surgicel, an oxidized cellulose and, **B,** Gelfoam, a gelatinous sponge.

inferior surface of the flap should not be overlooked. While waiting for the radiograph to be developed, the clinician can examine the area for latent bleeding and select the proper suture technique. If bleeding continues to be a problem, a number of steps can be taken:

1. The area can be infiltrated with anesthetic solutions having high vasoconstrictor concentrations (e.g., 1:50,000). This will only be effective when small vessels are involved.
2. The area can be packed with Avitene,* an absorbable topical hemostatic agent prepared from purified bovine collagen.
3. The area can be packed with gauze compressed with finger pressure for 5 to 10 minutes.
4. The bone cavity can be packed with bone wax.
5. The bone cavity can be packed with an artificial clotting agent (e.g., Surgicel or Gelfoam) (Fig. 18-23). The oxidized cellulose Surgicel and the gelatin sponge Gelfoam are inert and are eventually absorbed and replaced by connective tissue.
6. The bone cavity can be packed with an artificial bone ceramic (e.g., Synthograph). Synthos, a tricalcium phosphate complex product, forms a porous biocompatible ceramic mass in the presence of blood. Preliminary studies[11,12,30] suggest that it is inert and that as it is resorbed it acts as a matrix for osseous regeneration.

Once bleeding is under control, the flap is repositioned and cleaned. Precise flap placement is a prerequisite for healing. Various methods and materials have been used for closure, including tissue tacks, tissue adhesives, cyanoacrylates, and acrylic appliances, but sutures remain the standard.[18,27] A standardized suture setup (Fig. 18-24) should include a 3/8- to 1/2-inch half- to full-curve disposable atraumatic round or triangular cutting needle along with appropriate suture thread. Thread of 4-0 gauge is heavy enough for most mucosal and gingival flaps, but the palate may demand 3-0, and lip and cheek injuries should be closed with 5-0.

The two most often selected nonresorbable suture

*Avicon, Inc., Fort Worth, TX.

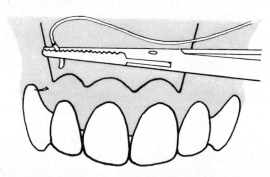

FIG. 18-24. A standardized sterile suture setup should include thin-tipped scissors, serrated hemostats, an atraumtic needle with attached 4-0 suture, cotton swabs, and 2 × 2 gauze squares.

FIG. 18-25. All suturing should begin by inserting the needle through the superficial surface of the unattached tissue before entering the inferior surface of the attached tissue.

threads are silk and monofilament.[18,19] Braided silk is the more popular, easiest to manage, easy to see in tissue, readily tied, and least expensive. However, it is easily penetrated by bacteria and food debris, which may evoke postoperative incision line infections (wicking effect).[58] For this reason oral hygiene must be emphasized and before silk sutures are removed, they should be cleansed with

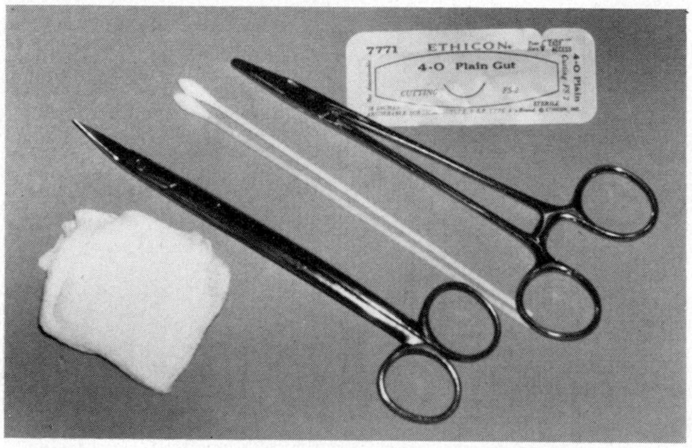

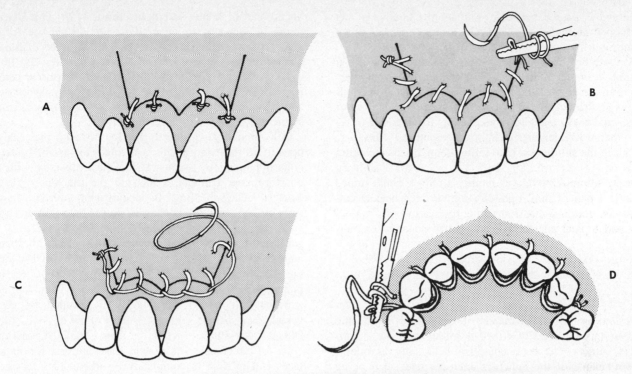

FIG. 18-26. Four suture techniques: **A,** Interrupted. **B,** Continuous mattress. **C,** Continuous blanket. **D,** Continuous sling.

a disinfectant. Monofilament (nylon, teflon-coated Dacron) is a product of the plastic age, and its advantage is its strength. It is inert and bacterially impenetrable, comes as a smooth strand, and will not break. However, it is difficult to tie when wet and when tightly pulled will cut through tissue much the way wire cuts cheese. This can become a problem during the first postoperative days, when the tissue becomes taut and distended from edema. The material is also very hard, and the cut ends can be sharp and irritating to the lip and cheek. The most common absorbable materials are catgut, collagen, and synthetic polyglycolic acid.[72] They are expensive and because they have a tendency to stretch are difficult to tie.

Their obvious advantage is absorbability, which eliminates the need for a suture removal appointment. This is particularly helpful to the debilitated or handicapped patient or the patient who must travel a considerable distance to come to the office. These materials are also advantageous for areas that are not easily accessible or when their removal may be painful, such as deep in the vestibule. A major concern is they do not always digest, leaving small fragments to delay healing.

Probably the greatest improvement in sutures has been the thread-to-needle attachment. The development of the atraumatic, knotless, eyeless needle enables the needle and the thread to pass effortlessly through the tissues. This minimizes the size of the hole; and because the needle requires little force to pull it through, it is less likely to tear the tissues.

Hemostats and scissors come in many shapes, sizes, and designs. As long as the hemostats can reach all areas of the oral cavity and have undamaged tight-fitting beaks, all marketed instruments will suffice. The surgical requirements for the scissors are the same as for the hemostats. It is extremely important to protect the tips of the scissors to preserve the sharpness and integrity of their points.

All suturing begins by inserting the needle through the superficial surface of the unattached tissue before entering the inferior surface of the attached tissue[57] (Fig. 18-25). This maintains the flap in position as the freed tissue is continually directed to the incision line. Such insertion direction also makes it easier to penetrate the free tissue.

To minimize tearing, the needle should be inserted at least 2 mm on either side of the incision line; the span between the sutures should not exceed 2 to 3 mm.

To prevent clefting, gingival crest sutures should not be placed in the thin radicular tissue at the necks of teeth but be directed into the papilla or lingual tissue or simply looped around the necks of the teeth.

There are basically four suture techniques: interrupted, continuous mattress, continuous blanket, and the continuous sling. The interrupted suture is a single loop ending in a surgeon's knot (Fig. 18-26, *A*). This is the simplest of all and the most commonly used. It is used when tissue position is not critical, when equal tension on both sides of the incision is required, or when a split incision requires a tie to the underlying periosteum. The continuous mattress suture begins as an interrupted one but continues to weave down the incision line until it terminates at the end of the cut with a surgeon's knot (Fig. 18-26, *B*). The continuous blanket suture varies from the mattress suture only in that each weave is an interlocking loop (Fig. 18-26, *C*). The continuous sling suture is also a weave, but with this technique the needle is inserted only in the free edge and the thread is passed between or under the contact points and looped around the tooth necks as it progresses down the incision line to its terminating knot (Fig. 18-26, *D*).

All these ties have advantages and disadvantages, and it becomes a matter of choice and experience as to preference. Whenever possible, it is advisable to select the continuous suture because it is faster, reduces the number of knots, enhances cleanliness, and seems to be easier to remove than a like number of interrupted sutures. However, a break in the suture or a knot failure jeopardizes the entire flap.

Sterile suture removal kits require a mirror; sharp-tipped scissors; a pair of thin, tight-closing, serrated beaked cotton pliers; cotton swabs for gentle application of disinfectants and topical anesthetics; and gauze squares for blotting.

Before and after removing sutures, it is advisable to swab the area with a disinfectant such as Gly-Oxide.

Surgery by area

Modern endodontic demands of the public require the clinician to be surgically skilled in all areas of the mouth. Apical surgery can be accomplished as long as one is knowledgeable of the radicular anatomy and surrounding major anatomic structures, possesses the ability to work in confined areas, is capable of reacting appropriately to surgical complications such as sustained bleeding and interrupted anesthesia, and has the self-assurance to manage the stress of arduous surgery complicated by limited access and visibility.

The surgical movements as described in this chapter are not specific for treating any particular segment of the mouth but can be applied to any area, regardless of the arch. However, each region presents unique anatomic variances for consideration.

Maxilla

The maxillary central incisors and cuspids are generally positioned within the alveolus at a near vertical posture. For this reason, the labial cortical plate of bone is usually very thin and the medullary bone generally absent. Because the palatal bone may be as much as 5 mm thicker than the labial at the apex, these teeth are more apt to have natural facial fenestrations and abscesses will normally drain to the labial. The apices of maxillary lateral incisors are commonly tipped palatally. As such, medullary bone is present labially and palatally and the pathologic destruction from a chronic inflammatory process can cause extensive osseous damage before it is discovered. A severe dilaceration to the distal is common and a large pathologic lesion will often come in contact with the mesial wall of the cuspid. Infected laterals may give rise to swelling or sinus tracts on either the labial or the palatal side or both simultaneously, depending on the severity and duration of the cause.

When large periapical lesions destroy both cortical plates (labial and palatal), the potential for complete remineralization following treatment is unlikely. Healing usually takes place following enucleation of the pathosis, but instead of bone, scar tissue forms.[4,70,87] This asymptommatic scar appears as a radiolucency in the area of the apex. Histologically it consists of a dense mass of fibrous connective tissue with coarse collagen bundles and fibrocytes. Although a definitive diagnosis of apical scar cannot be made without a biopsy, the history, signs, symptoms, and periodic radiographic assessments determine whether surgical exploration is necessary.

A technique suggested to develop a matrix that enables bone to fill these large defects involves the use of synthetic bone implantation. Studies at Indiana University with the nonresorbable Durapatite indicate the placement of the material delays healing. It appears that with the nonresorbable Synthograft, healing is slower than normal; however, the material appears to be gradually replaced by regenerated bone. Synthograft with a radiopacity similiar to bone is a form of β-tricalcium phosphate (hydroxyapatite).[11,12,30] Deposited as a slurry, the porous ceramic material is packed densely into the bony crypt. It quickly suffuses with blood and shortly is invaded by blood vessels and bone-forming tissue. Follow-up has shown that it does indeed act as a matrix with regenerating bone in direct apposition with the debrided lesion surfaces and in time is completely resorbed. This feature is its advantage over the nonresorbable ceramic bone materials.

There is usually 8 to 10 mm of attached gingiva in the anterior segment of the maxilla, offering the surgeon latitude in flap selection. Low-level muscle attachments can be avoided by choosing the triangular or trapezoidal flap designs and elevating beneath these fibers. The frenum should be circumvented or frenectomized. Since it is fibrous, its return when cut can be expected. When the mucobuccal fold is shallow the attached gingiva will be minimal to absent and the surgeon will be forced to incise and elevate the thick soft tissues of the free alveolar mucosa. Excessive capillary bleeding will be encountered and in proportion to the length of the roots and the extension of the lesion access and view will be limited. Concomitantly with a shallow fold, we will find a reduced vertical dimension of the anterior jaw. This will place the apices much closer to strategic anatomic structures including the floor of the nose, the maxillary sinus, and the nasopalatine canal. Postoperatively these patients can expect to experience swelling, pain, and possible nasal hemorrhage. Such complications could lead to hematoma or facial discoloration (ecchymosis). Accordingly, the patient should be alerted to potential problems and protected from infection by including along with the pre- and postoperative instructions a regimen of antibiotics and analgesics.

Because of their length, *maxillary cuspid* roots require elevation of the free mucosa, and the elevation and curettage come precariously close to the infraorbital vessels. The resultant bleeding at this level will most likely cause an ecchymosis. If an apical fenestration is discovered the root must be reduced to a level below the access cavity to allow new cortical bone to form over the root end. Attempting palatal surgery to gain access to the apices of the anterior teeth is difficult from both an access and a visibility standpoint.

However, when repair of perforation and resorptions demands a palatal approach, the flap procedure previously described in flap design is indicated. Elevation of the anterior palatal flap will be very laborious, as this thick leathery tissue is tenaciously attached to the bone. The patient should be instructed on the degree of difficulty; when the flap is to be extensive or when the vault is shallow, an impression for a palatal stent should be taken at the examination appointment. This appliance will hold the flap in contact with the palatal bone during the reattachment period, help prevent a hematoma from forming between the periosteum and the palate, and reduce the risk of sloughing.

The maxillary premolars are complicated by the variances in their root anatomy. (See Chapter 6.) Eighty-five percent of the maxillary first premolars have two roots, 14% have one, and a trace has three. Sixty percent of the maxillary second premolars have two roots, 40% have one, and it is extremely rare to have three.[35] Therefore, radiographic evaluation should be made from a number of films at different angulations. The triangular flap is the flap of choice and will provide ample access and convenience if unexpected problems are encountered. For the first premolar the vertical incision is made in the concavity between the cuspid and lateral and for the second premolar it can be either between the cuspid and lateral or cuspid and first premolar, depending on the bone eminence and location of the lesion. A relaxing incision distal to the first molar is advantageous. Single rooted teeth have a substantial amount of buccal and palatal bone but are easily located and reduced. The apices should be beveled at a 45-degree angle facing the surgeon's line of sight to facilitate the examination of the exposed root. These teeth should always be suspected of having "extra" canals. When a prior surgery has failed, a reverse fill must be seriously considered.[16,22] The divergence of two rooted premolars can create three problems. Similar to the cuspid, the buccal root is often naturally fenestrated and because of its inability to heal requires reduction beneath the opening in bone. The buccal and palatal roots may be so widely separated that the sinus or medullary bone is interposed between them. Rarely can the extent of divergence be predetermined radiographically. In order to gain access to the palatal root it may be necessary to radically reduce the buccal root and for this reason the buccal triangular flap is best. If the buccal root reduction has not solved the problem of locating or reaching the palatal root one can abort the buccal approach and incise and reflect a palatal flap. The double flap procedure may prove easier, less traumatic, and less frustrating since the palatal root can usually be reached without involving the major palatine vessels or the sinus. However, the cortical bone of the floor of the sinus may closely approximate the apices of premolars, therefore perforation of the schneiderian membrane is a risk.

The danger of a sinus perforation is the transporting of root tips, bone, root canal filling material, or root debris into the antrum. This is of particular concern when reverse filling materials are used. Special attention to surgical detail by the dental surgeon and the assistant will prevent such an occurrence. If this unlikely problem should occur, the sinus opening must be enlarged and carefully flushed and evacuated. A fiberoptic light is especially useful for examining the sinus cavity. If anesthesia is insufficient or the foreign body cannot be located and retrieved, then a referral to an otolaryngologist is indicated.

Very little has been reported in the literature about sinus communication and apicoectomy. However, proper selection and retraction of a flap will minimize complications because the sinus preforation will be closed by the flap after it is repositioned and affixed. As long as oral communication to the sinus defect is prevented, repair of the sinus membrane will begin immediately after the initial inflammation caused by the surgical insult subsides. As a prophylactic measure, the patient should be placed on an appropriate antibiotic regimen: amoxicillin (preferred), cephalexin, or erythromycin (for penicillin-sensitive patients), 500 mg every 6 hours. If acute sinusitis complications develop, the patient should be promptly referred to an otolaryngologist.

For *maxillary molars* the triangular flap with a short posterior relaxing incision is best. Because the tissue is generally thin and detaches with little resistance, soft tissue elevation of the maxillary posterior area is usually quite easy. Exostoses often exist on the buccal surface of the alveolar bone and, since the tissue covering them is extremely thin and fragile, it must be elevated carefully to prevent perforating or tearing. Once exposed, these bony protuberances are eliminated by grinding the bone surface smooth. The mesial buccal roots of maxillary first and second molars present similar problems to the maxillary premolars: root fenestrations and close apposition of the sinus.

Additional canals in the mesial buccal root of the maxillary first molar must always be suspected.[67,80,89] When this root is surgically treated, a reverse fill must be contemplated. The distal buccal root is usually deeper in bone and normally has a distal dilaceration. During surgery the antrum and the mesial buccal root of the second molar must be carefully avoided. It is very difficult to reach the apex of the palatal root from the buccal approach without perforating the sinus floor, therefore the palatal root is ordinarily approached via a palatal exposure. When placing the posterior relaxing incision, care must be used to prevent severing the posterior palatine neurovascular bundle. Severance would cause excessive bleeding and the patient would be left with numbness of that side of the palate.

Root resection of the maxillary second molars require the same flap requirements of access and convenience as the first molar. Although the roots are shorter, the antrum is often in close approximation. Unfortunately, the buccal roots are often fused and the buccal groove between the roots may traverse the entire buccal surface; curettage often results in an oral communication with the apex (similar to a dehiscence) and the case will fail. If during the surgery a sinus perforation occurs, in the presence of a large periodontal defect, communication to the sinus defect can lead to sinusitis. As a preventative, a suitable periodontal pack and an antibiotic regimen are indicated. A reverse fill of the second molar is complicated by the inability to gain a vertical approach to the root ends. The cheek, the angle of the roots, and the zygomatic process will allow only horizontal access. Therefore the slot technique must be used. If apical treatment must be compromised and the success of the case becomes questionable, intentional replantation should be considered a viable alternative.

Mandible

Mandibular central and lateral incisors have a very thin labial cortical layer of bone and dehiscences are frequent near the cervical crest. As the apex is approached the bone dimension increases dramatically, and a thick dense cortex with underlying medullary bone will be found inferior to midroot. Because dehiscences are so common, the submarginal Oschenbein-Luebke flap design is indicated. The literature reports multiple canals exist 35% to 40% of the time, so acute facial root bevels must be cut in order to examine the apex. A reverse fill is indicated, if the seal of the apex is in doubt, the root is an oval or dumb-bell shape, or an off-centered canal is noticed. The lingual tilt of the roots, the protuberance of the chin, the thickness of the root, and the tension of the mentalis and depressor muscles will all increase the difficulty of preparing the apex for a reverse fill. Hemorrhage can become profuse if the mentalis vessels are severed. Penetration into the floor of the mouth lingual to the apices while searching or reducing the root tips can also produce substantial bleeding problems.

Apical surgery via a lingual approach is rarely attempted, for it is extremely difficult. Intentional replantation is a viable alternative for treating major problems that exist on the lingual surface of mandibular central or lateral incisors.

The mentalis and depressor muscles make surgery to the apical area of the *mandibular cuspid* difficult and fatiguing. The origin of the depressor muscles increases the thickness of tissue covering the cuspid apex, and its elevation can cause difficulty in controlling bleeding problems, which interfere with access, convenience, and view. Depending on the amount of attached gingiva, either the submarginal or the triangular flap design is adequate. The angulation of the root must be carefully evaluated for fear that misorientation will direct the osseous opening toward the apex of the lateral incisor or the first premolar. The crown is normally in labial version, placing the apex in a most difficult position. Reverse fills require a horizontal approach and a slot preparation.

For *mandibular premolars,* a triangular flap with the vertical incision anterior to the cuspid should be quite effective for surgical treatment of the mandibular first or second premolar. A short vertical relaxing incision distal to the first molar will release flap tension. The buccal tissue in this area strips from bone easily and very little bleeding will be encountered.

However, as the vertical elevation continues, one approaches the neurovascular bundle at the mental foramen. The bundle is somewhat elastic and will elevate with the flap. By slowly drawing the flap buccally, the bundle will be stretched out of the foramen and become much more visible. The remaining elevation can continue while the bundle is kept in view. The position of the retractor is observed at all times. Damage from pressure, crushing, or excessive pulling can cause a temporary to permanent problem ranging from a disturbing tingling to paresthesia.

The mental nerve has the poorest chance of regenerating if severed because the flap of tissue containing the nerve will be very difficult to position over the foramen. Because of tissue and jaw movement, it would be impossible to maintain that position for a long enough period of time to allow a reunion and reinnervation. It is imperative these vessels be found, observed, and avoided throughout surgery. Inadvertently finding them, or curetting them in ignorance as part of the lesion, is inexcusable. The buccal window should be sufficiently enlarged to allow for identification of the root. The root tip is separated at a level at least 2 mm above the apex by a fissure bur and the tip is removed through the buccal opening. The lesion often retains its attachment to the root and is subsequently curetted along with the apex. If it separates from the root, a gentle curettage in the depth of the alveolus is performed while the bundle is kept in view. If the curette contacts the bundle within the bone, movement can be observed at the foramen. The depth and location of sutures now are quite risky because needle penetration into the bundle can also cause irreparable damage.

The difficulties of root surgery on *mandibular molars* are created by limited access, reduced vertical dimension from crest to shelf, long axis of the roots, presence of the mandibular canal, and thickness of the buccal cortical bone. For the mandibular first molar a triangular flap with the vertical incision placed anterior to the mental canal, again to observe its position throughout the surgery, is indicated. The flap offers little resistance to elevation, and the mental bundle is located and kept in view at all times.

A relaxing incision on the ridge distal to the last molar or extending into the retromolar pad will reduce flap tension and ease vertical elevation. A bony window that approximates the mid to lower third of the mesial root is prepared and a piece of x-ray lead foil is placed in the opening and radiographed. This will orient the dental surgeon to both lateral and vertical position.

Once orientation adjustments are made, the window is enlarged until the root is positively identified. At this point the root is beveled (45 to 55 degrees) until the canals are in view and examined. The lesion is curetted with knowledge the mandibular canal is directly inferior to the apex. The distal root is approached in the same manner but is usually located more lingual than the mesial root. Extensive buccal bone removal may be necessary. The difficulty of the mandibular second molars is increased because the external oblique ridge extends down to act like an additional cortical plate.[42] Entrance is eased if sterile high-speed drills are available, but their use also increases the potential danger. The neurovascular bundle courses through the mandibular canal and, although normally found inferior and slightly lingual to these teeth, can indeed be contiguous with or even superior to the apices. Apical surgery to any mandibular molar carries with it the risk of paresthesia. As long as one is aware of position at all times, this problem can be minimized. *The patient should be informed of this possibility before surgery.* Formal surgical consent forms are required in some states. We suggest they be used for everyone. A lingual approach to molars is deterred by the long axis of the teeth, the thickness of the plate, the concavity of the lingual bone, the presence of the tongue, and the fact the mandibular canal traverses from buccal to lingual as it extends from the mental canal to the ramus. If apical surgery is being considered for molars, the examination should include a panorex radiograph, and consent by the patient regarding risks, benefits, and alternatives, such as conventional retreatment, hemisection, and intentional replantation.

Midsurgical endodontics

As early as 1880 a technique was described[31,74] suggesting exposure of the root apex and removal of all existing pathosis before the initiation of root canal therapy. This technique is still popular with oral surgeons but over the years has lost favor with endodontists.

The procedure, which should more correctly be referred to as midsurgical endodontics, requires three phases of treatment[20]:

1. *Exposure phase*—includes the preparation of the operatory, doctor, patient, and tooth; the flap design; the incision, elevation, retraction, and osteotomy; and the curettage. The purpose of this phase is to expose the root tip, remove all pathologic tissue for biopsy, and whenever possible eliminate any obstruction from the canal.

2. *Endodontic phase*—includes cleaning, shaping, and if possible filling the canal with gutta-percha and sealer to the apex. When the apical foramen or any other known opening in the root cannot be sealed conventionally, an apical filling must be placed while the apex is exposed.

3. *Closure phase*—includes cleaning the surgical site of excess endodontic filling materials, bone wax, gauze, and blood and then positioning and suturing the flap in place. The patient is given postoperative instructions and any necessary prescriptions for pain and infection.

Seeing the root tip during the endodontic phase is a distinct advantage; but it may have some disadvantages, including

1. The root canal procedure is usually accomplished without a rubber dam, which increases the risk that the patient may aspirate or swallow an instrument.
2. Without the aid of the rubber dam, asepsis is difficult to maintain; and this increases the risk of failure.
3. Because bleeding is sometimes difficult to control, a dry canal may be unobtainable. Root canal sealers and cements will not function properly in the presence of moisture, which in turn invites failure.
4. Because a surgical and an endodontic setup are both exposed and used simultaneously, it is virtually impossible to maintain surgical asepsis.
5. The flap must be open for an extended time. Such repeated elevation, retraction, and curettage are traumatic; and these repeated insults are usually reflected postoperatively by increased swelling and pain.

Although the preceding arguments against the method are valid, they are predicated on the assumption that all teeth are endodontically treatable by a nonsurgical approach. This is not always the case, and for the following conditions this regimen may offer the only alternative to extraction:

1. When this technique was first reported, dentistry was without the advantage of x-ray equipment. To those who were dedicated to accuracy, exact root canal therapy could be accomplished only by midsurgical endodontics. Although this is not the case today, there are still occasions when such equipment is either unavailable or inaccessible—e.g., when endodontic procedures are performed in hospital operating rooms, surgical clinics, or other settings where general anesthetics are being administered to patients.

2. The size of a radiolucency is easily underestimated; and as a lesion is curetted, it is not uncommon to encounter an untreated adjacent root tip. If this occurs and the viability of the tip becomes suspect, the flap should be temporarily repositioned and the endodontic phase instituted on the newly involved tooth.

3. In treating teeth with large lesions, it is sometimes difficult to control the flow of purulence into the canal. Because root canal sealers and cements are influenced by moisture, best results are achieved when the fluid is eliminated surgically and the canal can be properly dried. A second moisture complication that may occur during treatment is the sudden emergence of blood. This often indicates a perforation, which may need to be corrected before the canal can be completed.

4. Often a canal becomes blocked by foreign objects such as particles of cement, alloy, tooth chips, dentin mud, ledges, and broken instruments. Exposure of the apex may offer a surgeon the opportunity to dislodge and remove such obstructions. When these canal restrictions are eliminated, the endodontic phase can proceed routinely.

5. Fractured roots offer many treatment options, all of which depend upon the location and direction of fracture and the survival of the pulpal tissue. Treatment of root fractures is described in detail in Chapter 15.

6. Although the aforementioned reasons for using this regimen are important, they represent only a small percentage of midsurgical procedures. The more common reasons involve the need to seal canal openings apically when they cannot be sealed by the nonsurgical canal approach:

a. Anatomic
   (1) Nonnegotiable dilacerated or curved roots
   (2) Extensive canal calcification
   (3) Nonnegotiable parallel canals
   (4) Nonnegotiable dens-in-dente
   (5) Impassable pulp stones

(6) Internal or external root perforations (when Ca[OH]$_2$ root repair fails)

(7) Immature apex development (when apexification fails)

b. Iatrogenic

(1) Difficult-to-remove posts and cores

(2) Failing cases with difficult-to-remove filling materials

(3) Broken instruments lodged in the canal that cannot be bypassed

(4) Root perforations that cannot be repaired internally

c. Inadequate seal of the apical foramen—a judgment decision made after the apex is examined clinically[7,15,25,61,78]

In midsurgical endodontics the fundamental surgical movements remain the same. However, the flap design may need to be altered because the access required is greater and increased visibility is imperative. Therefore it may be necessary to widen the flap laterally and select a nonconfining, nonfatiguing flap such as the trapezoid.

The apex is beveled at a 45-degree angle with a tapered fissure bur using high or low speed (Fig. 18-27). The re-

duction must provide a smooth flat surface facing the operator's line of sight. It must be wide enough to allow sufficient room for a Class I preparation yet provide a border of root relatively 2 mm wide. If the bevel is insufficient to provide proper examination of the root, as is the case in many molars, additional root or bone is removed. This is particularly important to examine C shape mesial molar roots. The debris within the isthmus between canals is the cause of many failures, as are the anatomic variances of the root ends of many teeth. After the apex has been reduced, a Class I cavity preparation approximately 3 to 5 mm deep and parallel with the long axis of the root is created in the center of the cut root surface. This preparation is made with a small round bur[5,7] and undercut with an inverted cone (33⅓ or 34) (Fig. 18-29). To avoid removing excessive bone for access, the cavity preparation should be made with microhead handpieces and microburs (Fig. 18-28). If the root location or its angle impedes the handpiece and prevents a parallel entrance, a modified preparation (referred to as the slot or Matzuri)[62] is recom-

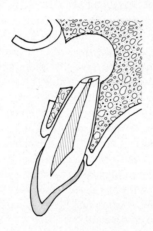

FIG. 18-27. When the apex is beveled at a 45-degree angle facing the surgeon, this affords the greatest opportunity to locate, examine, and operate on the remaining root surface.

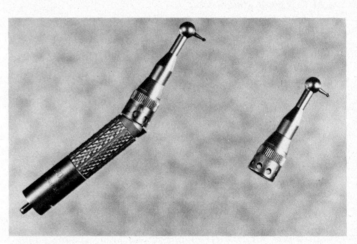

FIG. 18-28. To prepare the root end, miniature instruments are necessary. The minihead handpiece with miniburs requires only 10 mm of access.

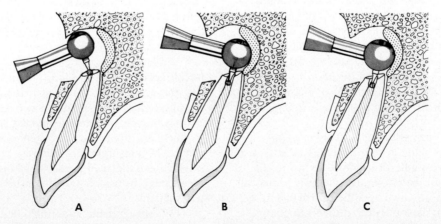

FIG. 18-29. A Class I cavity is prepared in the root end with a small round bur. Initially the handpiece head must be angled. **A,** Once parallel with the long axis, **B,** it continues to deepen the preparation to a depth of 3 to 5 mm. The preparation is then undercut, **C,** with an inverted cone for retention.

mended to lessen the risk of root perforation. For this technique the root bevel is prepared as usual (Fig. 18-30, *A*), but a tapered fissure bur is placed in the apical canal opening perpendicular to the long axis of the root (Fig. 18-30, *B*). A 3 to 5 mm grove or slot is prepared apically-gingivally in the root surface and undercut with a round or inverted cone (Fig. 18-30, *C* and *D*). This preparation will be particularly advantageous in mandibular incisors and molars.

To maintain a clear, dry field and capture any debris, the periapical area is packed with ¼-inch gauze or bone wax. Bone wax* consists of a highly purified beeswax, a softener, and a conditioner (isopropyl palmitate). The product has been used since 1963 in both medicine and dentistry. The literature suggests it is inflammatory if left in the bone, and there are claims that the material embolizes to the lung when pressed on bone marrow.[52] Its use was advocated for endodontic surgery as early as 1970 by Seldon. As the material is intended only as a barrier, it is to be removed before the area is closed. If bone wax is preferred, it must be packed into the area before the root preparation is made. This will prevent the material from lodging in the apex opening and interfering with the seal. Although somewhat more difficult to use than gauze, bone wax does offer a hemostatic advantage. Alternatively iodoform gauze strips can be packed behind and around the root tip after the preparation. For hemostasis the gauze can be saturated with Orastat or any other suitable liquid coagulant. Gauze is best used to block the sinus perforation during a reverse fill procedure. A single strip should be used, premeasured to allow it to extend out of the surgical site and prevented from being pushed completely through the defect.

In summary, both materials are relatively easy to use and simple to remove. The choice rests with the clinician. However, bone wax is *not* recommended when a sinus perforation is identified or suspected.

When the apical preparation is complete, the hemor-

---

*Ethicon, Inc., Summerville, NJ.

rhage controlled, and the root area clean and dry, attention is focused on the apical seal.

Gutta-percha is the standard for filling root canals.[7,41,77] It is not toxic, it is well tolerated by the tissues, it has fine working characteristics, it can be molded, flowed, and compressed, and it provides hermetic capabilities (as described in Chapter 8). Unless there are abuses in its use, it provides an ideal seal of the apical foramen. That quality is not lost when the well-condensed gutta-percha root is resected by a high-speed rotary instrument.[40] An apicoectomy by a high-speed handpiece does not adversely affect the seal and does not necessitate the placement of a retrograde material. Though obvious anatomic and iatrogenic indications appear to be the main reasons for reverse filling canals, the subjective clinical judgment of the seal becomes the responsibility of the dental surgeon.[7,25,61]

Throughout the years a gamut of materials have been selected as retrograde filling materials ranging from silver points, gutta-percha, gold foil, "Stailene," polycarboxylate cement, amalgam with and without zinc, copper cements and alloys, poly-HEMA, Cavit, Restodent, and other zinc oxide–eugenol mixtures.[44,49,69,94] Amalgam still appears to remain the most popular choice, even though it has some inherent deficiencies.

The following represents a summary of current studies relative to using amalgam for an apical retroseal:

1. Ormnell[68] first reported the incidence of a zinc carbonate precipitate. More recent studies provide strong evidence that zinc-containing and zinc-free amalgam are equally well tolerated by periapical tissues when placed in a dry preparation and a dry environment.[28,32,47]

2. Microleakage studies[46,60,64] indicate no significant differences between zinc-containing and zinc-free alloys when placed in a dry environment and kept dry during the initial set. Zinc-containing amalgam, if condensed in the presence of moisture, will expand as much as 4%.[55,94]

3. The sealing efficiency of a 3-mm amalgam thickness was significantly superior to a 1-mm thickness.

4. High copper-containing alloys have superior physical

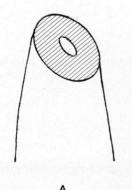
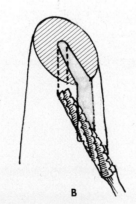
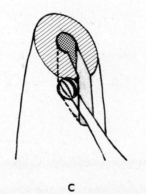
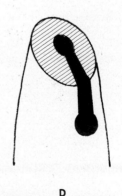

A   B   C   D

FIG. 18-30. When access is limited, the slot preparation is preferred. **A,** The root is beveled at a 45-degree angle. **B,** A tapered fissure bur cuts a 3 to 5 mm slot along the facial aspect of the exposed root. **C,** Then a round bur cuts retention. **D,** The final preparation gives the appearance of a keyhole.

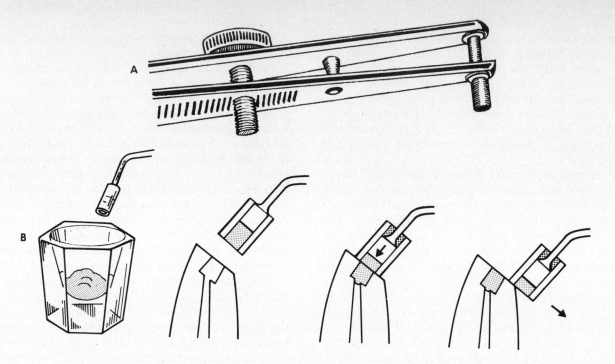

FIG. 18-31. Miniature carriers and pluggers afford greater control in confining the reverse fill material to the cavity preparation. Two efficient types are, **A,** the K-G carrier and, **B,** the Luebke carrier plugger.

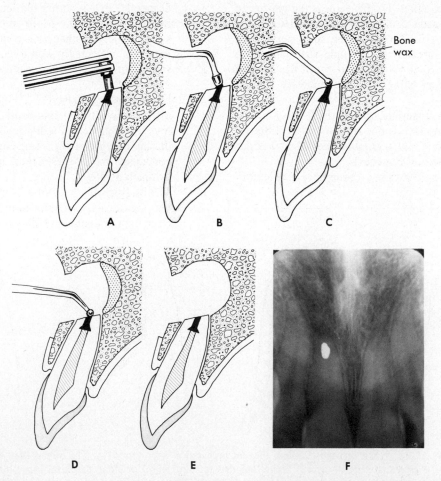

FIG. 18-32. When the preparation is complete, alternately, **A,** carry the amalgam to the opening, **B,** condense it with a miniplugger, and then, **C,** curette and, **D,** burnish until a smooth finish, **E,** is produced. Never place sutures until a radiographic examination, **F,** is completed and the bone wax is removed.

properties, resist corrosion, and have minimal cytotoxic effect.

5. Regardless of the amalgam selected, the placement of a cavity varnish in a dry field significantly improves the apical seal.

6. If a retrograde amalgam will be in contact with a metallic dowel post, an insulating layer of gutta-percha, zinc phosphate cement, Cavit, or zinc oxide–eugenol should be inserted between the two metals to prevent any electrochemical activity.

7. It has the pronounced discoloring effect on tissues and nonmetallic substitutes should be considered for larger repairs in the anterior maxillary segment.

Alternative to amalgam are zinc phosphate cement,[73,94] Poly-HEMA, Duralon,[8] Cavit,[14,32,44,90] Restodent,[14,69] gutta-percha, and zinc oxide–eugenol (U.S.P.).

Each material has advantages and disadvantages but the most recent literature supports the techniques involving cold packing or cold burnishing gutta-percha and zinc oxide–eugenol (U.S.P. pure or the commercially sold Restodent and I.R.M.)[14,69] These materials offer a good marginal seal, they are nondiscoloring, and they have minimal inflammatory potential.[28,61,78]

Stabholz et al[86] found Restodent* to be significantly superior to zinc phosphate cement, Cavit-W, Duralon, and amalgam in both marginal adaptation and sealability.

With the advent of the new gutta-percha "gun" (e.g., Obtura (also see p. 232), gutta-percha can be carried to the preparation, injected, and condensed to the walls. This method of delivering warm gutta-percha as an apical seal appears to be quite promising.

The introduction of minicarriers and pluggers (Fig. 18-31), as well as the efficiency of high-volume suction equipment, virtually eliminates excess material around the periapical area.[26] These instruments allow the clinician to carry and control minute amounts of filling material, and with care it is possible to confine *all* the material to the canal preparation. Each portion is injected into the preparation and condensed (Fig. 18-32, *A*) by a suitably sized plugger (Fig. 18-32, *B*). Alternately filling and condensing such small amounts will assure a good solid filling. Throughout the filling and condensing, marginal excess should be removed instantly (Fig. 18-32, *C*). A well-condensed amalgam should have a low residual mercury content. All materials should set to some degree before the final carving (Fig. 18-32, *D*). This will enable one to produce a smooth, flat, shiny finish and avoid saucering (Fig. 18-32, *E*). The bone wax or gauze is removed; and as suggested earlier, a clinical and radiographic examination is made *prior* to closure (Fig. 18-32, *F*). If the area appears clear, the tissue flap is repositioned and sutured in place. When a particle does appear to be displaced, an efficient inspection of the bone cavity and the undersurface of the flap is made. A fiberoptic light offers many benefits in this endeavor.

Some situations demand special attention.

1. The incidence of second canals (Fig. 18-33, *A*) in lower incisors, premolars, and the mesial-buccal root of maxillary first molars is considerable.[10,35,67,80,89] For this reason these teeth should be suspect when apicoectomies are performed. Their apices must be examined carefully for two canals. If the cut roots appear oval or dumbbell shaped, they probably have parallel canals. The apical preparation must then be altered from a single round opening to two round openings or an oval design combining both canals in a single preparation.

2. When the root has a severe dilaceration, it is possible to reduce the apex at a 45-degree angle and never contact the canal (Fig. 18-33, *B*). This can also happen when the roots are in lingual version (Fig. 18-33, *C*). Identification with the canal is imperative, and root reduction must be continued until the canal is confirmed.

3. In maxillary premolars, identifying and preparing the palatal root requires greater reduction of the buccal root. Because these teeth are usually short, attention must be focused on the remaining crown/root ratio and the amount of remaining cortical bone covering the buccal root surface.

4. Repairing wall perforations requires good judgment and commen sense. If the repair takes place deep in bone, uneventful healing should be expected; however, when excessive amounts of crestal bone must be removed to uncover the defect and an unfavorable periodontal condition results, the attempt is not warranted.[53,79] Root repair surgery should also be avoided if the adjacent teeth will be damaged or jeopardized in gaining access to the repair site. Intentional replantation might be a less traumatic alternative for such cases.[36] When repair of the damaged wall is accessible, the bone surrounding the margin of the root defect is removed until a 2-mm border of sound tooth structure is exposed. A Class I preparation within the root is made with an appropriately sized round bur. All efforts are made to remain within the existing opening and little if any enlargement of the defect is made. This may not be possible when additional access is required. If a post exists, it is reduced in length and a nonmetallic filling material will be selected. If a post is to be made, it is advisable to fabricate and seat the post at an appointment before or during the surgery. Possibilities of dislodging the reparative plug in the future should be eliminated.

The material and condensation techniques are similar to those of an apical reverse fill.

Root resection and hemisection

Root amputation and hemisection techniques were reported in the literature over 100 years ago.[75,85] Success in these cases depends on meticulous attention to endodontic, periodontal, and restorative detail. Poor execution of any phase can lead to ultimate failure.

Indications. There are number of reasons to select teeth for root resection[5,17,56]:

1. Uncorrectable periodontal disease with through-and-through furcal involvement
2. Periodontal conditions interproximally that are uncorrectable or unmaintainable

---

*Lee Pharmaceuticals, S. El Monte, CA.

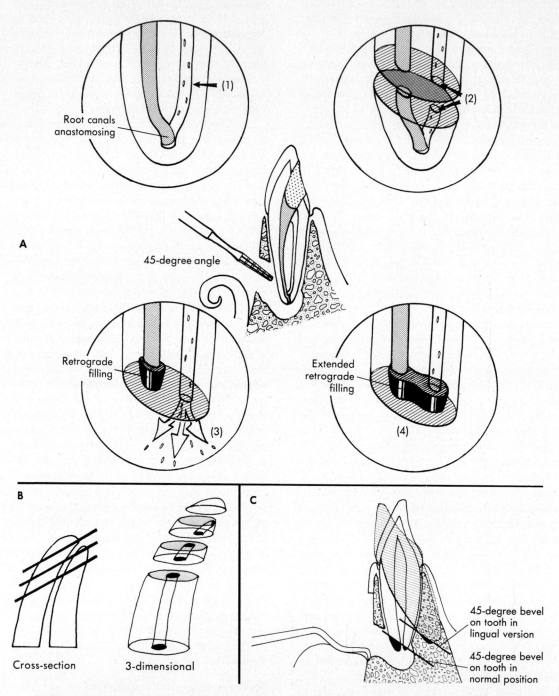

FIG. 18-33. Special situations demand special attention. **A,** Teeth with a high incidence of second canals *(1)* may actually be compromised by an apicoectomy that further exposes the untreated second canal *(2)*. For such teeth, sealing the treated canal will not discontinue the flow of toxins *(3)*. Therefore consideration should be given to this possibility by altering the preparation and sealing the entire apex *(4)*. **B,** With severe root curvatures beveled at a 45-degree angle the apical canal opening may not be exposed. **C,** A similar problem can arise with straight roots in severe lingual version. A 45-degree bevel, as shown on a tooth in normal position, may not expose the canal when the tooth is in lingual version *(striped)*.

3. Deep carious lesions along the root wall of a multi-rooted tooth making that section of the tooth unrestorable

4. Fracture, perforation, or severe resorption of one root of a multirooted tooth

5. Nonnegotiable canal in one root of a multirooted tooth not amenable to apical surgery

Before one decides on hemisection, the following should be considered:

1. Can the salvaged roots maintain stability, particularly if they are short and thin?

2. Will the remaining furcas in maxillary molars be sound and cleansable?

3. Does the patient have a poor oral hygiene history or a high caries index?

4. Are the remaining roots endodontically treatable and the crown restorable?

5. Is the location of the root furca accessible for separation?

6. Is the patient a medical risk?

7. Does the patient understand the treatment prognosis?

8. Will the patient accept the risk?

Regardless of the reasons for hemisecting mandibular molars, the basic objectives remain the same:

Separate the tooth in the furca.
Avoid damage to the retained root.
Remove as little bone as possible.

The surgical technique in cases indicated for periodontics will require a flap.[42,56,85] Because access to the apex is unnecessary, the gingival flap design with or without releasing incisions can be employed. For convenience it is best to release both labial and lingual tissue. This will not only uncover both aspects of the furca but also provide access to the depths of the periodontal pockets. Unless root structure has been destroyed below the gingival crest, most cases indicated for reasons other than periodontal do not require flaps.

Technique for hemisection

The chamber of the tooth is opened and cleaned and the canals in the half to be retained are instrumented (Fig. 18-34, A and B). After the canal is filled, all excess gutta-percha is removed from the chamber and the crown is filled with amalgam (Fig. 18-34, C). Consideration should be given to placing a preformed stainless steel post for crown reinforcement; amalgam can be condensed around the post. As the amalgam hardens, preparation is made for surgery.

When a mandibular molar is being sectioned, the crown height is initially reduced 2 to 4 mm to take the tooth out of occlusion. Reduction of the condemned coronal half will then continue until this segment is within 2 mm of the gingival crest (Fig. 18-34, D). This will eliminate all the weakened crown structure below the height of contour and allow full engagement of the root structure by the forceps beaks during extraction. When buccal and lingual grooves are present, they are used as guides for crown division. A radiograph is exposed to orient the vertical step of the crown division to the furca. All crown and root division can be accomplished with a no. 700 bur in a high-speed handpiece, accompanied by a copious water spray, and a high-volume aspirator.

Once oriented to the furca, a single vertical buccal-lingual cut is made 2 to 4 mm deep and no wider than the bur (Fig. 18-34, E). A second orientation radiograph is exposed. Any directional adjustments are made, and the vertical cut is continued until separation is complete (Fig. 18-34, F). This separation can be determined by:

1. *Feel*—There should be less resistance to the bur once it reaches bone.

2. *Radiographs*—The full cut should be apparent.

3. *Mobility*—The condemned half should be elevated without any movement to the other segment.

When separation is confirmed, elevation should continue until the root has at least a Class III mobility. The surrounding bone should provide the leverage for the elevators or root picks. No instrument should ever be wedged between the two segments either for elevation or to confirm or cause separation. When the condemned half is freed from the alveolus, the forceps beaks are positioned on the root body and minimal compressive forces are applied to the tooth as it is removed from its socket (Fig. 18-34, G). If during its removal the root refuses to release or breaks, a triangular flap is incised and reflected; buccal bone is removed from the condemned root surface, and the root is elevated and extracted. All sharp edges of the retained crown segment are reduced and, when necessary, a temporary crown is placed for protection. A final radiograph is exposed to examine the alveolus for root pieces or debris before the patient is dismissed (Fig. 18-34, H). If the original diagnosis was periodontal disease, the scaling or curetting procedures are accomplished on the remaining root. The flap is repositioned and appropriate sutures are placed. Depending on the diagnosis and one's clinical judgment, the patient is prescribed appropriate antibiotics and analgesics postoperatively.

Resection of the maxillary root or roots requires a full mucoperiosteal flap to provide sufficient access, increase visibility, and prevent damage to the remaining roots and furca. The removal of buccal roots from maxillary molars is relatively easy unless the patient has a small mouth. After the endodontic treatment has been completed, the crown is again packed with amalgam and the occlusal height is reduced. The mucosa is incised and reflected and the cortical bone is removed from the buccal surface of the root. When the offending root has been located and identified, the tapered fissure bur begins a cut at the cementum-enamel junction and passes in a medial and apical direction from the lateral surface of the root to the furca. Visibility should be good for maintaining orientation; but if there is doubt about one's position, a radiograph should be exposed. As one approaches the furca, caution is foremost to prevent cutting into the adjacent roots. After root separation is confirmed, the disconnected root is elevated from its alveolar socket. Additional bone, root, or the buccal surface of the crown may require further reduction to provide room for the root removal. The area is cleaned and radiographed, and the flap is sutured in place.[5,42]

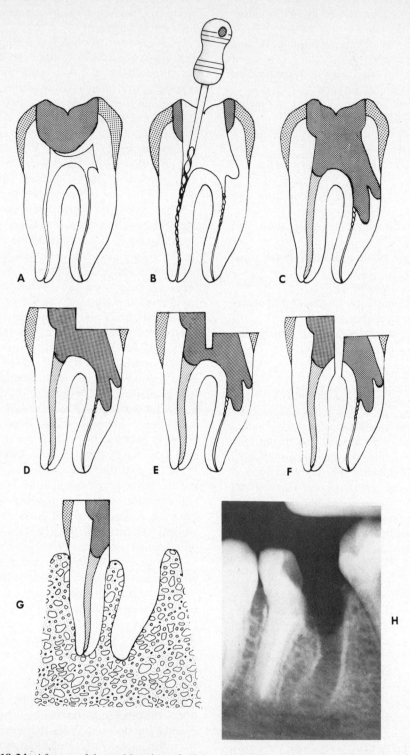

FIG. 18-34. After careful consideration of all the alternatives, when a tooth is selected for hemisection, the following will pertain: **A,** the bifurcation must be distinct and within an operable distance of the crest; **B,** the retainable root is instrumented; **C,** after the canal is filled with gutta-percha, the chamber is filled with amalgam; **D,** the crown height over the condemned half should be further reduced to within 2 mm of the crest and below the height of contour; **E,** initial separation is made with a fissure bur and radiographed for orientation; **F,** when oriented, the vertical cut is continued until separation is complete; **G,** the undersired root is removed; and, **H,** the remaining segment is shaped and radiographed.

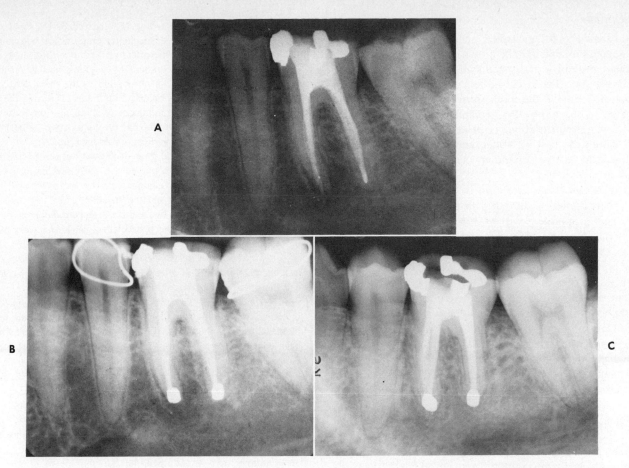

FIG. 18 35. A, Preoperative radiograph of a mandibular molar with a perforated mesial root tip at or near the mandibular canal. The patient was experiencing intense pain. B, The apices of the extracted tooth were filled with amalgam, and the tooth was replanted and splinted. C, Two-year postoperative radiograph. Healing with no detectable resorption.

A vertical triangulation technique has been advocated by Weine.[93] Vertical cuts are made through the crown up to the furca, with the crown and the root segment being removed simultaneously. The principles of hemisection are followed as the crown is reduced above the height of contour, and orientation radiographs are used during the cut. No flap is required; however, this technique should be used only when the root is being amputated for reasons other than periodontal. Because the restoration of hemisected or radisected teeth invites food impaction, excellent oral hygiene is required for the success of this procedure.

Intentional replantation

When radicular surgery would be difficult or traumatic, a seldom-used but potentially successful alternative is to extract the tooth, examine the root, correct the defect, and replant the tooth in its socket.[36] Nearly all dentists follow such treatment for traumatically avulsed teeth, and there is no reason why it should not be used for other situations.

The indications for intentional replantation are as follows:

1. The risk of permanent damage to strategic anatomic structures is high if apical surgery is attempted.

2. A foreign body that is near the inferior alveolar nerve must be removed by way of the socket.
3. The amount of bone between the root tip and the mucosal entry is exceptionally thick and dense.
4. The only access to a perforation is from an inoperable direction.
5. Idiopathic pain continues after seemingly successful endodontic treatment and apical surgery.
6. Endodontics cannot be performed on a tooth because of trismus, inability to keep the mouth open long enough, or inadequate interocclusal space.
7. There is suspected but unconfirmed damage to root structure (fracture, perforation).
8. The amount of bone removed to perform the task would leave the patient with an unmanageable periodontal pocket or adjacent tooth damage.

There are also contraindications:
1. The patient is a medical risk.
2. The crown is not restorable.
3. An advanced periodontal condition already exists.
4. The extraction is extremely difficult or traumatic, causing damage to the periodontal tissues or fracture of the cortical plates.
5. The patient does not understand or is unwilling to accept the risk of a guarded prognosis.

Technique

All canals should be cleaned, shaped, and filled to whatever degree possible and the crown should be restored with amalgam. Placing a preformed stainless steel post provides further support. The occlusal height should be reduced to temporarily remove the tooth from occlusal forces. Some elevation of the tooth after replantation should be anticipated, even when a splint is placed. Fluid pressure will build within the first 72 hours; and if the replanted tooth is allowed to receive continuous occlusal trauma, pain and failure are inevitable.

As in hemisection, elevation is the most important aspect. There should be no hurry in extracting this tooth. A slow, gentle approach will be kindest to the periodontal membrane. Because ankylosis and root resorption are sequelae of trauma to the healthy attachment apparatus, every precaution to preserve its integrity should be taken.

When the tooth is freed from the alveolar walls, the forceps are applied to the tooth, extractive forces are exerted, and the tooth is removed. The tooth, which will be held in the forceps throughout the procedure, is now gently bathed in a glass of warm sterile saline. The depth of the alveolus, but not the walls, may be curetted at this time. The roots are examined for damage and the apical 2 to 4 mm are trimmed. A tooth is ready for replantation when the gutta-percha fill is acceptable, when the apex is sealed with amalgam, when all evident root damage is repaired, and when the tooth has been cleansed of all debris by the swishing action of the saline. At no time is the root wiped clean with gauze or cotton, nor are the socket walls scraped, curetted, or aspirated.

The tooth is carried to its alveolus and replanted slowly into the socket. The unchanged forceps position guides the direction of insertion.

Alignment and occlusion are checked after insertion and, when necessary, a splint is fabricated. The splint is neeeded only when excessive mobility is apparent and should not be in place longer than 7 to 10 days. For stabilization, the acrylic acid-etch technique is best but periopacking or suturing across the reduced occlusal with 3-0 thread is adequate.

Appropriate antibiotics and analgesics are prescribed and the patient is periodically examined for any irreversible inflammatory reactions and root resorptions (Fig. 18-35).

POSTOPERATIVE INSTRUCTIONS

All patients should be carefully informed of the role played by postoperative care in healing.[4,70,87] These instructions should be *preprinted forms,* which can be handed to the patient after surgery. This will minimize a possible misunderstanding or misinterpretation. The information should be simply worded and should cover all potential problems. The following list of suggested rules covers the minor as well as the major complications:

1. *Bleeding*—A certain amount of bleeding should be expected. Mouth rinses should be avoided; however, a mild warm salt water rinse (½ tsp salt to 4 oz of warm water) can be used to freshen the mouth. If bleeding becomes excessive, locate the source and apply firm but steady finger pressure for 10 minutes. If bleeding continues, call the office or the home (after hours).

2. *Swelling*—A certain amount of swelling will be encountered after surgery. An ice pack applied to the facial area over the surgical site 10 minutes on and 20 minutes off during the first 24 postoperative hours will minimize swelling. For the following days until the sutures are removed, the application of heat will increase vascularity, relax tissues, and induce healing.

3. *Pain*—A long surgical procedure does not mean that postoperative pain is inevitable, nor does a short surgical encounter mean complete comfort is guaranteed. The ice packs will help reduce the pain possibility and the anesthetic will last for some time after surgery. Taking two aspirin or acetaminophens before the anesthetic wears off is suggested, since analgesics work better before pain begins.

A prescription for a stronger medication has been written in case the pain worsens. If after 48 hours the pain continues, please call the office or the home (after hours).

4. *Oral hygiene*—To reduce the possibility of postoperative infection, the mouth should be kept clean. Mouth washes (diluted) will reduce the bacterial flora; because only soft foods have been eaten, frequent toothbrushing is essential. All effort should be made to keep the bristles from injuring the gums.

5. *Infection*—Postoperative infection is unusual; but if symptoms such as chills, fever, pain, and excessive swelling are experienced after the third day, the office should be contacted.

6. *Diet*—Some loss of appetite may occur; however, it is important to take fluids, proteins, and supplemental vitamins high in B and C.

7. *Sutures*—An appointment has been made to remove the stitches. If the stitches loosen before this appointment, please call the office for an earlier appointment.

8. *Activities*—For the first day, talking, laughing, and other facial expressions should be minimized. The lips should not be stretched, to avoid separating the incision or tearing the stitches free. Normal activity can usually be continued on the second day.

REFERENCES

1. Abdal, A.K., and Retief, D.H.: The apical seal via the retrosurgical approach. I. A preliminary study, Oral Surg. **53**:614, 1982.
2. Abdal, A.K., Retief, H.D., and Jamison, H.C.: The apical seal via the retrosurgical approach. II. An evaluation of retrofilling materials, Oral Surg. **54**:213, 1982.
3. Aeschlimann, C.R., Robinson, P.J., and Kaminski, E.J.: Short term evaluation of periodontal surgery, J. Periodontol. Res. **14**:182, 1979.
4. Andreason, J.O., and Rud, J.: Modes of healing histologically after endodontic surgery in 70 cases, Int. J. Oral Surg. **1**:148, 1972.
5. Arens, D.E., Adams, W., and DeCastro, R.: Endodontic surgery, New York, 1981, Harper & Row, Publishers.
6. Barnes, I.E.: Surgical endodontics—introduction, principles, and indications. Dent. Update **8**:89, 1981.
7. Barry, G. Heyman, R., and Elias, A.: A comparison of apical sealing methods, Oral Surg. **39**:806, 1975.
8. Barry, G.N., et al.: Sealing quality of polycarboxylate cements when compared to amalgam as retrofilling material, Oral Surg. **42**:109, 1976.
9. Bender, I.B., and Seltzer, S.: Roentgenographic and direct observations of experimental lesions in bone, J. Am. Dent. Assoc. **62**:152, 1961.
10. Benjamin, K., and Dawson, J.: Incidence of two root canals in human mandibular teeth, Oral Surg. **38**:122, 1974.
11. Bhaskar, S.N., et al.: Biogradeable ceramic implants in bone, Oral Surg. **32**:336, 1971.

12. Bhaskar, S.N., et al.: Tissue reaction to intrabony ceramic implants, Oral Surg. **31**:282, 1971.

13. Black, C.V.: Special dental pathology, ed. 3, Chicago, 1924, Medico-Dental Publishing Co.

14. Blaney, T.D., et al.: Marginal sealing quality of IRM and Cavit as assessed by microbial penetrations, J. Endod **7**:453, 1981.

15. Block, R.M., and Bushell, A.: Retrograde amalgam procedures for mandibular posterior teeth, J. Endod. **8**:107, 1982.

16. Block, R.M., et al.: Endodontic surgical re-treatment—a clinical and histopathological study. J. Endod. **5**:101, 1979.

17. Bresterfeld, R.C., and Taintor, J.F.: Endodontic considerations related to hemisection and root amputation, Northwest-Dent. **57**:142, 1978.

18. Cassella, E.A., Pickett, A.B., and Chamberlin, J.H.: Unusual management problems in the treatment of a long standing destructive periapical cyst: report of a case, Oral Surg. **51**:93, 1981.

19. Castelli, W.A., et al.: Gingival response to silk, cotton and nylon suture materials, Oral Surg. **45**:179, 1978.

20. Chivian, N.: Surgical endodontics: a conservative approach, J. N.J. Dent. Soc. **40**:234, 1969.

21. Chivian, N.: Midsurgery endodontics. In Arens, D., Adams, W., and Castro, R., editors: Endodontic surgery, Philadelphia, 1983, Harper & Row, Publishers.

22. Citrome, G.P., Kaminski, E.J., and Heuer, M.A.: A comparative study of tooth apexficiation in the dog, J. Endod. **5**:200, 1979.

23. Clarke, M.A., and Bueltman, K.W.: Anatomical considerations in periodontal surgery, J. Periodont. **42**:610, 1971

24. Cohen, S., and Burns, H., editors: Pathways of the pulp, ed. 2, St. Louis, 1980. The C.V. Mosby Co.

25. Cunningham, J.: The seal of root fillings at apicectomy: a scanning electron microscope study, Br. Dent. J. **139**:430, 1975.

26. Curson, I.: Instruments for placing an amalgam apical seal, J. Dent. **1**:286, 1973.

27. Dahlberg, W.H.: Incisions and suturing in periodontal flap surgery, Dent. Clin. North Am. **13**:149, 1969.

28. Delivanis, P., and Tabibi, A.: A comparative sealability study of different retrofilling materials, Oral Surg. **45**:252, 1982.

29. Desirabode, A.M.: Nouveaux elements complets de la science et de l'art du dentist, Paris, 1943, Lobe.

30. Driskell, T.D., et al.: The sign of absorbable bioceramic in the repair of bone defects. Proceedings, 26th Annual Conference on Engineering, Medicine, and Biology, 1973.

31. Farrar, J.N.: Radical and heroic treatment of alveolar abscess by amputation of roots of teeth, Dent. Cosmos **26**:79, 1884.

32. Flander, D.H., et al.: Comparative histopathologic study of zinc-free amalgam and Cavit in connective tissue of the rat, J. Endod. **1**:56, 1975.

33. Frank, A.C., and Weine, F.S.: Non-surgical therapy for the perforative defect of internal resorption, J. Am. Dent. Assoc. **87**:863, 1973.

34. Goldsmith, J.P.: Salvaging teeth by molar apicoectomy, N. Y. J. Dent. **49**:324, 1979.

35. Green, D.: Double canals in single roots, Oral Surg. **35**:689, 1973.

36. Grossman, L.I.: Intentional replantation of teeth: a clinical evaluation, J. Am. Dent. Assoc. **104**:633, 1982.

37. Gutmann, J.I.: Principles of endodontic surgery for the general practioner, Dent. Clin. North Am. **28**:895, 1984.

38. Gutmann, J.I., and Harrison, J.W.: Posterior endodontic surgery: anatomical considerations and clinical techniques, Int. Endod. **18**:8, 1985.

39. Gutmann, J.I., and Hovland, E.: A critical reappraisal of the routine use of periradicular surgery in conjunction with endodontics, J. D. C. Dent. Soci. **53**:17-21, 1978.

40. Harrison, J., and Todd, M.: The affect of root resection on the sealing property of root canal obturations, Oral Surg. **50**:264, 1980.

41. Harty, F.J.: Endodontics in clinical practice, ed. 2, Bristol, 1982, John Wright & Sons.

42. Haskell, E.W., and Stanley, H.R.: Vital hemisection of a mandibular second molar; case report, J. Am. Dent. Assoc. **102**:503, 1981.

43. Ingle, J.: Endodontics, ed. 2, Philadelphia, 1976, Lea & Febiger.

44. Jew, C.R.: A histologic evaluation of periodontal tissues adjacent to root perforations filled with Cavit, Thesis, Chicaog, 1979, Loyola University.

45. Johnson, R.H.: Basic flap management, Dent. Clin. North Am. **20**:3, 1976.

46. Kaplan, S.D., et al.: A comparison of the marginal leakage of retrograde techniques, Oral Surg. **54**:583, 1982.

47. Kimura, J.: A comparative analysis of zinc and non-zinc alloys in retrograde endodontic surgery. Part 1: Apical seal and tissue reaction, J. Endod. **8**(8):359, 1982.

48. Koch, C.: History of dental surgery, vol. 1, Chicago, 1909, National Art Publishing Co.

49. Kopp, W.K., and Resberg, H.: Apicectomy with retrograde gold foil: a new technique, N.Y. State Dent. J. **39**:8, 1973.

50. Lang, N.P., and Loe, H.: The relationship between the width of keratinized gingiva and gingival health, J. Periodontol. **43**:623, 1972.

51. Lang, N.P., et al.: Longitudinal therapeutic effects on the periodontal attachment level and pocket depth in beagle dogs, J. Peridontol. Res. **14**:418, 1979.

52. Langeland, K., Dowden, W.E., and Tronstead, L.: Biologic aspects of endodontic implants, IADR Abstr. 1972.

53. Lantz, B., and Persson, P.A.: Periodontal tissue reactions after root perforations in dog's teeth: a histologic study, Odontol. Tedsk. **75**:209, 1967.

54. LeQuire, A., Cunningham, C., and Pelleu, G.: Radiographic interpretation of experimentally produced osseous lesions of the human mandible, J. Endod. **3**:274, 1977.

55. Liggett, W.R., et al.: Light microscopy, scanning electron microscopy, and microprobe analyses of bone response to zinc and non-zinc amalgam implants, Oral Surg. **49**:263, 1980.

56. Lost, C.: Hemisektionen und Wurzel amputationene. Alternative zur Extraktion spezlell nach endodontischen Misserfolgen, Zahnaerztl. Prax **31**:47, 1980.

57. Macht, S.D., and Krizek, T.J.: Sutures and suturing—current concepts, J. Oral. Surg. **36**:710, 1978.

58. Manor, A., and Kaffe, I.: Unusual foreign body reaction to a braided silk suture: a case report, J. Periodontol. **53**:86, 1982.

59. Marcotte, L.R., Dowson, J., and Rowe, N.H.: Apical healing with retrofilling materials amalgam and gutta-percha, J. Endod. **1**:63, 1975.

60. Marosky, J.E.: Marginal leakage of temporary sealing materials used between endodontic appointments and assessed by ^{45}Ca: an in vitro study, J. Endod. **3**:110, 1977.

61. Matloff, I.R., et al.: A comparison of methods used in root canal sealability studies, Oral Surg. **53**:203, 1982.

62. Matsura, S.J.: A simplified root-end filling technique, J. Michigan State Dent. Soc. **44**:40, 1962.

63. McGivern, B.F.: Temporary filling favored over alloy in retrograde root therapy, Clin. Dent. **2**:5, 1974.

64. Moodnik, R., et al.: Retrograde amalgam filling: a scanning electron microscopic study, J. Endod. **1**:28, 1975.

65. Münch, J.: Kieffer- und Schädeltrephanationen im Altertum, Quintessenz **18**:123, 1967.

66. Nelson, E.H., Funakoshi, E., and O'Leary, T.J.: A comparison of the continuous and interrupted suturing techniques, J. Periodontol. **48**:273, 1977.

67. Nosonorvitz, D., and Brenner, M.: The major canals of the mesiobuccal root of the maxillary first and second molars, N.Y. State J. Dent. **43**:12, 1973.

68. Omnell, K.A.: Electrolytic precipitation of zinc carbonate in the jaw; an unusual complication after root resection, Oral Surg. **12**:846, 1959.

69. Oynick, J. and Oynick, T.: A study of a new material for retrograde fillings, J. Endod. **4**:203, 1978.

70. Peacock, E.E., and van Winkle, W.: Surgery and biology of wound repair, ed. 2, Philadelphia, 1976, W.B. Saunders Co.

71. Peters, D.: Evaluation of prophylactic alveolar trephination to avoid pain, J. Endod. **6:**518, 1980.

72. Racey, G.L., et al.: Comparison of a polyglycolic-polylactic acid suture to black silk and plain catgut in human oral tissues, J. Oral Surg. **36:**766, 1978.

73. Retief, D.H., Austin, J.C., and Fatti, L.P.: Pulpal response to phosphoric acid, J. Oral Pathol. **3:**114, 1972.

74. Rhein, M.L.: Amputation of roots as a radical cure in chronic alveolar abscess. Dent. Cosmos **32:**904, 1880.

75. Ring, M.: Dentistry—an illustrated history, New York, 1985, The C.V. Mosby Co./Abrams.

76. Sargenti, A.: Apico-aeration made easy by a new instrument. J. Br. Endod. **6:**49, 1972.

77. Schilder, H.: Filling root canals in three dimensions, Dent. Clin. North Am. **11:**723, 1967.

78. Schommer, J.D.: Sealing root perforations by apicoectomy, J. Canad. Dent. Assoc. **37:**350, 1971.

79. Schwartz, S.F.: Treated perforations of the pulp chamber floor; histopathologic and technological study, Thesis, 1970, University of Texas Dental Branch at Houston.

80. Seidberg, B.H.: Frequency of two mesialbuccal root canals in maxillary first molars, J. Am. Dent. Assoc. **87:**852, 1973.

81. Seltzer, S., Sinai, I., and August, D.: Periodontal effects of root perforations before and during endodontic procedures, J. Dent. Res. **49:**332, 1970.

82. Serene, T.P., McKelvy, B.D., and Scaramella, V.M.: Endodontic problems resulting from surgical fistulation: report of two cases, J. Am. Dent. Assoc. **96:**101, 1978.

83. Shoha, R.R., Dawson, J., and Richards, A.G.: Radiographic interpretation of experimentally produced bony lesions. Oral Surg. **38:**294, 1977.

84. Simon, J.H.: Incidence of periapical cysts in relation to the root canal, J. Endod. **6:**845, 1980.

85. Smukler, H., and Tagger, M.: Vital root amputation: a clinical and histologic study, J. Periodontol. **47:**324, 1976.

86. Stabholz, X., et al.: Marginal adaptation of retrograde fillings and its correlation with sealability, J. Endod. **11:**5, 1985.

87. Stakiw, J.: Wound healing and its periodontal implications, J. Can. Dent. Assoc. **42:**35, 1976.

88. Tanzilli, J., Raphael, D., and Moodnik, R.: A comparison of the marginal adaptation of retrograde techniques: a scanning electron microscopic study, Oral Surg. **50:**74, 1980.

89. Thews, M.E., Kemp, W.B., and Jones, C.R.: Aberrations in palatal root and root canal morphology of two maxillary first molars, J. Endod. **5:**94, 1979.

90. Todd, M., and Harrison, J.: An evaluation of the immediate and early sealing properties of Cavit, J. Endod. **3:**362, 1979.

91. Trowbridge, H.O., and Emling, R.C.: Inflammation, a review of the process, Philadelphia, 1978, Distribution Systems, Inc.

92. Uchin, R.A.: Surgical endodontics, Dent. Clin. North Am. **23:**637, 1979.

93. Weine, F.S.: Endodontic therapy, ed. 3, St. Louis, 1982, The C.V. Mosby Co.

94. Zartner, R., James, G.: and Burch, B.: Bone tissue response to zinc polycarboxylate cement and zinc-free amalgam, J. Endod. **2:**203, 1976.

Self-assessment questions

1. Considerations prior to surgery include
   a. Medical condition of the patient
   b. Anatomic position of the tooth for access and vision
   c. Approximation of the major neurovascular supply to the area
   d. All of the above

2. Trephination
   a. Involves burring through the cortex and cancellous bone to relieve pain
   b. Is indicated when drainage is established through the pulp system
   c. Requires the use of antibiotics
   d. Requires prior obturation of the root canal space

3. A cellulitis is treated by
   a. Large doses of antibiotics
   b. The occasional necessity of an intraoral incision
   c. Closing the tooth if sufficient drainage from the incision is established
   d. All of the above

4. Marsupialization
   a. Eliminates the need for apical surgery
   b. Is intended to reduce the size of an apical lesion
   c. Requires long-term drainage through the open root canal
   d. Delays obturation of the root canal until evidence of bone deposition is noted

5. Anatomic complications requiring apical surgery include
   a. Asymptomatic calcified teeth with no evidence of periapical pathosis
   b. A well-filled dilacerated root canal
   c. Obturated canals with extensive root resorption showing evidence of healing
   d. Fenestrated roots of endodontically treated teeth with lingering symptoms

6. Which statement is correct with regard to the following flap designs?
   a. Semilunar offers ideal access and convenience to the operative site
   b. Luebke-Ochsenbein provides definitive landmarks for repositioning and suturing the flap
   c. Triangular is ideal in the presence of veneered crowns
   d. Trapezoidal has the disadvantage that the tension of the flap maximizes the pressure of retraction

7. The endodontic surgical incision
   a. Should create beveled edges for both the horizontal and the vertical component
   b. Is a continuous cut through the mucosa, connective tissue, and periosteum
   c. Is allowed to cross an existing or created body defect
   d. Should allow the vertical component to be placed over root prominences

8. The surgical flap
   a. Is elevated to leave the periosteum attached to the cortical bone
   b. Is detached from any underlying granulation tissue of the lesion by blunt dissection
   c. Is retracted by tissue impingement for proper access to the lesion
   d. May require additional anesthetic infiltration with a vasoconstrictor to control bleeding

9. The most reliable method of determining apical position for osteotomy is
   a. Measuring tooth from radiographs
   b. Placing a piece of aluminum foil over the approximate position and radiographing
   c. Estimating average lengths of the teeth
   d. Prior knowledge of root length

10. The following statement regarding curettage is true.
    a. If necessary, the soft tissue lesion is removed in fragments to minimize bone removal
    b. Ideally removal of all potentially pathologic tissue is unnecessary
    c. The bone access is enlarged to allow curettage of all sides of the bony crypt
    d. Sectioning the apex of the root for ease of curettage is contraindicated
11. Suturing of the flap requires
    a. Inserting the needle from attached tissue to the unattached flap
    b. Placing the suture at least 1 mm on either side of incision line
    c. Spacing sutures at least 4 mm apart
    d. Placing gingival crest sutures in the papilla or lingual tissues
12. Apically sealing the root canal by surgery requires
    a. An apicoectomy with the prepared surface perpendicular to the long axis of the tooth
    b. A flap design confined to the tooth involved
    c. A Class I cavity or a modified slot preparation of the canal
    d. The use of a zinc-containing amalgam or composite to seal the canal
13. Indications for a root resection are
    a. Correctable periodontal disease involving a through-and-through furca
    b. Restorable deep carious lesions along a root wall
    c. Perforation of one root in a multirooted tooth
    d. A nonnegotiable canal of a multirooted tooth amenable to apical surgery
14. Postoperatively, a patient should anticipate
    a. Excessive bleeding
    b. Pain requiring strong analgesics
    c. Mild swelling minimized by ice pack application
    d. Antibiotic therapy to prevent infection

19

THE MANAGEMENT OF PAIN AND ANXIETY

STANLEY F. MALAMED

The problem of managing pain and anxiety in the practice of dentistry is a significant one. Studies have demonstrated that the major reason why over 50% of adult Americans do not seek routine dental care is a fear of pain. Interviews with patients indicate that although they may not be in pain when they visit their dentist the overwhelming majority of patients truly believe that at some time during a typical dental appointment they will experience pain. The person most frequently cited as responsible for inflicting this discomfort is the dentist.

Pain and anxiety are entirely different problems, yet at the same time they are closely related. Pain produced by dental therapy can usually be minimized or entirely eliminated through careful patient management and the judicious use of the techniques of pain control, especially local anesthesia. Anxiety too can usually be managed effectively; however, before anxiety can be managed, it must first be recognized. Discovery of the cause of a patient's anxiety is a major factor in management of the problem. Once aware of the situation, the contemporary dentist has many techniques available to manage the patient.

In most areas of dental therapy, the problem of anxiety control is of greater importance than the management of pain. Pain control is usually readily achieved through local anesthetic administration. Once effective pain control has been established anxiety control usually becomes more readily achievable. In endodontic therapy, more than in any other specialty of dentistry, pain control often proves to be more difficult a problem than the management of anxiety. Because of this difficulty in achieving effective pain control, the patient undergoing endodontic therapy often looks upon the upcoming experience with a great deal of apprehension.

The following discussion will cover the problems of both pain control and anxiety control.

PAIN CONTROL

Although the achievement of adequate pain control for endodontic therapy is not usually difficult, there appear to be all too many instances when a satisfactory result eludes the doctor. The most likely explanation for this greater percentage of anesthetic failures in endodontics than in other dental therapy areas lies in the tissue changes that commonly develop in and around pulpally involved teeth. To help the doctor better understand the problems associated with pain control in endodontics, a review of the mode of action of local anesthetics is presented.

Local anesthetics—how they work

The commonly employed injectable local anesthetics are of a weakly basic nature and are poorly soluble in water. To make them clinically useful, they are combined with hydrochloric acid to form hydrochloride salts, which are soluble in water and acid in reaction.

When placed into solution, the salts of local anesthetic compounds exist in two forms: an uncharged molecule (RN) and a positively charged cation (RNH$^+$). The relative proportion of each form will depend on the pH of the solution in the cartridge and tissue and on the pK$_a$ of the specific anesthetic compound. The pK$_a$ is the pH value at which a compound contains equal amounts of un-ionized base form and ionized cation form.

The pK$_a$ for a given anesthetic agent is constant. The values for several local anesthetics are listed in Table 19-1. Because pK$_a$ is a constant, the relative proportion of free base (RN) and charged cation (RNH$^+$) in the local anesthetic solution will depend on the pH of the solution.

$$RNH^+ \rightleftharpoons RN + H^+$$

As the pH of a solution is decreased, the hydrogen ion (H$^+$) concentration is increased and the equilibrium in the equation shifts toward the charged cationic form. Proportionally more cation will be present than free base. If the pH of the solution is increased, the H$^+$ concentration is decreased and a proportionally greater percentage of the local anesthetic agent will exist in the free base form.

At a normal tissue pH of 7.4, it can be seen (Table 19-1) that there exists a greater proportion of anesthetic cation than of anesthetic base. Both forms of the anesthetic drug are essential for anesthetic activity.[26,27]

For years it was thought that the un-ionized base form of the anesthetic solution was solely responsible for producing nerve block. Studies demonstrated that local anesthetic agents were more effective when prepared as alkaline solutions.[25] The cationic form was thought to be merely a convenient water-soluble vehicle, devoid of any anesthetic properties, for dispersion of the solution through tissues. It has been demonstrated, however, that several factors are involved in the ultimate anesthetic profile of a compound. These include (1) diffusion of the compound through the lipid-rich nerve sheath (*pK$_a$* and *lipid solubility*) and (2) binding of the compound at the receptor site (*protein binding, nonnervous tissue diffusibility,* and *intrinsic vasodilator activity*).[9] (See Table 19-2.) Researchers[26,27] carried out studies evaluating the relationship between the pH of solutions, the presence or absence of a nerve sheath, and local anesthetic activity. They concluded that both forms of the anesthetic molecule are involved in the process of nerve sheath penetration and conduction block. The lipid-soluble uncharged (RN) base diffuses more easily through the nerve sheath than does the cationic (RNH$^+$) form. Clinically, local anesthetic agents with a lower pK$_a$ (more uncharged RN molecules) possess a more rapid onset of action than do agents with a higher pK$_a$ (Table 19-1).

TABLE 19-1. Dissociation constants (pK$_a$) of local anesthetics

Agent	pK$_a$	% base (RN) at pH 7.4	Approximate onset of action (min)
Mepivacaine	7.6	40	2 to 4
Etidocaine	7.7	33	2 to 4
Articaine	7.8	29	2 to 4
Lidocaine	7.9	25	2 to 4
Prilocaine	7.9	25	2 to 4
Bupivacaine	8.1	18	5 to 8
Tetracaine	8.5	8	10 to 15
Chloro-procaine	8.7	6	10 to 15
Procaine	9.1	2	14 to 18

The degree of lipid solubility appears to be important in determining the intrinsic anesthetic potency of a local anesthetic.

Table 19-3 lists the approximate lipid solubilities of various agents. Increased lipid solubility permits the anesthetic to penetrate the nerve membrane (which is 90% lipid) more easily.[5] This is reflected biologically as increased potency. Agents with greater lipid solubility produce more effective conduction blockade at lower concentrations than do the less soluble agents.

After penetration of the nerve sheath, a reequilibrium occurs between the base and the cationic forms. Now, at the cell membrane itself, the charged cation form binds to the protein receptor site. Protein binding of the anesthetic molecule is responsible for (1) suppression of the electrophysiologic events occurring in peripheral nerve block and (2) the duration of anesthetic activity. Proteins comprise approximately 10% of the nerve membrane. Local anesthetic agents (e.g., etidocaine and bupivacaine) that demonstrate a greater degree of protein binding (Table 19-4) than do others (e.g., procaine) appear to attach more securely to the protein receptor sites and possess a longer duration of action.

Fig. 19-1 illustrates the sequence of events involved in peripheral nerve block in normal tissues. At a normal pH of approximately 7.4, an anesthetic solution with a pK$_a$ of 7.9 will reach equilibrium with approximately 75% of its molecules in the charged cationic form and 25% in the base form. The base form can pass through the diffusion barrier represented by the nerve sheath (epineurium) more readily than can the cationic form. Once the nerve sheath has been penetrated, the RN molecules encounter a pH of 7.4 in the intracellular tissues surrounding the nerve membrane. The pH of the tissues within the epineurium and surrounding the nerve itself remains quite uniform even in the presence of marked changes in pH of extracellular tissues. This is due to the fact that the H$^+$, like the anesthetic cation, cannot easily penetrate tissues. The pH of extracellular fluid may therefore differ from the pH at the nerve membrane, and similarly the proportions of anesthetic base and cation at these sites may differ. In this environment reequilibrium occurs and approximately 75% of the base

TABLE 19-2. Summary of factors affecting local anesthetic action

Factor	Action affected	Description
pK$_a$	Onset	Lower pK$_a$ = More rapid onset of action; more RN molecules present to diffuse through nerve sheath; thus onset time is decreased
Lipid solubility	Anesthetic potency	Increased lipid solubility = Increased potency (Example: procaine = 1; etidocaine = 140) Etidocaine produces conduction blockade at very low concentrations whereas procaine poorly suppresses nerve conduction, even at higher concentrations
Protein binding	Duration	Increased protein binding allows anesthetic cations (RNH$^+$) to be more firmly attached to proteins located at receptor sites; thus duration of action is increased
Nonnervous tissue diffusibility	Onset	Increased diffusibility = Decreased time of onset
Vasodilator activity	Anesthetic potency and duration	Greater vasodilator activity = Increased blood flow to region = Rapid removal of anesthetic molecules from injection site; thus decreased anesthetic potency and decreased duration.

TABLE 19-3. Lipid solubility of local anesthetics

Agent	Approximate lipid solubility	Usual effective concentration (%)
Procaine	1	2 to 4
Mepivacaine	1	2 to 3
Prilocaine	1.5	4
Lidocaine	4	2
Bupivacaine	30	0.5 to 0.75
Tetracaine	80	0.15
Etidocaine	140	0.5 to 0.75
Articaine	—	—
Chloro-procaine	—	—

TABLE 19-4. Protein binding characteristics and duration of action

Agent	Approximate protein binding	Approximate duration of action (min)
Procaine	5	60 to 90
Prilocaine	55	100 to 240
Lidocaine	65	90 to 200
Mepivacaine	75	120 to 240
Tetracaine	85	180 to 600
Etidocaine	94	180 to 600
Bupivacaine	95	180 to 600
Articaine	95	—
Chloro-procaine	—	—

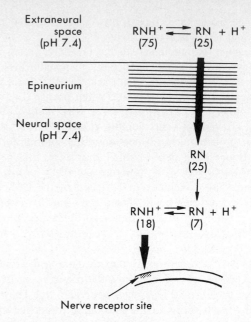

FIG. 19-1. Mode of action of a local anesthetic in normal tissue (pH 7.4). The anesthetic, with a pK_a of 7.9 is deposited in the extraneural tissues. Equilibrium occurs with approximately 75% of the molecules in the charged cationic form and 25% in base form. (Numbers in parentheses represent the proportion of anesthetic cation and base in extracellular and neurals compartments.)

reverts to the cation form, attaching to the receptor sites and producing neural blockade.

The pulpally involved tooth

The problem of inadequate pain control during endodontic therapy can be explained, in part, through alterations in periapical tissues. Pulpal and periapical pathologic conditions (inflammation and/or infection) lead to a decrease of the tissue pH in the region surrounding the involved tooth below what is normally found. Pus has a pH of 5.5 to 5.6. Because of its decreased pH, the dissociation of the anesthetic solution favors the formation of a much higher proportion of cation relative to free base (Fig. 19-2). About 99% of a given agent (with a pK_a of 7.9) will be in the cationic form. Unfortunately the electrically charged RNH^+ cations are unable to migrate through the neural sheath without the assistance of the uncharged anesthetic base, the form that is in very short supply in this situation. Therefore fewer anesthetic molecules reach the nerve membrane, where the intracellular pH remains normal and reequilibrium between base and cation can occur. Fewer cations are present, with a greater likelihood that incomplete anesthesia will develop.

Solutions

One possible method of obtaining more intense anesthesia in an area of infection would be to deposit a greater volume of anesthetic into the region. A greater number of free base molecules would be liberated, with greater diffusion through the nerve sheath and a greater likelihood that adequate pain control would develop.

Although this procedure is somewhat effective, injection of anesthetic solutions into areas of infection is undesirable because of the possibility of the spread of infection to a previously noncontaminated area. Deposition of the anesthetic solution into an area at a distance from the involved tooth is more likely to accomplish the goal of adequate pain control, because of the normal tissue conditions that exist there. Regional nerve block anesthesia will therefore be a major factor in pain control for endodontically involved teeth.

There are also occasions, fortunately rare, when even regional block anesthesia, at a distance from the infected tooth, will fail to produce adequate pain control. Omitting for a moment the most likely cause of this situation, improper injection technique, Najjar[23] has proposed that inadequate pain control may be due to the fact that morphologic changes (e.g., neurodegenerative changes in the axon or the presence of inflammatory mediators) are developing. He states that morphologic changes in inflamed nerve, even at a distance from the actual inflammatory site, appear to be a significant barrier for normal electrolyte exchange at the membrane level. The net result is a reinforcement of a nerve fiber's ability to generate action potentials. Studies[6,28] have demonstrated that inflammation produces a potentiation of peripheral nerve excitability.

Yet another situation, also unfortunate, in endodontic pain control relates to the inflamed tooth that when anes-

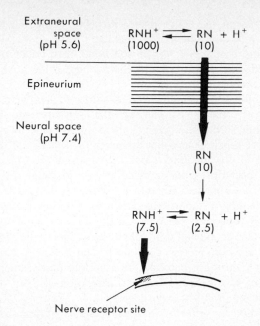

Extraneural space (pH 5.6)

$$RNH^+ \rightleftarrows RN + H^+$$
$$(1000) \quad (10)$$

Epineurium

Neural space (pH 7.4)

RN (10)

$$RNH^+ \rightleftarrows RN + H^+$$
$$(7.5) \quad (2.5)$$

Nerve receptor site

FIG. 19-2. Mode of action of a local anesthetic in an inflamed/infected area. The anesthetic, with a pK_a of 7.9, is deposited in the extraneural tissues (pH of 5.6). Equilibrium develops with approximately 99% of solution in the cationic form. Fewer anesthetic molecules pass through the epineurium to the neural space. The pH in the neural space is 7.4, and molecules reequilibrate. However, an insufficient number of molecules may be present to produce profound clinical anesthesia.

thetized becomes asymptomatic but, on attempts to gain access to the pulp chamber and canals, becomes exquisitely sensitive to manipulation. Although no entirely satisfactory explanation exists for this circumstance, it may be explainable on the basis of an increase in the rate of stimulation to the nerve endings that occurs with use of the high- or low-speed handpiece. The degree of neural blockade may be adequate for a lower level of stimulation prior to preparation, yet it proves inadequate to block completely the rapid flood of impulses arising with use of the handpiece. This is equivalent to the so-called "anesthetic window" seen in obstetric anesthesia following epidural nerve block during delivery. The degree of pain control is quite adequate except for the most intense muscular contractions. The same intense increase in the rate of neural stimulation is thought to be responsible for this phenomenon in endodontics.

Local anesthesia—techniques

The tissue changes and their possible actions on the effectiveness of local anesthetic solutions will influence the choice of local anesthesia to be used in attempts to prevent discomfort during therapy. Many methods are available for achieving pain control: local infiltration, regional nerve block, mandibular block, plus additional techniques.

Local infiltration (supraperiosteal injection). Local infiltration anesthesia may be described as a technique in which anesthetic solution is deposited *into* the area of treatment.[20] Small, terminal nerve fibers in the region are blocked and thus rendered incapable of transmitting impulses. Local infiltration anesthesia is commonly employed in attempts to achieve pulpal anesthesia of maxillary teeth. Because of the ability of local anesthetic solutions to diffuse through periosteum and the relatively porous cancellous bone of the maxilla this method of pain control will prove effective in endodontic procedures when infection (accompanied by local inflammation) is *not* present. Very often, however, when infection *is* present at the onset of an endodontic case and other techniques of pain control must be relied on initially, infiltration anesthesia may prove effective at subsequent visits provided effective cleaning and shaping of the root canals have been accomplished.

Infiltration anesthesia is rarely effective in the adult mandible posterior to the lateral incisors because of the inability of the anesthetic solution to penetrate the more dense cortical bone. It can be effective, however, in a significant number of adults in the central and lateral incisor region and, to a lesser degree, in the area of the canines.

In pediatric dentistry, infiltration anesthesia in the mandible is more successful. As a general rule, infiltration anesthesia in the mandible will be successful as long as the primary tooth remains. Once the tooth is replaced by a permanent tooth, regional block anesthesia should be considered.

In infiltration anesthesia the target area for deposition of the anesthetic solution is the apex of the tooth to be treated. Only 0.5 to 1 ml of solution need be deposited for adequate pain control. Approximately 3 to 4 minutes is allowed to elapse before starting the procedure. On rare occasion, adequate pulpal anesthesia, even on nonpulpally involved teeth, is not achieved following infiltration. From my clinical experience it appears that the most common cause of this is the failure on the part of the dentist to deposit the anesthetic solution at the apical region of the tooth. The maxillary central incisor and canine, with relatively long roots, are most frequently involved in this situation. A 27-gauge 1-inch needle is recommended.

Regional nerve block. Because of the nature of endodontically involved teeth, it is quite possible that infiltration anesthesia will prove ineffective in preventing the transmission of painful stimuli. In these situations regional nerve block anesthesia is recommended. Nerve block is defined as a method of achieving regional anesthesia by depositing a suitable local anesthetic solution close to a main nerve trunk, thus preventing afferent impulses from traveling centrally beyond that point.[20] Nerve block anesthesia is likely to be successful when infiltration has failed. This is because the anesthetic solution is being deposited some distance from the inflamed or infected tissue, where tissue pH and other factors are more nearly normal.

Several types of nerve block are useful in dentistry. Space does not allow for a detailed description of each of these, but a review of their effects does follow.

Maxillary anesthesia. Maxillary nerves that can be anesthetized include the posterior superior alveolar, the anterior superior alveolar, the greater palatine, the nasopalatine and the second division or maxillary.

The *posterior superior alveolar* (PSA) nerve block, also called the zygomatic or tuberosity block, is indicated when pulpal anesthesia is required for the maxillary third, second, and first molars, with the exclusion of the mesial-buccal root of the first molar. In addition, the underlying buccal alveolar process, periosteum, connective tissue, and mucous membranes are anesthetized. During endodontic therapy, palatal infiltration is usually required for anesthesia of the palatal soft tissues. Infiltration of 0.5 ml into the buccal fold above the mesiobuccal root of the first molar is required if the first molar is to be treated.

The *infraorbital* nerve block is an easy injection to administer and produces anesthesia of three nerves: the infraorbital, anterior superior alveolar, and middle superior alveolar. Dentally this block provides pulpal anesthesia for the central and lateral incisors, canine, premolars, and mesial-buccal root of the maxillary first molar, including the bony support and the soft tissues on the buccal surface. Palatal infiltration is usually required for anesthesia of the palatal soft tissues.

In both the posterior superior alveolar and the infraorbital blocks, 0.9 ml of anesthetic solution is deposited at the target area. A 25-gauge 1 5/8-inch needle is employed in the infraorbital nerve block while a 25- or 27-gauge, 1-inch needle is recommended for the PSA nerve block.

Palatal anesthesia is often required during endodontic therapy and is also needed around the gingival margins of the tooth to be clamped. An adequate level can be obtained by infiltrating 0.3 ml of anesthetic solution into the palatal gingiva 3 to 5 mm below the gingival margin.

Larger areas of the palate will seldom have to be anesthetized; but when required, two nerve blocks are readily available: the greater palatine and the nasopalatine.

The *greater* (or anterior) *palatine* nerve block provides anesthesia of both the hard and the soft tissues ranging from the third molar as far anterior as the first premolar. In the region of the first premolar, partial anesthesia may be encountered as branches of the nasopalatine nerve are met.

The *nasopalatine nerve* enters the palate through the incisive foramen, located in the midline just palatal to the central incisors and directly beneath the incisive papilla. It provides sensory innervation to the hard and soft tissues of the premaxilla as far distal as the first premolar, where fibers from the greater palatine nerve are encountered. A 27-gauge 1-inch needle is recommended for both injections.

Because of the density of the palatal soft tissues and their firm attachment to underlying bone, palatal injections are considered potentially traumatic. Palatal anesthesia can be produced with a minimum of discomfort if care is taken throughout the procedure to ensure adequate topical anesthesia, adequate pressure, slow penetration of tissues, continual slow deposition of solution, and injection of not more than 0.5 ml of solution.

A *maxillary* or *second division* nerve block, though rarely necessary, should be considered when other techniques of pain control prove inadequate because of infection accompanied by inflammation. This block provides anesthesia of the entire maxillary nerve peripheral to the site of injection: pulps of all maxillary teeth on the side of injection; buccal soft tissues and bone; hard palate on the injected side; and upper lip, cheek, side of the nose, and lower eyelid.

Two intraoral techniques are available to achieve a maxillary nerve block.[22,25] The *first*, the high tuberosity injection, follows the same path as the posterior superior alveolar nerve block except that the depth of needle insertion is greater in the maxillary block (1 1/4 inch vs. 1/2 to 3/4 inch in the posterior superior alveolar). A 25-gauge 1 5/8-inch needle is used, and 1.8 ml of solution is deposited. The *second* intraoral approach[22] involves entering the greater palatine foramen, which is usually located palatally between the second and third maxillary molars at the junction of the alveolar process and the palatal bone. A 1 5/8-inch 25-gauge needle is carefully inserted into the foramen to a depth of 1 1/2 inches. Following aspiration, 1.8 ml of anesthetic solution is slowly deposited.

Mandibular anesthesia. Management of pain in the mandible for pulpal anesthesia is normally achieved through the inferior alveolar nerve block. In addition, anesthesia of the buccal soft tissues and bone anterior to the mandibular molars is provided. The lingual nerve is usually anesthetized along with the inferior alveolar nerve. Anesthesia is achieved in the anterior two thirds of the tongue, the floor of the oral cavity, and the mucous membrane and mucoperiosteum on the lingual side of the mandible. A 25-gauge 1 5/8-inch needle is used and, following careful aspiration, 1.5 ml of anesthetic solution is deposited.

Successful inferior alveolar and lingual nerve block will provide anesthesia to all mandibular tissues except the buccal mucous membrane and mucoperiosteum over the molars. If anesthesia of this region is required, the buccal nerve must be blocked. The buccal nerve is not anesthetized during the inferior alveolar nerve block because it is a branch of the anterior division of the mandibular nerve; by contrast, the inferior alveolar and lingual nerves are branches of the posterior division. To block the buccal nerve, one uses a 25-gauge 1- or 1 5/8-inch needle and deposits 0.3 ml of anesthetic solution into the mucosa distal and buccal to the last molar in the arch.

In the absence of pulpal or periapical pathosis, inferior alveolar nerve block will be successful (adequate pain control achieved) 80% to 85% of the time. Its rate of success diminishes significantly when pathologic conditions exist. Because of the density of bone in the adult mandible, infiltration anesthesia is of little value posterior to the lateral incisors; thus block anesthesia becomes the primary avenue of achieving pain control. When block anesthesia proves ineffective, fewer alternative techniques are available. There are, however, other nerve blocks that may work in the mandible.

The incisive and mental nerves are terminal branches of the inferior alveolar nerve that arise at the mental foramen. The mental nerve, exiting from the mental foramen, provides sensory innervation to the skin of the lower lip and chin regions and the mucous membrane lining the lower lip; the incisive nerve, remaining within the mandibular canal, provides sensory innervation to the pulps of the premolars, canine, and incisors and the bone anterior to the mental foramen. Anesthesia of the region served by the *incisive nerve* should be considered when endodontic therapy is contemplated on a tooth anterior to the mental foramen. A 25- or 27-gauge 1-inch needle is employed, and 0.5 to 1 ml of anesthetic solution is deposited into the mental foramen. Finger pressure applied at the site of injection for 1 or 2 minutes following deposition ensures entry of solution into the mental foramen.

As mentioned previously, infiltration anesthesia is usually not effective in achieving pulpal anesthesia in the mandible. The sole exception is in the region of the lateral and central incisor, where up to 1 ml of anesthetic solution may be deposited into the mucobuccal fold at the level of the apex of the tooth. A 27-gauge 1-inch needle is recommended.

On occasion, adequate pain control is achieved in the mandible except in isolated areas. Usually the area involved is the mesial root of the first molar. Successful pulpal anesthesia of third molars is frequently difficult to achieve because of the multiplicity of accessory innervations that are thought to exist. Indeed, adequate anesthesia is easier to obtain for third molar extraction than for restorative or endodontic procedures.

The mesial portion of the mandibular first molar not uncommonly is sensitive to painful stimuli when all other portions of the same tooth and adjacent structures are insensitive. Although many theories (involving the cervical accessory and transverse neck nerves) have been put forward to explain this situation, the mylohyoid nerve (a branch of the posterior division of the mandibular nerve) appears to be the culprit.[10] The mylohyoid nerve branches off the inferior alveolar nerve well above the inferior alveolar's entry into the mandibular foramen. It passes along the lingual border of the mandible in the mylohyoid groove, sending motor fibers to the anterior belly of the diagastric muscle. It has been demonstrated to contain sensory fibers on occasion, that branch off and enter the body of the mandible through small foramina on the lingual border of the mandible at about the second molar. These fibers presumably pass anteriorly through the body of the mandible to the mesial root of the first molar.

Whether or not the mylohyoid nerve is responsible, the problem of sensitivity in the inflamed first molar pulp can be alleviated with a 27-gauge 1-inch needle and 0.5 ml of anesthetic solution deposited against the lingual side of the mandible at the level of the apex of the mandibular *second* molar. Within 2 to 3 minutes, adequate anesthesia should be present. Although most often observed with the first molar, the problem of partial anesthesia can occur with other teeth also. Management consists of depositing 0.5 ml of solution at the apex of the tooth immediately *distal* to the involved tooth.

Mandibular block. A true mandibular block injection, one that provides adequate anesthesia of all sensory portions of the mandibular nerve (buccal, inferior alveolar, lingual, mylohyoid), can be readily achieved through a technique called the *Gow-Gates mandibular block*.[13,15] The target area is higher than in the traditional inferior alveolar block technique: the lateral side of the neck of the mandibular condyle below the insertion of the lateral pterygoid muscle[13] (Fig. 19-3).

For this reason alone the success rate with the Gow-Gates mandibular block procedure can be expected to be greater than that with the traditional technique. Indeed, 97.25% of patients receiving the Gow-Gates block did not

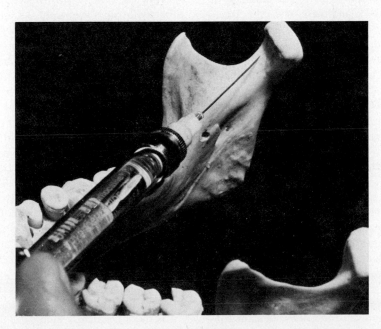

FIG. 19-3. Target area in the Gow-Gates technique is the lateral aspect of the neck of the condyle. (From Malamed, S.F.: Handbook of local anesthesia, ed. 2, St. Louis, 1986, The C.V. Mosby Co.)

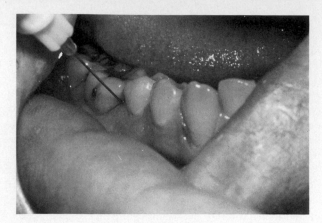

FIG. 19-4. To achieve anesthesia of the first molar, separate injections are required on the mesial and distal roots. (From Malamed, S.F.: Oral Surg. **53:**118, 1982.)

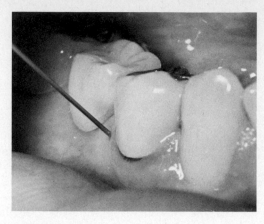

FIG. 19-5. In intraseptal injection a 27-gauge, 1-inch needle is inserted into the intraseptal bone distal to the tooth to be anesthetized. (From Malamed, S.F.: Handbook of local anesthesia, ed. 2, St. Louis, 1986, The C.V. Mosby Co.)

require supplemental anesthesia.[17] Other advantages of the Gow-Gates technique include a low positive aspiration rate (1.8%, compared with approximately 10% in the traditional technique) and no need for supplemental anesthesia (i.e., to the mylohyoid).

Two other techniques have been described that are effective in producing mandibular anesthesia, the PDL injection (described below) and the Akinosi technique. The Akinosi (closed mouth) technique permits mandibular anesthesia to be obtained reliably in patients with extremely limited mandibular opening. It has proved effective in patients with trismus and/or severe infection.

Akinosi technique.[1,14] Another novel approach to mandibular anesthesia was described in 1977 by Akinosi. This technique, a closed-mouth approach to mandibular anesthesia, is of particular importance in those situations in which limited opening of the mandible is possible, due to infection, trauma, trismus, or other causes. Significant in endodontic therapy because of the possible presence of edema and/or infection, the Akinosi technique employs a 25-gauge long dental needle held in the maxillary buccal fold on the side of injection. Needle insertion occurs in the soft tissue on the lingual aspect of the mandibular ramus at a site adjacent to the maxillary tuberosity. The needle passes almost parallel to the mandibular ramus for a distance of 25 mm, at which point aspiration is attempted, and if negative, 1.8 ml of anesthetic solution deposited. The primary disadvantage to the Akinosi technique is the absence of a bony contact to provide a landmark prior to injection of solution. However, the Akinosi mandibular block provides the clinician with a success rate approaching 80% to 85% in a situation (limited or no opening) in which failure was almost guaranteed in the past.

Additional local anesthetic procedures

On occasion, the local anesthetic techniques just described will fail to produce a desired degree of pain control. There are additional local anesthetic techniques that may then be employed to remedy the situation: the (1) periodontal ligament (PDL) injection, (2) intraseptal injec-

tion, (3) intrapulpal injection, and (4) intraosseous injection.

Periodontal ligament injection. The PDL (or intraligamentary) injection is frequently used in restorative dentistry whenever isolated areas of inadequate anesthesia are present.[31] It may also be used alone to achieve adequate pulpal anesthesia in isolated mandibular teeth.[18] Advantages to its use in this manner include adequate pulpal anesthesia with a minimal volume of solution (0.2 to 0.4 ml) and the absence of lingual and lower lip anesthesia.

This technique may also prove effective in endodontically involved teeth. A 27-gauge short needle is firmly placed between the periodontal ligament and the tooth to be anesthetized. With the needle bevel facing the root of the tooth, approximately 0.2 ml of anesthetic solution is deposited. Successful PDL anesthesia is usually indicated by resistance to the deposit of solution and by blanching of the tissues (ischemia) on injection. Multirooted teeth receive the injection (0.2 ml) on each root (Fig. 19-4).

Excessive volume of anesthetic can lead to complications, such as extrusion of the tooth.[24] Recently several devices (e.g., Ligmaject, Peripress) have been marketed to aid in this injection. Although they are effective, their success rate with this injection is equivalent to that with conventional-type syringes. The PDL injection is usually quite valuable as an adjunct to conventional nerve block techniques in endodontically involved teeth. Perhaps the only contraindication to its use would be insertion of the needle and deposition of anesthetic solution into an infected area.

Intraseptal injection. This injection, described by Saadoun and Malamed,[29] is a variation of the intraosseous injection.

A 27-gauge 1-inch needle is inserted into the intraseptal tissue in the area to be anesthetized (Fig. 19-5). Although it is more frequently employed than the intraosseous injection, its success rate is not as high. Because of the decreased bone density, it is more successful in younger patients. The needle must be firmly advanced into the

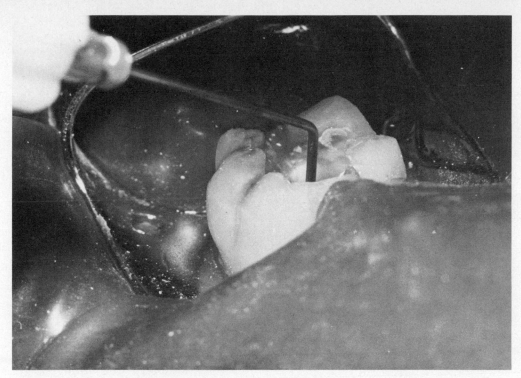

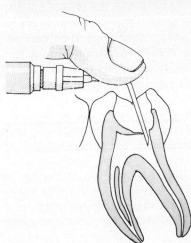

FIG. 19-6. In an intrapulpal injection the needle is inserted directly into the pulp chamber or a specific root canal. Ideally resistance is met and the solution is expressed under pressure.

cortical plate of bone. The soft tissues must be anesthetized prior to the needle insertion into bone. On injection, there must be considerable resistance to the advance of the plunger. Ease of administration usually means that the needle is located in the soft tissues, not bone. Resistance to injection as the solution is slowly forced under pressure into the cancellous bone is desirable. Enough solution must be administered to reach the periapical fibers (approximately 0.3 to 0.5 ml is recommended).

Intrapulpal injection. When the pulp chamber of a tooth has been exposed, either surgically or pathologically, the intrapulpal injection may be used to achieve adequate pain control.

A 25- or 27-gauge 1- or 1⅝-inch needle is inserted into the pulp chamber or specific root canal as needed. Ideally the needle will be firmly wedged into the chamber or canal (Fig. 19-6). On injection, significant resistance is met and

the solution must be inserted under pressure. Anesthesia is produced by the action of the anesthetic solution and by the applied pressure. There may be an initial brief period of sensitivity as the injection is started; but anesthesia usually occurs immediately thereafter, and instrumentation can proceed painlessly. When a snug fit of the needle in the canal is not possible, two procedures are used: (1) With the needle in the canal, warm white gutta-percha is inserted around it. After cooling, injection under pressure may proceed. (2) The anesthetic solution can be deposited in the chamber or canal, with anesthesia being produced by the chemical actions of the solution only. At least 30 seconds should elapse before an attempt is made to proceed with instrumentation. The former technique is preferred.

Intraosseous injection. Though rarely employed, the intraosseous injection can be effective in obtaining anes-

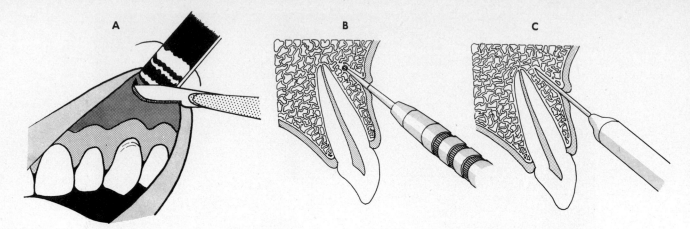

FIG. 19-7. An intraosseous anesthetic is used to obtain adequate pulpal obtundation only when other techniques have failed. The soft tissue over the site has previously been anesthetized through local infiltration. **A,** An incision is made down to the periosteum. **B,** By means of a small (½ or 1) round bur, a hole is opened in the cortical plate. **C,** A 25-gauge needle is placed in the opening, and anesthetic solution is deposited.

thesia adequate to permit opening of the pulp chamber, at which time intrapulpal anesthesia can be administered

To administer an intraosseous injection properly, the dentist must anesthetize the soft tissues and bone overlying the apical region of the tooth through local infiltration. A small incision (1 to 3 mm) is made down to the periosteum. By means of a small (no. ½ or 1) round bur, a hole is opened through the dense cortical plate of bone to the cancellous bone. Then with a 25-gauge (1-inch) needle in the opening, approximately 1 ml of anesthetic solution is deposited (Fig. 19-7).

On occasion, a patient will present with a truly "hot" tooth. Then local infiltration, regional block anesthesia, and the other techniques described may prove ineffective. Intrapulpal anesthesia cannot be utilized until the pulp chamber is opened, which may not be immediately possible. The following sequence of treatment may be of value in this situation:

1. If a high-speed bur proves highly traumatic, a low-speed bur (though more time consuming) may be less traumatic.
2. Inhalation or intravenous sedation may help to allay anxieties and moderate the patient's responses to painful stimuli.
3. When the pulp chamber has been opened, direct intrapulpal anesthesia usually can be administered and will prove effective.
4. If a high level of pain persists, preventing further instrumentation, I have taken a small cotton pellet saturated with a non-vasoconstrictor-containing local anesthetic solution (not topical anesthetic) and placed it loosely in the tooth preparation. After a 30-second delay the pellet is pressed more snugly into the area of the pulpal exposure. Some sensitivity may exist, but within 2 or 3 minutes the area becomes insensitive. The pellet is removed, and direct intrapulpal injection ensures adequate anesthesia.

Pain control—additional considerations

In the overwhelming majority of endodontic procedures, difficulty controlling pain usually exists at the first appointment only. When the canals have been located and tissues extirpated, the requirement for pain control becomes minimal. Soft tissue anesthesia may be necessary for rubber dam application; however, if adequate tooth structure exists, even this is unnecessary. Instrumentation within a thoroughly debrided canal seldom requires anesthesia. Overextension of files beyond the apical foramen may produce a sensitivity that serves as an indicator to the doctor. If the patient overresponds to instrumentation, local infiltration or direct intrapulpal injection can be used.

In the filling of canals, considerable pressure may be exerted during condensation of the filling materials and may produce patient discomfort and/or pain. Local infiltration anesthesia should be considered before this procedure is started.

The following sequence of anesthetic techniques will usually lead to effective pain control: (1) infiltration anesthesia (when possible), (2) regional nerve block anesthesia, (3) periodontal ligament injection, (4) intraseptal anesthesia, (5) intrapulpal anesthesia, (6) intraosseous injection, and (7) prayer.

"Electronic anesthesia" has recently gained attention in dental anesthesia. Devices modified from TENS (transcutaneous electrical nerve stimulators) have been used with considerable initial success in providing effective pain control in the oral cavity for a variety of dental procedures, including extirpation of tissue from pulpally involved teeth. These devices act by providing a constant mild stimulus of the nerve trunk, thereby "overloading" it so that noxious stimuli are unable to reach the cerebral cortex, where they are interpreted as painful by the patient. I have achieved successful anesthesia in mildly inflamed teeth in which endodontic procedures were to be initiated. Two such devices currently marketed include the H-wave Dental Unit* and The Comfort Machine.† Considerable clinical research remains to be done in evaluating this novel concept and these devices before any recommendation concerning their efficacy in endodontics can be forthcoming. However, these devices are especially attractive in providing clinical pain control for the "needle-phobic" dental patient.

Postoperative pain

Postoperative pain must also be considered. Quite frequently after endodontic treatment a patient will report varying degrees of discomfort. Most often the discomfort is described as a "soreness" that becomes less intense as time elapses. No treatment is normally required aside from a mild analgesic such as aspirin, acetaminophen, or a nonsteroidal anti-inflammatory agent.

If more intense pain develops in the postoperative period, the prudent doctor will prescribe two analgesics. One prescription is for a milder, nonnarcotic analgesic such as those just mentioned. The patient should be advised to take these medications for pain. In the event that the pain is not relieved by these agents, the second prescription, for a more potent narcotic containing analgesic, should be employed. Examples include aspirin or acetaminophen and codeine combinations and are listed in Table 12-3. Prescribing of these drugs *before* pain starts will go far to prevent many unnecessary middle-of-the night telephone calls from worried patients. An ounce of prevention is well worth a pound of cure.

Postoperative discomfort commonly becomes most bothersome when the patient attempts to go to sleep. During the day, with many activities interacting to occupy the patient's thoughts, there is less discomfort sensed. However, on retiring to bed, the patient is more free to consider the discomfort in the tooth. Pain becomes a greater problem at this time. With this in mind, the doctor should advise taking pain medications about an hour before retiring to bed. Most oral medications require at least 30 minutes to exert any action and approximately 60 minutes for maximal effect.

ANXIETY CONTROL

There are many causes of anxiety related to the dental situation; but that most frequently encountered is the fear of pain. As mentioned earlier, in no specialty of dentistry is the problem of pain control more acute than in endodontics. Because of this many patients are unusually apprehensive when encountering endodontic therapy.

Yet most adult patients will not openly express their fears to the doctor. Rather they will sit in the dental chair, undergo dental therapy, and "grin and bear it" or "take it like a man." Repression of these anxieties is not always innocuous. Indeed, many potentially life-threatening situations may be precipitated in this manner. Situations ranging from the hyperventilation syndrome and vasodepressor syncope to myocardial infarction have been encountered.

Although usually of a relatively benign nature, syncope and hyperventilation can, if improperly managed, lead to significant morbidity and possibly mortality.

Children, by contrast, do not have the inhibitions adults do concerning the expression of apprehension. A child faced with an unpleasant situation will verbalize: crying or screaming, perhaps even biting, kicking, or moving about in the dental chair. Significantly, healthy younger children rarely faint or hyperventilate.

Perhaps even more significant are the effects of unrecognized and unmanaged anxiety on the medically compromised patient. Patients with cardiovascular, respiratory, neurologic, and other metabolic disorders (thyroid disease, diabetes mellitus, adrenal disorders) cannot tolerate undue stress normally. They therefore represent an increased risk during dental therapy if they become apprehensive or feel pain.

Bennett[4] has stated, and I fully agree, that the greater the medical risk of the patient the more important it is to achieve adequate control of both pain and anxiety. The following discussion will present methods of recognizing anxiety in dental patients and will review the more common techniques of sedation, with special emphasis on their use during endodontic therapy.

Recognition of anxiety

Most patients do not admit to being apprehensive about their inpending dental treatment; therefore the task of exposing their anxiety becomes a form of detective work, the doctor and members of the office staff seeking clues to its presence.

A patient's previous dental history can aid in this regard. The patient with a history of many cancelled appointments for a variety of reasons may be hiding anxiety in this manner. In addition, the patient with a history of appointments for the emergency treatment of painful situations should be suspect. Once the emergency treatment is completed (e.g., extraction, pulpal extirpation) and the pain relieved, the patient does not reappear until the next episode of dental pain.

When the patient arrives in the dental office, he often times will sit in the waiting room and discuss his fears of dentistry with other patients or with the office receptionist. The receptionist should therefore become conscious of statements made by patients concerning fears of dentistry. It is a rare patient indeed who will express these same fears to the doctor. The receptionist should be trained to advise the "chairside personnel" (i.e., the assistant, the doctor) that "Mrs. Smith mentioned to me she was terrified of injections" or that "she heard root canal work is very painful." Armed with this knowledge, the doctor and staff are better able to manage this patient's anxieties.

When an apprehensive patient is seated in the dental chair, other clues can be noted that relate to anxiety. I believe the doctor should spend a period of time at each visit speaking with (not to) the patient. This permits the patient to speak up. Many patients complain that doctors do not allow (or do not seem to want) their patients to talk. Anxieties may be expressed at this time. Only a brief pe-

---

*Electronic Waveform Laboratory, Inc., Huntington Beach, CA.
†Pain Prevention Lab, Deerfield, IL.

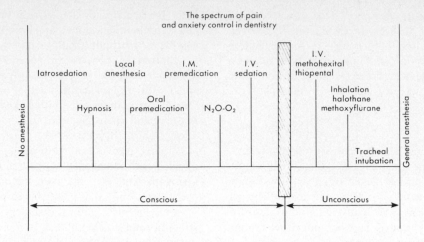

FIG. 19-8. Spectrum of pain and anxiety control in dentistry. Illustration of many of the techniques available in medicine and dentistry for patient management. Vertical bar represents the loss of consciousness. (From Malamed, S.F.: Sedation: a guide to patient management, St. Louis, 1985, The C.V. Mosby Co.)

riod need be devoted to this, but any time thus spent is time well spent.

Touch your patient. The feel of the skin of apprehensive patients when you shake their hand can tell much. Cold, wet palms usually indicate anxiety.

Watch the patient. Apprehensive patients do not stop watching the doctor. They are afraid they will be "snuck up on" and surprised (unpleasantly) with a syringe or some other equally unpleasant instrument. Look at the patient's posture in the chair. Nonanxious patients appear comfortable in the chair while apprehensive persons appear stiff, unrelaxed, on the verge of leaving the chair. The hands of nervous patients may be firmly gripping the armrest of the chair in what has come to be known as the "white knuckle syndrome." They may be clutching a handkerchief or shredding a tissue without even being aware of it.

The forehead and arms of nervous patients may be bathed in perspiration despite effective air conditioning. Patients may even be complaining about the warmth of the room.

When these methods of recognizing anxiety in a dental office are employed, the situation takes on the aspect of a game: Can the doctor detect the patient's anxiety? Will the patient successfully keep his fears hidden from the doctor so as not to appear "foolish"? Unfortunately, on many occasions the patient wins. Then the doctor, unaware of the patient's anxieties, proceeds with the planned dental treatment only to discover that the patient was indeed apprehensive and faints at the sight of a local anesthetic syringe or pushes the doctor's hand away at a critical time in a procedure. The anxiety is obvious at this point, but the ideal time to detect it is *before* dental treatment begins.

The medical history questionnaire is a device that may be used to assist in the recognition of anxiety at an early stage. Corah[8] and Gale[11] determined which factors involved in dental therapy are most anxiety inducing in patients. They created an anxiety questionnaire to help determine a patient's degree of anxiety. The School of Dentistry of the University of Southern California has included several questions from this anxiety questionnaire in its medical history form:

Do you feel very nervous about having dental treatment?
Have you ever had an upsetting experience in the dental office?
Has a dentist ever behaved badly toward you?
Is there anything else about having dental treatment that bothers you? If so, please explain.

These questions permit the patient to express feelings toward dentistry, perhaps for the first time. In our experience patients who would never verbally admit to anxiety will honestly answer these questions. The addition of one or more questions concerning dental attitudes to the patient's completed medical history form is highly recommended.

Anxiety toward dental therapy can readily be recognized through the use of the techniques just described. By so doing, the doctor is able to intervene and prevent the patient's anxiety from causing unwanted problems and complications during therapy.

Management of anxiety

A variety of techniques for the management of anxiety in dentistry are available. Together these techniques are termed a spectrum of pain and anxiety control (Fig. 19-8). They represent a wide range from nondrug modalities through general anesthesia. Although general anesthesia does maintain a useful place in this spectrum, its utilization today is quite limited outside the specialty of oral and maxillofacial surgery (and even within that specialty). Two reasons for decreased reliance on general anesthesia as a means of anxiety control have been (1) the introduction of the concept of sedation in dentistry and (2) the development within the past two decades of more highly effective agents for the management of anxiety.

From a practical viewpoint, sedation techniques present

relatively safe, reliable, and effective methods of controlling anxiety with little or no additional risk to the patient. *Sedation* is defined as the decrease or elimination of anxiety in a conscious patient.[2] *Conscious* is defined as the ability to respond appropriately to command with all protective reflexes intact, including the ability to clear and maintain a patent airway.[2] In viewing the spectrum chart the reader can see that there are essentially two major types of sedation: techniques involving the administration of drugs and techniques in which drug administration is not required. Techniques requiring drug administration are termed *pharmacosedation* and include oral sedation, intramuscular sedation, inhalation sedation, and intravenous sedation. The term *iatrosedation* is applied to nondrug techniques—hypnosis, biofeedback, acupuncture, electroanesthesia, and the not unimportant "chairside manner."

Iatrosedation*

Before discussing the techniques of pharmacosedation, I should like to consider the *nondrug* techniques. The techniques of iatrosedation are the building blocks from which all the pharmacosedative techniques grow. A relaxed and pleasant doctor-patient relationship will favorably influence the action of antianxiety drugs. Patients who are comfortable with a doctor either require a smaller dose of a given drug to achieve a desired effect or respond more intensely to the usual dose. This is in contrast to the patient who feels uncomfortable with a doctor. The greater anxieties and/or fears of the patient will cause him, either knowingly or unknowingly, to fight the effect of the drug and the result will be poor sedation and an unpleasant experience for both the patient and the doctor.

A determined effort must be made by all members of a dental office staff to help allay the anxieties of the patient.

Pharmacosedation

Although iatrosedation is the starting point for all sedative procedures in a dental office, the degree of anxiety present in many patients will prove too great to permit dental therapy to continue without the use of pharmacosedation. Fortunately several effective techniques are available to aid in relaxing the apprehensive patient.

What are the goals being sought when pharmacosedative techniques are used? Bennett[4] has listed them as follows: (1) The patient's mood must be altered. (2) The patient must remain conscious. (3) The patient must be cooperative. (4) All protective reflexes must remain intact and active. (5) Vital signs must be stable and within normal limits. (6) The patient's pain threshold should be elevated. (7) Amnesia may be present. These seven objectives comprise what might be considered ideal sedation for the dental patient.

There is, however, a second important component to ideal sedation that must always be considered: The level

of sedation must never reach beyond the level at which the doctor remains relaxed and capable of completing dental procedures of uncompromised quality. Indeed, the quality of the dentistry on a sedated patient should be at least as high as, if not higher than, the quality of the same treatment on a patient without the use of pharmacosedation. Drug utilization in dentistry must never become an excuse for inferior-quality dentistry. With adherence to these important criteria, the techniques discussed next may be employed safely and effectively.

Oral sedation. The most frequently employed technique of pharmacosedation, the oral route, offers some definite advantages over other techniques.

The oral route of drug administration is practically universally accepted by patients; and, in addition, it is one of the safest. Adverse drug reactions can and do arise following oral administration, but as a rule the intensity of the reaction is less than that seen following parenteral administration of the same drug.

The disadvantages of oral sedation tend to overshadow its advantages. Because of the following disadvantages, the goals of oral sedation should be kept within well-defined limits of safety: slow onset of action (approximately 15 to 30 minutes), maximum clinical effect in about 60 minutes, long duration of action (3 to 4 hours), inability to titrate patient to the ideal sedation level, inability to rapidly increase or decrease the sedation level if need be, and impaired status of the patient at the termination of the procedure (requiring an adult to accompany the patient home). As can be seen from these, the administrator has little control over the ultimate effect of a drug on a patient.

Because of this lack of control, it is recommended that the oral route of sedation not be employed to achieve more profound levels of sedation. Other, more controllable, techniques should be employed to achieve these levels. The uses to which oral sedation may safely be put include seeking a light level of sedation (a) 1 hour before a scheduled dental appointment to help lessen preoperative anxiety and (b) 1 hour before going to sleep the day before a dental appointment if anxiety is severe.

Many drugs are available for use via the oral route. I strongly recommend that the reader consult a textbook[19] before prescribing any oral antianxiety drug to a patient—to determine correct dosage, contraindications, precautions, and other important information. In my clinical experience the following agents have proved to be highly effective in reaching the goals just enumerated: diazepam (Valium), oxazepam (Serax), hydroxyzine (Atarax, Vistaril), and hexobarbital (Sombulex, Pre-Sed) for preoperative anxiety control; and flurazepam (Dalmane) or triazolam (Halcion) for hypnosis the night before dental treatment. Table 19-5 lists the commonly employed oral antianxiety and sedative hypnotic agents. Additional information regarding drugs for oral sedation can be found in Chapter 12.

It must be remembered that the dental patient receiving oral antianxiety agents should not be permitted to drive a motor vehicle either to or from the dental office.

*This term, introduced by Dr. Nathan Friedman of the University of Southern California School of Dentistry, is defined as relaxing of the patient through the doctor's behavior.

TABLE 19-5. COMMONLY USED ANTIANXIETY AND
SEDATIVE-HYPNOTIC DRUGS IN DENTISTRY

Drug group*	Proprietary	Dose† (mg)
Barbiturates		
Hexobarbital	Pre-Sed	250 to 500
	Sombulex	
Secobarbital	Seconal	100
Pentobarbital	Nembutal	50 to 100
Benzodiazepines		
Diazepam	Valium	5 to 10
Flurazepam	Dalmane	15 to 30
Oxazepam	Serax	15 to 30
Triazolam	Halcion	0.25 to 0.5
Others		
Chloral hy-drate	Noctec	500 to 1500
	Kessodrate	
	Felsules	
Hydroxyzine	Atarax	50 to 100
	Vistaril	

*Please see Chapter 12 for additional information.
†For a normal healthy 70 kg male. Patient response to these doses may vary; therefore the reader is advised to consult the drug insert for specific prescribing information before prescribing any drug.

Oral sedation may be required, especially at the first appointment, because of the preconceived ideas patients may harbor about endodontic therapy. Proper use of iatrosedation and pain control will commonly obviate the need for oral sedation at subsequent visits.

Intramuscular sedation. Intramuscular sedation is infrequently employed in dental practice.

Advantages of the intramuscular over the oral route include a more rapid onset of action for most drugs (approximately 10 to 15 minutes), maximum clinical effect within 30 minutes, and a more reliable drug effect for a given dose. Disadvantages include an inability to titrate to the ideal level of sedation, an inability to readily deepen the sedative effect if so desired, an inability to lighten the level of sedation, its long duration of action (3 to 4 hours for most drugs), and the need to administer an injection. The intramuscular route, like the oral route, lacks a degree of control that would be desirable. Therefore the level of sedation sought by IM sedation should remain light to moderate. Only doctors well trained in this technique and in airway maintenance should consider achieving more profound sedation via this route.

When a drug is to be injected into a patient, it should logically be administered directly intravenously, where its clinical action will be more controllable, than by the less reliable intramuscular route.

Narcotic analgesics such as meperidine (Demerol) and alphaprodine (Nisentil)* are frequently employed via the intramuscular route for sedation. Midazolam (Versed) and diazepam (Valium), (if injected *deeply* into muscle) are effective agents; however, if injected superficially diazepam is less effective than when taken orally.[3,12]

In endodontics IM sedation is not contraindicated. However, if an x-ray unit is not readily available at chairside, the patient will have to walk to the x-ray unit, possibly on several occasions; following IM injection he may require assistance in so doing. If the x-ray unit is present at chairside, no problem exists. Patients receiving any IM CNS depressants must have an adult available to escort them home from the dental office.

Inhalation sedation. Nitrous oxide (N_2O) and oxygen (O_2) inhalation sedation is a remarkably controllable technique of pharmacosedation and is currently employed by 35% of practicing dentists in the United States.[16]

Because of its advantages over other sedation techniques, inhalation sedation is usually the method of choice when sedation is required. The recognized advantages include its rapid onset of action (approximately 20 seconds, although 3 to 5 minutes may be required), the ability to titrate to the ideal level of sedation (N_2O is administered in 10% increments every 60 to 90 seconds until ideal sedation is achieved), the ability to rapidly lessen or deepen the level of sedation, total clinical recovery within approximately 3 to 5 minutes, and the ability to discharge most patients without any postoperative restrictions if the doctor so desires.

Disadvantages of this technique are few: the cost and size of the equipment plus the need for intensive education of both doctor and staff in using the technique and attendant emergency measures.

Because of the high degree of control maintained over inhalation sedation by the doctor, any level of sedation compatible with the doctor's degree of experience can be achieved.

Although nitrous oxide and oxygen inhalation sedation seems to be a nearly perfect technique, as with all drugs there will be times when the desired actions do not develop. Approximately 70% of all patients receiving N_2O-O_2 will be ideally sedated at a level between 30% and 40% N_2O, 15% will require less than 30% N_2O, and 15% will require more than 40%. Of this last 15% of patients, it may be said that some 5% to 10% will not be adequately sedated at any level of N_2O less than 70% to 75%. New inhalation sedation devices have a large number of safety features incorporated into them whose basic theme is to prevent the patient from ever receiving less than 20% oxygen. Therefore it is probable that approximately 5% of patients receiving inhalation sedation will never be adequately sedated. If we add to this patients who are unable to breathe through their nose and those who have very high levels of anxiety, it is entirely possible that a failure rate of 10% to 15% could occur with inhalation sedation.

I do not mean to denigrate this technique. My purpose in stressing the possibility of failures is to illustrate that no technique, even inhalation sedation, is a panacea. Failures can and will occur whenever drugs are administered to pa-

*Alphaprodine was removed from the market in July 1986.

tients. The drug administrator must know when to stop the administration. N_2O does not possess significant analgesic properties, although a degree of soft tissue analgesia develops in most patients at about 30% to 35% N_2O; therefore local anesthesia should be administered whenever it normally would have been.

Inhalation sedation is entirely compatible with endodontic therapy. Indeed, the use of rubber dam converts most patients into nose breathers, which facilitates administration of nitrous oxide-oxygen. Inhalation sedation with N_2O-O_2 is a highly effective, easy to use, and safe technique of pharmacosedation. It is most effective in patients with mild to moderate anxiety. Failures may be noted in unusually apprehensive individuals; but for these, other techniques are available.

In recent years several concerns have arisen relative to the use of nitrous oxide and oxygen in dentistry. The first involves the effects of long-term exposure to low levels of N_2O on dental personnel. The use of scavenger-type devices to remove exhaust N_2O from the environment is recommended, despite the paucity of definitive evidence of any danger to dental personnel.[7] Another concern that must be noted is the recreational abuse of N_2O by dental personnel. This has led to devastating effects, including peripheral sensory nerve deprivation.[21] N_2O is a potent anesthetic agent, not an innocuous vapor, and must not be abused. The third concern involves the use of any medication, especially N_2O, on a patient of the opposite sex. Cases have been reported[15] in which a doctor was accused of sexual improprieties while the patient was receiving N_2O-O_2. Two common threads appear: the patient received high concentrations of nitrous oxide (in excess of 60%); and the doctor treated the patient without the benefit of a second person (auxiliary) present in the treatment area. Accusations such as these may be prevented by simply titrating nitrous oxide to the ideal sedation level and having an auxiliary, preferably of the same sex as the patient, present in the treatment area at all times.

Intravenous sedation. The goal in the administration of any drug (except, obviously, local anesthetics) is to get an adequate level of the drug into the bloodstream. The delays in onset of action noted with the preceding techniques were due to the slow absorption of drugs from the gastrointestinal tract and from muscle into the blood. It is apparent, then, that the direct administration of a drug into the venous circulation will result in a much more rapid onset of action and a greater degree of control than are found with other pharmacosedative techniques.

Only inhalation sedation, in which the inhaled gases rapidly reach the alveoli and capillaries, has an onset of action approaching that of intravenous sedation. A drop of blood requires approximately 9 to 20 seconds to travel from the hand to the heart and then to the brain. Patients can thus be readily titrated to an ideal level of sedation. The length of time needed varies with the drugs employed: intravenous diazepam or midazolam may require up to 4 minutes whereas the Jorgensen technique may take 8 to 10 minutes. The level of sedation can easily be deepened if necessary, however, unlike inhalation sedation, it is impossible to lighten the level of intravenous sedation readily. Additional disadvantages to intravenous sedation include the possibility that potentially more dangerous situations will arise rapidly, especially if the techniques are improperly carried out, the requirement of additional training for both doctor and office staff if the technique is to be safely employed,[2] the need for a responsible person to escort the patient from the dental office, and a considerable increase in liability insurance costs.

Venipuncture is a learned skill, requiring practice and continued repetition if it is to be performed in an atraumatic manner. Once accomplished, the actual technique of intravenous sedation is quite simple to complete. Because of the degree of control maintained by the doctor the level of sedation sought can vary from light to profound depending on the experience of the doctor and the requirements of the patient.

Many techniques of intravenous sedation are available. Most involve the use of antianxiety agents and narcotic analgesics or sedative-hypnotics and narcotic analgesics. Although a great number of drugs fit into these categories and may be used successfully in intravenous sedation, several techniques have become quite popular in recent years: intravenous diazepam, diazepam and narcotics, and pentobarbital and narcotics. Midazolam (Versed) was recently introduced (July 1986) and promises to become a very important part of the IV sedation aramentarium.

1. Diazepam (Valium) is probably the most commonly used intravenous drug in dentistry. An antianxiety agent, diazepam in an average titrating dose of approximately 10 to 12 mg produced 45 to 60 minutes of excellent sedation. In 75% of our patients, an amnesic period of 10 to 15 minutes' duration accompanies sedation. During this period traumatic procedures can be completed, with the patient responding normally to them but having no recall at a later time. Diazepam possesses no analgesic properties, so patients must receive local anesthesia for pain control.

2. Narcotic agonists or narcotic agonist/antagonists may be combined with antianxiety agents to produce more profound sedation and add a degree of analgesia. Because of their potential side effects (i.e., nausea, orthostatic hypotension, respiratory depression), these agents should be used only when needed and by doctors trained in their use. In endodontic therapy, in which establishing adequate pain control may be difficult, the use of narcotics may, on occasion, be indicated. Narcotics affect the way pain is interpreted by the central nervous system and produce a milder response than might otherwise be experienced. In combination with local anesthesia, narcotics may help achieve adequate pain control in previously difficult situations.

3. Sedative-hypnotics (i.e., barbiturates) ought *not* to be employed as sole agents in intravenous sedation. While producing sedation these agents also *lower* the patient's pain reaction threshold, leading to an exaggerated response to any painful stimuli. Instead of grimacing, a patient may jump in the chair, creating an unpleasant or potentially dangerous situation. To overcome this handicap, narcotics are frequently injected along with the sedative hypnotics.

TABLE 19-6. Common routes of sedation in the dental office

Route of administration	Control		Recommended safe sedative levels
	Titrate	Rapid reversal	
Oral	No	No	Light only
Rectal	No	No	Light only
Intramuscular	No	No	Adults: light, moderate
			Children: light, moderate, profound
Intravenous	Yes	No (most drugs)	Children*: light, moderate, profound
		Yes (narcotics)	Adults: light, moderate, profound
Inhalation	Yes	Yes	Any level of sedation

From Malamed, S.F.: Handbook of medical emergencies in the dental office, ed 3, St. Louis, 1986, The C.V. Mosby Co.
*There is little need for intravenous sedation in normal healthy children. Most children who permit a venipuncture will also permit a local anesthetic to be administered intraorally. Intravenous sedation is of great benefit, however, in management of handicapped children.

Meperidine (combined with scopolamine) is injected following the sedative hypnotic pentobarbital (Nembutal) in a procedure termed the *Jorgensen technique*. For routine endodontic therapy this technique is too long-acting, pentobarbital having a clinical duration of approximately 4 hours.

Intravenous sedation, particularly the shorter-acting techniques (i.e., midazolam, diazepam, diazepam or midazolam and a narcotic) are ideally suited for endodontic therapy. If the x-ray unit is located some distance from the patient, it may be both difficult and inconvenient to move the patient to the unit. During the early phase of the procedure, immediately after injection of the drug(s) the patient may also have difficulty maintaining an open mouth. Bite blocks should be readily available for use at this time.

Table 19-6 summarizes the recommended levels of sedation for the techniques of sedation discussed in this chapter.

Combined techniques. On occasion it may be necessary to consider combining several of the techniques just described. Some words of caution are in order.

Quite frequently the patient who requires either inhalation or intravenous sedation will be apprehensive enough to need oral sedation either the night before or the day of dental therapy. There is no contraindication to this practice provided the level of oral sedation is not excessive *and* the inhalation or intravenous agents are carefully titrated. Because of the level of oral sedative already in the blood, the requirement for other agents will usually be decreased. If "average" doses of inhalation or intravenous drugs are used without titrating, an overdose may ensure. Titration is an important safety factor. When possible to titrate a drug, it is foolhardy not to.

The combination of intravenous and inhalation sedation should be avoided by all but the most experienced doctors. Too frequently reports are forthcoming of significant morbidity and, on occasion, mortality resulting from the ill-conceived conjoint use of these two potent techniques. Levels of sedation can vary rapidly; and unless constant effective monitoring is maintained, unconsciousness may develop with attendant airway problems before the doctor

ever becomes aware of it. Nitrous oxide–oxygen may be employed successfully at the same appointment as intravenous sedation in the following manner: when a patient requiring intravenous sedation is apprehensive about venipuncture, N_2O-O_2 may be used to aid in establishment of the intravenous infusion. Benefits of N_2O-O_2 in this situation include (1) a vasodilating effect, (2) anxiety-reducing actions, and (3) minor analgesic properties. After the establishment of an intravenous infusion, the patient must be placed on 100% oxygen and returned to the presedative state before any intravenous drug is administered.

Anxiety control—summary

Anxiety is a commonly encountered emotion during dental treatment in general and endodontic treatment in particular. Although iatrosedative procedures greatly aid in decreasing anxiety levels, the use of pharmacosedative techniques may become necessary. A number of effective techniques are available in dental practice. The least potent, most controllable technique that will allay anxiety should be used. Care must be observed, however, not to exceed the level of sedation at which the doctor feels capable of effectively and safely managing the patient. As a final note it should be remembered that no technique of sedation is always effective and that clinical failures are to be expected. When properly employed, the techniques of iatrosedation and pharmacosedation will permit the doctor to manage successfully approximately 95% of the patients seeking endodontic therapy without increasing the degree of risk to the patient.

REFERENCES

1. Akinosi, J.O.: A new approach to the mandibular nerve block, Br. J. Oral Surg. **15**:83, 1977.
2. American Dental Association, Council on Dental Education: Guidelines for teaching the comprehensive control of pain and anxiety in dentistry, J. Dent. Educ. **36**:62, 1972.
3. Baird, E.S.: Plasma level of diazepam and its major metabolic following intramuscular administration, Br. J. Anaesth. **45**:546, 1972.
4. Bennett, C.R.: Conscious sedation in dental practice, ed. 2, St. Louis, 1978, The C.V. Mosby Co.
5. Camejo, G., et al.: Characterization of two different membrane fractions isolated from the first stellar nerves of the squid Dosidicus gigas, Biochim. Biophys. Acta **193**:247, 1969.

6. Chapman, L.F., Goodell, H., and Wolff, H.G.: Tissue vulnerability, inflammation, and the nervous system. Read at American Academy of Neurology, April, 1959.

7. Cohen, F., et al.: Occupational disease in dentistry and chronic exposure to trace anesthetic gases, J. Am. Dent. Assoc. **101**:21, 1980.

8. Corah, N.: Development of dental anxiety scale, J. Dent. Res. **48**:596, 1969.

9. Covino, B.J.: Physiology and pharmacology of local anesthetic agents, Anesth. Prog. **28**:98, 1981.

10. Frommer, J., Mele, F.A., and Monroe, C.W.: The possible role of the mylohyoid nerve in mandibular posterior tooth sensation. J. Am. Dent. Assoc. **85**:113, 1972.

11. Gale, E.: Fears of the dental situation, J. Dent. Res. **51**:964, 1972.

12. Gamble, J.A.S.: Plasma levels of diazepam, Br. J. Anaesth. **45**:1085, 1973.

13. Gow-Gates, G.A.E.: Mandibular conduction anesthesia: a new technique using extraoral landmarks, Oral Surg. **36**:321, 1973.

14. Gustainis, J.F., and Peterson, L.J.: An alternative method of mandibular nerve block, J. Am. Dent. Assoc. **103**:33, 1981.

15. Jastak, J.T., and Malamed, S.F.: Nitrous oxide sedation and sexual phenomena, J. Am. Dent. Assoc. **101**:38, 1980.

16. Jones, T.W., and Greenfield, W.: Position paper of the ADA Ad Hoc Committee on trace anesthetics as a potential health hazard in dentistry, J. Am. Dent. Assoc. **95**:751, 1977.

17. Malamed, S.F.: The Gow-Gates mandibular block—evaluation after 4275 cases, Oral Surg. **51**:463, 1981.

18. Malamed, S.F.: The periodontal ligament injection—an alternative to mandibular block, Oral Surg. **53**:118, 1982.

19. Malamed, S.F.: Sedation: a guide to patient management, St. Louis, 1985, The C.V. Mosby Co.

20. Malamed, S.F.: Handbook of local anesthesia, ed. 2, St. Louis, 1986, The C.V. Mosby Co.

21. Malamed, S.F., et al.: The recreational abuse of nitrous oxide by health professionals, J. Calif. Dent. Assoc. **8**:38, 1980.

22. Malamed, S.F., and Trieger, N.T.: Intraoral maxillary nerve block: an anatomical and clinical study, Anesth. Prog. **30**:44, 1983.

23. Najjar, T.A.: Why can't you achieve adequate regional anesthesia in the presence of infection? Oral Surg. **44**:7, 1977.

24. Nelson, P.W.: Injection system (letter), J. Am. Dent. Assoc. **103**:692, 1981.

25. Poore, T.E., and Carney, F.M.T.: Maxillary nerve block: a useful technique, J. Oral Surg. **31**:749, 1973.

26. Ritchie, J.M., Ritchie, B., and Greengard, P.: Active structure of local anesthetics, J. Pharmacol. Exp. Ther. **150**:152, 1965.

27. Ritchie, J.M., Ritchie, B., and Greengard, P.: The effect of the nerve sheath on the action of local anesthetics, J. Pharmacol. Exp. Ther. **150**:160, 1965.

28. Rood, J.P., and Pateromichelakis, S.: Inflammation and peripheral nerve sensitization, Br. J. Oral Surg. **19**:67, 1981.

29. Saadoun, A.P., and Malamed, S.F.: Intraseptal anesthesia in periodontal surgery, J. Am. Dent. Assoc. **111**:249, 1985.

30. Shanes, A.M.: Electrochemical aspects of physiological and pharmacological action in excitable cells. II. The action potential and excitation. Pharmacol. Rev. **10**:165, 1958.

31. Walton, R.E., and Abbott, B.J.: Periodontal ligament injection: a clinical evaluation, J. Am. Dent. Assoc. **103**:571, 1981.

Self-assessment questions

1. Inadequate pain control with an inflamed or infected pulp is due to
   a. An increase in the tissue pH around the involved tooth
   b. A lower proportion of the cation
   c. A higher proportion of the free base
   d. The fewer cations available for binding at the neural receptor site

2. The ideal method of anesthetizing an area of infection would be to
   a. Use an anesthetic without a vasoconstrictor
   b. Infiltrate into the site of the infection
   c. Utilize the effect of a subperiosteal injection
   d. Use regional nerve block anesthesia

3. Local infiltration anesthesia is
   a. A technique in which the solution is deposited into the area of treatment
   b. Most effective in the presence of infection and local inflammation
   c. Effective in areas of dense cortical bone
   d. Less successful for primary teeth than permanent teeth in the mandibular arch

4. The infraorbital nerve block does not
   a. Anesthetize the posterior superior alveolar nerve
   b. Provide anesthesia to the maxillary premolars
   c. Provide anesthesia to the mesial-buccal root of the maxillary first molar
   d. Provide anesthesia to the maxillary canine

5. The maxillary or second division nerve block provides anesthesia for
   a. All maxillary teeth on the side of injection
   b. Buccal soft tissues and bone of the injected side
   c. Hard palate of the injected side
   d. All of the above

6. The Gow-Gates mandibular block
   a. Provides anesthesia to all sensory branches of the mandibular nerve
   b. Requires supplemental infiltration around the area of the involved tooth
   c. Has an injection site that is lower than in the traditional inferior alveolar block technique
   d. Has a high positive aspiration rate compared to the inferior alveolar block injection

7. The intrapulpal injection
   a. Provides anesthesia by action of the solution and applied pressure
   b. Requires placing a loose-fitting anesthetic needle into either the pulp chamber or the canal
   c. Does not create any period of discomfort during injection
   d. Usually provides anesthesia after 30 seconds of depositing anesthetic

8. One of the methods employed to recognize patient anxiety is
   a. Having a receptionist attuned to apprehensive patient statements
   b. Allowing the patient time to express himself
   c. Watching a patient's physical responses in the dental chair
   d. All of the above

9. The ideal pharmacosedation technique should
   a. Alter the patient's mood
   b. Lower a patient's threshold to pain
   c. Affect a patient's protective reflexes
   d. Render the patient unconscious

10. Which of the following drugs is not commonly used for antianxiety in dentistry?
    a. Secobarbital
    b. Oxycodone hydrochloride
    c. Hydroxyzine
    d. Diazepam

11. Which statement characterizes the oral route of drug administration?
    a. There is an inability to titrate to the patient's ideal sedation level
    b. Any adverse drug reaction is of greater intensity than the same drug administered by the parenteral route
    c. The onset of action is generally rapid (approximately 5 to 10 minutes)
    d. It is least accepted by patients compared to other routes of drug administration

12. A disadvantage of the intramuscular route of drug administration is
    a. Inability to titrate to the ideal level of sedation
    b. Inability to lighten the level of sedation
    c. Generally long duration of action (3 to 4 hours for most drugs)
    d. All of the above

13. Nitrous oxide and oxygen inhalation sedation
    a. Has significant analgesic properties, eliminating the need for local anesthesia
    b. Has a total clinical recovery period of 15 to 25 minutes
    c. Can be titrated to the ideal level of sedation
    d. Cannot be rapidly lessened or deepened

14. Intravenous sedation
    a. Has a relatively slow onset of action
    b. Requires no additional training for the dentist and staff
    c. Is readily titrated to the ideal level of sedation
    d. If too deep, is easily lightened

20

BLEACHING OF VITAL AND NONVITAL TEETH

RONALD E. GOLDSTEIN D.D.S.
RONALD A. FEINMAN D.M.D.

With careful diagnosis, case selection, treatment planning, and attention to technique, bleaching can change a patient's physical appearance dramatically. Sometimes this can be done in as little as one office visit, and almost always it is less invasive and less expensive than other esthetic procedures such as crowning or bonding. If considered as an adjunct to other procedures for correcting discoloration and other esthetic problems, bleaching holds out promise for an even larger group of patients who seek more attractive teeth.

Although the mechanisms by which bleaching removes discoloration are not fully understood and may be somewhat different for different types of stains, the basic process almost certainly involves oxidation, during which the molecules causing the discoloration are released. Consequently, the success of bleaching depends on the ability of the bleaching agent to permeate to the source of the discoloration and remain there long enough (and/or frequently enough) to overcome the intensity of the stain.

How well bleaching works—that is, the appropriateness of bleaching for any given patient—will depend in large part on the discoloration itself, its cause, and the length of time the discoloring agent has permeated the structure of the tooth.

More than 30,000 vital teeth have been bleached successfully over the past 18 years in our office and that of Dr. Donald Arens[2] without any sign of devitalization directly related to the bleaching procedures. Pulp studies to date indicate that careful vital bleaching does not elicit any permanent inflammatory responses.[4]

Nonvital bleaching, on the other hand, could initiate a cervical resorption response at the cementoenamel junction if it is not properly protected.[15]

DISCOLORATION

Discoloration of the teeth can occur by staining or damage to the enamel of the teeth, producing the familiar stains caused by tobacco, coffee or tea, or highly colored foods. Discoloration also occurs through the penetration of the tooth structure by some discoloring agent, whether medication given systemically such as the antibiotic tetracycline, excessive fluoride ingested during the development of tooth enamel, by-products of the body released into the dentinal tubules during illness (such as bilirubin involved with jaundice), trauma (primarily the breakdown of hemoglobin), or pigmentation escaped from the medicaments and materials used in dental repair. Often the discoloration is a combination of these and other genetic, environmental, medical, and dental factors.

For most patients, a good visual examination by a dentist familiar with the appearance of a wide variety of specific discoloration problems will suggest the etiology and consequently the appropriate technique and the likelihood of its success.[8]

Diagnosis

This diagnostic work-up should include an intensive prophylaxis to remove superficial staining that may be compounding more intrinsic discoloration. It also should be concerned with (1) establishing color baselines before treatment begins, (2) noting the condition of the teeth and mouth in general, (3) evaluating the patient's sensitivity, (4) taking a complete medical history, with a particular focus on diagnosis of any systemic problems or medications that might be affecting tooth coloration, and (5) determining any behaviors of the patient such as smoking or heavy caffeine use that may have contributed to the discoloration and which, if any, of these behaviors the patient is willing to modify in order to maintain the effect of treatment.

The major difference in bleaching technique depends on whether or not the tooth is vital or nonvital.

For vital teeth, in which the pulp remains alive, the bleaching agent must be applied to the outside of the teeth

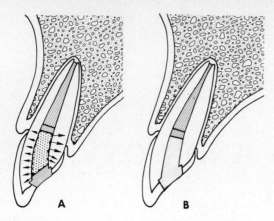

FIG. 20-1. Combination technique. **A,** After Superoxol has been heated on a cotton pellet in the chamber, it is mixed with sodium perborate into a paste and sealed within the access opening for 3 to 7 days. **B,** Final restoration.

while the patient remains immobile and his or her tissue and face are fully protected. With each treatment session, the bleaching agent permeates the appropriate structure of the discolored tooth or teeth—the enamel or the dentin—in order to release the molecules containing the discoloration. The use of high-intensity lighting and longer exposure times for the bleaching agent increases this permeation. Etching also may enhance the effects of bleaching by removing the pellicle or other surface organic substances and penetrating the enamel slightly, possibly exposing slightly deeper areas of enamel to the bleach. (See Plate 1, *I* and *J*.)

When the discoloration of a tooth comes from within the pulp chamber itself, whether from necrotic pulp tissue or from staining agents that are placed in the chamber as part of dental treatment, then the bleaching treatment must also take place within the chamber. This can be done in the dentist's office, using a special heat/light lamp to activate the bleaching agent packed in the pulp chamber. Alternatively, in an outpatient procedure aptly called the "walking bleach" method, the bleaching agent is left in for several days. This longer procedure may be more appropriate for discolorations of longer duration and more stubborn intensity (Fig. 20-1).

BLEACHING VITAL TEETH

The earliest efforts of bleaching go back more than a century and focused on the search for an effective bleaching agent that could be painted on discolored vital teeth. The reader interested in dental history should turn to the detailed article by Zaragoza.[23] By 1918 Abbot had introduced the forerunner of the combination used to bleach vital teeth today: a superoxol or hydrogen peroxide bleaching agent and an accelerated chemical reaction caused by heat and light devices. But only in the past decade, with the widespread application of bleaching to tetracycline stains of vital teeth, has bleaching moved toward becoming a basic part of esthetic dental practice. It seems appro-

priate, therefore, to begin our description of the problems amenable to improvement by bleaching with this relatively new dental problem that in turn helped create a new dental solution to many other problems.

Tetracycline discoloration. In the late 1950s and early 1960s, scientists and practitioners began to recognize the full impact of the new tetracycline antibiotics on tooth formation.[5,13,17,21,24] Children who had received tetracycline for as few as 3 days were faced with a lifetime of discolored teeth. Searching for a treatment that would counteract the discolorations caused by this (still) widely used antibiotic, dentists turned once again to bleaching. In 1970, Cohen and Parkins published a method for bleaching the discolored teeth of young adults who had undergone intensive, long-term tetracycline therapy for cystic fibrosis.[7] The results were promising, and in the next years other practitioners turned their energies to developing bleaching procedures that would improve not only tetracycline stains but other discolorations as well, both intrinsic and extrinsic.

Teeth are most susceptible to tetracycline discoloration during their formation, that is, the second trimester in utero to roughly 8 years of age. The tetracycline molecule appears to chelate with calcium and become incorporated into the hydroxyapatite crystal at the mineralizing front. The teeth thus take on the color of the mineralized tissue. This means that tetracycline staining is not confined to the enamel but instead predominantly involves the dentin, the matrix of which is being formed during the period in which the drug is taken.

The severity of stains—and the reason why tetracycline staining is so extremely variable in its extent, coloration, depth of stain, and location—depends on the time and duration of the drug administration, the type of tetracycline, and the dosage.

Mild yellow or gray tetracycline staining may respond well in three or fewer bleaching sessions, while darker yellow or gray staining will require twice as many sessions (Plate 1, *A* and *B*). Extensive tetracycline staining, with dark gray or blue staining and marked banding, responds but the bands are usually evident following even extensive treatment. Tetracycline-discolored teeth with marked banding may require bleaching in combination with some veneering technique.

Fluorosis staining. Mottled tooth enamel occurs when children ingest excessive fluoride during enamel formation and calcification, usually the third month of gestation through the eighth year of life. It is seen primarily in the southwest, with isolated reports from the east, in areas where drinking water contains natural fluoride concentration in excess of 1 part per million. When fluoride concentration exceeds 4 parts per million, a majority of the exposed young population can be expected to develop moderate to severe discoloration of the tooth surface.

The high concentration of fluoride is believed to cause a metabolic alteration in the ameloblasts, which results in a defective matrix and improper calcification. Histologic ex-

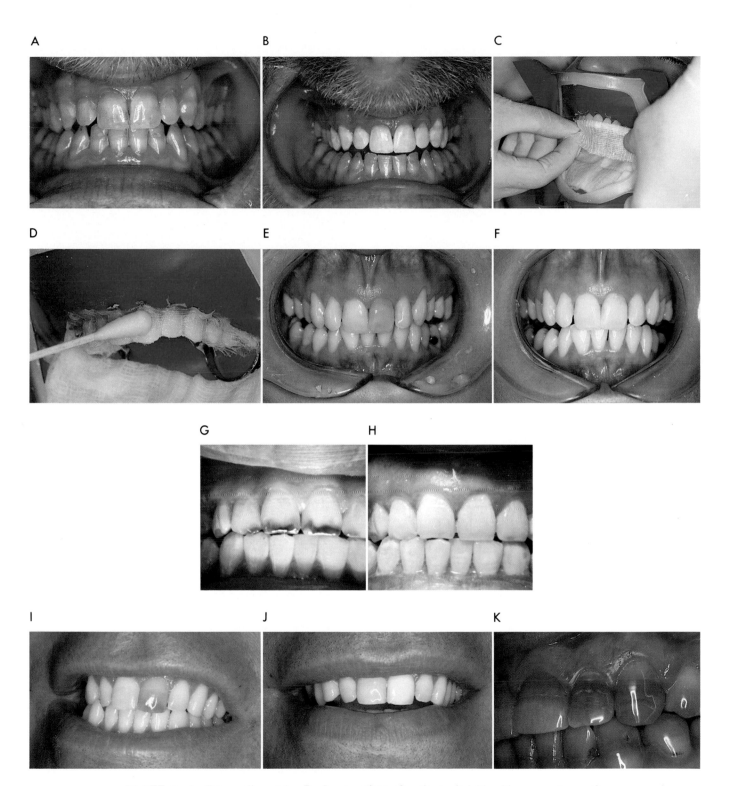

PLATE 1. A, Tetracycline stain. **B,** Same patient after three vital bleaching procedures. **C,** Application of gauze to anterior teeth that will be bleached. Dental floss is used to ligate each tooth that will be bleached. **D,** The gauze covering the surfaces of the teeth is continuously saturated throughout the procedure. **E,** Postendodontic discoloration, before treatment. **F,** Same patient after one in-office bleaching treatment. **G,** Endemic fluorosis stain. **H,** After the bleaching procedure. **I,** Vital discolored central incisor. **J,** Improved shade after one bleaching appointment. **K,** Heavily striated teeth are poor candidates for bleaching. (**G** and **H** courtesy Dr. P. Colon.)

INDICATIONS AND CONTRAINDICATIONS FOR BLEACHING VITAL TEETH

Indications	Contraindications
1. Mild tetracycline stains	1. Extremely large pulps
2. Fluorosis	2. Patient expectation too high
3. Aging	3. Very dark teeth
4. Yellow teeth	4. Sensitive teeth
5. Systemic diseases	5. Impatient patient

amination of the affected teeth will show a hypomineralized, porous subsurface enamel below a well-mineralized surface layer.

Most of the effects of fluorosis occur in permanent dentition, with premolar teeth most affected, followed by second molars, maxillary incisors, cuspids and first molars, and the mandibular incisors the least affected. Where fluoride concentration is very high, the primary teeth also may be involved.

The nature and the severity of fluorosis-related problems vary widely, depending on many factors such as genetic vulnerability, intensity and length of exposure, and the point in the development of the enamel at which excessive fluoride intake occurs. In general, there are two types of damage—discoloration and surface defects—for which bleaching is of differing value. Bleaching is an effective modality for most staining and discoloration problems of fluorosis, especially when the pigmentation appears on a smooth enamel surface. It is a useful adjunctive treatment for those teeth in which staining is accompanied by pitting and certain other surface defects. It is not appropriate for those teeth in which fluorosis has caused severe loss of enamel.

When contemplating bleaching for fluorosis or any other condition, the dentist should be on guard for white or opaque spots or multicolored staining, especially striates. (See Plate 1, *K*) Bleaching will lighten the teeth but only relative to the initial color, so that striated discoloration will be less discolored, but still striated. Teeth with white or opaque spots can seldom be bleached as light as the spots. In these cases, bleaching may more appropriately be used as a preparation for bonding, removing some or all of the dark stains or lightening the discrepancy of color before the veneer is placed on the teeth.

Extrinsic discoloration. Although bleaching works well and often quickly in discolorations caused by tobacco, coffee, tea, and highly colored foods, it has one major drawback: even extensive series of bleachings are no match for the continued application of the staining agent on the teeth, and the dentist must persuade the patient to change eating, drinking, and tobacco use habits that can undo the effect of bleaching.[8]

Breakdown and/or reflection of materials used in restorations

1. Tooth-colored restorations such as acrylics, silicate cements, or composites can cause the tooth to look grayer and discolored. These discolorations respond well to bleaching following the replacement of the degraded restorations.

2. Amalgams, even silver and gold, can reflect a discoloration through the enamel. In some cases, bleaching may be unnecessary if the materials can be changed to a less visible material. If not, bonding may be a preferable alternative.

3. Oils, iodines, nitrates, root canal sealers, pins, and other materials used in dental restorations can cause discoloration. The length of time these substances have been allowed to penetrate the dentinal tubules will determine the amount of residual discoloration and will, consequently, affect the success of bleaching (Fig. 20-2, *A* and *B*, p. 632).

4. Dental caries itself is a primary cause of ugly pigmentation and may be seen as an opaque white halo or a gray discoloration. The cause of discoloration should be removed before bleaching is attempted. An even deeper brown to black pigmentation can occur as a result of the bacterial degradation of food debris in areas of tooth decay or decomposing filling. If this breakdown is repaired and proper cleaning performed, bleaching may not be necessary.

By-products of illness causing discoloration of teeth by infusion of dentin during development. Although there are large numbers of these conditions, most are rare and infrequently seen. Some examples are as follows:

1. Bluish green or brown primary teeth may develop in children who suffered severe jaundice as infants. These stains are the result of postnatal staining of the dentin by bilirubin and biliverdin.

2. Erythroblastosis fetalis, a result of Rh factor incompatibility between mother and fetus, is characterized by destruction of an excessive number of erythrocytes. Among many other problems, the degradation of these blood cells causes an intrinsic pigmentation of the dentin of the infant's developing teeth.

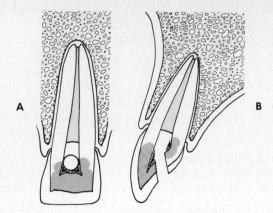

FIG. 20-2. A, Inadequate access opening provides a harbor for necrotic debris and root canal filling remnants. **B,** Trapped debris can extend into the dentinal tubules and cause discoloration.

3. Porphyria, an even rarer condition, causes an excess production of pigment that infuses the dentin and makes primary and permanent teeth appear purplish brown.

These conditions can sometimes be treated quite effectively with bleaching.

By-products of illness causing discoloration of teeth by interfering with normal matrix formation or calcification of enamel

1. Genetic conditions sometimes causing enamel hypocalcification or hypoplasia include amelogenesis imperfecta and clefting of the lip and palate.

2. Acquired illnesses with a similar effect include cerebral palsy, serious renal damage, and severe allergies. Brain, neurologic, and other traumatic injuries also can interfere with the normal development of the enamel.

3. Deficiencies of vitamins A, C, and D, calcium, and phosphorus during the formative period can cause enamel hypoplasia. (Such deficiencies do not affect adults similarly.)

If these conditions cause tooth deformity or white spots, the problems respond poorly to bleaching; bonding or crowning is more appropriate treatment.

Guide to bleaching vital teeth

The procedures for preparing and protecting the mouth are identical, whatever the cause of discoloration.

Before doing anything else, record the staining in the patient's mouth, using an instant or 35-mm camera. This provides an excellent data baseline from which to start and also an excellent record of pretreatment. Some patients may forget what their teeth looked like before treatment, especially if the change was an incremental, gradual one. The photographs also are valuable to determine needed follow-up.

Testing

1. Diagnosis should have been done recently enough to be completely accurate, especially in regard to any possi-

ble periapical or other pathologic condition, any possible caries or defective restorations that need repair or replacement before bleaching, and any enlargement of the pulp that might indicate that the teeth could be unusually sensitive to the heat process. Modern technology supplies the necessary tools. Radiographs and thermal and electric pulp tests are the only means of answering questions of pulp size and vitality that, in turn, will determine the procedures to be used in bleaching. Ultraviolet light is the only definitive method for diagnosing tetracycline staining; tetracycline depositions within the teeth will give off fluorescence. Transillumination techniques will enable the dentist to look at the teeth from different angles and observe the opacity, depth, and layers of any stains. Transillumination also can reveal caries, cracks, decalcified or hypocalcified areas, and areas of excess calcification, all of which may affect coloration and/or supply information essential for diagnosis of causative factors.

2. Verify the vitality of the teeth using an airstream, and compare the sensitivity of these teeth to the baselines recorded at the time of diagnostic examination.

Cleaning.

3. Normal prophylaxis pastes, even the very good ones, are simply not strong enough to take off deeply ingrained stain. A thorough prophylaxis using a Prophy-Jet* will free the teeth to be bleached of all surface stains as well as plaque. (Occasionally this thorough prophylaxis will restore an acceptable lightness to the patient's teeth. Much more often it will serve the dual purpose of allowing the dentist to see clearly the extent of deep stain and to better prepare the teeth for treatment.)

Isolating and protecting the teeth and mouth

4. Apply plain Orabase† to gingiva—labially, buccally, lingually, and interproximally—to protect the soft tissue of the mouth. No anesthetic is given to the patient, since it might dull the response of the patient and increase the inability to monitor the pulpal response.

5. Place the dam to isolate the teeth to be bleached and ligate all teeth with *waxed* dental floss. Form a protective pocket by turning the corners of the rubber and put Orabase on the lingual and linguoproximal surfaces only at the gingival areas to act as an additional seal to prevent leakage. Also put Orabase on any amalgams present to seal and help block out some of the heat that will be generated by the bleaching light.

Protecting the patient and the dental team

6. It is preferable not to use any local anesthesia during bleaching, for it is desirable to count on the patient's reflexes being fully intact so he or she can provide feedback if there is leakage on tissue or if the heat becomes too intense. Furthermore, an anesthetized patient will not feel a potential burn on the oral mucosa, lips, cheeks, or other tissue. However, there are a few patients who are so sen-

---

*Dentsply Int., York, PA.
†Colgate-Hoyt, Laboratories, Norwood, MA.

sitive to the procedures that they can not go through the mechanism of bleaching without anesthesia. For good management of these patients, some type of anesthesia may be needed. In such cases, a lower level of light should be utilized and an increased number of bleaching visits planned.

7. All members of the dental team should wear surgical rubber gloves and safety glasses.

8. The patient's hands and clothes should be well protected with a heavy plastic wrap, and the importance of the patient's wearing safety glasses throughout the entire procedure should be explained in detail.

9. Place a piece of gauze saturated with cold water under the rubber dam to protect the patient's upper lip and adjacent tissue. Also place gauze saturated with cold water over the clamps and the lower lip on top of the dam when bleaching maxillary teeth. Keep these gauze squares wet throughout the bleaching procedure, in order to protect the lips from the increased temperatures generated by the bleaching light.

10. Prepare the teeth to be bleached by first removing any excess varnish and jelly from the enamel surface and pumice each tooth to remove any excess Orabase or stain. Rinse thoroughly, and etch each tooth facially and lingually for 20 seconds, using 35% to 45% phosphoric acid. This will enhance the porosity of the enamel. Rinse thoroughly for 30 seconds, then dry the teeth. They should now appear chalky white.

11. Place on the dried teeth a piece of cotton gauze that has been saturated with Superoxol* or 35% hydrogen peroxide bleaching solution* (Plate 1, C).

12. Position a bleaching light approximately 13 inches from the teeth to be bleached, and shine the light as set above directly on the teeth. Begin with a rheostat setting of 5 and work your way upward as long as the patient feels no sensitivity. The best results are achieved at the highest light and heat intensitites, but overheating can cause tissue damage as well as pain. The rheostat on the light allows the dentist to adjust the precise temperature for the procedure. The bleaching temperature recommended for vital teeth is 115° to 140° for nonvital teeth up to the maximum of 160° (Fig. 20-3).

13. Keep the gauze over the teeth being bleached continually wet with the bleaching agent by dispensing fresh Superoxol from an eyedropper, and maintain contact of teeth to be bleached with a bleaching agent and light/heat for 30 minutes (Plate 1, D). Then remove gauze and flush teeth with copious amounts of warm water before carefully removing floss and rubber dam.

14. Polish the teeth with the yellow-banded polishing wheels.†

For teeth stained by coffee, tea, or other substances, a

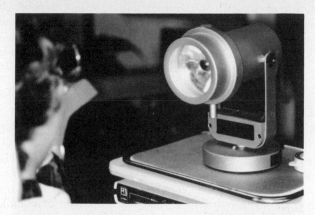

FIG. 20-3. The bleaching light is placed approximately 13 inches from the teeth for 30 minutes and adjusted to comfortable temperature through the rheostat.

dramatic difference may appear in only one or two visits. For tetracycline-stained teeth, five to ten visits are generally required for best results. It is best to prepare the patient for a longer sequence and to check carefully as the treatment proceeds, treating every 2 to 4 weeks. After the last treatment, you may want to refinish teeth with rotary polishers.*

Bleaching fluorosis-stained teeth

Unlike exogenous staining or teeth affected by tetracycline, fluorosis causes a much more heterogeneous pattern of staining. Only selected teeth may be affected, and they may have a mottled appearance rather than a consistent darkening. As a consequence, the method of attack for fluorosis staining is more selective. The dentist literally paints the bleach on the tooth directly, rather than blankets it with saturated gauze, in order to concentrate on the pattern of staining. For fluorosis-stained teeth, it is preferable to bleach the most discolored teeth first, proceeding to less discolored, and using the minimally discolored or unaffected teeth as a control.

Follow steps 1 through 9 for bleaching vital teeth.

10. Apply freshly made solution of bleaching agent† or Superoxol to the stained area of enamel of the teeth exposed through the rubber dam by using a cotton-tipped applicator. Allow to remain for 5 to 10 minutes.

11. Reapply mixture, and this time immediately disk enamel with fine cuttle disk.

12. Leave this mixture on the enamel, and bleach with light (Fig. 20-4, p. 634) for 5 minutes with a bleaching light set 13 inches from the teeth to be bleached. Set at rheostat setting of 5 and work up to temperature at which the patient is comfortable. As with tetracycline-stained teeth, the most effective bleaching will occur at highest

---

*Superoxol or Union Broach individual dose bleaching agent, Long Island, NY.

†Shofu Cosmetic Contouring Kit. Shofu Dental Corp., Menlo Park, CA.

*McInnes solution: 1 part diethyl ether, 5 parts 26% hydrochloric acid, 5 parts 30% hydrogen peroxide (Superoxol).

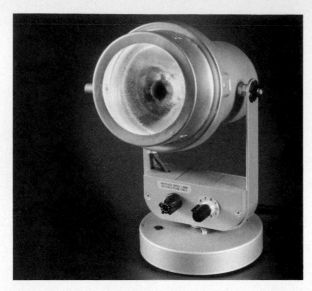

FIG. 20-4. Bleaching light (Union Broach) showing the reverse side with rheostat to control temperature *(right)* and replaceable fuse *(left).*

temperatures, but because the tooth is directly exposed to heat there is additional concern about possible injury to the pulp.

13. Repeat this sequence of application of bleach disking with sandpaper, and heating with light until desired shade is obtained, then neutralize by swabbing with 5.25% sodium hypochlorite and flushing with copious amounts of warm water before removing the rubber dam and any excess Orabase.

For fluorosis-stained teeth, a satisfactory treatment may result after only one or two visits. After the last treatment, the dentist may want to polish the bleached teeth with an impregnated rotary polishing wheel to achieve a high enamel luster.

The patient needs to be told that the teeth may appear chalky because of dehydration and that they will darken over the next few days after treatment, although to less than the previous shade. Some patients experience heightened sensitivity to cold for 24 to 48 hours and should avoid cold weather and cold drinks or food. Most patients are able to alleviate any discomfort in the period following the bleaching by taking two aspirin or acetaminophen tablets every 4 to 6 hours. The prognosis for fluorosis-stained teeth in one or two visits is excellent (Plate 1, *G* and *H*). The success of the response of the bleaching technique is directly related to the expectations of the patient. Often a lightening to a "mother-of-pearl" dull white consistency is a major improvement to the patient rather than a musty yellow color. All patients are cautioned that an annual "touch-up" bleach will usually be recommended for the removal of any new accumulated stain.

BLEACHING NONVITAL TEETH (Fig. 20-5, *A* to *G*)

Bleaching is often an excellent choice for a nonvital tooth that is discolored (Plate 1, *E* and *F*). The fact that the pulp

is already dead immediately removes one of the major concerns of bleaching—that the intense heat will cause damage to the pulp—and provides more maneuverability with temperature from the single tooth bleaching instrument. Caldwell estimates that a nonvital tooth can be heated to approximately 165° F without causing the patient discomfort.[6] This temperature will increase the rate at which the bleaching agent is effective about 200 times.[12]

In fact, it was the nonvital tooth's ability to withstand heat that made bleaching an acceptable, much less important, part of the armamentarium to correct the often drastic discoloration seen in nonvital teeth. Although Garretson published the results of an effort to bleach nonvital teeth in 1895,[13] the use of bleaching in pulpless teeth generally languished until the 1950s when the successes of the technique in vital teeth spurred dental researchers to turn renewed attention to its use with pulpless teeth. Dentists such as Pearson began trying to speed activation of bleaching in pulpless teeth by using chemicals that not only had bleaching capability but also oxygen-releasing capability; these would provide the same activation of bleaching as did the heat. Pearson left his bleaching agent, Superoxol, in the pulp chamber for 3 days.[19] Nutting and Poe carried such an approach one step further in 1967 with the "walking bleach" technique in which a mixture of Superoxol and sodium perborate is sealed in the pulp chamber for as long as a week.[18]

Contraindications

1. Extensive restorations with silicate or acrylic resins. (These teeth may not have enough enamel to respond properly to bleaching.)

2. Cracks and hypoplastic or severely undermined enamel.

3. Discoloration by metallic salts, particularly silver amalgam. (The dentinal tubules can become virtually saturated with these alloys and may cause staining, which no amount of bleaching with available products will significantly improve.)

Indications. Some types of stains of nonvital teeth can be removed with a surface bleach, since the nonvital teeth are as subject to external and other stains as the vital teeth, and these sources of discoloration may compound the problems specific to nonvital teeth. Certainly the nonvital teeth to be considered for bleaching must undergo the same thorough prophylaxis as described for vital teeth and all faulty restorations must be replaced.

But if, as is likely, the discoloration of a tooth has come from within the pulp chamber itself, then the bleaching treatment may also need to take place within the chamber. If a previous root canal has been done, this may afford the opportunity to bleach within the pulp chamber.

Discoloration of nonvital teeth due to pulp degeneration. The most common cause of discoloration in nonvital teeth is probably hemorrhage into the pulp chamber following severe trauma. The blood from the ruptured vessels is driven hydraulically into the dentinal tubules where the red blood cells undergo hemolysis, emitting hemoglobin. This released hemoglobin is then further degraded, releas-

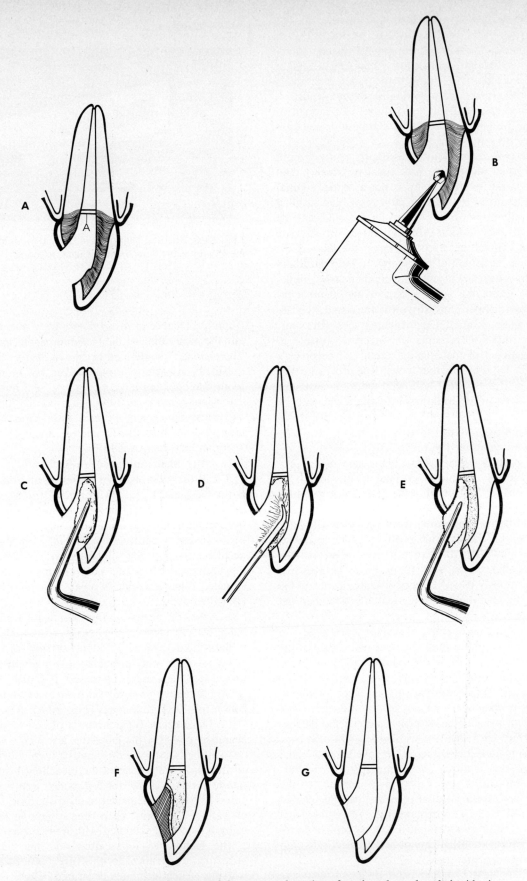

FIG. 20-5. A, Gutta-percha is removed from coronal portion of tooth and canal sealed with zinc phosphate cement 1 mm coronal to the cementoenamel junction *(A).* **B,** All debris and surface stains are removed. **C,** Cotton pellet saturated with 35% hydrogen peroxide is placed into pulp chamber. **D,** Heated tip from bleaching instrument is inserted into chamber. **E,** Remainder of pulp chamber is filled with cotton pellet impregnated with bleaching paste. **F,** With a double cement mix, impregnated cotton is sealed into pulp chamber. **G,** After desired color is reached, all bleaching material is removed and chamber is cleaned and filled with light shade of composite resin. (Courtesy Col. A.C. Goerig.)

ing iron, which forms a black compound by combining with hydrogen sulfide to become iron sulfide. The resulting grayish brown discoloration from the degradation products contained in the necrotic pulp is familiar to any dentist.

Pulp degeneration without hemorrhage also results in necrotic tissue, which contains various protein degradation products.

Incomplete root canal. Another common cause of tooth discoloration is an incomplete root canal in which pulpal debris is left in the tooth or there is not a proper coronal restoration. Failure to remove all pulp remnants, residual tissue in the pulp horns, filling material, and medicaments all can lead to discoloration (see Fig. 20-2). In all these conditions, the degree of discoloration in the teeth is directly related to the length of time between pulp death and treatment. The longer the discoloring compounds are in the chamber, the deeper the penetration into the dentinal tubules and the greater the discoloration—and, consequently, the more difficult the bleaching task. Discoloration of long duration presents the greatest obstacle to successful treatment of the nonvital tooth and becomes a major factor in deciding whether a chairside procedure will be sufficient or if the patient will need the more sustained exposure involved in the walking bleaching technique.

Guide to bleaching nonvital teeth
Entering and cleaning the tooth
1. Isolate, protect with Orabase, dam, and repeat protective measures as described for vital teeth, taking the same precautions for protection of the patient and members of the dental team.

2. As part of the diagnostic work-up, you will have thoroughly cleaned the external tooth in order to distinguish any compounding discoloration and to prepare the teeth for bleaching. Now, with the tooth to be bleached isolated, meticulously clean it internally. Any caries in the crown should be excavated and any leaking or washed out restorations replaced.

3. Establish a lingual opening of sufficient size to secure proper access to the entire pulp chamber and orifice of the root canal. All areas of the pulp chamber and pulp horns must be accessible to the bleaching agents (Fig. 20-5, *A*).

4. Remove all debris and a surface layer of dentin within the pulp chamber with a slow rotation bur. The freshened dentin permits easier penetration of the bleaching material (Fig. 20-5, *B*).

5. In endodontically treated teeth, remove the root canal filling material to a depth of 2 to 3 mm apical to the cervical line. Refill with zinc oxyphosphate cement, or the equivalent, 1 to 2 mm coronally to the cementoenamel junction (Fig. 20-5, *A*). This distance may be extended and modified if the gingival recession has been severe. If restored with a silver point that cannot be retreated, seal with 2 mm zinc oxyphosphate cement.[12a,15]

6. Remove any surface stains visible on the inside of the preparation with a bur. The seal should be checked and secured at this time.

7. Swab the entire preparation with chloroform or 70%

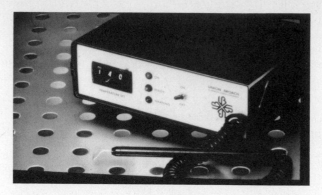

FIG. 20-6. Rheostat-controlled individual tooth bleaching instrument with exact temperature gauge. (Courtesy Union Broach Co.)

isopropyl alcohol to dissolve any fatty material and facilitate the penetration of the bleaching agent into the tubules. The chamber should then be blown dry.

NOTE: Bleaching should never be attempted on any tooth that does not have a complete seal in the root canal. The agent could escape through a porous root canal filling and cause the patient extreme discomfort, sometimes requiring heavy anesthetic and removal of the bleaching agent and the root canal filling.

In-office bleaching procedure
8. Fill the pulp chamber loosely with cotton fibers, and cover the labial surface with a few strands of cotton fiber in order to form a matrix for retaining the bleaching solution. Saturate this cotton matrix with 35% hydrogen peroxide, using a glass syringe fitted with a stainless steel needle. Discharge the solution slowly, thoroughly saturating the cotton inside the pulp chamber and on the labial surface. Wipe any excess away immediately (Fig. 20-5, *C*).

9. Apply the heated tip from the heating unit to the tooth being bleached (Figs. 20-5, *D*, 20-6, and 20-7); apply heat to the saturated gauze 5 minutes on and off.

10. A single tooth bleaching instrument that can be controlled for temperatures up to 160° F is placed in the chamber for 5-minute intervals on fresh, wet Superoxol soaked cotton for 20 to 30 minutes (Fig. 20-8). Remove cotton.

11. Once again, build a matrix of cotton within the pulp chamber, covering the labial surface with a few strands of cotton fiber. Saturate this matrix with the bleach. Once again, apply the heat from the bleaching instrument to the saturated cotton gauze for 5 minutes. Remove the cotton.

12. Repeat this sequence four to six times, or for a total of 20 to 30 minutes, each time removing the cotton and using new cotton saturated with fresh bleach.

The techniques for sealing and the final seal after bleaching are identical for this office procedure and for the walking bleach technique described below.

Out-of-the-office or "walking" bleach technique for nonvital teeth
8. On a glass mixing slab, prepare a bleaching paste of

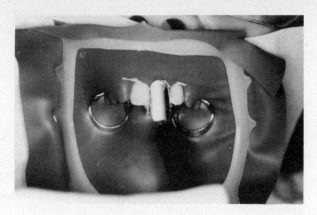

FIG. 20-7. Heated tip from individual bleaching instrument is curved to fit labial surface.

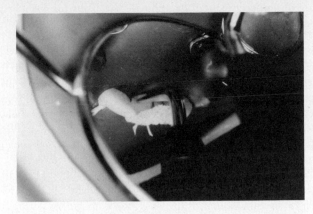

FIG. 20-8. Straight tip within the pulp chamber itself.

sodium perborate (Amosan)* and enough 35% hydrogen peroxide to form a thick white paste.

9. Fill the entire chamber of the tooth with this paste, leaving adequate space to place a temporary restoration and sealer (Fig. 20-5, E).

10. Seal by applying a solvent around the enamel margin, flowing a medium-stiff mix of zinc phosphate cement to close the area, and finally asking the patient to bite on a cotton roll with a plastic strip over the cotton (Fig. 20-5, F).

11. Have the patient return in 5 days or earlier, if there are any problems.

Final Seal After Either Office or Out-of-Office Bleaching Procedures

12. Remove the temporary seal with a no. 2 or 4 carbide bur.

13. Remove the cotton or bleaching paste and swab the preparation thoroughly with chloroform.

14. Air dry, clean, wash, and diffuse unfilled resin internally and throughout the bleached crown to seal the dentinal tubules. Use several coats and polymerize to prevent recurrence of coronal stain.

15. Etch the marginal walls with 35% phosphoric acid to assure good mechanical bonding. The entire restoration is placed at one time and finished properly to assure good marginal adaptation.

16. Fill the cavity with composite resin restorative material of the lightest shade esthetically compatible with the tooth (Fig. 20-5, G).

Sending the patient home

As with the bleaching of vital teeth, the dentist aims for slight overbleaching because the teeth will tend to darken slightly after the final bleach. This should be explained to the patient, as should the steps to be taken if he or she

experiences heightened sensitivity to cold or discomfort.

The single episode of bleaching in office or the 5 days of walking bleach will be adequate, in many cases, to achieve the desired effect. If the response was significant but inadequate, one may elect rebleaching for further improvement.

NONVITAL BLEACHING TECHNIQUES FOR VITAL TEETH

Abou-Rass advocates what he calls "intentional endodontics"—that is, the removal of the healthy pulp in order to be able to place the bleach inside severely discolored vital teeth.[1] While we are ot the school that believes in doing no harm to a healthy tooth, we recognize that occasionally teeth do not respond to repeated bleaching and that this may be a viable alternative in selected cases. Fields has a case history of endodontic treatment of tetracycline-stained teeth that failed to respond to repeated vital bleaching.[9]

CONCLUSION

Esthetic dentistry, like plastic and reconstructive surgery, is no longer considered as primarily a last resort of the desperately disfigured whose desire is to look normal. Though both esthetic and reconstructive surgery continue to treat these patients, often working miracles of appearance and personality, the more typical patient of the restorative dentist today is a perfectly normal-appearing person who wishes to look better, younger, and healthier and who believes, usually rightly, that his or her dental problems stand in the way of this goal. Bleaching is an important tool for these purposes.

But it is a relatively new addition to our collection of tools and we have few carefully controlled long-term studies of its effectiveness. Such work is needed, both to assess the permanency of the effects produced by bleaching and to compare the advantages and disadvantages of bleaching compared to other treatment modalities and of bleaching used alone or in conjunction with other treatments. A necessary first step for the accumulation of such

*Coopercare, Inc., Palo Alto, CA.

a literature will be a mechanism to assess, quantify, and describe discoloration before and after treatment. A next step will look more closely at the mechanism by which bleaching works, allowing us to better predict for which patients it will be most successful and to better understand the reasons why the length of its effect is variable and unpredictable for any individual patient. Most bleachings, whether vital or nonvital teeth, will require touch-ups within 1 to 3 years.

But simultaneously with these scientific and clinical advances, we need to give both professionals and prospective patients a broader, better awareness of the possibilities of bleaching and the limitations of these procedures.

REFERENCES

1. Abou-Rass, M.: The elimination of tetracycline discoloration by intentional endodontics and internal bleaching, J. Endod. 8(3):101, 1982.
2. Arens, D.: Personal communications, Oct. 1985.
3. Arens, D.E., Rich, J.J., and Healey, H.J.: A practical method of bleaching tetracycline-stained teeth, Oral Surg. 34:812, 1972.
4. Baumgartner, J.C., Reid, D., and Pickett, A.: New and pulpal reactions to the modified McInnes bleaching technique, J. Endod. 9:12, 1983.
5. Bevelander, G.: The effect of the administration of tetracycline on the development of teeth, J. Dent. Res. 49:1020, 1961.
6. Caldwell, C.B.: Heat source for bleaching discolored teeth, Ariz. Dent. J. 13:18, 1967.
7. Cohen, S., and Parkins, F.M.: Bleaching tetracycline stained vital teeth, Oral Surg. 29:465, 1970.
8. Feinman, R.A., and Goldstein, R.E.: Bleaching, Chicago, 1986, Quintessence Publishing Co.
9. Fields, J.P.: Intracoronal bleaching of tetracycline-stained teeth: a case report, J. Endod. 8:512, 1982.
10. Garretson, J.E.: A system of oral surgery, ed. 6, Philadelphia, 1985, J.B. Lippincott Co.
11. Goldstein, C.: Bleaching—advanced prosthodontics, University of Southern California, Presentation June 30, 1985.
12. Goldstein, R.E.: Esthetics in dentistry, Philadelphia, 1976, J.B. Lippincott Co.
12a. Harrington, G.W., and Natkin, E.: External resorption associated with bleaching of pulpless teeth, J. Endod. 5:344, 1979.
13. Jordan, R.E., et al.: Conservative vital bleaching treatment of discolored dentition, Comp. Cont. Ed. 5(10):803, 1984.
14. Kehoe, J.C.: Bleaching today, Fla. Dent. J. 55:12, 1984.
15. Lado, E.A., Stanley, H.R., and Weisman, M.I.: Cervical resorption in bleached teeth, Oral Surg. 55:78, 1983.
16. Ledoux, W.R., et al.: Structural effects of bleaching on tetracycline-stained vital rat teeth, J. Prosth. Dent. 54(1):55, 1985.
17. Mello, H.S.: The mechanism of tetracycline staining in primary and permanent teeth, J. Dent. Child. 478, 1967.
18. Nutting, E.B., and Poe, G.S.: A new combination for bleaching teeth, Dent. Clin. North Am. 655, 1967.
19. Pearson, H.H.: Bleaching of the discolored pulpless tooth, J. Amer. Dent. Assoc. 56:64, 1958.
20. Robertson, W.D., and Melfi, R.C.: Pulpal response to vital bleaching procedures, J. Endod. 6(7):645, 1980.
21. Shwachman, H., and Schuster, A.: The tetracyclines: applied pharmacology, Pediatr. Clin. North Am. 3:295, 1956.
22. Zach, L., and Cohen, G.: Pulp response to externally applied heat, Oral Surg. 19(4):515, 1965.
23. Zaragoza Torres, V.M.: "Blanqueamiento de dientes con vitalidid: Metodologia" (Bleaching of Vital Teeth—Technique), Madrid, 1984, Estomodeo.
24. Zegarelli, E.V., et al.: Discoloration of the teeth in patients with cystic fibrosis of the pancreas, N.Y. State Dent. J. 27:237, 1961.

Self-assessment questions

1. Agents causing discoloration include
   a. Tetracycline antibiotic
   b. Fluoride
   c. Hemoglobin breakdown
   d. All of the above
2. Bleaching of vital teeth
   a. Causes an irreversible pulpitis
   b. Utilizes the "walking bleach" technique
   c. Could initiate a cervical resorption response
   d. Affects both the enamel and the dentin
3. Bleaching nonvital teeth
   a. Is limited to the enamel surface of the tooth
   b. Is strictly an inpatient procedure
   c. Can be done by means of an outpatient "walking bleach" method
   d. Is successful regardless of the discoloring agent
4. The definitive method for diagnosing tetracycline staining is by
   a. History
   b. Vitality testing
   c. Ultraviolet light
   d. Visual examination
5. The procedure for vital bleaching *does not* include
   a. Orabase protection of the soft tissues
   b. Routinely anesthetizing the patient
   c. Using Superoxol or 35% hydrogen peroxide
   d. A lighted adjustable heat source
6. Contraindications to bleaching nonvital teeth include:
   a. Extensive silicate or acrylic restorations
   b. Cracks and hypoplastic or severely undermined enamel
   c. Discoloration by silver amalgam
   d. All of the above
7. Prior to bleaching application in a nonvital tooth
   a. Establish access to all parts of the pulp chamber
   b. Remove the root canal filling material to a depth of 2 to 3 mm apical to the cervical line
   c. Swab the prepared surface with chloroform or 70% isopropyl alcohol
   d. All of the above
8. The out-of-office or "walking" bleach technique
   a. Is a heat treatment procedure
   b. Uses a mixture of sodium perborate and 35% hydrogen peroxide
   c. Requires the patient to return in 24 hours
   d. Can be used in a poorly obturated root canal

21

POSTENDODONTIC RESTORATION

HAROLD F. EISSMANN
RYLE A. RADKE, Jr.

Current oral rehabilitation concepts are oriented toward a ''tooth-supported'' occlusion, which offers the biomechanical and physiologic benefits of fixed prosthetic therapy. Masticatory efficiency, tooth stabilization, maintenance of vertical dimension, and conservation of supporting tissues are major advantages of the tooth-supported prosthesis over the mucosa-supported prosthesis. Considering the advantages of the tooth-supported prosthesis in terms of the technical simplifications in design and fabrication and the psychologic advantages derived from patient comfort, one should be able fully to appreciate oral rehabilitative therapy as an interdisciplinary composite of periodontal, orthodontic, endodontic, and restorative techniques directed toward the retention of strategic abutment teeth.

The importance of periodontal and orthodontic procedures leading to the correction of lesions, contours, and levels of inverting and supporting periodontal tissues cannot be overemphasized. This chapter, however, will focus on the interdependence of restorative and endodontic procedures.

INDICATIONS FOR PRERESTORATIVE TREATMENT

Endodontic treatment prior to restorative procedures is indicated when:
1. There is irreversible damage to the pulp.
2. The loss of retentive coronal tooth structure due to caries, trauma, or abrasion cannot be substituted by a pin-retained core addition.
3. The occlusal or axial realignment of teeth that are malposed would endanger the integrity of the pulp.
4. The crown/root ratio of teeth with inadequate periodontal support is to be improved by the use of endodontic stabilizers.[13]
5. Overdenture techniques require the retention of roots as anchors for bar and stud attachments.[21]
6. Grossly defective teeth with a guarded pulpal prog-

nosis would pose difficulties in postrestorative endodontic intervention.

A prospective abutment tooth that has been endodontically treated will retain an unaltered periodontal attachment; biologically, there are no additional requirements in restorative treatment planning.[2,14] Biomechanically, however, special precautions are indicated because of changes within the dentin.[2,24]

GENERAL CONSIDERATIONS FOR RESTORATION
Brittleness of tooth structure

The loss of dentinal resiliency is the most important factor for consideration in the reinforcement of teeth with a small cervical circumference.

Mineralization and dehydration of the dentinal tubules result in an increasing loss of dentin resiliency.[2,24] Forces of occlusion as well as lever forces caused by the attachment of a prosthesis will cause a deformation by flexing. The stress generated may become excessive and lead to fractures of unprotected cusps or coronal fracture in the area of smallest circumference—the cervical area.

Loss of tooth structure

For molars (i.e., for multirooted teeth) the loss of coronal tooth structure substantially reduces fracture resistance. Tooth structure may be lost because of caries, fracture, or abrasion; operative alignment necessitating endodontic intervention; or the removal of dentin to gain access for endodontic cleaning and shaping.

Discoloration of tooth structure

With the loss of resilient dentin, a definite change in the tooth appearance can be expected. Even if there is no gross discoloration, there is certainly an altered light refraction potential due to a more opalescent dentin. In the cosmetic region of the mouth, these changes may warrant full coronal coverage. If a delicate gingival architecture allows the transmission of root discoloration, a shoulder margin should be extended 1.5 mm into the gingival sulcus. The porcelain restoration should have a gentle cervical prominence. The porcelain surface is prepared with a disk, a rubber wheel, pumice, and a natural glaze.

BASIC COMPONENTS USED IN RESTORATION

The goal in restoring endodontically treated teeth is the design and fabrication of the final restoration. The objectives of restoration can be stated as 3 R's: reinforcement, replacement, and retention. To meet these objectives, the restorative effort must include the use of such basic components as a dowel, core, and coping.

Reinforcement of the remaining tooth structure is achieved with the dowel and coping.

Replacement of missing tooth structure is achieved with the core.

Retention is supplied by the dowel for the core, and the core supplies retention for the final restoration.

The *dowel* is a post extending approximately two thirds the length of the root canal to provide reinforcement and retention. The design objective for the dowel, core, and coping is to distribute stress, generated by torque, throughout the remaining tooth structure. Without the use of a dowel of the proper length, this stress would tend to be concentrated at the area of the gingival margin. Isotope investigation with radioactive phosphorus has indicated that metabolic processes in the pulpless tooth decrease more rapidly in the coronal dentin, with a corresponding loss of elasticity. This process is noticed less in the dentin of the root, as long as a healthy periodontium is maintained.[2]

Dowel retention is affected by length, taper, diameter, and surface configuration of the dowel. Length and taper show the most dramatic means of increasing retention.[4] The biologic and structural limits on the dowel length are root morphology and the need to ensure an apical seal with 4 mm of gutta-percha. A general rule based on average tooth sizes[14a] would show that nearly all teeth can accept an 8-mm dowel while leaving 4 mm of apical seal. Radiographic verification of root curvature, wall thickness, and root length also must be included in the process of determining dowel length.

Dowel diameter should be assessed to avoid unnecessary removal of dentin. Most studies have shown that as the dowel diameter increases, the resistance of the tooth to fracture decreases. The diameter that provides adequate reinforcement for the core without endangering the root should allow more than 1 mm of tooth structure around the post and should have a diameter varying from 0.7 mm on mandibular incisors to 1.7 mm on maxillary incisors.[25]

Experience has shown that an inadequate diameter leaves the restoration vulnerable to failure because it will not be able to withstand masticatory forces. Therefore, either a tapered design that follows the shape of the canal or a two-stage instrumentation of the canal, as shown in Fig. 21-6, *D,* can be recommended.

Because the design objective makes the use of a coping mandatory for stress distribution, additional features for re-

sisting rotational forces are unnecessary in the dowel. The tooth structure contained within the walls of the coping is never circular; consequently, rotational displacement of the restoration cannot take place.

The *core* is an addition to the preparation to provide optimum length for retention. The core may be a coronal extension of the dowel, a pin-retained gold casting, a pin-retained amalgam addition, or a pin-retained composite.

The dowel and core are considered a foundation restoration. As such they become an integral part of the abutment preparation. The final restoration is subsequently constructed and seated as a routine procedure. Because the oral cavity presents an ever changing environment, the design of the restoration must provide for the removal of the retainer in an uncomplicated and noninjurious manner. This requirement is satisfied by making the fabrication of the dowel and core and the construction of the final restoration two separate procedures.

The *coping* is a band of metal approximately 2 mm in width. It surrounds the root at the margin with a ferrule effect and may be part of the core or formed by the final restoration.

A recent study indicates that the coping increases the resistance of root to vertical fracture.[22a]

The gingival margins of the final restoration are so placed in tooth structure that a cosmetic advantage can be gained without severe tooth reduction. The marginal adaptation of the core to tooth structure is not critical, since these margins are within the outline of the final restoration form. An exception would be in cases with severe loss of coronal tooth structure or when multiple abutment splinting is planned. Then the restoration of the individual tooth remnant with dowel, core, and coping may offer the most precise results.

A venting technique (i.e., a channel along the length of

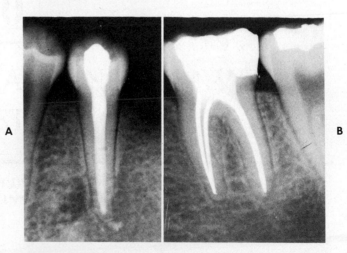

FIG. 21-1. Two prospective abutment teeth representing the two major concepts in restorative treatment. **A,** Single-rooted tooth with adequate coronal tooth structure for optimal preparation design. The small cervical circumference, however, indicates the need for dowel reinforcement. **B,** Multirooted tooth with a large cervical circumference. No dowel reinforcement against fracture was required.

the dowel) can substantially decrease hydraulic pressure and allow for proper seating of the coping during cementation. The integrity of each abutment tooth and surrounding marginal gingiva is safeguarded during prolonged restorative treatment.

Illustration of use

The restoration of endodontically treated teeth is not a standardized procedure. Such variables as the amount of remaining coronal tooth structure and the tooth circumference at the cervical area necessitate a skillful application of basic design principles to satisfy individual requirements.

For example, the premolar shown in Fig. 21-1, *A*, has retained its entire axial enamel surface. The root canal is large, and the cervical constriction pronounced. The tooth

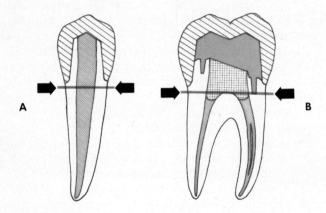

FIG. 21-2. The need for reinforcement of a single-rooted tooth against fracture depends on the cervical circumference. **A,** A small circumference needs dowel reinforcement. **B,** A larger circumference does not need reinforcement.

circumference is too small for this tooth to function as an abutment without dowel reinforcement against fracture at the cervical area (Fig. 21-2, *A*). A subsequently placed abutment retainer, full veneer design, will provide a coping effect. Adequate coronal tooth structure is present for optimum design.

The molar in Fig. 21-1, *B*, shows extensive loss of coronal tooth structure. The cervical circumference is large enough to resist fracture (Fig. 21-1, *B*). Dowel reinforcement is unnecesssary. The major concern is to gain retentive preparation walls. This is accomplished by a core addition. The obturation of the root canals with silver points and the difficulty of dowel preparation in a multirooted tooth make pin retention a more practical choice. Here the core may be a parallel pin casting or a nonparallel amalgam. A composite core is contraindicated because of the proximity of the core margin to the retainer margin on the distal tooth surface. A well-adapted gold core margin or amalgam ensures greater marginal integrity. In addition, a metal core allows better visualization in difficult access areas.

The restorative approach to endodontically treated teeth has undergone countless transitions. A profusion of techniques are available for consideration. A review of restorative failures often reinforces our determination to seek improvements.

The five most common failures of restorative techniques (Fig. 21-3) are as follows:

1. *No reinforcement dowel.* When no reinforcing dowel is placed, there is the potential for fracture at the cervical area of a tooth with a constricted circumference.
2. *Dowel of inadequate length.* A dowel of inadequate length will not alleviate this fracture potential, be-

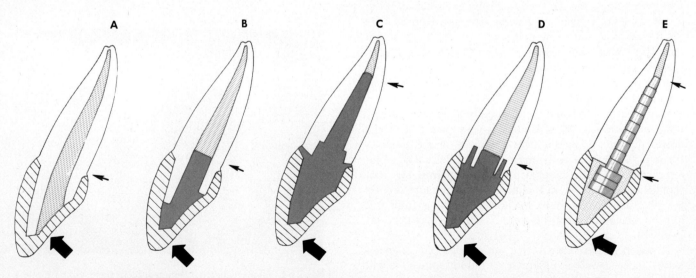

FIG. 21-3. Five most common causes of failure in restorative techniques. Small arrows indicate the level of potential fracture. Large arrows indicate the direction of force. **A,** No reinforcement dowel. **B,** Dowel of inadequate length. **C,** No ferrule effect in coping. **D,** Pin retention substituted for dowel placement. **E,** Preformed post with insufficient dentinal walls to support composite core.

cause it will not distribute stress throughout the remaining root structure.

3. *No ferrule effect.* A dowel of optimum length may offer retentiveness but will not reinforce against fracture of the root unless the coronal portion of the root is contained by the ferrule effect of the coping.

4. *Pin retention substituted for dowel placement.* Pin retention as a substitute for forming and duplicating dowel channels is oriented toward technique rather than based on principle. (One clinician boasted of his ability to negotiate 12 parallel pins around the orifice of a canine canal.) Failure is as inevitable as if a dowel of improper length had been constructed.

5. *Preformed post with insufficient dentin to support the core material.* This can result in failure of the restoration as shown in Fig. 21-7.

A wooden tent pole may be used as an illustration of the basic design principle employed in the restoration of a pulpless tooth. A metal dowel inserted into the pole would readily cause the pole to split if a metal ferrule were not affixed. The ferrule around a tooth protects against splitting when lever forces act against the inserted dowel.

Similar ferrule-type protection is required in the pulpless root (Fig. 21-4). A lightly chamfered preparation with walls 2 mm in length and with a 2-degree taper surrounds the coronal aspect (Fig. 21-4). The canal is instrumented to within two thirds of the length of the root. The general morphologic form of the canal is maintained. The foundation restoration is a composite of the ferrule or coping, the retention and reinforcement dowel, and the core. The core is shaped to the specific abutment preparation requirement. Once this foundation restoration is firmly cemented to the pulpless root, basic design criteria are satisfied.

In Fig. 21-5, *D,* all coronal dentin was lost and a complete foundation dowel-core-coping is indicated. Crown-lengthening procedures should be instituted either surgically or orthodontically to provide for a proper coping on these teeth.

RESTORATION OF SINGLE-ROOTED TEETH: DOWEL-AND-CORE TECHNIQUES

The fabrication of a dowel, or post, is the most readily abused step in the procedure for restoration of a pulpless

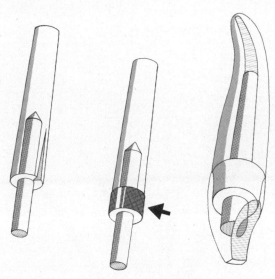

FIG. 21-4. Basic principle for a foundation restoration for the single rooted abutment tooth. Splitting of a wooden tent pole is prevented by the addition of a metal ferrule *(arrow).* A single-rooted abutment tooth requires similar ferrulelike protection (with dowel, coping, and core) against fracture.

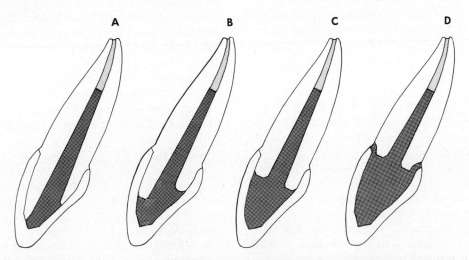

FIG. 21-5. Various methods by which a single-rooted tooth can be reinforced. Notches indicate the amount of tooth structure lost and the necessary core additions. **A,** Adequate coronal dentin precludes the use of a core. **B,** One third of the coronal dentin was lost and replaced with a core addition to the dowel. **C,** Two thirds of the coronal dentin was lost and replaced with a core addition to the dowel. **D,** All coronal dentin was lost. A complete foundation (dowel-core-coping) restoration is needed. Crown-lengthening procedures have to be considered in these cases if a 3 mm coping cannot be placed.

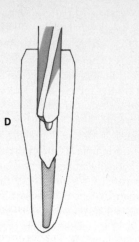

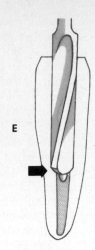

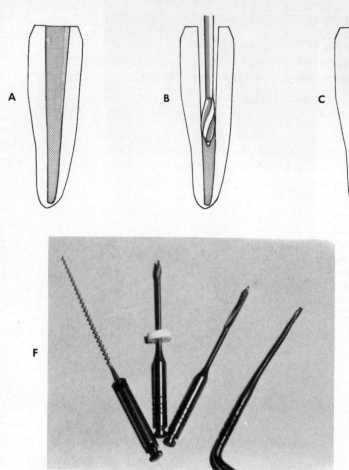

FIG. 21-6. Instrumentation for dowel space. **A,** Warm root canal plugger softens gutta-percha. **B,** Gates-Glidden bur removes softened gutta-percha to proper depth (4 mm from apex). Only gutta-percha is removed in this step. **C,** Peeso reamer is introduced to shape canal walls to proper depth. Slight amount of dentin is removed to smooth internal undercuts. **D,** If needed, Peeso reamer of larger diameter is introduced into coronal portion only to develop parallel sided walls for added retention in coronal third. Bur is stopped at point where dentin is removed. **E,** Abusive overinstrumentation of canal unnecessarily weakens apical portion of canal *(arrow)*. **F,** Instruments for dowel space preparation, impression, and cementation. *Left to right:* Lentulo spiral, Gates-Glidden with stop in place, Peeso reamer, root canal plugger used to soften gutta-percha for instrumentation.

tooth. The preparation of an adequate channel is difficult, and fear of perforation often leads to the acceptance of a foreshortened channel. In addition, reproducing the length and form of the channel requires considerable skill. There is no universal technique suitable for every tooth or to every clinician's skill; however, a discussion of the most widely employed techniques may be helpful.

Armamentarium for preparation of the dowel channel

A radiograph is used to ascertain root curvature, length, and wall thickness. A dowel length of 8 mm is practical for most teeth.

However, some teeth require special attention when preparing a dowel space. Occasionally, some maxillary and mandibular central and lateral incisors have roots too short to accept a dowel length of 8 mm and still maintain a 4-mm apical seal of gutta-percha. The maxillary first premolar is also difficult to properly build up because of short roots combined with minimal root diameter. When the radiograph reveals longer than usual roots, advantage should be taken of the opportunity for added dowel length for retention and reinforcement of the dowel and core.

The preparation of the dowel space obturated with gutta-percha can be accomplished safely by means of the following procedure.

First, the gutta-percha is warmed with a root canal plugger and then a Gates Glidden drill introduced (Fig. 21-6), using a size that will remove the majority of the gutta-percha without removing dentin. If resistance is felt, the drill must not be forced. It must be removed and the gutta-percha rewarmed before one can proceed. Four mm of gutta-percha is left for an apical seal. It is prudent to use a stop on the Gates Glidden, as shown in Fig. 21-6, *F.*

Next, after the proper length of the dowel space has been obtained with the Gates Glidden drill, the final shaping of the canal is done with a Peeso reamer of the same number (Fig. 21-6). It will bind slightly when introduced into the canal. When this step of preparation is completed, all gutta-percha and root canal sealant should be removed from the walls of the dowel space. This step will help determine the type of dowel to be used (i.e., preformed or cast dowel and core) (Fig. 21-24).

It is important that excessive dentin not be removed in preparation of the dowel space. More than 1 mm of dentinal walls must remain to resist masticatory forces.[28,31] The post diameter would vary from 0.7 mm on mandibular incisors to 1.7 mm on maxillary incisors.[25]

The Peeso reamer that will give an adequate dowel space for proper reinforcement would fall between the no. 3 and 4 reamer or a diameter of 1.1 through 1.3 mm,

FIG. 21-7. Failures of composite core foundations due to lack of dentinal support and coping. **A,** Teeth 7, 8, and 10 were restored with a preformed post and a composite core. There was insufficient coronal dentin and coping to resist the forces of mastication. The arrow indicates the preformed post remaining on tooth 10. To restore these teeth, crown lengthening and a cast post and core were necessary to gain sufficient reinforcement and retention for new restorations. **B,** Loss of restoration and fracture of root from lack of proper reinforcement. Arrow indicated root fracture. **C,** Insufficient dentinal walls remaining to support a fixed bridge with preformed post and composite core.

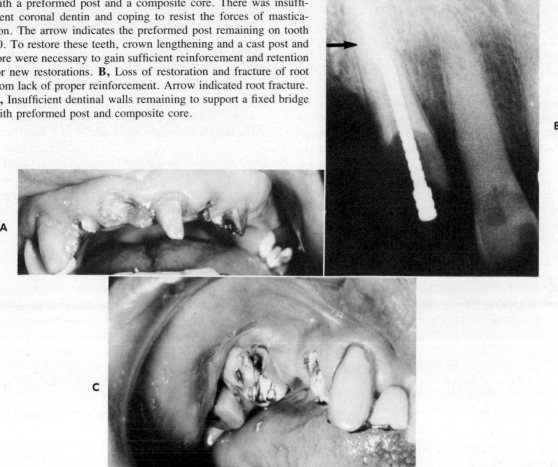

depending on the availability of tooth structure. The smaller diameter no. 2 Peeso would ordinarily be used only for mandibular anterior teeth, maxillary first premolars, buccal roots of maxillary molars, and mesial roots of mandibular molars. When the coronal portion of the canal size is such that a no. 4 or larger Peeso reamer is required to reach sound dentin, then the canal should be tapered in form and a custom cast post used in order to conserve the apical dentin. The dentin remaining in the apical third is most important to prevent root fracture in this area (Fig. 21-6, *E*).

Another approach to the root with a large orifice would be to instrument the dowel space in two stages (Fig. 21-6, *D*). The apical portion of the canal is instrumented with the smaller Peeso reamer and the occlusal portion with the large no. 4 or 5 to establish a clean dowel channel without overinstrumentation. An additional benefit of two-stage instrumentation is that it results in a parallel sided channel that greatly enhances the retention of the post.[27]

Root canals obturated with silver points present a most difficult problem (Fig. 21-8, *B*). Techniques for removing silver cones are described in Chapter 8. Silver points that resist removal should not be reduced by grinding. The

risks of grinding against a silver point include root perforation and loss of the cement seal leading to possible apical inflammation. To minimize these risks, the clinician would be forced to settle for dowel of inadequate length. The prudent operative compromise would be to cement three to four retention pins to retain a core addition and prepare for a 3-mm coping effect.

Cementation of the dowel

The considerations when cementing a dowel are as follows:

1. Fit of the dowel
2. Cleaning and surface preparation of the canal
3. Cleaning and surface preparation of the dowel
4. Selection of the luting agent, or cement

The dowel, whether cast or preformed, should not be forced into place but should fit loosely in the canal. If there is a possibility of hydraulic pressure building up, a small relief channel should be placed the length of the post for cement escape. The dowel should be placed only with finger pressure. No biting force or tapping to place with a mallet should be used.

The canal walls should be free of all restorative materials. The properly prepared canal should have no gutta-percha or root canal sealant present. As recommended by Goldman,[10] the canal walls should be cleansed with the chelating agent 17% ethlendiamine-tetra-acetic acid (EDTA), followed by rinse with 5.25% sodium hypochlorite. The canal walls are then rinsed with water and dried with paper points. This procedure will help remove the

"dentinal smear layer," which lessens the retentive properties of the luting agents.

The surface configuration of the dowel has been shown to greatly affect retention. Serrated posts are reported to be as much as 4.3 times more retentive than smooth-walled posts.[4] The surface of a cast post can be altered with air abrasives or with a coarse diamond to simulate a serrated surface and thereby increase the retentive properties.[20]

The luting or cementing agents that seem to have the best results are the zinc phosphate and glass ionomer cements.[29] Epoxy and composite cements are being developed, but results obtained with these cements appear not to be advantageous at this time.

Techniques with premanufactured components

Kurer crown anchor system. The advantage of the Kurer crown anchor system (Fig. 21-9) is the ease by which the dowel and core can be obtained.

Basically the components are supplied as a screw (dowel) with an elongated head (core). The assortment of core sizes ranges from 2.5 to 4 mm diameter, and the core can be shaped to a preparation form of adequate circumference for a limited number of single-rooted teeth. The retentive capability of a tooth preparation is proportional to the length, taper, and circumference of its preparation walls. This is especially true of preparations supporting porcelain jacket crowns, which resist fracture best near or within 1.5 mm of the cement interface. Optimum preparations for maxillary central incisors and canines therefore may have diameters of 5 to 7 mm and walls extending 2 to 4 mm farther than the core supplied; such preparations may be a contraindication to this system's use.

The Kurer system specifies that the canal entrance re-

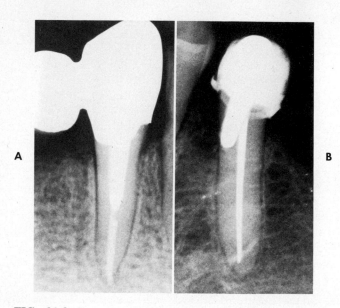

FIG. 21-8. Improper clinical judgment in obturating the root canal should not be compounded by an inadequate restorative effort. **A,** Dowel of adequate length for a short-span bridge. An additional 3 mm in dowel length is optimal for bridges with a two- or three-pontic span. **B,** Silver points should be removed and the apical third of the root canal obturated with gutta-percha to avoid root perforation during dowel preparation.

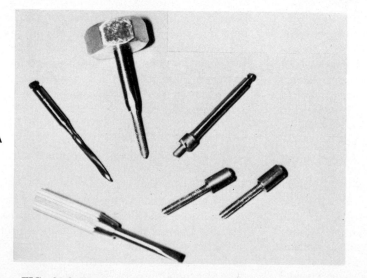

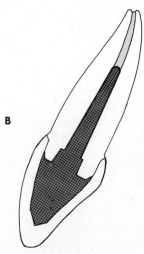

FIG. 21-9. Kurer crown anchor system. **A,** Armamentarium *(clockwise beginning at bottom):* screwdriver, Girdwood bur, root canal tap, root frazer, and dowels with core additions. **B,** Core addition shaped to resemble the preparation of a maxillary incisor. The size of the core is proportioned to offer optimal retention for the final restoration. A recess in the coronal end of the root is made with the root frazer to gain a positive seat for the core. The ferrule-type circumferential preparation, a most important feature, has been omitted in this illustration.

ceive a well-type recess, accomplished with a root facer. The recess provides a positive seat for the core. Next, the canal is tapped. The dowel and core can now be trial seated and adjusted for proper length. For the final seating procedure the dowel is dipped into cement and rotated into the canal until the core is firmly seated within the recess. Since the core represents the screw head, it can be shaped to the desired preparation only after cementation is accomplished. The technique should specify use of a ferrule-type coping instead of a gingivally inclined shoulder on the labial and lingual aspects to resist rotation of the final restoration.

A successful application of the Kurer system must include the following precautions.

1. Ensuring that the tooth size compares favorably with available core sizes
2. Ensuring that the morphology of the canal orifice is adaptable to a circular dowel preparation without sacrifice of mesial and distal root dentin
3. Ensuring that the root dentin is sufficiently resilient to resist fracture during cementation
4. Controlling heat and trauma during core shaping
5. Surrounding the root with a 2 mm ferrule-type preparation so the final restoration will provide coping protection

The disadvantage of the Kurer crown anchor system is the removal of a considerable amount of dentin. Accordingly, root perforation and/or a split root are risks the clinician must consider before selecting this technique.

Whaledent dowel system. As with the Kurer system, a complete armamentarium is available in kit form for the Whaledent dowel system (Fig. 21-10). The circular dowel is threaded; however, the intent is only for greater cement retention, not for the dowel to serve as a screw.

A groove extending the length of the dowel acts as an escape channel to lessen hydraulic pressure during cementation. An ingenious paralleling instrument may be used for drilling supplemental pin channels parallel with and at selected distances from the dowel channel. Metal pins are supplied and become an integral part of a plastic core addition to the dowel. Nylon pins are used for a cast-gold core addition technique. The intended function of the supplemental pins is to resist rotation of the core, which is attached to a circular dowel, and to offer some protection against root fracture. There should be little doubt that coping protection provides these functions far more effectively.

The longitudinal cement escape channel of the dowel is a commendable feature; however, the cylindrical shape of the dowel raises concern. A dowel should extend two thirds the length of the root into a naturally tapered channel. The use of a cylindrical dowel necessitates excessive removal of root dentin at the apical end of the orifice or selection of an undersized dowel, which would fit loosely at the coronal entrance.

Stutz pivot system. The Stutz pivot system consists of a shell 14 mm long and a matching dowel (Fig. 21-11). This system offers a simple approach to dowel-and-core fabrication and minimizes the hazard of cementation (Fig. 21-12).

The root orifice is enlarged with a Stutz or Ackerman bur. The shell is then trial seated and cemented. A carrier tool is provided to facilitate the introduction of the shell into the canal and to prevent the flow of cement into the shell. For all practical purposes, there should be no detrimental hydraulic pressures generated in the cementing of the shell. Its walls are tapered, and only reasonable accuracy of seating is required. The dowel may now be seated

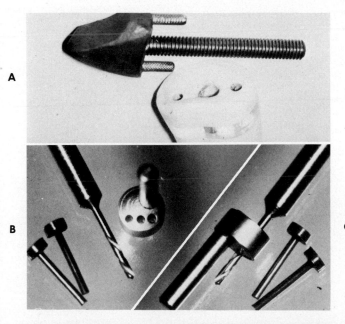

FIG. 21-10. Whaledent dowel system. **A,** Plastic core pattern with dowel and parallel auxiliary metal pins. **B,** Armamentarium *(from left):* plastic pins, twist drill, and paralleling device for pin channels, which can be placed 1, 2, or 3 mm from the root canal. **C,** Twist drill inserted into the paralleling device. When the plunger is anchored in the root canal, the auxiliary pin channels can be readily made parallel with the root canal.

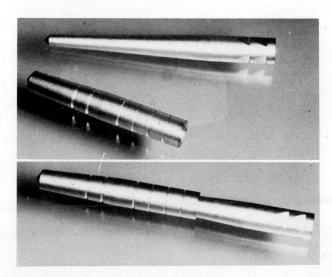

FIG. 21-11. Major components employed with the Stutz pivot system: dowel and shell.

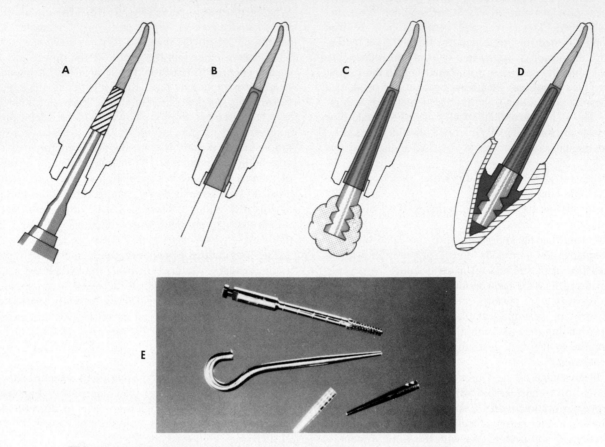

FIG. 21-12. Procedure and armamentarium for the Stutz pivot system. **A,** Preparation of the dowel channel. **B,** Cementation of the sleeve. **C,** Dowel with wax retention for the indirect impression technique. **D,** Dowel with core addition cemented. Final restoration seated for verification. **E,** Dowel and sleeve, sleeve-seating instrument, and calibrated tapered fissure bur.

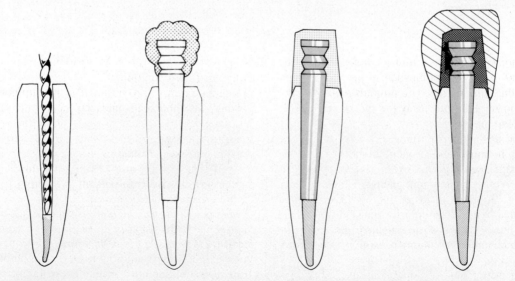

FIG. 21-13. Steps for developing a cast post and core with the Unitek BCH post system. This system has excellent versatility due to the large selection of posts in varying diameters and lengths. The system is calibrated to the Peeso reamers.

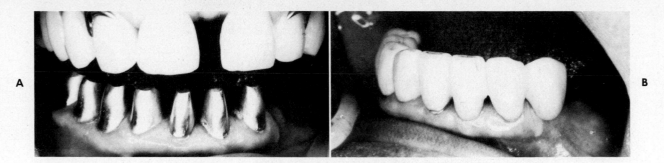

FIG. 21-14 Foundation restorations fabricated with the Kerr Endopost system, **A,** and a subsequently constructed porcelain-bonded-to-metal splint, **B.**

FIG. 21-15. Unitek BCH endodontic post system.

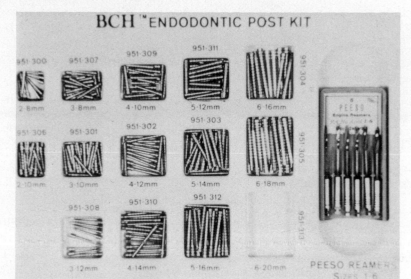

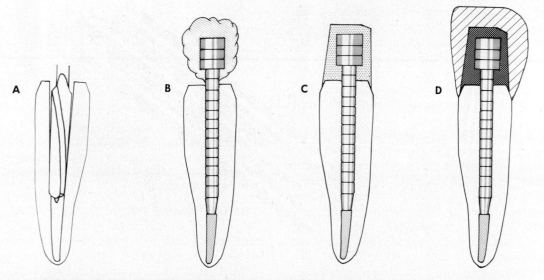

FIG. 21-16 Procedure with the Kerr Endopost system. **A,** Initial removal of gutta-percha has been done with a Gates-Glidden bur. Final instrumentation of the dowel channel is achieved with a Kerr Endofile. **B,** Kerr Endopost, calibrated to the Endofile, seated in the root canal channel and furnished with sticky wax retention for the indirect impression technique. **C,** Kerr Endopost with wax or plastic core addition ready for processing by the direct core technique. **D,** Laboratory fabrication of an entire foundation restoration, Kerr Endopost, core, and coping.

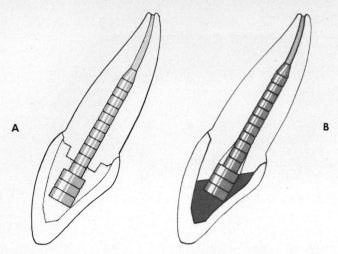

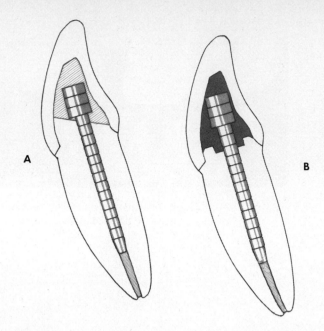

FIG. 21-17. A, Maxillary incisor with a Unitek post retaining a cast core. The direction of the occlusal force against the maxillary anterior tooth calls for the use of a cast core when half or more of the preparation is replaced by a core addition. **B,** Maxillary incisor with cast post and core.

and a plastic core pattern shaped. (Plastic is preferred to wax, because the dowel fits snugly into the shell and there is less chance for distortion of the core pattern when the dowel is withdrawn.)

For the indirect technique a large bulk of plastic must be added to the dowel so it will be retained in the impression material. Once the core has been cast to the dowel, the dowel and core may be cemented accurately and the tooth preparation finalized.

Kerr Endopost system. The Kerr Endopost system (Figs. 21-13 and 21-14) provides a simple procedure for the fabrication of dowel-and-core foundations for small single-rooted teeth with nearly circular root canal orifices. The armamentarium offers a selection of reamers of various diameters and matching Endoposts.

The canal orifice is reamed to the desired depth and the dowel fitted. The procedure for fabricating a core-and-coping addition is identical to the one described for the Stutz pivot system.

Unitek BCH endodontic post system. The Unitek BCH endodontic post system and the knurled wire system (Figs. 21-15 to 21-22) provide the operator with a wide selection of dowel lengths and diameters. For convenience the BCH system is calibrated to the Peeso reamers. The knurled wire system gives excellent versatility in dowel form and length. It is useful in developing direct patterns of post and cores and allows the core addition to be cast directly to the knurled wire retention post. (Fig. 21-17, *B*).

Whaledent para-post system. Para-posts are obtainable in various diameters and are of sufficient length for most clinical situations (Fig. 21-23, *A*). The form of the para-post is optimized for retention, with parallel sides and a serrated surface. The serrations are for retention, and the post is not screwed into place but is passively cemented. The system also provides plastic patterns carefully calibrated to Whaledent drill sizes, allowing the operator excellent casting patterns for cast posts and cores.

FIG. 21-18. A, Mandibular incisor with a Unitek post retaining a composite core. The composite core is adequate for a single-tooth restoration when half or more of the dentinal walls remain. **B,** Mandibular incisor with a Unitek post and cast core. A cast core is indicated because of loss of tooth structure.

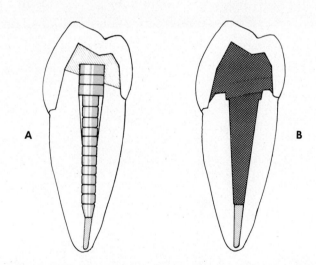

FIG. 21-19. A, Manibular premolar with a Unitek post retaining a composite or amalgam core. When half of the core is remaining dentin, this is an excellent buildup. **B,** Manibular premolar with a cast dowel and core.

Starlite Endowel system. Starlite Endowels (Fig. 21-24) are plastic tapered dowel pins that are color coded and calibrated to match endodontic files or reamers of sizes 80, 90, 100, 120, and 140.

When the dowel preparation has been finalized with file or reamer instrumentation, an equivalent-sized Endowel is inserted to serve as a ready dowel pattern for either the direct or the indirect core buildup technique.

Noteworthy is the longitudinal V groove on either side of the Endowel, which, when reproduced in the final casting, allows excess cement to escape coronally.

Parkell calibrated instrument system. The armamentarium for the Parkell calibrated instrument system in-

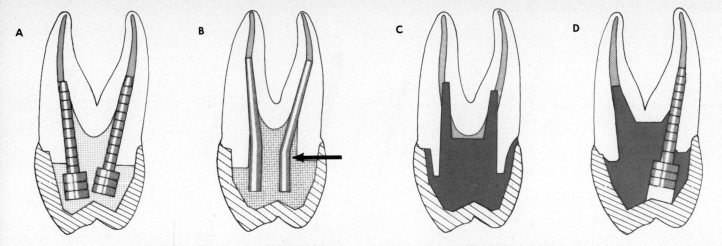

FIG. 21-20. A, Maxillary first premolar with Unitek posts retaining a composite or amalgam core. This procedure is adequate for the support of a single-tooth restoration. To serve as a bridge abutment, the tooth should be rebuilt with a cast dowel and core. **B,** Maxillary first premolar with Kerr Endopost or knurled wire. Post is bent *(arrow)* to give the composite or amalgam the best distribution around it. Three-pronged clasp bending pliers are useful for this procedure. **C,** Maxillary first premolar with parallel cast post canals are instrumented as deeply as possible without endangering the root. **D,** Maxillary first premolar with non-parallel cast post. The Unitek pin seats through a hole in the casting at cementation. This gives maximum length for posts in each canal without danger of overinstrumentation.

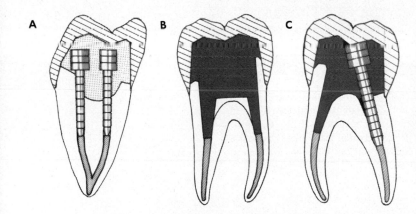

FIG. 21-21. A, Mesial view of a mandibular molar with Unitek posts cemented into the canals of a mesial root and retaining a composite or amalgam core. **B,** Mandibular molar with parallel cast dowel and core buildup. **C,** Mandibular molar with nonparallel cast dowel and core with a Unitek post placed in a hole in the casting for the nonparallel canal. This procedure allows maximum length for the dowels without danger of overinstrumentation. This buildup would provide maximum retention and reinforcement for a bridge abutment.

FIG. 21-22. A, Maxillary molar with a Unitek post cemented into the mesiobuccal, distobuccal, and palatal root channels to retain and support a composite or amalgam core. **B,** Maxillary molar with a cast nonparallel dowel and core. This type of reinforcement works very well for the maxillary molar with widely divergent roots and little or no coronal dentinal support.

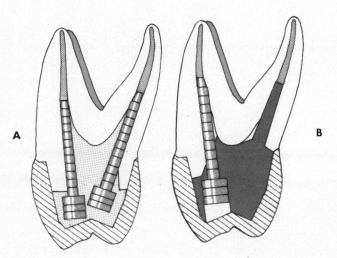

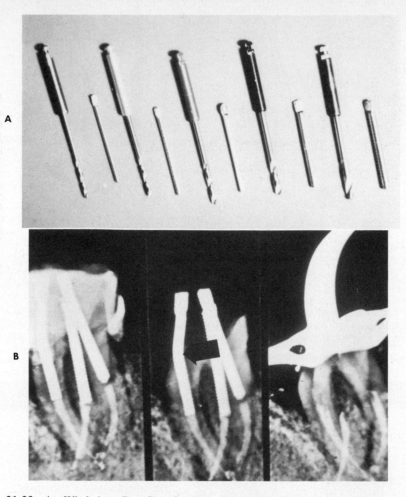

FIG. 21-23. A, Whaledent Para-Post-System. Color-coded drills of various diameters with matched metal posts. Excellent system for amalgam or composite buildups. This system also provides precisely calibrated casting patterns that match the drills. B, Posts in place for a composite buildup. Note bend in Para-Post in palatal canal to properly space posts for buildup material. Posts should be spaced to keep a uniform thickness of core material around all surfaces of the post. (B courtesy Dr. Ronald Nicholson.)

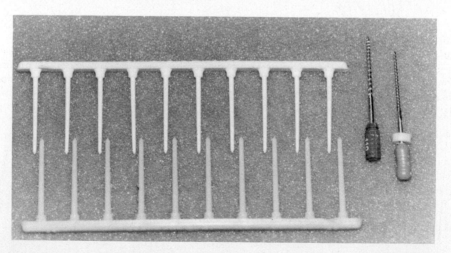

FIG. 21-24 Starlite Endowels of various diameters. The file or reamer is used to prepare the dowel preparation.

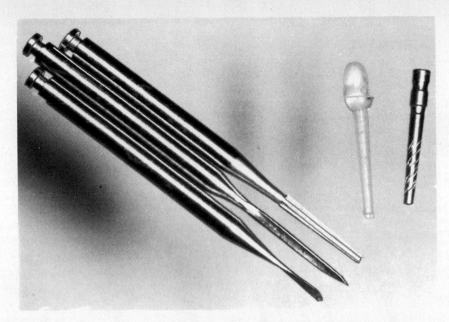

FIG. 21-25. Parkell calibrated instrument kit. *From left,* Double-bladed bur, reamer bur, tapered fissue bur, and plastic and metal dowel pins.

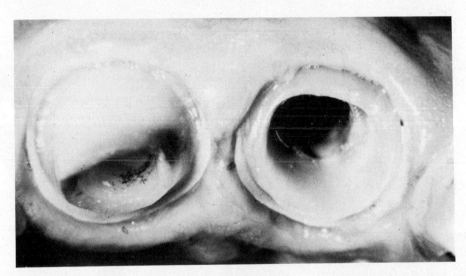

FIG. 21-26. Large and/or irregular canal orifices, necessitating the fabrication of individual dowels.

cludes burs and dowel pins of equivalent sizes (Fig. 21-25).

The dowel preparation is initiated with a two-bladed bur. A reamer bur is then used to establish the length of the dowel channel. The preparation is finished with a tapered fissure bur calibrated to match the plastic and stainless steel dowel pins. When the tapered stainless steel dowel post is cemented with zinc oxyphosphate cement, a suprastructure is provided upon which composite resins or amalgam can be adapted. This then acts as a base for a permanent restoration.

The plastic dowel pins are used for the direct dowel-and-core technique; that is, the core buildup with self-curing resin or inlay wax is accomplished in the mouth. The stainless steel dowel serves as a transfer pin when the in-direct dowel-and-core technique is preferred (laboratory fabrication). The metal pin is lubricated before the impression is poured; the pin is then removed from the stone cast and replaced by a plastic dowel pin. The core addition can now be waxed. The stainless steel dowel pin may also retain an interim plastic crown.

Techniques with components fabricated by the dentist

Indirect dowel-and-core technique. The indirect dowel-and-core technique is most versatile in its application, particularly for teeth with large or irregular canal orifices (Figs. 21-26 and 21-27). The indirect technique also should be applied to damaged teeth with little remaining tooth structure and to posterior teeth with nonparallel roots that need core additions.

When the canal and initial tooth preparation has been

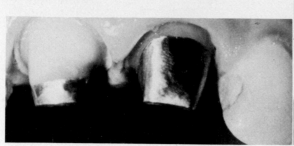
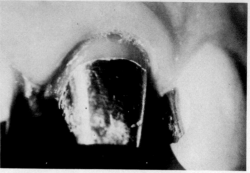

FIG. 21-27 Dowel-retained core additions of varying sizes according to the amount of missing coronal tooth structure in need of replacement for optimal preparation form. For cosmetic reasons the margin for the final restoration should be in tooth structure. A cement margin, as revealed by the enlarged view, is acceptable. The cementation of the dowel and core is not critical; this margin will be protected by the final restoration, which will extend farther gingivally by at least 2 mm.

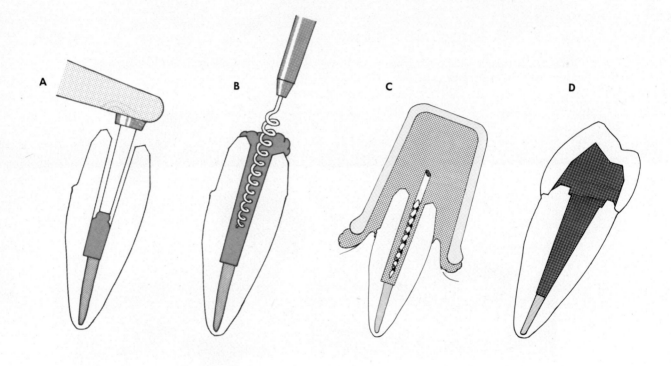

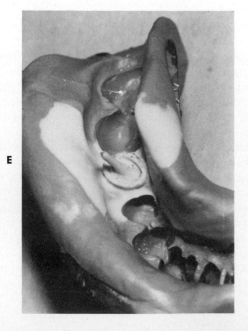

FIG. 21-28. A, Impression material is carried as far into the canal as possible with syringe tip. **B,** Lentulo spiral removes air bubbles and prevents voids in impression. **C,** A broken file is introduced into the impression material for reinforcement of post. Care must be taken that the segment of file does not touch the impression tray. **D,** Finished dowel and core in place with final restoration. **E,** Impression with 3M polysiloxane Express.

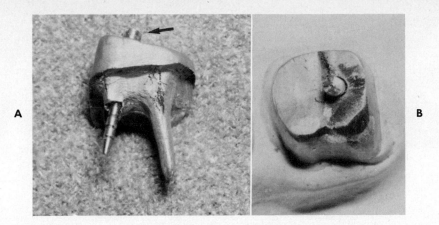

FIG. 21-29. A, The restoration of a molar with divergent roots where a complete core foundation is necessary. The Unitek post is shown partially withdrawn from the casting *(arrow).* **B,** Assembled post and core with Unitek post in place. The Unitek post is cemented at the same time as the casting.

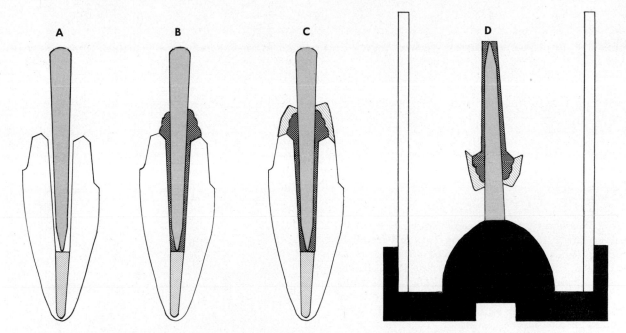

FIG. 21-30. Direct technique for dowel-and-core fabrication. **A.** Plastic dowel pin loosely fitted to the canal channel. **B,** Autocuring resin applied. **C,** Final core pattern carved in wax. **D.** Dowel-and-core pattern invested for casting. There is no asbestos liner.

accomplished, the impression material of choice is injected into the canal orifice.

The vinyl polysiloxane elastomeric material Express* gives a superior impression of the post space. The syringe material is introduced into the canal with Lentulo spiral (Fig. 21-28, *B).*

The polysiloxane can be reinforced with a segment of a no. 50 or 60 endo file that has been shortened to fit the canal. It is imperative that the reinforcing segment of the file not protrude. If the impression tray touches the file, it

will be placed under tension and will hopelessly distort the impression of the post space.

For large-diameter posts (1.2 mm or larger), reinforcement of the polysiloxane has not been necessary because of the strength and accuracy of this material. The main purpose of the reinforcment is to prevent deflection of the canal impression during pouring of the stone cast.

When the cast is ready for waxing, it must be thoroughly lubricated. The wax is carried into the canal with a hot instrument and all voids removed by heating a PKT no. 1 waxing instrument or a root canal plugger until red and inserting it to the bottom of the dowel space. A section of an endo file is heated and place to the bottom of the

---

*Express and its automixing system for the syringe material were developed by the 3M Co., St. Paul, MN.

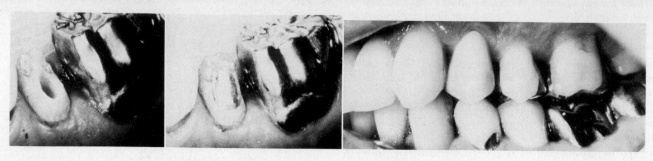

FIG. 21-31. Application of the direct dowel-and-core technique.

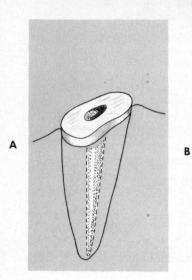

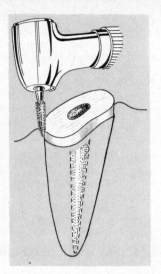

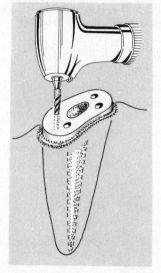

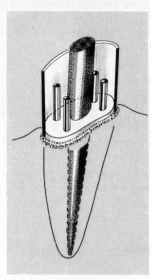

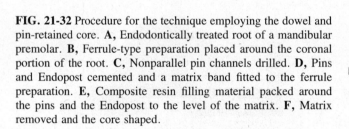

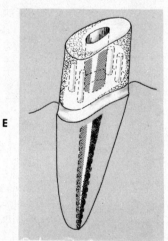

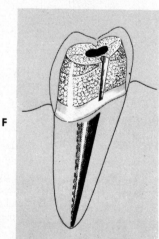

FIG. 21-32 Procedure for the technique employing the dowel and pin-retained core. **A,** Endodontically treated root of a mandibular premolar. **B,** Ferrule-type preparation placed around the coronal portion of the root. **C,** Nonparallel pin channels drilled. **D,** Pins and Endopost cemented and a matrix band fitted to the ferrule preparation. **E,** Composite resin filling material packed around the pins and the Endopost to the level of the matrix. **F,** Matrix removed and the core shaped.

wax pattern for reinforcement. The file becomes a convenient means of removing the pattern without breakage or distortion. The file also allows pumping of the pattern several times to ensure easy withdrawal before completing the core addition. At burnout, the file reinforcement is removed with a hemostat before casting.

The custom cast dowel should be slightly undersized to avoid internal stress on the root during cementation and try-in. This is easily accomplished using 50 gm of Lustercast* investment with 18 ml of water and no liner for the

*Kerr Sybron Company, Romulous, MI.

casting ring during the investment procedure. A cast dowel and core on teeth with nonparallel roots that need extensive restoration can be restored using the following procedure. A casting is made in the larger root, which is integral with the core addition. A lubricated Unitek post is incorporated into the wax-up and withdrawn, leaving the post channel (Fig. 21-29, *A*). (For illustrations of techniques for mandibular and maxillary molars, see Figs. 21-21, *C,* and 21-22, *B*.) To maintain patency of the hole during the casting procedure, a graphite plug should be placed in the channel. After casting, the graphite is removed with a bur.

Construction of the dowel-and-core foundation and subsequent final restoration on one cast is not advocated as a procedure of choice; there is no allowance for minor discrepancies that may occur in the cementing of the dowel and core. Should the need for only one cast arise, it is suggested that a die spacer be formed over the core before the final restoration is waxed. The minute space gained should compensate for discrepancies and ensure marginal integrity of the final restoration.

Direct dowel-and-core technique. A direct approach to dowel-and-core construction is preferred by many clinicians because it avoids the impression procedure.[26]

A plastic dowel pin is loosely fitted to the prepared and lubricated canal channel (Fig. 21-30, A). The pin should be 10 mm longer than the core addition to serve as a handle and sprue. A pattern of the canal channel is obtained when the pin is relined with autocuring resin (Fig. 21-30, B). During setting of the resin, the pattern is pumped frequently to ensure withdrawal. Excess resin is roughly shaped to serve as a matrix for the core addition, but the final core pattern is added and carved in wax (Fig. 21-30, C). Wax can be manipulated with greater ease than resin. Protection of the tongue and lower lip with a 2 × 2 inch gauze sponge is a simple precaution when hot wax is carried to the tooth by a beavertail burnisher or by cotton pliers. The completed dowel-and-core pattern is withdrawn by its pin handle and invested for casting (Fig. 21-30, D).

The direct dowel-and-core technique can be a time-saver in cases requiring minimal core addition to the preparation (Fig. 21-31). Large core additions, core-and-coping combinations, or multiple dowel-and-core foundations can be carved and finished with greater accuracy and ease by the indirect technique. Casting mishaps cannot be rectified when the direct approach is used, however.

Endopost with pin-retained core technique. A dowel-and-core foundation may be fabricated in one appointment by a technique suggested by Sapone[24]:

1. A 2 to 3 mm ferrule-type preparation is placed around the coronal portion of the root. The field may now be isolated with a gingival retraction cord and rubber dam (Fig. 21-32, B).
2. The canal orifice is cleared to within 5 mm of the apex and an Endopost is fitted accurately.
3. The canal orifice is obstructed with cotton while four nonparallel pin channels are drilled (Fig. 21-32, C) and the pins cemented (Fig. 21-32, D). Cemented pins are preferred over threaded pins in the treatment of brittle, pulpless teeth. A threaded pin offers six times greater retention potential[8]; however, pins cemented into 3 to 4 mm deep channels should offer adequate retention.
4. The Endopost is cemented and a matrix band is fitted to the ferrule-type preparation (Fig. 21-32, D).
5. A composite resin filling material is packed around the pins and Endopost to the level of the matrix (Fig. 21-32, E).
6. After a sufficient hardening time, the matrix is removed and the core shaped (Fig. 21-32, F).
7. The rubber dam is removed, the retraction cord retrieved, and the impressions taken for the final restoration.

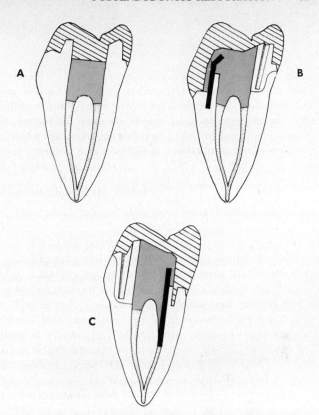

FIG. 21-33 Various methods for the restoration of mandibular molar with partial veneer coverage. **A,** Mesial-occlusal-distal onlay. B, Nonparallel pin supporting a composite or amalgam core for a reverse three-quarter crown. **C,** Pins in the root canal supporting a composite or amalgam core for a three-quarter crown.

RESTORATION OF MULTIROOTED TEETH

The large circumference of a multirooted tooth generally precludes the necessity for a reinforcement dowel.[8] Core additions are retained by the existing coronal tooth structure through the use of retention pins.

These pins are cemented rather than threaded into the brittle dentin. When there is a lack of coronal dentin, core retention must be gained from the nearly parallel walls of the prepared pulp chamber and from short parallel dowels extending into the divergent root canals. Because the cosmetic requirement is not critical in the posterior region of the dental arches, a number of molar teeth may be prepared to receive partial veneer retainers. The objective is to design the retainer with the potential to protect the tooth against fracture. Tooth preparation following the principles of extracoronal resistance and complete occlusal protection can accomplish this.

Mandibular molar abutment

A tooth with sound, prominently contoured, axial enamel surfaces and in favorable occlusal-axial alignment may be prepared to receive a mesial-occlusal-distal-type onlay retainer (Fig. 21-33, A) to serve as an abutment for a short-span fixed bridge.

The bulbous pulp chamber is filled with an amalgam or composite base. Both buccal and lingual cusps are hooded

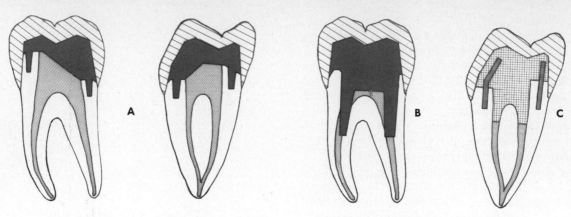

FIG. 21-34 Various methods of core additions to a mandibular molar in preparation for full crown coverage. **A,** Cast gold core addition utilizing the parallel pin technique. **B,** In cases of insufficient tooth structure, retention is gained from within the pulp chamber and by the placement of short dowel pins. **C,** Nonparallel pin-supported composite or amalgam core extending into the pulp chamber.

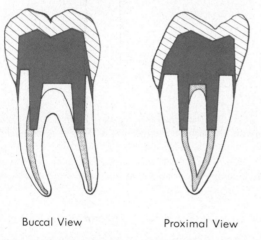

Buccal View   Proximal View

FIG. 21-35. Use of an entire foundation restoration (dowel, core, and coping) for a grossly defective mandibular molar. The combination of internal and circumferential retention and a resistance form provides optimal protection for this abutment tooth. The nonparallel post and core technique also can be used in the event of widely divergent roots, as shown in Fig. 21-29.

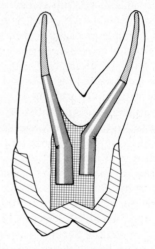

FIG. 21-36. Reinforcement of maxillary molar with preformed posts, Endoposts, or Unitek posts with composite resin supporting a full veneer crown. Note that the posts are shaped *(arrow)* with three-pronged clasp pliers to gain the optimum space for the composite core.

sufficiently to gain reciprocating walls of 2 to 3 mm length. The action of these walls tend to contain the tooth structure within the retainer and counteract wedgelike stress generated with intracoronal retainers by the lever action of the bridge span on the abutment.

Fig. 21-33, *B,* shows a tooth with a fractured buccal cusp but a sound prominently contoured lingual enamel surface. Two to three nonparallel pins are cemented into the buccal root dentin to aid in the retention of a silver alloy or composite resin core. The preparation for a reverse three-quarters crown retainer will best preserve the remaining coronal tooth structure. Adequate hooding of the lingual cusp substantially adds to the protection potential of the retainer and allows for the occlusal realignment of teeth with a lingual-axial inclination. Mesial and distal retention grooves must be placed entirely in dentin, never in core material; otherwise, the circumferential protection of extracoronal retainers cannot be achieved.

A tooth with a fractured mesial-lingual cusp but with a sound enamel surface is presented in Fig. 21-33, *C.* A pin is cemented into the lingual canal of the mesial root to aid in the retention of the silver alloy or composite resin core. The tooth is prepared to receive a three-quarter crown retainer with extensive hooding of the buccal cusps; additional retention from the lingual root dentin is provided through the use of parallel pins.

The occlusal third of the tooth preparation in Fig. 21-34, *A,* was lost and replaced with a cast-gold core. The margins of the final full veneer restoration are placed 2 mm below the farthest gingival extension of the core to gain optimum marginal integrity.

Should an inadequate bulk of dentin prevent the placement of pins, the walls of the pulp chamber may be prepared with a slight taper and short dowels extended into the double-rooted canals. This method will provide adequate retention for the core addition (Fig. 21-34, *B*).

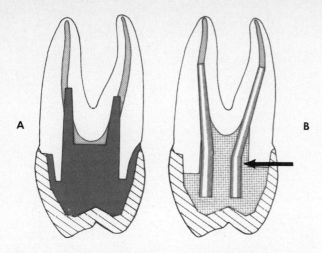

FIG. 21-37. Reinforcement and restoration of a maxillary first premolar. **A,** Cast cores supporting a full veneer crown. **B,** Two Endoposts with composite resin supporting a full veneer crown.

The use of nonparallel pins combined with the retention potential of the pulp chamber will greatly enhance the strength of an amalgam or composite core addition. However, the area of greatest resistance to dislodgement of the full veneer crown is near its gingival extension; the final restoration therefore should always encompass not less than 2 mm of tooth structure beyond the core addition (Fig. 21-34, *C*).

When there is a gross defect of coronal tooth structure or when extensive restorative treatment is planned, the pulpless tooth should be protected with a core-and-coping combination (Fig. 21-35). Internal retention can be gained by instrumenting the walls of the pulp chamber and extending short dowels into the root canals. External retention and circumferential protection result from the ferrule effect of the coping. The gingival margins of the bridge retainer are formed by the core-coping and are usually placed at or slightly above the gingival margin. This procedure greatly facilitates not only tooth protection and tissue management during prolonged treatment periods but also the fabrication and insertion of multiabutment restorations.

Maxillary molar abutment

In general, the techniques described for the restoration of mandibular molars are applicable to maxillary molars as well. Minor modifications are dictated by a cosmetic requirement. For example, it may be desirable to preserve the prominent mesial-buccal enamel surface of a maxillary molar that has suffered loss of a lingual cusp. Tooth reduction to accommodate a cosmetic veneer would tend to weaken the remaining coronal tooth structure.

The fabrication of a seven-eighths, partial veneer crown presents a simple solution. The loss of retention on the lingual aspect is compensated by the placement of retention pins, and the mesial-buccal groove offers resistance against lingual displacement of the retainer. Hooding of the buccal cusp for additional protection and a resistance form is cosmetically undesirable; however, a 1 mm occlusal reverse bevel is placed for protection as a compromise.

A reverse three-quarter crown retainer may be chosen for a tooth with loss of buccal tooth structure. This design will best preserve the remaining coronal dentin.

Reinforcement and support of brittle coronal dentin are accomplished with individual Endoposts cemented into the three canals and by obturation of the pulp chamber with a composite resin (Fig. 21-36). This technique permits the retention of fragile tooth structure as preparation walls.

Maxillary first premolar

The restoration of the maxillary first premolar presents more challenges than does that of any other tooth. First, it is a small-diameter tooth and therefore warrants dowel reinforcement; second, it is a multirooted tooth with divergent root canals; and third, it is a tooth with a high cosmetic requirement, usually necessitating a buccal cosmetic veneer. Two techniques commonly used to restore the maxillary first premolar are shown in Fig. 21-37.

When the major portion of coronal dentin is lost, a cast-gold foundation is the treatment of choice (Fig. 21-37, *A*). Parallel dowel preparations are extended as far as possible into the root canals. Additional retention for the core is provided by the walls of the pulp chamber and by the external walls of the remaining tooth structure.

The problem of loss of significant coronal dentin can also be resolved with two Endoposts cemented into the root canal and a composite core addition (Fig. 21-37, *B*). If the premolar is to be used as an abutment tooth, the coping effect should be provided by dentin walls with a 3 mm or more circumference. A further precaution is to use torque-minimizing (nonrigid) connectors to reduce the lever action potential of the fixed bridge span.

SPECIAL RESTORATIVE PROBLEMS
Traumatic injury of a maxillary central incisor

Figs. 21-38 to 21-40 illustrate the procedure for restoration when traumatic injury has occurred in a cosmetic region.

The injury in Fig. 21-38 resulted from a football accident. Over half the coronal tooth structure was lost. Clinical examination revealed an oblique lingual fracture line extending to 3 mm above the alveolar crest (Figs. 21-39 and 21-40, *A*). Access for tooth preparation was gained by gingivectomy and alveolectomy. Sufficient lingual bone was removed to establish a core margin 2 mm coronal to the alveolar crest for the reorganization of the epithelial attachment. The apical third of the canal was obturated with gutta-percha; the remaining facial tooth surface was then reduced axially, and a shoulder was established 1.5 mm subgingivally. The shoulder extended interproximal to the fracture site.

At this point a lightly chamfered finish line was prepared 1.5 mm apical to the shoulder and following the fracture line around the lingual root surface to the opposing shoulder extension. The gingival preparation margin consisted of a facial shoulder and a more apically placed lingual chamfer. When mesial and distal grooves were placed at the junction of the shoulder and chamfer, the facial axial wall was hooded for additional resistance. The lingual half of the tooth resembled the preparation for a

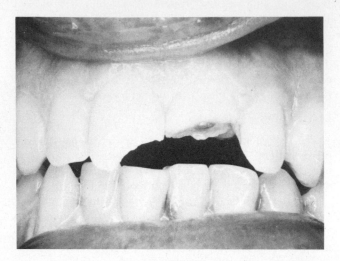

FIG. 21-38. Fracture of maxillary central incisors.

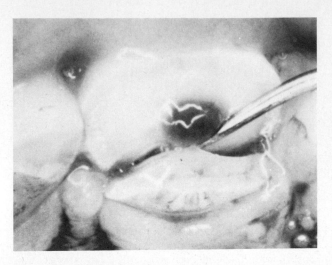

FIG. 21-39. Longitudinal fracture of the maxillary left central incisor in Fig. 22-38.

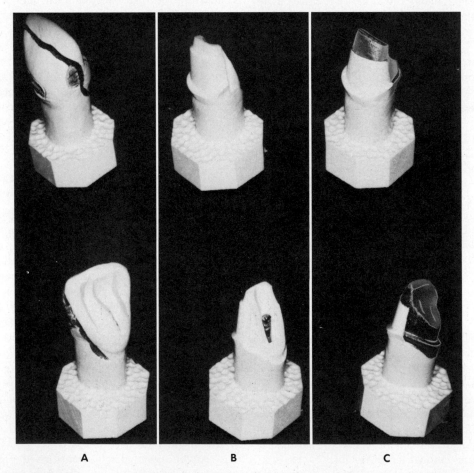

A   B   C

FIG. 21-40. Method of fabricating a foundation restoration in a cosmetic region. **A,** Oblique fracture of a maxillary central incisor extending 2 to 3 mm apical to the alveolar crest. **B,** Preparation design for the dowel and core. The core replaces the lingual tooth structure. It is retained by proximal grooves, a reverse bevel, and the dowel. **C,** This core design allows the placement of a cosmetic gingival margin for the final restoration.

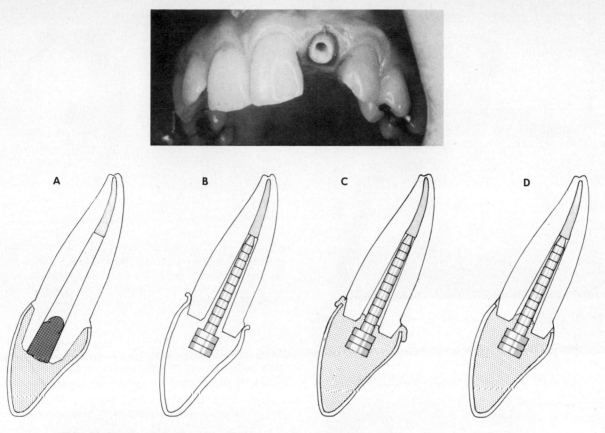

FIG. 21-41. *Top,* Maxillary lateral incisor with a fractured clinical crown prepared for interim coverage. *Bottom,* **A,** Dowel channel obturated with a wax plug to prevent the intrusion of plastic or of temporary cement. **B,** Insufficient tooth structure indicates the need for a retention dowel. The interim dowel pin should be seated loosely in the dowel channel. **C,** As the crown matrix is relined with autocuring resin, the dowel pin becomes an integral part of the crown. **D,** After cementation with a modified temporary cement, the occlusion is adjusted. A light centric contact only and hypocclusion in all excursions are maintained. The root lacks ferrule-type protection during this interim coverage stage.

three-quarters crown. A platinized wire was fitted to serve as a dowel and became an integral part of the core casting (Fig. 21-40, *B*).

The foundation restoration, once cemented, completed the tooth preparation requirements for a porcelain jacket crown or a porcelain-fused-to-metal crown (Fig. 21-40, *C*). The lingual margin was fashioned into the core metal continuous with the facial margin, giving an esthetic result. With the placement of the lingual chamfer apical to the facial shoulder, a continuous shoulder margin could be effected in the core metal without the need for overcontouring at the core-root margin.

Interim restorations

When adequate retentive dentin walls remain, the method of temporization for endodontically treated teeth differs from that for vital teeth only insofar as protection of exposed dentin is not essential.

The temporary coverage can be purposefully short of the marginal gingiva to allow these tissues to heal more favorably. When the preparation extends into a bifurcation area or the gingival outline of the preparation form has been altered due to root amputation, the contour of the interim restoration must reflect an understanding of the principles of physiologic design. This design must afford optimal cleaning and stimulating action for the gingiva. Restorations fabricated with autocuring resins permit better flexibility in shaping the temporary coverage to closely resemble the contour of the final restoration. (See Root amputation, p. 669).

When a tooth is prepared for a cast pin-retained core, the short preparation may be protected with an aluminum shell, tightly adapted at the margins and only high enough to cover the tooth remnant. The pin channels are closed with cotton before the aluminum shell is seated with a temporary zinc oxide—engenol cement.

In cosmetic areas, or where the interim restoration must be in occlusal function, retention can be enhanced by the addition of a plastic or metal dowel into the autocuring resin crown. This procedure is illustrated by the case shown in Figs. 21-41 to 21-43.

The patient had suffered the loss of the clinical crown of the maxillary left lateral incisor. The tooth had been endodontically treated and the canal obturated with gutta-

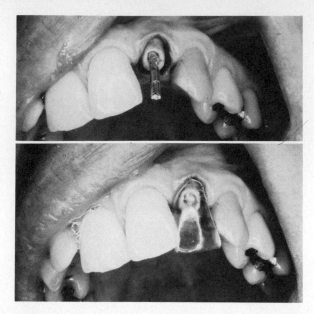

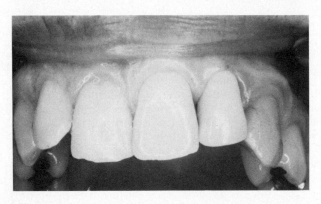

FIG. 21-42. Interim retention dowel fitted and celluloid matrix adapted.

FIG. 21-43. Interim restoration contoured to allow for the reorganization of healthy gingival tissues.

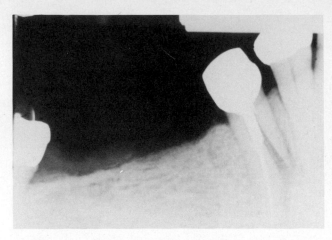

FIG. 21-44. Catastrophic failure of premolar abutment on bridge. Tooth had no coping and the dowel was of insufficient length due to silver point. Solderless connector at the distal of the premolar could potentially prevent this type of failure by providing stress release.

percha. There was no radiographic evidence of apical involvement. The canal was opened to the apical third with a Gates-Glidden bur and smoothly instrumented with a no. 701 Busch long-shanked fissure bur (Fig. 21-41, *top*). The canal orifice was temporarily closed with a soft wax plug (Fig. 21-41, *bottom, A*). A smooth, flame-shaped diamond instrument was used to prepare the coronal 2 mm of the root for a coping. Simultaneously the sulcular epithelium was abraded because of the necessary apical extension of the preparation to gain the coping effect. A small retraction cord saturated with resin epinephrine was gently introduced into the expanded sulcus.

When the preparation length is 3 mm or more, a plastic crown form may be fitted and simply relined with autocuring resin. In this case the preparation length was inadequate (Fig. 21-41, *bottom, B*). An orthodontic wire was loosely fitted into the root canal. A celluloid crown form was then selected, contoured to the gingiva, and perforated in the mesial and distal contact areas (Fig. 21-42). The celluloid serves only as a matrix for autocuring resin and

will be removed. When contact areas in the matrix are relieved, proper tooth contacts are subsequently obtained.

Autocuring resin was used because the patient's tooth color could not be matched with a premanufactured carboxylate crown; this resin is often used for interim restorations since unimpaired cosmetic function is one of the objectives of such restorations and autocuring resin allows the clinician to blend body and incisal colors to harmonize with most tooth shades.

Before the actual fabrication of the dowel-retained temporary crown, the tissue retraction cord was removed and impressions taken. The direct dowel-and-core technique was not indicated. The shortness of the preparation walls called for a complete foundation restoration; in addition, the low lip line allowed a 0.5 mm gingival metal margin.

The completed interim restoration was contoured submarginally to be inoffensive to the reorganization of the marginal gingiva (Fig. 21-43). The occlusal contacts were kept light and the incisal length adjusted to avoid contact in a lateroprotrusive excursion. Occlusal adjustment was most important, since the crown was being retained by a dowel (orthodontic wire); however, the coronal portion of the root was still unprotected by a properly adapted metal coping. Hyperocclusion against this temporary crown could fracture the root.

Structurally weakened abutment tooth

When a structurally weakened tooth is used as an abutment for a bridge, allowance for movement through the use of a solderless connector is indicated. This type of a joint allows independent movement of the abutment tooth and sudden application of force can be dissipated through the movable segments. The more severe the damage, the more important this feature becomes for the preservation of the tooth remnants (Fig. 21-44).

The solderless connector is indicated when the following types of teeth are used for abutments:

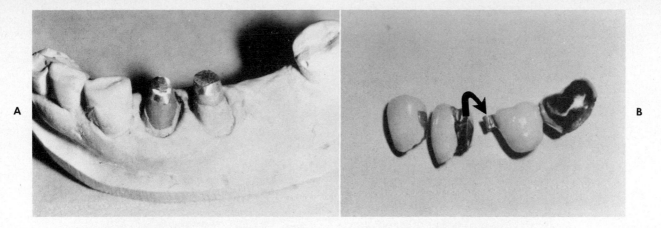

FIG. 21-45. Structurally weakened teeth incorporated into a fixed bridge. **A,** Working cast of reinforcing posts and cores. Note that castings are shown as cast after removal from sprue. **B,** The final restoration is constructed with a solderless connector *(arrow)*. The first premolar is a single restoration. The original bridge was rigid and double abuted. The first and second bicuspids fractured under load after less than 1 year of service.

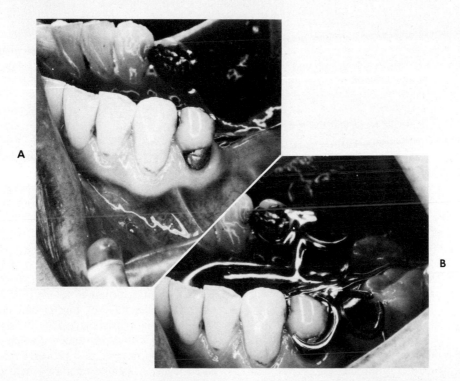

FIG. 21-46. Restoration of an abutment tooth to an existing removable partial prosthesis. **A,** Tooth inspected for defects. Missing portions of the clinical crown are temporarily replaced with a soft wax. **B,** Partial denture trial seated to verify the contour of any wax additions. The improper adaptation of the buccal clasp arm can be corrected during fabrication of the plastic pattern.

Teeth with little remaining coronal structure and the potential for minimal coping even after crown elongation procedures. These teeth have very little resistance to lateral and torquing forces (Fig. 21-44).

Teeth that cannot be reinforced properly with an adequate dowel because of a silver point and teeth with perforations or roots that have been shortened through apicoectomies. These teeth are potentially weakened in their ability to withstand the forces of mastication.

Splinting these structurally weakened teeth to sound teeth is not recommended, as the increased lever arm can magnify potentially damaging forces (Fig. 21-45).

Restoration of an abutment tooth to an existing removable partial prosthesis

An existing, functional, removable partial prosthesis utilizing abutment teeth that have become grossly defective, requiring restoration of all coronal surfaces, is a common occurrence.

The treatment procedure of choice should reestablish

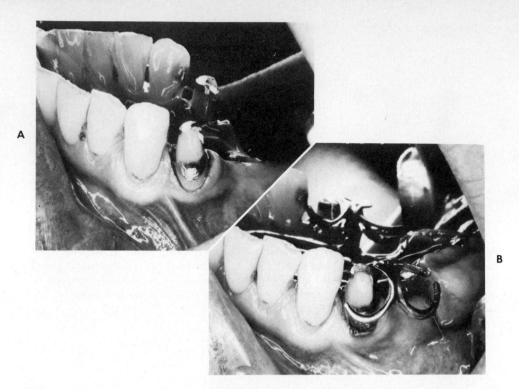

FIG. 21-47. Tooth preparation and verification of axial and occlusal reduction. **A,** Additional reduction in the occlusal rest area. **B,** Clearance between the clasp and dentin.

optimum function of the abutment teeth and the prosthesis, allowing the patient to function with the prosthesis throughout the therapy. Such a treatment procedure is illustrated in Figs. 21-46 to 21-49.

The patient had suffered the loss of a second premolar; the first premolar had been endodontically treated. The tooth required extensive coronal restoration and a dowel reinforcement because of a small cervical circumference.

The full-coverage restoration had to be contoured to fit the clasp design of the existing partial denture. Subsequently, the missing second premolar was added and the appliance rebased. Cosmetically a cast-gold crown was satisfactory.

Such a crown may be fabricated by the following procedure:

1. The tooth is inspected for missing portions: fractured restorations or tooth enamel. Any missing part of the coronal crown form is replaced with a soft utility wax (Fig. 21-46, *A*).

2. A sectional alginate impression is taken and placed in a humidor.

3. The tooth is prepared for full coverage. Additional reduction in the occlusal rest area is a wise precaution (Fig. 21-47, *A*). The partial denture is trial seated. If necessary, the clasp arms may be slightly expanded at this time to minimize reduction of critical tooth structure. There should be a clearance of over 1 mm between the clasp and the dentin (Fig. 21-47, *B*).

4. The retraction cord may be placed into the gingival sulcus.

5. The root canal is opened to within one third of the

apex by means of a Girdwood or Gates-Glidden bur. A metal dowel is selected, trimmed to fit the canal channel, longitudinally grooved with a Joe Dandy disk, and cemented.

6. The alginate is trimmed along the periphery and cleared of interproximal projections to facilitate reinsertion; once free of excess moisture, its surface in the area of the abutment tooth is moistened with a monomer to give the plastic crown a smoother surface. The abutment tooth impression area is filled with autocuring resin; when the resin is of a slightly doughy consistency, the surface is covered with petrolatum to prevent evaporation of the monomer. The bulk of plastic can now reach evenly a heavy doughy consistency. This consistency is constantly tested with a dull instrument; when it is reached, the impression is inserted and properly oriented to the unprepared teeth. A sample of plastic held quietly in the palm of the clinician's hand will serve as the setting index. If the alginate is kept at room temperature prior to insertion, the sample held in the hand will set faster than that in the mouth.

7. Once the setting index reaches a rubber stage, the alginate is removed from the mouth. If the plastic stays on the preparation, it is rubberlike. It is removed gently, and scissors are used to cut off any excess. (If the plastic is still in the impression, it is tested for the rubber stage and snapped out with cotton pliers; the excess is then trimmed.) The plastic is reseated on the preparation and the partial denture placed. The patient bites in centric position and holds. As the plastic polymerizes, the partial denture and plastic pattern are seated and then unseated.

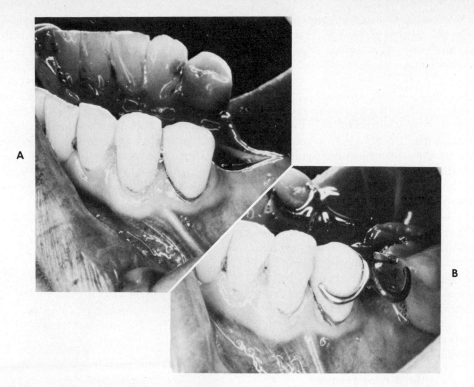

FIG. 21-48. Plastic crown pattern corrected for proper contour. **A,** Seated on the preparation. **B,** Function with the removable partial denture clasp verified.

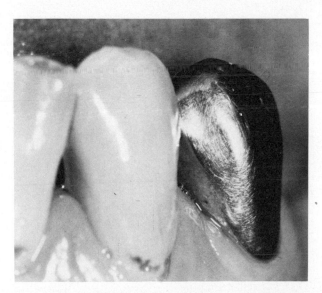

FIG. 21-49. Final gold coverage restoration.

When the plastic has sufficiently hardened, it will probably be retained by the clasps; the partial denture is set aside.

8. A sectional impression can be taken while the plastic pattern hardens completely. It is necessary only to obtain a die of the prepared tooth, because the plastic pattern takes the place of the wax pattern. On the die, only the marginal adaptation needs to be accomplished.

9. The hardened plastic pattern is pushed out of its clasp confinement and trimmed to the indentations caused by the clasp arms. The gingival extension is trimmed to be 2 mm

short of the preparation margin; this constitutes the area for margin adaptation with casting wax. The shape of the plastic pattern, occlusion, and seating of the partial denture are verified (Fig. 21-48).

In the event that a distortion is noticed, the area of the occlusal rest and areas of clasp contact can be relieved on the plastic pattern, soft casting wax added, the clasp arms gently warmed, and the partial denture inserted. The displaced wax is then carved away.[30]

Before the plastic pattern is seated on the die, the clinician vents it with a no. 6 round bur to allow for visual verification of proper seating of the pattern on the die. The attachment of the sprue will obturate the opening; in addition, with the insertion of the metal sprue into the plastic pattern, a more secure attachment is achieved; this prevents possible separation of sprue and pattern during the investing procedure.

10. The plastic pattern is now ready for the addition of 2 mm of inlay wax for proper adaptation to the die margin

The casting itself will be an unpleasant surprise. The plastic does not have the smoothness of a polished wax pattern and consequently a rough casting results. Diligent finishing will produce a cast-gold restoration to meet the patient's (and the clinician's) highest expectations (Fig. 21-49).

11. A second plastic crown is fabricated to provide the patient with an interim restoration that allows him to function comfortably with his removable prosthesis.

In the foregoing described treatment procedure a metal restoration could be readily constructed and be functionally adequate. For many patients, however, the reproduction of the buccal cusp of a mandibular first premolar in gold would be cosmetically unsatisfactory. Thus the procedure is somewhat altered, and more chair time is required to attain a buccal porcelain surface properly adapted to the clasp arm.

With the altered procedure a plastic pattern is fabricated and a working cast constructed with a removable die.

In the laboratory the buccal axial surface of the plastic pattern is reduced to resemble the design of a porcelain-fused-to-metal crown. Care must be taken not to alter the occlusal rest area and lingual surface.

Margin adaptation, investing, and casting are completed as for all bake-on restorations.

The ceramicist will add additional bulk to the buccal surface and return the crown in a bisque state.

The crown is adjusted in the mouth for proper occlusal contact. The partial denture is repeatedly fitted with thin articulating paper or typewriter ribbon between the buccal clasp arm and the porcelain surface. By these methods and with patience, the porcelain surface can be reduced and contoured to optimal axial form.

The porcelain is then glazed, and the restoration is ready for cementation.

Restored pulpless tooth without reinforcement

Fractures of restored pulpless teeth without reinforcement are a familiar dilemma to the clinician. As a rule, the fracture occurs at or slightly coronal to the finish line because the instrumentation of a shoulder or a chamfer constitutes a stress concentration point.

Various procedures have been suggested to cope with this problem; the following case discussions present three typical treatment approaches for a fractured maxillary central incisor previously restored with a porcelain-bonded-to-metal crown.

Patient no. 1 felt cosmetically impaired and decided to have the maxillary incisors restored. One central incisor had been endodontically treated. Twelve months later, she was dissatisfied again because a central incisor had fractured (Fig. 21-50, *bottom, left*). Material research has provided a means to reinforce porcelain by the bake-on technique; common sense tells us to treat the tooth with similar concern.

A dowel preparation was prepared; three nonparallel pin channels were placed; and an Endopost and three pins were cemented.

The tooth fragments were removed from the ceramic restoration; a trial seating was tested for interference by the dowel or pins in the proper orientation of the restoration to the previous finish line. The pins had to be bent toward the dowel. The previous restoration was then filled with composite, which was also injected around the dowel and pins. The crown was seated and properly aligned.

After excess resin material was carefully removed and the margin area polished, the occlusion was adjusted. All occlusal porcelain contacts were polished with a rubber wheel only. Hopefully by this method the restoration would readily wear the opposing teeth into harmony with the wear pattern of the remaining dentition, thus preventing a potential traumatic occlusion against a tooth that had been "fixed" only, not soundly restored.

The three pins placed aid in the retention of the core material; they are not, however, a substitute for a coping.

Patient no. 2 also appeared for treatment with a central incisor crown in hand. Unfortunately the root canal had been obturated with a silver point that could not be removed (Fig. 21-50, *bottom, right*).

Nonparallel pins were cemented around the canal orifice. The previous restoration was recemented with a composite. This should be considered as a temporary treatment procedure until time permits the construction of a fixed partial prosthesis.

Patient no. 3 presented a situation quite similar to that of patient no. 1. The treatment procedure was the same,

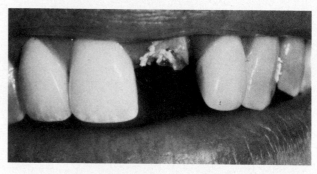

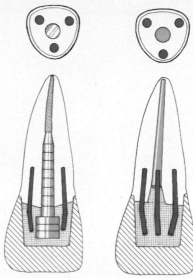

FIG. 21-50. Emergency treatment procedure for a fractured maxillary central incisor. *Top.* Fracture of an unreinforced central incisor previously restored with a porcelain-bonded-to-metal crown. *Bottom,* Two widely used methods of repair both demonstrate basic deficiencies. *Left,* A composite core addition is retained by a dowel and three nonparallel pins. The previous crown was used as a matrix for the core addition. However, the crown does not surround an adequate amount of remaining tooth structure to provide a ferrule effect. *Right,* The root canal has been obturated with a silver point that resisted removal attempts. The composite core addition is retained by three nonparallel pins and molded to fit the previous crown. The "repair" lacks dowel-and-ferrule-type reinforcement and must be considered only temporary.

but the previous crown was liberally lubricated with hot petrolatum before the composite resin core addition was made. The crown was then reprepared to gain the ferrule-like coping effect by a newly constructed restoration, giving the patient the comfort of optimal reinforcement and restoration of a previously questionable tooth.

Fractured abutment for a removable partial prosthesis

Abutment teeth with full-coverage restorations may demonstrate an accelerated rate of pulpal degeneration due to previous carious lesions that necessitated the restoration, iatrogenic insults during the fabrication of the restoration, or increased functional demands on the abutment tooth.[14] The resulting remineralization of the dentin, with a loss of resiliency, may weaken the abutment tooth sufficiently to cause it to fracture at the area of smallest circumference near the margin of the restoration. Frequently the occurrence of root caries contributes to the fracture.

The procedure described in the following case history

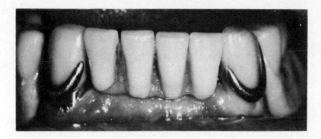

FIG. 21-51. Removable partial prosthesis before the mandibular canine ceramic crown fractured at the gingival line.

offers a technique to reorient the severed abutment crown to the endodontically treated root. The technique is equally applicable to fractured abutment teeth of fixed and removable partial prostheses. It has been successfully used in numerous fracture cases, the majority involving crowns with precision attachments.

A 75-year-old patient functioned comfortably with a removable partial prosthesis stabilized in part by his only remaining teeth, the mandibular canines (Fig. 21-51). Both canines had been beautifully restored with ceramic crowns. The tooth structure fractured at the level of the finish line (Fig. 21-52).

The procedure used in this case is as follows:

At the *first appointment,* dowel preparation, preparation

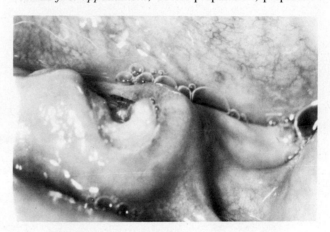

FIG. 21-52. Root remnant of the fractured mandibular canine abutment.

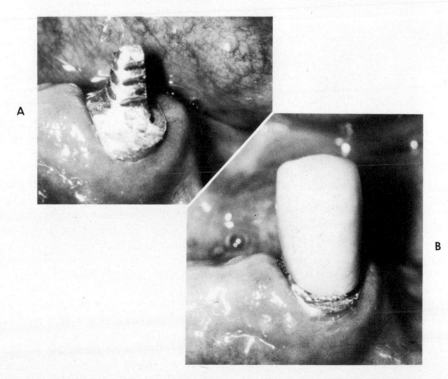

FIG. 21-53. A, Dowel, coping, and primary core seated on endodontically treated root. **B,** Previous crown verified.

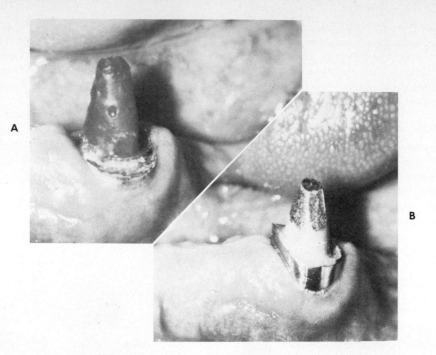

FIG. 21-54. Primary core with autocuring plastic addition. **B,** Completed foundation restoration.

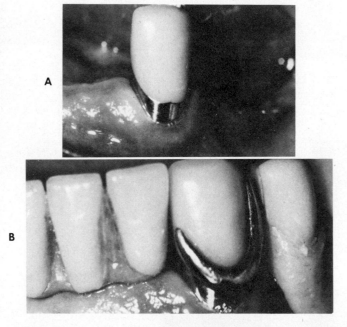

FIG. 21-55. A, Previous crown and foundation restoration cemented. **B,** Removable partial prosthesis inserted.

for the coping effect, and tissue retraction and impression are accomplished. A plastic temporary crown is fabricated to enable the patient to wear the partial denture. The laboratory procedure includes the waxing and casting of a dowel, coping, and primary core. (The primary core is merely the sprue extension.)

At the *second appointment* the dowel, coping and primary core are seated on the endodontically treated root (Fig. 21-53, *A*). The previous crown, internally cleaned and smoothed, is trial seated on the primary core (Fig. 21-53, *B*). Some adjustments may need to be made to the core, coping, and margins of the crown. There should be no contact between the crown and foundation restoration. Any metal contact would tend to interfere with the orientation of the crown to the occlusion and the partial denture. The final verification is made by placing soft utility wax in the crown, seating the crown on the primary core, inserting the partial denture, and asking the patient to close and hold in centric position. When the crown is removed, there should be no metal penetration through the wax and the margins of the crown should be at least 1 mm above the coping.

The wax is now removed; the crown is lubricated with heated petrolatum; the primary core is notched to later firmly anchor the new plastic lining; and the foundation restoration is properly seated on the root.

The lubricated crown is filled with autocuring resin; the notched primary core is also coated with resin and periodically moistened with a monomer.

As the resin within the crown reaches a heavy doughy consistency, the crown is seated on the primary core (Fig. 21-54), *A*). The heavy, doughy consistency of the plastic offers slight resistance as the partial denture is inserted and the patient is asked to close in centric and hold. The resistance of the plastic will ensure proper orientation of the crown to the partial denture and opposing teeth; the crown cannot slump.

The patient holds the centric position until the plastic has set. The appliance is then removed, as is the crown, which will be joined to the foundation restoration.

In the *laboratory* the dowel is held with pliers; as the pliers are tapped with a metal instrument, the crown will lift off the plastic core addition.

The margins are cleared of plastic and adapted with in-

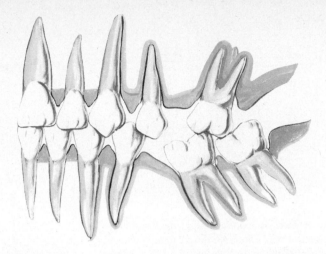

FIG. 21-56. Posterior bite collapse. The maxillary second molar is a questionable abutment because of an unmanageable periodontal lesion involving the distal-buccal root.

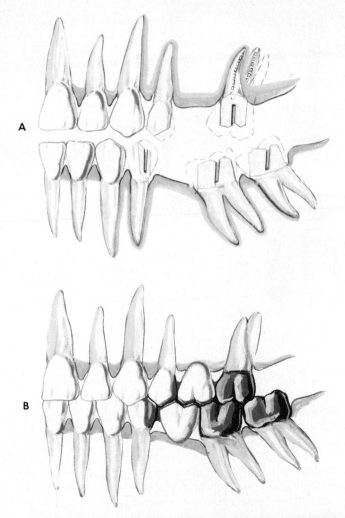

FIG. 21-57. A, Amputation of the distal-buccal maxillary molar root and surgical correction of tissue architecture in addition to, **B,** orthodontic alignment of the abutments enhanced the treatment prognosis. Unfortunately the mandibular third molar was retained. This compromised the axial alignment of the second molar and future hygienic maintenance.

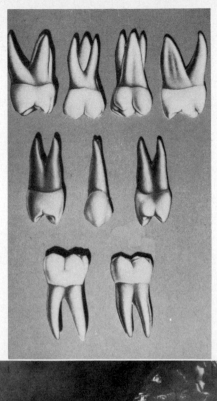

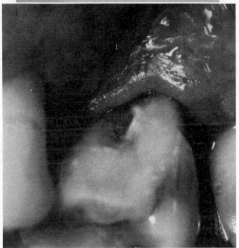

FIG. 21-58. A, Various bifurcations and trifurcations that may be rendered maintainable after amputation of one root. **B,** The subsequent restorative effort can be as simple as the placement of a Class I amalgam or composite resin.

lay wax. A sprue is attached to the plastic core, and the relined foundation restoration is invested (Fig. 21-54, *B*). Gold will readily cast to gold; no soldering will be required (Fig. 21-55).

Root amputation
Abutment tooth

Root amputation (Chapter 17) can offer the chance to retain a portion of a multirooted tooth to serve as an abutment in a maintainable state—a state relatively immune to disease (Figs. 21-56 and 21-57).

Following endodontic treatment the root with the most

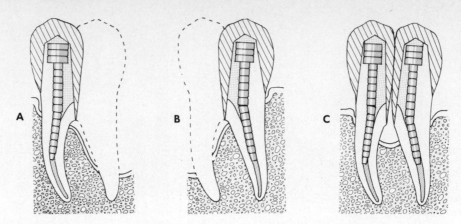

FIG. 21-59. Hemisected mandibular molar and bicuspidization. **A,** Amputation of the distal root. Note the dowel reinforcement. **B,** Amputation of the mesial root. Note the dowel reinforcement. **C,** Bicuspidization. Each remaining root should be dowel reinforced. Note that dowel is shaped with three-pronged clasp bending pliers.

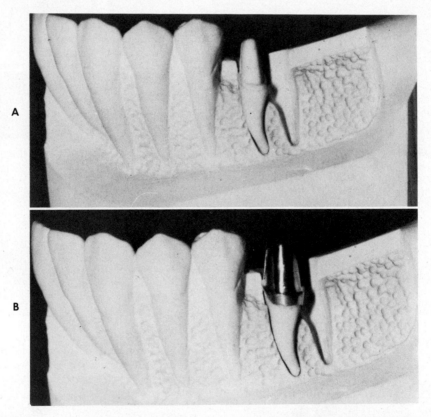

FIG. 21-60. A, Dowel-reinforced mesial root of a mandibular hemisected first molar. **B,** Entire foundation restoration necessitated by inadequate coronal tooth structure.

severe periodontal involvement is removed. The alveolar bone at the amputation site is so contoured that during healing the gingiva can conform to an accentuated interproximal festoon. This actually creates a sluiceway that prevents debris and plaque retention at the base of the clinical crown where the root was severed. To further enhance hygienic convenience, the crown form is fluted to complement the festooned gingiva.

In the case shown in Fig. 21-58, *B,* only a composite restoration needed to be placed to close the exposed pulp chamber. However, when an abutment tooth with an amputated root is being restored, the outline form of the tooth preparation and the contour of the final restoration must show a real awareness for convenience of hygienic maintenance.[2] The management of occlusal stress must reflect the understanding that the periodontal support area is minimized.

The abutment tooth altered by root amputation should

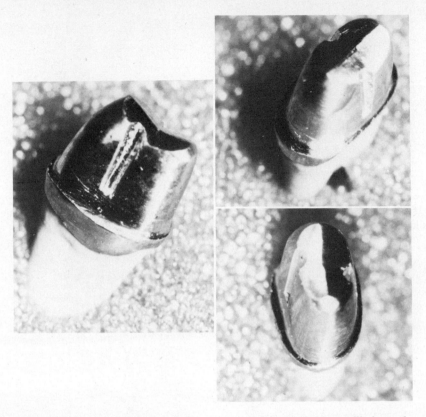

Fig. 21-61. Countour of an entire foundation restoration for a retained mandibular molar root.

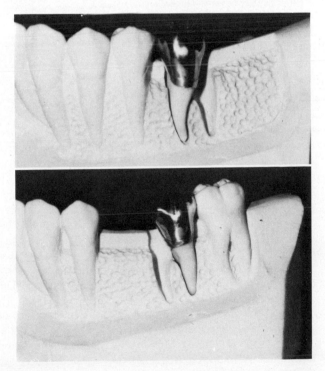

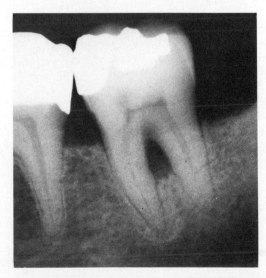

FIG. 21-62. Full crown restoration, resembling the anatomy of a premolar after hemisection, for a retained mesial or distal molar root.

FIG. 21-63. Limitations of bicuspidization when mesial and distal roots are not sufficiently divergent.

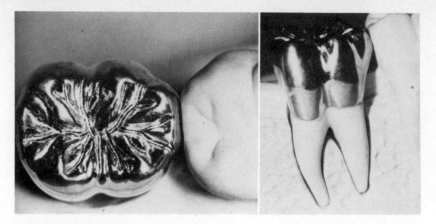

FIG. 21-64. Molar abutment with severed gingival extension of the preparation demonstrating the principles of physiologic crown contouring.

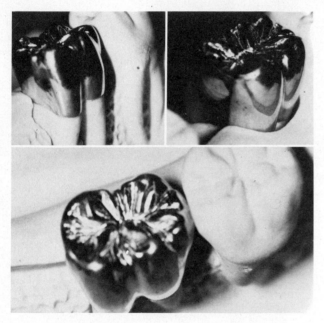

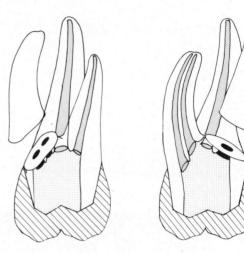

FIG. 21-66. Mesial-buccal and distal-buccal root amputation of a maxillary molar.

FIG. 21-65. Buccal and lingual fluting and the arrangement of sluiceways permit stimulation of the gingival tissues, rendering this restoration conviently hygienic.

be treated as a minimal abutment tooth. In questionable cases a provisional plastic splint may be seated for periods up to 12 months. The load force, received by the resilient plastic surface and transmitted favorably to the supporting tissues, will effect optimal biologic adaptation of these tissues to occlusal stress.

The occlusal surfaces of the final restoration must be so formed and aligned that the intensity, direction, and distribution of the occlusal stress are well within the limits for biologic adaptation of the periodontal ligaments and the alveolar bone. Without question, this design principle can be optimally satisfied by the use of medium-hard gold occlusal surfaces.

Mandibular molar

The periodontal involvement necessitating root amputation (or hemisection) of a mandibular molar usually affects

the bifurcation area, or in the most posterior tooth the distal root (Fig. 21-59, A). Less frequently the mesial root has an untreatable bony lesion that necessitates its removal (Fig. 21-59, B). In a large number of cases, mesial or distal roots of mandibular molars have been retained, dowel reinforced as required for single-rooted pulpless teeth, and have been restored to function as premolars individually or as abutment teeth with a highly satisfactory prognosis.

Figs. 21-60 to 21-65 demonstrate the advantage of retaining the mesial root of a mandibular first molar. The tooth remnant should be dowel reinforced (Fig. 21-53, A). The need for any core addition depends on the amount of coronal dentin. If because of trauma or decay most of the coronal tooth structure is missing, a complete foundation restoration is indicated (Figs. 21-60, B, and 21-61, see also Fig. 22-5, D). The restoration of a mesial root may well be a superior choice to such alternatives as a cantilevered fixed splint, a unilateral removable partial prosthesis, or an implant anchor (Fig. 21-62). The restoration of a distal root may serve as an abutment for a short-span fixed partial prosthesis; or, as illustrated in Fig. 21-62, the

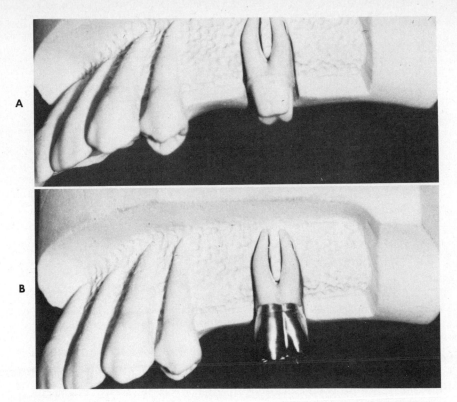

FIG. 21-67. Utilization of both buccal roots of a maxillary molar. The palatal root was amputated by decay and subsequent lost. **A,** Abutment tooth preparation. **B,** Completed restoration of the bridge abutment.

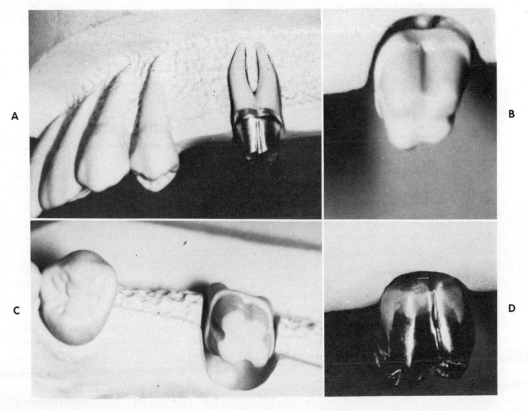

FIG. 21-68. Preparation design, coping, and full veneer crown on a maxillary molar with an amputated palatal root. **A,** Buccal view of the coping. **B,** Lingual view of the preparation. **C,** Occlusal view of the preparation. **D,** Lingual contour of the abutment crown.

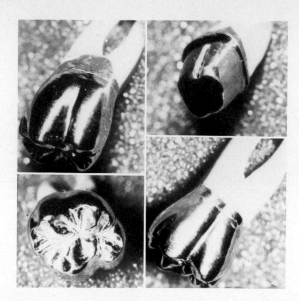

FIG. 21-69. Contour of the final restoration supported by both buccal roots of a maxillary molar. The crown contour is determined, to a large degree, by the preparation contour. Gold was used in this preparation because of a core addition.

root may be splinted to a second molar that also has lost considerable support. This will shorten the pontic span and increase the area of periodontal support for the prosthesis.

A bifurcation involvement can be treated with coagulum grafts if lateral bony walls are present. Such procedures should always be explored before restorative compromises are undertaken. In bicuspidization of the tooth (Fig. 21-59, *C*), for example, it is hoped that mesial and distal roots can be restored with premolar crowns (usually connected by soldering). The bifurcation will be covered by an interdental papilla. With an interdental brush the patient can maintain this area as conveniently as he does the interdental embrasure in the premolar region. However, these results can be obtained only in rare cases when the molar tooth shows a wide divergence of mesial and distal roots (Fig. 21-63). Bicuspidizing is successful only when a large interdental embrasure space can be formed for the organization of an interdental papilla and for hygienic convenience.

Any narrow embrasure constitutes a debris-trapping crevice. Orthodontic movement to gain additional root separation can be considered; however, this has infrequent application. A more practical procedure is to drastically invaginate the buccal and lingual preparation walls above the bifurcation (Figs. 21-64 and 21-65). The subsequent crown form will show accentuated fluting in these areas, which will substantially enhance the maintenance prognosis.

Maxillary molar

Root amputation in the maxillary molar opens an unmanageable trifurcation into an accessible bifurcation. Any one of the three molar roots may be amputated (Fig. 21-66).

The decision is based on a detailed periodontal evaluation; in difficult cases the final determination should be made at the time of periodontal surgery, when the bone support can be visually examined.

Palatal root amputation is illustrated in Figs. 21-67 to 21-69. The palatal root had been severed by decay. The two buccal roots were endodontically treated. The cervical circumference was large and did not warrant dowel reinforcement. The coronal tooth structure had sufficient defects to require a coping; and, prepared in this manner, the tooth has served successfully as an abutment for a short-span bridge for over 20 years.

Mesial-buccal root amputation is illustrated in Figs. 21-70 to 21-72. Root amputation was necessary to render the trifurcation area maintainable. Osseous recontouring was complemented by the tooth preparation form, which showed a pronounced indentation of the mesial-buccal surface. Both the tooth preparation and the coping are illustrated in Fig. 21-71. The use of a coping depends on the quality of the remaining tooth structure and on the extent of restorative treatment. In cases of extensive splinting, the protection of the individual abutment tooth (especially a pulpless tooth, which could be sufficiently reduced) with a coping does establish better margin integrity. An additional benefit is the favorable control of gingival tissues during treatment. The contour of the final restoration is in harmony with the altered gingival architecture (Fig. 21-72).

The patient can approach the bifurcation conveniently from a mesial-buccal direction and with an interdental brush can maintain cleanliness and health in this area.

Distal-buccal root amputation is illustrated in Figs. 21-73 to 21-75. The prognosis for amputating a distal-buccal root in the presence of an adjacent tooth is, at best, guarded. The patient's oral hygiene potential must be cautiously assessed; once the area has been altered by amputation and a recontoured gingival architecture, it is difficult to maintain. The convenience of a mesial-buccal approach

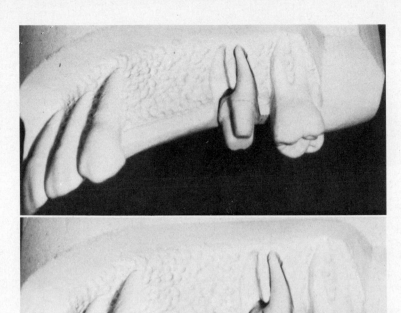

FIG. 21-70. Preparation and restoration of a maxillary molar with an amputated mesial-buccal root.

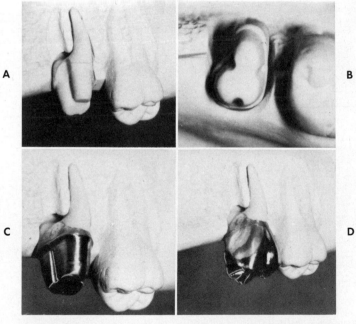

FIG. 21-71. Preparation, coping, and final restoration of a maxillary molar with an amputated mesial-buccal root. **A,** Buccal view. **B,** Occlusal view. **C,** Buccal view with coping. **D,** Final restoration.

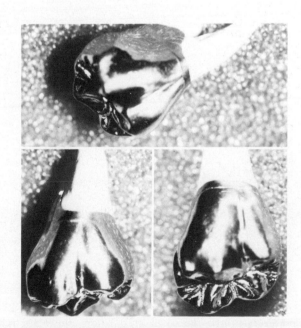

FIG. 21-72. Physiologic contouring for the full veneer crown of a maxillary molar with an amputated mesial-buccal root.

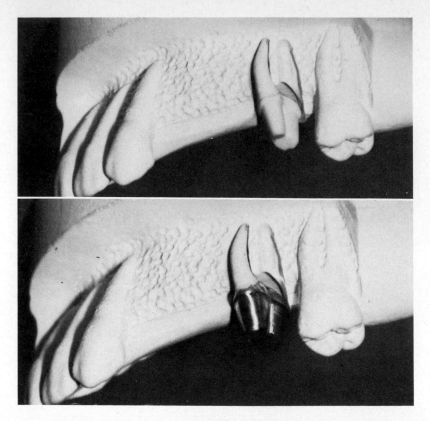

FIG. 21-73. Maxillary molar with an amputated distal-buccal root.

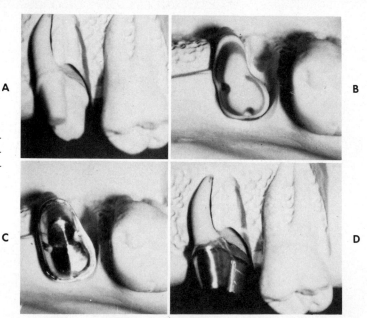

FIG. 21-74. Preparation and coping design for a maxillary molar with an amputated distal-buccal root. **A,** Buccal view. **B,** Occlusal view. **C,** Occlusal view with coping. **D,** Buccal view with coping.

does not exist in this situation. Figs. 21-74 and 21-75 demonstrate how the tooth preparation allows for maximum embrasure space, as reflected by optimal physiologic contouring of the final restoration.

Root amputations are most frequently necessitated by the loss of supporting tissues due to periodontal disease. An alteration of tooth form and gingival architecture is an inevitable result. In the restoration of these teeth, then, it

is important that the physiologic design principles be applied with the highest degree of imagination and skill to render these restorations conveniently hygienic.

Root preservation for overdenture support

The root-supported overdenture gains the advantage over the conventional mucosa-supported overdenture insofar as it has better denture base stability, positive retention

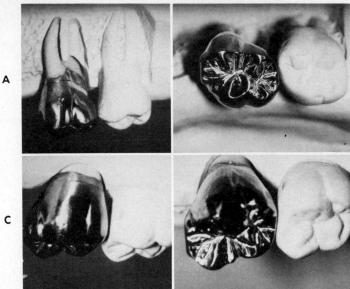

FIG. 21-75. Physiologic contouring for the full veneer crown of a maxillary molar with an amputated distal-buccal root. **A,** Buccal view. **B,** Occlusal view. **C** and **D,** Palatal views.

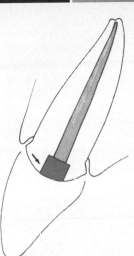

FIG. 21-76. The root surface is dome-shaped, 1 to 3 mm above the gingival margin. The coronal 2 mm is obturated with amalgam *(arrow)*. The bearing area around the periphery of the tooth is relieved to minimize encroachment on the gingival tissue and to provide a release in shearing forces on the tooth. The root remnant should only be expected to resist vertical forces.

due to preserved alveolar architecture or attachments, improved proprioception and mastication, and more favorable acceptance by the patient.[9,19]

The predictable and continuous resorption of the alveolar bone once the teeth are lost has led to efforts to retain maintainable roots.[1,3,11,15] Retention of these roots contributes to the preservation of alveolar bone, attached gingiva, and proprioception.[15,19,23]

Overdenture therapy is used when the remaining dentition is periodontally weakened sufficiently to present an undesirable crown/root ratio for any prospective abutment tooth. In this situation, removal of the clinical crown effectively reduces lever action and contributes to tooth stability.[16,32] Corrective periodontal and endodontic treatment precedes any operative procedure.

Abutment selection

An anterior or a posterior tooth can be altered for overdenture support if sufficient bone is present, if the roots can be treated endodontically, and if the patient's interest and oral hygiene make treatment desirable. Corrective periodontal therapy is implemented to gain physiologic gingival contours with minimal pocket depth and adequate attached gingiva. Multirooted teeth may be hemisected, bicuspidized, or root amputated.[23]

Tooth preparation

Reduction of the root to within 1 to 3 mm above the marginal gingiva will not compromise the periodontal tissues. The root surface is contoured to a dome shape; 2 mm of the root canal filling material is replaced with dental amalgam (Figs. 21-76 to 21-78); and the polished, exposed root surface is treated with a fluoride preparation for chemical protection. Daily application of minimal amounts of a fluoride gel into the root recess of the prosthesis may provide continued protection.[15,16,19]

Roots requiring a more extensive restoration because of defects or caries susceptibility will receive a dome-shaped gold protection. This root coping gains resistance and retention form from a 4 to 8 mm long dowel (multiple dowels for multirooted teeth) and a ferrule that surrounds the coronal 2 mm of the root protectively (Fig. 21-79).

An all-acrylic resin overdenture is indicated for root coping or polished root surfaces. The acrylic resin is slightly relieved to avoid impingement of the marginal gingiva; excessive relief could allow tissue proliferation (Fig. 21-80). The advantages of the all-acrylic resin denture base are its ease of fabrication and its simplicity of maintenance; also its stability, support, and positive retention are rarely compromised in tooth-supported complete dentures. In fact, a facial-lingual undercut can be so pronounced in the alveolar architecture that a resilient denture material must be used there. A tooth-supported removable partial denture will sustain the saddle area as well as can

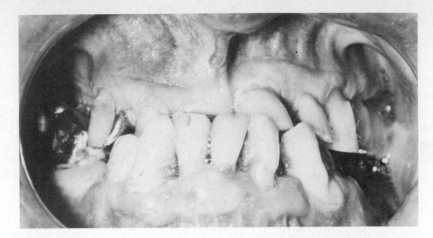

FIG. 21-77. The patient is prognathic, and the dentition is periodontally weak.

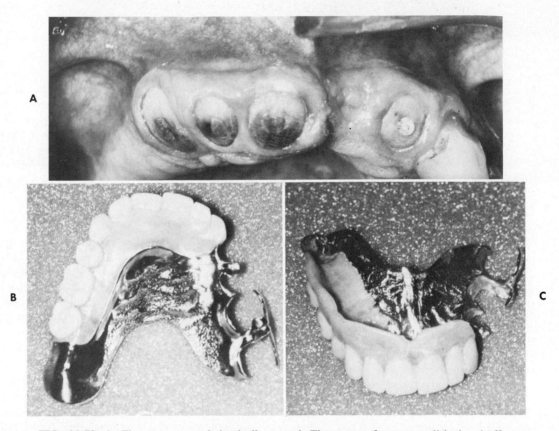

FIG. 21-78. A, The roots are endodontically treated. The root surfaces are polished and effectively contribute to the support of the removable partial denture. **B,** Occlusal view. **C,** Palatal view.

be done by the occlusal rests if the root recess is lined by a convex metal surface (Figs. 21-81 to 21-84). A convex surface can contact the root coping or dome-shaped root surface only at a point located so the force is directed axially. The intent is to equalize the support points within the prosthesis, not the retention.

Bar and stud fixation

When positive denture retention cannot be effected by the remaining ridge form, an attachment fixation should be considered. Dolder[5] and Gilmore separately popularized bar-type attachments. Connecting two or more roots with a rigid metal bar enhances the stability of periodontally weakened roots. Cross-arch splinting can be readily provided with bar connectors to which the overdenture is attached by metal clips embedded in the denture base. The main disadvantage of bar fixation is hygiene. To minimize nonaxial forces against the splinted roots, the bar should be close to the ridge tissue; however, this compromises

Text continued on page 683.

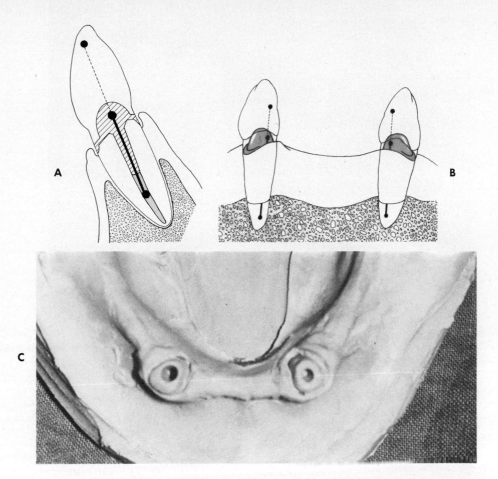

FIG. 21-79. A, Root copings gain retention and resistance form from a 4 to 8 mm long dowel and a ferrule that protectively surrounds the coronal 2 mm of the root. **B,** The crown/root ratio is improved by the use of root copings. **C,** The labial undercuts maintained by root preservation will contribute to denture retention.

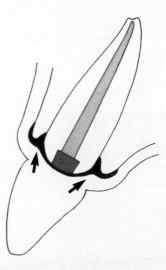

FIG. 21-80. The root recess in the denture base is slightly relieved to avoid impingement of the marginal gingiva.

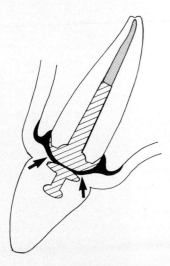

FIG. 21-81. A tooth-supported removable partial denture will gain stability for the saddle area from convex metal surfaces embedded in the denture base. Arrows indicate areas of relief.

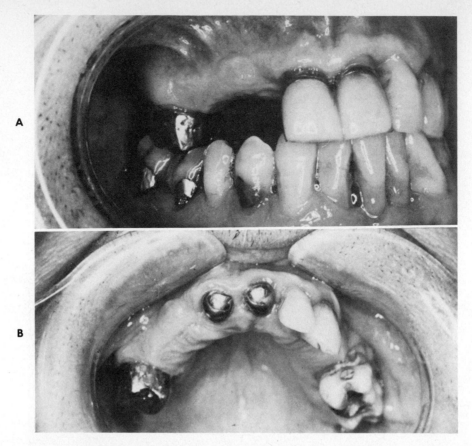

FIG. 21-82. **A,** The crowns of the central incisors, which are periodontally weak, are removed. **B,** Root copings are placed to gain improved support for the prosthesis.

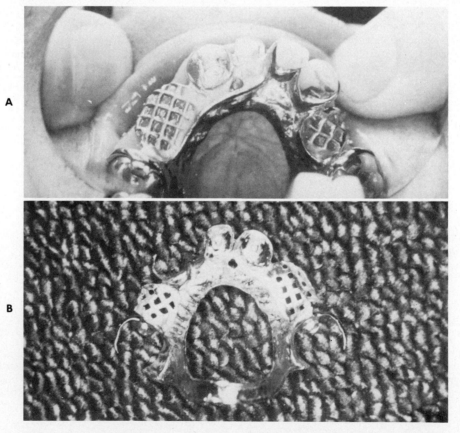

FIG. 21-83. **A,** The framework for the removable partial denture is trial seated. **B,** Palatal view. The convex surfaces will be in point contact with the root copings.

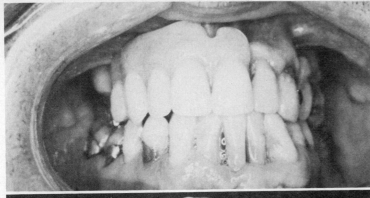

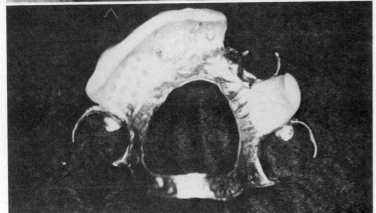

FIG. 21-84. A, Finished prosthesis. B, Finished removble partial denture, palatal view.

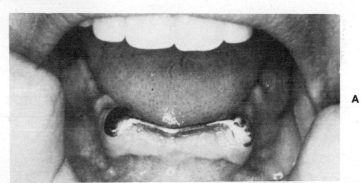

FIG. 21-85. A, A bar-type attachment placed close to the edentulous ridge can compromise oral hygiene. B, Denture base with retention clips, C, Root copings with a bar-type attachment prior to insertion.

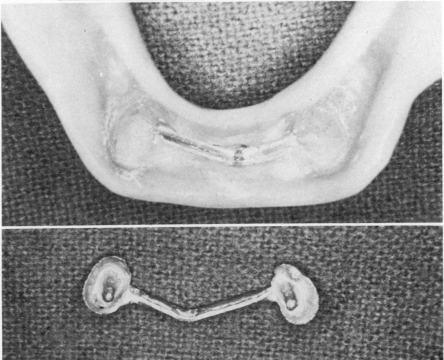

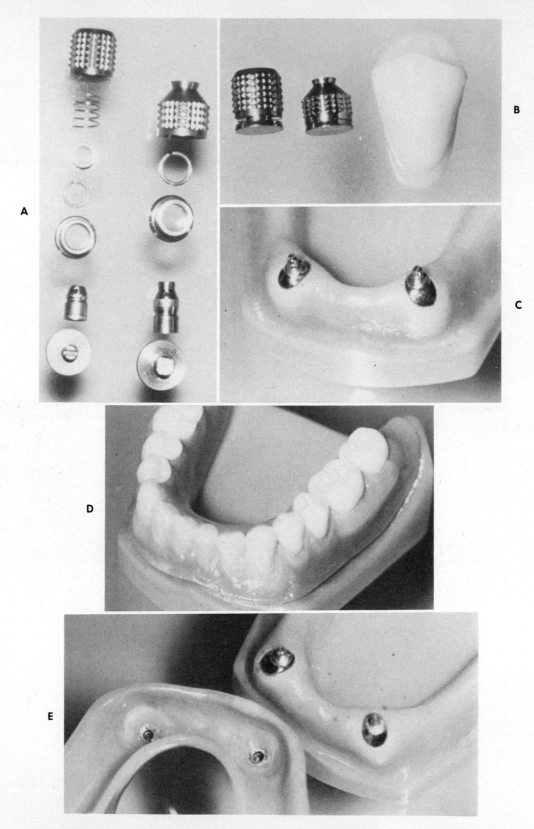

FIG. 21-86. A, Components of a stud-type attachment (Gerber). **B,** Size comparison with a denture tooth. **C,** Stud-type attachments inserted. **D** and **E,** Overdenture with additional retention by stud-type attachments supported by retained roots and retention rings embedded in the denture base.

tissue health, especially at the junction of the bar and the root coping (Fig. 21-85). Fenner et al.[9] advocated the use of stud fixation for overdentures (Fig. 21-86). These attachments provide effective denture retention and are conveniently hygienic.

When stable roots are present, the choice of bar or stud fixation rests entirely with the clinician. Both attachments will allow vertical and hinging motions of the denture base. The inherent advantages and disadvantages, when understood,[3,5,7,15] will lead to a prudent selection for a given patient. Attachments require difficult and time-consuming technical and clinical procedures that are not justified when adherence to the basic principles of denture design can provide adequate stability of the overdenture.

REFERENCES

1. Atwood, D.A.: Reduction of residual ridges in the partially edentulous patient, Dent. Clin. North Am. **17**:747, 1973.
2. Boyle, P.E.: Kronfeld's histopathology of the teeth, ed. 4, Philadelphia, 1955, Lea & Febiger.
3. Brewer, A.A., and Morrow, R.M.: Overdentures, ed. 2, St. Louis, 1980, The C.V. Mosby Co.
4. Colley, I.T., Hampson, E.D., and Lehman, M.L.: Retention of post crowns: an assessment of the post of different shapes and sizes, Br. Dent. J. **124**:63, 1968.
5. Dolder, E.J.: The bar joint mandibular denture, J. Prosthet. Dent. **11**:689, 1961.
6. Eissmann, H.F., Radke, R.A., and Noble, W.H.: Physiological design criteria for fixed dental restorations, Dent. Clin. North Am. **15**:543, 1971.
7. Fenner, W., Gerber, A.A., and Mühlemann, H.R.: Tooth mobility changes during treatment with partial dentures, J. Prosthet. Dent. **6**:520, 1956.
8. Frank, A.L.: Protective coronal coverage of the pulpless tooth, J. Am. Dent. Assoc. **39**:895, 1959.
9. Franz, W.R.: The use of natural teeth in overlay dentures, J. Prosthet. Dent. **34**:135, 1975.
10. Goldman, M., et al.: Effect of the dentin smear layer on tensile strength of cemented posts, J. Prosthet. Dent. **52**:485, 1984.
11. Henderson, D., and Steffel, V.L.: McCracken's removable prosthodontics, ed. 6, St. Louis, 1981, The C.V. Mosby Co.
12. James, R.: Personal communication.
13. Judy, W.: Improved technique of endodontic stabilization, Quintessence Int. **6**:1, 1975.
14. Leicester, H.M.: Biochemistry of the teeth, St. Louis, 1949, The C.V. Mosby Co.
14a. Linek, H.A.: Tooth carving manual, Los Angeles, 1949, University of Southern California.
15. Lord, J.L., and Teel, S.: The overdenture: patient selection, using of copings, and follow-up evaluation. J. Prosthet. Dent. **32**:41, 1977.
16. Mensor, M.C.: Attachment fixation for overdentures, J. Prosthet. Dent. **37**:366, 1977.
17. Miller, P.A.: Complete dentures supported by natural teeth, J. Prosthet. Dent. **8**:924, 1958.
18. Moffa, J.P., Rassano, M.R., and Doyle, M.G.: Pins—a comparison of their retentive properties, J. Am. Dent. Assoc. **78**:529, 1969.
19. Morrow, R.M., et al.: Tooth supported complete dentures: an approach to preventative prosthodontics, J. Prosthet. Dent. **21**:513, 1969.
20. Newburg, R.E., and Pameijer, C.H.: Retentive properties of post and core systems, J. Prosthet. Dent. **36**:636, 1976.
21. Noyes, F.B.: Noyes' oral histology and embryology, ed. 7 (revised by I. Schour), Philadelphia, 1953, Lea & Febiger.
22. Preiskel, H.W.: Precision attachments in dentistry, ed. 3, St. Louis, 1980, The C.V. Mosby Co.
22a. Radke, R.A., and Barkhordar, R.A.: A study of the role of the coping in root fracture, J. Endod. In press.
23. Richard, G.E., et al.: Hemisected molars for additional overdenture support, J. Prosthet. Dent. **38**:16, 1977.
24. Sapone, J.: Personal communication.
25. Schillingburg, H.T., and Kessler, J.C.: Restoration of the endodontically treated tooth, Chicago, 1982, Quintessence Publishing Co.
26. Sheets, C.E.: Dowel and core foundations, J. Prosthet. Dent. **23**:58, 1970.
27. Sorensen, J.A., and Martinoff, J.T.: Clinically significant factors in dowel design, J. Prosthet. Dent. **52**(1):28, 1984.
28. Standlee, J.P., et al.: Analysis of stress distribution in endodontic posts, Oral Surg. **33**:952, 1972.
29. Standlee, J.P., Caputo, A.A., and Hanson, E.C.: Retention of endodontic dowels: effects of cement, dowel length, diameter, and design, J. Prosthet. Dent. **39**:401, 1978.
30. Thurgood, B.W., Thayer, K.E., and Lee, R.E.: Complete crowns constructed for an existing partial denture, J. Prosthet. Dent. **29**:507, 1973.
31. Tjan, A.H.L., and Whang, S.B.: Resistance to root fracture of dowel channels with various thickness of facial dentin walls, J. Prosthet. Dent. **53**:496, 1985.
32. Waller, M.I.: The root rest and the removable partial denture: a clinical investigation, J. Prosthet. Dent. **34**:16, 1975.

Self-assessment questions

1. The most common failures of restorative technique include:
   a. No reinforcement dowel
   b. Dowel of inadequate length
   c. No ferrule effect
   d. All of the above
2. A proper-length dowel
   a. Distributes stress to the area of the gingival margin
   b. Extends at least one-fourth the length of the root canal
   c. Provides both reinforcement and retention
   d. Leaves at least 2 mm of gutta-percha for the apical seal
3. The ferrule effect
   a. Prevents horizontal fractures of the clinical crown
   b. Reinforces against vertical root fracture
   c. Gives stability to the coronal restoration
   d. Provides retention of the dowel
4. The dowel diameter
   a. Does not affect the resistance of the tooth to fracture
   b. Should ideally allow more than 1 mm of tooth structure around the post
   c. Should be at least 0.5 mm in diameter for maxillary incisors
   d. Is designed to resist rotational forces

5. According to the authors, what is the most abused step affecting the restoration of a pulpless tooth?
   a. Endodontic obliteration of the canal
   b. Fabrication of the dowel
   c. Perfection of the gingival margins
   d. Selection of the proper restorative materials

6. Why do canals obliterated with silver points present difficult problems in preparing the dowel space?
   a. They may be difficult to remove
   b. Burring against the silver point may disrupt the apical seal
   c. The risk of perforation is increased when one is burring out a silver point
   d. All of the above

7. If silver points resist removal, what would be the best compromise for restoring an endodontically treated tooth requiring additional support?
   a. Cement three or four retention pins to retain a core addition
   b. Use the silver point as the dowel support
   c. Bur out the silver point for post and core
   d. Extract the tooth

8. A single-rooted endodontically treated tooth with severe cervical destruction is best resotred by
   a. Preparing the remaining tooth structure for a full crown
   b. Pin-retained composite core with a full cast crown
   c. Dowel and core with a full cast crown
   d. Cemented parallel pin cast coping with a cast crown

9. Restoration of a multirooted tooth
   a. Does not necessarily require a reinforcement dowel
   b. Requires the use of threaded rather than cemented pins
   c. Requires long parallel dowels for core retention
   d. Should follow the principles of extracoronal resistance and occlusal protection

10. A hemisected retained root of a mandibular molar
    a. Does not require dowel reinforcement
    b. Is restored to function as a premolar
    c. Is an inferior choice over a cantilever fixed splint
    d. Cannot serve as an abutment for a short-span fixed partial prosthesis

22

PEDODONTIC-ENDODONTIC TREATMENT

JOE H. CAMP

Despite water fluoridation and emphasis on the prevention of caries, premature loss of primary and young permanent teeth continues to be common. The total prevention of caries is the ultimate goal of dentistry; but meanwhile, procedures must be utilized to preserve the primary and young permanent teeth ravaged by caries. This chapter deals with preservation of the primary and young permanent teeth that are pulpally involved. The objective of pulpal therapy is conservation of the tooth in a healthy state functioning as an integral component of the dentition.

Preservation of arch space is one of the primary objectives of pedodontics. Premature loss of primary teeth may cause aberration of the arch length, resulting in mesial drift of the permanent teeth and consequent malocclusion. Whenever possible, the pulpally involved tooth should be maintained in the dental arch—provided, of course, that it can be restored to function, free of disease.

Other objectives of preserving primary teeth are to aid in esthetics and mastication, prevent aberrant tongue habits, aid in speech, and prevent the psychologic effects associated with tooth loss.

Loss of pulpal vitality in the young permanent tooth creates special problems. Since the pulp is necessary for the formation of dentin, if the pulp is lost before root length is completed the tooth will have a poor crown/root ratio. Pulpal necrosis before the completion of dentin deposition within the root leaves a thin root more prone to fracture in the event of trauma. This situation also creates special problems in endodontic treatment since endodontic techniques are usually not adequate to obturate the large blunderbuss canals. Additional procedures of apexification or apical surgery often become necessary to maintain the pulpless immature permanent tooth; the prognosis for permanent retention of the tooth is poorer than for the completely formed tooth.

In this chapter emphasis is on maintenance of pulpal vitality in the primary and young permanent teeth whenever possible to avoid many of the problems discussed elsewhere in this book.

Successful pulpal therapy in the primary dentition requires a thorough understanding of primary pulp morphology, root formation, and the special problems associated with resorption of primary tooth roots. Differences in the morphology of the primary and permanent pulps, in root formation, and in primary root resorption are covered later in this chapter. The reader is referred to Chapter 10 for a complete description of pulp and dentin formation.

Differences in primary and permanent tooth morphology (Fig. 22-1)

According to Finn[46] and Wheeler[205] the basic differences between the primary and the permanent teeth are as follows:

1. Primary teeth are smaller in all dimensions than the corresponding permanent teeth.
2. Primary crowns are wider from mesial to distal in comparison to their crown length than are permanent crowns.
3. Primary teeth have narrower and longer roots in comparison to crown length and width than do permanent teeth.
4. The facial and lingual cervical thirds of the crowns of anterior primary teeth are much more prominent than those of permanent teeth.
5. Primary teeth are markedly more constricted at the dentin-enamel junction than are permanent teeth.
6. The facial and lingual surfaces of primary molars converge occlusally so the occlusal surface is much narrower in the facial-lingual than the cervical width.
7. The roots of primary molars are comparatively more slender and longer than the roots of permanent molars.
8. The roots of primary molars flare out nearer the cervix, and they flare more at the apex, than do the roots of permanent molars.

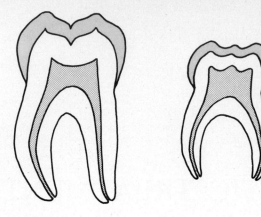

FIG. 22-1. Cross section of primary and permanent molars.

9. The enamel is thinner, about 1 mm, on primary teeth than on permanent teeth and it has a more consistent depth.
10. The thickness of the dentin between the pulp chambers and the enamel in primary teeth is less than in permanent teeth.
11. The pulp chambers in primary teeth are comparatively larger than in permanent teeth.
12. The pulp horns, especially the mesial horns, are higher in primary molars than in permanent molars.

A detailed discussion of the anatomy of the individual primary root canals is presented later in this chapter.

Diagnosis

Before the initiation of restorative procedures on a tooth, a thorough clinical and radiographic examination must be concluded. The case history and any pertinent medical history must be thoroughly reviewed. A comprehensive coverage of diagnosis is to be found in Chapter 1, and the reader is referred to that chapter for a more in-depth discussion.

Good periapical and bite-wing radiographs are essential to complete the diagnosis. Examination of the soft and hard tissues for any apparent pathosis is a routine part of the examination.

In the event that pulp therapy is required, the preoperative diagnosis is of utmost importance and should dictate the type of treatment to be carried out. If the pulpal status is not determined before operative procedures are begun and pulp therapy becomes necessary during the treatment, an adequate diagnosis may be impossible.

There are no reliable clinical diagnostic tools for accurately evaluating the status of the pulp that has become inflamed. An accurate determination of the extent of inflammation within the pulp cannot be made short of histologic examination.[180] Diagnosis of pulpal health in the exposed pulp of children is difficult, and the correlation between clinical symptoms and histopathologic conditions is poor.[116]

Although the diagnostic tests are admittedly poor for evaluating the degree of inflammation within the primary and young permanent pulp, they must always be performed to obtain as much information as possible to aid in the diagnosis before treatment is rendered. The recommended diagnostic tests for use in primary and young permanent teeth are discussed next.

Radiographs

Current radiographs are essential to examining for caries and periapical changes. Interpretation of radiographs is complicated in children by physiologic root resorption of primary teeth and by incompletely formed roots of permanent teeth. If one is not familiar with diagnosing radiographs of children or does not have radiographs of good quality, these normally occurring circumstances can easily lead to misinterpretation of normal anatomy for pathologic changes.

The radiograph does not always give evidence of periapical pathosis when present, nor can the proximity of caries to the pulp always be accurately determined. What may appear as an intact barrier of secondary dentin overlying the pulp may actually be a perforated mass of irregularly calcified and carious dentin overlying a pulp with extensive inflammation.[116]

The presence of calcified masses within the pulp is important to making a diagnosis of pulpal status (Fig. 23-2). Mild, chronic irritation to the pulp will stimulate secondary dentin formation. When the irritation is acute and of rapid onset, the defense mechanism may not have a chance to lay down secondary dentin. When the disease process reaches the pulp, the pulp may form calcified masses away from the exposure site. These calcified masses are always associated with advanced pulpal degeneration in the pulp chamber and inflammation of the pulp tissue in the canals.[104,116]

Pathologic changes in the periapical tissues surrounding primary molars are most often apparent in the bifurcation or trifurcation areas rather than at the apices as in permanent teeth (Figs. 22-2 and 22-3, *A*). Pathologic bone and root resorption is indicative of advanced pulpal degeneration that has spread into the periapical tissues. The pulpal tissue may remain vital even with such advanced degenerative changes.

Internal resorption occurs frequently in the primary dentition following pulpal involvement. It is always associated with extensive inflammation[65] and usually occurs in the molar root canals adjacent to the bifurcation or trifurcation area. Because of the thinness of primary molar roots, once the internal resorption has become advanced enough to be seen radiographically there is usually a perforation of the root by the resorption (Fig. 22-3, *B*). After perforation of the primary tooth root by internal resorption, all forms of pulpal therapy are contraindicated. The treatment of choice is extraction.

Pulp tests

The electric pulp tester is of little value in the primary dentition or in young permanent teeth with incompletely developed apices. Although it may indicate vitality, it will not give reliable data as to the extent of inflammation within the pulp. Many children with perfectly normal teeth do not respond to the electric pulp tester even at the higher settings. Added to these factors is the unreliability of the

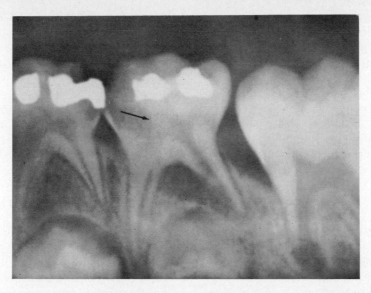

FIG. 22-2. Calcified mass in the pulp chamber. There is internal and external root resorption. The calcified mass *(arrow)* is an attempt to block a massive carious lesion. Because of resorption, this tooth should be extracted. Note the bone loss in the bifurcation area.

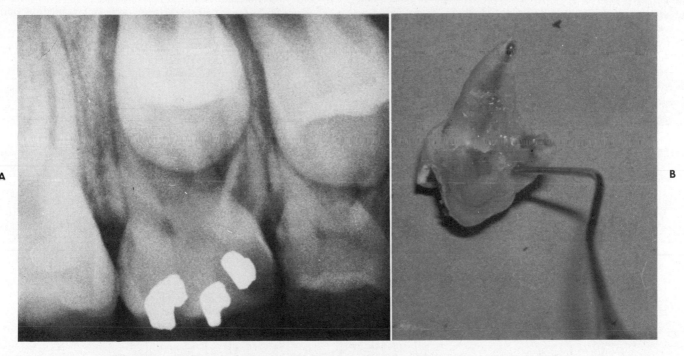

FIG. 22-3. Internal resorption due to inflammation from carious pulp exposure. **A,** Note the bone loss in the trifurcation and the internal resorption in the mesial root. **B,** Extracted tooth. Note the perforation of internal resorption. The probe is extended through the resorption defect.

response in the young child because of apprehension, fear, or management problems.

Thermal tests are also generally unreliable in the primary dentition for determining pulpal status.

Percussion and mobility

Teeth with extensive pulpal inflammation usually exhibit tenderness to percussion; however, this test is not very reliable in primary teeth of young children because of the psychologic aspects involved.

Tooth mobility is also not a reliable test of pulpal pa-

thosis in primary teeth. During phases of active physiologic root resorption, primary teeth with normal pulps may have varying degrees of mobility. Furthermore, teeth with varying degrees of pulpal inflammation may have very little mobility.

Pulpal exposures and hemorrhage

It has been reported that the size of the exposure, the appearance of the pulp, and the amount of hemorrhage are important factors in diagnosing the extent of inflammation in a cariously exposed pulp. A true carious exposure will always be accompanied by pulpal inflammation.[116,180] (See Chapter 14.)

The pinpoint carious exposure may have pulpal inflammation varying from minimal to extensive to complete necrosis. However, the massive exposure will always have widespread inflammation or necrosis and will not be a candidate for any form of vital pulp therapy. Excessive hemorrhage at an exposure site or during pulp amputation is evidence of extensive inflammation. These teeth should be considered candidates for pulpectomy or extraction.

History of pain

A history of spontaneous toothache is usually associated with extensive degenerative changes in the pulp of a primary tooth[65]; nevertheless, absence of pain cannot be used as a factor in judging pulpal status, since varying degrees of degeneration or even complete necrosis of the pulp are seen without any history of pain.

Guthrie et al.[65] attempted to use the first drop of hemorrhage from an exposed pulp site as a diagnostic aid for determining the extent of degeneration within the pulp. A white blood cell differential count (hemogram) was made for each of 53 teeth included in the study. A detailed history, including percussion, electric pulp test, thermal tests, mobility, and history of pain, was obtained. The teeth were extracted and histologically examined. Upon correlation of the histologic findings with the hemogram and a detailed history, it was determined that percussion, electric and thermal pulp tests, and mobility were *unreliable* in establishing the degree of pulpal inflammation. The hemogram did not give reliable evidence of pulpal degeneration, even though teeth with advanced degeneration of the pulp involving the root canals did have an elevated neutrophil count. A consistent finding of the study, however, was advanced degeneration of pulpal tissue in teeth with a history of spontaneous toothache.

Primary teeth with a history of spontaneous, unprovoked toothache should not be considered for any form of pulp therapy short of pulpectomy or extraction.

INDIRECT PULP THERAPY

Indirect pulp therapy is a technique for avoiding pulpal exposure in the treatment of teeth with deep carious lesions in which there exists no clinical evidence of pulpal degeneration or periapical pathology. The procedure allows the tooth to utilize the natural protective mechanisms of the pulp against caries. It is based on the theory that a zone of affected demineralized dentin exists between the outer infected layer of dentin and the pulp. When the infected dentin is removed, *the affected dentin can remineralize and the odontoblasts form reparative dentin* thus avoiding a pulp exposure.[30]

Disagreement exists as to whether the deep layers of the carious dentin are infected. Several studies[93,100] showed deep carious lesions to be infected, whereas another[57] reported an area of softened and discolored dentin far in advance of bacterial contamination in acute caries. Still others[168,206] found that most organisms had been removed after the removal of the softened dentin although the incidence of bacterial contamination was higher in primary teeth than in permanent teeth; however, some dentinal tubules still contained small numbers of bacteria.

Kopel[96] summarized the results of various studies of the carious process and identified three distinct layers in active caries: necrotic soft dentin not painful to stimulation and grossly infected with bacteria, firm but softened dentin painful to stimulation but containing fewer bacteria, and slightly discolored hard sound dentin containing few bacteria and painful to stimulation.

In indirect pulp therapy the outer layers of carious dentin are removed. Thus most of the bacteria are eliminated from the lesion. When the lesion is sealed, the substrate upon which the bacteria act to produce acid is also removed. Exposure of the pulp occurs when the carious process advances faster than the reparative mechanism of the pulp. With the arrest of the carious process, the reparative mechanism is able to lay down additional dentin and avoid a pulp exposure.

Although carious dentin left in the tooth probably con-

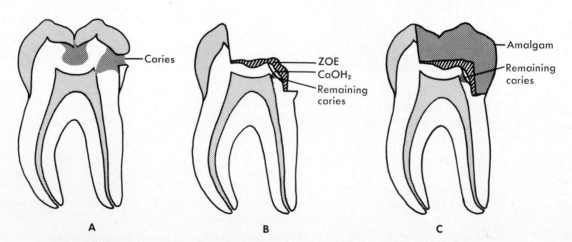

FIG. 22-4. Indirect pulp therapy. **A,** The pulp would probably be exposed if all caries were removed. **B,** All decay is eliminated except that just overlying the pulp. Calcium hydroxide–ZOE is placed over the remaining caries and deep carious excavation. (Ca[OH]₂ may be deleted and only ZOE placed.) **C,** The tooth is sealed with amalgam.

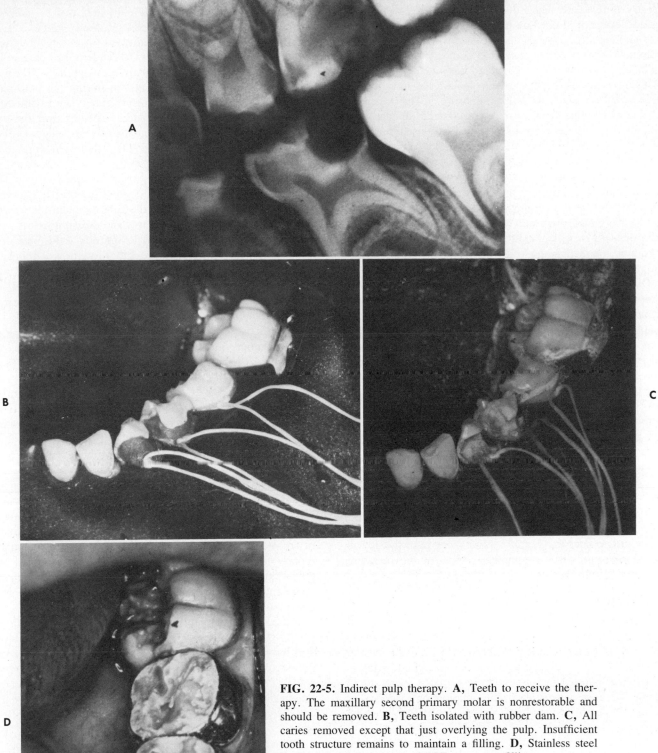

FIG. 22-5. Indirect pulp therapy. **A,** Teeth to receive the therapy. The maxillary second primary molar is nonrestorable and should be removed. **B,** Teeth isolated with rubber dam. **C,** All caries removed except that just overlying the pulp. Insufficient tooth structure remains to maintain a filling. **D,** Stainless steel bands placed for retention of ZOE temporary fillings.

tains some bacteria, the number of organisms can be greatly diminished when this layer is covered with zinc oxide—eugenol or calcium hydroxide.[44,93]

The reparative and recuperative powers of the dental pulp have long been recognized in dentistry. In the middle eighteenth century Pierre Fauchard advised that all caries in deeply carious sensitive teeth should not be removed because of the danger of pulpal exposure.[96] The principles of indirect pulp therapy were recognized as early as 1850.[67,81,208] These early investigators proposed leaving a layer of partially softened dentin to avoid exposure of the pulp and suggested that recalcification of areas of soft decalcified dentin could occur when the softened dentin was sealed under a filling. All these early investigators attributed their success to proper selection of cases. The techniques suggested were only for teeth without a history of pain or teeth in which slight inflammation was suspected. Although the techniques were empirical, the treatment was judged successful.

Dimaggio and Hawes[35,36] selected primary and permanent teeth that were free of clinical signs of pulpal degeneration and periapical pathosis and that appeared radiographically to have a pulp exposure if all the decay were removed. Upon removal of all decay, pulp exposure occurred in 75% of the teeth. In another group of teeth judged clinically to be the same as the first group, the authors achieved 99% success in avoiding pulp exposures with indirect pulp therapy. Reporting on an expanded number of teeth observed from 2 weeks to 4 years, their success rate remained at 97% for the indirect pulp therapy technique.[68]

Indirect pulp therapy has proved to be a very successful technique when cases are properly selected. Numerous other reports[71,92,103,132,193] show successes ranging from 74% to 99%. Differences in case selection, length of study, and type of investigation are responsible for the variations in success. Frankl's report[50] of pulp therapy in pedodontics provides a complete review of the literature on indirect pulp therapy.

Indirect pulp therapy technique

Indirect pulp therapy is utilized in teeth in which pulpal inflammation has been judged to be minimal and complete removal of caries would probably cause a pulp exposure (Fig. 22-4, *A*). Careful diagnosis of the pulpal status is completed before the treatment is initiated. Any tooth judged to have widespread inflammation or evidence of periapical pathosis should receive endodontic therapy or be extracted.

The tooth is anesthetized and isolated with a rubber dam. All the caries except that immediately overlying the pulp is removed. Care must be taken to eliminate all the caries at the dentin-enamel junction. Because of its closeness to the surface, caries left in this area will likely cause failure. If there is communication of the caries with the oral cavity, the carious process will continue, resulting in failure.

Care must also be taken in removing the caries to avoid exposure of the pulp. A large round bur is best to remove the caries. The use of spoon excavators when approaching the pulp may cause an exposure by removal of a large segment of decay. Nevertheless, if used judiciously a spoon excavator is not contraindicated for removing caries near the dentin-enamel junction. All undermined enamel is not removed, for it will help retain the temporary filling.

After all caries except that just overlying the pulp has been removed, a sedative filling of either zinc oxide–eugenol (ZOE) or calcium hydroxide is placed over the remaining carious dentin and areas of deep excavation. The tooth may then be sealed with ZOE or amalgam (Fig. 22-4, *B* and *C*).

If the remaining tooth structure is insufficient to retain the temporary filling, a stainless steel band or temporary crown must be adapted to the tooth to maintain the dressing within the tooth (Fig. 22-5). If the dressing is lost and the remaining caries reexposed to the oral fluids, the desired effects cannot be achieved and a failure will occur.

If this preliminary caries removal is successful, the inflammation will be resolved and deposition of reparative dentin beneath the caries will allow subsequent eradication of the remaining caries without pulpal exposure.

The sedative dressing to be used in indirect pulp therapy may be either calcium hydroxide or ZOE. Studies have shown both materials to be effective and no compelling evidence has been presented that calcium hydroxide is superior to ZOE.[40,92,184,193]

The treated tooth is reentered in 6 to 8 weeks, and the remaining caries extirpated. The rate of reparative dentin deposition has been shown to average 1.4 μm per day following cavity preparations in dentin of human teeth. The rate of reparative dentin formation decreases markedly after 48 days.[177] The greatest rate at which reparative dentin is laid down occurs during the first month following indirect pulp therapy and then diminishes steadily with time. Pulpal floor depth reportedly has little effect on the amount of reparative dentin formed.[193] By contrast, another report[158] has stated that dentin formation is accelerated by thin dentin, that more dentin formation occurs with longer treatment times, and that greater dentin formation is observed in primary than in permanent teeth.

If the initial treatment was successful, when the tooth is reentered the caries will appear to be arrested. The color will have changed from a deep red rose to light gray or light brown. The texture will have changed from spongy and wet to hard, and the caries will appear dehydrated. Practically all bacteria are destroyed under ZOE and calcium hydroxide dressings sealed in deep carious lesions.[2,93]

Following removal of the remaining caries, the tooth may be permanently restored. The usual procedure of pulpal protection with adequate bases is, of course, mandatory before placement of permanent restorations.

DIRECT PULP CAPPING AND PULPOTOMY

Direct pulp capping and pulpotomy involve the application of a medicament or dressing to the exposed pulp in an attempt to preserve vitality. Pulpotomy differs from pulp capping only in that a portion of the remaining pulp is removed before application of the medicament. These procedures have been employed for carious, mechanical, and traumatic exposures of the pulp—with reported high incidence of success as judged radiographically and by the absence of clinical signs and symptoms. Histologic examinations, however, have shown the presence of chronic inflammation under many carious pulp caps and diminished success rates.

Orban[135] described the histopathology of the pulp and concluded that the cells of the pulp were the same as those of loose connective tissue. He believed these cells could differentiate and healing could occur in the dental pulp. In subsequent years much experimentation has taken place, with advocates both for and against pulp-capping and pulpotomy procedures.

Although disagreement exists concerning pulp capping and pulpotomy as permanent procedures in mature secondary teeth, it is universally accepted that vital technique must be employed in teeth with incompletely formed roots with exposed pulps. Once root formation has been completed, routine endodontic treatment may be performed.

Cvek[26] has reported that pulp capping and partial pulpotomy with calcium hydroxide on *traumatically exposed pulps* are successful 96% of the time. He found that the time between the accident and treatment was not critical as long as the superficially inflamed pulp tissue was removed prior to capping. The size of the exposure had no bearing on success or failure. The study included both mature teeth and teeth with incompletely formed roots. Continued calcification of the pulp following pulp capping was not a consistent finding, and when it occurred, it was usually within the first year. These findings have been substantiated by subsequent studies.[28,52,94]

Because of the normal aging of the dental pulp, chances of successful pulp capping diminish with age. Increases in fibrous and calcific deposits and a reduction in pulpal volume may be observed in older pulps. With age the fibroblast proliferation observed in the teeth of young animals is significantly reduced.[166]

Teeth with calcifications of the pulp chamber and root canals are not candidates for pulp capping procedures. These calcifications are indicative of previous inflammatory responses or trauma and render the pulp less responsive to vital therapy.[9, 27]

Agreement generally exists concerning pulp caps in young permanent teeth with blunderbuss apices, but there is disagreement as to whether mature permanent teeth should be pulp capped after a carious pulp exposure. Pulp capping after carious pulp exposure is widely accepted as the treatment of choice. Many clinicians believe that to obtain good results teeth must be carefully selected; pulp capping should be done only in the absence of a history of pain and when there is little or no bleeding at the exposure site.[116] However, other clinicians recommend extirpation of all cariously exposed pulps except those with incompletely formed apices, believing that although there may be no pain enough toxic products remain in the pulp to maintain the inflammation.[101]

These long-standing inflammations with circulatory disturbances are frequently accompanied by apposition and resorption of the canal walls and calcification in the pulp. The inflammation, calcification, apposition, and resorption may thrive under pulp caps regardless of which material is used as the pulp-capping agent. In teeth with blunderbuss apices, some clinicians recommend pulp extirpation and filling of the canals after a pulp cap as soon as the apical foramen has closed because continued calcification may eventually render the canals nonnegotiable.[101]

Little disagreement exists that the ideal treatment for all carious pulp exposures on mature permanent teeth should be pulpal extirpation and endodontic treatment. It is unrealistic, however, to believe that this can be achieved in all cases. Extirpating the pulp is economically unfeasible in many cases and is time consuming and difficult to accomplish in certain teeth. If vital pulp therapy fails, one usually still has the option of endodontic treatment.

Agreement exists that carious exposures on primary teeth should *not* be pulp capped. *Pulp-capping procedures in primary teeth should be reserved for teeth with mechanical exposures.* The pulpotomy procedure for primary teeth (see p. 694) has been shown to be much more successful than pulp capping, and the time requirements for performing the procedures are similar. Therefore *it is recommended that carious pulp exposures on primary teeth not be pulp capped.*[104,179,180]

According to Seltzer and Bender[166] pulp capping should be discouraged for carious pulp exposures since microorganisms and inflammation are invariably associated. Macroscopic examination of such exposures is difficult, and areas of liquefaction necrosis may be overlooked. Because of accelerated aging processes in carious teeth and in teeth having undergone operative procedures, they are poorer candidates for pulp caps than are noncarious teeth; and because of diminished blood supply, periodontally involved teeth are poor risks for pulp capping.

There is general agreement[30,106,116,166] that the larger the area of carious exposure the poorer the prognosis for pulp capping. With a larger exposure more pulpal tissue is inflamed and there is greater chance for contamination by microorganisms. With larger exposures there is also greater damage from crushing of tissues and hemorrhage causing a more severe inflammation. However, when exposure occurs as a result of traumatic or mechanical injury to a healthy pulp, the size of the exposure does not influence healing.[26,138]

Location of the pulp exposures is an important consideration in the prognosis. If the exposure occurs on the axial wall of the pulp, with pulp tissue coronal to the exposure site, this tissue may be deprived of its blood supply and undergo necrosis, causing a failure. Then a pulpotomy or pulpectomy should be performed rather than a pulp cap.[176]

If pulp capping or pulpotomy is to be done, care must be exercised in removal of caries and/or dentin over the exposure site to keep to a minimum the pushing of dentin chips into the remaining pulp tissue. Studies have shown decreased success when dentin fragments are forced into the underlying pulp tissue.[9,89] Inflammatory reaction and formation of dentin matrix are stimulated around these dentin chips. In addition, microorganisms may be forced into the tissue. The resulting inflammatory reaction can be so severe as to cause failure.

Experiments on germ-free animals have shown the importance of microorganisms in the healing of exposed pulp tissues; injured pulpal tissue contaminated by microorganisms did not heal whereas tissue in germ-free animals did heal regardless of the severity of the exposure.[88] Pulp procedures should always be carried out with rubber dam isolation and aseptic conditions to prevent introduction of microorganisms into the pulp tissue.

Marginal seal over the pulp capping or pulpotomy procedure is of prime importance. The suggestion has been made[112] that major considerations for healing are respect for living tissue and the establishment of a tight marginal seal to prevent ingress of bacteria and reinfection. Healing and the formation of secondary dentin are inherent properties of the pulp. If allowed to do so, the pulp, like any connective tissue, will heal itself. Healing following pulp amputation has been shown to be essentially the same as initial calcification events that occur in other normal and pathologic calcified tissues.[69] Factors promoting healing are conditions of the pulp at the time of amputation, removal of irritants, and proper postoperative care such as proper sealing of the margins.

After mechanical exposure of the pulp, an acute inflammation occurs at the exposure site. Blood vessels dilate, edema occurs, and polymorphonuclear leukocytes accumulate at the injury site. If the initial tissue damage is too severe, the pulp will become chronically inflamed, with eventual necrosis of the pulp. It has been shown, however, that repair can occur after pulp exposure. Mechanical exposures have a much better prognosis than do carious exposures because of the lack of previous inflammation and infection associated with the carious exposures. Repair depends on the amount of tissue destruction, the presence of hemorrhage, the patient's age, the resistance of the host, and other factors involved in connective tissue repair.[166]

After pulpal injury, reparative dentin is formed as part of the repair process. Although formation of a dentin bridge has been used as one of the criteria for judging successful pulp capping or pulpotomy procedures, bridge formation can occur in teeth with irreversible inflammation.[195] Moreover, successful pulp capping has been reported without the presence of a reparative dentin bridge over the exposure site.[159,202]

Pulp-capping agents

Many materials and drugs have been employed as pulp-capping agents. Materials, medicaments, antiseptics, anti-inflammatory agents, antibiotics, and enzymes have been utilized as pulp capping agents; but *calcium hydroxide is generally accepted as the material of choice for pulp capping*.[27,116,166]

Prior to 1930, when Hermann[74] introduced calcium hydroxide as a successful pulp-capping agent, pulp therapy had consisted of devitalization with arsenic and other fixative agents. Hermann demonstrated the formation of sec-

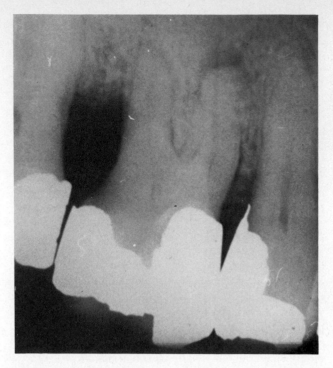

FIG. 22-6. Calcification of pulp chambers and root canals after calcium hydroxide pulp capping. The pulp chamber is completely obliterated, and the root canals partially obliterated. Because of calcification after the pulp capping, the root canals are extremely difficult to locate and negotiate.

ondary dentin over the amputation sites of vital pulps capped with calcium hydroxide.

In 1938 Teuscher and Zander[189] introduced calcium hydroxide in the United States; they histologically confirmed complete dentinal bridging with healthy radicular pulp under calcium hydroxide dressings. Further reports[62,209] firmly established calcium hydroxide as the pulp-capping agent of choice. After these early works many studies have reported various forms of calcium hydroxide used, with success rates ranging from 30% to 98%.[50] The dissimilar success rates are attributed to many factors, including selection of teeth, criteria for success and failure, differences in responses among different animals, length of study, area of pulp to which the medicament was applied (coronally or cervically), and the type of calcium hydroxide employed.

When calcium hydroxide is applied directly to pulp tissue, there is necrosis of the adjacent pulp tissue and an inflammation of the contiguous tissue. Dentin bridge formation occurs at the junction of the necrotic tissue and the vital inflamed tissue. Although calcium hydroxide works effectively, the exact mechanism is not understood. Compounds of similar alkalinity (pH of 11) cause liquefaction necrosis when applied to pulp tissue. Calcium hydroxide maintains a local state of alkalinity that is necessary for bone or dentin formation. Beneath the region of coagulation necrosis, cells of the underlying pulp tissue differentiate into odontoblasts and elaborate dentin matrix.[166]

Occasionally, in spite of successful bridge formation,

the pulp remains chronically inflamed or becomes necrotic. Internal resorption is a sometime occurence following pulp exposure and capping with calcium hydroxide. In other cases complete dentin mineralization of the remaining pulp tissue occludes the canals to the extent that they cannot be penetrated for endodontic therapy if necessary. For these reasons pulpal extirpation and canal filling have been recommended as soon as root formation is completed after the use of calcium hydroxide[101,166] (Fig. 22-6). However, in view of the low incidence of this occurrence, it does not seem to be routinely justified unless necessary for restorative purposes.

It was postulated[209] that calcium would diffuse from a calcium hydroxide dressing into the pulp and participate in the formation of reparative dentin. Experiments with radioactive ions, however, have shown that calcium ions from the calcium hydroxide do *not* enter into the formation of new dentin. Radioactive calcium ions injected intravenously were identified in the dentin bridge. Thus it was established that *the calcium for the dentin bridge comes from the bloodstream.*[4,141,161]

Different forms of calcium hydroxide have been shown to produce marked differences when applied to a pulp exposure.*

Commercially available compounds of calcium hydroxide in modified forms are known to be less alkaline and thus less caustic on the pulp. It has been demonstrated that the dentin bridge forms directly under Dycal or Life.[75,84,143,176,188,194] The chemically altered tissue created by Dycal or Life application is resorbed first, and the bridge is then formed in contact with the capping material. With calcium hydroxide powder (or Pulpdent) the bridge forms at the junction of the chemically altered tissue and the remaining subjacent vital pulp tissue. The altered tissue degenerates and disappears, leaving a void between the capping material and the dentinal bridge. This is the reason a bridge can be seen better radiographically with calcium hydroxide powder or Pulpdent than with Dycal or Life. The quality of the dentin bridging was equally good with either material.

Conflicting evidence has been reported on the success of Hydrex.† The resin catalyst in Hydrex caused pulpal necrosis when used as a direct pulp-capping agent.[163] MPC, a variation of Hydrex, has been shown to be a poor pulp-capping agent.[75,142] Reolit, another hard-setting calcium hydroxide base, has proved unsuccessful in pulp capping, probably because of its neutral pH.[188]

The combination of calcium hydroxide in a methyl-cellulose base and metacresylacetate was shown to consistently produce bridging of regular reparative dentin with normal, uninflamed pulp tissue below the calcific barrier.[50,202]

The incorporation of antibiotics into pulp-capping agents to reduce or eliminate pulp infections has led to varying responses. Generally the antibiotic was ineffective in reducing inflammation or stimulating reparative dentin deposition.* Dangers exist in the use of antibiotics as pulp-capping agents. Immunologic sensitization through pulp canals has been demonstrated. The induction of a hypersensitivity reaction may be a dangerous sequel to topically applied antibiotics.[166]

Corticosteroids have been incorporated into pulp-capping agents in attempts to reduce pain and inflammation.[15,20,47] Reparative dentin formation is inhibited by corticosteroids unless they are incorporated with calcium hydroxide. Reports have pointed out that although pain usually disappeared when the corticosteroids were used these agents might have merely disguised and conserved a chronic inflammation and thus were not beneficial but just postponed the degeneration.[101,166] Combinations of corticosteroids and antibiotics have likewise proved of no value as pulp-capping agents.[80]

Isobutyl cyanoacrylate has been reported to be an excellent pulp-capping agent because of its hemostatic and bacteriostatic properties; at the same time it causes less inflammation than does calcium hydroxide.[12,14] Severe inflammation with N-butyl cyanoacrylate has occurred, however.[133]

Polycarboxylate cements have been reported to be well tolerated by pulp tissue, but they are initially irritating and do not stimulate formation of a dentin bridge.[41,117,156]

Other materials used as pulp-capping agents have included dentin,[198] albumin,[119] acid and alkaline phosphatase,[166] chondroitin sulfate,[166] chondroitin sulfate and collagen,[166] calcium-eugenol cement,[79] calcitonin (a calcium-regulating hormone),[171] barium and strontium hydroxide,[78] and native enriched collagen solution.[16,55]

An absorbable form of tricalcium phosphate ceramic has been reported to produce dentinal bridging when used as a pulp-capping agent in monkeys. The formation of a dentin bridge was enhanced when compared with that in a control using calcium hydroxide, and pulpal inflammation was minimal.[72]

The use of ZOE applied directly to pulp tissue is a controversial issue. As compared with calcium hydroxide, ZOE produced favorable results according to some researchers[98,162,202] but allowed chronic inflammation and eventual necrosis of pulp tissue to persist according to others.[65,114,164] Dentin bridge formation does not normally occur under ZOE pulp caps although it has been reported.[148]

Although capping inflamed pulps is not recommended, ZOE has been shown to be a more beneficial agent than calcium hydroxide under these circumstances.[195] Calcium hydroxide placed on acutely inflamed pulps leads to necrosis.

The ideal treatment for all carious exposures, except those in teeth with incompletely formed roots, might be pulp extirpation and root canal filling; nevertheless there are still indications for direct pulp capping. Economics, time, and difficulty of achieving root canal filling in certain teeth are a few of the reasons one may choose pulp capping over another form of pulp therapy. *The pulp cap-*

---

*References 11, 32, 77, 98, 140, 143, 160, 163, 176, 188, 194, 202.
†References 32, 77, 160, 163, 176.

*References 6, 20, 59, 117, 173.

ping material of choice at the present time remains calcium hydroxide. If pulp capping is considered, one must consider all the factors discussed in this section to determine the prognosis of each case. In the event of failure of direct pulp capping, there is usually the option of endodontic therapy.

Pulp capping should *not* be considered for primary carious pulp exposures or for permanent teeth with a history of spontaneous toothache, radiographic evidence of pulpal or periapical pathosis, calcifications of the pulp chamber or root canals, excessive hemorrhage at the exposure site, or exposures with purulent or serous exudates.

PULPOTOMY

The pulpotomy procedure involves removing pulp tissue that has inflammatory or degenerative changes, leaving intact the remaining vital tissue, which is then covered with a pulp-capping agent to promote healing at the amputation site or an agent to cause fixation of the underlying tissue. The only difference between pulpotomy and pulp capping is that additional tissue is removed from the exposed pulp. Traditionally, the term "pulpotomy" has implied removal of pulp tissue to the cervical line. However, the depth to which tissue is removed is determined by clinical judgment. All tissue judged to be inflamed should be removed in order to place the dressing on healthy, uninflamed pulp tissue. In multirooted teeth, the procedure may be simplified by removing tissue to the orifices of the root canals.

The difficulties in assessing the extent of inflammation in cariously exposed pulps have been previously discussed (see p. 686). However, several studies[28,70,199] have shown that inflammation is confined to the surface 2 to 3 mm of the pulp when traumatically exposed and left untreated for up to 168 hours. In experimental animals, the results were the same whether the crowns were fractured or ground off. Direct invasion of vital pulp tissue by bacteria did not occur, even though the pulps were left exposed to the saliva. Under the same circumstances with cavity preparations into the teeth that left areas to impact food, debris, and bacteria in contact with the pulp, the inflammation ranged from 1 to 9 mm with abscess and pus formation.[28,70] The same results have been obtained in permanent teeth with incompletely formed roots as well as those with mature ones. Pulpotomy procedures for primary teeth are discussed later in this chapter.

Pulpotomy procedures using the carbon dioxide laser[167] and electrosurgery[154] have been reported. The advantages of these techniques are the lack of hemorrhage and less mechanical damage to the underlying pulp. While these areas appear promising, not enough research has been done to determine their validity.

Calcium hydroxide pulpotomy on young permanent teeth

While vital pulp capping and pulpotomy procedures for cariously exposed pulps in teeth with developed apices remain controversial, it is universally accepted that vital techniques be employed in those teeth with incompletely developed apices. While many materials and drugs have been used as pulp capping agents (see p. 690), the application of calcium hydroxide to stimulate dentinal bridge formation in accidentally or cariously exposed pulps of young permanent teeth continues to be the treatment of choice.

The indirect pulp therapy technique should be used whenever possible with deep carious lesions in order to avoid exposure of the pulp (see p. 692). Every attempt should be made to maintain the vitality of these immature teeth until their full root development has been completed. Loss of vitality before root completion leaves a weak root more prone to fracture. Loss of vitality before completion of root length may leave a poor crown/root ratio and a tooth more susceptible to periodontal breakdown because of excessive mobility. If necessary, the remaining pulp tissue can be extirpated and conventional endodontic therapy completed when root formation has been completed.

Endodontic treatment is greatly complicated in teeth with necrotic pulps and open apices. Although apexification procedures have been perfected for these teeth, the treatment is extensive and costly for the patient and the resulting root structure is weaker than in teeth with fully developed roots. If the calcium hydroxide pulpotomy is not successful, the apexification procedure or surgical endodontics may still be performed.

Technique

After the diagnosis is completed, the tooth is anesthetized. If possible, pulpal procedures should always be performed under rubber dam isolation and aseptic conditions to prevent further introduction of microorganisms into the pulpal tissues. Care must be taken when placing the rubber dam on a traumatized tooth. If any loosening of the tooth has occurred, the rubber dam clamps must be applied to adjacent uninjured teeth. If this is impossible because of lack of adjacent teeth or partially erupted ones that cannot be clamped, careful isolation with cotton rolls and constant aspiration by the dental assistant may be utilized to maintain a dry field (Fig. 22-7).

In traumatically exposed pulps, only tissue judged to be inflamed is removed. Cvek[26] has shown that with pulp exposures resulting from traumatic injuries, regardless of the size of the exposure or the amount of lapsed time, pulpal changes are characterized by a proliferative response with inflammation extending only a few millimeters into the pulp. When this hyperplastic inflamed tissue is removed, healthy pulp tissue is encountered.[26] In teeth with carious exposure of the pulp, it may be necessary to remove pulpal tissue to a greater depth to reach uninflamed tissue.

The instrument of choice for tissue removal in the pulpotomy procedure is an abrasive diamond bur utilizing high speed and adequate water cooling. This technique has been shown to create the least damage to the underlying tissue.[63] Care must be exercised to assure removal of all filaments of the pulp tissue coronal to the amputation site; otherwise, hemorrhage will be impossible to control. Following pulpal amputation, the preparation is thoroughly washed with physiologic saline or sterile water to remove all debris. The water is removed by vacuum and cotton

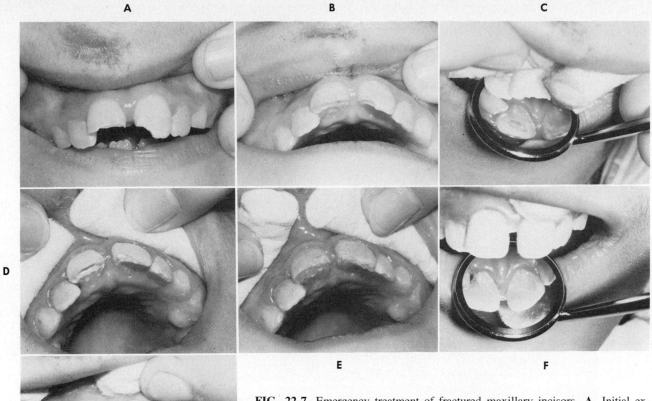

FIG. 22-7. Emergency treatment of fractured maxillary incisors. **A,** Initial examination 4 days after the trauma. **B,** Right central incisor with pulp exposure, left central with dentin exposure. **C,** Pulpotomy preparation after hemorrhage has been controlled with a moistened cotton pellet. **D,** Application of Dycal to the pulpal stump and exposed dentin. **E,** Acid-etching of enamel. **F** and **G,** Completed acid-etch resin restoration.

pellets. Air should not be blown on the exposed pulp since it will cause desiccation and tissue damage.

Hemorrhage is controlled by slightly moistened cotton pellets (wetted and blotted almost dry) placed against the stumps of the pulp. Completely dry cotton pellets should not be used since fibers of the dry cotton will be incorporated into the clot and, when removed, will cause hemorrhage. Dry cotton pellets are placed over the moist pellets and slight pressure is exerted on the mass to control the hemorrhage. Hemorrhage should be controlled in this manner within several minutes (Fig. 22-7, *C*). It may be necessary to change the pellets to control all hemorrhage. If hemorrhage continues, one must carefully check to be sure that all filaments of the pulp coronal to the amputation site were removed and that the site is clean.

If hemorrhage cannot be controlled, amputation should be performed at a more apical level. Should it become necessary to extend into the root canals, a small endodontic spoon or round abrasive diamond bur may be used to remove the tissue on anterior teeth with single canals (Fig. 22-8). On posterior teeth, the use of endodontic files or reamers may be necessary if tissue is being amputated

within the canals. *Obviously, extension of the amputation site is carried into the root canals only in teeth with blunderbuss apices.*

On teeth with blunderbuss apices, if tissue removal has been extended several millimeters into the root canals and hemorrhage continues, a compromise treatment should be considered. The hemorrhage is controlled with chemicals such as aluminum chloride or other hemostatic agents. Once hemorrhage is controlled, calcium hydroxide is placed in the canal against the pulp stump and the tooth is sealed. These compromised teeth must be closely monitored for development of pathologic conditions. If necrosis of the remaining pulp tissue occurs, apexification procedures are instituted. If vitality is maintained, further root development with dystrophic calcification usually occurs. In these compromised cases, once the apex has formed, the tooth is reentered and conventional endodontic therapy is completed with gutta-percha obliteration.

In the normal pulpotomy procedure, once the hemorrhage has been controlled, a dressing of calcium hydroxide is placed over the amputation site (Fig. 22-7, *D*). If the pulpal amputation extends into the tooth only a few milli-

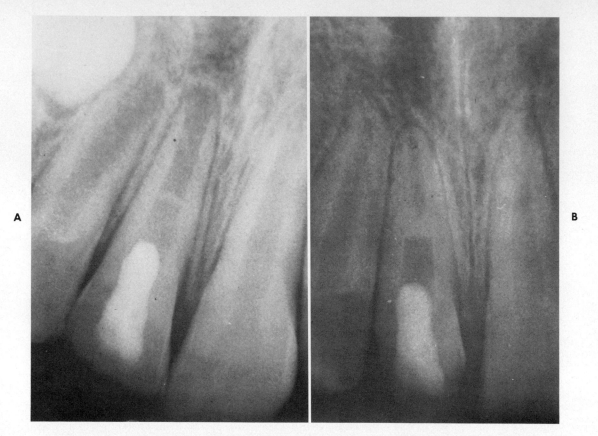

FIG. 22-8. Deep calcium hydroxide pulpotomy. **A,** Central incisor with an immature apex 10 weeks after a traumatic exposure of the pulp and a calcium hydroxide pulpotomy. Note the dentin bridge. **B,** Three years after pulpotomy. Note the thickening of the dentin bridge and the completion of root development. The tooth remained asymptomatic. No further endodontic treatment is indicated at this time.

meters, the use of a hard setting material (e.g., Dycal or Life) is usually easiest. However, for deeper amputation, calcium hydroxide powder carried to the tooth in an amalgam carrier is the easiest method of application. The amalgam carrier is tightly packed with powder; then all but one fourth to one third of the pellet is expressed from the carrier and discarded. The remaining calcium hydroxide in the carrier is then expressed into the preparation site. The pellet of calcium hydroxide powder is carefully teased against the pulp stump with a rounded end plastic instrument. The entire pulp stump must be covered with a thin layer of calcium hydroxide. Care must be taken not to pack the calcium hydroxide into the pulp tissue, as this will cause greater inflammation and increase the chances of failure, or if pulpotomy is successful, there will be increased calcification of the remaining pulp tissues around the particles of calcium hydroxide.

Pulpdent (calcium hydroxide in a methylcellulose base) may also be utilized for the pulpotomy procedure. If commercial preparations of calcium hydroxide are used, care must be taken to avoid trapping air bubbles when applying the material.

After the calcium hydroxide has been applied to the pulp stumps, a creamy mix of ZOE or other cement base must be flowed over the calcium hydroxide and allowed to set completely. When a composite resin restoration is to be utilized, eugenol-containing compounds must be avoided since these interfere with the setting reaction of the composite. In these cases, a second layer of Dycal or Life is placed. After setting, the cement base layer should be thick enough to allow for condensation of a permanent restoration to effectively seal the tooth.

A permanent type of restoration should always be placed in the tooth to ensure the retention of the calcium hydroxide–cement base dressing. Unless a crown is necessary, amalgam is the material of choice for posterior teeth, and a composite restoration (Fig. 22-7, *E* to *G*) is preferred for anterior teeth.

Follow-up after pulp capping and pulpotomy

After pulp capping and pulpotomy, the patient should be recalled periodically for 2 to 4 years to determine success. Although the normal vitality tests such as electric and thermal sensitivity are reliable after pulp capping, they are usually not helpful in the pulpotomized tooth. Although histologic success cannot be determined, clincial success is judged by the absence of any clinical or radiographic signs of pathosis; the verification of a dentin bridge both

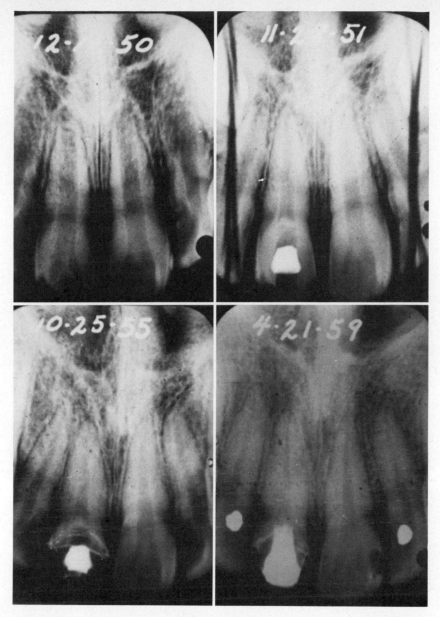

FIG. 22-9. Calcium hydroxide pulpotomy on a permanent incisor with an immature (or blunder-buss) apex. Traumatic exposure of the pulp of the central incisor was treated with a calcium hydroxide pulpotomy. The tooth at 1 year, 5 years, and 8½ years after pulpotomy remained asymptomatic. Root formation was completed, and the root canal appears to be of similar size to that of the adjacent incisor. (Courtesy Dr. Ralph McDonald.)

radiographically and clinically, and the presence of continued root development in teeth with incompletely formed roots.

Controversy exists as to whether the pulp should be reentered after the completion of root development in the pulpotomized tooth. Some researchers[101,166] believe that pulp capping and pulpotomy procedures invariably lead to progressive calcification of the root canals. After successful root development, they advocate extirpation of the remaining pulp tissue and endodontic treatment. They recommend endodontic therapy because of the high incidence of continued calcification, which would render the canals

nonnegotiable at some future time when endodontic therapy might be required because of disease. However, it has been my experience and others[26,94,99,148] that with good case selection, if a gentle technique is used in removal of pulp tissue, care is taken to avoid contamination of the pulp with bacteria and dentin chips, and the dressing of calcium hydroxide is not packed into the underlying pulp tissue, the progressive calcification of the pulp is an infrequent sequela of pulpotomy (Fig. 22-9).

In a follow-up study of clinically successful pulpotomies previously reported,[26] researchers[29] removed the pulps 1 to 5 years later for restorative reasons and found histologi-

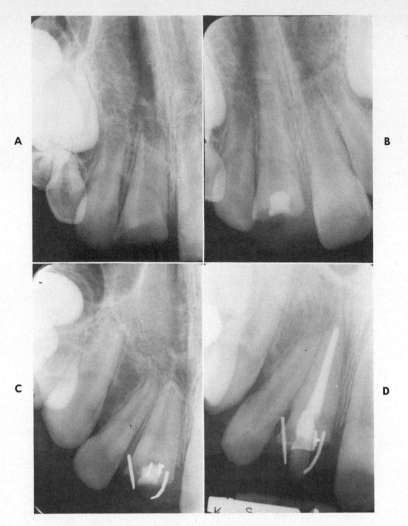

FIG. 22-10. Apexogenesis following calcium hydroxide pulpotomy. **A,** A traumatic injury has exposed the pulp in the maxillary central incisor before formation of the root was completed. **B,** Two months after calcium hydroxide pulpotomy, a dentin bridge has formed. **C,** Two and a half years after the pulpotomy, the root has completed its development. Note the lack of further pulpal calcification and a misplaced pin for retention of a temporary composite restoration. **D,** Root canal treatment has been completed so that the tooth may be permanently restored with a post and core and crown.

cally normal pulps. They concluded that changes seen in the pulps do not represent sufficient histologic evidence to support routine pulpectomy after pulpotomy in accidentally fractured teeth with pulp exposures. Thus the routine reentry to remove the pulp and place a root canal filling after completion of root development is contraindicated unless dictated by restorative considerations such as the necessity for retentive post placement. Nevertheless, canal calcification, internal resorption, and/or pulp necrosis are potential sequelae of pulp capping and pulpotomy procedures. Although unlikely, they are possible and the patient should be clearly informed.

In posterior teeth, where surgical endodontics is difficult, if continued calcification of the canal is observed following root closure, reentry of the tooth for endodontic therapy is recommended. In anterior teeth, if calcification of the canal has made conventional endodontics impossible, surgical endodontics may be performed with relative ease. Therefore, in anterior teeth, routine endodontic therapy following completion of root development is contraindicated unless clinical signs and symptoms of pathosis are present or unless it is necessary for restorative procedures (placement of a post for retention of a crown because of missing tooth structure) (Fig. 22-10).

Formocresol pulpotomy on young permanent teeth

Because of the reported clincial and histologic success with the formocresol pulpotomy on primary teeth, there has been much interest in this technique on young permanent teeth. Evidence of continued apical development following formocresol pulpotomy procedures on young permanent teeth with incompletely developed apices has been reported.* Several authors have reported better results with

---

*References 45,54,123,139,157.

diluted formocresol. However, they reported a high incidence of internal resorption which increased in severity with longer periods of time.[54,139]

The formocresol procedure has appeal because there is a lack of calcification of the remaining pulp tissue as is sometimes seen with calcium hydroxide pulpotomy. After root completion, the tooth can easily be reentered, the pulp extirpated, and routine endodontic therapy performed. Contrary to these findings, one group of researchers[3] has shown calcification of the canals by continuous apposition of dentin on the lateral walls with equal frequency whether using calcium hydroxide or formocresol. The only common denominator to this reaction was the presence of dentin chips that had accidentally been pushed into the radicular pulp tissue.

Other studies[90,122] have shown complete replacement of the pulp tissue with granulation tissue and the formation of osteodentin along the walls of the canals in permanent teeth following formocresol pulpotomies. The reaction was described as a healing rather than destructive process, but persistent chronic inflammation was noted.

Although this treatment has been reported to be partly successful, it cannot be routinely recommended until further research showing the technique to be successful has been completed.

Formocresol pulpotomy procedures have been reported as temporary treatments on permanent teeth with necrotic pulps. Clinical success after 3 years has been reported.[192] The formocresol pulpotomy was performed rather than extraction when routine endodontic therapy could not be completed because of financial considerations. Complete endodontic treatment was advocated at a later date, with the formocresol pulpotomy used only as a *temporary* treatment.

Formocresol pulpotomy on primary teeth

The use of formocresol in dentistry has become a controversial issue since reports of wide distribution of the medicament following systemic injection[124] and the demonstration of an immune response to formocresol-fixed autologous tissue implanted in connective tissues or injected into root canals.[17,190] However, the formocresol pulpotomy continues to be the treatment of choice for primary teeth with vital carious exposures of the pulp in which inflammation and/or degeneration are judged to be confined to the coronal pulp. The last reported survey of North American dental schools in 1968[175] showed a majority of pedodontic departments advocated the formocresol pulpotomy technique. Currently it is still widely taught and utilized in clinical practice. The current formocresol pulpotomy technique is a modification of that reported by Sweet in 1930.[186]

Histologic studies[111,113] have demonstrated the effects of formocresol on pulps of primary and permanent human teeth. Formocresol-saturated cotton pellets caused the surface of the pulp to become fibrous and acidophilic within a few minutes. After exposure to the formocresol for a period of 7 to 14 days, three distinct zones became evident: (1) a broad acidophilic zone of fixation, (2) a broad pale-staining zone with diminished cellular and fiber definition (atrophy), and (3) a broad zone of inflammatory cells concentrated at the pale-staining zone junction and diffusing apically into normal pulp tissue. There was no evidence of an attempt to wall off the inflammatory zone by fibrous tissue or calcific barrier. After 60 days to 1 year, the pulp was progressively fixed and the entire pulp ultimately became fibrous.

Subsequent investigations[42] showed that the effect of formocresol on the pulp varies depending on the length of time the drug is in contact with the tissue. After 5 minutes there was a surface fixation blending into normal pulp tissue apically. Formocresol sealed in contact with the pulp for 3 days caused calcific degeneration, and the technique was termed vital or nonvital according to the length of time of the application. As a part of this report, the clinical data from Sweet's files were compiled and showed a 97% success rate.

The ingrowth of fibroblasts in tissue underlying formocresol-pulpotomized noncarious human primary canines has been reported.[33] At 16 weeks the entire pulp had degenerated and was being replaced with granulation tissue. Mild inflammation and some calcific degeneration were noted.

Doyle et al.[37] compared calcium hydroxide and formocresol pulpotomies on mechanically exposed, healthy, primary dental pulps. A formocresol pellet was sealed in place 4 to 7 days, and the histologic study was conducted from 4 to 388 days. Of the 18 teeth in the calcium hydroxide group, only 50% were judged histologically to be successful; of the 14 teeth treated with formocresol, 92% were histologically successful. Radiographically the success rates were 64% and 93% whereas the clinical success rates were 71% and 100% (calcium hydroxide versus formocresol pulpotomy). The authors were able to identify vital tissue in the apical third of the root canals after treatment with formocresol pulpotomies.

Studies of the effect of adding formocresol to the ZOE filling over the 5-minute–formocresol-pulpotomized primary tooth[7,197] have shown no appreciable differences between when formocresol was included in the cement and when it was not; and histologic investigations[149,174,197] have reported no significant differences between the two-appointment and the one-appointment (5-minute) formocresol pulpotomies.

Accumulation of formocresol has been demonstrated in the pulp, dentin, periodontal ligament, and bone surrounding the apices of pulpotomized teeth.[56,126] Formaldehyde was shown to be the component of formocresol that interacts with the protein portion of cells. The addition of cresol to formaldehyde appears to potentiate the effect of formaldehyde on protein.[128]

Application of radioactive formocresol to amputated pulp sites has been shown to result in immediate absorption of the material. The systemic absorption was limited to about 1% of the applied dose regardless of the amount of time the drug was applied. It was shown that formocresol compromised the microcirculation, causing vessel thrombosis, which limited further systemic accumulation.[126]

Animal experiments[17,190] have demonstrated that in vivo

formocresol-fixed autologous tissue will produce an immune response when implanted into connective tissues or injected into root canals. The tissue became antigenically altered by formocresol and activated a specific cell-mediated lymphocyte response.

Other studies have demonstrated no evidence of this response in nonpresensitized animals,[169] while presensitized animals showed only a weak allergic potential.[196] This is in agreement with researchers[34] who have shown that formaldehyde demonstrated a low level of antigenicity in rabbits and as such would be an acceptable pulp medicament in regard to immunologic potential. Other investigators[107] studied lymphocyte transformation induced by formocresol-treated and untreated extracts of homologous pulp tissue in children with varying past experience with formocresol pulpotomies. Significant transformation responses were noted in over half the children, but they were unrelated to a clinical history of formocresol pulpotomy. Sensitization to pulp-related antigens was a common finding in the study. The authors concluded that formocresol pulpotomy does not induce significant immunologic sensitization to extracted antigens of homologous pulp or to pulp antigen altered by treatment with formocresol and therefore does not support other animal studies in which intense immunization schedules were used.[107] Clinical use of formocresol for many years without reports of allergic reactions has quite obviously substantiated this finding.

After systemic administration of formocresol in experimental animals, it is distributed throughout the body. Metabolism and excretion of a portion of the absorbed formocresol occur in the kidneys and lungs. The remaining drug is bound to tissue predominately in the kidneys, liver, and lungs. When administered systemically in high dosages, acute toxic effects (including cardiovascular changes, plasma and urinary enzyme changes, and histologic evidence of cellular injury to the vital organs) were noted. The degree of tissue injury appeared to be dose related, with some of the changes being reversible in the early stages. The authors[124] were careful to point out that the administered dosages were far in excess of those used clinically in humans and should not be extrapolated to clinical dental practice. In another study, the same authors emphasized that the quantities of formaldehyde absorbed systemically via the pulpotomy route were small and did not contraindicate the use of formocresol.[137]

A subsequent study[125] in which 16 pulpotomies (5-minute application of full-strength formocresol) were performed on a dog displayed early tissue injury to the kidneys and liver. However, cellular recovery could be expected since there was no evidence of the onset of an inflammatory reaction. In animals subjected to only one of four pulpotomies, there was no injury to the kidneys or liver. The heart and lungs of all the animals were normal. The authors pointed out that 16 pulpotomies on a small dog presents a much higher exposure to systemic formocresol than would be experienced clincially in a human with several pulpotomies. They further concluded that no clinical implications regarding the toxicity of absorbed formocresol should be drawn from this study. Other

investigators[58] have shown the effect of formocresol on pulp tissue is controlled by the quantity that diffuses into the tissue and the quantity can be controlled by the length of time of application, the concentration used, the method of application, or a combination of all these factors.

Implantation of undiluted formocresol-fixed tissue in animals causes necrosis of the surrounding connective tissues,[19] and dilution of the formocresol decreases the tissue irritation potential.[60] Investigations utilizing one-fifth concentration formocresol for pulpotomies have noted little difference as related to the initial effects on tissue fixation; however, an earlier recovery of enzyme activities was apparent with the diluted formocresol as compared to the undiluted. Postoperative complications are reduced, and there is an improvement in the rate of recovery from the cytotoxic effects of formocresol when diluted.[108,109,185] It has been reported clinically that the same success is achieved with the diluted formocresol as with the undiluted.[53,120,121] *Therefore it is recommended that one-fifth concentration formocresol be utilized for pulpotomy procedures since it is equally effective as and less damaging than the traditional preparation.*

One-fifth concentration formocresol is prepared in the following manner. The dilute solution is prepared by mixing 3 parts glycerin with 1 part distilled water. One part formocresol is then thoroughly mixed with 4 parts diluent.[121]

A histologic study on teeth with induced pulpal and periapical pathosis[91] showed no resolution of inflammation or periapical pathosis after a 5-minute pulpotomy procedure. Canals with vital tissue exhibited more internal resorption than was reported by other researchers, and more apical resorption was seen in teeth with periapical and furcal involvement that was seen in teeth with vital pulps. Ingrowth of tissue was not observed in canals with necrotic tissue. Also noted was the lack of evidence of formocresol fixation of either apical or furcal lesions. Despite extensive inflammatory reactions around the apices of primary teeth close to the permanent tooth germs, no ill effects were observed on any tooth germs from the formocresol. Formocresol fixation was confined within the canals in all instances. Since the authors[91] concluded that the formocresol pulpotomy is an unacceptable procedure on teeth with pulpal and periapical pathosis, this study points out the importance of confining formocresol pulpotomies to primary teeth containing vital tissue in the root canals.

The fear of damage to the succedaneous tooth has been offered as an argument against formocresol pulpotomy on primary teeth. Studies have shown conflicting findings, ranging from the same incidence of enamel defects in treated and untreated contralateral teeth[153] to an increase in defects and positional alterations of the underlying permanent tooth.[118] It should be pointed out that studies of this nature are follow-up studies long after treatment, without knowledge of the existing status of the pulp prior to pulpotomy. Also no one has devised a study to ascertain the effects of the condition that necessitated the pulpotomy procedure. If the strict criteria outlined in this section are followed, the incidence of defects to the permanent teeth does not increase after formocresol pulpotomy.

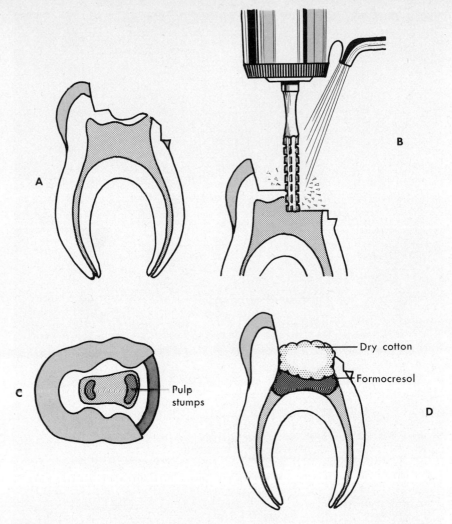

FIG. 22-11. Formocresol pulpotomy. **A,** Carious pulp exposure in the primary tooth. **B,** Removal of the roof of the pulp chamber. **C,** Pulp stumps after hemorrhage controlled. **D,** Formocresol application for 5 minutes. After fixation of the pulp stumps, a base ZOE is applied and the tooth is permanently restored.

Indications and contraindications

The formocresol pulpotomy is indicated for pulp exposure on primary teeth in which the inflammation and/or infection are judged to be confined to the coronal pulp. If inflammation has spread into the tissues within the root canals, the tooth should be considered a candidate for pulpectomy and root canal filling or extraction. The contraindications for formocresol pulpotomy on a primary tooth are (1) a nonrestorable tooth, (2) a tooth nearing exfoliation or with no bone overlying the permanent tooth crown, (3) a history of spontaneous toothache, (4) evidence of periapical or furcal pathology, (5) a pulp that does not hemorrhage, (6) inability to control hemorrhage following a coronal pulp amputation, (7) a pulp with serous or purulent drainage, and (8) the presence of a fistula.

Technique (Fig. 22-11)

The formocresol pulpotomy is utilized on primary teeth whose roots are judged to be free of inflammation and/or infection. Compromise on this principle will lead to a di-

minished success rate and possible damage to the succedaneous tooth. Therefore the importance of a proper diagnosis cannot be overstressed.

After the diagnosis has been completed, the primary tooth is anesthetized and isolated with a rubber dam. All caries is removed. The entire roof of the pulp chamber is cut away with a high-speed bur and copious water spray. All the coronal pulp is removed with a bur or spoon excavator. Care must be exercised to extirpate all filaments of the coronal pulp. If any filaments remain in the pulp chamber, hemorrhage will be impossible to control. The pulp chamber is thoroughly washed with water to remove all debris. The water is removed by vacuum and cotton pellets.

Hemorrhage is controlled by slightly moistened cotton pellets (wetted and blotted almost dry) placed against the stumps of the pulp at the openings of the root canals. Completely dry cotton pellets should not be used since fibers of the cotton will be incorporated into the clot and, when removed, will cause hemorrhage. Dry cotton pellets

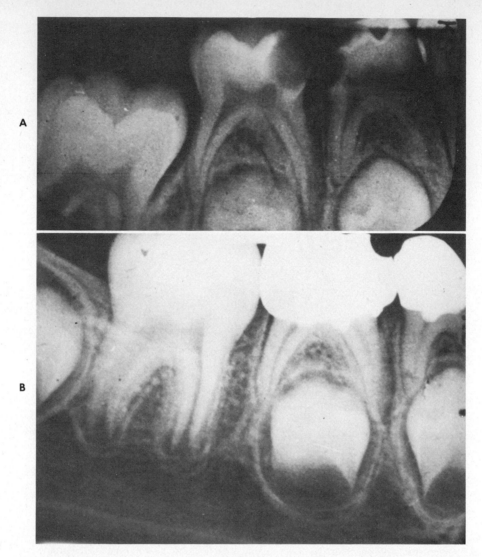

FIG. 22-12. Formocresol pulpotomy. **A,** Primary first and second molars with carious pulp exposures. **B,** Eighteen months after formocresol pulpotomy. Note the eruption of the permanent first molar.

are placed over the moist pellets, and pressure is exerted on the mass to control the hemorrhage. Hemorrhage should be controlled in this manner within several minutes. It may be necessary to change the pellets to control all hemorrhage. If hemorrhage occurs, carefully check to be sure that all filaments of the pulp were removed from the pulp chamber and that the amputation site is clean.

If hemorrhage cannot be controlled within 5 minutes, the pulp tissue within the canals is probably inflamed and the tooth is not a candidate for a formocresol pulpotomy. The clinician should then proceed with pulpectomy, or the tooth should be extracted.

When the hemorrhage has been controlled, one-fifth dilution formocresol on a cotton pellet is placed in direct contact with the pulp stumps. Fixation will not occur unless the formocresol is in contact with the stumps. The cotton pellet is blotted to remove excess formocresol after saturation and before the tooth is entered. Formocresol is

caustic and will create a severe tissue burn if allowed to contact the gingiva.

The formocresol is left in contact with the pulp stumps for 5 minutes. When it is removed, the tissue will appear brown and no hemorrhage should be present. If an area of the pulp was not contacting the medication, the procedure must be repeated for that tissue. Small cotton pellets for applying the medication usually work best since they allow closer approximation of the material to the pulp.

A cement base of ZOE is placed over the pulp stumps and allowed to set. The tooth may then be restored permanently. The restoration of choice is a stainless steel crown for primary molars. On anterior primary teeth a composite tooth-colored restoration is the treatment of choice unless the tooth is so badly broken down that it requires a crown.

With the formocresol, no dentin bridge formation occurs as with the calcium hydroxide pulpotomy (Fig. 22-12).

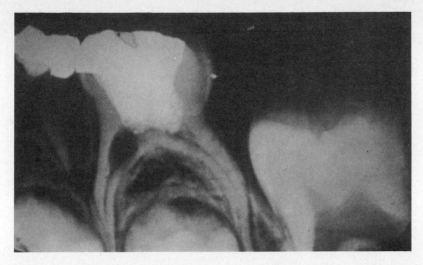

FIG. 22-13. Formocresol pulpotomy failure. Note the internal resorption in the mesial root and the radiolucency in the bifurcation.

Failure of a formocresol pulpotomy is usually detected radiographically (Fig. 22-13). The first signs of failure are often internal resorption of the root adjacent to the area where the formocresol was applied. This may be accompanied by external resorption, especially as the failure progresses. In the primary molars a radiolucency develops in the bifurcation or trifurcation area. In the anterior teeth a radiolucency may develop at the apices or lateral to the roots. With more destruction the tooth will become excessively mobile. A fistula usually develops. It is rare for pain to occur with the failure of a formocresol pulpotomy. Consequently, unless patients receive follow-up checks after a formocresol pulpotomy, failure may go undetected. When the tooth loosens and is eventually exfoliated, the parents and child may consider the circumstances normal.

Glutaraldehyde pulpotomy

Numerous studies* have reported the use of glutaraldehyde as a substitute medicament for pulpotomy procedure on primary teeth. The application of 2% aqueous glutaraldehyde has been shown to produce a rapid surface fixation of the underlying pulpal tissue while its depth of penetration is limited. Unlike the varied response to formocresol, a large percentage of the remaining pulp tissue remained vital. A narrow zone of eosinophilic-stained and compressed fixed tissue was found directly beneath the area of application, which blended into vital normal-appearing tissue apically.

Investigators[97] have shown that, with time, the glutaraldehyde-fixed zone is replaced through macrophagic action with dense collagenous tissue, thus the entire root canal tissue is vital. Since glutaraldehyde does not perfuse pulp tissue to the apex, it will not demonstrate systemic distribution as seen with formocresol.[31,105,203,204]

It is because of these biochemical effects on pulp tissue

that glutaraldehyde has been proposed for use in pulpotomies on primary teeth rather than formocresol. However, glutaraldehyde has been shown to produce antigenic products in much the same manner as formocresol,[147] Also, purified solutions of glutaraldehyde have been shown to be unstable.[146] Therefore, other researchers[147] have concluded that minimal evidence exists to justify the change from formocresol to glutaraldehyde as a pulpotomy agent.

PULPECTOMY IN PRIMARY TEETH
Primary root canal anatomy

To complete endodontic treatment on primary teeth successfully, the clinician must have a thorough knowledge of the anatomy of the primary root canal systems and the variations that normally exist in these systems; and to understand some of the variations present in the primary root canal systems requires understanding root formation.

Root formation

According to Orban[136] development of the roots begins after enamel and dentin formation has reached the future cementum-enamel junction. The epithelial dental organ forms Hertwig's epithelial root sheath, which initiates formation and molds the shape of the roots. Hertwig's sheath takes the form of one or more epithelial tubes (depending on the number of roots of the tooth, one tube for each root). During root formation the apical foramen of each root has a wide opening limited by the epithelial diaphragm. The dentinal walls taper apically, and the shape of the pulp canal is like a wide open tube. Each root contains one canal at this time, and the number of canals is the same as the number of roots. When root length is established, the sheath disappears but dentin deposition continues internally within the roots.

Differentiation of a root into separate canals, as in the mesial of the mandibular molars, occurs by continued deposition of dentin; this narrows the isthmus between the walls of the canals and continues until there is formation

*References 31,97,155,187,203.

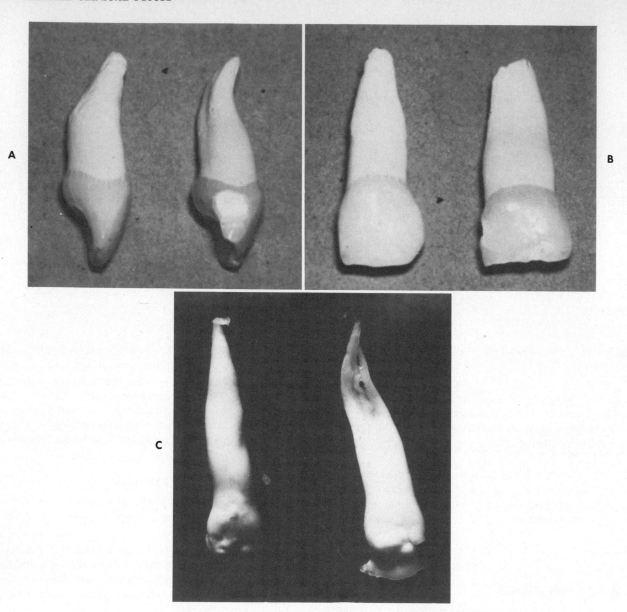

FIG. 22-14. Primary central incisors and silicone models of the pulp canals. **A,** Beginning resorption of the roots on the apical third of the lingual surfaces. **B,** Facial surfaces. **C,** Models. The pulp canals were injected with silicone and the tooth structure decalcified away, leaving a model of the root canal systems. Note the division of the canal on the right.

of dentin islands within the root canal and eventual division of the root into separate canals. During the process communications exist between the canals as an isthmus, then as fins connecting the canals. The reader is referred to Chapter 10 for a complete description of pulp and dentin formation.

As growth proceeds, the root canal is narrowed by continued deposition of dentin and the pulp tissue is compressed. Additional deposition of dentin and cementum closes the apex of the tooth and creates the apical convergence of the root canals common to the completely formed tooth.

Root length is not completed until 1 to 4 years after a tooth erupts into the oral cavity. In the primary teeth the

root length is completed in a shorter period of time than in the permanent tooth because of the shorter length of the primary roots.

The root-to-crown length of the primary teeth is greater than that of the permanent teeth. The primary roots are more narrow than the permanent roots. The roots of the primary molars diverge more than do those of the permanent teeth. This feature allows more room for the development of the crown of the succeeding premolar.[205]

The primary tooth is unique insofar as resorption of the roots begins soon after formation of the root length has been completed. At this point in time, the form and shape of the root canals roughly correspond to the form and shape of the external anatomy of the teeth. Root resorption

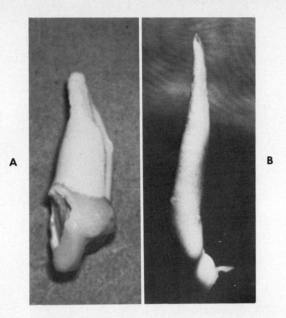

FIG. 22-15. Maxillary primary canine and silicone model of the root canal. **A,** Mesial surface. **B,** Model of the root canal.

and the deposition of additional dentin within the root canal system, however, significantly change the number, size, and shape of the root canals within the primary tooth.

It should be noted that most of the variations within the root canals of primary teeth are in the facial-lingual plane and that dental radiographs do not show this plane but show the mesial-distal plane. Therefore, when we view radiographs of the primary teeth, many of the variations present are not visible.

Primary anteriors (Figs. 22-14 and 22-15)

The form and shape of the root canals of the primary anterior teeth resemble the form and shape of the exteriors of the teeth. The permanent tooth bud lies lingual and apical to the primary anterior tooth. Due to the position of the permanent tooth bud, resorption of the primary incisors and canines is initiated on the lingual surface in the apical third of the roots (Fig. 22-14, A).

Maxillary incisors. The root canals of the primary maxillary central and lateral incisors are almost round but somewhat compressed. Normally these teeth have one canal without bifurcations. Apical ramifications or accessory canals and lateral canals are rare but do occur[210] (Fig. 22-14).

Mandibular incisors. The root canals of the primary mandibular central and lateral incisors are flattened on the mesial and distal surfaces and sometimes grooved, pointing to an eventual division into two canals. The presence of two canals is seen less than 10% of the time. Occasionally lateral or accessory canals are observed.[210]

Maxillary and mandibular canines. The root canals of the maxillary and mandibular canines correspond to the exterior root shape, a rounded triangular shape with the base toward the facial surface. Sometimes the lumen of the root canal is compressed in the mesial-distal direction. The

canines have the simplest root canal systems of all the primary teeth and offer few problems when being treated endodontically. Bifurcation of the canal does not normally occur. Lateral canals and accessory canals are rare[210] (Fig. 22-15).

Primary molars (Fig. 22-16)

The primary molars normally have the same number of roots and position of the roots as do the corresponding permanent molars. The maxillary molars have three roots, two facial and one palatal; the mandibular have two roots, mesial and distal. The roots of the primary molars are long and slender compared with crown length and width, and they diverge to allow for permanent tooth bud formation.

The deposition of secondary dentin in primary teeth has been reported.[13,76,82] When formation of the roots of the primary molars has just been completed, only one root canal is present in each of the roots. After root formation the basic morphologic pattern of the root canals may change, producing variation and alterations in the number and size of the root canals due to the deposition of secondary dentin. This deposition begins at about the time root resorption begins. Variations in form are more pronounced in teeth showing evidence of root resorption.[76]

The most variation in the morphology of the root canals is found in the mesial roots of both maxillary and mandibular primary molars. These variations originate in the apical region as a thinnning of the narrow isthmus between the facial and lingual extremities of the apical pulp canal. Subsequent deposition of secondary dentin may produce a complete separation of the root canal into two or more individual canals. Many fine connecting branches or lateral fibrils form a connecting network between the facial and lingual aspects of the root canals.

The variations found in the mesial roots of the primary molars are also found in the distal and lingual roots but to a lesser degree. Accessory canals, lateral canals, and apical ramifications of the pulp are common in primary molars—occurring in 10% to 20%.[76,210]

In the primary molars, resorption usually begins on the inner surfaces of the roots next to the interradicular septum. The effects of resorption on canal anatomy and root canal filling on the primary teeth is discussed in detail later in this chapter.

Maxillary first primary molar. The maxillary first primary molar has from two to four canals that roughly correspond to the exterior root form with much variation. The palatal root is often round and longer than the two facial roots. Bifurcation of the mesial-facial root into two canals occurs in approximately 75% of maxillary first primary molars.[76,210]

Fusion of the palatal and distal-facial roots occurs in approximately one third of the maxillary primary first molars. In most of these teeth, two separate canals are present with a very narrow isthmus connecting. Islands of dentin may exist between the canals, with many connecting branches and fibrils (Fig. 23-16, A).

Maxillary second primary molar. The maxillary primary molar has two to five canals roughly corresponding

A   B   C

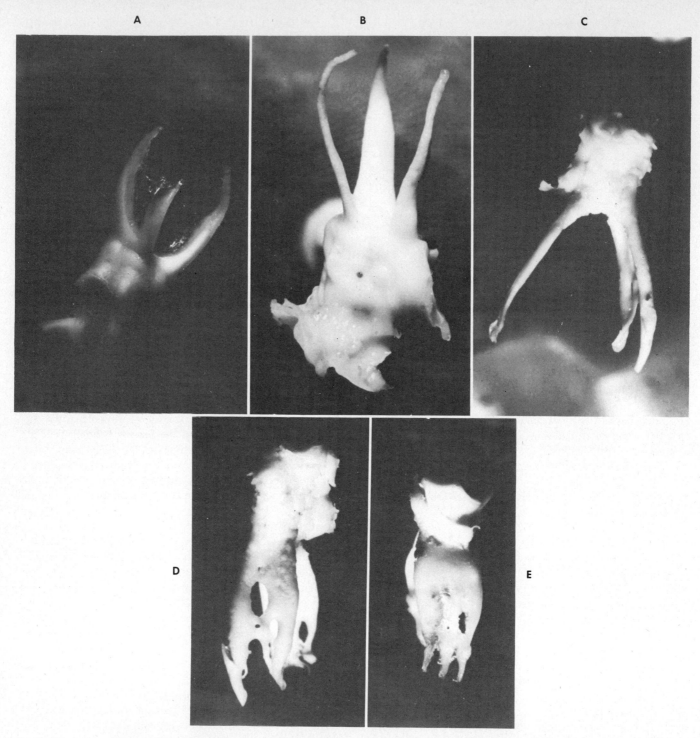

D   E

FIG. 22-16. Silicone models of the root canal systems of primary molars. **A,** Maxillary first molar. Note the fused distal and palatal roots. Note the thin fin connecting the roots. **B,** Maxillary second molar, facial surface. **C,** Mandibular first molar, facial view. **D,** Same tooth from the mesial surface. Note the connecting fibrils between the facial and lingual canals. **E,** Mandibular second molar, distal view. Three canals are present.

to the exterior root shape. The mesial-facial root usually bifurcates or contains two distinct canals. This occurs in approximately 85% to 95% of maxillary second primary molars[76,210] (Fig. 22-16, *B*).

Fusion of the palatal and distal-facial roots sometimes occurs. These fused roots may have a common canal, two distinct canals, or two canals with a narrow connecting isthmus of dentin islands between them and many connecting branches or fibrils.

Mandibular first primary molar. The mandibular first primary molar usually has three canals roughly corresponding to the external root anatomy but may have two

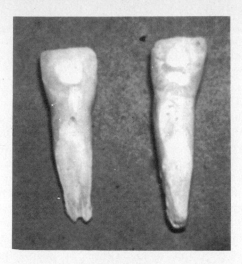

FIG. 22-17. These two primary mandibular incisors have lingual and apical resorption. Note that the left incisor has the apical foramen just beneath the cervical line whereas the right has its apical foramen at the apex of the root.

to four canals. It is reported that approximately 75% of the mesial roots contain two canals whereas only 25% of the distal roots contain more than one canal[76,210] (Fig. 22-16, C and D).

Mandibular second primary molar. The mandibular second primary molar may have two to five canals but usually has three. The mesial root has two canals approximately 85% of the time whereas the distal root contains more than one canal only 25% of the time[76,210] (Fig. 22-16, E).

ROLE OF RESORPTION ON CANAL ANATOMY AND APICAL FORAMINA

In the newly completed roots of the primary teeth, the apical foramina are located near the anatomic apices of the roots. After the deposition of additional dentin and cementum, there are multiple apical ramifications of the pulp as it exits the root just as in the mature permanent tooth.

Because of the position of the permanent tooth bud, physiologic resorption of the roots of the primary incisors and canines is initiated on the lingual surfaces in the apical third of the roots. In the primary molars, resorption usually begins on the inner surfaces of the roots near the interradicular septum.

As resorption progresses, the apical foramen may not correspond to the anatomic apex of the root but be coronal to it. Therefore radiographic establishment of the root canal length may be erroneous. Resorption may extend through the roots and into the root canals, creating additional communications with the periapical tissues other than through the apical foramina or lateral and accessory canals (Fig. 22-17).

Permanent tooth bud

The effects of primary endodontic therapy on the developing permanent tooth bud should be of paramount concern to the clinician.

Manipulation through the apex of the primary tooth is contraindicated since the permanent tooth bud lies immediately adjacent to the apex of the primary tooth. Overextension of root canal instruments and filling materials must be avoided. If signs of resorption are visible radiographically, it is advisable to establish the working length of endodontic instruments 2 or 3 mm short of the radiographic apex. The use of the radiographic paralleling technique with a long cone for maximum accuracy when measuring canal lengths is recommended.

Anesthesia is usually necessary for pulp extirpation and enlargement of the canals but is rarely needed when primary teeth are filled at a subsequent appointment. The response of the patient can sometimes be used as a guide to the approach to the apex and as a check to the length of the canal that was previously established radiographically. Hemorrhage after pulp removal indicates overextension into the periapical tissues.

The filling material utilized to obliterate the root canals on primary teeth must be absorbable so it can be absorbed as the tooth resorbs and so it offers no resistance or deflection to the eruption of the permanent tooth. *Materials such as gutta-percha or silver points are contraindicated as primary root canal fillers.*

Pulpectomy

Pulpectomy and root canal filling procedures on primary teeth have been the subject of much controversy. Fear of damage to developing permanent tooth buds and a belief that the tortuous root canals of primary teeth could not be adequately negotiated, cleaned, shaped, and filled have led to the needless sacrifice of many pulpally involved primary teeth.

Much has been written regarding potential damage to the developing permanent tooth bud from root canal fillings. While magnifying these dangers, many authors have advocated extraction of pulpally involved primary teeth and placement of space maintainers. However, there is no better space maintainer than the primary tooth. Also, nothing has been written concerning the damage of space maintainers on existing teeth in the mouth. Many space maintainers are placed and adequate follow-up is not achieved due to carelessness of either the patient or the clinician. Decalcification and rampant caries are frequent sequelae from loosened bands retained for extended periods of time. Poor oral hygiene around space maintainers contributes to increased decay and gingival problems. Deflection of erupting permanent teeth because of too long retention of space maintainers is sometimes encountered. Loss of space maintainers with resulting space loss can occur if the patient delays returning for treatment. These are a few of the problems that may be avoided by retention of the pulpally involved primary tooth when possible.

Economics has been advanced as an argument against endodontic treatment of primary teeth, but it is not a reasonable argument when compared to the cost of space maintainers including the required follow-up treatment. In fact, endodontic treatment is probably the less expensive of the two alternatives when the entire treatment sequence is considered.

Success of endodontic treatment on primary teeth is judged by the same criteria as are used on permanent teeth. The treated primary tooth must remain firmly attached in function without pain or infection. Radiographic signs of furcal and periapical infection should be resolved, with a normal periodontal attachment. The primary tooth should resorb normally and in no way interfere with the formation or eruption of the permanent tooth.

The usual means of studying root canal filling on primary teeth has been clinical and radiographic. There exists a great need for histologic study in this area.

Early reports of endodontic treatment on primary teeth usually involved devitalization with arsenic in vital teeth and the use of creosote, formocresol, or paraformaldehyde pastes in nonvital teeth. The canals were filled with a variety of materials usually consisting of zinc oxide and numerous other additions.[39,61,86,178]

The first well-documented scientific report of endodontic procedures on primary teeth was published by Rabinowitch in 1953.[145] A 13-year study of 1363 cases of partially or totally nonvital primary molars was reported. Only seven cases were failures. Most patients were followed for 1 or 2 years clinically and radiographically. Fillings of ZOE and silver nitrate were placed only after a negative culture was obtained for each tooth. Periapically involved teeth required an average of 7.7 visits to complete treatment; teeth with no periapical involvement required an average of 5.5 visits. Rabinowitch listed internal resorption and gross pathologic external resorption as contraindications to primary root canal fillings.

Another well-documented study reported a success rate of 95% in both vital and infected teeth using a filling material of thymol, cresol, iodoform, and zinc oxide.[1]

The reader is referred to Bennett[8] for a review of the techniques of partial and total pulpectomy.

In a well-controlled clinical study of primary root canals utilizing Oxpara paste as the filling material,[102] five preexisting factors were reported to lessen the prognosis: perforation of the furca, excessive external resorption of roots, internal resorption, extensive bone loss, and periodontal involvement of the furca. When teeth with these factors were eliminated, a clinical success rate of 96% was achieved. When all symptoms of residual infection were resolved before filling of the canals, the success rate improved. No radiographic evidence of damage to the permanent teeth was noted.

After reviewing the literature on root canal fillings on primary teeth, one is impressed with the lack of histologic material in this area. There exists a great need for further research on the subject.

Contraindications for primary root canal fillings

Except for the following situations, all primary teeth with pulpal involvement that has spread beyond the coronal pulp are candidates for root canal fillings whether vital or nonvital:

1. A nonrestorable tooth
2. Radiographically visible internal resorption in the roots

3. Teeth with mechanical or carious perforations of the floor of the pulp chamber
4. Excessive pathologic root resorption involving more than one third of the root
5. Excessive pathologic loss of bone support with loss of the normal periodontal attachment
6. The presence of a dentigerous or follicular cyst

Internal resorption usually begins just inside the root canals near the furcation area. Because of the thinness of the roots of the primary teeth, once internal resorption has become visible radiographically, there is invariably a perforation of the root by the resorption (Fig. 23-3). The short furcal surface area of the primary teeth leads to rapid communication between the inflammatory process and the oral cavity through the periodontal attachment. The end result is loss of the periodontal attachment of the tooth and ultimately further resorption and loss of the tooth.

Mechanical or carious perforations of the floor of the pulp chamber fail for the same reasons.

ACCESS OPENINGS FOR PULPECTOMY ON PRIMARY TEETH
Anterior teeth

Access openings for endodontic treatment on primary or permanent anterior teeth have traditionally been through the lingual surface. This continues to be the surface of choice except for the maxillary primary incisors. Due to problems associated with the discoloration of endodontically treated primary incisors, it has been recommended to use a facial approach followed by an acid-etch composite restoration to improve esthetics[110] (Fig. 22-18). Bleaching techniques which are quite successful in permanent teeth are unsuccessful in primary teeth.

Many maxillary primary incisors requiring pulpectomy have discoloration caused by the escape of hemosiderin pigments into the dentinal tubules following a previous traumatic injury. Subsequent to pulpectomy and root canal filling, most primary incisors discolor.

The anatomy of the maxillary primary incisors is such that access may successfully be made from the facial surface. The only variation to the opening is more extension to the incisal edge than with the normal lingual access in order to give as straight an approach as possible into the root canal.

The root canal is filled with ZOE (see below), then the ZOE is carefully removed to near the cervical line. A liner of Dycal or Life is placed over the ZOE to serve as a barrier between the composite resin and the root canal filling. The liner is extended over the darkly stained lingual dentin to serve as an opaquer. The access opening and entire facial surface are acid-etched and restored with composite resin (Fig. 22-18).

Posterior teeth

Access openings into the posterior primary root canals are essentially the same as those for the permanent teeth. (Chapter 6 contains a detailed description of access openings.) Important differences between the primary and permanent teeth are the length of the crowns, the bulbous

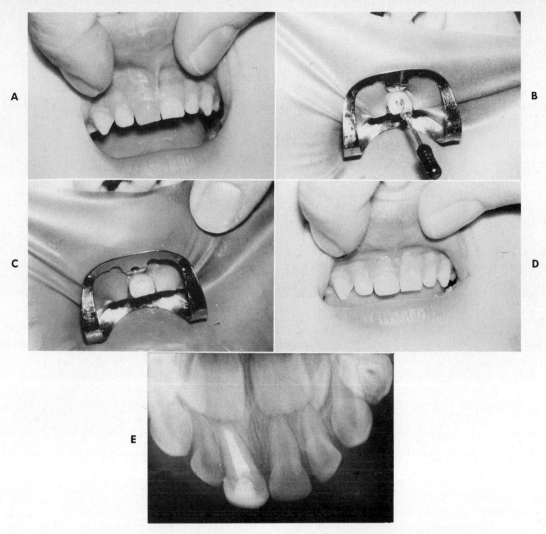

FIG. 22-18. Primary anterior root canal treatment using a facial approach. **A,** Discolored primary central incisor with a necrotic pulp. **B,** Tooth during root canal cleansing. **C,** Root canal filling with ZOE has been completed. The ZOE was removed to the cervical line and a Dycal liner was placed over the dentin. The tooth has been acid-etched. **D,** Composite resin has been bonded over the facial surface to achieve esthetics. **E,** Post-operative radiograph showing the completed procedures.

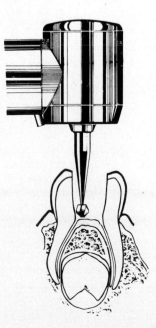

FIG. 22-19. Access opening in primary molar. A no. 4 round bur has been used to remove the roof of the pulp chamber and the dentin ledges over the canal orifices. Note the minimal length of the bur needed to penetrate to the pulpal floor. Caution must be exercised to avoid perforation of the pulpal floor. (From Goerig, A.C., and Camp, J.H.: Pediatr. Dent. **5**:33, 1983.)

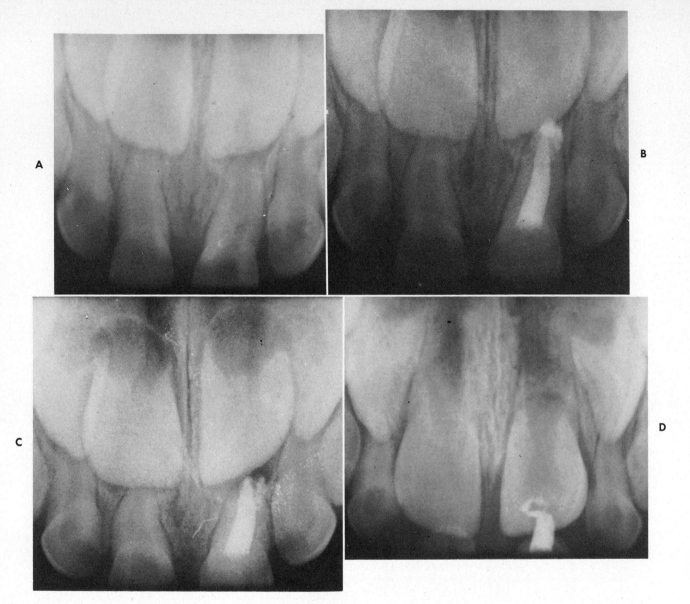

FIG. 22-20. Pulpectomy and root canal filling with ZOE in central incisor. **A,** Primary tooth with pulpal necrosis. **B,** Root canal filled, slight overfill. **C,** One year later. **D,** Three years later, ready for exfoliation. Note that the tooth resorbs slightly ahead of the absorbing ZOE.

shape of the crowns, and the very thin dentinal walls of the pulpal floors and roots. The depth necessary to penetrate into the pulpal chamber is quite less than that in the permanent teeth. Likewise, the distance from the occlusal surface to the pulpal floor of the pulp chamber is much less than in permanent teeth. In the primary molars, care must be taken not to grind on the pulpal floor since perforation is likely (Fig. 22-19).

When the roof of the pulp chamber is perforated and the pulp chamber identified, the entire roof should be removed with the bur. Since the crowns of the primary teeth are more bulbous, less extension toward the exterior of the tooth is necessary to uncover the openings of the root canals than in the permanent teeth.

Canal cleaning and shaping

Use of the rubber dam is essential in any endodontic procedure. As in permanent endodontic therapy, canal cleaning and shaping is one of the most important phases of primary endodontic therapy. The principles and techniques for permanent teeth described in detail in Chapter 7 are also advocated for primary teeth. The main objective of the chemical-mechanical preparation of the primary tooth is debridement of the canals. Although an apical taper to the canals is desirable, it is not necessary to have an exact shape to the canals as is necessary for gutta-percha fillings.

The importance of establishing a correct working length has been discussed (Chapter 7). To prevent overextension

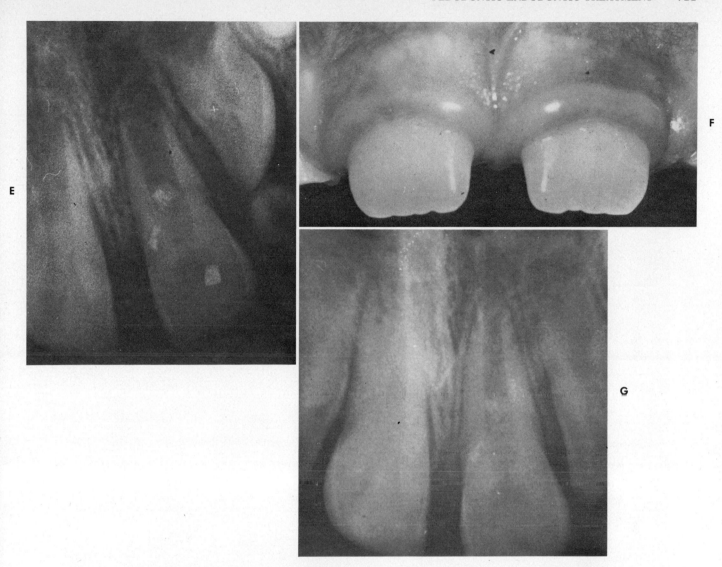

FIG. 22-20, cont'd. **E,** Permanent teeth, small traces of ZOE remaining in the soft tissues. These will be absorbed. **F,** The permanent central incisors newly erupted. Note that no defects are present on the crown even though there was a slight overfill of the primary root canal filling. **G,** Five years after pulpectomy and root canal filling. Note the normal apical closure and the almost total absorption of the ZOE remnants.

through the apical foramen, it is suggested that the working length be shortened 2 or 3 mm short of the radiographic root length, especially in teeth showing signs of apical root resorption.

When working length is established, the canal is cleaned and shaped as described in Chapter 7. The use of the Gates-Glidden drills is contraindicated; or if the drills are used, they must be confined simply to flaring the opening into the canals. Gates-Glidden drills should not be used in the canals because of the danger of perforation.

Instruments should be gently curved to help negotiate canals, as described in Chapter 7. Shaping of the canals proceeds in much the same manner as is done to receive a gutta-percha filling. Care must be taken not to perforate the thin roots during cleaning and shaping procedures. The

canals are enlarged several file sizes past the first file that fits snugly into the canal, with a minimum size of 30 to 35.

Since many of the pulpal ramifications cannot be reached mechanically, copious irrigation during cleaning and shaping must be maintained (Chapter 7). Debridement of the primary root canal is more often accomplished by chemical means than by mechanical means.[96] This statement should not be misinterpreted as a deemphasis of the importance of thorough debridement and disinfection of the canal. The use of sodium hypochlorite to digest organic debris and RC-Prep to produce effervescence must play an important part in removal of tissue from the inaccessible areas of the root canal system.

After canal debridement the canals are again copiously

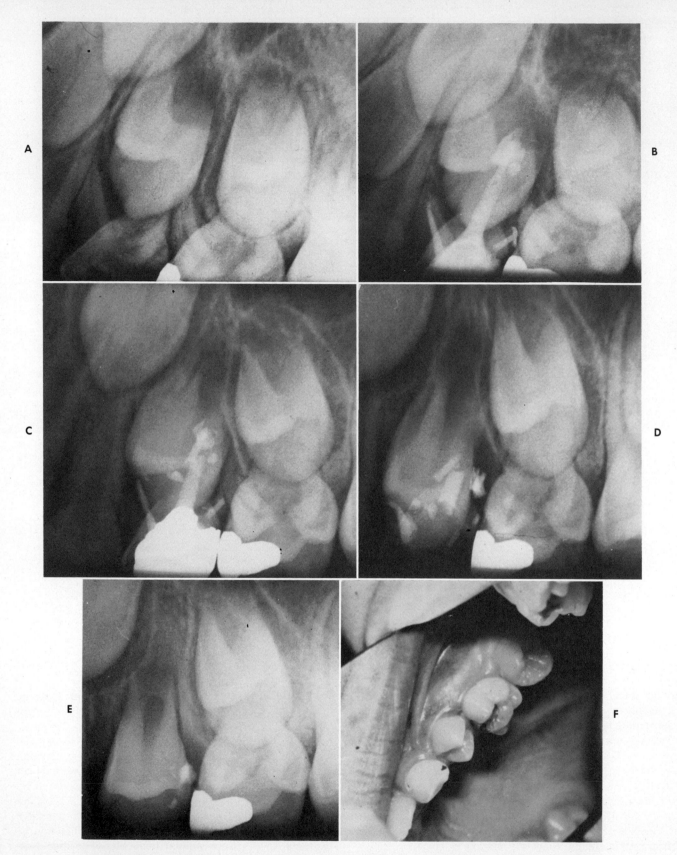

FIG. 22-21. Pulpectomy and root canal filling with ZOE in a maxillary posterior tooth. **A,** Carious exposure of a primary first molar. **B,** Root canals filled with ZOE. **C,** One year later. **D,** Two and one half years later. The tooth is ready to exfoliate. **E,** Erupted permanent premolar. Note the slight amount of ZOE retained in the soft tissue. The ZOE will undergo absorption. **F,** Note the permanent crown, free of defects.

flushed with sodium hypochlorite and are then dried with sterile paper points; a pellet of cotton is barely moistened with camphorated parachlorophenol and sealed into the pulp chamber with a temporary cement.

At a subsequent appointment the rubber dam is placed and the canals reentered. As long as the patient is free of all signs and symptoms of inflammation, the canals are again irrigated with sodium hypochlorite and dried preparatory to filling. If signs or symptoms of inflammation are present, the canals are recleaned and remedicated and the filling procedure delayed until a later time.

Filling of the primary root canals

As previously discussed, the filling material for primary root canals must be absorbable so it will absorb as the roots resorb and will not interfere with the eruption of the permanent tooth. *The filling material of choice is ZOE without a catalyst.* The lack of a catalyst is necessary to allow adequate working time for filling the canals. The use of gutta-percha or silver points as primary root canal fillers is contraindicated.

The filling of the primary tooth is usually performed without a local anesthetic. This is preferable if possible so the patient's response can be utilized to indicate approach to the apical foramen. It is, however, sometimes necessary to anesthetize the gingiva with a drop of anesthetic solution to place the rubber dam clamp without pain.

The ZOE is mixed to a thick consistency and is carried into the pulp chamber with a plastic instrument or on a Lentulo. The material may be packed into the canals with pluggers or the Lentulo. A cotton pellet held in cotton pliers and acting as a piston within the pulp chambers is quite effective in forcing the ZOE into the canals. The endodontic pressure syringe[10,64] is also effective for placing the ZOE in the root canals.

Regardless of the method utilized to fill the canals, care should be used to prevent extrusion of the material into the periapical tissues. The adequacy of the obturation is checked by radiographs (Figs. 22-20 and 22-21).

In the event a small amount of the ZOE is inadvertently forced through the apical foramen, it is left alone since the material is absorbable.

When the canals are satisfactorily obturated, a fast-set temporary cement is placed in the pulp chamber to seal over the ZOE canal filling. The tooth may then be restored permanently.

In the primary molars it is advisable to place stainless steel crown as the permanent restoration to prevent possible fracture of the tooth.

Follow-up after primary pulpectomy

As previously stated, the rate of success following primary pulpectomy is high. However, these teeth should be periodically recalled to check for success of the treatment and to intercept any problem associated with a failure. While resorbing normally without interference with the eruption of the permanent tooth, the primary tooth should remain asymptomatic, firm in the alveolus, and free of pathosis. If evidence of pathosis is detected, extraction and conventional space maintenance are recommended.

It has been pointed out[181] that pulpally treated primary teeth may occasionally present a problem of overretention. After normal physiologic resorption of the roots reaches the pulp chamber, the large amount of ZOE present may impair the absorption and lead to prolonged retention of the crown. Treatment usually consists of simply removing the crown and allowing the permanent tooth to complete its eruption.

APEXIFICATION

A thorough knowledge of normal root formation is necessary to help understand the processes involved in treating the pulpless permanent tooth with a wide-open immature apex.

Endodontic management of the pulpless permanent tooth with a wide-open blunderbuss apex has long presented a challenge to dentistry. Prior to the introduction of apical closure techniques, the usual approach to this problem was surgical. Although the surgical approach was successful, the mechanical and psychologic aspects offered many contraindications. In the pulpless tooth with an incompletely formed apex, the thin fragile dentinal walls made it difficult to achieve an apical seal. When a portion of the root was removed to obtain a seal, the crown/root ratio was poor. Since this situation was usually present in the child patient, a less traumatic approach was desirable.

Many techniques have been advocated to manage the pulpless permanent tooth with an incompletely developed apex. The canals are cleaned and filled with a temporary paste to stimulate the formation of calcified tissue at the apex. The temporary paste is later removed after radiographic evidence of apical closure has been obtained and a permanent filling of gutta-percha is placed in the canal. The term apexification is used to describe this procedure.[182]

Many materials have been reported to successfully stimulate apexification. The use of calcium hydroxide for apexification in the pulpless tooth was first reported by Kaiser in 1964.[87] The technique was popularized by the work of Frank.[49] Since that time *Ca(OH)$_2$ alone or in combination with other drugs has become the most widely accepted material to promote apexification.*

The calcium hydroxide powder has been mixed with camphorated parachlorophenol (CMCP), metacresyl acetate, cresanol (a mixture of CMCP and metacresyl acetate), physiologic saline, Ringer's solution, distilled water, and anesthetic solution. Although some of these materials appear to enhance the action of the Ca(OH)$_2$ better than others, all have been reported to stimulate apexification. Most reports in the American literature have advocated mixing the Ca(OH)$_2$ with CMCP or Cresanol, whereas reports from other parts of the world show the same success using distilled water or physiologic saline as the vehicle with which the Ca(OH)$_2$ is mixed.*

Materials like ZnO pastes,[23] antibiotic pastes,[6,73] Walkoff's paste,[18] and Diaket[51] have also been reported to promote apexification successfully. Similar results have been

---

*References 21,25,38,49,66,87,115,127,182,183.

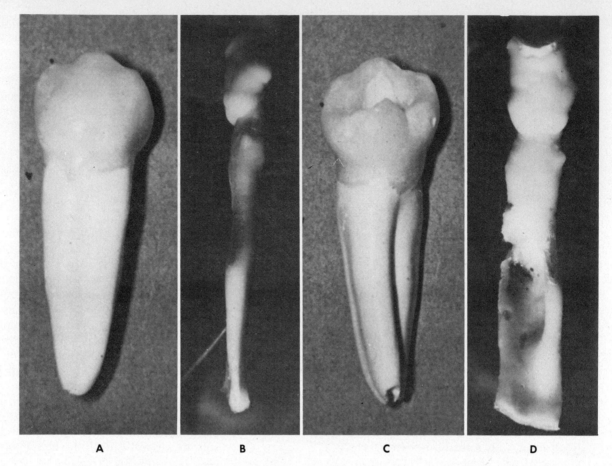

FIG. 22-22. Extracted mandibular premolar and silicone model of the root system. **A,** Facial view. **B,** Model from the facial surface. Note that the root canal diverges apically, which would correspond to a radiograph view of the tooth in the mouth. **C,** Lingual view. **D,** Model from the proximal view, apically divergent canal. With further development the root canal sytem will divide into two canals.

achieved after bleeding into the canal was stimulated by laceration of granulation tissue outside the canal.[134]

Attempts at apexification with calcium chloride[83] and barium hydroxide[172] have proved unsuccessful. However, the addition of barium sulfate to calcium hydroxide to enhance radiopacity has been shown to produce apexification. The recommended ratio of barium sulfate in 1 part added to 8 parts calcium hydroxide.[200,201] Diatrizoate (organic iodine) has also been effectively utilized as a radiopaquer.[170] An endodontist's report[200] on apexification provides a better review of this literature.

In the teeth of humans and primates, tricalcium phosphate promotes apexification similar to that found with $Ca(OH)_2$.[95,152] The material has also been packed into the apical 2 mm of the canal to act as barrier against which gutta-percha is condensed.[24] The treatment was achieved in one appointment. Using radiographic assessment, the authors reported successful apexification comparable to that achieved in multiple appointments with $Ca(OH)_2$.[24]

Collagen-calcium phosphate gel has been reported to produce apexification faster than $Ca(OH)_2$ in animals and humans. Various forms of hard and soft tissues were shown revitalizing pulpless root canals within 12 weeks.

Formation of cementum, bone, and reparative dentin was noted within the connective tissue ingrowths, a normal periodontal ligament and the absence of ankylosis were also noted. The gel appears to function as an absorbable matrix, supporting hard tissue growth into the debrided root canals.[129,130,131] In contrast to this, however, another investigator[22] showed that collagen-calcium phosphate gel inhibits the reparative process, with extensive destruction of periapical tissues and no evidence of apexification. Despite the fact that this area of research shows promise for the future, at present it must be considered experimental.

Although apexification will occur with many materials, it has been reported even without the presence of canal filling material after removal of the necrotic pulp tissue.[43] The most important factors in achieving apexification seem to be thorough debridement of the root canal (to remove all necrotic pulp tissue) and sealing of the tooth (to prevent the ingress of bacteria and substrate). It has been noted that apexification will not occur when the apex of the tooth penetrates the cortical plate. To be successful, the apex must be completely within the confines of the cortical plates.[201]

Although highly successful, apexification should be the

treatment of last resort in the tooth with an incompletely formed root. Attention should be focused on the maintenance of vitality within these teeth so that as much root length and dentin formation within the root as possible can occur. Indirect pulp therapy and vital pulp capping and pulpotomy techniques have proved to be successful aided by the tremendous blood supply present with the open apex. These procedures should be the treatment if choice if the possibility of success exists with any of them. When the tooth with an incompletely formed apex becomes pulpless or periapical disease has developed, apexification is the preferred treatment.

Determination of the extent of apical closure is many times difficult to ascertain. Radiographic interpretation of apical closure is often misleading. It must always be remembered that the dental radiograph is a two-dimensional picture of a three-dimensional object. Under normal conditions the dental radiograph shows the mesial-distal plane of the tooth rather than the facial-lingual plane. The facial-lingual aspect of the root canal, however, is usually the last to become convergent apically as the root develops. Therefore it is possible to have a dental radiograph showing an apically convergent root canal while in the facial-lingual plane the root canal is divergent (Fig. 22-22).

In teeth with vital tissue remaining in the root canal, techniques to maintain the vitality, rather than pulpectomy, should be utilized until complete root formation has occurred.

Technique

Diagnosis of pulpal necrosis in the tooth with an incompletely formed apex is sometimes difficult unless a frank exposure of the pulp chamber exists.

The usual cause of endodontic involvement in a tooth with an incompletely developed root is trauma. A detailed history of any injury is of prime importance from both a diagnostic and a treatment point of view as well as documentation for insurance and dental-legal reasons.

Radiographic diagnosis of disease is complicated in these teeth because of the normal radiolucency occurring at the apex as the root matures. Comparison of root formation with that in contralateral teeth should always be considered.

The electric pulp tester usually will not provide meaningful data in teeth with incompletely formed roots. Thermal tests are more reliable for ascertaining vitality but may be complicated by the reliability of the response in the young child.

The presence of acute or chronic pain, percussion sensitivity, mobility, and any discoloration of the crown should be considered in the diagnosis.

In the tooth without a pulp exposure—if any doubt persists after all the foregoing tests have been completed—take a watch-and-wait approach before entering the tooth endodontically to be certain that conclusive evidence of pulpal necrosis exists. If dentin exposure is present, the tooth must be restored in such a manner as to prevent any further pulpal irritation.

In the apexification technique the canal is cleaned and sanitized in the routine endodontic manner. (See Chapter 7 for an in-depth discussion of this technique.) As with any endodontic procedure, the use of the rubber dam is mandatory.

The access opening is made as usual but may require some extension, especially in the anterior teeth, to accomodate the larger-sized instruments necessary to clean the root canals.

The length of the canal is established radiographically and the canal is cleaned as thoroughly as possible. Frequent irrigation with sodium hypochlorite helps remove debris from the canal. Since the coronal half of the root canal is of smaller diameter than the apical half, root canal instruments that are smaller than the canal space must be utilized. Thus, while mechanically cleaning and shaping the canal, lean the instruments toward each surface of the tooth to contact all surfaces of the root because the canal diverges apically.

After thorough debridement the canal is dried and just *barely* medicated with camphorated parachlorophenol (CMCP) or some other suitable intracanal medicaments. It is then sealed with a temporary cement.

If symptoms persist or any signs of infection are present at a subsequent appointment, or if the canal cannot be dried, the debridement phase is repeated.

When the tooth is free of signs and symptoms of infection, the canal is dried and filled with a stiff mix of $Ca(OH)_2$ and CMCP. The filling procedure is usually performed without the use of local anesthetic. This is preferable if possible so the patient's response can be utilized to indicate approach to the apical foramen.

The material should be spatulated as little as possible since spatulation decreases the working time and may cause the material to set into a hard mass before the filling procedure is completed. If this happens, the canal may contain voids and should be recleaned and the filling procedure repeated.

The paste may be carried into the canal with an amalgam carrier, Lentulo spiral, disposable syringe, or endodontic pressure syringe. Pluggers are helpful for packing the material to the apex. The addition of some dry $Ca(OH)_2$ powder within the canal by means of an amalgam carrier will aid in condensing the paste of the apex. The canal should ideally be completely filled with the paste but should not be overfilled. The response of the patient is used as a guide in approaching the apex; however, because of differences in patient response, this method is not wholly reliable. Radiographic checks of the depth of the filling are essential to verify an adequate filling. The addition of small amounts of barium sulfate to the paste aids in radiographic interpretation without altering the response of the material.

It has been reported that successful apexification can occur with an overfill of material; in fact, it has been reported that an overfill is preferable to an underfill.[21] In the event of an overfill, the material (being absorbable) is not removed from the apical tissues. The presence of an overfill rarely causes postoperative pain.

After the canal is filled, the access opening must be sealed with a permanent filling material. If the outer seal is defective, the calcium hydroxide paste is lost and recon-

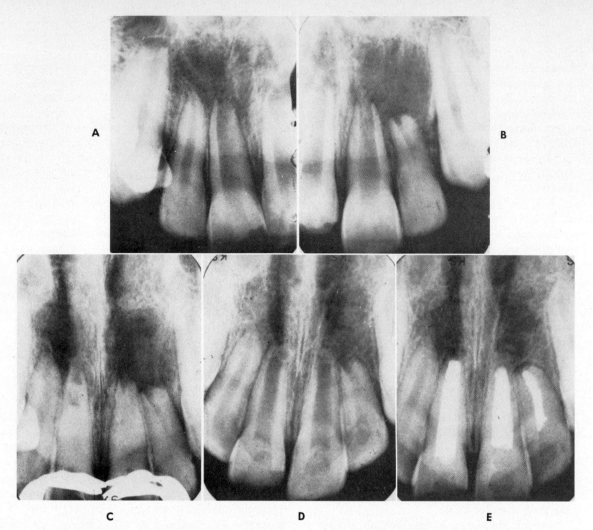

FIG. 22-23. Apexification in three permanent incisors, using calcium hydroxide—CMCP filling material. **A** and **B,** Open apices of the three incisors with periapical pathosis. Note the calcification that has occurred in the lateral incisor before pulpal necrosis. **C,** Calcium hydroxide—CMCP filling placed in two teeth. Note the void in the left incisor requiring further filling. **D,** Radiographic appearance of apexification a year later. **E,** Permanent root canal filling of gutta-percha after apexification.

tamination of the canal will result. For this reason temporary-type cements should never be used to seal the tooth after the filling procedure. Composite resin or silicate cement is recommended for anterior teeth and amalgam for posterior teeth.

Periodic recall

The usual time required for apexification is 6 to 24 months. During this time the patient is recalled at 3-month intervals for monitoring of the tooth.

If any signs or symptoms of reinfection or pathology occur during this phase of treatment, the canal is recleaned and refilled with the $Ca(OH)_2$ paste. The patient is recalled until radiographic evidence of apexification has become apparent. Then the tooth is reentered and clinical verification of apexification is made by the failure of a small instrument to penetrate through the apex after removal of the

$Ca(OH)_2$ paste. If apexification is incomplete, the canal is repacked with the $Ca(OH)_2$ paste and the periodic recall continued (Fig. 22-23).

Histologic of apexification

The calcified material that forms over the apical foramen has been histologically identified as an osteoid (bone-like) or cementoid (cementum-like) material by investigators who have done apexification following periapical involvement of the treated teeth.* The formation of osteodentin after the placement of calcium hydroxide paste immediately on conclusion of a vital pulpectomy has also been reported.[38]

Histologic studies consistently report the absence of

---

*References 21,66,95,129,152,183,200.

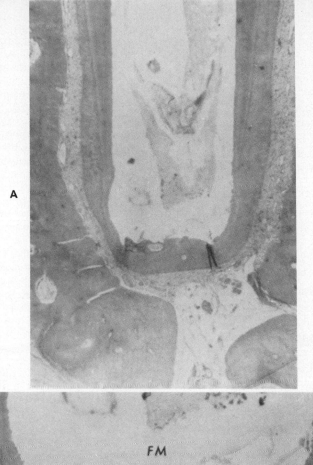

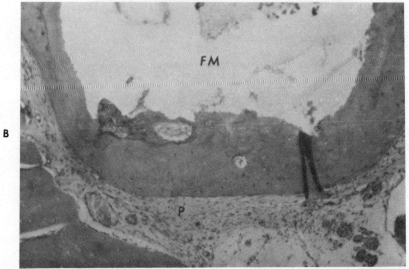

FIG. 22-24. Histologic sections of a dog's mouth after apexification. **A,** Cementum-like calcified tissue is closing the wide open apical foramen. Note the presence of debris within the canal due to inadequate cleaning of the canal before filling. **B,** Higher magnification showing cellular detail. The periodontal ligament, *P,* is free of inflammation. The filling material, *FM,* calcium hydroxide—CMCP, was lost during processing. Note the presence of tissue communication through the calcified tissue. (H & E stain.)

Hertwig's epithelial root sheath. Normal root formation usually does not occur following apexification. Instead, there appears to be a differentiation of adjacent connective tissue cells into specialized cells; there is also deposition of calcified tissue adjacent to the filling material. The calcified material is continuous with the lateral root surfaces. The closure of the apex may be partial or complete but

consistently has minute communications with the periapical tissues (Fig. 22-24). For this reason apexification must always be followed by filling of the canal with a permanent root canal filling of gutta-percha.

Various types of apical closure have been reported in clinical studies of apexification. In view of the histologic evidence of subsequent studies, it would appear that these types of apical closure simply relate to the level to which the filling material was placed within or beyond the apical foramen.

Many of the failures of apexification have been shown histologically to arise from the difficulty of adequately cleaning and sanitizing the wide-open canals. The tooth with an apically divergent root canal is much more difficult to clean thoroughly than is the mature tooth, which becomes increasingly smaller as the apex is approached.

Although the formation of calcified tissue was noted in the presence of mild inflammation, the results were consistently better in specimens free of inflammation. It is recommended therefore that the cleaning and filling procedure be done at separate appointments rather than in a single appointment. Likewise, ideally all signs and symptoms of infection and inflammation should be absent before the $Ca(OH)_2$ paste is placed.

Obturation with gutta-percha

After verification of successful apexification, the canal is thoroughly cleaned, care being taken not to damage the calcific barrier at the apex. The canal is then obturated with gutta-percha in the usual manner. Due to the large size of the canal, it may be necessary to prepare a customized gutta-percha point as described in Chapter 8. While the apexification procedure is highly successful, the root of such a tooth is weak and prone to fracture with subsequent injuries. Therefore apexification should be a treatment of last resort after all attempts at vital therapy have failed.

REFERENCES

1. Andrew, P.: The treatment of infected pulps in deciduous teeth, Br. Dent. J. **98**:122, 1955.
2. Aponte, A.J., Hartsook, J.T., and Crowley, M.C.: Indirect pulp capping success verified, J. Dent. Child. **33**:164, 1966.
3. Armstrong, R.L., et al.: Comparison of Dycal and formocresol pulpotomies in young permanent teeth in monkeys, Oral Surg. **48**:160, 1979.
4. Attala, M.N., and Noujaim, A.A.: Role of calcium hydroxide in the formation of reparative dentin, J. Can. Dent. Assoc. **35**:267, 1969.
5. Baker, G.R., and Mitchell, D.F.: Topical antibiotic treatment of infected dental pulps of monkeys, J. Dent. Res. **48**:351, 1969.
6. Ball, J.S.: Apical root formation in a non-vital immature permanent incisor, Br. Dent. J. **116**:166,1964.
7. Beaver, H.A., Kopel, H.M., and Sabes, W.R.: The effect of zinc oxide-eugenol cement on a formocresolized pulp, J. Dent. Child. **33**:381, 1966.
8. Bennett, C.G.: Pulpal management of deciduous teeth, Pract. Dent. Monogr., p. 1, May-June, 1965.
9. Berk, H., and Krakow, A.A.: A comparison of the management of pulpal pathosis in deciduous and permanent teeth, Oral Surg. **34**:944, 1972.
10. Berk, H., and Krakow, A.A.: Endodontic treatment in primary teeth. In Goldman, H.M., et. al., editors: Current therapy in dentistry, Vol. 5, St. Louis, 1974, The C.V. Mosby Co.
11. Berk, H., and Stanley, H.R.: Pulp healing following capping in human sound and carious teeth, J. Dent. Res. **37**:66, 1958.
12. Berkman, M., et al.: Pulpal response to isobutyl cyanoacrylate in human teeth, J. Am. Dent. Assoc. **83**:140, 1971.
13. Bevelander, G., and Benzer, D.: Morphology and incidence in secondary dentin in human teeth, J. Am. Dent. Assoc. **30**:1079, 1943.
14. Bhasker, S.N., et al: Pulp capping with isobutyl cyanoacrylate, J. Am. Dent. Assoc. **79**:640, 1969.
15. Bhaskar, S., Cutright, D.E., and Van Osdel, V.: Tissue response to cortisone-containing and cortisone-free calcium hydroxide, J. Dent. Child. **36**:1, 1969.
16. Bimstein, E., and Shoshan, S.: Enhanced healing of tooth-pulp wounds in the dog by enriched collagen solution as a capping agent, Arch. Oral Biol. **26**:97, 1981.
17. Block, R.M., et al.: Cell-mediated immune response to dog pulp tissue altered by formocresol within the root canal, J. Endod. **3**:424, 1977.
18. Bouchon, F.: Apex formation following treatment of necrotized immature permanent incisor, J. Dent. Child. **33**:378, 1966.
19. Brian, J.D., et al.: Reaction of rat connective tissue to unfixed and formaldehyde-fixed autogenous implants enclosed in tubes, J. Endod. **6**:628, 1980.
20. Brosch, J.W.: Capping pulps with a compound of calcium phosphate, neomycin and hydrocortisone, J. Dent. Child. **32**:42, 1965.
21. Camp, J.H.: Continued apical development of pulpless permanent teeth following endodontic therapy (thesis), Indiana University School of Dentistry, 1968.
22. Citrome, G.P., Kaminski, E.J., and Heuer, M.A.: A comparative study of tooth apexification in the dog, J. Endod. **5**:290, 1979.
23. Cooke, C., and Rowbotham, T.C.: Root canal therapy in nonvital teeth with open apices, Br. Dent. J. **108**:147, 1960.
24. Coviello, J., and Brilliant, J.D.: A preliminary clinical study of the use of tricalcium phosphate as an apical barrier, J. Endod. **5**:6, 1979.
25. Cvek, M.: Treatment of non-vital permanent incisors with calcium hydroxide, Odontol. Rev. **23**:27, 1972.
26. Cvek, M.: A clinical report on partial pulpotomy and capping with calcium hydroxide in permanent incisors with complicated crown fractures, J. Endod. **4**:232, 1978.
27. Cvek, M.: Endodontic treatment of traumatized teeth. In Andreasen, J.O.: Traumatic injuries of the teeth, ed. 2, Philadelphia, 1981, W.B. Saunders Co.
28. Cvek, M., et al.: Pulp reactions to exposure after experimental crown fracture or grinding in adult monkey, J. Endod. **8**:391, 1982.
29. Cvek, M., and Lundberg, M.: Histological appearance of pulps after exposure by a crown fracture, partial pulpotomy, and clinical diagnosis of healing, J. Endod. **9**:8, 1983.
30. Dannenberg, J.L.: Pedodontic-endodontics, Dent. Clin. North Am. **18**:367, 1974.
31. Davis, M.J., Myers, R., and Switkes, M.D.: Glutaraldehyde: an alternative to formoscresol for vital pulp therapy, J. Dent. Child. **49**:176, 1982.
32. Delaney, J.M., and Seyer, A.E.: Hard set calcium hydroxide as a sole base in pulp protection, J. Dent. Child. **33**:13, 1966.
33. Dietz, D.: A histological study of the effects of formocresol on normal primary pulpal tissue (thesis), School of Dentistry, University of Washington, 1961.
34. Dilley, G.J., and Courts, F.J.: Immunological response to four pulpal medicaments, Pediatr. Dent. **3**:179, 1981.
35. Dimaggio, J.J., and Hawes, R.R.: Evaluation of direct and indirect pulp capping (abstract), J. Dent. Res. **40**:24, 1962.
36. Dimaggio, J.J., and Hawes, R.R.: Continued evaluation of direct and indirect pulp capping (abstract), J. Dent. Res. **41**:38, 1963.
37. Doyle, W.A., McDonald, R.E., and Mitchell, D.F.: Formocresol versus calcium hydroxide in pulpotomy, J. Dent. Child. **29**:86, 1962.
38. Dylewski, J.J.: Apical closure of non-vital teeth, Oral Surg. **32**:82, 1971.
39. Easlick, K.A.: Operative procedures in management of deciduous molars, Int. J. Orthod. **20**:585, 1934.
40. Ehrenreich, D.W.: A comparison of the effects of zinc oxide and eugenol and calcium hydroxide on carious dentin in human primary molars, J. Dent. Child. **35**:451, 1968.
41. El-Kafrawy, A.H., et al.: Pulp reaction to a polycarboxylate cement in monkeys, J. Dent. Res. **53**:15, 1974.
42. Emmerson, C., et al.: Pulpal changes following formocresol applications on rat molars and human primary teeth, J. South. Calif. Dent. Assoc. **27**:309, 1959.

43. England, M.C., and Best, E.: Noninduced apical closure in immature roots of dogs' teeth, J. Endod. **3:**411, 1977.

44. Fairbourn, D.R., Charbeneau, G.T., and Loesche, W.J.: Effect of improved Dycal and I.R.M. on bacteria in deep carious lesions, J. Am. Dent. Assoc. **100:**547, 1980.

45. Feltman, E.M.: A comparison of the formocresol pulpotomy techniques and dycal pulpotomy technique in young permanent teeth (thesis), School of Dentistry, Indiana University, 1972.

46. Finn, S.B.: Morphology of the primary teeth. In Finn, S.B., et al., editors: Clinical pedodontics, ed. 3, Philadelphia, 1967, W.B. Saunders Co.

47. Fiore-Donno, G., and Baume, L.J.: Effects of capping compounds containing corticosteroids on the human dental pulp, Helv. Odontol. Acta **6:**23, 1962.

48. Foster, H.R.: The pulpless deciduous teeth, J. Am. Dent. Assoc. **23:**2057, 1936.

49. Frank, A. L.: Therapy for the divergent pulpless tooth by continued apical formation, J. Am. Dent. Assoc. **72:**87, 1966.

50. Frankl, S.N.: Pulp therapy in pedodontics, Oral Surg. **34:**293, 1972.

51. Friend, L.A.: The root treatment of teeth with open apices, Proc. R. Soc. Med. **59:**1035, 1966.

52. Fuks, A.B., Bielak, S., and Chosak, A.: Clinical and radiographic assessment of direct pulp capping and pulpotomy in young permanent teeth, Pediatr. Dent. **4:**240, 1982.

53. Fuks, A.B., and Bimstein, E.C.: Clinical evaluation of diluted formocresol pulpotomies in primary teeth of school children, Pediatr. Dent. **3:**321, 1981.

54. Fuks, A.B., Bimstein, E., and Bruchim, A.: Radiographic and histologic evaluation of the effect of two concentrations of formocresol on pulpotomized primary and young permanent teeth in monkeys, Pediatr. Dent. **5:**9, 1983.

55. Fuks, A.B., et al.: Enriched collagen solution as a pulp dressing in pulpotomized teeth in monkeys, Pediatr. Dent. **6:**243, 1984.

56. Fulton, R., and Ranly, D.M.: An autoradiographic study of formocresol pulpotomies in rat molars using ^{3}H-formaldehyde, J. Endod. **5:**71, 1979.

57. Fusayama, T., Okuse, K., and Hosoda, H.: Relationship between hardness, discoloration and microbial invasion in carious dentin, J. Dent. Res. **45:**1033, 1966.

58. García-Godoy, F., Novakovic, D.P., and Carvajal, I.N.: Pulpal response to different application times of formocresol, J. Pedodont. **6:**176, 1982.

59. Gardner, D.E., Mitchell, D.F., and McDonald, R.E.: Treatment of pulps of monkeys with Vanocomycin and calcium hydroxide J. Dent. Res. **50:**1273, 1971.

60. Gazi, H.A., Nayak, R.G., and Bhat, K.S.: Tissue-irritation potential of dilute formocresol, Oral Surg. **51:**74, 1981.

61. Gerlach, E.: Root canal therapeutics in deciduous teeth, Dent. Surv. **8:**68, 1932.

62. Glass, R.L., and Zander, H.A.: Pulp healing, J. Dent. Res. **28:**97, 1949.

63. Granath, L.E., and Hagman, G.: Experimental pulpotomy in human bicuspids with reference to cutting technique, Acta Odontol. Scand. **29:**155, 1971.

64. Greenberg, M.: Filling root canals of deciduous teeth by an injection technique, Dent. Dig. **67:**574, 1964.

65. Guthrie, T.J., McDonald, R.E., and Mitchell, D.F.: Dental hemogram, J. Dent. Res. **44:**678, 1965.

66. Ham, J.W., Patterson, S.S., and Mitchell, D.F.: Induced apical closure of immature pulpless teeth in monkeys, Oral Surg. **33:**438, 1972.

67. Harris, C.A.: The principles and practice of dental surgery, ed. 4, Philadelphia, 1850, Lindsay & Blakiston.

68. Hawes, R.R., Dimaggio, J.J., and Saygeh, F.: Evaluation of direct and indirect pulp capping (abstract). J. Dent. Res. **43:**808, 1964.

69. Hayashi, Y.: Ultrastructure of initial calcification in wound healing following pulpotomy, J. Oral Pathol. **11:**174, 1982.

70. Heide, S.: Pulp reactions to exposure for 4, 24 and 168 hours, J. Dent. Res. **59:**1910, 1980.

71. Held-Wydler, E.: "Natural" (indirect) pulp capping, J. Dent. Child. **31:**107, 1964.

72. Heller, A.L., et al.: Direct pulp capping of permanent teeth in primates using a resorbable form of tricalcium phosphate ceramic, J. Endod. **1:**95, 1975.

73. Herbert, W.E.: Three cases of disturbance of calcification of a tooth and infection of the dental pulp following trauma, Dent. Pract. **9:**176, 1961.

74. Hermann, B.W.: Dentinobliteration der Wurzelkanale nach der Behandlung mit Kalzium, Zahnaertzl. Rund. **39:**888, 1930.

75. Heys, D.R., et al.: Histological considerations of direct pulp capping agents, J. Dent. Res. **60:**1371, 1981.

76. Hibbard, E.D., and Ireland, R.L.: Morphology of the root canals of the primary molar teeth, J. Dent. Child. **24:**250, 1957.

77. Hirschfeld, Z., Sela, J., and Ulmansky, M.: Hydrex and its effect on the pulp, Oral Surg. **34:**364, 1972.

78. Holland, R., et al.: Histochemical analysis of the dogs' dental pulp after pulp capping with calcium, barium and strontium hydroxides, J. Endod. **8:**444, 1982.

79. Hørsted, P., El Attar, K., and Langeland, K.: Capping of monkey pulps with Dycal and a Ca-eugenol cement, Oral Surg. **52:**531, 1981.

80. Hume, W.R., and Testa Kenney, A.E.: Release of ^{3}H-triamcinolone from Ledermix, J. Endod. **7:**509, 1981.

81. Inglis, O.E.: Can recalcification of dentin occur? A proposition, Pacific Dent. Gaz. **8:**763, 1900.

82. Ireland, R.L.: Secondary dentin formation in deciduous teeth, J. Am. Dent. Assoc. **28:**1626, 1941.

83. Javelet, J., Torabinejad, M., and Bakland, L.K.: Comparison of two pH levels for the induction of apical barrier in immature teeth of monkeys, J. Endod. **11:**375, 1985.

84. Jerrell, R.G., Courts, F.J., and Stanley, H.R.: A comparison of two calcium hydroxide agents in direct pulp capping of primary teeth, J. Dent. Child. **51:**34, 1984.

85. Johansson, B.I., Persson, I., and Mancra, P.: Histologic effects of collagen and chondroitin sulfate as capping agents in amputated rat molar pulps, Arch. Oral Biol. **8:**503, 1963.

86. Jordon, M.E.: Operative dentistry for children. New York, 1925, Dental Items of Interest Publishing Co.

87. Kaiser, J.H.: Management of wide-open canals with calcium hydroxide. Presentaion at the American Association of Endodontics, Washington, D.C., April 17, 1964. Cited by Steiner, J.C., Dow, P.R., and Cathey, G.M.: Inducing root end closure of non-vital permanent teeth, J. Dent. Child. **35:**47, 1968.

88. Kakehashi, S., Stanley, H.R., and Fitzgerald, R.T.: The effects of surgical exposures of dental pulps in germ-free and conventional laboratory rats, Oral Surg. **20:**340, 1965.

89. Kalnins, V., and Frisbie, H.E.: Effect of dentin fragments on the healing of the exposed pulp, Arch. Oral Biol. **2:**96, 1960.

90. Kelley, M.A., Bugg, J.L., and Skjonsby, H.S.: Histologic evaluation of formocresol and oxpara pulpotomies in rhesus monkeys, J. Am. Dent. Assoc. **86:**123, 1973.

91. Kennedy, D.B., et al.: Formocresol pulpotomy in teeth of dogs with induced pulpal and periapical pathosis, J. Dent. Child. **40:**44, 1973.

92. Kerkhove, B.C., et al.: A clinical and television densitometric evaluation of the indirect pulp capping technique, J. Dent. Child. **34:**192, 1967.

93. King, J.B., Crawford, J.J., and Lindahl, R.L.: Indirect pulp capping: a bacteriologic study of deep carious dentine in human teeth, Oral Surg. **20:**663, 1965.

94. Klein, H., et al.: Partial pulpotomy following complicated crown fracture in permanent incisors: a clinical and radiographic study, J. Pedodont. **9:**142, 1985.

95. Koenigs, J.F., et al.: Induced apical closure of permanent teeth in adult primates using a resorbable form of tricalcium phosphate ceramic, J. Endod. **1:**102, 1975.

96. Kopel, H.M.: Pediatric endodontics. In Ingle, J.I., and Beveridge, E.E., editors: Endodontics, ed. 2, Philadelphia, 1976, Lea & Febiger.

97. Kopel, H.M., et al.: The effects of glutaraldehyde on primary pulp tissue following coronal amputation: an in vivo histologic study, J. Dent. Child. **47**:425, 1980.

98. Kozlov, M., and Massler, M.: Histologic effects of various drugs on amputated pulps of rat molars, Oral Surg. **13**:455, 1960.

99. Krakow, A.A., Berk, H., and Grøn, P.: Therapeutic induction of root formation in the incompletely formed tooth with a vital pulp, Oral Surg. **43**:755, 1977.

100. Langeland, K.: Management of the inflamed pulp associated with deep carious lesion, J. Endod. **7**:169, 1981.

101. Langeland, K., et al.: Human pulp changes of iatrogenic origin, Oral Surg. **32**:943, 1971.

102. Laurence, R.P.: A method of root canal therapy for primary teeth (thesis), School of Dentistry, Emory University, 1966.

103. Law, D.B., and Lewis, T.M.: The effect of calcium hydroxide on deep carious lesions, Oral Surg. **14**:1130, 1961.

104. Law, D.B., Lewis, T.M., and Davis, J.M.: Pulp therapy. In Law, D.B., et al., editors: An atlas of pedodontics, Philadelphia, 1969, W.B. Saunders Co.

105. Lekka, M., Hume, W.R., and Wolinsky, L.E.: Comparison between formaldehyde and glutaraldehyde diffusion through the root tissues of pulpotomy-treated teeth, J. Pedod. **8**:185, 1984.

106. Lewis, T.M., and Law, D.B.: Pulpal treatment of primary teeth. In Finn, S.B., et al., editors: Clinical pedodontics, ed. 3, Philadelphia, 1967, W.B. Saunders Co.

107. Longwill, D.G., Marshall, F.J., and Creamer, H.R.: Reactivity of human lymphocytes to pulp antigens, J. Endod. **8**:27, 1982.

108. Loos, P.J., and Han, S.S.: An enzyme histochemical study of the effect of various concentrations of formocresol on connective tissues, Oral Surg. **31**:571, 1971.

109. Loos, P.J., Straffon, L.H., and Han, S.S.: Biological effects of formocresol, J. Dent. Child. **40**:193, 1973.

110. Mack, R.B., and Halterman, C.W.: Labial pulpectomy access followed by esthetic composite resin restoration for nonvital maxillary deciduous incisors, J. Am. Dent. Assoc. **100**:374, 1980.

111. Mansukhani, N.: Pulpal reactions to formocresol (thesis), College of Dentistry, University of Illinois, 1959.

112. Massler, M.: Pulp protection and preservation, Pract. Dent. Monogr., p. 3, January, 1958.

113. Massler, M., and Mansukhani, H.: Effects of formocresol on the dental pulp, J. Dent. Child. **26**:277, 1959.

114. Masterson, J.B.: The healing of wounds of the dental pulp of man, Br. Dent. J. **120**:213, 1966.

115. Matsumiya, S., Susuki, A., and Takuma, S.: Atlas of clinical pathology, Vol. 1, Tokyo, 1962, The Tokyo Dental College Press.

116. McDonald, R.E., and Avery, D.R.: Treatment of deep caries, vital pulp exposure, and pulpless teeth in children. In McDonald, R.E., and Avery, D.R., editors: Dentistry for the child and adolescent, ed. 3, St. Louis, 1978, The C.V. Mosby Co.

117. McWalter, G.M., El-Kafrawy, A.H., and Mitchell, D.F.: Pulp capping in monkeys with a calcium hydroxide compound, an antibiotic and a polycarboxylate cement, Oral Surg. **36**:90, 1973.

118. Messer, L.B., Cline, J.T., and Korf, N.W.: Long-term effects of primary molar pulpotomies on succedaneous bicuspids, J. Dent. Res. **59**:116, 1980.

119. Molven, O.: Dental pulp lesions covered with albumin, Oral Surg. **30**:413, 1970.

120. Morawa, A.P., et al.: Clinical studies of human primary teeth following dilute formocresol pulpotomies (abstract), J. Dent. Res. **53**:269, 1974.

121. Morawa, A.P., et al.: Clinical evaluation of pulpotomies using dilute formocresol, J. Dent. Res. **42**:360, 1975.

122. Müniz, M.A., Keszler, A., and Dominguez, F.V.: The formocresol technique in young permanent teeth, Oral Surg. **55**:611, 1983.

123. Myers, D.R.: Effects of formocresol on pulps of cariously exposed permanent molars (thesis), College of Dentistry, University of Tennessee, 1972.

124. Myers, D.R., et al.: Acute toxicity of high doses of systemically administered formocresol in dogs, Pediatr. Dent. **3**:37, 1981.

125. Myers, D.R., et al.: Tissue changes induced by the absorption of formocresol from pulpotomy sites in dogs, Pediatr. Dent. **5**:6, 1983.

126. Myers, D.R., et al.: Distribution of ^{14}C-formaldehyde after pulpotomy with formocresol, J. Am. Dent. Assoc. **96**:805, 1978.

127. Natkin, E.: Diagnosis and treatment of traumatic injuries and their sequelae. In Ingle, J.I., editor: Endodontics, Philadelphia, 1965, Lea & Febiger.

128. Nelson, J.R., et al.: Biochemical effects of tissue fixatives on bovine pulp, J. Endod. **5**:139, 1979.

129. Nevins, A.J., et al.: Revitalization of pulpless open apex teeth in rhesus monkeys, using collagen-calcium phosphate gel, J. Endod. **2**:159, 1976.

130. Nevins, A., et al.: Induction of hard tissue into pulpless open-apex teeth using collagen–calcium phosphate gel, J. Endod. **4**:76, 1978.

131. Nevins, A., et al.: Hard tissue induction into pulpless open-apex teeth using collagen-calcium phosphate gel, J. Endod. **3**:431, 1977.

132. Nirschl, R.F., and Avery, D.R.: Evaluation of new pulp capping agent in indirect pulp therapy, J. Dent. Child. **50**:25, 1983.

133. Nixon, G.S., and Hannah, C.M.: N-butyl cyanoacrylate as a pulp capping agent, Br. Dent. J. **133**:14, 1972.

134. Nygaard-Øtsby, B.: The role of the blood clot in endodontic therapy: an experimental histologic study, Acta Odontol. Scand. **19**:323, 1961.

135. Orban, B.: Contribution to the histology of the dental pulp and periodontal membrane with special reference to the cells of defense of these tissues, Am. Dent. Assoc. J. **16**:965, 1929.

136. Orban, B.J., editor: Oral histology and embryology, ed. 4, St. Louis, 1957, The C.V. Mosby Co.

137. Pashley, E.L., et al.: Systemic distribution of ^{14}C-formaldehyde from formocresol-treated pulpotomy sites, J. Dent. Res. **59**:603, 1980.

138. Pereira, J..C., and Stanley, H.R.: Pulp capping: influence of the exposure site on pulp healing—histologic and radiographic study in dogs' pulp, J. Endod. **7**:213, 1981.

139. Peron, L.C., Burkes, E.J., and Gregory, W.B.: Vital pulpotomy utilizing variable concentrations of paraformaldehyde in rhesus monkeys (abstract no. 269), J. Dent. Res. **55**:B129, 1976.

140. Phaneuf, R.A., Frankl, S.N., and Ruben, M.: A comparative histological evaluation of three calcium hydroxide preparations on the human primary dental pulp, J. Dent. Child. **35**:61, 1968.

141. Pisanti, S., and Sciaky, I.: Origin of calcium in the repair wall after pulp exposure in the dog, J. Dent. Res. **43**:641, 1964.

142. Pitt Ford, T.R.: Pulpal response to MPC for capping exposures, Oral Surg. **50**:81, 1980.

143. Pitt Ford, T.R.: Pulpal response to a calcium hydroxide material for capping exposures, Oral Surg. **59**:194, 1985.

144. Pruhs, R.J., et al.: Relationship between formocresol pulpotomies on primary teeth and enamel defects on their permanent successors, J. Am. Dent. Assoc. **94**:698, 1977.

145. Rabinowitch, B.Z.: Pulp management in primary teeth, Oral Surg. **6**:542, 1953.

146. Ranly, D.M.: Glutaraldehyde purity and stability: implications for preparation, storage, and use as a pulpotomy agent, Pediatr. Dent. **6**:83, 1984.

147. Ranly, D.M., and Lazzari, E.P.: A biochemical study of two biofunctional reagents as alternatives to formocresol, J. Dent. Res. **62**:1054, 1983.

148. Ravn, J.J.: Follow-up study of permanent incisors with complicated crown fracture after acute trauma, Scand. J. Dent. Res. **90**:363, 1982.

149. Redig, D.F.: A comparison and evaluation of two formocresol pulpotomy techniques utilizing Buckley's formocresol, J. Dent. Child. **35**:22, 1968.

150. Reynolds, R.L.: The determination of pulp vitality by means of thermal and electric stimuli, Oral Surg. **22**:231, 1966.

151. Ritchey, W.H.: A very simple technique for abscessed deciduous teeth, Texas Dent. J. **82**:5, 1964.

152. Roberts, S.C., Jr., and Brilliant, J.D.: Tricalcium phosphate as an adjunct to apical closure in pulpless permanent teeth, J. Endod. **1:**263, 1975.

153. Rølling, I., and Poulsen, S.: Formocresol pulpotomy of primary teeth and occurrence of enamel defects on the permanent successors, Acta Odontol. Scand. **36:**243, 1978.

154. Ruemping, D.R., Morton, T.H., Jr., and Anderson, M.W.: Electrosurgical pulpotomy in primates—a comparison with formocresol pulpotomy, Pediatr. Dent. **5:**14, 1983.

155. 's-Gravenmade, E.J.: Some biochemical considerations in endodontics, J. Endod. **1:**233, 1975.

156. Safer, D.S., Avery, J.K., and Cox, D.F.: Histopathologic evaluation of the effects of new polcarboxylate cements on monkey pulps, Oral Surg. **33:**966, 1972.

157. Sanchez, Z.M.C.: Effects of formocresol on pulp-capped and pulpotomized permanent teeth of rhesus monkeys (thesis), University of Michigan, 1971.

158. Sayegh, F.S.: Qualitative and quantitative evaluation of new dentin in pulp capped teeth, J. Dent. Child. **35:**7, 1968.

159. Sayegh, F.S.: The dentinal bridge in pulp-involved teeth. I, Oral Surg. **28:**579, 1969.

160. Sayegh, F.S., and Reed, A.J.: Correlated clinical and histological evaluation of Hydrex in pulp therapy, J. Dent. Child. **34:**471, 1967.

161. Sciaky, I., and Pisanti, S.: Localization of calcium placed over amputated pulps in dogs' teeth, J. Dent. Res. **39:**1128, 1960.

162. Sekine, N., Hasegawa, M., and Saijo, Y.: Clinicopathological study of vital pulpotomy, Bull. Tokyo Dent. Coll. **1:**29, 1960.

163. Sela, J., Hirschfeld, Z., and Ulmansky, M.: Reaction of the rat molar pulp to direct capping with the separate components of Hydrex, Oral Surg. **35:**118, 1973.

164. Sela, J., and Ulmansky, M.: Reaction of normal and inflamed dental pulp to Calxyl and zinc oxide-eugenol in rats, Oral Surg. **30:**425, 1970.

165. Seltzer, S.: Advances in biology of the human dental pulp, Oral Surg. **32:**454, 1971.

166. Seltzer, S., and Bender, I.B.: Pulp capping and pulpotomy. In Seltzer, S., and Bender, I.B., editors: The dental pulp, biologic considerations in dental procedures, ed. 2, Philadelphia, 1975, J.B. Lippincott Co.

167. Shoji, S., Nakamura, M., and Horiuchi, H.: Histopathological changes in dental pulps irradiated by CO_2 laser: a preliminary report on laser pulpotomy, J. Endod. **11:**379, 1985.

168. Shovelton, D.S.: A study of deep carious dentin, Int. Dent. J. **18:**392, 1968.

169. Simon, M., van Mullem, P.J., and Lamers, A.C.: Formocresol: no allergic effect after root canal disinfection in non-presensitized guinea pigs, J. Endod. **8:**269, 1982.

170. Smith, G.N., and Woods, S.: Organic iodine: a substitute for $BaSO_4$ in apexification procedures, J. Endod. **9:**153, 1983.

171. Smith, H.S., and Soni, N.N.: Histologic study of pulp capping in rat molars using calcitonin, Oral Surg. **53:**311, 1982.

172. Smith, J.W., Leeb, I.J., and Torney, D.L.: A comparison of calcium hydroxide and barium hydroxide as agents for inducing apical closure, J. Endod. **10:**64, 1984.

173. Soldali, G.D.: Pulp capping with antibiotics, Fla. Dent. J. **46:**18, 1975.

174. Spedding, R.H.: The one-appointment formocresol pulpotomy for primary teeth, J. Tenn. Dent. Assoc. **48:**263, 1968.

175. Spedding, R.H.: Pulp therapy for primary teeth—a survey of the North American dental schools, J. Dent. Child. **35:**360, 1968.

176. Stanley, H.R., and Lundy, T.: Dycal therapy for pulp exposures, Oral Surg. **34:**818, 1972.

177. Stanley, H.R., White, C.L., and McCray, L.: The rate of tertiary (reparative) dentine formation in the human tooth, Oral Surg. **21:**180, 1966.

178. Stanton, W.G.: The non-vital deciduous tooth, Int. J. Orthod. **21:**181, 1935.

179. Starkey, P.E.: Methods of preserving primary teeth which have exposed pulps, J. Dent. Child. **30:**219, 1963.

180. Starkey, P.E.: Management of deep caries of pulpally involved teeth in children. In Goldman, H.M., et al., editors: Current therapy in dentistry, vol. 3, St. Louis, 1968, The C.V. Mosby Co.

181. Starkey, P.E.: Treatment of pulpally involved primary molars. In McDonald, R.E., et al., editors: Current therapy in dentistry, vol. 7, St. Louis, 1980, The C.V. Mosby Co.

182. Steiner, J.C., Dow, P.R., and Cathey, G.M.: Inducing root end closure of non-vital permanent teeth, J. Dent. Child. **35:**47, 1968.

183. Steiner, J.C., and Van Hassel, H.J.: Experimental root apexification in primates, Oral Surg. **31:**409, 1971.

184. Stewart, D.J., and Kramer, I.R.H.: Effects of calcium hydroxide on the unexposed pulp, J. Dent. Res. **37:**758, 1958.

185. Straffon, L.H., and Han, S.S.: Effects of varying concentrations of formocresol on RNA synthesis of connective tissue in sponge implants, Oral Surg. **29:**915, 1970.

186. Sweet, C.A.: Procedure for the treatment of exposed and pulpless deciduous teeth, Am. Dent. Assoc. J. **17:**1150, 1930.

187. Tagger, E., and Tagger, M.: Pulpal and periapical reactions of glutaraldehyde and paraformaldehyde pulpotomy dressing in monkeys, J. Endod. **10:**364, 1984.

188. Tagger, M., and Tagger, E.: Pulp capping in monkeys with Reolite and Life, two calcium hydroxide bases with different pH, J. Endod. **11:**394, 1985.

189. Teuscher, G.W., and Zander, H.A.: A preliminary report on pulpotomy, Northwest. Univ. Dent. Res. Grad. Q. Bull. **39:**4, 1938.

190. Thoden Van Velzen, S.K., and Feltkamp-Vroom, T.M.: Immunologic consequences of formaldehyde fixation of autologous tissue implants, J. Endod. **3:**179, 1977.

191. Tomes, J.: A system of dental surgery, Philadelphia, 1859, Lindsay & Blakiston.

192. Trask, P.A.: Formocresol pulpotomy on (young) permanent teeth, J. Am. Dent. Assoc. **85:**1316, 1972.

193. Traubman, L.: A critical clinical and television radiographic evaluation of indirect pulp capping (thesis), Indiana University School of Dentistry, 1967.

194. Tronstad, L.: Reaction of the exposed pulp to Dycal treatment, Oral Surg. **38:**945, 1974.

195. Tronstad, L., and Mjor, I.A.: Capping of the inflamed pulp, Oral Surg. **34:**477, 1972.

196. van Mullen, P.J., Simon, M., and Lamers, A.C.: Formocresol: a root canal disinfectant provoking allergic skin reactions in presensitized guinea pigs, J. Endod. **9:**25, 1983.

197. Venham, L.L.: Pulpal responses to variations in the formocresol pulpotomy technique: a histologic study (thesis), College of Dentistry, The Ohio State University, 1967.

198. Walsh, M.: Pulp reaction to anorganic bovine dentin (thesis), Indiana University School of Dentistry, 1967.

199. Watts, A., and Patterson, R.C.: Migration of materials and microorganisms in the dental pulp of dogs and rats, J. Endod. **8:**53, 1982.

200. Webber, R.T.: Apexogenesis versus apexification, Dent. Clin. North Am. **28:**669, 1984.

201. Webber, R.T., Schwiebert, K.A., and Cathey, G.M.: A technique for placement of calcium hydroxide in the root canal system, J. Am. Dent. Assoc. **103:**417, 1981.

202. Weiss, M.B. and Bjorvatn, K.: Pulp capping in deciduous and newly erupted permanent teeth of monkeys, Oral Surg. **29:**769, 1970.

203. Wemes, J.C., et al.: Histologic evaluation of the effect of formocresol and glutaraldehyde on the periapical tissues after endodontic treatment, Oral Surg. **54:**329, 1982.

204. Wemes, J.C., et al.: Diffusion of carbon-14-labeled formocresol and glutaraldehyde in tooth structures, Oral Surg. **54:**341, 1982.

205. Wheeler, R.C.: A textbook of dental anatomy and physiology, ed. 4, Philadelphia, 1965, W.B. Saunders Co.

206. Whitehead, F.I., MacGregor, A.B., and Marsland, E.A.: The relationship of bacterial invasions of softening of the dentin in permanent and deciduous teeth, Br. Dent. J. **108**:261, 1960.

207. Willard, R.M.: Radiographic changes following formocresol pulpotomy in primary molars, J. Dent. Child. **43**:414, 1976.

208. Williams, J.L.: The non-removal of softened dentine before filling, Int. Dent. J. **20**:210, 1899.

209. Zander, H.A.: Reaction of the pulp to calcium hydroxide, J. Dent. Res. **18**:373, 1939.

210. Zurcher, E.: The anatomy of the root canals of the teeth of the deciduous dentition and of the first permanent molars, New York, 1925, William Wood & Co.

Self-assessment questions

1. A primary objective in preserving primary teeth is
   a. Maintaining arch length
   b. Aid in esthetics and mastication
   c. Prevent aberrant tongue habits
   d. All of the above

2. The most reliable correlation of advanced pulp degeneration is
   a. The response to the electric pulp tester
   b. History of spontaneous, unprovoked toothache
   c. The response to thermal testing
   d. The degree of mobility

3. Indirect pulp therapy
   a. Removes all the layers of carious dentin
   b. Removes all the bacteria from the carious lesion
   c. Is successful with teeth having clinical evidence of pulpal or periapical pathosis
   d. Is dependent on remineralization of affected dentin and reparative dentin formation

4. Pulp capping should *not* be considered for
   a. Carious exposures of primary teeth
   b. Permanent teeth with a history of spontaneous pain
   c. Excessive hemorrhage at the exposure site
   d. All of the above

5. Calcium hydroxide
   a. Is the material of choice for pulp capping
   b. Does not enter into the formation of the dentin bridge
   c. Many cause complete dentin mineralization of the remaining pulp tissue
   d. All of the above

6. The formocresol pulpotomy for primary teeth is indicated when
   a. There is evidence of periapical or furcal pathologic conditions
   b. A fistula is present
   c. Inflammation and/or infection are judged to be confined to the coronal pulp
   d. The tooth is nearing exfoliation

7. The formocresol pulpotomy technique for primary teeth includes
   a. Removing the pulp tissue to the midroot level
   b. Controlling hemorrhage with dry cotton pellets
   c. Leaving the formocresol in contact with the pulp stump for 15 minutes
   d. Using a cement base of ZOE over the pulp stump

8. The formocresol pulpotomy for young permanent teeth
   a. May be considered as a temporary measure if extraction is the other choice
   b. Is the recommended treatment of choice with mechanical exposures
   c. Will cause calcification of the remaining pulp tissue
   d. May be utilized as a permanent procedure with necrotic pulps

9. The calcium hydroxide pulpotomy for young permanent teeth
   a. Is indicated for treatment of necrotic pulps
   b. Is an attempt to maintain pulp vitality
   c. Is indicated when there is a traumatic exposure and fully developed roots
   d. Is temporarily restored until the pulp status can be assessed

10. Roots of primary teeth have the following characteristic:
    a. A root/crown ratio less than that of the permanent teeth
    b. A divergence in primary molars less than that in permanent molars
    c. Resorption beginning soon after completion of root length
    d. Variations within the root canals, usually in a mesiodistal plane

11. General considerations for endodontic treatment of primary teeth include
    a. The possible coronal repositioning of the apical foramen during resorption
    b. Prevention of overinstrumentation and possible damage to the permanent tooth bud
    c. Utilization of an absorbable filling material to obliterate the root canal system
    d. All of the above

12. One of the following is not a contraindication for root canal therapy of primary teeth:
    a. Mechanical or carious perforation of the floor of the pulp chamber
    b. Presence of a dentigerous or follicular cyst
    c. Apical resorption involving the roots
    d. Radiographic evidence of internal resorption in the roots

13. The filling of choice for primary root canals is
    a. Cavit
    b. Chloropercha
    c. ZOE without a catalyst
    d. $Ca(OH)_2$ paste

14. Apexification technique is the treatment of choice for a permanent tooth with a wide-open apex when
    a. There is a history of spontaneous pain with a caries exposure
    b. The tooth is pulpless or periapical disease is evident
    c. There is a fracture of the clinical crown exposing the pulp for less than 24 hours
    d. There is a large mechanical exposure with profuse bleeding of the pulp

23

FAILURES IN THERAPY

PAUL EUGENE ZEIGLER
THOMAS P. SERENE

INTRODUCTION

DUDLEY H. GLICK

Many authors display a propensity to reduce complex problems involving success and failure to terms so simple that a casual reader, with little effort, can expand a narrow grasp of the subject into a broad, convenient misunderstanding.

Not long ago a recent graduate, employed by a local union group and arbitrarily designated as their "endodontist," told me he had treated about 1000 patients in 2 years without a single failure. In fact, he felt "endo was such a breeze" that he would soon leave the union and limit his practice to endodontics. (Ah youth!) This outstanding statistic impressed me because I have never had such remarkable clinical success, not even with my first 100 patients. I asked for his percentage of recalls and whether the radiographs had disclosed any pathologic manifestations, such as periapical lesions. Quite candidly he replied he did not know; however, like an experimental nihilist, he added that all symptoms had subsided shortly after treatment and his patients voiced no complaints—and that's what really counted!

This young dentist had reduced criteria for success of treatment to a very narrow definition: absence of pain. How convenient it would be if his concept could be totally accepted; unfortunately absence of pain is not a completely reliable measure for good health or success in endodontic treatment. Needless to say, he has since confided to me that he has become more introspective and even concedes to an occasional failure.

Countless people are living today with some disease in its pain-free stage; the bodily defenses are capable of handling the disease until a tissue stress situation occurs. Endodontic treatment apparently succeeds in some cases in spite of, not necessarily because of, our best efforts. This fortunate circumstance can also be attributed to the tremendous capacity of the body's natural defenses to cope with infections and to enhance the body's survival rate.

Practicing endodontists know that lack of pain is not the sole criterion of success, but they would be hard pressed to present universally acceptable criteria for success or failure. This is evidenced by the plethora of research and clinical studies in the literature, replete with conjectures, hypotheses, and conclusions. A review of the literature reveals the complexity of success and failure; their ultimate causes cannot be reduced to a few simple statements or be assessed unequivocally.

Following is a list of some of the factors that influence success of failure of endodontic treatment:

Age and sex of the patient
Health and general systemic status of the patient
Radiographic interpretation
Canal infection (revealed by cultures)
Use of the rubber dam
Type of treatment
Morphologic considerations
Cleaning and shaping
Procedural mishaps (e.g., broken instruments or perforations)
Filling technique (material used and apical level of the obturating material)
Linear crown and root fracture
Periodontal condition
Resorption
Idiopathic cause of failure
Final restoration
Lingering postoperative pain (recalcitrant and inexplicable)

The list is endless, so it would be impossible to expound on all factors in depth.

In 1973 Frank and Weiner[6] attempted to investigate and evaluate criteria that make up successful endodontic treatment. Research designs were outlined, and pertinent characteristics and hypotheses were established. The studies succeeded only in raising new issues and variables requiring further definitive answers instead of resolving previous questions. The studies continued on at length but (mercifully) ended in futility.

The final suggestions included *criteria for treatment evaluation:*

1. Success
   a. Affected tooth is asymptomatic, functional, and firm in its alveolus.
   b. Soft tissue appears normal and responds normally to manual examination.
   c. Radiographs reveal a normal lamina dura.
2. Failure
   a. Affected tooth is symptomatic or has an abnormal appearance.
   b. Soft tissue responds abnormally to manual examination.
   c. Radiographs reveal that
      (1) A lesion has remained the same or has only diminished in size, but total repair has not occurred.
      (2) A lesion appears subsequent to endodontic treatment, or a preexisting lesion increases in size.
      (3) There are conflicting findings with respect to symptoms, tissue response, and radiographic evaluation.

Like many other previous researchers on the subject of successful therapy, Frank and Weiner concluded that diagnosis of symptoms and evaluation of radiographs merit the highest priorities in determining success.

Endodontic success is not a myth. The millions of happy people walking around with pain-free results will agree. However, slipshod techniques should not be considered successful because the patient has no overt symptoms.

Visible evidence of successful results can be related from clinician to clinician by radiographs. However, it is possible that the patient is pain free after treatment in spite of a valid radiographic interpretation of apparent pathologic conditions. Conversely, there may be a persistence of pain and swelling and the formation of a sinus tract but a normal-appearing radiograph. How are success and failure determined in such instances?

An examination of studies for success and failure must be carefully evaluated because there is an overabundance of self-serving criteria. To add to the confusion, many statistics of success and failure are based on case selection.

Goldman et al.[7,8] did a clinical study on the subjective variability of radiographic interpretations. It appears that the radiograph is also a questionable means for determining success and failure, inasmuch as six examiners agreed on less than half the cases and three "specialists" agreed only 65% of the time. (Too often one sees what one wants to see when it comes to interpreting radiographs.) In this study the radiologist (skeptic) gave a lower incidence of success than did the endodontist (enthusiast) who had treated the teeth, which suggests that clinicians may be the least reliable in radiographic interpretations of their own treatment.

Bender et al.[2] showed that it is possible to have a "normal" radiograph while histologically there is chronic inflammation and proliferation of epithelial cells. These authors demonstrated that an apical lesion can start

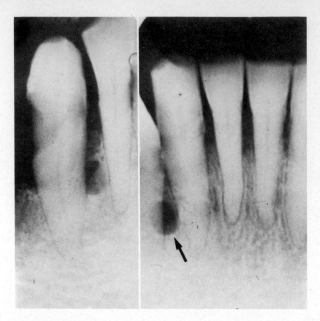

FIG. 23-1. Lateral peridontal cyst *(arrow)* associated with a vital mandibular canine.

developing long before there is pulp necrosis and evidence of rarefaction. They recommended, as have many others, a reappraisal of "traditional" criteria for success.

Whether we would really benefit from a remeasuring of the standards of success and failure is questionable. Perhaps we are our own worst critics and have set up too rigid criteria of success based on the radiograph. The physician accepts such rates as a 5-year success rate for cancer and a 3- to 5-year success rate for hip prosthesis. Are these arbitrary figures? Are they valid? Do physicians want to consider them valid if a majority of their patients fall into that 3- to 5-year class? Similarly, should we look for short-range success or anticipate long-range failure in dentistry?

We should not delude ourselves; failures do and will occur in spite of outstanding efforts and the best available techniques. Our aims might be noble and high; yet our ability to achieve them may fail miserably—in part because we are dealing with human tissues, which do not always follow the text.

However, there are certain variable factors that do contribute significantly to success or failure. This chapter explores a few.

FAILURES CAUSED BY INCORRECT DIAGNOSIS*

Initially failures can occur because of an incorrect diagnosis. This may be related to the fact that many oral lesions appear similar to endodontic lesions. Although an accurate diagnosis is not always possible, regardless of the test used, the diagnostic tests and procedures listed in Chapter 1 are necessary to prevent a misdiagnosis. Moreover, when making a diagnosis, the clinician should al-

*We gratefully acknowledge the special contributions of Drs. John Andrews, Thomas Higginbotham, Robert Krasny, and Gene Palmer.

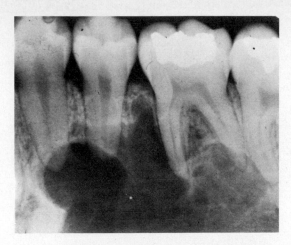

FIG. 23-2. Ameloblastoma in the mandible, confirmed by biopsy. Note the areas of bone destruction. All teeth tested vital.

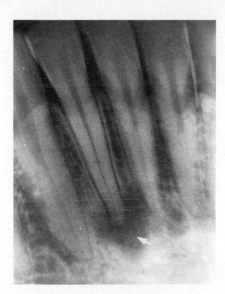

FIG. 23-3. Periapical osteofibrosis (cementoma) associated with a mandibular lateral incisor. All teeth tested vital. Note the uniform periodontal ligament space around the root apex. (Courtesy Drs. James R. Jensen and Thomas P. Serene.)

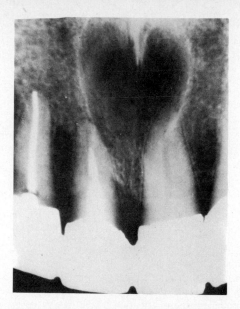

FIG. 23-4. Incisive canal cyst was confirmed by biopsy. The diagnosis was complicated by previous endodontic therapy.

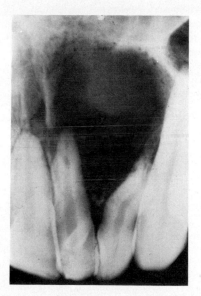

FIG. 23-5. Globulomaxillary cyst confirmed by biopsy. All teeth tested vital.

ways rely on a *combination* of tests rather than a single test.

Misinterpretation of oral lesions

Odontogenic lesions. Odontogenic lesions (cysts) often resemble lesions of endodontic (pulpal) origin. Whereas some appear to be associated with several teeth, others appear almost identical to an apical radiolucency involving a single nonvital tooth. Usually, all teeth having odontogenic lesions are *vital and asymptomatic*.

The lateral periodontal cyst is a rare entity of uncertain cause[21] (Fig. 23-1). If such a cyst becomes infected, it may manifest itself clinically as a lateral periodontal abscess. The ameloblastoma is a true neoplasm of enamel organ-type tissue that does not undergo differentiation to the point of enamel formation (Fig. 23-2). Cementomas,

as classically described, are rather common lesions (Fig. 24-3). Some theorists believe their origin is from odontogenic tissue; others that they represent only an unusual reaction of periapical bone.[21]

Developmental lesions. Developmental lesions (cysts) can also resemble endodontic lesions.

The median anterior maxillary cyst, which lies in or near the incisive canal, is the most common type of maxillary developmental or fissural cyst[21] (Fig. 23-4). Median mandibular developmental cysts occur in the midline of the mandible and are extremely rare. The globulomaxillary cyst is found within bone at the junction of the globular portion of the medial nasal process and the maxillary process, usually between the maxillary lateral and canine teeth

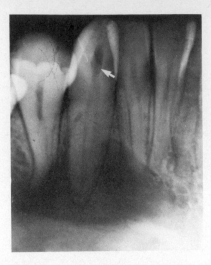

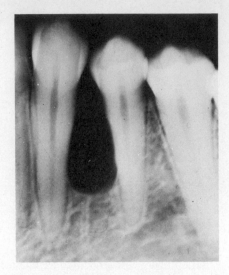

FIG. 23-6. Central giant cell reparative granuloma confirmed by biopsy. The patient presented with partial numbness of the lower lip and throughout the distribution of the mental nerve. An intraoral swelling extended from the mandibular lateral incisor to the second premolar anteroposteriorly and downward from just below the gingiva to the lower border of the mandible. *Note:* The canine was previously opened *(arrow)*. Although all teeth (central and lateral incisors, canine, first premolar) tested nonvital, hemorrhagic tissue was encountered in the root canals of these teeth during prophylactic endodontic therapy.

FIG. 23-7. Neurofibroma confirmed by biopsy. Note the similarity to a lateral periodontal lesion. All teeth tested vital.

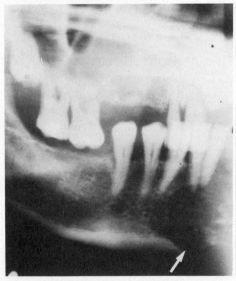

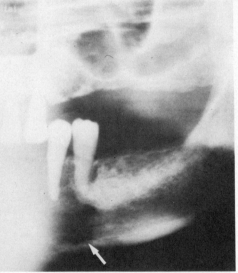

FIG. 23-8. Squamous cell carcinoma confirmed by biopsy. Note the areas of bone destruction in the mandible *(arrows)*.

(Fig. 23-5). The diagnosis of incisal canal and globulomaxillary cysts can be made, in part, on their location and appearance. Again, the teeth involved are usually *vital and asymptomatic.*

Oral tumors. Oral tumors are often associated with one or more teeth.

The central giant cell reparative granuloma may involve either jaw; however, the mandible is most often affected (Fig. 23-6). The neurofibroma, a tumor of nerve tissue origin, may give the appearance of an endodontic-periodontal lesion (Fig. 23-7). Squamous cell carcinomas are the most common malignant neoplasms of the oral cavity[21] (Fig. 23-8). The final diagnosis of all oral tumors must be (and can only be) confirmed by biopsy.

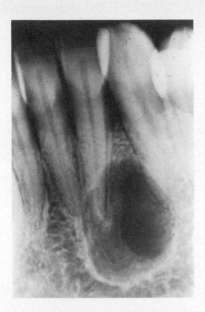

FIG. 23-9. Traumatic bone cysts in the mandible confirmed by biopsy. All teeth tested vital.

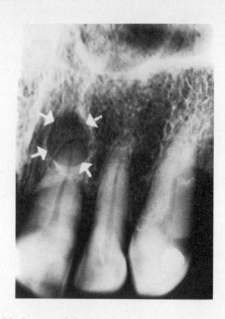

FIG. 23-11. Image of the incisive canal *(arrows)* superimposed over the apex of the maxillary central incisor. Note the continuity of the periodontal ligament space around the apex. All teeth were tested vital.

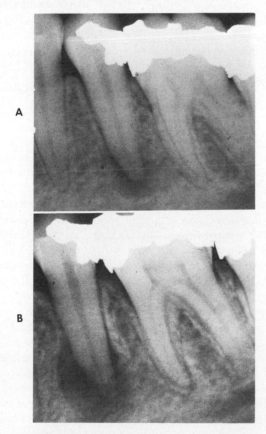

FIG. 23-10. A, Image supposedly of the mental foramen superimposed over the apex of the mandibular premolar. No diagnostic tests were performed. **B,** one year later. Note the enlargement of the apical radiolucency. The premolar tested nonvital. Vitality tests could have prevented this misinterpretation.

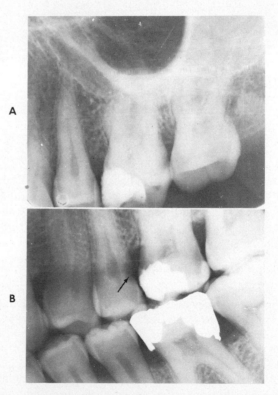

FIG. 23-12. A, Maxillary first molar referred for endodontic therapy because of pain and discomfort. This radiograph was sent with the patient. **B,** Bite-wing radiograph taken on the day of referral, since the maxillary second premolar was severely painful to percussion and thermal testing. The pain was due to a carious lesion in the premolar *(arrow).*

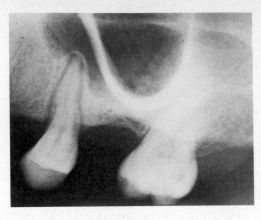

FIG. 23-13. Pain and thickened periodontal ligament space due to traumatic occlusion. The tooth tested vital. (Courtesy Drs. James R. Jensen and Thomas P. Serene.)

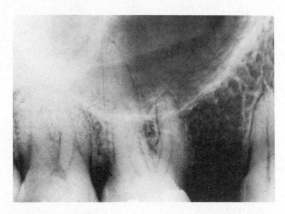

FIG. 23-14. Maxillary first molar (with routine restoration) slightly sensitive to percussion and thermal change because of maxillary sinus involvement. No endodontic therapy was necessary since symptoms gradually disappeared.

Physical injury of bone. Physical injury of bone, such as the traumatic bone cyst, is an unusual lesion that occurs with disturbing frequency in the jaws as well as in other bones of the skeleton (Fig. 23-9). Radiographically this lesion can appear very similar to a chronic apical periodontitis.

Misinterpretation of anatomic landmarks

The radiographic superimposition of anatomic landmarks over the apices of the teeth presents problems when one is attempting to formulate a diagnosis. The landmarks most often misinterpreted are the mental foramen and the incisive canal (Figs. 23-10 and 23-11).

In addition to the usual diagnostic tests, radiographs taken at different angles are often helpful in confirming the diagnosis. Radiographically an intact lamina dura may help the clinician to differentiate the anatomic landmark from a periapical pathosis.

Incorrect diagnosis of pain

Pulpal pain can usually be diagnosed best with a thermal stimulus (hot or cold), especially in the case of dental car-

ies (Fig. 23-12). Abnormal responses from inflamed pulps can usually be categorized into three groups:

1. Pain that lasts as long as the stimulus is applied but is of more intense character than in "normal" teeth (reversible pulpitis)
2. Pain that is brought on by the stimulus and continues after the stimulus has been removed (irreversible pulpitis)
3. Pain present that is made worse by the application of the stimulus (a more advanced stage of irreversible pulpitis)

Occasionally pulpal pain is associated with periodontal problems, or it may be referred from other structures (Figs. 23-13 and 23-14). Pulpal pain in many instances is severe (sharp or dull throbbing) whereas periodontal pain is usually not so acute. Pain can be indicative of tissue damage; however, its severity cannot always be correlated with the severity of tissue damage.

FAILURES CAUSED BY ANATOMIC VARIATIONS

Endodontic failures can occur as a result of failure to locate, clean and shape, or fill the complete root canal system (Fig. 23-15). Knowing the variations in root canal morphology is helpful in predicting the presence of an "extra" canal in the system. "Extra" canals exist most frequently in mandibular incisors, maxillary second premolars, mesial-buccal roots of maxillary first molars, mandibular premolars, and distal roots or mandibular molars. In general, teeth with short broad roots tend to have "extra" canals.

Multiple canals and foramina

Mandibular incisor. According to most anatomic studies* mandibular incisors have a labial and a lingual canal about 40% of the time (Fig. 23-16). Fortunately only about 1% of the teeth have two canals with independent foramina.

Failure to locate one of the two canals with a common foramen may affect the long-term prognosis if percolation occurs from a lateral canal into the untreated area. Failure is certain when the clinician fails to treat one canal in the small percentage of teeth that have two apical foramina. Therefore, if a lesion develops on a mandibular incisor following endodontic treatment, the possibility of a second canal should be considered. Radiographs taken from a mesial or distal angle may reveal a second canal. An attempt to locate the canal is best made by altering the access preparation (extending it more to the lingual) to allow exploration of the chamber floor. Only when this proves fruitless should a surgical approach to the apex be attempted.

Maxillary second premolar. The maxillary second premolar has a significant percentage of multiple canals (about 25%) and one or more foramina at the apex[9] (Fig. 23-17). A careful study of diagnostic radiographs may give the clinician an indication of the presence of a second canal.

---

*References 3, 10, 15, 16, 25.

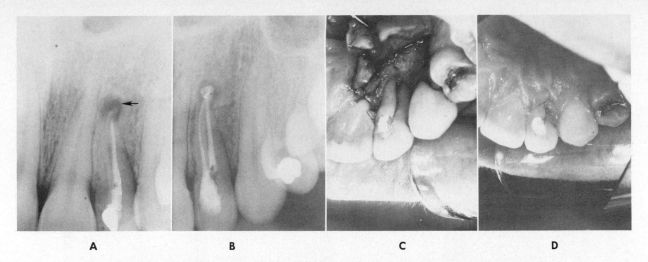

FIG. 23-15. Failure of a maxillary lateral incisor due to an unfilled additional root. **A,** Initial radiograph showing the failure *(arrow).* **B,** Endodontic re-treatment. **C,** Palatal view of the defect. **D,** Postsurgical healing. (Courtesy Drs. Irving L. Fried and Alan A. Winter.)

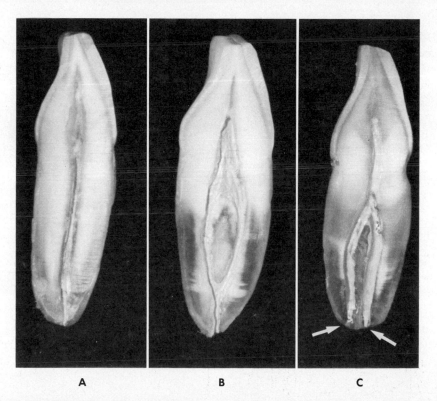

FIG. 23-16. Mandibular incisor canal system. **A,** Single canal with a single foramen. **B,** Two canals with a common foramen. **C,** Two canals with two separate foramina *(arrows).*

If the root canal disappears or becomes less distinct radiographically, it may be a broad canal that is dividing into two finer canals (Fig. 23-18). Often the main canal will again appear distinct near the apex, indicating that the accessory canals have merged (Fig. 23-19). Green[9] used the term "lateral septum" to describe such canals (Fig. 23-17). Occasionally the septum is quite short and can be eliminated during the cleaning and shaping of the canal system thus producing one broad (buccal-lingual) canal.

Mesial-buccal root of the maxillary first molar. In anatomic studies of the maxillary first molar[9,17-19] the mesial-buccal root shows evidence of two canals about 50% of the time.[18] The number of second mesial-buccal canals found in clinical work is usually less.

The fact that there is a low failure rate for treatment of the maxillary first molar indicates either that the second canal merges with the primary canal (Fig. 23-20, *B*) or that secondary dentin so reduces the pulpal space as to prevent

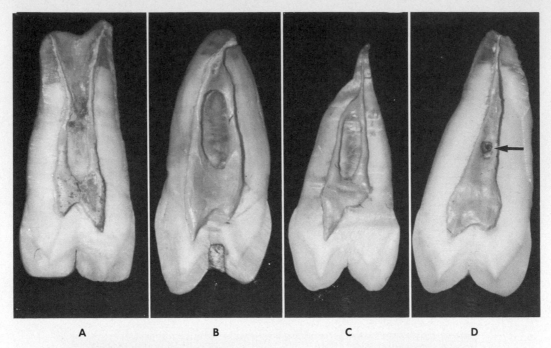

FIG. 23-17. Maxillary second premolar canal system. **A,** Two canals with two separate foramina. **B,** One canal with a large lateral septum. **C,** One canal with a large lateral septum. **D,** One canal with a small lateral septum *(arrow)*.

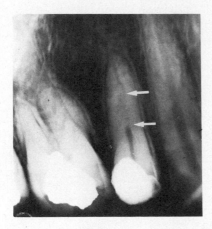

FIG. 23-18. One canal dividing into two by a lateral septum; indicated by a sudden narrowing of the canal. Arrows show where the main canal divides into two finer canals that then rejoin into one canal apically.

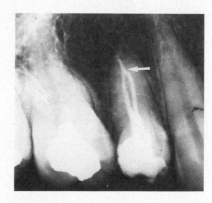

FIG. 23-19. Two canals with a common foramen *(arrow)*. (Same tooth as in Fig. 23-18. This is a posttreatment radiograph.)

percolation from creating an apical inflammatory lesion within the usual 2-year recall period. The long-term success, however, may be less favorable if these canals are not filled. In a radiographic study of the mesial-buccal root of the maxillary first molar[17] about 30% of the roots had two canals with two apical foramina and another 12% had single canal configurations with two distinct apical foramina.

With such a high percentage of roots having two canals and two foramina, a search for the "extra" canal in the mesial-buccal root should be a routine part of the treatment procedure of the maxillary first molar. Although surgical access to the mesial-buccal root is usually not complicated,

the patient is far better off if a search for the possible orifice of the second canal is attempted before a retrofilling is considered. A small percentage of maxillary first molars have well-developed fourth roots associated with the mesial-buccal root (Fig. 23-21). The fourth root can usually be identified with radiographs, but gaining straight line access to the canal may be a problem.

Mandibular premolar. Anatomically the mandibular premolars can be the easiest or the most complicated teeth in the dental arch to treat.

The canal morphology (as illustrated in Chapter 6) shows a wide variety of shapes (Fig. 23-22). In a radiographic study of 1393 first premolars,[27] about 70% had

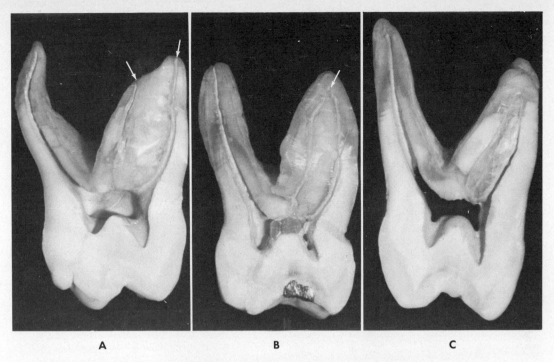

FIG. 23-20. Maxillary first molar mesial-buccal root canal system. **A,** Two canals with two separate foramina *(arrows)*.**B,** Two canals with a common foramen *(arrow)*. **C,** Single ribbon-shaped canal.

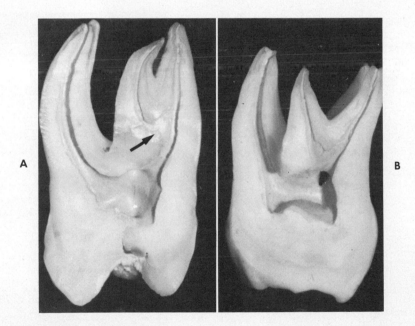

FIG. 23-21. Maxillary first molar with four roots. **A,** Two mesial-buccal roots. Arrow shows a septum between the two canals. Direct line access is very difficult. **B,** Two mesial-buccal roots. Direct-line access here is readily possible.

one canal, 23% had two canals, and less than 1% had three canals. Approximately 8% of the first premolars had open apices. Of 938 second premolars, 85% had one canal, 12% had two canals, and less than 1% had three canals.[27] Open apices were present in less than 4% of the teeth examined in the mandibular second premolar group

(Fig. 23-23, *B*). Most mandibular premolars have single roots, but some have two distinct apices (Fig. 23-22, *D*).

Gaining access to the canal orifices when a broad oval canal divides into two canals can be a problem that requires adjusting the access preparation (Fig. 23-24). If straight line access cannot be gained, the instrument will

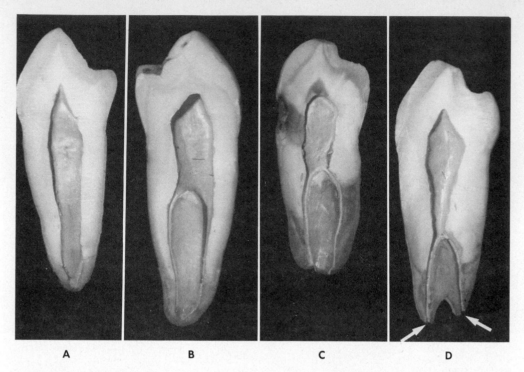

FIG. 23-22. Mandibular second premolar canal system. **A,** Single ribbon-shaped canal. **B,** Two canals with a common foramen. **C,** Two canals with two separate foramina. **D,** Two canals with two apices *(arrows).*

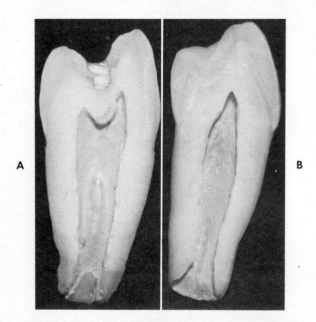

FIG. 23-23. Mandibular premolar canal system. **A,** Wide ribbon-shaped canal with two separate foramina. **B,** Wide ribbon-shaped canal with an open apex.

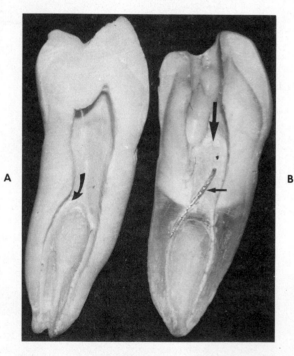

FIG. 23-24. A, Lingual canal *(arrow)* in which direct-line access would be difficult. **B,** Canal in which an instrument has separated *(arrow).*

bend in the oval section of the canal as apical pressure is applied. Instrument separation can occur under these circumstances if the file is severely rotated.

Distal root of a mandibular molar. A small percentage of distal roots of mandibular molars have two canals and two apical foramina[9,22] (Fig. 23-25).

If the first file placed in the canal points to the buccal or lingual side, the presence of a second orifice should be suspected. Furthermore, if two canals are present, each will be smaller in diameter than a single canal (Fig. 23-26). Additional films taken from a different angle will aid in confirming the presence of an extra canal. If a lesion

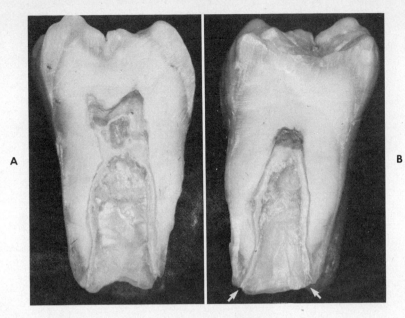

FIG. 23-25. Mandibular first molar with four canals. **A,** Mesial root. **B,** Distal root. Arrows mark the distal foramina.

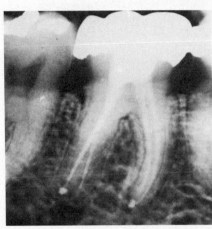

FIG. 23-26. Mandibular first molar with four canals. When four canals are present, all have roughly the same diameter. When three canals are present, the distal canal is markedly larger than the mesial canals.

FIG. 23-27. Bone loss in the furca area with an apical lesion on the mesial root. Arrows show the extent of bone loss before endodontic therapy.

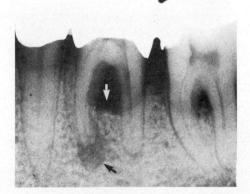

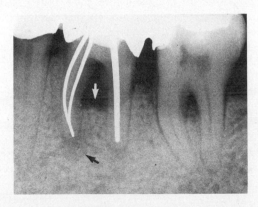

FIG. 23-28. Failure of bone loss repair in the furca area after endodontic treatment. The apical lesion healed. Inadequate sealing of the communicating accessory canals in the furca contributed partly, or entirely, to this failure. Arrows show the extent of bone loss and healing after endodontic therapy.

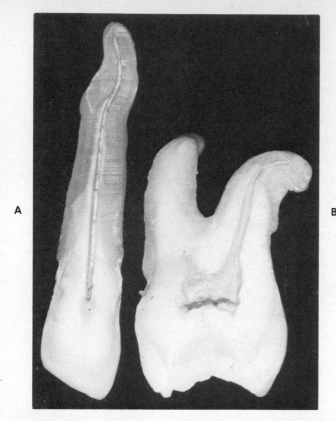

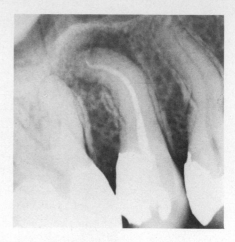

FIG. 23-30. Canal filled around a sickle-shaped curve.

FIG. 23-29. Canal curvatures. **A,** Premolar with a light S-shaped curvature. **B,** Molar palatal root with a sickle-shaped curvature.

persists after complete obliteration of the distal canal, a search for a possible second canal should be considered.

Accessory canals

The presence of accessory canals in the furcation area of maxillary and mandibular molars has been well established. In a study of 22 maxillary molars,[14] 55% of the teeth had accessory canals in the furca and middle third of the root. Of 24 mandibular molars, 63% demonstrated the presence of accessory canals in the same anatomic areas.[14] In another study of 95 maxillary molars[5] there were one or more accessory canals in the furca region of about 77% of the teeth; furthermore, 76% of 100 mandibular molars had accessory canals.

Accessory canals play a definite role in the prognosis after treatment. They can affect the prognosis if the coronal seal is not adequate (Figs. 23-27 and 23-28). Posttreatment damage to the bone in the furca usually occurs if the coronal seal is lost before completion of the permanent restoration. If a delay in placement of the permanent restoration is anticipated, it would be well to place a temporary alloy or composite restoration.

Sickle-shaped, dilacerated, and S-curved canals

Roots with severe curvatures are difficult to correctly clean and shape (Fig. 23-29). Sickle-shaped curves and dilacerated curves can usually be enlarged and shaped if instruments are used properly. The S-shaped curvature,

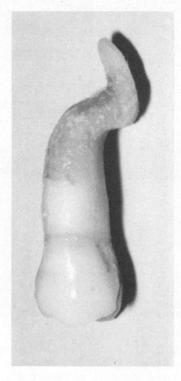

FIG. 23-31. Premolar with a pronounced S-shaped curve. This tooth would be difficult to properly clean and shape to the apical foramen.

however, is far more difficult to negotiate completely. If the prognosis for complete root canal filling is questionable, the patient should be advised that careful observation is necessary (Figs. 23-30 and 23-31).

Fortunately most of the roots with extreme curvatures can be treated surgically. The root can be amputated apical to the curvature, and a retrofilling can be placed to seal off the canal.

FAILURES CAUSED BY ALTERED CANAL SPACE
Calcification

Calcifications that alter the root canal space can make canal cleaning, shaping, and filling difficult. Developmen-

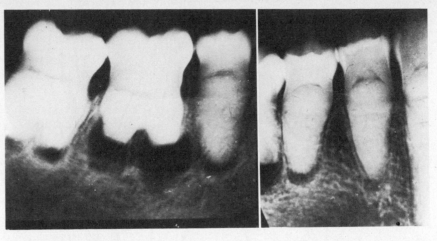

FIG. 23-32. Dentinal dysplasia in mandibular teeth.

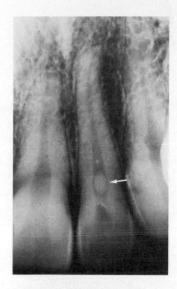

FIG. 23-33. Denticle (pulp stone) *(arrow)* in a maxillary lateral incisor.

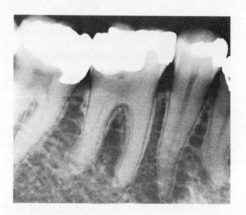

FIG. 23-34. Mandibular first molar with a calcified pulp chamber and calcified canals due to a previous pulp-capping procedure. *Note:* Should endodontic therapy now become necessary, it would probably require the use of a calcium-chelating agent.

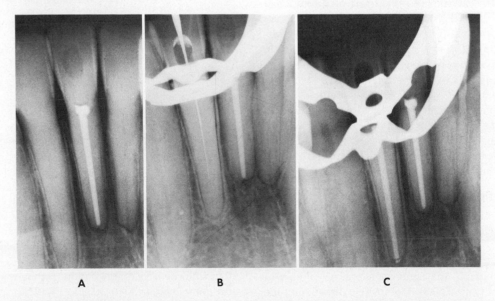

A   B   C

FIG. 23-35. Mandibular lateral incisor with a history of trauma. Since the tooth required endodontic therapy, a chelating agent was necessary to find and negotiate the heavily calcified canal. *Note:* Several appointments were necesary just to reach the working length. **A,** First appointment. **B,** Second appointment. **C,** Immediately after placement of the root canal filling.

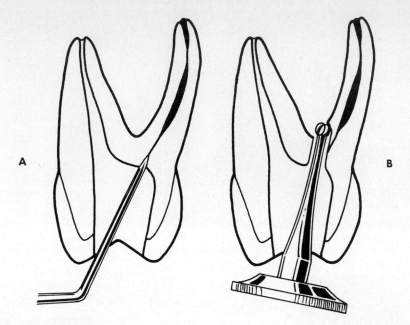

FIG. 23-36. A, Endodontic explorer in a chelated canal. **B,** Perforation of the chamber floor with a bur.

tal diseases, such as dentinal dysplasia and dentinogenesis imperfecta, cause a constriction of the existing space with secondary dentin (Fig. 23-32).

Diffuse calcification can occur when long fibrillar structures in the connective tissue walls of blood vessels in the pulp calcify. Occasionally these become large enough to block cleaning and shaping of the canal. Denticles (pulp stones) often occur in the pulp chamber and may be attached to the dentin wall or exist unattached in the pulp tissue (Fig. 23-33). Calcification in the pulp is a response to caries or the irritation from restorative procedures (Fig. 23-34). Endodontic problems arise clinically when pulps become nonvital or symptomatic; such calcifications preclude cleaning and shaping of all or part of a root canal sytem. The use of EDTA (a chelating agent) may soften the calcification enough to make cleaning and shaping possible (Fig. 23-35). If the canals cannot be completely cleaned and shaped, a retrofilling is usually possible.

Calcified canals should be managed with a sharp explorer or small file along with a chelating solution.[20] Burs tend to ledge chamber floors and lead to perforation (Fig. 23-36). When the use of a bur is necessary, it is wise to expose a bite-wing radiograph first without the clamp. This view usually gives the most accurate picture of the existing chamber and canal orifices.

Internal resorption

Internal resorption (Chapter 16) is a highly destructive form of inflammatory response by the pulp to injury. It is insidious because it is usually asymptomatic until the root has been perforated. Early diagnosis (which can be made only with a radiograph) may prevent lateral perforation of the root or crown (Fig. 23-37). Complete extirpation of the pulp is necessary to arrest further resorption of the dentin.

Thorough chemical-mechanical debridement of the canal

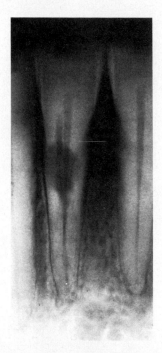

FIG. 23-37. Internal resorption perforating the external root surface.

is complicated by the presence of inflammatory tissue within the "harbor" area of dentin resorption. Gaining access to the resorbed area is much easier if the canal space coronal to the resorbed area is enlarged first with files and then with Gates-Glidden burs. Inflammatory tissue can be removed with a precurved file and copious use of sodium hypochlorite irrigating solution. Filling the canal space can be completed in two stages: (1) The apical segment is filled with laterally condensed gutta-percha and the gutta-percha is removed from the coronal segment of the root.

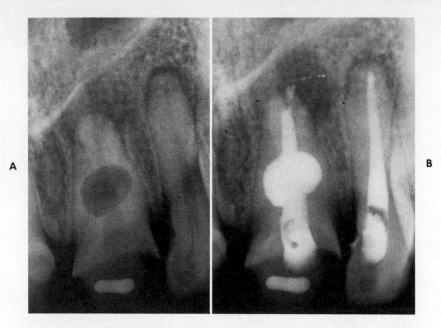

FIG. 23-38. A, Internal resorption. B, Filled.

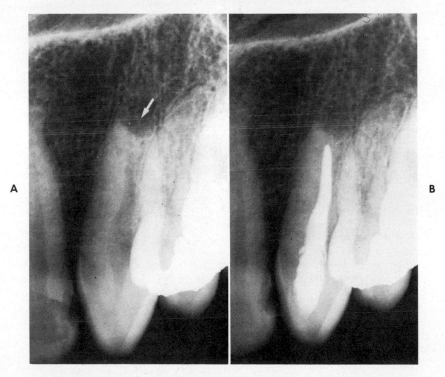

FIG. 23-39. A, Crater-shaped external resorption at the apex *(arrow)*. B, Preparation of a stop in the dentin allows complete obliteration of the canal space without overfilling.

(2) Warmed gutta-percha is vertically condensed to fill the irregularities in the resorbed area (Fig. 23-38).

External resorption

External resorption may alter the canal space by perforating the root or destroying the natural canal constriction at the apex. Root end resorption usually produces a cup-shaped crater, as viewed from the external portion of the root. When the resorption involves the apical foramen of the tooth, the canal constriction is destroyed, and proper filling is then difficult. Such canals should be cleaned and shaped *short* of the radiographic apex so a ''stop'' can be formed in the dentin. If a stop cannot be created, overextension of the filling may result (Fig. 23-39).

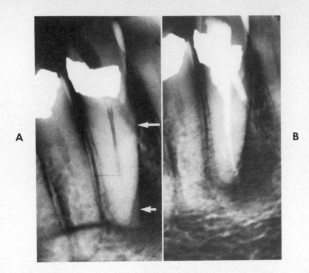

FIG. 23-40. A, Mesial root perforation due to a failure of the access preparation *(top arrow)*. Note the bifurcated root canal system *(bottom arrow)*. B, Perforation filled along with the root canal. This tooth will most likely fail periodontally and require surgical intervention.

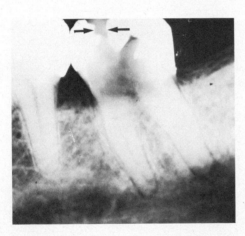

FIG. 23-41. Pulp chamber with the floor destroyed by underextended but overzealous preparation. Because of the inevitable sequelae of periodontal inflammation in the furca area, the endodontic prognosis is poor. Arrows indicate the underextension of this access opening.

FAILURES CAUSED BY TECHNICAL DIFFICULTIES
Access preparation

Perforation. The most common causes of failures related to access preparations are openings that are misaligned from the long axis of the tooth and are also small and/or incorrectly placed on the tooth surface. (See Chapter 6 for an illustrated discussion of root perforation.) An access opening that is misaligned and underextended will most often cause root or furca perforations and tooth loss unless surgically corrected (Figs. 23-40 to 23-42).

Stripping is a type of lateral perforation of the root that most often occurs in the mesiobuccal or mesiolingual canals of the mandibular first molars (Fig. 23-43, *A*). The

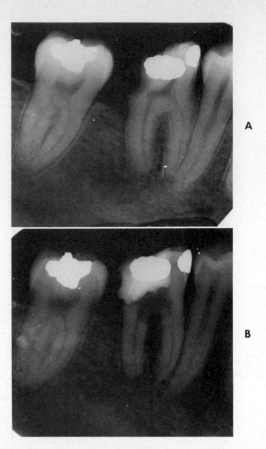

FIG. 23-42. Failure of an access opening prepared during an emergency visit. A, Initial radiograph. B, Excessive access opening with furcation perforation.

mesial root of the mandibular first molar has a concavity on the distal surface that places the canals closer to the surface than they appear on the radiograph (Fig. 23-43, *B* and *C*). When there are curvatures in the coronal third of the canal, there is a tendency for the root canal file to remove more dentin from the inside of the curvature. Kessler, Peters, and Lorten[12] have shown the use of anticurvature filing, rather than circumferential filing, will keep the canal preparation clear of the distal surface of the root. Care should also be taken in the use of the Gates-Glidden bur to flare the canal preparations. Once the perforation has occurred, it can be detected by the presence of hemorrhage on the paper point used to dry the canal (see Fig. 6-18, *D* and *G*). As with any perforation, prompt sealing of the area should be done. Once an inflammatory lesion develops in the area, the use of calcium hydroxide in the canal will sometimes allow bone repair.

Underextended preparation. Underextended access openings do not necessarily lead to failure of treatment, but they certainly complicate therapy. The most common problems are failure to gain straight line access to the canals and failure to thoroughly debride the pulp horns, resulting in coronal discoloration or continual contamination of the canal. The prevalence of additional canals in certain roots has been well demonstrated.[23] Without adequate vi-

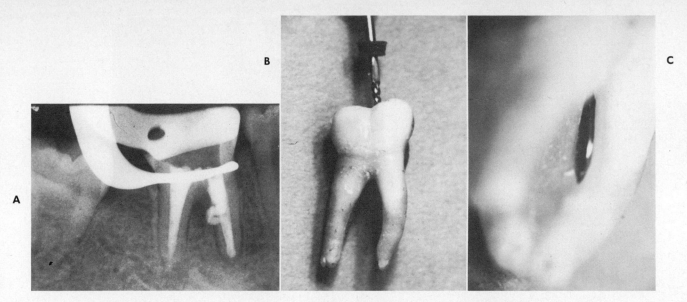

FIG. 23-43. Stripping perforation. **A,** Lateral perforation on the mesial root of the mandibular first molar. **B** and **C,** Extracted tooth showing perforation with a reamer in place.

sual access to the pulp chamber, additional canals can easily be missed and failure results.

Overextended preparation. Overextended preparations are generally not as disastrous as underextended preparations; however, they can so weaken the clinical crown that a simple postendodontic restoration is no longer possible and complicated fixed prosthetic procedures become necessary (Fig. 23-44).

The preoperative radiograph must be carefully examined to determine whether any conditions present would make the clinician suspect that the canals may be difficult to locate. If so, the access preparation must be enlarged or otherwise altered to minimize the chances of a perforation. In other words, both visual access and instrumental access must be increased.

Some conditions requiring a larger access preparation are secondary dentin obliterating the pulp chamber, a full-coverage restoration, teeth drastically inclined in their long axis, and the suspicion that extra roots or canals may be present.

Canal preparation

Endodontic failures are usually considered to have occurred when teeth fail to respond to treatment or there is evidence of failure on a recall visit after the canals have been sealed. An important category of failure which is frequently overlooked or underemphasized includes teeth that can never be brought to the filling stage because symptoms never subside; in these teeth surgical intervention may be the only option.

It has been proved that teeth may respond to treatment in spite of the clinician's failing to adhere to sound treatment procedures. However, for a reasonably high rate of predictable success to be achieved, the principles for sound treatment cannot be ignored.

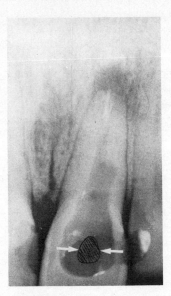

FIG. 23-44. Excessive coronal tooth loss as a result of overextended preparation. Arrows indicate the outline of a more conservative access opening.

Length determination

Of primary significance is the principle of locating *all* canals and determining their lengths and curvatures. Failure to properly measure the actual working length of the canal precludes the ability to properly clean and shape the canal. A tooth that is filled to improperly measured and shaped canals is an open invitation to ultimate failure: asymptomatic teeth can suddenly become symptomatic or symptoms in symptomatic teeth can refuse to abate.

Successful endodontic treatment requires the recleaning and reshaping of all canals whose unfilled spaces and foramina could be a source of periradicular infection. To prevent failure, one can modify the shape of the canal to fa-

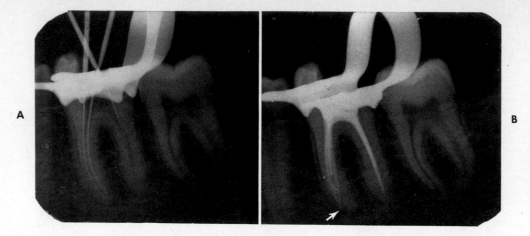

FIG. 23-45. Failure caused by not following the canal curvature. The result was an underextended filling. **A,** Length determination. **B,** Completed filling, well short of the apical foramen. There is a near perforation here *(arrow).*

cilitate the introduction of a filling substance that should obliterate the original as well as the modified canal space. If the modified canal space inhibits the sealing of the original canal, one can expect failure to lurk in the unfilled spaces. Inadequate cleaning and shaping make the filling procedure difficult and stir up, rather than evict, the microbial inhabitants. On the other hand, overinstrumentation can lead to root perforation, microbial inoculation, and patient aggravation. Fig. 23-45 shows the result of failing to follow the curvature and retain working length in mesial canals. Although length determination in the canals was acceptable, preparation failure probably occurred because of one or more of the following:

1. Failure to keep the correct working length with small precurved instruments
2. Failure to use each instrument to its fullest before proceeding to the next larger size
3. Failure to use the serial filing technique with recapitulation

Separated instruments

From time to time, even the most careful clinician will have an endodontic instrument fracture during root canal preparation. The patient *must* be advised of the presence of the instrument fragment, how it will affect the course of treatment, and what the ultimate prognosis for the tooth will be. The information should be given in such a manner as not to alarm the patient unduly. For this reason the endodontist refers to a fractured root canal file as a "separated" instrument. Fortunately today's stainless steel root canal instruments resist corrosion relatively well and can be incorporated into the finished root canal filling. The long-term prognosis depends on how well the canal can be sealed around the separated instrument.

Instruments with smaller diameters (nos. 10 to 25) may separate if they have been stressed in a previous operation. Therefore any of these instruments that have been used previously should be carefully checked with a magnifying class for a tendency of the flutes to "unwind." Most files

and reamers have triangular or square stock twisted into spiral flutes. Forcing the instrument into a small canal while rotating eventually unwinds and weakens the blade. Overheating the instrument during sterilization destroys the temper of the metal and makes the instrument more subject to fracture during use. Because loss of temper is difficult to detect, close attention should be given to the sterilization technique. Any instrument that has been bent sharply during use should be discarded immediately.

As the clinician progresses to the larger-diameter instruments (nos. 30, 35, 40), fracture may occur when the instrument is rotated in a curved canal. Instrument separation in the less flexible sizes can be prevented by straight line filing (i.e., avoiding the quarter turn that locks the instrument flutes in the dentin).

When an instrument separates in a canal, if it is lodged in the apical third, there is little likelihood it can be successfully removed from the canal. Occasionally it can be bypassed (Fig. 23-46). Enlarging the canal with small round burs to retrieve the instrument will frequently cause lateral perforation of the root. The use of barbed broaches to engage the fractured segment often will fracture the broach. Some of these separated instruments can be removed with a Masserann Kit.*

The safest method for removing a separated instrument is to attempt to bypass the segment with a no. 10 file after softening the dentin in the area with the calcium chelating agent EDTA. To administer an effective quantity of EDTA requires the canal be enlarged as far as the separated segment by a series of files or Gates-Glidden burs (Fig. 23-46, *A*). Before using EDTA, the clinician should dry the canal with paper points to eliminate any sodium hypochlorite that might be present. EDTA is a weak acid; and the presence of any strong base alters its pH, making it ineffective. The chelating agent should be left in the canal for 5 minutes before attempts are made to negotiate around the

---

*Medidenta Co., Woodside, N.Y.

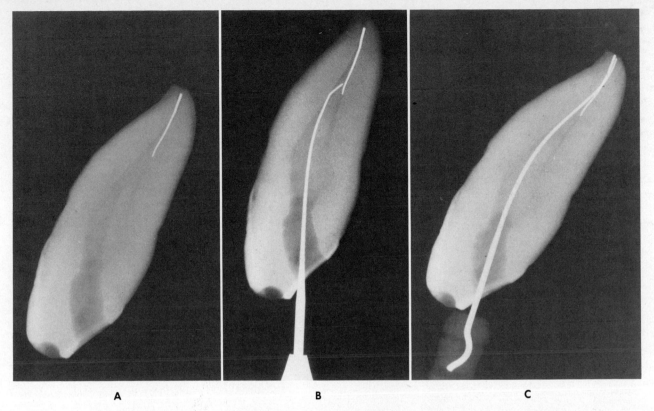

FIG. 23-46. A, Canal in which a file has separated. **B,** After use of no. 10 and no. 15 files, a no. 20 K-type file tip is bent to bypass the separated file. **C,** The separated file bypassed.

fractured instrument. A no. 10 file with a gentle bend at the tip is placed in the canal and with light apical pressure is rotated on quarter of a turn until the tip engages any slight space left between the canal wall and the separated instrument (Fig. 23-46, *B*). Gradually enlarging this space may allow the no. 10 file to pass around the fractured instrument segment (Fig. 23-46, *C*). To continue enlarging the space, the clinician selects a new no. 10 file and removes 1 mm of the instrument tip with a sharp nail clipper. Removing the tapered tip makes the working end of the file equivalent to a no. 15 file in diameter while retaining the flexibility of a no. 10 file. Removing the sharp tip also reduces the danger of the instrument's perforating the canal wall laterally. Once the blunted instrument goes to the working length, a no. 15 file can be used to enlarge the bypass. Use of the larger-diameter file in the bypass should not be attempted because severe canal distortions may result. Filling the canal with a warmed gutta-percha technique (Chapter 8) can be done once a no. 20 file goes to the working length.

Prognosis for teeth with separated instruments

In the apical third. The prognosis for teeth with separated instruments depends on several factors. If the instrument separates and obliterates the apical third of the canal, the prognosis may be quite good, particularly if the fragment is bypassed (Fig. 23-46, *C)* and warmed of diffused gutta-percha is condensed around it. If the stainless steel fragment cannot be bypassed, it may still effectively fill the canal if it lodges tightly and dentin shavings are packed ahead of it. To avoid possible litigation in the future, the dentist must advise the patient of the presence of the fractured instrument and the guarded prognosis.

In the middle third. When the instrument fractures in the middle third of the canal and canal space exists apical to the segment, the prognosis is much less favorable if the bypass cannot be accomplished. When the separation occurs in a root with two canals and the second canal is successfully bypassed, there is a chance for success if the canals have a common apical foramen. If an apical lesion develops later and the area can be approached surgically, a retrofilling procedure can be used.

Beyond the apical foramen. If the instrument separates beyond the apical foramen, the periapical portion should be removed. The protruding fragment acts like a mechanical irritant each time occlusal pressure is applied to the tooth (Fig. 23-47).

The apical third of the root is exposed through a surgical approach. When removing the bone, the clinician must exercise care not to engage the instrument protruding through the apical foramen with the bur. If he is able to see the separated instrument, he can sometimes force it back coronally into the canal by grasping it with a mosquito hemostat. The fragment may then be teased out of the canal access preparation with a small Hedström file. If the instrument cannot be forced back into the canal, the temptation to attempt to withdraw it apically should be resisted.

The taper on the instrument generally prevents such an apical withdrawal. A slot preparation is cut down to the instrument on the labial surface of the root apex with a no. ½ round bur (Fig. 23-48). Once its surface is visualized in the apical section, the instrument is bent labially and cut at the base of the preparation with the no. ½ round bur. The apex of the tooth is slightly beveled and the slot preparation completed before filling with amalgam. Warmed gutta-percha can be condensed around the fragment remaining in the canal through the coronal access.

Occasionally the separated instrument will lodge in the periapical region, as when the length determination has been inaccurate and the instrument tip becomes separated in the bone around the tooth apex. More often the separated instrument will be forced periapically from the canal

during the bypass procedure or while the root canal filling is being condensed. If periapical surgery is feasible, the instrument may be recovered during the curettage. Filling the root canal should be done prior to the curettage. If the quality of the root canal filling is questionable, retrograde filling can be included in the surgical procedure. When the separated instrument is associated with root apices where surgery is not advisable, the instrument tip can be left in

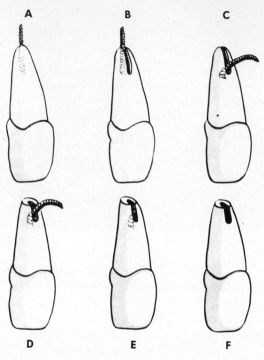

FIG. 23-48. A, Separated file protruding through the apical foramen. B, Slot preparation cut down to the instrument. C, Labial bendings. D, Beveled apex. E, Instrument cut off in the base of the slot preparation. F, Cavity preparation filled with amalgam.

FIG. 23-47. A, Separated file protruding through the apical foramen. B, File removed and the apex sealed with amalgam.

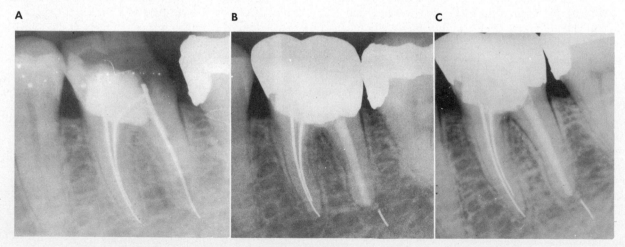

FIG 23-49 A, Mandibular molar with an overextended silver point. B, In attempting to solve the problem, the clinician left a fragment of silver point in the periapical region and filled the canal with gutta-percha. C, Eight months later the fragment appears to be encapsulated.

place. The stainless steel tip acts like a foreign body and becomes encapsulated with fibrous tissue. In the cases we have seen, migration of the instrument has not taken place. The patient should be advised that the area is to be checked radiographically on a regular basis.

Fig. 23-49 illustrates an attempt to re-treat a mandibular molar with an overextended silver point. Upon reinstrumentation of the distal canal, a separation of the section extending beyond the apical foramen took place. Since the 2 mm segment could not be recovered, the canal was filled with gutta-percha and the fragment of silver point was left in place (Fig. 23-49, *A* and *B*). An 8-month follow-up radiograph (Fig. 23-49, *C*) showed the encapsulated foreign body stabilized in the periapical region.

Canal filling

Failures caused by inadequacies in filling the canal are usually related to deficiencies in canal preparation, because well-cleaned-and-shaped root canals can be filled accurately. When complications are encountered in preparing the canal, the space often cannot be filled completely.

Underextension. Fillings that are short of the apical foramen fail for several reasons. The most obvious failures occur in teeth whose canals cannot be cleaned properly and organic debris left in the space. If the canal was originally cleaned but incompletely filled, tissue fluid breakdown products from the area can cause a chronic inflammatory response in the periapical tissue (Fig. 23-50).

Root canal fillings that are short can usually be readily

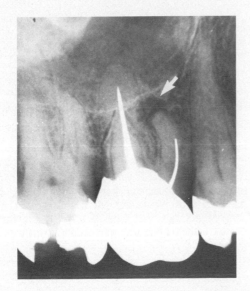

FIG. 23-50. Underfilled canal. The result was a periapical lesion *(arrow).*

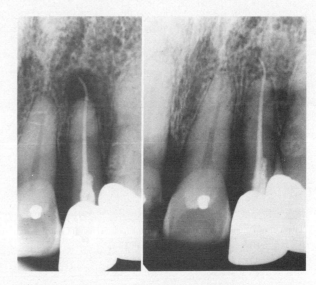

FIG. 23-51. Healing around an overextended gutta-percha filling.

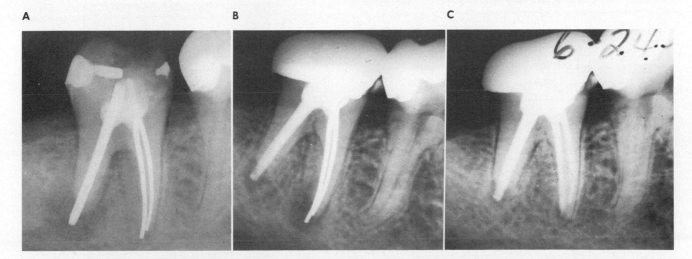

FIG. 23-52. A, Distal root with a periapical lesion resulting from an overextended silver point. **B,** The canal has been re-treated and filled with gutta-percha. The distal apical lesion is healing, but the periapical lesion around the mesial root (which is still filled with silver cones) is enlarging. **C,** Two years later. The mesial roots were re-treated and filled with gutta-percha. The periapical tissue is repairing well.

identified on the radiograph. If a lesion fails to heal or appears on the follow-up radiograph, re-treatment should be the first consideration. Gutta-percha can be removed with the aid of a solvent such as xylene; however, care must be exercised not to force the irritating solvents into the periapical tissue. To avoid forcing irritating fluids through the apical foramen, the clinician should leave a short section of gutta-percha intact in the apical third of the canal. This section can then be extracted with a file after all solvents are removed from the canal with paper points. Once the gutta-percha has been extracted, the canal should be completely cleaned and shaped. Refilling should be delayed until the clinician is sure there is no inflammatory response in the periapical tissues from the canal preparation.

Difficulties can be encountered in removing an inadequate root canal filling. For example, a firmly seated silver cone sometimes cannot be removed. A surgical approach

to the root apex may then be necessary to correct the short root canal filling.

Overextension. This is to be avoided whenever possible because it limits the biologic repair in the periapical region. Slight overextension with gutta-percha delays but usually does not prevent periapical healing (Fig. 23-51). If the surgical approach is not complicated, gross overextensions can be removed by apical curettage.

Overextension of silver points is a more serious deterrant to apical healing (Fig. 23-52). Silver points are usually extruded beyond the apical foramen because the master cone did not fit properly. Frequently teeth with silver points extending beyond the apical foramen are really underfilled because space exists between the canal walls and the silver cone (Fig. 23-53). An attempt should be made to remove the silver cone and reprepare the canal (Fig. 23-54).

Silver cone removal can be done by first working a no.

A

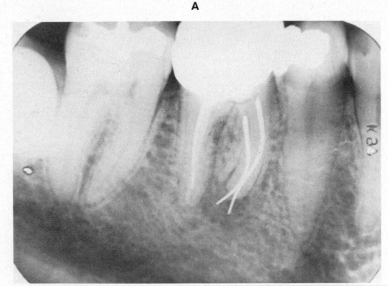

FIG. 23-53. Failure of treatment in the mesial-buccal root of a mandibular first molar probably due to overextension of (not overfilling with) silver cones. In addition, another foramen is demonstrated. **A,** Radiograph of the failure. **B,** Extracted root. **C,** View of the root apex with an additional foramen *(arrow)*. **D,** Radiograph demonstrating the foramen *(arrow)*.

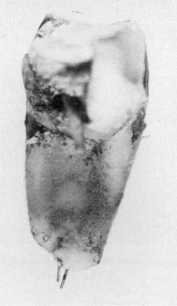

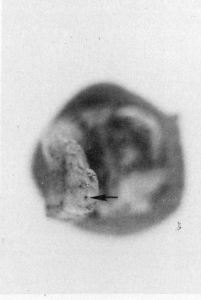

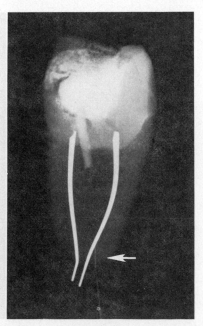

B   **C**   **D**

15 file alongside the silver point. In mandibular anteriors with oval canals the bypass can be readily accomplished. The Endosonic unit is used with a no. 15 file to break up the seal and elevate the silver point (Fig. 23-55, *A* and *B*). The canal system is reprepared and filled when the tooth is asymptomatic (Fig. 23-55, *C*). If attempts to remove the silver cone are fruitless, apical curretage and a retrofilling should be considered.

Master cone selection. Failures can occur when gutta-percha appears to fill the canal to the apical foramen but does not obliterate the canal space laterally. This type of failure can usually be traced back to a master cone that binds tightly in the coronal or middle third of the canal but fails to fill the apical third. The tugback resistance in these cases originates in the wrong area. Attempts to correct the situation by lateral condensation fail because accessory cones cannot be accurately passed into the apical third of the canal.

Fortunately failures of this type can be corrected by removing the gutta-percha and properly flaring the canal preparation. Fig. 23-56 shows an exaggerated case in which the master silver cone failed to fit all the dimensions of the canal.

Roots will occasionally split (vertical fracture) during the lateral or vertical condensation phase of endodontic treatment, usually with teeth that are being re-treated several years after the original root canal filling. Lateral or vertical condensation pressure with gutta-percha should not be excessive. Condensation in the coronal third likewise should be accomplished with caution. When a root splits, extraction is usually necessary.

Retrofilling technique for the palatal root of the maxillary first premolar

When an endodontic failure occurs on the palatal root of the maxillary first premolar, access to the area from a buccal approach often requires amputation of the buccal root. This is necessary for visualization of the buccal surface of the palatal root. The amputation should be performed in the middle third of the buccal root (Fig. 23-57).

With the buccal root tip removed, curettage of the palatal root lesion can be attempted. A conventional root canal cavity preparation is usually difficult on palatal roots. The slot preparation can be adapted when access to the area is limited. If the palatal root apex cannot be beveled, the slot may be prepared on the buccal surface of the root. The preparation is carried through the canal, and an alloy filling is placed to block the canal coronal to the apex.

Poor or faulty post technique

The preservation of internal tooth structure is very important when one is considering postendodontic restora-

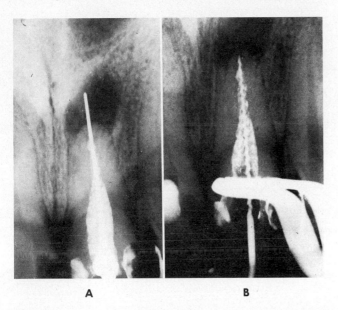

FIG. 23-54. A, Underfilling of the canal and an overextended silver point. **B,** Silver point removed from the canal. A Hedström file is used to remove old sealer.

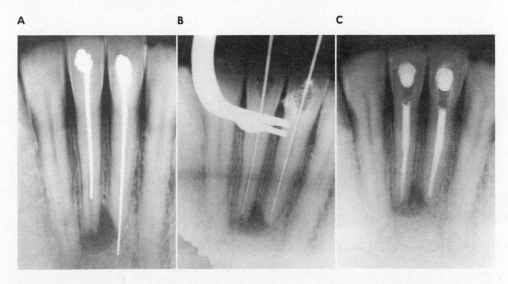

FIG. 23-55. Silver cone removal with the endosonic unit. **A,** Over- and underfilled canals with silver point. **B,** Points removed and length determination film. **C,** Canals refilled.

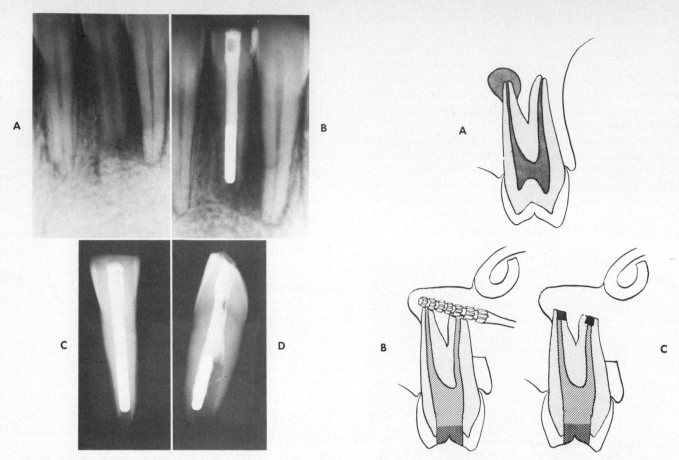

FIG. 23-56. A, Nonvital pulp with arrested root development. **B,** Tooth endodontically treated with silver point and zinc oxide–eugenol paste. **C,** Labiolingual view. **D,** Mesiodistal view. Note the open space lingual to the silver point. Tugback was obtained *only* in the mesial-distal dimension.

FIG. 23-57. A, Periapical lesion on the palatal root. **B,** Slot preparation made after apices beveled. **C,** Alloy fillings.

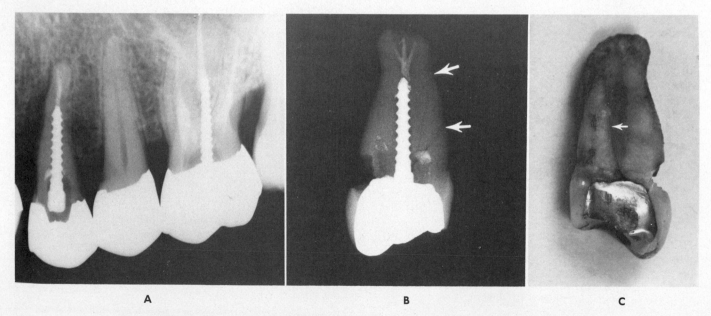

FIG. 23-58. Fractured maxillary first premolar. **A,** Note the extensive bone loss along the root extending almost to the apex. There was extensive mobility. **B,** Distal view showing a screw post and the resulting fractures *(arrows)* along with the trifurcation of the canal at the apex. **C,** Crack along the distal root surface *(arrow).*

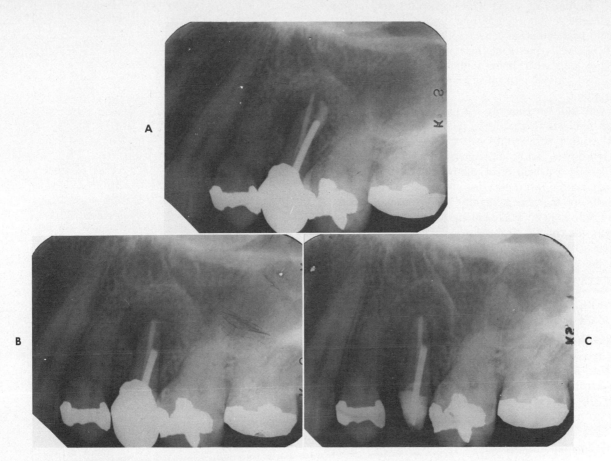

FIG. 23-59. Improper post placement in a maxillary second premolar due to perforation with a motor-driven instrument. **A,** Post perforation and excess filling material. **B,** Surgical intervention. No apparent defect after beveling of the post. **C,** One year postoperative healing.

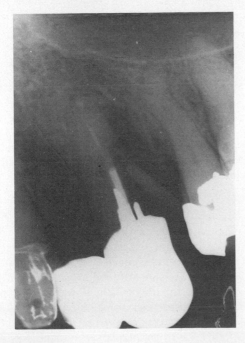

FIG. 23-60. Fracture of a maxillary canine with a short post and pin buildup.

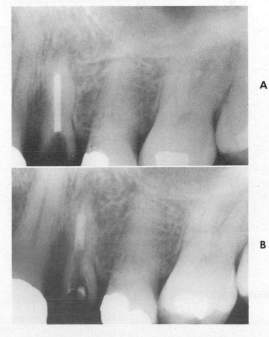

FIG. 23-61. Dowel removal with the endosonic unit. **A,** Fractured dowel. **B,** Dowel removed and canal retreated.

tions.[19] Failures can occur with large posts and improper post placement (Figs. 23-58 and 23-59). In addition, inadequate post extension can be source of failure (Fig. 23-60). It is usually preferable to employ heated instruments and large files and reamers initially to create post depth. Then motor-driven instruments can be used to refine the preparation.

Dowels will occasionally fracture within the canal and require removal (Fig. 23-61, *A* and *B*). Since they are placed with a permanent cement rather than sealer, the fractured dowel can be difficult to remove. Use of an ultrasonic unit can help break the cement seal. Placing the tip of a Cavitron instrument directly on the silver point butt may break up the cement slightly. Once the seal is broken, a no. 15 file may be worked alongside the dowel to further break up the cement. If the dowel cannot be grasped with a hemostat, a no. 35 inverted cone bur can be used to notch the dowel; the notched dowel can then be caught with an excavator and elevated out of the root canal.

FAILURES FROM OTHER CAUSES
Traumatic injury

Teeth that require endodontic treatment after traumatic injury have a higher failure rate than do teeth with pulpal problems of other origin. Severely luxated teeth, teeth replanted following avulsion, and teeth with root fractures in which the coronal segment is displaced are especially prone to fail despite satisfactory endodontic treatment. (See Chapter 15). Failure is related to injury of the attached apparatus that results in root resorption (Fig. 23-62).

Before treatment is instituted on traumatically injured teeth, the patient should be informed of the guarded prognosis and this fact should be recorded in the patient's treatment record.

The highest failure rate is encountered in teeth that have been completely avulsed and then replanted more than 30 minutes after the traumatic incident. With the destruction of the periodontal ligament, healing usually results in ankylosis. When the periodontal ligament does not intervene between the alveolar bone and the root cementum, resorption of cementum and dentin takes place. The rate at which this resorption occurs depends on whether it is an inflammatory or a replacement resorption: in the former, cementum and dentin are lost and inflammatory tissue remains in the void (Fig. 23-63); in the latter, bone replaces the lost tooth structure. (For further information regarding causes and treatment of root resorption, see Chapter 16).

Replacement resorption is a much slower process. Unfortunately the more rapid type of resorption seems to take place in the teeth of younger patients. The rapidity of resorption in the younger age group may be related to the higher metabolic rate in the tissues around the tooth. Any tooth that has been luxated presents similar problems in varying degrees. Again, the resorption depends on the extent of the damage to the periodontal ligament.

The incomplete vertical root fracture is one of the most difficult to diagnose. Radiographic evidence of the fracture usually is not demonstrated until bone resorption has had

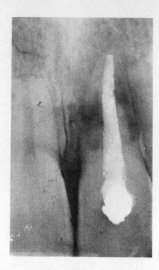

FIG. 23-62. Inflammatory resorption after replantation of a traumatically avulsed central incisor.

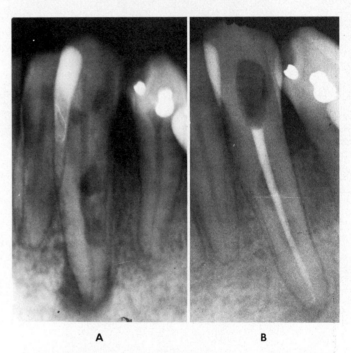

A   **B**

FIG. 23-63. A, Combined external resorption and apical inflammatory lesions. **B,** Endodontic treatment completed. External resorption has not perforated the canal space.

time to develop in the area of the fracture (Fig. 23-64). If pulpal symptoms develop in a tooth and no reason for symptoms can be found, an incomplete vertical fracture in the root system should be considered. If the tooth is more tender when released abruptly from occlusal pressure, it may mean that the periodontal ligament is being pinched as the fracture closes after being opened slightly by the occlusal pressure. The response to pressure is the basis for the glass bead test for an incomplete vertical root fracture. Extirpating the pulp (if it is vital) will reduce the symptoms of pulpitis but will not solve the basic cause for the pulpitis. If the tooth continues to be sensitive to pressure,

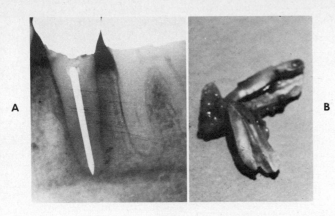

FIG. 23-64. A, Incomplete vertical fracture. Note the typical halolike bone resorption pattern. **B,** Extracted tooth. Note the fracture.

the root canal treatment should not be completed. Often the fracture will develop to the point where a part of the crown becomes mobile. The clinician should extract the mobile segment and attempt to restore the remaining tooth structure. If coronal restoration is not feasible, extraction of the tooth is the only alternative (Fig. 23-65).

Paste root canal fillings cannot be placed with the same degree of accuracy as solid core fillings. Overfilling can easily occur when the apical foramen is transported (Fig. 23-66). When the paste material is toxic, acute inflammation in the periapical tissues often occurs. The ZOE paste containing paraformaldehyde and steroids advocated by Sargenti has been shown to be strongly cytotoxic in tissue culture studies and biopsy material taken from the periapical tissues of overfilled canals.[1,4,13]

Endodontic-periodontal lesions

Treatment of teeth in which there appears to be both pulpal and periodontal disease is difficult. When an apical lesion extends along a root to the alveolar crest, it is necessary to determine whether the primary disease was pulpal or periodontal. The causes, diagnosis, and treatment of endodontic-periodontal lesions are described in Chapter 17.

Failures in this category can usually be attributed to an incorrect diagnosis or treatment of the primary and secondary factors associated with an endodontic-periodontal lesion.

Intentional replantation

There are times when re-treatment of a failure by routine or surgical endodontic therapy is extremely difficult. After all other treatment modalities have been considered and excluded, intentional replantation may be attempted.

Because the incidence of external resorption is high in replanted teeth, the success rate is lower than for conventional endodontic therapy. However, resorption seems to occur less rapidly in older age groups and when the tooth is out of the alveolus for only a few minutes. Since the tooth must be delivered from the socket intact, careful case selection is necessary.

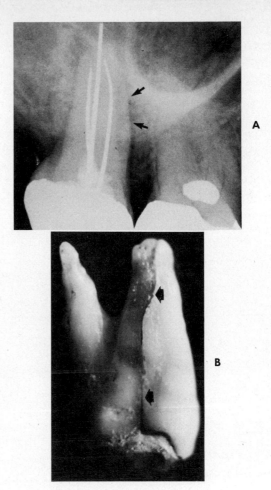

FIG. 23-65. Incomplete vertical fracture. **A,** Slight halolike radiolucency on the mesial-buccal root *(arrows)* indicating incomplete fracture of the root. **B,** Extracted tooth. Note the extent of the fracture *(arrows).*

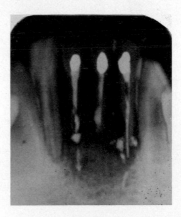

FIG. 23-66. Overfill with paraformaldehyde-steroid paste.

Fig. 23-67 illustrates a case of intentional replantation. Perforations were present in the apical third of the root and in the cervical area. The tooth was extracted, and repair of the perforations was accomplished effectively. Before replantation the cervical epithelial attachment was excised to prevent the tissue from proliferating apically during healing (''creviculectomy''). Once the tooth was replaced in the socket, it was splinted with a periodontal dressing and checked for occlusal interferences. Healing was uneventful.

Unknown causes

Occasionally failures will appear even after what might be considered ideal therapy. Some cases may fail after a relatively short time (Fig. 23-68); others may be successful for many years and then fail (Fig. 23-69). The etiology of these failures is difficult to rationalize and often open to speculation.

SUMMARY

We have discussed some of the more significant factors that contribute to endodontic failures. We hope the informed clinician will avoid these pitfalls and be able to enjoy the personal gratification of predictably successful endodontic treatment.

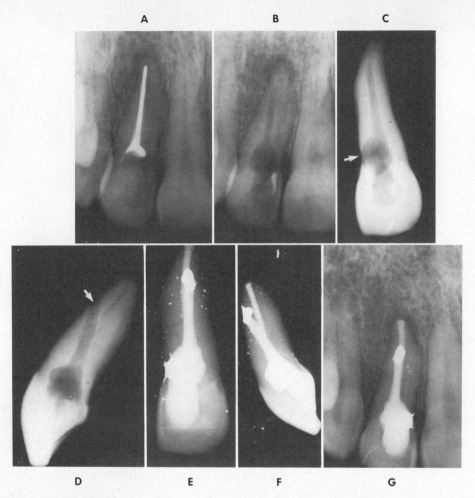

FIG. 23-67. Intentional replantation for endodontic failures. **A,** Maxillary lateral incisor filled with silver point. Development of an apical lesion indicates failure. **B,** Silver point removed. Perforation is apparent in the apical third of the root and the cervical area. **C,** Labial-lingual view. Arrow shows the cervical perforation. **D,** Mesial-distal view, arrow showing the apical perforation. **E** and **F,** Perforations repaired and the canal filled. **G,** Tooth replanted. (**B** courtesy Dr. Francis Howell.)

FIG. 23-69. Mandibular first molar with eventual failure of treatment in the distal root (after 30 *years* of success). **A,** Following completion of the initial endodontics performed approximately 30 years previously. A chronic abscess with a sinus tract was now clinically evident at the distal root apex. **B,** Following apicoectomy in the oral surgery office. The sinus tract reappeared after several months because the surgeon had failed to place an apical seal. **C,** Following removal of the silver points the sinus tract would not resolve itself even with Ca(OH)$_2$ therapy. It was speculated that there was a defect or crack in the root. A decision was made to complete the root canal filling and do another apicoectomy. Root canals were filled with gutta-percha and sealer. **D,** Immediately after the second apicoectomy. **E,** One year postoperative, healing complete.

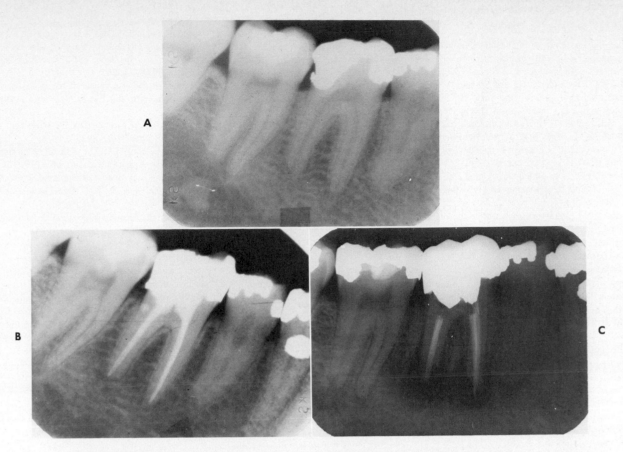

FIG. 23-68. Mandibular first molar of a 20-year-old man requiring endodontic therapy due to vital pulp expoxure. **A,** Initially. **B,** Immediately postoperative. **C,** Five years postoperative. Note the extreme apical resorption of both roots. Biopsy confirmed the diagnosis of periapical granulomas.

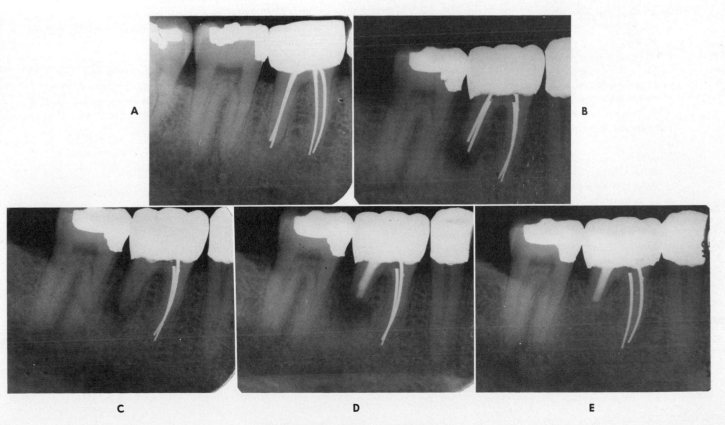

FIG. 23-69. For legend see opposite page.

REFERENCES

1. Antrim, D.: Evaluation of the cytotoxicity of root canal sealing agents on tissue cells in vitro: Grossman's sealer, N_2 (permanent), Richert's sealer and Cavit, J. Endod. **2:**111, 1976.
2. Bender, I.B., Seltzer, S., and Soltanoff, W.: Endodontic success—a reappraisal of criteria, Oral Surg. **22:**780, 1966.
3. Benjaminm, K., and Dowson, J.: Incidence of two root canals in human mandibular incisor teeth, Oral Surg. **38:**122, 1974.
4. Block, R.M., Pascon, E.A., and Longeland, K.: Paste technique retreatment study: a clinical, histopathologic and radiographic evaluation of 50 cases, Oral Surg. **60:**76, 1985.
5. Burch, J.G., and Hulen, S.: A study of the presence of accessory foramina and the topography of molar furcations, Oral Surg. **38:**451, 1974.
6. Frank, A.L., and Weiner, J.M.: Clinical studies in endodontics, University of Southern California, 1973. (Unpublished data.)
7. Gelfand, M., Sundeman, E.J., and Goldman, M.: Reliability of radiographical interpretations, J. Endod. **9:**71, 1983.
8. Goldman, M., Pearson, A.H., and Darzenta, N.: Endodontic success—who's reading the radiograph? Oral Surg. **33:**432, 1972.
9. Green, D.: Morphology of the pulp cavity of permanent teeth, Oral Surg. **8:**743, 1955.
10. Green, D.: A stereomicroscopic study of the root apices of 400 maxillary and mandibular anterior teeth, Oral Surg. **9:**1224, 1956.
11. Grossman, L.I., editor: Transactions, Fifth International conference on Endodontics, Philadelphia, 1973, University of Pennsylvania.
12. Kessler, J., Peters, D., and Lorten, L.: Comparison of the relative risk of molar root perforations using various endodontic instrumentation techniques, J. Endod. **9:**439, 1983.
13. Langeland, K., Debate: Is N_2 an acceptable method of treatment? Transactions of the Third International Conference on Endodontics, Philadelphia, 1963.
14. Lowman, J.V., Burke, R.S., and Pelleu, G.B.: Patent accessory canals: incidence in molar furcation region, Oral Surg. **36:**580, 1973.
15. Madeira, M.C., and Hetem, S.: Incidence of bifurcations in mandibular incisors, Oral Surg. **36:**589, 1973.
16. Mueller, A.H.: Anatomy of the root canals of the incisors, cuspids and bicuspids of the permanent teeth, Am. Dent. Assoc. J. **20:**1361, 1933.
17. Pineda, F.: Roentgenographic investigation of the mesiobuccal root of the maxillary first molar, Oral Surg. **36:**253, 1973.
18. Pomeranz, H.H., and Fishelberg, G.: The secondary mesiobuccal canal of maxillary molars, J. Am. Dent. Assoc. **88:**119, 1974.
19. Seidberg, B.H., et al.: Frequency of two mesiobuccal root canals in maxillary permanent first molars, J. Am. Dent. Assoc. **87:**852, 1973.
20. Serene, T.: Technique for the location and length determination of calcified canals, J. Calif. Dent. Assoc., October, 1976.
21. Shafer, W.G., Hine, M.K., and Levy, A.B.: A textbook of oral pathology, ed. 4, Philadelphia, 1983, W.B. Saunders Co.
22. Skidmore, A.E., and Bjorndal, A.M.: Root canal morphology of the human mandibular first molar, Oral Surg. **32:**778, 1971.
23. Slowey, R.R.: Radiographic aids in the detection of the extra root canals, Oral Surg. **37:**762, 1974.
24. Trabert, K.C., Caputo, A.A., and Abou-Rass, M.: Tooth fracture—a comparison of endodontic and restorative treatment, J. Endod. **4:**341, 1978.
25. Vertucci, F.J.: Root canal anatomy of the mandibular anterior teeth, J. Am. Dent. Assoc. **89:**369, 1974.
26. Weine, F.S.: Endodontic therapy, ed. 3, St. Louis, 1982, The C.V. Mosby Co.
27. Zillich, R., and Dowson, J.: Root canal morphology of mandibular first and second premolars, Oral Surg. **36:**738, 1973.

Self-assessment questions

1. In formulating a diagnosis, one must remember that
   a. A combination of tests rather than a single test is more reliable
   b. Many oral lesions appear similar to endodontic lesions
   c. Generally, nonendodontic lesions present teeth that are usually vital and asymptomatic
   d. All of the above
2. What percent of mandibular incisors have two canals with independent foramina?
   a. 1%
   b. 10%
   c. 20%
   d. 30%
3. What is the most common neoplasm in the oral cavity?
   a. Osteosarcoma
   b. Fibrosarcoma
   c. Squamous cell carcinoma
   d. Adenocarcinoma
4. If an "extra" canal is suspected, what can the clinician do to confirm its presence?
   a. Take an additional radiograph from a mesial or distal horizontal angulation
   b. Alter the access opening in an apical direction
   c. Increase the radiographic angle in the vertical plane
   d. Evaluate a bite-wing radiograph of the pulp chamber
5. Canal calcification
   a. Generally indicates a poor prognosis for retention of the tooth
   b. Is generally managed with burs
   c. Is most frequently observed with developmental diseases
   d. May require the use of a chelating agent for treatment
6. Sudden narrowing of the root canal in the radiograph generally indicates
   a. Obliteration of the canal
   b. A branching or dividing canal
   c. Artifact on the radiograph
   d. Dystrophic calcification
7. Treatment of internal resorption
   a. Is deferred until symptoms develop
   b. Is arrested by pulpotomy and calcium hydroxide therapy
   c. Is complicated by the inflammatory tissue within the resorbed area
   d. Requires lateral condensation of gutta-percha to fill the resorbed area
8. An underextended access preparation
   a. Provides adequate access to all canals
   b. Prevents straight line access to the canals
   c. Allows for adequate debridement of the pulp chamber
   d. Allows adequate vision for possible additional canals

9. Fracture of a root canal file can be minimized by
   a. Not stressing the file and allowing the flutes to "unwind"
   b. Using full turns (360-degree rotation) within the canal
   c. Using the instrument numerous times
   d. Sharply bending the instrument before inserting it into the canal

10. The prognosis for nonsurgical intervention for teeth with broken instruments is good when
    a. The instrument fragment is in the middle third and cannot be bypassed
    b. The instrument fragment obliterates the apical third of the canal
    c. The instrument fractures beyond the apical foramen
    d. The instrument is smaller than a no. 20

11. Failures caused by inadequate filling of the canal can result from
    a. Underfilling and leaving organic debris in the unfilled space
    b. Overextending and underfilling a canal with silver points
    c. Obtaining master cone reistance in the wrong area
    d. All of the above

12. Which statement describes the failure rate following traumatic injuries?
    a. Failure is related to injury of the pulp
    b. The lowest failure rate is in teeth that have been completely avulsed and replanted
    c. Failure is generally in the form of inflammatory or replacement resorption
    d. Resorption progresses slower in younger patients

13. Incomplete vertical root fractures
    a. Can be demonstrated radiographically in their early stages
    b. Present no difficulty in diagnosis
    c. Should be considered when pulpal symptoms develop from no apparent cause
    d. Are solved by extirpating the symptomatic pulp

14. Intentional replantation
    a. Has a success rate equal to conventional endodontic therapy
    b. Has a low incidence of external resorption
    c. Requires careful case selection since the tooth must be extracted intact
    d. Is considered as a routine endodontic procedure

PART FOUR

HISTORY AND PHILOSOPHY OF ENDODONTICS

24

HISTORY

JAMES L. GUTMANN

So, when disease invades the arch,
And strides in anguish on his angry march,
His burning touch, like the electric flame
Flashes through every fibre of the frame

Solyman Brown, *Dentologia*, 1840[15]

DERIVATION OF "DENTIST"

Early history tells us that physicians, other medical practitioners, and barbers were identified with the practice of dentistry. Weinberger[76] relates that as long ago as 3000 BC, the Egyptians suggested that physicians who were more adept in the treatment of dental disease should be distinguished from other physicians. They were identified in Egyptian hieroglyphics by an eye followed by a tusk (representing a tooth) or by a bird and a tusk. These symbols have been translated as "treater or maker of teeth," "tooth worker," and "great one of the toothers." Later, Greek writers used the term "dental physician" (and Latin used *dentalis medicus* or *dentarius medicus,* meaning the specialized medical practitioner).[71]

The first definition of a dental practitioner appears in a book written in 1687 by Charles Allen of York; today this work is designated as the first English dental book (Fig. 24-1). On the cover appears the inscription *The Operator for the Teeth* with a claim by the author that he was the "professor of the same."[71]

In 1622 the title of "surgeon dentist" was given by the French to Gillies and several other men. A slight change to "dental surgeon" was introduced in 1840, when the Baltimore College of Dental Surgery graduated its first class (of two surgeons). The bestowed degree was Chirurgiae Dentium Doctor, which abbreviated would be C.D.D., although the translated initials D.D.S. have always been used. Now, in the twentieth century, the degree of Doctor of Dental Medicine (D.M.D.) is thought by some to be more appropriate.

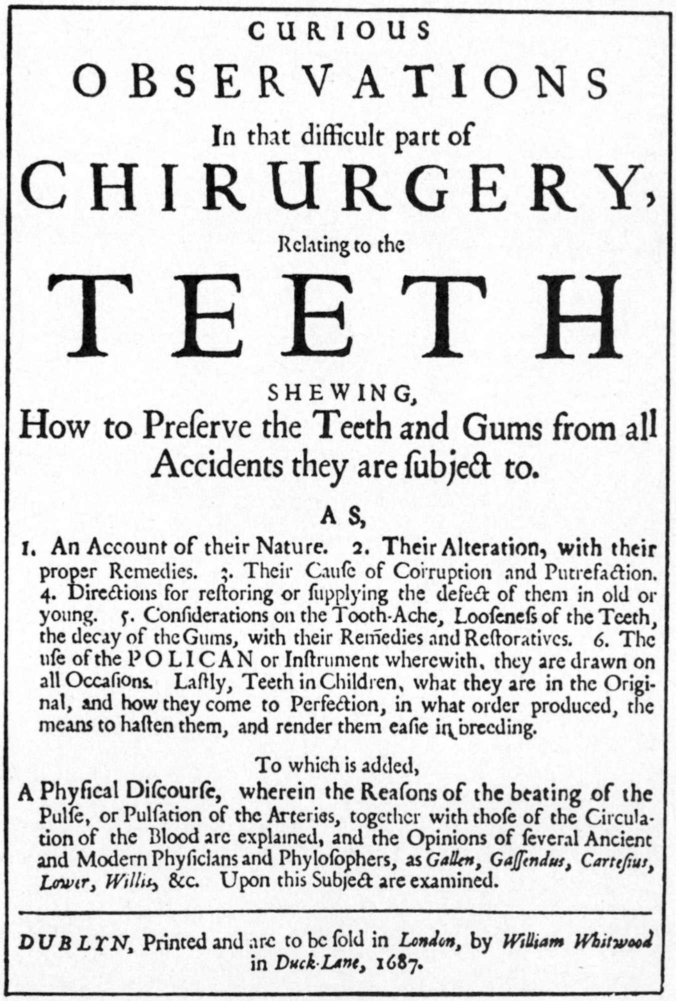

CURIOUS
OBSERVATIONS
In that difficult part of
CHIRURGERY,
Relating to the
TEETH
SHEWING,
How to Preserve the Teeth and Gums from all Accidents they are subject to.

A S,

1. An Account of their Nature. 2. Their Alteration, with their proper Remedies. 3. Their Cause of Corruption and Putrefaction. 4. Directions for restoring or supplying the defect of them in old or young. 5. Considerations on the Tooth-Ache, Looseness of the Teeth, the decay of the Gums, with their Remedies and Restoratives. 6. The use of the POLICAN or Instrument wherewith, they are drawn on all Occasions. Lastly, Teeth in Children, what they are in the Original, and how they come to Perfection, in what order produced, the means to hasten them, and render them easie in breeding.

To which is added,

A Physical Discourse, wherein the Reasons of the beating of the Pulse, or Pulsation of the Arteries, together with those of the Circulation of the Blood are explained, and the Opinions of several Ancient and Modern Physicians and Phylosophers, as *Gallen, Gassendus, Cartesius, Lower, Willis,* &c. Upon this Subject are examined.

DUBLYN, Printed and are to be sold in *London,* by *William Whitwood* in *Duck-Lane,* 1687.

FIG. 24-1. Reproduction of the title page of a pamphlet on dental surgery by Charles Allen, published in London in 1687. (From Weinberger, B.W.: An introduction to the history of dentistry, vol. 1, St. Louis, 1948, The C.V. Mosby Co.)

756

DERIVATION OF "ENDODONTICS"

In the latter part of the nineteenth and the first part of the twentieth century, endodontics was referred to as root canal therapy or pathodontia.[42] Dr. Harry B. Johnston, of Atlanta, Georgia, was well known in the early twentieth century as a lecturer and clinician in root canal therapy, and for his lectures and demonstrations of a modified version (his own) of the Callahan root canal treatment and filling, which became known as the Johnston-Callahan technique. In 1928 he terminated his association with Dr. Thomas Hinman and began his own practice; this was the first practice to be "limited to endodontics." Johnston coined the term endodontics, from the Greek *en,* in or within, and *odous,* tooth: the process of working within the tooth.

Formation of the American Association of Endodontists

In 1943 when a group of men met in Chicago to form an association of dental practitioners interested in root canal therapy, they used the term "endodontics" and called the organization the American Association of Endodontists. They envisioned endodontics as becoming a special area of dental practice. In an editorial that appeared in the first issue of the *Journal of Endodontia* in 1946, Dr. Balint Orban highlighted the need for the pursuit of quality within this emerging specialty.[57]

Today after much work and thought, things are looking brighter. The "endodontist" is not any more a rebel against the ruling of "science" but a recognized specialist of dentistry. The technique has been refined to such a degree that it gives standing to the dentist even in the eyes of the medical profession, and safety to the patient. Since root canal treatment has been elevated to the status of a specialty, those who intend to do this work must adequately prepare themselves for it.

By 1963, more than 200 dentists were limiting their practice to endodontics.[37] Because of the remarkable growth and development of endodontics during the previous 25 years, and because of the untiring efforts of leaders in the American Association of Endodontists, the American Dental Association recognized endodontics as a special area of dentistry in 1963. The first examination and certification of diplomates occured 2 years later, in 1965.[50]

ENDODONTICS—ITS DEFINITION AND SCOPE OF ACTIVITY

The current definition and scope of the specialty of endodontics[1] is as follows:

That branch of dentistry which is concerned with the morphology, physiology, and pathology of the human dental pulp and periradicular tissues. Its study and practice encompass the basic and clinical sciences including the biology of the normal pulp, and the etiology, diagnosis, prevention, and treatment of diseases and injuries of the pulp and associated periradicular conditions.

Included in the scope of knowledge and skill in the clinical discipline of endodontics are: the differential diagnosis of pain of pulpal and/or periapical origin as well as other maxillofacial, cephalic or chest pains referred to the oral region; the control of pain emanating from the pulp and/or periapical region,; treatment by pulp capping or pulpotomy as well as by pulpectomy, canal debridement and preparation, and obturation of the root canal space; selective surgical removal of pathological tissues resulting from pulpal pathosis; replantation; hemisection; root amputation; endodontic implants; and the bleaching of discolored teeth.

Endodontics as an academic discipline is also responsible for the advancement of endodontic knowledge through research, the transmission of information concerning advances in biologically acceptable procedures and materials, and the education of the public and profession as to the importance of endodontics in keeping the dentition in a physiologically functional state for the maintenance of oral and systemic health.

While this definition has undergone periodic scrutiny and updating, and the reader can fully comprehend its ramifications, it is often the roots of these concepts that have remained an enigma. It is for this reason that an overview and, sometimes, an in-depth exploration of our early beginnings are in order. Oftentimes humorous, yet painfully serious, it is from these anecdotal records that a true appreciation of the art and science of modern endodontics is gained. To this end, let us begin.

CURE OF TOOTHACHE

> For there was never yet philosopher
> That could endure the toothache patiently
>
> Shakespeare, *Much Ado About Nothing*
> Act V, Scene I, Lines 35-36

As recorded in medical history, toothache has been the scourge of the ages. Many unusual remedies have been described; and it is quite evident that necessity, instinct, and mere chance have taught civilizations the means to usual and unusual "cures." On Egyptian tablets, in Hebrew Bibles, and from Chinese, Greek, and Roman medical writings are recorded descriptions and causes of this scourge.

The Ebers papyrus,[21] written about 1500 BC, contained the recipe for a medicament for "curing the gnawing of the blood in the tooth." The ingredients to be used included

The fruit of the Gebu plant—one thirty-second part
Onion—one sixty-fourth part
Cake—one sixteenth part
Dough—one eighth part
Anest plant—one thirty-second part
Water—one-half part

This was left to stand and then chewed for 4 days.

Pliny, a noted Roman writer, offered many popular methods for dealing with a toothache[67]:

In the fuller's thistle, an herb which grows near rivers, is found a small worm which has the power of curing dental pains, when the said worm is killed by rubbing it on the teeth, or when it is closed up with wax in the hollow teeth.

It is considered very beneficial for toothache to bite off a piece from wood which has been struck by lightening, and to touch the sick tooth with it; but whilst biting off the little piece of wood, it is necessary to keep both hands behind the back

A remedy for toothache is to touch the diseased teeth with the tooth of a Hyena . . . or to scratch the gums with the tooth of a hippopotamus which has been taken from the left side of the jaw.

It is beneficial against tooth to chew the root of panax, and to wash the teeth with its juice. It is also useful to chew the root of hyoscyamus soaked in vinegar, or else that of polemonium.[29]

It is said that if senecio be taken from the earth, and the aching tooth be touched three times with it, spitting alternatively three times, and then the herb be replanted in the same spot, so that it may continue to live, the tooth will never give pain any more.[29]

The pain on the teeth is lessened by picking the gums with the bones of the sea dragon. It is also very beneficial to pick the gums with the sharp bone of the puffin. If the same be pounded together with white hillebore, and the mixture thus obtained be rubbed on the diseased teeth, they may be made to fall out without pain. The ashes, also, of salt fish burnt in an earthen vase, with the addition of powdered marble, is a remedy against toothache. Frogs are also boiled in a hemina (0.274 liter) of vinegar, the decoction being then used to wash the teeth with; but this however, must be kept in the mouth for some time. In order to render this remedy less nauseous, Sallustium Dianisius used to hang several frogs, by their hind feet, over a vase in which he boiled the vinegar, so that the juices of the animals might drip into this from their mouths . . . 36 hearts of frogs are well boiled in a sextary of old oil, in a copper vessel, and the oil is then used against toothache, dropping it into the ear, on the side of the pain. Some, after having boiled the liver of frog, pound it with honey, and smear it on the sore teeth. If the teeth are decayed and fetid, many counsel the drying of a hundred frogs in an oven, leaving them there for one night, then the addition of an equal weight of salt, reducing the whole to powder, and rubbing the teeth with it.[29]

Archigenes of Apamea (a Syrian city), who lived in Rome in the latter part of the first century, was well known as a physician and operator and distinguished himself with his daring trepanations.[29] He recommended various remedies for odontalgia, including a mouthwash made by boiling gallnuts and hallicacabum in vinegar, and a concoction of roasted earthworms and spikenard ointment mixed with crushed eggs of spiders. His principal statement regarding dentistry was that odontalgia, in certain cases, was related to a disease in the anterior part of the tooth.

From the Middle Ages are recorded accounts of many "improved" methods of relieving the aching tooth. There was still a strong belief during this time that tooth decay was caused by presence of tooth "worms."

In an ancient Babylonian epic,[39] the worm comes weeping to the goddess Ea, asking what is to be its food and, on being told that it is to have fruits for sustenance, cries out[41]:

> Me! What are these ripe figs to me,
> and soft pomegranates?
> Lift me up, between the teeth and the
> jaw bone set me,
> That I may destroy the blood of the teeth,
> And ruin their strength,
> Grasp the prong and seize the root.

The priest-physician Andrew Boorde,[12] who achieved fame in the late fifteenth century, described his own unique "deworming technique":

And if it (toothache) do come by wormes, make a candell of waxe with Henbane sedes and lyght it and let the perfume of the candell entre into the toth and gape over a dyshe of cold water and than you may take the wormes out of the water and kyll them on your nayle.

Abulcasis (1050-1122)—known as abir-al-Qasim Khalaf ibu ('Abbas al-Zahrowi)—controlled toothaches through the use of cautery. He inserted a red-hot needle into the pulp through a tube which was designed to protect the surrounding structures.[66] Guy de Chauliac, a famous medieval surgeon, used a mixture of camphor, sulfur, myrrh, and asafetida as a filling material to cure toothache caused by worms.[76] In Bohemia in the eleventh century the Regimen Sanitatis Salernitarium contained the following verse (recommending the use of Henbane):

Sic dentes serva, porrorum college grana,
Ne careas thure cum hyoscyamo ure,
Sicque per embotum fumum cape dente remotum.

The 1607 English version follows:

If in your teeth you hap to be tormented
By meane some little wormes therein to breed,
Which pain (it need be tane) may be prevented,
By keeping cleane your teeth, when as you feede;
Burn Francomsence (a gum no evil sented),
Put Henbane unto this; and Onyon seed,
And with a funnel to the tooth that's hollow
Convey the smoke thereof, and ease shall follow.[39]

In the later Middle Ages, French anatomist Ambrose Paré (1517-1592) wrote:

Toothache is, of all others, the most atrocious pain that can torment a man, being followed by death. Erosion [caries] is the effect of an acute and acrid humor. To combat this, one must recourse to cauterization . . . By means of cauterization . . . one burns the nerve, thus rendering it incapable of again feeling or causing pain.[29]

The physician for the Imperial Baths at Carlsbad, Johann Stephan Strabelbergen (1630), used oil of vitriol or a concoction made of a frog cooked in vinegar to kill worms in teeth. Lazarre Rivierre was the first to recommend a remedy that is still being used for toothache: placing a small piece of cotton moistened with oil of cloves in the cavity. He altered this with oil or camphor of oil or boxwood.[76]

John Aubrey (1626-97), in his book *Brief Lives,* reflects on bits of folklore designed to cure the toothache[22]:

To cure the Tooth-ach, Take a new Nail, and make the Gum bleed with it, and then drive it into an Oak. This did Cure William Neal, Sir William Neal's Son, a very stout Gentleman, when he was almost Mad with the Pain, and had a mind to have Pistoll'd himself.

A history of the remedies used to combat toothache

would be incomplete if it did not include the suggestions of the "founder of modern dentistry," Pierre Fauchard.

Guerini[29] translates from *Le Chirurgien Dentiste*, written in 1728 by Fauchard:

Some pretend to cure toothache with an elixer of some special essence; others with plaster; others by means of prayers and signing of the cross; others with specifics for killing the worms which are supposed to gnaw the tooth and so cause pain; others pretend to be so clever that they can cure the most inveterate toothache by merely touching the tooth with a finger dipped into or washed with some rare and mysterious liquid; finally, they promise to cure every kind of toothache by scarifying the ears with a lancet or cauterizing them with a hot iron.

Finally, Fauchard speaks of another remedy, assuring his readers that with this remedy many persons who have had almost all of their teeth decayed and who suffered very often from toothache have found great relief:

It consists of rinsing the mouth every morning and also before going to bed with a spoonful of one's own urine immediately after it has been emitted, always provided the individual be not ill. One is to hold it in the mouth for some time and the practice ought to be continued. This remedy is good, but undoubtedly not pleasant, except so far that it produces great relief. It is rather difficult in the beginning to accustom one's self to it. But what would not one do to secure his health and repose.

To explain the virtue of the urine as a remedy, Fauchard explains its chemical composition and then adds:

The rectified spirit of urine [liquid ammonis] could be substituted for the human urine and one should then take two drams of this substance and mix it with two or three ounces of aqua vital, or water of cresses, or of cochlearea. Sal volatile [ammonium carbonate] has the same virtues. Those who wish to make use of it should dissolve fifteen or thirty grains of it in the same quantity of the same liquid.

Fauchard goes on to speak of trepanation of the teeth when they are worn away or decayed and causing pain. He begins by saying: "Most of the varieties of pain caused by the canines and the incisors when worn away, or decayed, cease after the use of the trepan." He uses the word trepan in a wide sense, meaning any instrument (even a needle or a pin) with which "one penetrates into the inner cavity of the teeth."

In 1756 L.B. Lenter, a German, wrote a pamphlet in which he recommended electricity as a means of curing toothache.[29] Other writers recommended the use of a magnet as an alternative.

In 1770 Thomas Berdmore published his *Treatise on the Disorders and Deformities of the Teeth and Gums*. In it he addressed various causes of toothache and its cure. When the toothache was caused by "obstructions and inflammation of the nerves and vascular parts of the tooth," the treatment indicated was "counter-impression" and sedatives—primarily to divert the mind from the "disordered nerve." In practice the burning of the ear with a hot iron was performed to serve as a "counter-impression." To Berdmore, however, this treatment was unacceptable:

For my own part, I do not approve of such treatment. I know it is not often attended with success; and even where it is, the relief is only for a moment: for it is owing to the terror and agitation of mind naturally connected with the idea of burning, more than to any pretend connection of nerves: and I have, in my own practice, seen people relieved of pain on the appearance of the surgeon, and by the dread of the operation, as often as any man can pretend to have (been) cured by the actual cautery applied in such a manner. I would never advise, therefore, to amuse the patient with such a precarious experiment, whilst more rational and more effectual methods may be used. . . .[7]

In his book published in 1794, Raniere Gerbi, a professor at the University of Pisa, recommended a very singular cure for a violent toothache. Under the name circulio anteodontalgicies [*sic*] he described an insect living habitually in the flowers of the *Cardisus spinosimus* that could be used to great advantage against a toothache in the following manner:

One crushes fourteen or fifteen larvae of the insect between the thumb and forefinger, and then rubs the two fingers together until the matter remaining upon them is entirely absorbed. Instead of the larvae, one may use fully developed insects. One then applies the two fingers that have crushed the insects, or their larvae, upon the decayed and aching tooth. If the pain is of a nature to be cured by this means, it diminishes almost spontaneously and ceases altogether in a few minutes. It is said that the fingers preserve their healing power for a great length of time, even a whole year.[29]

Other medical practitioners of this era in other countries described similar procedures using different types of insects.

Dental "scientists" were still pursuing the elusive "tooth worm"; while no scientific accounts actually exist which support its presence, the Chinese dentists, especially, are said to understand how to make superstitions pay. When a patient with the toothache presents himself, they (the dentists) are in the habit of making an incision into the gums "to let the worms out." For this purpose they employ an instrument that has a hollow handle filled with artificial worms. When the incision is made, the operator, by a dexterous turn of the instrument, drops the worms into the mouth; the excitement of the patient and the loss of blood cause at least a temporary relief. The worms were then collected, dried and ready to be taken out of the next patient's gum.[51] (Entrepreneurism at its finest!)

In 1883 F.H. Balkwill of England attempted to scientifically explain the causes of pain in teeth without pulps that exhibited "no evidence of pericemental irritation."[5]

. . . these used to be regarded as teeth of especial suspicion. The conditions of danger are, I think, pretty generally recognised. The pulp chamber is occupied by a fluid in a state of putrescent fermentation, as sufficiently evidenced by its smell, with the presence of bacteria. If any of the putrescent fluid is retained in the apices of the pulp cavity when the tooth is stopped, matter is formed in the periosteum commencing at these apices, which having no outlet, forms an abscess with the attending inflammation. It has been often stated in our current literature that decomposition going on in the putrescent fluid, liberates gas, which escaping by the apical foramen, adds to, if it does not excite, the inflammation. I was under this impression myself, but having performed the following experiment to verify the fact, am somewhat staggered in this opinion.

I took two teeth, extracted for alveolar abscess, having putrescent pulp cavities, cleaned out the cavities of decay, without disturbing the pulp cavities, and filled them up with gutta percha to act as a cork, and then coated the teeth all but the apices of the roots with melted resin and wax. These were then placed roots uppermost in the bottoms of two jam pots full of water which had been boiled, and two small wide-mouth bottles full of water inverted over them: it will be clear that any bubbles arising from the foramina at the apices of the roots would be retained by the bottles; but up to the present time none have appeared. The bottles were placed over the teeth on July the thirtieth, and kept in the upper part of a greenhouse for the sake of warmth. I will now pass them around for inspection. (This was written on August 21st; the two following days were very warm, and when the paper was read, and the experiment exhibited, two extremely small bubbles were just perceptible in each bottle.)

There is no doubt that history is replete with highly questionable concepts and treatments regarding the toothache. However, the one major unswerving constant in this malady is pain and its effect on the patient, as Robert Burns so well stated in 1795[22]:

. . . the delightful sensations of an omnipotent Tooth-ach so engross all my inner man, as to put it out of my power even to write Nonsense.

REPLANTATION/TRANSPLANTATION

Replantation/transplantation operations were common 10 centuries ago. The practice was used as a treatment for odontalgia; at that time, with few instruments and no anesthetics available, it must have been crude and painful.

An early treatise on the subjects was written by the great Arabian surgeon Abulcasis (1050-1122). As physician to Emir Hakam II, he authored the treatise ''Al-Tasrif'' (The Method)—a portion of which was translated into Latin as ''De Chirurgen.''

Sometimes when one or two teeth have fallen out, they are replaced in the socket and bound in aforesaid manner (ligatures or gold wire to the adjacent teeth) and remain there. The operation must be carried out with great delicacy and ability, by skillful hands.[29]

He also was the first who asserted that the teeth could be transplanted or taken from the jaws of one person and placed into those of another, and yet maintain their ''living principle.''[16] It was in making this statement that Dr. Harvey Burdell in 1839 severely criticized the concepts held by Albucasis.

The doctrine of transplanting teeth, so as to render them as healthy as the original ones, is an absurd theory, for it is impossible, and contrary to the laws of physical science, to revive a living principle between the nerve of a tooth thus transplanted and the jaw bone, and it is doubted whether a healthy tooth can

be extracted and replaced again, into the socket of the jaw of the same person, without destroying its vitality, although the celebrated Hunter was of a different opinion.

Being a humble scientist, Dr. Burdell continued by citing a case of Ambrosie Paré (1561), allowing him to relate the circumstance of transplantation himself:

A princess was obliged to have a diseased tooth extracted, and on applying to a surgeon, she brought with her one of her waiting maids, who stood by the side of her mistress, and when the tooth of the mistress had been extracted, a sound one also was taken from the jaw of the girl and placed into the socket of the jaw of the former, which took root and became sound and healthy.

Paré also advised that immediacy in transplanting and ''binding it to a neighboring tooth'' were critical for success.[29]

In his book Fauchard suggested that whenever the wrong tooth is extracted by accident it should be immediately replanted; the same should be done when violent pain necessitates extraction of a sound tooth.[29]

In his famous *Natural History of the Human Teeth*, published in 1778, the English anatomist John Hunter suggested:

In cases where the cavities penetrate some depth, without, however, the destruction of the crown so extensive as to render it useless, the best mode of treatment is extraction and replantation, after having subjected the tooth to boiling in order to cleanse it perfectly and to destroy its vitality entirely.[29]

According to Hunter this treatment would prevent further destruction of the tooth, which, once dead, could no longer be the seat of any disease.

If however one wishes to have recourse to cauterization of the nerve, it is necessary to reach as far as the apex of the root which, however, is not always possible.[29]

Hunter was the first to suggest that pulp destruction was indispensable for the retention of the tooth.

In 1778 in his *Practical Treatise on the Diseases of the Teeth,* John Hunter set down very clear criteria for the transplantation of teeth.[36]

Although this operation is in itself a matter of no difficulty, yet, upon the whole, it is one of the nicest of all operations, and requires more chirurgical and physiological knowledge than any that comes under the care of the dentist. There are certain cautions necessary to be observed, especially if it be a living Tooth which is to be transplanted; because in that case it is meant to retain its life, and we have no great variety of choice. Much likewise depends upon the patient: he should apply early, and give the dentist all the time he thinks necessary to get a sufficient number of Teeth that appear to be of a proper size, etc. Likewise he must not be impatient to get out of his hands before it is adviseable.

The *incisores, cuspidati,* and *bicuspides,* can alone be changed, because they have single fangs. The success is greatest in the *incisores* and *cuspidati* than the *bicuspides;* these last having frequently the ends of their fangs forked, from which circumstance the operation will become less perfect.

It is hardly possible to transplant the grinders, as the chance of fitting the sockets of them is very small. When indeed a grinder is extracted, and the socket sound and perfect, the dentist may, perhaps, be able to fit it by a dead Tooth.

He went on to discuss at length the replacement of a tooth that had been extracted (drawn) by mistake.

It sometimes happens, that a Tooth is drawn on an idea that it is diseased, because it gives pain, but appears after the extraction to be perfectly sound. In such a case I would recommend the replacing it, that there may be no loss by the operation; and the seat of the pain will probably be removed to the next Tooth. A Tooth beat out by violence, should be replaced in the same manner. This ought to be done as soon as possible; however, I would even recommend the experiment twenty-four hours after the accident, or as long as the Socket will receive the Tooth, which may be for some days.

If the Tooth be replaced at any time before its life is destroyed, it will re-unite with the cavity of the Socket, and be as fast as ever.

No tooth is excepted from this practice; for although in the Grinders there are more fangs than one, yet these fangs will as readily go into their respective Sockets as one fang would; and most probably when the Tooth has been beat out, the Sockets are enlarged by their giving way.

However, the Grinders are not so subject to such accidents as the fore Teeth, both from their situation, and from their firmness in the Sockets.

Where a Tooth has been only loosened, or shoved out in part, the patient must not hesitate, but replace it immediately. As a proof of the success to be expected from replacing Teeth, I will relate the following case.

A gentleman had his first *bicuspis* knocked out, and the second loosened. The first was driven quite into his mouth, and he spit it out upon the ground; but immediately picked it up, and put it into his pocket. Some hours afterwards he called upon me, mentioned the accident, and shewed me the Tooth. Upon examining his mouth, I found the second *bicuspis* very loose, but pretty much in its place. The Tooth, which had been knocked out, was not quite dry, but very dirty, having dropped on the ground, and having been some time in his pocket. I immediately put it into warm water, let it stay there to soften, washed it as clean as possible, and then replaced it, first having introduced a probe into the Socket to break down the coagulated blood which filled it. I then tied these two Teeth to the first grinder, and the cuspidatus with silk, which was kept on some days, and then removed. After a month they were as fast as any Teeth in the head; and, if it were not for the remembrance of the circumstances above related, the gentleman would not be sensible that his Teeth had met with any accident. Four years have now passed since it happened.

Shortly after Hunter's exposé, Dr. M.N. Dubois De Chemant wrote his *Dissertation on Artifical Teeth,* in which he severely attacked the transplantation of teeth, citing the potential of systemic disease transmission.[19] Although the account is lengthy, its content is most interesting, especially when one notes with particular interest that De Chemant converted Hunter to his way of thinking.

INOCULATION OF PARTICULAR DISEASES

Which have been the consequence from the cruel operation of the transplanting of human teeth, whether they be extracted from the living subject or taken from the dead body.

I shall not endeavor to trace the origin of that unnatural and dangerous operation of the transplanting of human teeth, recently extracted from unfortunately poor persons, believed to be healthy, whose necessities being taken advantage of, are mutilated in order to contribute to the vain gratification of others in affluent circumstances. Neither shall I attempt to state when the disgusting use of the teeth of dead persons commenced. I shall confine myself to expose the absurdity of the opinions of those who transplant them; and some of the diseases which they inoculate, which will prove that this horrible method is far more dangerous than that of making teeth of the other animal substances of which I have already shewn the great inconveniences.

Notwithstanding what may have been said by some practitioners, and received by great numbers, I think I can state that transplanted teeth can never recover life. Being placed in the sockets, they always remain there as extraneous bodies which can never take root. In order that they should partake of that principle of life which preserves the natural teeth, it is necessary that the nerve, the artery, and the vein, which belong to the teeth which are extracted, should exactly meet the vessels of those which are transplanted, so as to restore in them the circulation of the blood and the nervous influence. But this is impossible, because a contraction of the vessels takes place immediately after the extraction of the tooth. Experience proves that transplanted teeth, being thus deprived of all nourishment, are more liable than all others to fall into a state of disease, either in becoming carious, or turning yellow or black. The examination which I have made of teeth which have been transplanted for six months, has convinced me that there has been no union of nerve to nerve, of artery to artery, or of vein to vein. I have cut several through, both in length and breadth, without discovering the least trace of vessels in the cavity. Transplanted human teeth are therefore very inferior to teeth made of sea-horse, ivory, etc.

Mr. John Hunter, who used to be consulted on the diseases occasioned by artificial teeth, and of whom I have already spoken, thought, at one time, that transplanted natural teeth might be substituted for those which are decayed: he recommended, and was present several times at this operation, and it was not until after he had observed that these transplanted teeth inoculated diseases, that he renounced this cruel practice, and became, I may take the liberty to observe, an enthusiast to my discovery. In his treatise on the venereal disease, he relates the following six cases.

The first case is that of a lady who had one of the bicuspidati transplanted, which fastened very well. About a month after, she danced til five or six o'clock in the morning, caught cold and had a fever in consequence, which lasted near six weeks. In this time, ulceration in the gum and jaw took place, though it was not then known; and when she was beginning to recover, it was found that not only the gum and socket of this tooth were diseased, but also those of the tooth next to it. The two teeth were taken out, and the sockets of both afterwards exfoliated; but the parts were very backward in healing. This gave rise to various opinions, the principal of which was, that it was venereal.

The second case was also in a young lady; the transplanted tooth fastened apparently well, and continued so for about a month, when the gum began to ulcerate, leaving the tooth and socket bare. The ulcer continued, and blotches appeared upon the skin, and ulcers also in the throat. The disease was treated as venereal, the complaints gave way to this course, but they re-

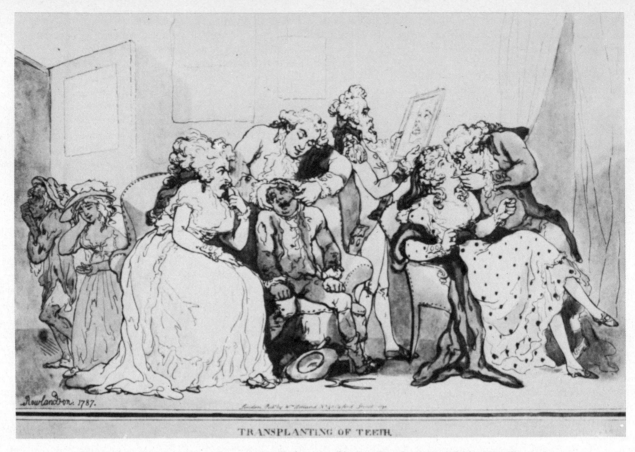

TRANSPLANTING OF TEETH.

FIG. 24.2. Reproduction of an early caricature by Thomas Rowlandson (1756-1827) illustrating the extracting of teeth from the mouths of the poor to be sold to the well-to-do for transplantation. (From Weinberger, B.W.: An introduction to the history of dentistry, vol. 1, St. Louis, 1948, The C.V. Mosby Co.)

curred several times after severe courses of mercury; however she at last got well.

The third case was of a gentleman, where the transplanted tooth remained without giving the least disturbance for about a month, when the edge of the gum began to ulcerate, and the ulceration went on till the tooth dropped out. Some time after, spots appeared almost every where on the skin; they had not the truly venereal appearance, but were redder, or more transparent.

The fourth case was that of a young lady, who had a tooth transplanted and about the same distance of time after it, as mentioned in the former cases, the gum began to ulcerate, and the ulceration was making considerble progress. The surgeon who was consulted, desired mercury to be given immediately. I was afterwards desired to see her, and advised that mercury should not be had recourse to, that we might ascertain the nature of the case, but to extract the tooth. The tooth was drawn and the gum healed up as fast as any common ulcer, and has ever since continued well.

The fifth case was that of a young lady, eighteen years of age, who had one of the incisors transplanted, which fastened tolerably well; but six or seven weeks after the operation an ulceration of the gum took place; the tooth was immediately ordered to be removed, and the bark was given without any other medicine, and she got well in a few weeks.

The sixth case was that of a gentleman, aged twenty-three, a native of the West Indies, who had the two front incisors transplanted, and about the same time after the operation as in the former cases, an ulceration of the gum took place, which increased to a very great degree, and the edges of the gum sloughed off. An eminent surgeon was consulted, who ordered the bark; and the patient without taking any other medicine, got well in nearly the same time as the ladies in cases four and five, who had their teeth taken out. The gums recovered themselves perfectly, but were considerably shorter.

To these cases I could add a number of others, related by different practitioners; but the preceding will, without doubt, suffice to convince the reader of the danger of transplanting teeth. Indeed, if all the symptoms or accidents mentioned in those cases were produced by healthy teeth, taken from persons who had never had any venereal or scrofulous affection, it is then certain, that there exists in some constitutions hidden seeds of disease, which we can only discover by the effects they produce; and also, that irritation alone might, in this case, produce inflammation of the gums, in the throat, etc. and caries in the socket; for a tooth newly transplanted produces greater irritation, as it is impregnated with different blood. If then, it be proved that the transplanting of one or several teeth may communicate the venereal poison, or scrofulous infection which existed in the mass of the blood of the person from whom the teeth were taken, it is clear that we ought for ever to banish from the profession of the dentist the dangerous practice of transplanting teeth, and even the use of them in any other manner, whether with pivots or otherwise.

It may be easily thought that those who have not made the

human structure their particular study, may have been made to believe that teeth recently extracted, of the requisite size might unite with the sockets into which they were inserted; but it seems difficult to conceive how any one can conquer the aversion caused by the disgusting and horrible idea of ornamenting the mouth with the teeth of dead people. I should pardon this attempt if these were not, like those made of corruptible materials, liable to putrefaction, and even to inoculate diseases, as the following case proves.

A dentist of Paris had the opportunity of obtaining such teeth as he wanted from the persons who died in the hospital called the Hotel-Dieu. One day he took the teeth of a young man who had died of the small-pox; these teeth were washed and infused in spirit of wine; they were afterwards fixed upon a base made of the sea-horse tooth; but notwithstanding these precautions, these teeth inoculated the small-pox to the baroness of W. The disease was particularly violent about the mouth, which disfigured her so much that she could scarcely be recognised.

The use of dead teeth can only be attributed to ignorance or cupidity, because they do not require that skill and dexterity which is requisite to prepare artificial ones.

Benjamin Bell, another contemporary of Hunter's, also cautioned operators to be wary in transplantation because contagious maladies of a serious nature (syphilis) could be communicated from one patient to another[29] (Fig. 24-2).

In the late 1800s Dr. H.N. Wadsworth[73] keenly and humorously alerted the profession to the usefulness of replantations, in addition to providing sound clinical guidelines for the clinical management of these cases:

Hundreds and thousands of patients of intelligent, discriminating, appreciative minds and plethoric purses, who would gratefully accept almost any alternative rather than resort to an artificial tooth, are yet doomed to do so in cases quite unnecessary because unaware of a remedy; because many of us as a profession have not yet seized hold of and applied a principle that nature is constantly illustrating for us, that every little while the country clown is practically and successfully applying for our imitation.

Look back on any of our dental records, and call to mind the number of teeth and roots that have lost their original position; that are at the time we remove them entirely changed from their original location; that are to all intents and purposes dead internally, and externally, nerves and blood vessels, some even lying at right angles with their former position, i.e. flat on the gum, and yet, when we examine them, evincing a remarkable evidence of health action, and requiring a considerable amount of lancing to free them from their attachment to the gum, and of force to remove them.

We see a country clown who has received a kick from a horse or mule, a blow from any of the thousand and one sources from which they emanate, and a front tooth is knocked out. It is picked up, pushed into its place, and with no attention whatever returns to its duty and becomes a valuable and useful member.

With these useful practical hints of what nature is doing to correct the ravages of disease, of what uneducated boors can do to remedy the disfiguring results of a painful accident, what are we doing as an educated body of scientific men to meet these forlorn hopes in our practice? In applying these principles that

nature on the one hand and ignorance on the other have thrust before us, to awaken our dormant ideas and shame our boasted skill as professional men?

In summary his guidelines for replantation were as follows:

1. Fill the root canal first
2. Splint to prevent movement
3. Do not remove any healthy periosteum
4. Rinse with warm water
5. Work as rapidly as possible

Advertisements appearing in American newspapers in the late eighteenth century indicated that transplantation was an important part of some dental practices in America (Fig. 24-3).

Here again Dr. Wadsworth[75] provided the practitioner with sound guidelines for what he termed a manipulation that required skill but resulted in greater reward:

Having disposed of one branch of our subject, we come to another and much more difficult one, requiring a much higher order of talent for success, the utmost skill and watchfulness in its manipulations, and far greater honor and reward in its success. Let us examine and inquire into the peculiar surroundings of "transplanting."

In choosing a tooth for transplanting, it should be from the mouth of a young and healthful person, thoroughly healthy, lest we transplant also a dangerous subtle disease, of the same temperament, if possible; of smaller organization physically, that as far as possible we may avoid having to reduce the size or change the shape of the tooth to have it fit. I look upon any cutting, or even scratching or bruising, as so many wounds to injure and render less certain the result; and every portion of periosteum remaining on the tooth should be carefully encouraged to remain, as it is of vital importance.

The procedure itself was to be performed after the nerve was "carefully" killed and the canal was filled "thoroughly to the apex." Speed in the procedure was of utmost importance after extraction.

If not absolutely necessary, I would not change the external surface of the tooth in any particular whatever. I would not wipe a drop of blood from its surface, but instantly insert it in its new location and at once apply the splint after the blood has ceased to flow.

The patient was instructed to eat only an "unstimulating diet," and the splint was removed in 10 days "in the most delicate manner."

A rather unusual case of transplantation is related by Dr. W.J. Younger,[77] of San Francisco:

In October, 1886, I was presented with a number of teeth which had been extracted at various periods, more or less remote. One of these teeth, a central, I transplanted in a lady's mouth in Dr. Kingsley's office, New York. On the following day I discovered a perpendicular crack in the tooth extending from the cutting edge to the cervical margin, which promised to disfigure the tooth. So I removed it and substituted another in its place. On July 31, 1889, two years and nine months later, I implanted this same cracked tooth in the mouth of a physician of San Francisco.

A

> # T E E T H
>
> ANY Perſon that is willing to diſpoſe of their FRONT TEETH, may hear of a purchaſer, by applying to No. 28, Maiden Lane, for which a generous price will be given.
>
> *N. B. Four Guineas will be given for every Tooth.*

B

> DR. Le MAYEUR, Dentiſt who tranſplants TEETH, at No. Maiden-Lane, will leave this City on 2d of February, and will not return till May next.

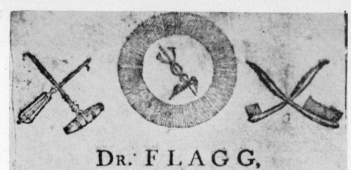

C

> # DR. FLAGG,
>
> *Continues his* PRACTICE, *as* SURGEON DENTIST *the moſt ſucceſsful of the profeſſion, in all its branches,*
>
> FOR the extracting of the firſt teeth in children, and the regular arrangement of the ſecond ſett ; for the preſerving, drawing, mending, curing, making or tranſplanting of teeth, for the adult. All who may require his aſſiſtance, and wiſh a confidence in him, are at liberty to bring their phyſician or ſurgeon with them, as he is emulous of giving perfect ſatisfaction.
>
> He confidently aſſerts, that the ſenſation, or nerves of the teeth in the head, can be *extracted*, by a ſimple, ſafe and eaſy proceſs, with inſtruments, and the teeth ſtill preſerved and prevented from a further decay. On the truth of what he aſſerts in this, or his hand-bill he riſques his profeſſional reputation.
>
> ☞ Caſh is given for ſound live Teeth, at his Room, near the corner of *Winter-Street, two doors from Fauſt's Statue, Marlborough Street.*
>
> ⤙✦✦◉◎◉✦✦⤚
>
> EXPLANATION
>
> of the Caducies, (Mercury's ſimbol of peace) which he arrogates as Surgeon's arms. The healing art, winged with a ſpeedy cure, and encompaſſed with the rays of light, knowledge or experience.
>
> The Field *azure* is charged with a Caducies *argent;* encircled with the rays of light—Or—The Dental types on the dexter chief are two bruſhes, which refer to cleanlineſs, and the inſtruments in the ſiniſter are emblematical of that laſt reſort or cure, for the anguiſh which is occaſioned by imprudent neglect or obſtinate reſiſtance to dental remedy.

FIG. 24-3. A, Advertisement placed in the *New York Royal Gazette* in August, 1782, by Jean Pierre Le Mayeur, who arrived in New York from France in 1781. (One guinea was equivalent to $5.00.) **B,** Advertisement by Le Mayeur in the February, 1784, edition of the *Independent Journal* announcing his departure from the city for a time. **C,** Advertisement placed in the *Massachusetts Magazine* in 1795 by Josiah Flagg, Jr., explaining the nature of his practice. (From Weinberger, B.W.: An introduction to the history of dentistry in America, vol. 2, St. Louis, 1948, The C.V. Mosby Co.)

It was one of three teeth that I implanted, the gentleman having had the two centrals and the left lateral knocked out by a piece of an exploding gun in a charge during the war. He had therefore worn a partial gold plate for over twenty-five years. This central was the only tooth that would match, and the doctor did not mind the crack, as he said, "It is not for beauty but for service that I want the teeth."

The tooth lasted approximately 2 years before completely splitting in two. The physician then proceeded to tie the two segments of his tooth together with silk ligature. Three months later the tooth was extracted and microscopically "on the portion of the root grasped by the forceps I [Dr. Younger] discovered a thick covering of pericementum. . . ."

Today research in transplantation and replantation of teeth continues, but "new discoveries" are often merely repetitions of old axioms.

DENTAL ANESTHESIA

As civilization progressed through the centuries, clinicians had new thoughts on ways to stop dental pain. From earliest recorded history we learn of the wide use of arsenic as an obtundent of pain. One of the earliest recorded mentions of this drug was in a translation of a 500 BC Chinese manuscript with the following formula: "Arsenic (gr. 1.80), huangtou [soybeans] (gr. 3.60); pulverize, mix with water, and with part of the mass form a small pill, which put close to the aching tooth or in the ear. If afraid of the arsenic, then sleep. Cure certain."[10]

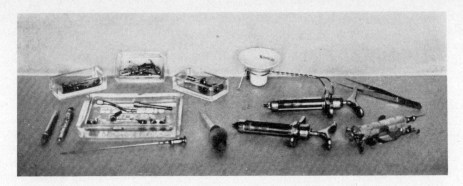

FIG. 24-4. Armamentarium that was needed for preparation of the novocaine solution prior to manufacture of the Carpule. The cup was used to prepare the solution. The proper amount of distilled water was placed in the cup and brought almost to a boil. One or two tablets of novocaine were introduced, and the solution was allowed to cool. It was then drawn into the syringe, of which several types are portrayed. (From Kells, C.E.: Three score years and nine, New Orleans, 1926, published by author.)

How could they miss? From this operation might have originated: "This operation was a success, but the patient died."

The earliest possible recorded method of producing general anesthesia is translated from the manuscript of Guy de Chauliac (1300-1368):

Some prescribe medicaments which send the patient to sleep, so the incision may not be felt, such as opium, the juice of Morel, hyoscyamine, mandrake, ivy, hemlock, and lettuce. A new sponge is soaked by them in these juices and left to dry in the sun. When they have need of it, they put the sponge in warm water and they hold it under the nostrils of the patient until he goes to sleep, then perform the operation.[79]

Guerini[29] comments: "It seems that the narcosis thus obtained was sufficiently intense, since Guy also speaks of the means used to awaken the patient. These consisted in applying another sponge, soaked in vinegar, under the nose, or dropping into the nostrils and ears the juice of rue or fennel."

The era of cocainization of patients began at the end of the eighteenth century.[43] In 1884 Karl Koller, a Viennese physician, introduced cocaine as an anesthetic. Hall and Halstead demonstrated the surgical value of neural cocainization in 1884 by experiments tried on themselves and others. Hall anesthetized the infraorbital for the maxillary teeth, and Halstead's experiments were on the inferior dental nerve; he obtained complete anesthesia of the tissues of the jaw with an injection of 9 minims of a 4% solution.

The use of a local anesthetic for removing the pulp "was first brought to notice in this country by publication in the Medical Record of October 11, 1884, of a letter from Dr. Noyes of New York, then studying in Germany," according to George Maxfield.[48]

On November 13 following, I read a paper on "Hydrochlorate of Cocain" before the Connecticut Valley Dental Society, one sentence of which I quote: "What has already been accomplished with cocain leads us to believe that by its use we can banish arsenic from our practice, for if placed on an exposed pulp it should so benumb it as to allow its removal to be a painless operation."

What brave and determined men! It is not too late to give belated thanks to these men to whom we are indebted for one of the greatest blessings of humanity: painless dentistry!

Now, in the era of modern dentistry, one of our greatest blessings has been the invention of novocaine (procaine hydrochloride) by Alfred Einhorn and his associates in 1905[47] (Fig. 24-4).

In March of 1905, Einhorn, a research chemist, announced his invention of the wonderful drug. Strangely enough, although his discovery has become the most widely used anesthetic in the world, Einhorn himself is all but forgotten. The men responsible for various general anesthetics have been heralded in many books and been recipients of numerous awards; plaques have been placed in universities commemorating their efforts; their names have been duly recorded in scientific halls of fame. Yet Alfred Einhorn is not mentioned in a standard encyclopedia and remains virtually unknown—a shadowy figure whose sole recognition consists of a few lines in some textbooks on anesthesia.

Before the advent of novocaine the narcotic cocaine, introduced by Koller, was used for local anesthesia. Although it was highly efficient, it possessed many undesirable characteristics. Not only was there the risk of addiction with its use, but also it had a rather formidable degree of toxicity. These undesirable properties, together with its high cost, created a demand for substitute. Einhorn believed that an ideal anesthetic should be nontoxic, nonhabiting forming, nonirritating to human tissue, stable enough to permit sterilization by boiling, of low cost, and soluble in isotonic salt solution.

There are several possible reasons for Einhorn's failure to receive acclaim. First, his discovery occurred at an inopportune time, since World War I coincided with the period of novocaine's increasing acceptance throughout the world. In addition, Einhorn's Germanic origin may have tempered the enthusiasm of its reception. An interesting sidelight is that before the war, Germany possessed a virtual monopoly on the production of the drug. However, with the advent of hostilities the U.S. Government released the formula to American pharmaceutical houses with the provision that their product be called procaine, presumably to afford some degree of protection to the German-registered trademark. This distinction, retained for some time after the war, eventually became pointless; today the terms novocaine and procaine are used interchangeably. Another reason for Einhorn's failure to receive recognition might be the nature of the man himself. Primarily a quiet and unassuming research chemist, he made no effort to exploit his discovery. Having achieved his goal, he immediately turned to new fields to conquer.

In tandem with the development of anesthetics came the development of anesthetic techniques. It was not until 1906 that the method of nerve blocking known as conductive anesthesia was introduced by Noguie of Paris.

PULP CAPPING

In 1756, Phillip Pfaff, the German dentist to Frederick the Great, first mentioned a pulp capping procedure. He fashioned a piece of metal, gold or lead, to "...die Figur einer halben Hulse von einer Erbse, diren unterster Theil eine Vertiefung haben soll." (...the shape of half a peapod, so that the lower surface should have a concavity.) In that way the metal would be prevented from contacting the living and therefore sensible pulp.[24]

In 1826 Leonard Koecker published his *Principles of Dental Surgery,* from which an excerpt was taken by the editor of the *American Journal of Dental Science* for the first volume (1839). In doing so, the editor was hoping to elicit "from some of our correspondents, an article on the same subject invalidating or confirming the doctrines therein advanced." The excerpt is entitled "Of treating the lining membrane of the tooth when exposed."[45]

I require for this the following apparatus: 1. A small iron wire, fastened to an ivory handle. The extremity of this wire I file to the size of the exposed surface of the nerve, and bend the wire in such a direction as to enable me to touch the exposed part of the membrane, without touching any other part of the tooth or the mouth. 2. A thick tallow candle, with a large wick.

I direct the patient to discharge all the saliva he may have in his mouth, and then to incline his head backwards against the head support of my operating chair. I put the candle into his left hand, and direct him to hold it in such a position that the flame of it may be on a level with his mouth, and about eight inches from it; I now place myself on the right side of the patient, and, holding his lips sufficiently open with my left hand, to prevent the instrument from touching them, I again dry the cavity as perfectly as possible with a lock of cotton fastened to the point of the cauterizing wire. Having effected this, I throw away the cotton from the extremity of the wire, and make it red hot in the flame of the candle. With the wire thus heated, I touch the exposed part very rapidly, so that its surface contracts, without, however, suffering it to penetrate deeply into the nerve, or to touch any part of the bony structure; as this would inevitably

bring on suppuration and destruction of the whole lining membrane. The bleeding spot must be touched very quickly with the hot wire, which is sometimes necessary to be repeated two or three times before the parts are sufficiently contracted. The wire should be perfectly red hot, for in this state the cautery acts suddenly, and almost entirely without pain; but when heated to any temperature short of that redheat, much pain and inflammation are generally produced. This operation is, indeed, so slightly painful, that I have been solicited by my patients to repeat it, although they had required much persuasion to induce them in the first instance to suffer its application. It, however, must be performed very adroitly, and without any loss of time. To prevent the flow of saliva to interfere, the patient must be desired not to close his lips, but to keep his mouth wide open, until the whole of the operation is finished, which he is capable to do for a certain time only.

When the hemorrhage has been arrested in this way, and an artificial cicatrix formed, I wash the cavity, as before the cauterization with warm water. I carefully remove every particle of the ashes or matter that may have been left by the cauterization, taking great care not to wound the membrane again.

The nerve, which, before cauterization, had a fleshy appearance, is, after this operation, like a black point. I take care not to disturb this point, for if the black scar be removed, a new wound will be formed and bleeding again will ensue; but I leave the future healing altogether to nature, and only caution my patient against using such things as might interfere with its salutary operations.

Having thus far removed all possible cause of future disease and irritation, in order to prevent any unnecessary exposure of the nerve, by which inflammation and destruction of it might be produced, I now terminate the operation by fulfilling the third indication, that is, to protect the nerve against injurious impressions from without, by filling up the cavity of the tooth with metal. Having again perfectly dried the cavity, I now take a small plate of very thin lead leaf, and lay it upon the exposed nerve, and on the immediately surrounding bony parts. I next carefully fill up the whole cavity with gold. The dressing of the cavity and the firm insertion of the two different metals also, must be completed before the patient can be allowed to close his mouth, which is not unfrequently very difficult.

In the 1800s a conflict existed regarding the appropriate medicament for pulp capping. The two most common were arsenic and creosote. Issac Greenwood wrote a letter in 1841 to the editor of the *American Journal & Library of Dental Science* extolling the virtues of an arsenic (3 parts) and acetate morphine mixture placed on the exposed pulp.[27]

When a patient applies to me for the cure of tooth-ache, I examine the tooth, and clean out the cavity, endeavouring to make bare the nerve, if practicable, with a small instrument. If the nerve bleeds, so much the better. I then wipe out the cavity with raw cotton, steeped in essence of peppermint, laudanum, or alcohol. After which I take raw cotton of sufficient size to stop up three-fourths of the cavity of the tooth. I dip the point into laudanum, so as somewhat to saturate the cotton with it, that the mixture I shall mention below may adhear to it. I then take up upon the point of it, by touching the mixture, about the size of a large pin's head, and in no instance do I ever use more, however large the cavity in the tooth; but sometimes a smaller quantity. This I place in the cavity of the tooth, immediately in contact, if I can, with the nerve, and stop up the cavity with mastic, composed of Venice turpentine, heated, and mixed with calcined plaster of Paris and chalk. Feuchtwanger's Prussian cement for the teeth, will answer, placed upon the raw cotton in the tooth and sometimes mixed up with it so as to fill up the cavity, charging the patient to take it out in three days exactly, and in no wise to masticate on that side during the time. If a patient will come to me, which they generally will do, I take it out for them, which I prefer to do, and wash out the cavity with alcohol. The tooth is by this time cured...The symptoms of the efficacy of the cure are these, viz: the pain, after commencing, will endure for three or four hours, sometimes more, according to the irritability of the patient. After the acute pains have passed away, a soreness will continue for some time, accompanied by a looseness of the organ, occasioned by the inflamed state of the periosteum. This gradually dies away, and by the second or third day, in almost every case, disappears. If, when the raw cotton and the mastic are removed on the third day, the patient takes cold water in the mouth, and no pain arises from it, the cause is removed. This is the proof in all cases. I have been thus prolix, in order that you may be supported by one who has tested its efficacy for years with success, and, indeed, I make use of no other remedy.

On the other side of the ledger, Dr. W.H. Atkinson, speaking at a meeting of the Brooklyn Dental Association in 1867, highlighted the use of creosote for treating dental pulps.[3]

When a pulp is exposed and aches, I remove all extraneous matter from the part; if this does not arrest the pain I dry out the cavity by applying pieces of bibulous paper until it is perfectly dry.

I then apply pure creosote and hold a dry napkin around the tooth for a minute, and if the pain continues I remove the napkin and syringe the cavity with tepid water, washing out all the creosote, and then apply a fresh napkin and proceed as before; then apply the best chloroform upon a pledget of cotton.

If this does not succeed repeat it again, and apply the tincture of aconite. In most cases it will not be necessary to repeat this process. I next proceed to prepare the cavity for the filling. I apply the napkin, or sheet rubber to keep dry and then delicately, fragments of bibulous paper until all moisture is removed, when I place a drop of creosote on the exposed part and then put a soft mass of osteo-plastic over the creosote.

I wait for the osteo-plastic to firmly set, then remove the excess and fill boldly.

In 1883, W.E. Harding of Shrewsbury, England, astutely differentiated between the capping of an accidental exposure and a carious exposure (like a good wine, Harding claimed that a cariously exposed pulp had a certain "nose" to it).[30]

In the "good old days," the treatment of an exposed pulp was the extraction of the tooth, but that mode of procedure has long been exploded by the progress of Dental Science.

The first question the dental surgeon of to-day asks himself is not,—Can I save the tooth, but can I save the pulp? This, gentlemen, has added much to our labour and anxieties, but it has also contributed much to our professional usefulness to mankind.

We all know how easily and successfully cases of accidental exposure can be treated. My usual plan is to swab out the cavity with carbolic acid, which will arrest the bleeding, then place over the point of exposure a small piece of court plaster, or blotting of Fletcher's artificial dentine. This can be applied in a more plastic state than the phosphate fillings, and unlike oxychloride of zinc it is non-irritant and easily removed if necessary. When this has hardened the permanent filling may be proceeded with at the same sitting.

The reason these cases are so easily dealt with is that the pulp is quite healthy, and if covered with a non-conductor at once, so as to exclude the germs of micro-organisms, it will heal by first intention.

But in those cases where the exposure results from caries the difficulties are vastly greater, as the pulp is almost sure to be inflamed, and probably suppurating. My experience of these cases treated by capping is the reverse of satisfactory, the percentage of successful cases being small, and on this point I hope some of the gentlemen present will give us the benefit of their experience.

The first point to determine is the condition of the pulp. The history of the case is often deceptive, for if the cavity is in such a position as not to be exposed to the impact of food it may not have given much pain, and yet be suppurating; but in the odour we have a certain means of diagnosis. If that peculiar phosphatic odour is present, I very much doubt the possibility of saving the pulp, and think any attempt at capping will result in its death, and eventually in a chronic abscess; in such cases the destruction of the pulp is, I think, by far the best treatment.

Should capping be determined upon, the application to the exposed surface of iodoform and eucalyptus oil has generally proved the most successful. It may then be covered with artificial dentine—and in these cases it is always safer to put in a temporary filling for a few weeks, which can be removed in case of pain. Hill's gutta percha over the artificial dentine answers very well.

PULP EXTIRPATION

> If then the teeth, designed for various use
> Decay and ache, 'tis only from abuse,
> And low, triumphant art can well ensure,
> At least a remedy, if not a cure.
>
> Solyman Brown, *Dentologia*, 1840[15]

In years past, removing the pulp was truly an "unnerving" experience. Snell, a nineteenth-century writer, related the use of acetate of morphine and actual cautery for the destruction of inflamed and sensitive pulps (1832).[71] He improved on the red-hot iron by devising a steel instrument with a bulb at the end from which projected a platinum wire. Heat was retained in the steel bulb for a sufficient time to allow the platinum wire to do its work of destruction in the root canal.

The first use of arsenious acid (arsenic trioxide) for pulp destruction was recommended by Shearjashub Spooner in 1836. Spooner contributed to American dental literature by writing his *Guide to Sound Teeth* and *A Popular Treatise on Teeth*. He recommended a fortieth or fiftieth part of arsenious acid to be mixed with an equal quantity of sulfate of morphia and applied to an exposed pulp. This would destroy the pulp's vitality in 3 to 7 hours after application but not without pain.

An excellent description of what could almost be considered as a modern technique for pulp extirpation was given by E. Baker in 1839[4]:

When the nerve of a front tooth, or the nerve of one of the bicuspides, is from the depth of the decay, unavoidably exposed, it is less objectionable, and I believe, is the practice adopted by the most successful dentists at this time, to proceed to destroy the nerve directly, by running a small instrument up the cavity of the tooth as high as where the nerve commences to go through the foramen at the end of the root. The instrument there meeting with resistance from the diminished size of the canal, cuts off the nerve at that point. The nerve being taken out the internal cavity after having been made perfectly clean and dry, should be immediately filled with gold to its highest point. There is seldom little, and often, no inflammation in a tooth after being treated in this manner, and what is of very great importance, there is very seldom a gum boil, provided the operation has been performed with competent skill. The late Mr. Hudson of Philadelphia, who certainly has not been excelled, if equalled, as an operator, followed this practice more than thirty years since, and teeth treated by him in this manner, remain to this time.

Solyman Brown, in 1839, described his arsenic and creosote treatment for the "destruction of living nerve" tissue.[14]

To a carious opening which is the immediate cause of toothache, as well as to one in which a living nerve must be destroyed in order to prepare the tooth for stopping, the arsenic should be applied on the extremity of a lock of cotton, steeped in creosote instead of water. The effect of the creosote is to allay the pain which the arsenic along would produce when acting on the living nerve... In all these cases it will be well to apply the remedy in the early part of the day, in order that the patient may be able to use proper caution in preventing the removal of the cotton, and also be careful to keep the mouth free from any portion of the medicine which may make its escape. Excoriations of the lips, tongue and gums, may be the unpleasant consequences of applying the remedy in the after part of the day, in case, during sleep, the cotton should be displaced. It need scarcely be remarked that a powerful and dangerous remedy like this, should be used with the utmost care.

In 1867, Andrew B. Bookins' treatise on "Root Filling" was a severe indictment of the "quackery" that was being used to devitalize pulp tissue.[13]

What can I say with reference to the devitalization of dental nerves that has not already been said by those, something my seniors, both in practice and in years? Or what shall we do that has been left undone in the treatment of this class of cases, preparatory to the introduction of gold in the canals and crown cavities?

Among the practitioners of General Medicine, we have the infinitisimal Homoeopathy, the heroic Allopathy, and the so-called Eclectic; the latter assuming the assurance of the first, the thunder of the second, with ostensible result of the trio.

In 1884 Cassius M. Richmond introduced the Richmond crown and also suggested an "in vogue" method of filling root canals at one sitting without previous treatment. The method he used to remove a live pulp from a single-rooted tooth was by knocking it out with a tapered orangewood stick and applying phenol.

A friend of Dr. Richmond, Dr. G.A. Mills,[52] was very interested in the origins of this technique and attempted to answer the question, "Who did it first?"

Dr. C.M. Richmond tells me that Dr. George Lawrence, son of Dr. Ambrose Lawrence, of Lowell, Mass., made a practical use of this operation of "pulp-knocking" in the mouth of his brother, Dr. A.S. Richmond, in Chicago, September, 1878, upon a superior central incisor, for a crown setting. This practice had been in use by Dr. A. Lawrence for twenty-five years. Who did it before this, let some one else answer. At the union meeting held in Springfield during this month, this "pulp-knocking" was detailed by Dr. J.L. Williams in connection with his remarks, illustrated, upon how the root of a tooth receives its nourishment after the removal of the pulp, and Dr. Searle stated that he had often resorted to a method of plunging a sharp stick into the pulp, and that the patient said it seemed (as I should think it would) that a broom-handle had been thrust up through his head. My impression at that time was this: that they failed to catch the idea that it could be done comparatively painlessly, and that it could be made a humane operation. I will only add, that report says "pulp-knocking" has been patented.

In 1866 Dr. J.H. M'Quillen[54] recommended the use of an ether spray to numb the pulp during removal:

Apply in the first place a pledget of cotton saturated with chloroform for a few seconds, and then direct the etherial spray into the carious cavity (the first dash of which without such precaution would be likely to cause intense pain), and while the current is maintained by an assistant, carefully enlarge the opening into the pulp cavity, and as soon as the pulp can be touched without any painful manifestations, pass a barb broach into the cavity, rotate rapidly, and remove the pulp.

In 1900 Harlan[31] advocated pulpal digestion through the use of natural enzymes (papain):

I desire to call your attention to a process for the liquefaction of pulp-tissue in small tortuous roots and those not easily accessible . . . In the year 1881 Van Antwerp, of Kentucky, discovered that the fresh leaves of pawpaw, or Carica papaya, would digest fresh meat, beefsteak, and other animal flesh. The pulp, as is well known, consists of blood-vessels and other tissues, and is dissimilar to any other formation in the body. It is capable of coagulation, and will undergo putrefaction after death, the same as others of the soft tissues. This being granted, we must at once concede that there are teeth having very attenuated and twisted roots where it is almost a physical impossibility to remove all the dead pulp-tissue before the putrefactive process begins. To relieve us of this operative procedure, I have long been interested in the digestion of such tissues . . .

I find that pulp-tissue is digested more rapidly if the surface has been lightly painted with one to two hundred sodium fluosilicate, or a solution of borate of soda, one to two hundred; carbonate of soda or magnesia may be used, but not in excess. If one gram of papain is made into a thick paste with glycerol and a drop of hydrochloric acid solution, one to three hundred, is added it always acts well.

In the mouth, clinically, the papain will act more rapidly, four days being usually sufficient to digest small fragments of pulp-tissue. If a large mass of pulp-tissue remains in a tooth the papain paste must be reapplied at the end of the second day, and occasionally for a third time. I have found from repeated experiments that it is best to remove all tissue in sight, and then pack the roots and pulp-chamber full of the paste and seal with oxysulfate or oxyphosphate of zinc, and let it remain without interference five to eight days. In this way the patient suffers no uneasiness, and there is no risk of pericemental irritation.

Often events occur within the development of a discipline or technique that are not sufficiently appreciated. It was to this end that Dr. R. Ottolengui[58] addressed his editorial "An Era in Dentistry" in 1903. The thrust of his exposé was twofold: (1) to point out the apprehension expressed by practitioners in the use of arsenic compounds to devitalize pulps and (2) to alert the profession to a new and totally predictable method for pulpal anesthesia prior to removal.

In the presence of these difficulties many experiments have been made in the direction of immediate pulp removal under anesthesia, general or local. Before the discovery of cocaine, some administered gas and so painlessly removed the pulp tissue. But at once a new obstacle was found. Hemorrhage! After an application of arsenic there is usually little if any hemorrhage, but following the removal of a living, healthy pulp the hemorrhage is always considerable, and in those of anaemic temperament often copious and troublesome. For a time, therefore, arsenic again held sway. With the advent of cocaine a new series of attempts were made. Some reported success by slow hyperdermatic injections, but this attracted little credence or following. Then followed cataphoresis, and this was very successful, but very slow, and after a time cataphoric appliances lost their place in the dental armamentarium. Pulp removal under cataphoretic application of cocaine likewise met with the troublesome hemorrhage, but by this time the peroxide of hydrogen preparations were at our disposal and because of their haemostatic action were helpful. Still as has been noted, cataphoresis has lost its popularity, and so arsenic became dominant again. But during the discussions on cataphoresis an important suggestion was made, with the final result that pulp treatment has been solved.

The important suggestion was to dissolve cocaine in guiacol sulfuric ether and apply this mixture to the pulp under pressure to achieve anesthesia. This discovery was attributed to Dr. William J. Morton in 1897; and coupled with the practices of Dr. Clyde Davis, an efficient pressure anesthetic with hemostatic properties was made available and the use of arsenic could be abolished.

The proposition of Dr. Morton was almost immediately adopted. A prominent drug house within a few months marketed a solution of this character which was used for obtunding sensitive dentine and remarkable results were reported. Practitioners soon found that the pressure produced by the evaporation of the ether was not always efficient, but the word being suggestive,

mechanical pressure was also used and the problem was solved, at least so far as the anaesthetizing and removal of the pulp was concerned. For several years the removal of pulps by pressure anaesthesia has been coming into more and more general use. There still remained, however, the occasional trouble with hemorrhage, and this was not confined to the mere flow of blood during the sitting. Too often after treatment the patient would return the severe pain caused by the blood pressure of the apex, due to an uncontrolled hemorrhage. At this juncture the papers of Dr. Clyde Davis appeared, recommending the use of adrenalin in connection with the cocaine pressure anaesthesia, and any further use of arsenic should be a very rare requirement. The adrenalin not only acts as a haemostatic, but appears to violently contract the pulp, thus enabling the operator to fully uncover it . . .

For the present, it suffices to congratulate the profession that the suggestion of Dr. Morton and his discovery of pressure anaesthesia, culminating in the method of pulp removal outlined by Dr. Davis, absolishes arsenic and its unpleasant sequences.

DENTAL RADIOGRAPHY

> . . . I set you up a glass, where you may see the inmost part of you.
>
> *Hamlet,* Act III, Scene 4

Before the discovery of x rays endodontic techniques were empirical. Project yourself to those times and attempt to guess what your chances of endodontic diagnosis, treatment, and success would be without the use of radiographs. Put succinctly by Dr. W.A. Price[12] in 1901, the x-ray or dental skiagraphy brought to light our inability to perform adequate root canal treatment:

> We now turn our attention to the dentists' graveyard, root canal fillings, where so many cover up defective, careless work, trusting it will never come to light, and often reminding the patient that when his tooth gives trouble again it will have to be extracted. Humanity should thank God for a new light that will go into these dark places and show up what is often criminally careless or willfully bad work in filling roots.

On November 8, 1895, after many years of experimentation with Crookes' tubes, Wilhelm Conrad Röntgen, the German physicist, announced the discovery of a "new kind of light," which he called "x-ray," probably because the rays were of a kind then unknown.

It is interesting to note that the dental profession was quick to experiment with new discoveries. German literature reports that 14 days after the announcement of the discovery, the science of dental radiodontics was founded by the taking of the first radiograph. Walkoff, a German dentist, lay on the floor for 25 minutes to make the exposure. The processing of this film took 1 hour.[69]

Probably the first dental radiograph in the western hemisphere was taken by William Herbert Rollins, D.D.S., M.D. Born in 1852 in Charleston, Mass., Rollins plunged his inventive abilities into the development of an intraoral cassette and an intraoral fluoroscope; he also designed and built an x-ray apparatus for dental use (Fig. 24-5). His inventions were described in dental literature 9 months following the announcement of the "discovery" of x-rays in the United States. His contributions to dental radiology did

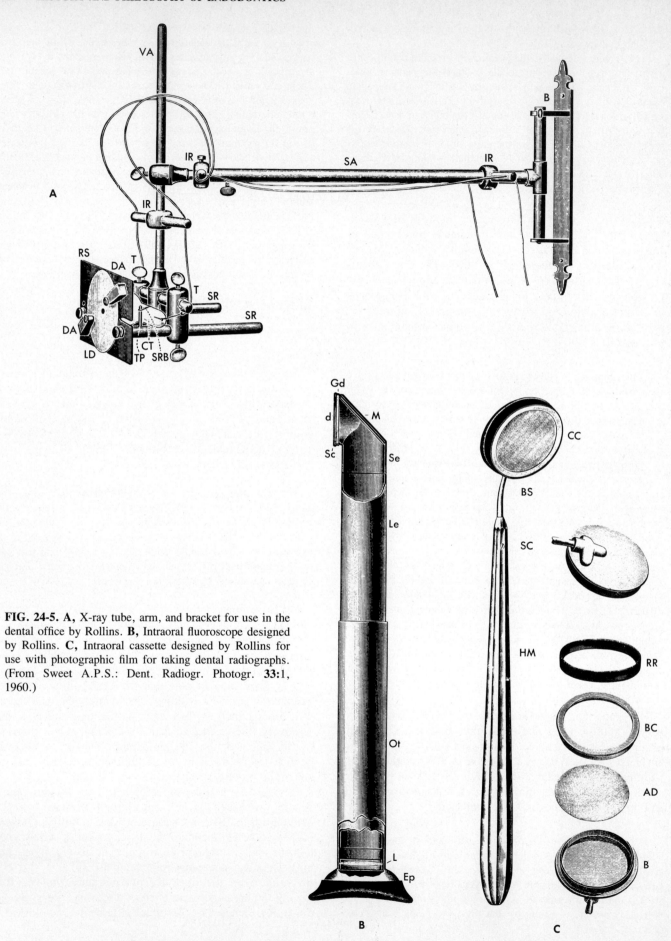

FIG. 24-5. A, X-ray tube, arm, and bracket for use in the dental office by Rollins. **B,** Intraoral fluoroscope designed by Rollins. **C,** Intraoral cassette designed by Rollins for use with photographic film for taking dental radiographs. (From Sweet A.P.S.: Dent. Radiogr. Photogr. **33:**1, 1960.)

not stop there; he recorded improvements and inventions in radiographic technique and equipment.[71]

The x-ray apparatus (tube, arm, and bracket) built by Rollins during 1896 was apparently the first dental x-ray apparatus. It is interesting to note that many of the present x-ray tubes still retain some of the original form. Rollins did not patent his inventions; thus his name does not appear on any of his many contributions to the dental, medical, and electronic professions.

Another member of the dental profession who contributed to the knowledge of dental radiography, Dr. C. Edmund Kells, of New Orleans, a pioneer in research and experimentation, sacrificed his life that we could "see." After he lost one arm because of radiation, it was found that the other arm needed to be amputated. Dr. Kells chose death instead.

In his writings, Kells[43] reported on a clinic he had presented in 1896 before the Southern Dental Association, demonstrating the taking of a skiagraph (from the Greek *skia*, shadow). He was so enthusiastic in his research of the x-ray that he transported his Tesla coil and bulky equipment from New Orleans to Ashville, N.C., for this demonstration.

To take the skiagraph, he had to devise a means of getting the object as close as possible to the plate on which the shadow was to be produced. His device was a film holder containing a pocket for the film and an articulating surface for the teeth to bite down on; this was held steady for a long exposure. He made his film holder from rubber, gutta-percha, and aluminum.

The demonstration had to be presented in the evening because in those times there was no electric current during the day. The demonstration created quite a sensation in the hotel at which it was presented; people from other meetings crowded into the room.

Kells did not use vulcanite film holders for long, because he discovered that he could enclose the film in black dental velum rubber clamped on an aluminum plate and embedded in an occlusal bite surface of modeling compound. The exposure time would take from 5 to 15 minutes. Three years later, because of some of the improvements mentioned before, the exposure time was reduced to 1 or 2 minutes.

ROOT CANAL ANTISEPSIS

The history of the methods and manner of canal preparation is fascinating. The investigation of writings on dental therapeutics, however, is puzzling, because of the many conflicting statements as to the source of the medications.

The introductions of creosote by Reichenbach in 1830 and phenol by Runge in 1834[65] were the earliest of the significant discoveries that became favorites for use as antiseptics, caustics, and obtundents. In many combinations, they occupied an important part in dentistry for the treatment of diseases of the pulp during the nineteenth and twentieth centuries.

In the treatment of pulp tissues, phenol enjoyed the greater popularity. When combinations were discovered,

metacresylacetate (Cresatin) became popular. Monochlorophenol, introduced by Salkoff in 1891 (he later added camphor, which reduced the coagulant action), became the leader during an era of much activity in remedial research.[65]

In 1894 formocresol was introduced. Credit for its origin is given to a list of researchers: Marion (1895), Lepkowski (1895), Schroder (1896), Witzel (1898), Bonnecker (1898), Prinz (1898), and Gysi (1899). Following its introduction before the Fourth International Dental Congress in 1904 by Buckley, formocresol took a prominent part in endodontic therapy.[61]

Combinations of chemicals that, when introduced separately into the canal, would produce an explosion were also known. Sodium combined with potassium was widely used and was thought to be a reliable sterilizing agent because it produced intense heat in the root.

The use of sodium and potassium was first demonstrated in the United States by Emil Schrier of Vienna at the World's Columbian Dental Congress (1893) in Chicago.[68] Following that introduction, the mixture became popular and at first was imported from Vienna. It was put in glass vials shaped like test tubes; the sodium and potassium, appearing like an amalgam, had a cover of paraffin. At the time of introduction into the root canal, a hole was punctured in the paraffin and a broach inserted; when removed, the broach was covered with the amalgamlike mass. This was then immediately introduced into the canal (the compound rapidly oxidizes when exposed to air), where it produced an explosion, breaking up calcific materials and forcing them into the open. Syringing with peroxide of mercury into which mercury bichloride was mixed (1:500) was used as an aftertreatment.[59] Interestingly, this same technique was advocated by Waas in 1948.[74]

It is a curious phenomenon in these days of world wars and atom bombs that so many endodontists have acquired a fear complex. They seem to be afraid of the very occasional infinitesemal spark or the almost inaudible "fff-sst" sound reaction resultant from the use of Sodium and Potassium in root canal therapy...the metallic agent tracks down the slightest evidence of moisture. Even though the user is not aware of it he will succeed in opening any multiple accessory apical foramenae present and also any branching side foramenae present. Furthermore as the drug is a metallic paste and used only in the most minute particles at each application, it is impossible to have the material run through the apical foramen and destroy a large amount of periapical tissue. It is self-limiting in its action.

While this "burning issue" is interesting, this concept is undoubtedly destined for a permanent resting place in the forgotten archives of "irrationalized endodontics."

Exploding chemicals stimulated the inventive minds of the profession and must have inspired Dr. John Ross Callahan. In 1893 he presented a paper, "Sulfuric Acid for Opening Root Canals," before the Ohio State Dental Society.[17] He claimed he had discovered a means of opening difficult roots, even though the use of so strong a solution appeared to be heroic. Callahan's method was to use a 20% to 50% aqueous solution of the acid on a pledget of cotton sealed in the tooth for 24 to 48 hours.

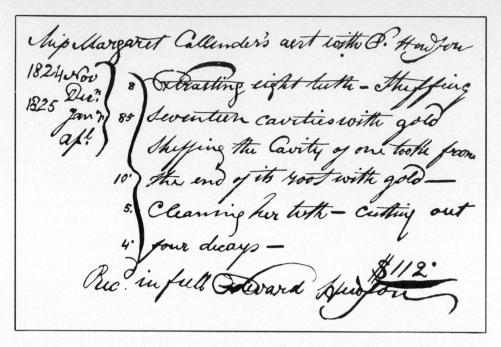

FIG. 24-6. Statement rendered by Dr. Edward Hudson. Among members of the dental profession of that era, Hudson was a recognized leader and originator of dental techniques. He was reputed by his colleagues to be the originator of the root canal filling. (From Koch, C.R.E., and Thorpe, B.L.: A history of dental surgery, vol. 2, Fort Wayne, Ind., 1909, National Art Publishing Co.)

I confess that at first sight the application of so strong a solution as fifty percent looks to be rather heroic; but four years' constant use has proved to me that there is little or no danger of injuring the tooth or the surrounding tissue, if the operation be controlled by any part of common sense.

On removal of the stopping the cavity was washed out with water and the acid solution pumped into the canal with a Donaldson root canal cleanser until the canal was open to the apex. The acid was said to attack the tooth substance vigorously, breaking up the lime salts. To neutralize the acid and force the debris to the surface, a saturated solution of bicarbonate of soda was introduced into the tooth opening, producing an explosive effervescent reaction.

We do not hesitate to use arsenic or nux vomica, aconite, argenti nitras, cocain, and scores of other poisonous drugs. We can have the action of the acid under perfect control. I always keep a saturated solution of bicarbonate soda on my case, so that I may stop the action of the acid at any moment. In but few cases is it probable that the acid will go through the apical foramen in quantities or strength sufficient to have any corrosive effect, for the reason that neutralizing agents in the dentine will have materially weakened the acid before it can pass through the extremely small opening at the apex of the root. If there be an abscess present, the foramen is likely to be larger, and the condition of the tissues about the apex of the root will be materially benefited by the presence of the acid even if in the full strength of the solution. In my mind there could be no better agent for the breaking down of the diseased tissues and the positive destruction of all germ life.

In recent years other effervescent combinations have been suggested. Since the successful use of Dakin's solution (sodium hypochlorite) during World War I, many chlorine solutions have been suggested. Hydrogen peroxide, introduced in 1818 as oxygenated water by Thenardin, was used after the chlorinated solution to produce the desired effervescence.

As root canal therapy progressed, clinicians became suspicious of the presence of bacteria in the canals. Experiments relative to electrosterilization (ionization) in the canal were made as early as 1883 (Cohn and Mendelsohn), 1890 (Apostali and Laquerrier), 1895 (Rhein), and 1900 (Lehman). These pioneers presumed that with electrosterilization they could destroy pathogenic tissue in the periapical region. Many types of electrolytes and metal electrodes were experimented with.[63]

ROOT CANAL FILLING MATERIAL

Prior to the nineteenth century there is very little recorded to indicate that dental practitioners removed pulps from root canals and substituted filling materials. In his book Fauchard referred to filling a cavity in a tooth with lead and then inserting a pivot (probably in the pulp chamber) to retain an artificial crown.[29]

Fig. 24-6 is a reproduction of a bill rendered by Dr. Edward Hudson (1783-1833), of Philadelphia. Dated 1825, the bill includes a charge of $20.00: "One tooth; one stuffed canal, with gold, $20.00." A recognized leader and originator of dental techniques, Hudson was reputed by his colleagues to be the originator of root canal filling.

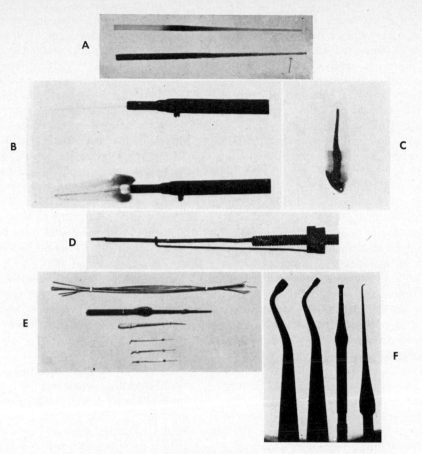

FIG. 24-7. **A,** Orangewood points saturated with silver nitrate and used as root canal fillings. The upper point as received from the manufacturer (S.S. White); the lower point after fitting and preparation for the final canal filling. **B,** Holder made by Kells for fitting the orangewood point and a radiograph of the fitted point. **C,** Radiograph of a tooth showing the orangewood point cemented in place. **D,** Root canal gauge and plugger made by Kells for filling the canal with gutta-percha points. The length of the canal was ascertained by means of iridoplatinum attached to the end of the plugger. Kells termed this "the precision method" but claimed there could be only "apparently" satisfactory results because of the inconsistency of the radiographic picture. **E,** Iridoplatinum wire used to fill canals and the holder for fitting the points. Points manufactured by the Young Manufacturing Co. **F,** Instruments used for filling canals with iridoplatinum points. (From Kells, C.E.: Three score years and nine, New Orleans, 1926, published by author.)

Although Hudson's bill is one of the earliest recordings of the filling of a root canal with gold, earlier writers such as Bourdet (1757) and Townsend (1804) referred to this mode of filling canals. Later much invention and practice with using other canal filling materials occurred—for example, various metals, oxychloride of zinc, paraffin, and amalgam.[44]

Gutta-percha

During this period of search, a material first used in filling teeth and later as a root canal filling material was introduced: gutta-percha.

Gutta-percha is a product made from the latex of trees of the genus *Payena* found mainly in the Malaya Peninsula, Indonesia, and Brazil. It is the earliest known molding material. The main polymer of gutta-percha is a polymer of isoprene (C_5H_8), with a weight of 30,000. It differs structurally from natural rubber insofar as it is the *trans*-isomer of the polymer whereas rubber is the *cis*-isomer.

Gutta-percha was not introduced into the dental profession by chance. The story of its beginning is one of great frustration and labor by Dr. Asa Hill.[44]

After obtaining his education by personal reading and study and a preceptorship in a dental office, Hill began the practice of dentistry in Danbury, Conn. In 1840 there arose within the dental profession a debate on the use of amalgam in place of gold for filling teeth. The profession had just experienced the organization of the American Society of Dental Surgeons. The "amalgam war," as it was known, became so intensified among the Society members that it caused the eventual dissolution of the Society.

A search began for a plastic filling material. To inspire research, the French Academy, setting forth many exacting specifications, offered a large prize for such a discovery.

Hill entered the competition and began what turned out to be years of laborious and frustrating experimentation. After using many substances concocted into mixtures of all types and after many failures, he finally thought he had hit on the right formula: a mixture he brought out in 1847 as "Hill's stopping." The preparation consisted principally of bleached gutta-percha and carbonate of lime and quartz; it was very crude at first introduction in 1848 under a patent. The dental profession became hostile about the patent and columns of protest appeared in the dental literature. After weathering many accusations, Hill lived to see almost universal acceptance of "Hill's stopping."

In 1867 Dr. G.A. Bowman made claim before the St. Louis Dental Society of the first use of gutta-percha for canal filling in an extracted first molar.[56] The demonstration must have produced much interest, for the molar was exhibited at a number of dental meetings in Europe and is now said to be in the museum at Northwestern University. With Dr. C.F. Allen, Bowman invented the Bowman-Allen rubber dam forceps in 1873.

References to the use of gutta-percha for root canal filling prior to the turn of the century were very few and very vague. An early reference was in a paper read before the New York Odontological Society by Dr. Safford G. Perry in 1883.[60] Perry claimed that he had been using a pointed gold wire wrapped with soft gutta-percha. He also began using gutta-percha rolled into a point and packed into the canal. He prepared the points by cutting baseplate gutta-percha into slender strips, warming them with a lamp, laying them on his operating case, and rolling them with another flat surface. He then used shellac warmed over a lamp and rolled into a point of the desired size. Before placing the final point, he saturated the tooth cavity with alcohol; capillary attraction let the alcohol run into the canal, softening the shellac so it could be packed.

Richmond, whose method of knocking out pulps is described earlier in this chapter (p. 768), used a similar point, carbolized, to fill the canal.[43]

Kells[48] also claimed the use of a similar point made of orangewood. Later, when he used radiographs to check the filling, he found the orangewood point to be radiolucent. He learned that dipping the points into a saturated solution of silver nitrate and exposing them to the sunlight would make them radiopaque. Later, the impregnated points were manufactured by S.S. White Manufacturing Company (Fig. 24-7, A).

S.S. White began manufacture of gutta-percha points in 1887.[42] In 1893 William Herbert Rollins introduced a new type of gutta-percha to which he added vermillion.[76] There were critics of this, because vermillion is pure oxide of mercury and dangerous in the quantities suggested.

In our century, new techniques and materials have been developed for the filling of root canals.

The use of radiographs to check the final filling was begun. Consequently it became evident that the canal was not cylindrical, as earlier imagined, and that additional filling material was necessary to fill in the voids.

At first, hard-setting dental cements were used but these proved unsatisfactory. It was also thought that the cement should have strong antiseptic action. Thus many formol-type pastes were developed. Later these pastes were found to be harmful if they penetrated beyond the apical foramen.[39]

Callahan[18] recommended a solution of rosin in chloroform as a filling material in which gutta-percha might be dissolved. The mixture was absorbable. Other absorbable pastes were introduced by Walkoff (1928), Hellner (1932), Munch (1932), and Muller (1936).

Root canal points of various metals, description, and manufacture were used through the years and abandoned; the most popular of these was silver. A pioneer in research into the use and manufacture of the silver point was Dr. Elmer Jasper, who in 1930 was convinced that if silver points could be standardized to the size of the root canal instruments the result would be a more desirable canal filling. He appealed to the Young Dental Manufacturing Company of St. Louis to make these points (Fig. 24-7, E). This company began by hand processing the points at the rate of eight to ten per week. More economical means of production evolved when a swaging machine was engineered.[38]

Calcium hydroxide

Although the earliest reference to the use of $Ca(OH)_2$ is attributed to Nygren,[55] its development in current practice situations is often attributed to Hermann[35] in 1930 and Zander[79] in 1939. $Ca(OH)_2$ as a dressing for vital pulpotomies in teeth with open apices (apexogenesis) was advocated by Eastlick[20] in 1943.

Rapid calcification has followed the use of calcium hydroxide as a pulp chamber paste, and completion of uncalcified root ends has followed the employment of the vital pulpotomy technique.

In 1959 Granath[26] described the use of $Ca(OH)_2$ *(rotbehandling med kalciumhydroxid)* to stimulate apexification following trauma to an incompletely formed upper central incisor. In the United States its use for apexification procedures was popularized by Kaiser[40] and Frank[25] in 1964. Since then $Ca(OH)_2$ has been advocated to manage many procedural or pathologic problems associated with pulpless teeth.[34]

TRAUMATIC INJURIES TO TEETH

The historical management of traumatic tooth injuries has had little review in previous articles on the history of endodontics, save replantation following avulsion. One of the first recordings on the management of trauma is found in Thomas Berdmore's writings[7] in 1770.

When a tooth is loosened by violence, but not moved out of its socket (luxation), ligature alone, and stringent washes to brace the gums, are sufficient for the cure. In this case the pain ceases with the looseness of the teeth; but if it be violent in the beginning, sedatives must be applied.

He astutely identified the fact that in the case of loosened teeth, "...teeth that are pushed inward (intrusion), or outward (luxation), or to the side (lateral luxation) by violence," the nerve may be severed. "The nerve of the tooth is in this case generally broken off, and the tooth-ache, which attends it, is owing to the pressure of the point of the root on the lacerated nerve at the bottom...''[7]

In 1806, Joseph Fox, in his *Diseases of the Teeth, The Gums, and The Alveolar Processes,* outlines a rather modern clasification and approach to the management of traumatic tooth injuries.[23]

The teeth are liable to be fractured by blows, which may be inflicted either by accidents, or from malicious intentions. The incisors of the upper jaw are the most exposed to these accidents: boys, in their various amusements, occasionally receive blows in the mouth, which not unfrequently occasion fractures of the front teeth.

In falling upon the face, the teeth are sometimes struck against a stone; in throwing of stones at each other, one may be received against the teeth; in an incautious attempt to catch a cricket ball, the force of which is not sufficiently spent, it may come with violence against the mouth: in these, and other similar ways, persons are subjected to fractures of the teeth: also, in the mastication of food, hard substances, such as a splinter of bone, or a small stone, or a shot in game, may unexpectedly be bitten upon, at which time the muscles of the lower jaw, being in very strong action, exert a force sufficiently powerful to fracture a perfectly sound tooth.

The treatment of these cases will depend much upon the extent of the injury. If a small piece be broken off from the point of a tooth, nothing more will be necessary than with a fine file to make the rough edge smooth. (Class I fracture)

A tooth rarely becomes carious in consequence of an accident of this kind; for, if there be no predisposition in a tooth to decay, the mere removal of a small portion of it will not cause caries.

A fracture of a tooth occasions inconvenience in proportion to the injury done to the cavity of the tooth. If it should extend nearly into the cavity, having left only a thin piece of bone to cover it, the person will be subject for some time to pain on exposure to cold air; this, however, is generally cured by a deposit of bone taking place within the cavity, by which the nerve is defended, and the tooth may remain during life without exciting further trouble. (Class II fracture)

If the fracture should extend into the cavity, the membrane will immediately be exposed, and inflammation will follow. In this case the treatment must be regulated by the age and peculiar circumstances of the patient. If the accident should have happened to a youth under fifteen or sixteen years of age, it would be better to extract the tooth, because the teeth on each side will gradually approach each other, so that when he is arrived at maturity the loss may never be observed...(Class III fracture)

When a blow has been received upon a tooth so as to loosen it, if the person be young, it will become fast again; but it gradually loses the whiteness of its colour, and at length acquires a bluish tinge...

If a blow be inflicted with sufficient violence to remove a tooth from its socket, it may be returned again; and, if secured to the other teeth by a ligature, it will become fast in a few days. I have known a case in which a tooth had remained out of the socket for six hours, and yet, when returned, became again perfectly united. It will be necessary when a tooth has been out of the socket for some time to introduce a probe, and remove the coagulated blood, the fang may then be inserted with ease, and inflammation will be avoided. But when the teeth have been loosened or beaten out by a blow, and the alveolar process have been injured, or fractured, the teeth will never become perfectly fast; inflammation arises, and nothing but extraction will effect the cure.

In his 1839 *Treatise,* Harris questioned the value and ability to retain avulsed teeth.[32] In doing so, he has provided us some interesting case reports.

I have, on several occasions, replaced teeth that had been knocked from their sockets; but in only one instance was the operation attended with any thing like success. A healthy boy, of about thirteen years of age, while playing bandy, received a blow from the club of one of his playmates, which knocked the left central incisor of the upper jaw entirely out of its socket. I saw the boy about fifteen minutes after the accident. The alveolus was filled with coagulated blood. This I sponged out, and, after having bathed the tooth in tepid water, carefully and accurately replaced it in its socket, and secured it there by silk ligatures attached to the adjacent teeth. On the following day, the gum around the tooth was considerably inflamed; to reduce which, I directed the application of three leeches to the gum, and a frequent use of diluted tinct. myrrh as a wash for the mouth. At the expiration of four weeks, the tooth became firmly fixed in its socket, but from the effusion of coagulable lymph, the alveolar membrane was thickened, and the tooth, in consequence, somewhat protruded. A slight soreness, on taking cold, has ever since been experienced.

Dr. E. Noyes, an eminent dentist of this city, a few days ago, mentioned to me a case somewhat similar in its character. The subject of it was a boy of about ten years of age. One of his front teeth, by a fall, was forced from its socket. On its being replaced shortly after, it, in a few weeks, became again firm in its alveolus... The alveolar processes and jaw-bones are often much injured by mechanical violence. About five years ago, I was requested by the late Dr. Baker, of this city, to visit, with him, a lady who, by the upsetting of a stage between Washington and Baltimore, had her face severely bruised and lacerated. All that portion of the lower jaw, which contained the six anterior teeth, was splintered off, and only retained in the mouth by the gum and integuments, with which it was connected. The wounds of her face, having been properly dressed, the detached portion of the jaw was carefully adjusted and secured by a ligature passed round the front teeth and first molars, and by a bandage on the outside, passed round the chin and back part of the head. Her mouth was washed, five or six times a day, with diluted tinct. myrrh. The third day after the accident by the direction of Dr. B., she lost twelve ounces of blood; and, in about five or six weeks, with no other treatment than the dressing of the wounds, she perfectly recovered.

By 1848, John Tomes, in his *Dental Physiology and Surgery,*[73] provided us with a complete classification of trauma with detailed discussions of recommended treatment. Beyond the previous descriptions provided by his predecessors, he did identify and discuss root fractures as being a classification of trauma.

The root of a tooth, you are aware, is invested with periosteum, and fracture may occur without that membrane being detached, except at the line where the fracture has taken place. The tooth may, therefore, be retained in its place. If, however, the force causing the injury has been great, the fractured part may have been knocked out. The alveolus, by the same blow, may have been fractured, in which case there may be great displacement of the tooth, and in some instances without detachment from its socket. The direction of the fracture may be either transverse or oblique, and may itself be either simple or comminuted.

It has been believed that union of a fractured tooth could never occur, but the preparation which I am enabled to show you, through the kindness of my friend Mr. Saunders, whose property it is, shows that union not only can, but in this instance has, taken place. The tooth is a central incisor of the upper jaw; the fracture extended obliquely through the middle of the fang, and was obviously attended with slight displacement, in which position perfect union has taken place. Several small nodules of dentine mark the line of union, the oblique direction of which, together with the displacement, are so well marked, that there can be no doubt of the producing cause of the present appearance of the tooth—namely, fracture and subsequent union.

A second case of union is recorded in the American Journal of Dental Science, vol. i., where you will see a woodcut representing an incisor fractured near the neck, with the crown bent at a right angle with the fang, and in that position united.

It will not be difficult to understand how a tooth fractured through the fang may be united, supposing the pulp be not destroyed, by the injury of the dentine. You have seen that, when the surface of a tooth is worn, the pulp forms dentine in the cavity opposite to the worn external surface, and I shall show you that, when a tooth becomes decayed, the pulp will, in some cases, form dentine in the pulp-cavity, opposite to the seat of the disease situated on the external surface. The process of development in the two cases is similar to that engaged in the formation of the dentine of the body of the tooth. In each case we recognise reparative attempts, and also an unquestionable proof that where there is dental pulp there we may have, under favourable circumstances, dentine developed. If, then, a tooth be fractured through the fang, and the pulp be not destroyed, a process may be set up similar in every respect to that effecting the union of fractured bones.

Mr. Owen describes and figures a specimen—the inferior canine tusk of the Hippopotamus, in which a fracture completely through the tooth, near its base, is perfectly reunited, and the reunion effected by the development of secondary dentine, or osteo-dentine, as he calls it.

If we examine osseous union, we shall be able to trace the following steps up to the completion of the process. Thus, the immediate consequence of fracture of a bone is the effusion of blood from the lacerated vessels of the injured part; this is followed by effusion of liquor sanguinis, or lymph; the formation of cartilage between the fractured extremities then succeeds, and after awhile the cartilage is converted into bone, and the union is complete. Similar action would no doubt arise when dental union takes place, but instead of cartilage we should have dental pulp, which would be converted into dentine. Numerous specimens of hypertrophy of the cementum attest that, whenever there is dental periosteum, there may be formed dental bone or cementum. The bony layer of the fang may, therefore under favourable circumstances, be united.

Treatment. — If the fracture be situated about the middle of the fang, or near the neck, and the body of the tooth be knocked out, the remainder of the root, if painful, should be extracted;

but if a small portion of the fang only remain in the alveolus, it is not well, unless it be painful or loose, to attempt the removal, as the operation would be attended with considerable pain. A small piece of root very seldom gives any inconvenience, and is, after a time, by the deposition of bone in the alveolus, brought towards the surface and thrown off, or it may be impacted in bone, and there remain without giving any evidence of its existence. . . .

Again, a small portion of the fang of a fractured tooth may wholly or in part be absorbed. It must not be denied, however, that, in a few cases, the remaining part of the fang of a fractured tooth will produce inflammation, and subsequently a gum-boil, which had the stump been removed, would probably have been avoided. . . .

If, then, after fracture the crown be not detached, but yet feels very loose in the gums, it should be removed; or, if the gum be inflamed, it should be removed, whether loose or not. Should, however, the fractured tooth be tolerably free from pain, and the gum from inflammation, and at the same time be held tolerably well in its place, we may attempt to get a union of the fractured surfaces. If we could insure perfect absence of motion in the tooth, it seems probably, judging from the specimen before us, that union might be effected. It will however, be extremely difficult to ensure perfect rest in the parts, and we know that even a bone will not unite unless there is total absence of motion between the fractured extremities, and much less would a tooth, when the nature of the new tissue, namely dental pulp, is much less firm, and therefore more readily injured than cartilage. From these circumstances our chances of success will, I fear, be small, though I think the chance worth the trial.

If several teeth with their alveoli are fractured, and there is displacement, the whole should be brought back to the proper position, and the patient should be enjoined to avoid all causes of motion in the injured part, which should be fomented, by taking into the mouth the hot poppy-head fomentation, which should be renewed as soon as it cools. The general health should also be attended to, and aperients given if necessary.

USE OF THE RUBBER DAM

Treating teeth in a dry operative field was a problem of great concern to clinicians for several centuries. Many devices and inventions were attempted—including gold bands with tapering flanges, plaster of Paris dams, and even bibulous paper surrounding the area of operation. Cotton, rubber tubing, coffer dams of wax and gutta-percha, and finally the original saliva ejector (a pump operated by squeezing rubber bulbs) were used. Most of these attempts must have been cumbersome, frustrating, time consuming, and of brief success.[6]

A young dentist of Monticello, N.Y., conceived the idea of using a sheet of rubber to dam the saliva. He demonstrated this technique to some of his colleagues in New York City, who accepted his suggestion with enthusiasm. This generous gentleman, Dr. Sanford Christie Barnum (Fig. 24-8), gratuitously donated his discovery to dentistry.

Barnum was born in 1838 in Oakland Valley, N.Y., where he received his early education and attended Monticello Academy. His uncle, Dr. Joseph Clowes, practiced dentistry in New York City and took Barnum into his of-

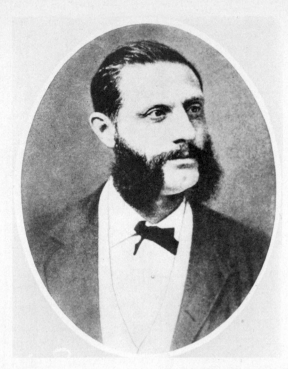

FIG. 24-8. Dr. Sanford Christie Barnum, inventor of the rubber dam. (From Koch, C.R.E., and Thorpe, B.L.: A history of dental surgery, vol. 2, Fort Wayne, Ind., 1909, National Art Publishing Co.)

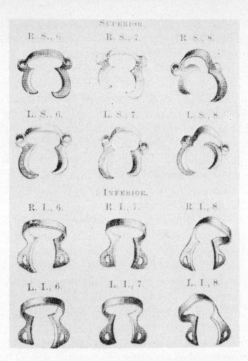

FIG. 24-9. Twelve of the 32 clamps devised by Dr. Delous Palmer (From Latimer, G.S.: Dent. Cosmos 6:13, 1864.)

fice as a dental student at the age of 18. After 4 years, Barnum left his uncle's office and started his own practice in Monticello. Finding he needed more scientific education, he attended the New York College of Dentistry and received his degree of Doctor of Dental Surgery. In 1868 he was one of the first students to graduate from that institution. After returning to his uncle's practice, he gained a fine reputation in prosthetic and operative dentistry.[72]

Barnum first tried the rubber dam in 1862; at this time he was practicing in Monticello. In 1864 he demonstrated the use of the rubber dam to his uncle, who was most impressed with the idea. His uncle successfully urged Barnum to freely offer his invention to the profession. The response of the dental profession to his invention plus his generosity in foregoing remuneration gave him worldwide recognition.

After the introduction of the rubber dam, various techniques were developed for its placement and retention.

A hand-pressured hollow was devised to form holes—the dam to be placed on a block of tin or a piece of boxwood. A hot instrument was also tried for this purpose. In 1882 S.S. White introduced a punch resembling the one used today.

Many means of attaching the rubber dam to the tooth were tried, including cotton spunk, twine, wedged thread and silk ligatures, silver wire, bibulous paper, a string of beads, even dental cement.

In 1882 Dr. Delous Palmer introduced a set of metal clamps for each tooth (Fig. 24-9). This inspired the invention of numerous types of clamps—rubber dam screw clamp, root clamp, lever clamp, festoon clamp, broad-flange clamp, beaked molar clamp, dens-sap clamp, reach-o-rounds clamp, hinge-and-joint clamp, universal clamp.

INVENTORS OF DENTAL INSTRUMENTS

When it was discovered that the tooth had a pulp (instead of a "worm"), inventors put their minds to the task of fashioning instruments to work in these tiny canals. Very little is recorded in dental publications regarding the inventors and their products. When inventions were placed in the hands of a manufacturer, usually the name of the designer was not disclosed. According to custom, if the inventor was a professional man (as most were) he was generous and shared his discovery without patent or remuneration.

One such inventor, unknown and forgotten by the profession, was W.H. Rollins. After developing an interest in dentistry, he spent 3 years as a preceptor in a dental office. Later he entered Harvard, attaining a D.M.D. degree in 1873 and an M.D. degree in 1879. His curiosity and inventiveness remained unabated, and he published many ideas in professional journals.[69]

There may be several reasons why the profession has forgotten Rollins. A modest man with a strong personality, he was shy and had few friends. He refused to attend dental meetings, where he could have introduced his discoveries. Instead, he mailed his reports to now defunct dental magazines. He believed his inventions should be given freely to the various professions. When a manufacturer placed his wares on the market, the name of Rollins was never mentioned.

William H. Rollins was responsible for hundreds of inventions and improvements in radiology, medicine (he was the first to secure radium and advocate its use in cancer treatment), dentistry (he invented dental materials, techniques, and dental instruments, and made new improvements in old materials), physics, genetics and radio reception.

For endodontics, Rollins invented rubber dam clamps with rubber edges to protect teeth and give a firmer grip (1889), saws for cutting roots (1889), a new anesthetic—arsenite of cocaine (1891), an improved gutta-percha with vermilion added (1893), formaldehyde in solid form (1898), and a root canal drill (used in a dental engine with a motor and controlled by a foot switch; the engine speed was reduced by a worm gear to 100 rpm to prevent breakage of the small-diameter drill) (1889) (Fig. 24-10).

Rollins' greatest interest after dental inventions was discoveries in photography. He made camera film and invented the first steroscopic camera. Before his death in 1929, he wrote that the new radio he had created was greatly superior to any on the market.[70]

Edward Maynard, A.M., M.D., D.D.S. (Fig. 24-11), was another inventor who attained great renown for his inventions outside the profession. Born in Madison, N.Y., in 1813, he received his early education at Hamilton Academy. In 1835 he entered the field of dentistry.

During those times dental instruments were not systematized and clinicians designed instruments for personal use. This was no hardship to Maynard, who was an able mechanic.

Maynard was the first to recognize that there were such things as dental fibrils and that during cavity preparation these could be cut with less pain, depending on the direction of the cutting. From his research he contributed techniques to avoid injury to adjacent tissues.

In 1838 Maynard advocated pulp removal and became quite expert in filling premolar and molar canals with gold foil. For the removal of pulp tissue, he invented the barbed broach. These broaches were made from the untempered steel of watch springs filed down to the fineness of a horse hair and were barbed on one side.

Besides pulp removal, he also advocated the use of his "watch spring" instruments, made into probes, for determining the length of the "fang"[53]:

It must be a self-evident fact that it is a matter of vital importance preparatory to attempting to fill the fangs of teeth where the foramen are large, to determine the exact length of the roots; in accomplishing this object, Dr. Maynard employs a very delicate probe with a hooked extremity, made from a watch-spring, and marked at regular intervals upon the sides. On passing this along the pulp cavity, if it passes out through the foramen, a sensation similar to that experienced when the gum is pricked by instruments will be felt; and on attempting to draw the probe back, in place of coming away easily, the hooked extremity will be most likely to catch on the edge of the foramen. As Dr. M. suggests, if, on rotating the probe, it is found to catch all around, there can be no question that it is arrested by the edge of the foramen; but if it catches on one side only, it is most likely due to some prominence or depression on the side of the pulp cavity. Having determined beyond a question of doubt that the probe has caught on the edge of the foramen, by means of the marks on

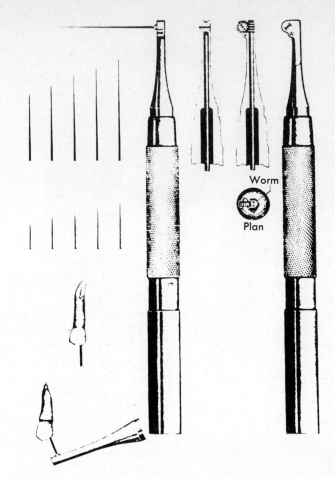

FIG. 24-10. Root canal drill designed by Rollins. (From Sweet, A.P.S.: Dent. Radiogr. Photogr. 33:1, 1960.)

the sides of the probe the exact length of the fang can be ascertained.

Maynard's reputation reached the European continent. He received an invitation to exhibit his dental dexterity in the Court of St. Petersburg, Russia. This demonstration was followed by an appointment as dentist to the royal family. Emperor Nicholas offered to appoint him "actual dentist to his Majesty," with the rank of major, if he would remain in Russia for another 10 years to teach and practice. He refused.

The name of Edward Maynard does not have as great an attachment to dental science as it should, but it is of great importance in the field of military arms; the well-received Maynard rifle has enjoyed worldwide use.[44]

Maynard made reamers from piano wire and filed them to the desired shape.[61] Fine reamers had four corners; large reamers had three corners. He claimed that piano wire had perfect temper and was almost impossible to break, no matter how fine.

An individual often overlooked in the development of endodontic instruments was Dr. Robert Arthur[2] of Baltimore. In 1852 he described how to make a fine root canal file, and he also provided guidelines for its mechanical properties:

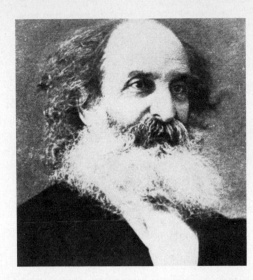

FIG. 24-11. Edward Maynard, A.M., M.D., D.D.S. (From Koch, C.R.E., and Thorpe, B.L.: A history of dental surgery, vol. 3, Fort Wayne, Ind., 1909, National Art Publishing Co.)

But in regard to instruments intended for this purpose there are several particulars to be observed. They must be small enough to pass into the canal of the fang, to the very extremity—they must have some elasticity, enough to take the slight curves presented by many fangs coming under treatment, and that formed by the relative position of the fang to the opening from the external cavity—they must also possess sufficient strength and toughness to prevent them from breaking when used for the purpose in question—and must be given such form as will enable them to seize hold of the pulp and draw it out. The best material for these instruments, which I have yet found, is fine steel, well annealed. The best steel for the purpose, of which I have any knowledge, is piano wire.

After annealing the wire, cut into the proper lengths for the instruments, it is fitted into suitable sockets. For this purpose I generally use steel wire with a socket drilled in it, into which the wire for the instrument is cemented. But any convenient form which may suggest itself to the operator will, of course, answer. It will be found convenient to have a considerable number so that there may be at hand, instruments of a variety of sizes, thus saving the necessity of frequently changing them.

When securely fastened into the sockets, they may be filed down to the required size. It is advisable for those who have never practiced this operation to prepare teeth of the several classes, and make the instruments of such size that they will readily pass into the smallest fangs. In order to obtain the most desirable form, and to preserve as much body as possible to the instruments, it has been suggested (by Dr. White) that they should be square, except in cases where it is necessary that they should correspond with the form of the fang. After they are reduced to the desired size, they should be well burnished (a suggestion of Dr. Maynard); this will give them a slight temper, and increase the little elasticity they have acquired in the process of filing. There should now be cut upon them with a sharp knife, small barbs, looking toward the handle of the instrument. Care must be observed, too, that the points of these little instruments should be made sharp, so that they will pass alongside of the pulp in the fang, and not push it upward in the attempt to take it away. The use of these instruments is too obvious to need any

elaborate description; they pass readily into the fang and will draw out the pulp as they are withdrawn.

If, by accident, the instrument used should break—and this is an accident which careful handling should made very rare—it will sometimes be found difficult, and it may be impossible, to remove. If not jammed in the fang so as to be immovable, it may, in many cases, be withdrawn by rendering a small instrument magnetic, and passing gently up till it comes into contact with the fragment to be removed. The use of a magnetized instrument was suggested some time ago by the late Dr. John Harris, for a similar purpose. Once or twice during my practice I have found it impossible to remove the broken fragment of the instrument from the fang, and was obliged to fill without regard to it. I have observed no unfavorable results in these cases which I could attribute to this cause.

All this is hard to believe as we struggle with modern "standardized" instruments.

The standardization of root canal instruments and filling material received serious discussion 25 years ago. The Research Committee of the American Association of Endodontists, inspired by the reports of Dr. John Ingle, recommended that dental manufacturers of endodontic supplies standardize their products.[50] The result was the instruments we have presently available—no models of perfection but a step in the right direction.

USE OF LEECHING

Leeches, which were widely used by the medical profession, also were used for the treatment of an abscessed tooth. They were applied with the object of drawing out the "bad blood." They probably eased the pain by relieving the congested tissues of some of the swelling.

In the days when leeching was popular, youngsters would appear fascinated by the jar containing these black monsters on display in "drugstore" windows with the large jars of chemically colored water that were lighted by an incandescent lamp at night.

Leeching had great popularity before the "wonder drugs." One of the advocates of leeching was Kells,[43] who described the manner of application. Following is a condensed version of this description:

The treatment usually takes 20 to 30 minutes, during which time the patient and the operator must not budge. The buccal gum in the apical area of the affected root should be dry when it is scarified lightly with a rapidly revolving abrasive wheel. The leech is applied to the area while in a leech tube; the tube looks like a bent glass liquid dropper but has a larger opening at the curved application end (Fig. 24-12). The leech has a similar appearance at both ends; therefore, one must determine the "business end," which is always free and lively. The leech is placed in the leech tube, and the curved end is rapidly applied to the scarified area. The process of application requires much study; the difficulty is in getting the leech to begin biting the scarified tissue and suck the blood. This procedure may be as hard to learn as it is to sell the patient experiencing it (shades of Dracula!).

The leech at the time of application is a long, slender creature; following the blood-sucking procedure, however,

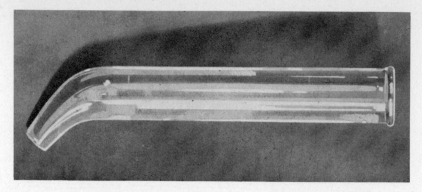

FIG. 24-12. Tube for holding a leech. (From Kells, C.E.: Three score years and nine, New Orleans, 1926, published by author.)

it is thick enough to fill the tube. At this time it lets go of the tissue and, by slight movement of the tube, can be removed and destroyed.

To prolong the bleeding of the affect gum tissue, the patient is supplied with hot water to be held in the mouth and changed frequently; this practice is to be continued for 5 to 20 minutes. Continuous bleeding is the "success" of the procedure.

Kells[43] mentioned that in his day this was the only way to treat postoperative root-filling problems.

The root-canal problem is—or rather should be —the dental problem of today, and of the future. Whatever success I reach in dealing with root-canals, I feel sure is due entirely to two things- the one, the use of leeches; the other assimilating their qualities and sticking to my patient "like a leech."

The moment I have completed a root-canal filling, I throw a life-line around the patient, and I hold on to my end like "grim death."

Assuming a case: I fill a root-canal at nine o'clock. The tooth "feels comfortable" says the patient. Everything looks lovely; there is no reason to expect trouble. Now here's my long suit. While there is no reasons to expect trouble, I fear it all the same. That's why I possibly will win out.

The tooth is filled. I am very careful to relieve the occlusion. If I fail to do this, I may as well cut my life-line. I have made my first great inexcusable mistake. I then say to my patient, "Now listen, if the tooth feels the least bit sore during the day, you must phone me right away." Should I get the message, an appointment is made, and, believe me, I see that it is kept all right. I find that the tooth is a little sore on pressure. The very first thing to do is to again look after the occlusion. Then a leech is applied.

When the patient is now discharged, the life-line is still about him. I tell him that if his tooth is not a whole lot better by eight o'clock, he must apply slippery elm poultices for one hour by the clock, and he must apply anti-phlogistine to his face and keep it on all night. Failing to carry out these instructions, and an abscess forming, I wash my hands of the case; or words to that effect—or more so. This is no time for flim-flamming.

At nine o'clock another pull on the line. I ring him up and find out how he is, and if necessary, prescribe pyramidon or codein, in addition to what he has already done. With these directions faithfully carried out, he will probably answer (another pull

on the life-line) an early ring at seven or seven-thirty the following morning with the reply that he slept all night and his tooth is comfortable. If that's the case, the life-line is cast off, because if this incipient peridental inflammation is checked, the game is won. Thus, you see, I have in fact stuck to him "like a leech" and that's why I got the result.

Now let's take the same case and handle it differently.

I fill a root-canal at nine o'clock. Upon completion, the tooth is comfortable, so I do not look after the occlusion, but I say, "If the tooth gets sore, call in the morning." Next day, the patient calls and says the tooth is pretty sore; cannot close on it without pain. I try to grind it down, but it hurts so much I give it up (twenty-four hours too late). I paint the gum with aconite and iodin (just that much aconite and iodin wasted; might as well pour water on a duck's back) and tell the patient to take some aspirin if it does not get any better.

The usual story. All day it feels fairly comfortable, but "Watchman what of that night?" About nine o'clock it begins to get worse. Maybe his doctor gives him some codein and he sleeps, or maybe he passes a sleepless night; and the next morning he comes to the office in a frightfully bad fix with his face swollen, and then I apply a leech. Vain effort—twenty-four hours, or possibly thirty-six hours, too late. Besides the leeching, I do everything else imaginable, but to no avail. The abscess must run its course, or possibly the tooth is extracted.

These are two pictures of extreme cases, I will admit. There are all kinds of degrees between the two

Now this is the way I look at it. I don't care how well the canal is filled, and how fine it looks in the skiagraph, if the dentist allows his patient to go thru one or more days of suffering thru indifference and because he did not do the right thing at the right time, I call him, a pretty poor dentist, as far as filling root-canals is concerned.

I don't mean to say that I can always avert postoperative pain after a root-canal filling, because that is not the truth. I don't believe anybody can do that. But what I do mean is that I use every means known to me to prevent this pain, and once I fill a root-canal, that patient "has the call" for the next forty-eight hours. That's what I mean. I believe that's why I am fairly successful with my immediate root-canal problems.

At any time would my office hours be prolonged and dinner missed—and many a time this has been done—rather than take a chance.

I fancy I hear that hardhearted Brother McGee calling "the count" on me, so I reckon I'd better quit right here.

THE LESSONS OF HISTORY

Now that we have had a brief overview of the empirical development of endodontics (occasionally intertwined with some scientific basis) it is necessary to step back again, in the not too distant past, to carefully review the astute words of one of the twentieth-century pioneers of endodontics, Dr. James Roy Blayney.

It is time to stop the exchange of personal opinions and to make an analytical survey of the work that has been completed in order to base further studies upon facts that have been definitely established. Not only is this the proper procedure for those interested chiefly in research, but the clinician should follow the same course and base his plan of treatment upon the principles that may be recognized and accepted today.[8]

It is apparent that until recent times, pulp canal therapy has been practiced upon an empirical basis, and that paper either read or published presented only the author's opinion and did not submit evidence established by a critical investigative program to support his statements.[11]

I believe society will be better served if the rank and file of the profession will place pulp-canal therapy on a biologic basis.[10]

Whenever pulp is removed and the canal treated and filled in a manner that is compatible with or favorable to a physiologic reaction, we may expect a satisfactory percentage of success. Also, whenever treatment is carried on in such a way as to antagonize biologic processes of repair, we will continue to have many failures. As we see the question, it does not materially matter if an operator uses one style of an instrument, while another prefers a broach of different pattern, provided each will do the task for which it was designed. The crying need is not a new technic, a new drug or the like, but a better and more keen appreciation of the processes by which nature repairs traumatic injury or overcomes an infectious process.[9]

Failing to heed this futuristic exhortation, we may be faced with crying out the words of Giles McQuiggin—"expunge, expunge!"

THE ACHING TOOTH[49]

Why art thou so rebellious, raging tooth?
Why break the peace that pleasantly prevailed,
And raise such warfare in thy warm abode?
There's room enough for thee, and chance as fair
As any of thy fellows may possess;
And there you all might dwell, a happy band
In the firm brotherhood that Nature formed,
When she permitted you to take the place
Of that confederacy which she had tried,
And proved too weak to stand the powerful test
Of spreading bone and sinew: —on the soil
Where reigned and ruled the Aborigines
That were your predecessors, you have pow'r
To cluster unmolested; succeeding foes
May never push you from your gifted rights.

You form a compact,—leagued for life and death;
There you should stand in undivided strength,
And hail the friendly visitant that comes
To nourish and sustain you; and repel
With greater energy, the foreign foe
That dares intrude on your domestic peace.

What cause have you for quarrel in your ranks?
What party feuds to rouse you up for fight?
Or why should Cuspidatus ask a right
That to Incisor he'd refuse to grant?
Or why Incisor, seek a place of pow'r
To which his friend Molar might not aspire?
'Tis vain to talk of preference or place,
In a society so firmly bound,
And in such close connexion; —one and all,
Should spurn the nullifier's hated cause,
And stick to *union* to the very last.

And what are names or offices to you?
Or what care you for principle or laws,
Save those which Nature in her wisdom gave
To regulate her household; —they belong
As well to you, as to unnumbered throngs,
That pass through being's changes to decay.
The badge of honor that the Whig may wear,
Or title that the Democrat may boast,
Hath no high preference for you to claim;
You have no principle for which to fight,
As ever changing politicians have,
Who madly sacrifice a thousand times
In saving once, from foul pollution's touch,
The principle they quarrel to sustain.

Your only dread need be the heartless quack,
That like a greedy Vampire, seeks to draw
Blood from your mangled socket, and to thrust
His plundering talons in your owner's purse.
Or it may be, perchance, that he may drive
A plug of composition through your crown,
Or closely pack his tin, deep in your heart;
And for the wretched deed, demand his price,
And nothing less than gold will suit his taste.

Now seeing these are truths, that I have sung,
A few of multitudes that might be told,
Why may you not all live in peace and love
And help each other in your daily toil?
You'd better do it; —and you aching one,
I warn you once again; —your raging stop,
Or by your hopes of custard, I declare,
That I shall turn against you, and raise up
With all my might, the cry, *expunge! expunge!!*

ACKNOWLEDGMENT

Special thanks is given to Dr. Vincent Milas for his generous assistance in preparing this chapter.

REFERENCES

1. American Association of Endodontics: An annotated glossary of terms used in endodontics, ed. 4, Chicago, 1984, The Association.
2. Arthur, R.: Treatment of dental caries complicated with disorders of the pulp and peridental membrane, Am. J. Dent. Sci. 2:505, 1852.
3. Atkinson, W.H.: Treatment of dental pulps, Am. J. Dent. Sci. 1:103, 1867.
4. Baker, E.: On the treatment of the nerves of the teeth, Am. H. Dent. Sci. 1:170, 1839.
5. Balkwill, F.H.: On the treatment of pulpless teeth, Br. Dent. J. 4:588, 1883.
6. Barbakow, A.Z.: The rubber dam; a 100 year history, J. Am. Acad. Gold Foil Operators 8:1, 1965.

7. Bermore, T.: Treatise on the disorders and deformities of the teeth and gums, London, 1770.

8. Blaney, J.R.: The biologic aspect of root canal therapy, Dent. Items. Int. **49:**681, 1927.

9. Blaney, J.R.: What teeth should be extracted: a report based upon further studies of root-canal therapy, J. Am. Dent. Assoc. **15:**1217, 1928.

10. Blaney, J.R.: Fundamentals governing pulp-canal therapy, Dent. Cosmos **74:**635, 1932.

11. Blaney, J.R.: The progress of pulp-canal therapy, Proc. Dent. Centenary Celebration, P. 646, March 18-20, 1940.

12. Boorde, A.: The breviare of helth, London, 1552, Thomas East Co.

13. Brookins, A.B.: Root filling, Am. J. Dent. Sci. **1:**168, 1867.

14. Brown, S.: Cure of tooth-ache, Am. J. Dent. Sci. **1:**227, 1839.

15. Brown, S.: Dentologia: a poem in the diseases of the teeth and their proper remedies, New York, 1840.

16. Burdell, H.: Observations on the anatomy, suture, physiology, and diseases of the teeth, Am. J. Dent. Sci. **1;**66, 1839.

17. Callahan, J.R.: Sulfuric acid for opening root canals. Dent. Cosmos **36:**329, 1894.

18. Callahan, J.R.: Rosin, solution for the sealing of the dental tubuli and as an adjuvant in the filling of root canals, Allied Dent. J. **9:**53, 110, 1914.

19. DeChemant, M.N.D.: Dissertation; artificial teeth, London, 1804.

20. Eastlick, K.A.: Management of pulp exposure in the mixed dentition, J. Am. Dent. Assoc. **30:**179, 1943.

21. Ebers, G.M.: Ebers papyrus, vol. 2, Leipzig, 1975, Engleman.

22. Foley, G.H.: Foley's footnotes, Wallingford, PA, 1972, Washington Square East.

23. Fox, J.: Diseases of the teeth, the gums and the alveolar processes, London, 1806, James Swan.

24. Francke, O.C.: Capping of the living pulp: from Philip Pfaff to John Wessler, Bull. Hist. Dent. **19:**17, 1971.

25. Frank, A.L.: Clinical presentation at the American Association of Endodontists meeting, Washington, D.C., April, 1964.

26. Granath, L.E.: Några synpunkter på behandlingen av traumatiserade incisiver påbarn, Odontol. Rev. **10:**272, 1959.

27. Greenwood, I.I.: Letter to the editor. Am. J. Lib. Dent. Sci. **2:**138, 1841.

28. Grossman, L.I.: Endodontics 1776-1976: a bicentennial history against the background of general dentistry, J. Am. Dent. Assoc. **93:**78, 1976.

29. Guerini, V.: History of dentistry, Philadelphia, 1909, Lea & Febiger.

30. Harding, W.E.: A few practical observations on the treatment of the pulp, J. Br. Dent. Assoc. **4:**318, 1883.

31. Harlan, A.W.: Pulp digestion, Dent. Cosmos **42:**1272, 1900.

32. Harris, C.A.: The dental art; practical treatise on dental surgery, Baltimore, 1839, Armstrong J. Berry.

33. Harris, C.A.: A dictionary of dental science, bibliography and medical terminology, Philadelphia, 1849, Lindsay & Blakiston.

34. Heithersay, G.S.: Calcium hydroxide on the treatment of pulpless teeth with associated pathology, J. Br. Endod. Soc. **8:**74, 1975.

35. Hermann, B.W.: Dentinobliteration der Wurzelkanale nach der Behandlung mit Kalzium, Zahnaerztl. Rund. **39:**888, 1930.

36. Hunter, J.: Practical treatise on the diseases of the teeth. Part II, London, 1778.

37. Ingle, J.: Endodontics, Philadelphia, 1965, Lea & Febiger.

38. Jasper, E.A.: Personal correspondence, Maryland Heights, Mo. 1973, Young Dental Manufacturing Co.

39. Juge, H.: Absorbable pastes for root canal fillings, Int. Dent. J. **9:**462, 1959.

40. Kaiser, J.H.: Presentation at the American Association of Endodontists meeting, Washington, D.C., April, 1964.

41. Kanner, L.: Folklore of the teeth, New York, 1928, Macmillan Co.

42. Keane, H.C.: A century of service to dentistry, Philadelphia, 1944, S.S. White Dental Manufacturing Co.

43. Kells, C.E.: Three score years and nine, Chicago, 1926, Lakeside Press.

44. Koch, C.R.E., and Thorpe, B.L.: A history of dental surgery, vols. 2 and 3, Fort Wayne, Ind., 1909, National Art Publishing Co.

45. Koecker, L.: Of treating the living membrane of the tooth when exposed, Am. J. Dent. Sci. **1:**135, 1839.

46. Latimer, G.S.: Barnum's rubber dam, Dent. Cosmos **6:**13, 1864.

47. Link, W.J.: Alfred Einhorn, discoverer of novocaine, Dent. Radiogr. Photogr. **32:**1, 1959.

48. Maxfield, G.A.: Methods of destroying dental pulps, Dent. Cosmos **36:**870, 1894.

49. McQuiggin, G.: The aching tooth, Am. J. Dent. Sci. **1:**77, 1839.

50. Milas, V.B.: A history of the American Association of Endodontists, Chicago, 1968, General Printing Co.

51. Miller, W.D.: The microorganisms of the human mouth, Philadelphia, 1890, S.S. White Dental Manufacturing Co.

52. Mills, G.A.: Who did it first?, Dent. Cosmos **25:**447, 1883

53. M'Quillen, J.H.: Fang filling, Dent. Cosmos **2:**225, 1861.

54. M'Quillen, J.H.: Local anaesthesia in extirpation of the dental pulp, Dent. Cosmos **8:**225, 1866.

55. Nygren, J.A.: Rådgivare angående bästa sättet att vårda och bevara tändernas friskhet, Stockholm, 1838.

56. History of dentistry in Missouri, Fulton, Mo., 1938, The Ovid Press, Inc.

57. Orban, B.: Editorial, J. Endod. **1:**1, 1946.

58. Ottolengui, R.: An era in dentistry, Dent. Items Int. **25:**870, 1903.

59. Ottolengui, R.: Table talks on dentistry, vol. 2, Brooklyn, 1935, Dental Items of Interest Publishing Co.

60. Perry, S.G.: Preparing and filling the roots of teeth, Dent. Cosmos **25:**185, 1883.

61. Perry, S.G.: Gutta-percha points for sealing root canals, Dent. Cosmos **53:**1122, 1911.

62. Price, W.A.: Practical progress in dental skiagraphy, Dent. Item Int. **23:**458, 1901.

63. Prinz, H.: Electrosterilization of root canals, Dent. Cosmos **59:**374, 1917.

64. Prinz, H.: Diseases of the soft tissue and their treatment, Philadelphia, 1937, Lea & Febiger.

65. Prinz, H., et al: Pharmacology and dental therapeutics, ed. 9, St. Louis, 1945, The C.V. Mosby Co.

66. Ring, M.E.: Dentistry: an illustrated history, St. Louis, 1985, The C.V. Mosby Co.

67. Rowe, A.H.R.: An historical review of materials used for pulp treatment up to the year 1900, J. Br. Endod. Soc. **2:**30, 1968.

68. Schreier, E.: Die behandlung inficirter wurzelcanale mit kaliumnatrium, Trans World's Columbian Dental Congress, Chicago, 1894, Knight, Leonard & Co., p. 589.

69. Sweet, A.P.S.: Some historical aspects of radiodontics, Dent. Radiogr. Photogr. **15:**2, 1942.

70. Sweet, A.P.S.: William Herbert Rollins, D.D.S., M.D., dentistry's forgotten man, Dent. Radiogr. Photogr. **33:**1, 1960.

71. Taylor, J.A.: History of dentistry, Philadelphia, 1922, Lea & Febiger.

72. Thorpe, B.L.: Sanford Christie Barnum, Dent. Rev. **17:**779, 1903.

73. Tomes, J.: Dental physiology and surgery, London, 1848, J.W. Parker.

74. Waas, M.: Use of sodium and potassium in root canal therapy, J. Endod. **3:**14, 1948.

75. Wadsworth, H.W.: Resetting and transplanting teeth, Dent. Cosmos **18:**577, 1876.

76. Weinberger, B.W.: An introduction to the history of dentistry, St. Louis, 1948, the C.V. Mosby Co.

77. Younger, W.J.: Some of the latest phases in implantation and other operations, Dent. Cosmos **35:**102, 1893.

78. White, T.C.: On the conservative treatment of exposed pulp, J. Br. Dent. Assoc. **4:**164, 1883.

79. Zander, H.A.: Reaction of pulp to calcium hydroxide, J. Dent. Res. **18:**373, 1939.

25

QUESTIONS/ANSWERS AND LINGERING CONTROVERSIES

Question:

Should pastes containing paraformaldehyde, lead tetroxide, phenylmercuric borate, and steroids be used for filling root canals?

Answer:

Howard Martin

The science of endodontics has made great advances in the past several years. Endodontics now has a predictable, reproducible, biologically oriented basis for therapy.

The use of a paraformaldehyde paste falls into the category of a questionable procedure. The paste materials presently in use, referred to as N-2 or by similar names (e.g., RC-2B, RET-B, RC-2 White), are all comparable in formulation. The purpose of the paste is to achieve an antiseptic obturation of the canal, a sclerotic zone to maintain apical vitality, and ease of manipulation.

The N-2–type pastes contain formaldehyde, lead tetroxide, titanium dioxide, steroids, phenylmercuric borate, and zinc oxide.

As shown on the preprinted prescription forms, 6.5% of the paste is paraformaldehyde, a highly caustic fixative generally used in inanimate disinfection; it is too irritating to be placed in contact with periapical tissues. The original concept in the 1940s had been to use a 3% paraformaldehyde paste on denuded roots for *desensitization*. Bringing the paste in direct contact with periapical tissues creates a coagulative necrosis and tissue fixation. The fixed tissue eventually acts as an irritant to the surrounding vital tissue and has the potential for future breakdown. Paraformaldehyde often leads to poor healing and failure.

Lead compounds are used in the N-2 formulation primarily to make the paste radiopaque; however, even in the *absence* of lead compounds, the paste is still basically radiopaque. Lead compounds have absolutely no therapeutic function in the paste formulation. Lead has a definite toxic effect on cells and internal organs.

Steroids in the paste are primarily for the alleviation of pain and other symptoms. However, steroids reduce the normal inflammatory action necessary for wound healing.

If placed in necrotic areas, they exacerbate an active infection. The use of steroid compounds may be good for certain types of endodontic problems; however, the indiscriminant use of a potentially good drug for *all* patients, without any consideration of indications or contraindications, is of questionable value. If less caustic paste materials were used and proper adherence to cleaning and shaping procedures followed, there would be no need for steroids.

Phenylmercuric borate is a weak antiseptic and is irritating to connective tissue. It has been shown to play only a minor *and unnecessary* role in the proper cleaning, shaping, and obturation of the root canal system.

Tissue culture reactions.[11,21,23-27] The N-2 pastes cause a severe derangement of the cells. The cells cannot multiply; thus their regenerative and reparative ability is decreased. Lead, mercury, and titanium dioxide prevent cell multiplication whereas paraformaldehyde causes cellular degeneration. As the N-2 pastes are absorbed into the periapical tissues, their cytotoxicity remains because the toxic components are water soluble. The N-2 pastes, in their state, continue to cause degeneration of cells, affecting cellular respiration, leading to chronic inflammation, and inhibiting growth and repair.

Connective tissue reactions.* The N-2–type pastes have an overall *long-lasting* inflammatory action. Reactions to these slowly absorbed pastes have been ankylosis, resorption, and necrosis. The dispersion of the particles in the paste indicates a lack of stability. As time passes, the resorption and disintegration of N-2 generate an even greater coagulative necrosis and inflammatory reaction.[4]

Because N-2–type pastes are highly irritating, an additional burden is placed on the defense mechanism of the periapical tissues. The type of healing that may occur is questionable, and the fixed cells have the potential to break down into a focus of necrotizing material. Follow-up stud-

---

*References 1, 4, 7, 12, 16, 21, 32.

ies of the periapical tissue response to inflamed pulps treated by the N-2 method show the development of lesions ranging from apical periodontitis to osteomyelitis.

Bone reactions.[3] Bone reactions have been sequestration, long-standing chronic inflammation, ankylosis and necrosis. There is reduced healing and a concurrent production of osteoclasia and resorption. N-2–type pastes have been found in the granules of macrophages. This indicates the material's constant but slow absorbability.

Reactions to lead.[9,20,22] Lead compounds have been demonstrated to be bone seekers and quite toxic. Lead absorbed from the root canal paste is present in increased amounts in the blood, adrenal glands, kidney, spleen, and bone. The possibility of an increased toxicologic burden on the body must also be considered. The prudent clinician, considering the duration and nature of the patient's exposure to lead, should select as alternatives the safer and more predictable materials that are widely available.

Reactions to paraformaldehyde.* Paraformaldehyde is an effective antiseptic only in high concentrations, but it is toxic in all concentrations. As used in the N-2–type pastes, its "antiseptic" efect is available for approximately 7 to 10 days because of a marked decrease in formaldehyde content at body temperature, the change being independent of the location of the cement. Paraformaldehyde creates an intravitam fixation of tissue. The fixed tissue breaks down because of the loss of paraformaldehyde concentration. This decrease in paraformaldehyde leads to a reversible effect that results in complete necrosis of the fixed tissue. The necrotizing action creates a zone of degenerated material that may act as a constant source of chronic inflammation and potential breakdown. As a "fixing agent" it also affects periodontal structures and thus creates probable ankylosis and resorption.

A further consequence of fixation is to make the contents of the pulp cavity noxious, leading to a chronic inflammatory reaction in the periapical tissue. In addition, antigenicity and the formation of autoantibodies through sensitization by formaldehyde-treated pulp has been demonstrated. In such cases N-2–fixed tissue becomes an immunogen leading to antigen-antibody reactions in the periapical tissue.

Antigenic reactions.† The goal of cleaning and shaping the root canal system is to remove pulp tissue, pulpal remnants, organic predentin, and infected or necrotic dentin. To rely on chemical paste fixation to accomplish this all-important task fails in the biologic concept of proper wound debridement.

N-2 fixation of remaining tissue in the root canal has been shown to cause the fixed material to develop antigenic properties and elicit a humoral response. Antibodies have developed in response to pulp tissue fixed and altered by these pastes. N-2 paste therefore may be a hapten. The concept that N-2 paste acts like a hapten and the remaining noxious tissue like a protein carrier develops; and a cell-mediated immunologic reaction is thus actuated.

As has been amply demonstrated, tissue reactions to N-2–type pastes are highly inflammatory. Development and continuance of granulomatous reactions are evidenced by the irrational products found in macrophages. N-2 granules and dispersion particles are found in the inflammatory cells.

The fixation of the remaining canal tissue and periapical tissue and the N-2 paste itself all lead to an antigenic reaction. A pathway develops from the canal directly to the surrounding connective tissue, which acts as a spillway for the cascading immunologic reaction and thus perpetuates the periapical inflammatory lesion. Formaldehyde fixation changes the autologous tissue into a foreign material that elicits an immune response. This provides additional justification for not using formaldehyde-type pastes in endodontic therapy.

Reactions in the sclerotic zone.[27] Histologically the sclerotic zone has been shown to be necrotic in *all* cases in which N-2–type pastes have been used. As such, it must be regarded as a potential focus of constant irritation and a potential source of breakdown. Apical to this zone the tissue undergoes metaplasia. Sequelae have been chronic inflammation, resorption, foreign body reactions, absorbed N-2 particles, ankylosis, and necrosis. As a "barrier," the sclerotic zone is ineffective and is, by its presence, destructive to surrounding tissues.

Three-dimensional solid obturation is necessary for proper healing and success. N-2–type pastes are absorbable and exhibit a lack of stability through dispersion. These unacceptable characteristics lead to voids in the pseudo-obturation of the canal. Voiding within the obturator or sealer is a major cause of failure (i.e., an incompletely filled root canal).

The N-2 pastes, loosely packed or placed in the canal system with a Lentulo spiral, are difficult to control. Because they occasionally penetrate the apical tissue and cause acute exacerbations,[6,19] the prudent clinician using them should carefully consider the components of these pastes, especially when they may come into contact with neurovascular bundles. Several cases[10] of paresthesia with utilization of N-2–type paste compounds have been reported in the literature following overextension of the paste beyond the apical foramen in mandibular premolars. (Additional cases are reported by Dr. Zinman on the next page.) A case of maxillary sinus infection resulting from N-2, leading to a Caldwell-Luc procedure, has been confirmed.[18]

The proper approach to the treatment of a patient with an endodontic problem includes an aseptic technique, cleaning and shaping of the entire canal system and its contents, careful irrigation with a sanitizing solution, and three-dimensional obturation of the root canal system with a sealer and inert solid core. A therapy based on sound, proved biologic principles will ensure patient comfort and the greatest success.

---

*References 13, 15, 17, 27, 30, 31.
†References 2, 5, 15, 28, 29.

REFERENCES

1. Asano, S.: Clinico-pathological study of direct pulp capping and immediate root canal filling after vital pulp extirpation with N2 and "calvital," Shikwa Gakuho **73:**989, 1973.

2. Block, R., et al.: Antibody formation to dog pulp tissue altered by N2-type paste within the root canal, J. Endod. **3**:309. 1977.

3. Brewer, D.: Histology of apical tissue reaction to overfill, J. Calif. Dent. Assoc. **3**:58, 1975.

4. Brown, B., Kafrawy, A., and Patterson, S.: Studies of Sargenti technique of endodontic—reaction to the materials, J. Endod. **4**:238, 1978.

5. Campbell, A., et al.: Cell-mediated response to endodontic cements: research report, J. Endod. **4**:147, 1978.

6. Ehrmann, E.: N2 root canal treatment, Aust. Dent. J. **8**:434, 1963.

7. Engstrom, B., and Spångberg, L.: Effect of root canal filling material N2 when used for filling after partial pulpectomy, Sven. Tandlak. Tidskr. **62**:815, 1969.

8. Garry, J.: President's message, Am. Endod. Soc. Newsletter, September 1973.

9. Goodman, L.: and Gilman, A.: The pharmacological basis of therapeutics, ed. 3, New York, 1965, The Macmillan Co.

10. Grossman, L.: Paresthesia from N2, Oral Surg. **46**:700, 1978.

11. Keresztesi, K., and Kellner, G.: Biological effect of root filling materials, J. Fed. Dent. Int. **16**:222, 1966.

12. Langeland, K., et al.: Methods in the study of biologic responses to endodontic materials: tissue response to N_2, Oral Surg. **27**:522, 1969.

13. Lawrence, C., and Block, S.: Disinfection, sterilization and preservation, Philadelphia, 1971, Lea & Febiger, Chapters 32 and 41.

14. Makkes, P., Thoden van Velzen, S., and Vanden Hoff, A.: Response of the living organism to dead and fixed dead enclosed homologous tissue, Oral Surg. **46**:296, 1978.

15. Makkes, P., Thoden van Velzen, S., and Wesselink, P.: Reactions of the living organism to dead and fixed dead tissue, J. Endod. **4**:17, 1978.

16. Muruzabal, M.: Process of healing following endodontic treatment in molar of the rat, Transactions, Fifth International Conference on Endodontics, Philadelphia, 1973, University of Pennsylvania.

17. Nishida, O., et al.: Investigation of homologous antibodies to an extract of rabbit dental pulp, Arch. Oral Biol. **16**:733, 1971.

18. Norris, J.P.: Personal communication, 1976.

19. Orlay, H.: Overfilling in root canal treatment, two incidents with N2, Br. Dent. J. **120**:8, 1966.

20. Oswald, R. and Cohn, S.: Systemic distribution of lead from root canal fillings, J. Endod. **1**:59, 1975.

21. Rappaport, H., Lilly, G., and Kapsimalis, P.: Toxicity of endodontic filling materials, Oral Surg. **18**:785, 1964.

22. Shapiro, I., et al.: Blood-lead levels in monkeys treated with a lead-containing (N-2) root canal cement; a preliminary report, J. Endod. **1**:294, 1975.

23. Spångberg, L.: Biological effects of root canal filling materials. VI. The inhibitory effect of solubilised root canal filling materials on respiration of HeLa cells, Odontol. Tidskr. **77**:121, 1969.

24. Spångberg, L.: Biological effects of root canal filling materials II. Effect in vitro of water-soluble components of root canal filling materials on HeLa cells, Odontol. Rev. **20**:133, 1969.

25. Spångberg, L.: Biological effects of root canal filling materials. IV. Effect in vitro of solubilised root canal filling materials on HeLa cells, Odontol. Rev. **20**:289, 1969.

26. Spångberg, L.: Biological effects of root canal filling materials. V. Toxic effect in vitro of root canal filling materials on HeLa cells and human skin fibroblasts, Odontol. Rev. **20**:427, 1969.

27. Spångberg, L.: Biological effects of root canal filling materials. Effect on bone tissue of two formaldehyde-containing pastes: N2 and Riebler's paste, Oral Surg. **38**:934, 1974.

28. Spector, W., and Heesom, N.: The production of granulomata by antigen-antibody complexes, J. Pathol. **98**:31, 1969.

29. Thoden van Velzen, S., and Keltkramp-Vroom, T.: Immunologic consequences of formaldehyde fixation of autologous tissue implants, J. Endod. **3**:179, 1977.

30. Sato, H., and Tsutsumi, S.: Tissue course changes in formaldehyde content of cement and paste containing paraformaldehyde, Bull. Tokyo Dent. Coll. **20**:1, 1979.

31. Brian, J., Jr., Ranly, D., Fulton, R., and Madden, R.: Reaction of rat connective tissue to unfixed and formaldehyde-fixed autogenous tissue enclosed in tubes, J. Endod. **6**:628, 1980.

32. Newton, C., Patterson S., and Kafrawy, A.: Studies of Sargenti's technique of endodontic treatment: 6-month and one-year responses, J. Endod. **6**:509, 1980.

Question:

What is the legal status of the formaldehyde-containing pastes?

Answer:

Edwin J. Zinman

N-2 paste and similarly compounded formaldehyde-containing pastes *continue* to remain nonapproved drugs by the United States Food and Drug Administration.[1] Regulations adopted pursuant to the Federal Food, Drug, and Cosmetic Act mandate that no "new drug" may be distributed in interstate commerce unless first approved by the Food and Drug Administration for both safety and efficacy.[2]

A "new drug" application for N-2 submitted in 1962 was withdrawn in 1967 after failing to substantiate the efficacy and safety of N-2 with well-documented clinical and animal studies rather than testimonial evidence.[3] The Food and Drug Administration's Dental Drug Products Advisory Committee concluded its November, 1975 hearing by finding that "insufficient scientifically valid data are available to permit a judgment that N-2 and RC-2B [formaldehyde-containing pastes] can be generally recognized as safe and effective. Moreover, the Committee is concerned that the safety and therapeutic value of some of the ingredients in the materials has not been established."

State drugs laws provide separate penalties and prohibitions in addition to the federal drug laws and regulations. Violation of either federal or state law may constitute negligence per se.[4]

Statutory "grandfather" exceptions to these regulations are drugs generally recognized by qualified scientific experts of the dental profession to be safe and effective.[5] Grossman's root canal cement, Kerr pulp canal sealer, PCA root canal sealer, and gutta-percha would probably qualify for the aforesaid exemption because of their accepted usage in the instruction programs of American schools of dentistry for many years.

A 1978 opinion of the California Attorney General concluded:

Neither state nor federal drug laws prohibit a pharmacist from compounding or dispensing N-2 or RC-2B substances pursuant to a bonafide prescription order of a dentist, if the substance N-2 or RC-2B is determined by the dentist to be appropriate in the treatment of the condition or which he attends a patient and if the component elements of such materials in any combination or singly have not been banned by state and federal law or regulation.[2]

Although a cursory reading of the California Attorney General's opinion appears to allow California dentists to prescribe and use N-2-type pastes, the opinion does not constitute a complete legal exculpation for N-2 usage.

First, the Attorney General's opinion is only advisory

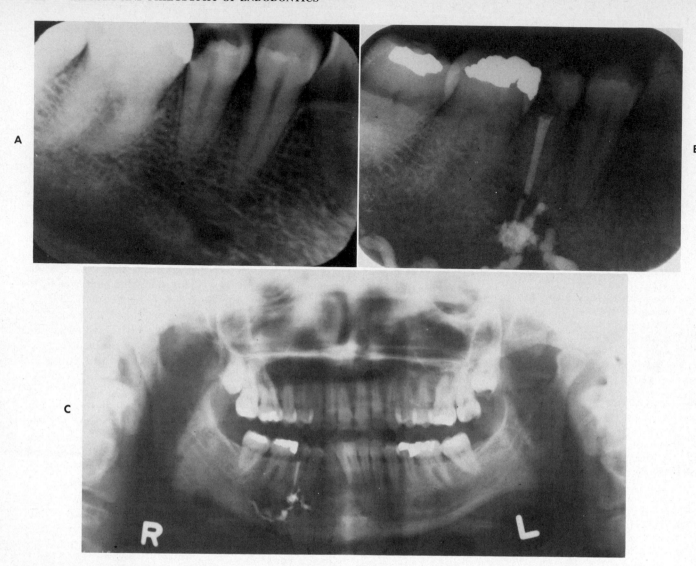

FIG. 25-1. Settled litigation in which a 33-year-old woman received N-2 paste treatment for a mandibular right second premolar. **A,** June, 1974, immediately preoperative. **B,** February, 1976. **C,** February, 1976.

and not a decision. Consequently the courts are not required to follow the opinion. To the extent that the opinion interprets California' Sherman Food, Drug, and Cosmetic Act, it would not be a precedent decision regarding jurisdictions outside California for interpreting another state's drug law.

Second, the opinion shifts any liability from the pharmacist to the dentist pursuant to a "written prescription of a dentist, for an individual patient's needs."[7] Therefore a dentist could be required to provide copies of an individual written prescription for each patient; moreover, ordering N-2 or RC-2B in bulk as a chemical compound does not legally protect the dentist since a federal court has ruled that a bulk order of the drug does not constitute a prescription for individual patients.[8]

Third, the opinion specifically cautioned "[N]or do we imply that the prescribing of a new drug or the dispensing of a new drug may not constitute negligence." As an ex-

ample of negligence the opinion stated, "Informed consent on the part of the patient is necessary before dental treatment can be begun[9] and any dental treatment given without informed consent exposes the dentist to an action in negligence. . . . the patient (must) be apprised of the medicines which will be prescribed for his condition and their use and effect, both beneficial and harmful."[10]

Irrespective of any drug law, a cause of action will lie for negligent administration of N-2. Dr. Sargenti[11] has warned that "over-instrumentation and overfilling in using the N-2 method cannot be condoned." Several examples of negligent misuse of N-2 follow:

Case one (Fig. 25-1). This case involved a 33-year-old woman who had received N-2 paste treatment for tooth 29. Almost 8 years postoperatively the paresthesia persists. Prior to trial the case was settled for $80,000 (including a contribution of $12,500 from the manufacturer of RC-2B).[12]

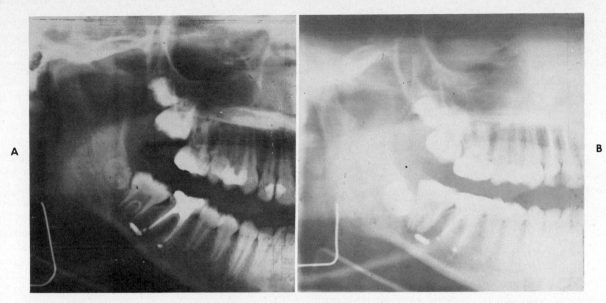

FIG. 25-2. Case in which the mandibular left first molar was overfilled with a formaldehyde-containing paste. **A,** One month postoperative. **B,** Two years later. Note the apparent distal migration of the paste. Paresthesia has persisted as of this date.

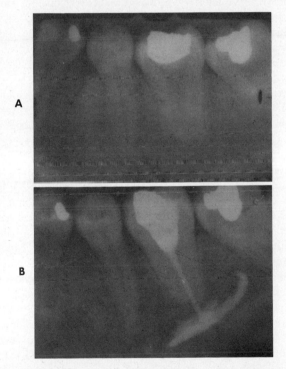

FIG. 25-3. Case in which the mandibular left first molar was grossly overfilled in a 26-year-old woman. **A,** Preoperative. **B,** Postoperative.

Case two (Fig. 25-2). This case had dental records that revealed an overfilling of a formaldehyde-containing paste in tooth 19 of 9-year old boy.

Case three (Fig. 25-3). This case illustrates a gross overfill of tooth 19 in a 26-year-old woman. Paresthesia has persisted 3 years. The case was eventually settled for a considerable sum of money.

Drug manufacturer's liability for distributing para-formaldehyde-containing pastes. A manufacturer of a product, such as a drug, is strictly liable for any personal injuries resulting from its defective design. The doctrine of strict liability does not require proof of negligence but rather a showing of some design defect.[13] Design defect is broadly interpreted; and numerous product liability precedents demonstrate that the defect or defectiveness concept has embraced a great variety of injury-producing deficiencies, from products causing injury because they deviate from the manufacturer's intended result (e.g., the one soda bottle in ten thousand that explodes without explanation[14]) to products which, though "perfectly" manufactured, are unsafe because of the absence of a safety device (e.g., a bulldozer without rear view mirrors[15]) and including products that are dangerous because they lack adequate warnings or instructions (e.g., a telescope that contains inadequate instructions for assembling a "sun filter" attachment[16]).

Virtually all manufacturers of formaldehyde-containing pastes provide no labeling instructions for proper dosage, mixture, or administration; nor do they give any warnings regarding harmful sequelae. Accordingly numerous lawsuits have been filed against the drug manufacturers of formaldehyde-containing pastes under the doctrine of strict liability[17] and at least one verdict for $150,000 has resulted.[18]

Similarly a strict liability suit has been settled against the manufacturer of the Fistulator, recommended for use in conjunction with N-2 pastes for trephination, under the strict liability allegation of failure to provide directions to the dentist regarding proper use of the Fistulator and/or warning of any harmful sequelae arising from its misuse.[19]

Case four. This case concerns a paresthesia secondary to N-2 method therapy and subsequent fistulation. In answer to interrogatories, the defendant dentist opined that fistulation after canal obturation with a paraformaldehyde-containing paste had mechanically injured the mental nerve, resulting in paresthesia. The paresthesia has continued 10 years postoperatively.

Recent court decisions have broadened the doctrine of strict liability.

After the plaintiff makes a prima facie showing that the injury was proximately caused by the product's design, the burden or proof may shift to the manufacturer to show that, on balance, the benefits of the challenged design outweigh the risk of danger inherent in such design.[19]

When the "risk vs. benefit" standard is applied, the feasibility and cost of alternative designs may be considered by the jury as relevant factors. Moreover, although the manufacturer took reasonable precautions in an attempt to design a safe product or otherwise acted in a reasonably prudent way to absolve himself of liability under a negligence theory, this fact would not preclude the imposition of liability under the doctrine of strict liability, if, upon hindsight, the trier of fact concluded the product's design was unsafe to consumers.[20]

Thus the manufacturer of an N-2–type paste would be required to prove that the risks arising from usage of the paste outweighed the benefits of using conventional endodontic pastes. Germane to such evidentiary proof is that there appears to be a greater incidence of adverse side effects secondary to N-2 usage than occurs with conventional pastes.[21] For example, there have been no published documented cases of permanent paresthesia related to filling root canals with conventional endodontic pastes whereas numerous instances of paresthesia secondary to N-2 usages have been published.[22] In the first reported case of N-2–induced paresthesa, no recovery has yet occurred after 19 years.[23]

In conclusion, the benefit of the generally recognized wide margin of safety and time-proved efficacy of conventional endodontic sealers outweighs the potentially greater risk inherently associated with formaldehyde-containing paste.

Dubious defenses to usage of formaldehyde-containing pastes

Customary practice. Customary practice not consonant with reasonably prudent care under the same or similar circumstances does not constitute a defense to professional negligence.[24]

For instance, one study of 2423 California dentists concluded that 30% of dentists responding to the survey have used Sargenti paste in their practice.[25] Nevertheless, whether the usage of N-2 in endodontic therapy represents a negligent custom rather than a standard of practice is a jury question since customary practice does not conclusively prove that the standard of care has been met irrespective of the numbers who follow a particular modality.

In a precedent case[26] the Washington Supreme Court held the physician-defendant negligent as a matter of law although virtually all other ophthalmologists customarily failed to perform the simple and well-known test for glau-

coma on patients under 40. In rendering its decision the court relied on an earlier legal precedent that "courts must in the end say what is required; there are precautions so imperative that even their universal disregard will not excuse their omission."

Alternative method of therapy. The difference of dental opinion concerning the desirability of one particular dental procedure over another does not establish negligence in the choice of treatment so long as the less favored method is observed by a respectable minority of practitioners.[27]

However, whether a *respectable* minority would follow a technique (e.g., the N-2 method) that is not taught as a recognized modality of endodontic therapy in any American school of dentistry and remains nonapproved by the United States Food and Drug Administration is debatable. Accordingly the issue to be decided by the trier of fact, whether judge or jury, is not whether conventional endodontic therapy also bears risk of failure or complication but rather whether a reasonably prudent practitioner would forego usage of formaldehyde-containing pastes because of the increased hazard of untoward complications such as paresthesia.

Much like the Ford Pinto,* N-2 may be a convenient and inexpensive alternative, until an accident occurs. Due to a design defect inherent in both these products, catastrophic injury is more likely to occur from their use. For example, the paraformaldehyde content of N-2, which spreads chemically far beyond the point of initial contact, has caused numerous permanent paresthesias.[22]

Consequently the American Dental Association's Council on Dental Therapeutics specifically warns of "severe postoperative complications that not infrequently accompany these [Sargenti] materials when inadvertently extruded past the apex."[28]

Contributory Negligence. A patient has a legal duty to follow the instructions of the treating dentist, but failure to do so does not constitute contributory negligence unless the defendant produces expert testimony to show that the alleged contributory negligence of the patient was a substantial factor contributing to the patient's injuries. Since the same result to the patient might have occurred regardless of plaintiff's conduct by not adhering to the dentist's instructions, the defendant bears the burden of proof of proximate causation of contributory negligence.[29]

Duty to refer to an endodontist. Several recent decisions have required the general dentist to exercise the same amount of skill and degree of care as an endodontist diagnosing endodontic disease[30] and performing endodontic therapy.

---

*A. Nanda v. Ford Motor Co., 509 F.2d 213 (1974); 36 A.T.L.A. Law J. 98 (1976); Comment: The liability of an automobile manufacturer for failure to design a crashworthy vehicle, 10 Willamette Law J. 38 (1973); Grimshaw v. Ford Motor Co., Orange Co. California Superior Court, no. 19-77-61 ($127,500,000 verdict, remititur granted $6.2 million, pending appeal); Norton v. Ford Motor Co., Circuit Court of Arlington Co. Virginia. Law no. 17856, 17857, and 17858. (Date of accident, 5/11/73.)

In *Simpson v. Davis*[31] the general dentist'e endodontic treatment fell below the requisite standard of care because he failed to use a rubber dam as a precautionary measure against aspiration whereas all endodontists would have employed a rubber dam under similar circumstances. Since the N-2 technique has not required a rubber dam, injury arising from failure to use a rubber dam in performing endodontic therapy may constitute a deviation from the standard of dental practice. Thus both the general dentist and the specialist must conform to the higher level of care required of a specialist in endodontics.[32]

Fraudulent Concealment. Allegations of fraudulent concealment will extend the statute of limitations beyond the time period prescribed for dental negligence since fraud ordinarily involves a longer statute of limitations.[33] Fraudulent allegations have been filed in litigation concerning undisclosed fractured endodontic instruments[34] as well as the suppression of the fact that N-2–type drugs were unapproved by the United States Food and Drug Administration.[35] Proof of fraud may subject the defendant to punitive damages, which would not ordinarily be covered by professional negligence insurance since most states bar insurance coverage for fraud as contrary to public policy.[36] In fact, juries have awarded punitive damages for fraudulent misrepresentation and fraudulent concealment.[37]

Conclusion. In conclusion, the benefit of the generally recognized wide margin of safety and time-proved efficacy of conventional endodontic filling materials outweighs the potentially greater risks associated with formaldehyde-containing endodontic pastes.

REFERENCES

1. Congressional hearing on Sargenti drug, J. Endod. **2**:6, 1976.
2. 21 U.S.C.A., § 355.
3. Eleventh report by the Committee on Government Operations, House report no. 94-787, January, 1976.
4. *Toole v. Richardson-Merrell, Inc.*, 60 Cal. Rptr. 398 (1967); 251 Cal. App. 2d 689.
5. Federal Food, Drug, and Cosmetics Act, 21 U.S.C.A. §321 (p). See also Drug Amendment Act of 1962, §107(c) (4) Pub. Law 87-781.
6. California Attorney General's opinion, CV 76/212, CV 77/236.
7. California Attorney General's opinion, supra, p. 28.
8. California Dental Association: Membership letter, June 26, 1978. See also *Cedars N. Towers Pharm., Inc., v. U.S.A.*, Florida Fed. Dist. Ct. no. 77-4965 (Aug. 18, 1978).
9. *Cobbs v. Grant*, 8 Cal. 3d 229, 242–244.
10. California Attorney General's opinion, supra, p. 31.
11. Sargenti, A.: The Sargenti N-2 method, Dent. Surv., October, 1978.
12. *Knapp v. Stein*, Los Angeles County Superior Court, §15813 (Norwalk), J. Am. Dent. Assoc., Section on litigation, September, 1977.
13. Traynor, R.J.: The ways and means of defective products and strict liability, Tenn. L. Rev. **32**:363, 1965; *Cronin v. J.B.E. Olson Corp.* (1972), 8 Cal. 3d 121; 104 Cal. Rptr. 433 (1973); 501 P. 2d 1153; *Barker v. Lull Engineering, Inc.*, 143 Cal. Rptr. 225 (1978).
14. *Escola v. Coca Cola Bottling Co.*, 24 Cal. 2d 453, 150 P. 2d (436) (1944).
15. *Pike v. Frank G. Hough Co.*, 2 Cal. 3d 465; 85 Cal. Rptr. 629 (1970); 467 P. 2d 229 (1970).
16. *Midgley v. S.S. Kresge Co.*, 55 Cal. App. 3d 67; 127 Cal. Rptr. 217 (1976).
17. Personal files of the author and communications with other attorneys.
18. *Pierce v. Moore Drug*, 83-22181, U.S. District Court, Colorado (1986).
19. *Porter v. Hoyt and Medidenta et al.*, San Francisco, California Superior Court no. 741033.
20. *Barker v. Lull Engineering Co., Inc.*, 143 Cal. Rptr. 225 (1978); 20 Cal. 3d 413; 573 P. 2d 443. See also *Henderson v. Ford Motor Co.* (Tex. 1974) 519 S.W. 2d 87, 92; *Welch v. Outboard Marine Corp.* (5th Cir. 1973) 481 F 2d 252, 254.
21. American Dental Association, Council on Dental Therapeutics: Guide to dental materials and devices, ed. 8. Chicago, 1977, The Association, p. 187.
22. Ehrmann, E.H.: Root canal treatment with N-2, Aust. Dent. J. **8**:434, 1963; Orlay, H.G.: Overfilling in root canal treatment, Br. Dent. J. **120**:376, 1966; Serene T.: Endodontic problems resulting from surgical fistulation; report of two cases, J. Am. Dent. Assoc. **96**:101, 1978.
23. Ehrmann, E.H.: Personal communication.
24. *Hooper, T.J.* (2nd Cir. 1932, Hand, L.J.) 60 F. 2d 737, 740, cert., den. sub. non. *Eastern Transportation Co. v. Northern Barge Corp.*, 287 U.S. 662, 53 Sup. Ct. 220; 77 Law Ed. 571 (1932); Prosser, W.L.: Law of torts, §33, St. Paul, Minn., 1971, West Publishing Co., pp. 166-168; *Barton v. Owens*, 139 Cal. Rptr. 494 (1977)
25. Marketing Research Bureau report, September, 1978.
26. *Helling v. Carey*, 83 Wash. 2d 514; 519 P. 2d 981 (1974).
27. Witkin, B.: Summary of California Law, ed. 8, Vol.. 4. Torts, §515, *Hubbard v. Calvin*, 147 Cal. Rptr. 905 (1978).
28. American Dental Association, Council on Dental Therapeutics, supra (ref 21), p. 197.
29. *Barton v. Owens* (1977), 139 Cal. Rptr. 494 (1977); *LeMons v. Regents of the University of California* (1978), 21 Cal. 3d 874; 148 Cal. Rptr. 355 (1978).
30. *Evans v. Ohanesian*, 39 Cal. App. 121; 112 Cal. Rptr. 236 (1974).
31. *Simpson v. Davis* (Kan. 1976) 219 Kan. 584; 549 P. 2d 950.
32. *Simpson v. Davis*, supra 957; Komensky, A.M.: Dental professional liability prevention. 2. Council on insurance, J. Am. Dent. Assoc. **97**:1008, 1978.
33. *Sanchez v. Valley View Hospital and Medical Center* (Colo. App.) 521 P. 2d 1290; *Layton v. Allen* (Sup.) 246 A. 2d 794; *McCluskey v. Thraraw*, 31 Wis. 2d 245; 142 N.W. 2d 787.
34. *Wallace v. Garrett*, Marin Co., California Superior Court, Case no. 80946 (1978).
35. *Billings v. Uzelac*, Contra Costa Co., California Superior Court, Case no. 179095 (1978).
36. California insurance code, §533.
37. *Sinopoli v. Issvoran*, Alameda Co., California Superior Court, Case no. H-43098-0 ($20,000 punitive damages). See also *Smith v. Courter*, 535 S.W. 2d 199 (1974).

26

FUTURE

STEPHEN COHEN
RICHARD C. BURNS

The privilege of preparing this fourth edition has given us the opportunity to stand among the giants in our field. Introspection and insights gained during this experience have also provided us a glimpse into the promise of the future.

To paraphrase the late George Bernard Shaw, "Some look at the future and say why; others look and say why not." As we write this last chapter, we feel a stirring that this is indeed a commencement for a new order of endodontics. We dentists are most fortunate to bear witness to the accelerating rate of change within our field—a heralding call to the exciting challenge we face as we are thrust into the future.

The doctoral student of the 1980s is performing routine endodontics without a preconceived sense of inadequacy. The recent dental graduate is better trained to complete almost all phases of routine endodontic treatment. The "mystique" of endodontic therapy continues to wither and fade as uncomplicated endodontics becomes incorporated within the general scope of dental health care.

The need for restorative dentistry will most likely diminish, along with the continued decline of dental caries, resulting from widespread use of topical and systemic fluorides, adhesive sealants, and the soon-to-be announced anticaries vaccine. Accordingly, we expect that general practitioners will devote more of their time to preventive dental procedures because of the already observable dramatic reduction in the number of teeth afflicted by caries.

The endodontist will, because of his educational background, continue to be the most knowledgeable and skillful provider of endodontic therapy. Therefore, complex endodontic procedures will be performed by him while uncomplicated endodontic procedures will be performed routinely within a matter of minutes by the restorative dentist. An increased public awareness that endodontic treatment is desirable and almost always painless will encourage patients to seek the benefits of root canal therapy. Conse-quently extractions will be as unusual in the future for patients who care about their teeth as endodontics was 40 years ago, when patients seldom had a choice.

It is evident that one era is coming to an end and a new one is beginning. Is this merely a statement of high hopes, or is it based on facts? We will discuss some of the more salient categories of endodontics, illustrating the emerging trends, and allow the reader to decide.

In the field of diagnosis there will be *less* reliance on radiographs because of the emerging technologies of ultrasonics, infrared sensors, magnetic resonance imaging, and transillumination to detect early changes in the texture, temperature, and composition of hard and soft tissues. When radiographs are needed, the quality of diagnostic films will be enhanced, with less radiation, by the use of intensifying screens and xeroradiographs. Electronic canal-measuring devices will rapidly provide the length of the root canal system, thereby further reducing the need for x radiation.

Even today radiographic clarity can be improved enormously by computer enhancement. Further technologic development, along with miniaturization, to provide numerical values to shapes and densities, resulting in a film that has color, will become commercially feasible. Indeed, prototypes are available today that can show a three-dimensional color image on a video screen, thereby further reducing the need for films of any type.

Sophisticated vitality testers that quantifiably measure patient responses to thermal and electric stimuli will become available commercially (Fig. 1-12, *E*).

Pain control will be more predictable than ever before. With the widespread use of intraligamental injections as a supplement to conventional anesthetic techniques, the need for intrapulpal anesthesia will be virtually eliminated. Even today there are electrical devices available to the dentist that alter or reduce painful stimuli, thereby reducing the need for local anesthetics.

Preserving a healthy pulp when restorative considerations do not apply will continue to be paramount. All indications point to the likelihood that when endodontic treatment is necessary the majority of teeth will be treated completely in one visit. Furthermore, during treatment planning, the clinician will weigh the risks and guarded prognoses for questionable pulp caps and pulpotomies in permanent teeth against the high degree of predictability of root canal therapy, making the choice of endodontic treatment almost irresistable.

Total debridement of the root canal system will be completed within minutes by the use of rotary-reciprocating or ultrasonic devices in concert with efficient hand instruments. Through the application of computer-enhanced fiberoptic images on a video screen, the dentist can actually look around the entire root canal to assure thorough debridement. The precise location of apical foramen will be ascertained with ultrasensitive temperature gauges. If complete treatment cannot be provided in one visit, thorough canal debridement will obviate the need for potentially irritating and antigenic intracanal medications. Mild biocompatible solutions will be used instead of harsh irrigants.

Following debridement, the root canal system will be filled within seconds by polymeric materials having qualities similar or superior to those of gutta-percha. These biocompatible materials will be introduced into the canal systems by injection, thermoplasticization, or compaction. It is technologically possible that controllable dentin welding of the apical foramen with a laser beam will make overextensions of filling materials a problem of the past. Demographic studies reveal that the population is living longer and the "baby boom" is over. Accordingly, the general dentist and the endodontist will be required to have more diverse knowledge and clinical skills to diagnose and treat the endodontic problems commonly found in an aging population.

Following canal obturation there will be increased emphasis placed on coronal reinforcement for posterior teeth. Precast hard metal posts available in a variety of lengths, widths, and tapers will replace many of today's cast dowels. Furthermore, there will be a heightened appreciation of the need for full cuspal protection for all posterior teeth to avoid crown fracture. For the greater good of saving a tooth, the pulp occasionally must be considered an expendable organ when sound coronal retention requires incorporating the restoration into the pulp chamber or beyond. The ease, speed, and success of endodontic treatment will allow the clinician to consider the pulp chamber merely as an extension of the restorative zone.

The continued improvement of nonsurgical endodontic therapy will significantly diminish the need to perform apical surgery except for cases of canal obstruction or other aberrations. When retrograde obturation is necessary, nonirritating, *nonmetallic* sealing materials that bond to dentin will be used routinely.

The number of iatrogenically discolored teeth will continue to decline rapidly. Closer attention to properly extended access openings, wider use of nondiscoloring filling materials, less reliance upon potentially discoloring intralcanal medicaments, and alternatives to amalgam for sealing access cavities in anterior teeth will all contribute to virtually eliminating the disfigurement of the dark tooth. Endodontics and esthetics will embrace. Today the medical and dental professions are both keenly aware of the cause/effect relationship between systemic tetracycline administration during the tooth-formative years and discolored (but caries resistant) vital teeth. Accordingly, vital teeth discolored as a result of chemotherapy will be a rarity.

Endodontics will continue to reach out for high technology; indeed, high technology has already been incorporated into clinical practice. But no technology can replace tactile sense and common sense. We hope dentists will continue to maintain control over modern mechanical devices and not be mesmerized by the bells, chimes, gongs, whistles, and glitter—which are no substitute for clear, sound thinking.

With ever increasing speed, simplicity, and reliability imparted to endodontic treatment, nostrums of the past for canal obturation (which are periodically resurrected as pharmacologic panaceas under the guise of new names) will disappear. Pastes imbued with almost mystical qualities will be viewed as merely footnotes in our dental history.

As a greater percentage of routine endodontic cases are treated by the general practitioner, there will be a continued need for graduate endodontists to provide diagnosis and treatment for difficult cases. Some postgraduate endodontics programs will be terminated. However, postgraduate programs will still be essential to prepare highly qualified teachers, researchers, and clinical endodontists needed by the public as well as the profession.

Better oral protection devices for individuals engaging in organized sports, along with coaches insisting that the player, as well as the play, is important, will significantly reduce the number of dental injuries. There will be less need for endodontic treatment caused by contact sports.

As we reach the end of this text, we hope it is evident that today's reach is within tomorrow's grasp. Not everyone will want to seize the moment. There will be resistance to change.

But our professional future is inevitable. What happens next is up to us. The readiness and the resolve are all, for the ultimate goal of endodontics is to conquer the inner space of the Pathways of the Pulp.

ANSWERS TO SELF-ASSESSMENT QUESTIONS

SHANNON WONG
CHARLES J. CUNNINGHAM

1—Diagnostic procedures

1b	5d	9a	13a
2a	6b	10b	14c
3b	7d	11c	
4a	8c	12b	

2—Endodontic emergencies

1a	5a	9d	13b
2d	6c	10b	14a
3c	7a	11c	
4b	8b	12d	

3—Case selection and treatment planning

1a	5b	9c	13b
2c	6c	10b	14a
3b	7d	11a	
4a	8d	12d	

4—Preparation for treatment

1b	5d	9b	13b
2c	6b	10d	14d
3d	7c	11a	
4a	8a	12c	

5—Endodontic armamentarium and sterilization

1a	5c	9c	13b
2b	6b	10a	14d
3c	7d	11d	
4b	8a	12c	

6—Access openings and tooth morphology

1c	5b	9b	13b
2a	6a	10d	14d
3d	7d	11c	
4b	8c	12a	

7—Cleaning and shaping of the root canal system

1b	5d	9a	13a
2d	6b	10c	14a
3d	7c	11d	
4a	8c	12a	

8—Obturation of the root canal system

1b	5c	9c	13d
2d	6d	10d	14a
3b	7a	11c	
4a	8b	12a	

9—Records and legal responsibilities

1d	5c
2d	6a
3c	7d
4a	8b

10—Pulp structure and function

1c	5d	9b	13d
2a	6b	10a	14a
3b	7c	11d	
4a	8b	12c	

11—Pathology

1a	5c	9b	13b
2c	6a	10a	14d
3a	7d	11d	
4b	8b	12a	

12—Microbiology and pharmacology

1b	5c	9d	13b
2a	6a	10c	14d
3d	7c	11b	
4a	8b	12a	

13—Instruments and materials

1b	5c	9b	13c
2a	6c	10a	14a
3d	7a	11a	
4b	8d	12d	

14—Pulpal reactions to caries and dental procedures

1c	5d	9b	13a
2b	6b	10a	14b
3d	7a	11d	
4a	8d	12a	

15—Traumatic injuries

1d	5a	9a	13d
2a	6b	10d	14d
3c	7b	11b	
4c	8b	12a	

16—Root resorption

1c	5c	9c
2d	6a	10b
3d	7d	11b
4d	8a	12a

17—Periodontal-endodontic treatment

1d	5d	9d
2b	6d	10d
3b	7a	11d
4d	8c	12c

18—Surgical endodontics

1d	5d	9b	13c
2a	6b	10c	14c
3d	7b	11d	
4b	8d	12c	

19—The management of pain and anxiety

1d	5d	9a	13c
2d	6a	10b	14c
3a	7a	11a	
4a	8d	12d	

20—Bleaching of vital and nonvital teeth

1d	5b
2d	6d
3c	7d
4c	8b

21—Postendodontic restoration

1d	5b	9d
2c	6d	10b
3b	7a	
4b	8c	

22—Pedodontic-endodontic treatment

1d	5d	9b	13c
2b	6c	10c	14b
3d	7d	11d	
4d	8a	12c	

23—Failures in therapy

1d	5d	9a	13c
2a	6b	10b	14c
3c	7c	11d	
4a	8b	12c	

INDEX

T indicates table.